DIAGNOSTIC PATHOLOGY OF PARASITIC INFECTIONS
WITH CLINICAL CORRELATIONS

Diagnostic Pathology of Parasitic Infections with Clinical Correlations

Second Edition

YEZID GUTIERREZ, M.D., M.P.H. & T.M., Ph.D.

Adjunct Staff, Department of Clinical Pathology
The Cleveland Clinic Foundation
Cleveland, Ohio

New York   Oxford
OXFORD UNIVERSITY PRESS
2000

Oxford University Press

Oxford   New York
Athens   Auckland   Bangkok   Bogotá   Buenos Aires   Calcutta
Cape Town   Chennai   Dar es Salaam   Delhi   Florence   Hong Kong   Istanbul
Karachi   Kuala Lumpur   Madrid   Melbourne   Mexico City   Mumbai
Nairobi   Paris   São Paulo   Singapore   Taipei   Tokyo   Toronto   Warsaw

and associated companies in
Berlin   Ibadan

Library of Congress Cataloging-in-Publication Data
Gutierrez, Yezid.
Diagnostic pathology of parasitic infections with clinical correlations/
Yezid Gutierrez.—2nd ed.
p.   cm.   Includes bibliographical references and index.
ISBN 0-19-512143-0
1. Parasitic diseases—Diagnosis.   2. Diagnostic parasitology.
3. Parasitic diseases—Histopathology.
I. Title.
[DNLM: 1. Parasitic Diseases—diagnosis.   2. Parasitic Diseases—physiopathology.
3. Parasites.
WC 695 G984d 1999]   RC119.G87   2000
616.9′6075—dc21   DNLM/DLC   for Library of Congress   98-52783

The science of medicine is a rapidly changing field. As new research and clinical experience broaden our knowledge, changes in treatment and drug therapy do occur. The author and the publisher of this work have checked with sources believed to be reliable in their efforts to provide information that is accurate and complete, and in accordance with the standards accepted at the time of publication. However, in light of the possibility of human error or changes in the practice of medicine, neither the author, nor the publisher, nor any other party who has been involved in the preparation or publication of this work warrants that the information contained herein is in every respect accurate or complete. Readers are encouraged to confirm the information contained herein with other reliable sources, and are strongly advised to check the product information sheet provided by the pharmaceutical company for each drug they plan to administer.

1 3 5 7 9 8 6 4 2

Printed in the United States of America
on acid-free paper

PREFACE

The second edition of *Diagnostic Pathology of Parasitic Infections with Clinical Correlations* preserves the spirit of the first edition in regard to its orientation as a tool for the anatomic pathologist. However, the entire text has been rewritten, incorporating new information regarding the most important molecular and immunologic aspects of parasitic diseases in humans. The recent explosion in our knowledge of the Microspora, especially the several species described in immune-suppressed patients and their morphologic diagnosis, has resulted in an entirely new chapter. *Pneumocystis*, now considered a fungus, is not discussed. The newest classification of the protists, the capillariids, and *Trichinella* is followed in this text, and the discussion of the basic biologic aspects of parasitism has been greatly expanded. This book, which could also be called *The Biologic Basis of Medical Parasitology*, is useful to all students of parasitic diseases of humans. Almost all of the illustrations from the first edition are included, with better resolution, and numerous new photographs, including 16 color plates, have been added. References have been considerably increased and classical works cited, the knowledge of which is necessary to comprehend the biology of parasitism in humans.

The medical library of the Cleveland Clinic provided constant support by obtaining numerous references not available in the area. Their patience, and understanding were unfailing. My indebtedness to them is great,

and thanks are not sufficient to express my appreciation to the staff of the interlibrary loan department. M. D. Little at the School of Public Health and Tropical Medicine of Tulane University provided parasitic material not included in the first edition from his collection and from the collection of the late P. C. Beaver. Much help was also provided by M. D. Little regarding some aspects of the classification of helminths and the clarification of controversial issues. The book is also enhanced by new material kindly sent by colleague pathologists from many institutions around the world. I thank all of them, too numerous to mention, for their academic interest and their desire to clarify esoteric findings that usually are of a benign nature. The excellent and warm collaboration of the staff of Oxford University Press, especially my editor, Lauren Enck, is very much appreciated. They committed themselves to publish the book with better reproduction of the illustrations and to correct and clarify the prose of a non-English-speaking author. All correspondence to the author should be addressed to: Dr. Yezid Gutierrez, 14280 Sweetbriar Lane, Novelty, Ohio 44072. Telephone: (440) 338-8656, Fax: (440) 338-8656, E-mail: ygutierrez@pol.net.

Novelty, Ohio   Y. G.
August 1999

Preface to the First Edition

This book has been written with the anatomic pathologist in mind. It deals with both the pathologic processes of parasitic infections in man and with the diagnostic characteristics of parasites in tissue sections. Clinicians interested in human parasites will find clinico-pathologic correlations useful for the understanding of these infections as they occur in man. Because of this orientation, all aspects dealing with diagnosis in the clinical laboratory are only briefly mentioned, and then only regarding diagnostic stages found in body fluids or stool samples from those organisms recovered from tissues. Often these diagnostic stages are illustrated for the sake of completion. This means, for example, that the diagnosis of malaria in blood samples is cursorily mentioned, and only *Plasmodium falciparum* found in tissues is fully discussed.

The purpose of the book is to serve as a diagnostic tool for those confronted with the problem of determining the identity of a parasite in a tissue section. The parasitologic aspects have been kept to a minimum and are mentioned only to provide a basis for the understanding of the infection and the diagnosis of parasites in tissues. A few adult stages of helminths are illustrated, because they may be recovered during autopsies or during the gross examination of surgical specimens. The book is all-inclusive, which means that all parasites described until now in the tissues of man have been covered: a great majority of these are illustrated. The illustrations are mainly of diagnostic stages and are intended to depict the morphologic characteristics of each parasite. Because the book is all-inclusive, dealing with many esoteric organisms, or organisms that have been rarely described in man, was unavoidable. Diagnosticians not familiar with basic parasitologic aspects may find it difficult to follow the descriptions of parasites, especially helminths in cross-sections, but I hope that this work will clarify some of these concepts and that this neglected area of pathology will become more familiar through the use of this book. One aspect not covered is that of dealing with the numerous artifacts that are often mistakenly diagnosed as parasites. However, a summary presented in tables organized by organ systems at the end of the book contains a list of all parasites found in human tissues. This list should simplify the diagnostic process.

This book was written in the old fashioned way; a single author toiling alone for several years and exploring the literature published during the last 100 years. This is reflected in the references at the end of each chapter, where key articles are cited, even if very old by modern standards. This does not mean that help from several individuals was not at hand: M.D. Little and P.C. Beaver from the School of Public Health and Tropical Medicine at Tulane University, New Orleans, were very kind with their time, suggestions, material from their vast collection of cases, and, more importantly, their constant encouragement. M.D. Little read the entire manuscript; P.C. Beaver read a large portion until health problems did not allow him to continue. Without their collaboration, this work would probably not have come to light; my indebtedness to both is too great to express with words.

I would also like to thank other people: my students and residents who always ask more questions than I can answer; the numerous individuals who sent me their material in consultation; the personnel at the Allen Memorial Medical Library of Cleveland, especially Mrs. D. Komarjanski for her constant help with the literature searches; my secretary, Mrs. P. Ragin, for her dedication to the many drafts of the manuscript; my wife, Teresa, an academic widow, who zealously protected my time for writing; and finally, all the people at Lea & Febiger, for their outstanding collaboration.

Cleveland, Ohio   Y. Gutierrez

CONTENTS

DIAGNOSTIC PATHOLOGY OF PARASITIC INFECTIONS
WITH CLINICAL CORRELATIONS

1

INTRODUCTION

Parasitology is the study of the association between organisms that live on or in another, larger animal known as the *host*, from which they derive their sustenance. This definition applies in a general sense to all groups of organisms (bacteria, fungi, viruses, spirochetes, rickettsiae, and others) inhabiting all animals and humans. Parasitology, as it is understood today, is the branch of medicine that deals with the study of animal forms (protists, helminths, and arthropods) living in humans, animals, or plants. *Medical parasitology* is the branch of parasitology concerned with all parasitic forms using humans as their host and studies all aspects of this association, both at the individual level and at the community level.

The biologic association between the host and its parasites results in different forms of cohabitation, depending on the effects they have on each other. If no harm occurs to the host, the association is called *commensalism*. If both the parasite and the host benefit, it becomes *mutualism*; a much closer relationship, in which neither parasite nor host cannot survive alone, is referred to as *symbiosis*. Hosts are classified on the basis of which stages of the parasite they harbor; in a *definitive host* the sexual development of the parasite occurs, such as humans for *Schistosoma*. An interme-

diate host is one in which the larval stages develop, for example *Echinococcus granulosus* in humans. Depending on the degree of adaptation to a parasitic life, the host can be *obligate* when the parasite cannot survive alone, for example all tapeworms. A *facultative* host is used by parasites that are naturally free-living organisms, such as occurs when *Acanthamoeba* and *Naegleria* become parasitic. A *spurious* host is one that temporarily harbors parasitic forms ingested in food. These parasitic forms are evacuated unchanged in the stools, where they may be found, as occurs with *Fasciola hepatica* when humans consume infected animal liver. Hosts are *specific* when the parasite has only one species as its host and cannot survive in any other, for example *Taenia solium*, which requires humans for its existence. By contrast, hosts are *inespecific* when many species of host will do, as in *Clonorchis sinensis*.

Homo sapiens has its own determined set of parasites found in no other animals. These are the parasites acquired during the dawn of humanity and that evolved together with humans, for example, *Enterobius vermicularis*, *Wuchereria bancrofti*, and *Taenia solium*, among many others. These parasites are well adapted to their host, usually producing few or no serious clinical consequences. The number of species found parasitizing humans is about 270 and growing, but only 16% are core human parasites that cannot survive without humans. It was long thought that the evolutionary aim of adaptation of parasitic associations was to become true commensals. Recently this concept has been revised, and now it is believed that the development of an intermediate degree of virulence serves better the multiplication of the parasite. In general, in evolutionary terms, the newer a parasite is to its host, the more harmful it is, for example *Naegleria*, which produces an almost invariably fatal infection. Humans can acquire parasites from animals (*zoonosis*), usually accidentally, for example when a mosquito carrying the infective larvae of *Dirofilaria immitis* bites a human, rather than a dog, and passes the larva to this unnatural host. Other parasites occur with equal frequency in animals and humans, such as *Schistosoma japonicum* and *Clonorchis sinensis*, in which case we speak of *euzoonosis*. We refer to *zooanthroponoses* when a parasitic infection of humans passes accidentally to animals, as when dogs acquire *Strongyloides stercoralis*. The term *zoonosis* and all combinations of it have been criticized for being strictly anthropocentric and lacking scientific validity.

Parasites may occur in tissues and internal organs, producing *infections*, and on the skin, hair, and clothes, producing *infestations*. Infestations usually are produced by arthropods (*ectoparasites*), such as *Pediculus humanus* and *Phthirus pubis*. Based on the idea that the intestinal lumen is actually "outside the body," it was once thought that intestinal worms produce infestations, an idea discarded long ago. As defined above, the terms *infection* and *infestation* have long been accepted as the correct manner in which to refer to these two states of parasitism. Yet, *infestation* is still commonly used to denote infections produced by internal parasites. Bad habits die hard!

Parasites that produce disease (a yes-or-no phenomenon) are *pathogens*. This means that if one organism produces disease once, either in *Homo sapiens* or in a species of animal, it becomes a pathogen for that species. The severity of symptoms a pathogen produces is termed *virulence*. The reactive processes provoked in the host by a pathogen, and the dynamics of this process, result in *disease* and are often referred to as *pathogenesis*.

Hosts are continuously exposed to their parasites, and when they acquire them, they suffer the consequences of the infection, which depend on the virulence of the parasite. The infection may produce no consequences, or may cause morbidity or even mortality. Sometimes parasites are acquired and lost spontaneously. Hosts thrive without their pathogenic para-

sites, but parasites cannot exist without their hosts. In recent history, infections with *Cryptosporidium* and *Enterocytozoon* were found first in immune-deficient individuals because the disease was amplified in these hosts. Soon after immune-competent hosts were found to be infected with them, it was relatively easy to understand that those organisms had been acquired eons ago by humans and that they produce limited disease. In this sense they are not new or emergent but just newly recognized.

Since parasites need their hosts for survival, it is obvious that they have to be readily available in the milieu in which their hosts live. Therefore, parasites have developed diverse specific methods of entering their hosts. The most common route of entry is the mouth; parasites gain access with food normally ingested. Consumed foods may come from animals, which are normal intermediate hosts for the parasite; for example, the larval stage of *Taenia solium* occurs in pork. The fecal-oral route, referred to as *contamination*, is another common pathway by which parasites enter the host. This process occurs when feces or other body fluids containing infective stages reach drinking water or food, as with most intestinal protozoa. Soil is a common vehicle, especially for organisms that have an obligatory phase of development in the environment. The *soil-transmitted* helminths *Ascaris lumbricoides*, *Trichuris trichiura*, and *Toxocara canis* are acquired by ingestion of soil laden with infective eggs of the parasite. Since small children have a proclivity to ingest soil, they suffer from these infections in greater percentages, and because they acquire large numbers of parasites, they suffer greater morbidity. In contrast, adults may ingest small amounts of soil when food is accidentally contaminated with soil, and thus they have subclinical infections. The hookworms and *Strongyloides stercoralis* are also soil transmitted, but their infective larval stages enter actively through the skin and sometimes are ingested with water; adults are more prone to this type of infection. Some parasites need snails as intermediate hosts. Living within these hosts, the parasites develop and multiply the number of infective stages. These parasites include all species of trematodes or flukes, the *snail-transmitted* helminths. Other parasites are acquired *percutaneously*, a process that requires a hematophagous arthropod. The arthropod ingests the parasite during a blood meal taken from an infected host; the parasite develops to the infective stages in the arthropod, which then inoculates the parasite to a new host, as with *Leishmania*, *Trypanosoma*, and *Plasmodium*. Sometimes the arthropod deposits the infective stages on the skin of the host because of its proclivity to defecate during its blood meal, as in

Trypanosoma cruzi. In these instances, the feces of the vector contain the infective stages, which gain access to the tissues through the mucosa or abrasions in the skin. Similarly, the filarial worms have infective larvae that develop in mosquitoes and locate in their mouthparts to migrate to the skin of the host during the mosquito's blood meal. These larvae penetrate the skin and gain access to the internal organs. Transfused blood can transmit trypanosomiasis, malaria, and toxoplasmosis; the same infections can be passed from the mother to the fetus.

Once the parasite gains access to the new host by any of the routes described above, it migrates to the location where it normally resides. Many parasites of the gastrointestinal tract acquired by the oral route pass through the stomach and develop in the area of the intestine to which they are adapted. Examples include *Giardia* and *T. solium* in the small intestine and *Entamoeba histolytica*, *Trichuris trichiura*, and *Enterobius vermicularis* in the colon. Other parasites move through the lungs before locating in the intestine, such as *Ascaris lumbricoides*. Parasites inoculated by arthropods through the skin often began to multiply at the inoculum site (*Leishmania* and *Trypanosoma*) and then spread to other organs. Or, if inoculated directly into the bloodstream (*Plasmodium*), they are carried to the liver, where they develop stages capable of parasitizing the erythrocytes. Some species of filarial worms enter the skin to develop in the subcutaneous tissues, where they remain (*Loa loa*, *Onchocerca volvulus*). Other species develop temporarily in the subcutaneous tissues before reaching the internal organs (*Dirofilaria immitis*, *Wuchereria bancrofti*, and species of *Brugia*). Many parasites with obligatory migration through the tissues may find wrong (*ectopic*) sites where they eventually perish. *Fasciola hepatica* normally migrates from the intestine into the peritoneal cavity and then to the biliary system, but it may lodge anywhere in the body. The schistosomes and the paragonimids are also well known for their ectopicity.

The period between acquisition of the infection and the beginning of clinical manifestations is the *incubation period*. This period is variable; for example, in *Leishmania donovani*, it may be up to 25 years. The period between acquisition of the parasite and the time when eggs, larvae, or microfilariae are shed is known as the *prepatent period*. The period during which these diagnostic stages are shed in the body or body fluids is referred to as the *patent period* or *patency*. Often, the prepatent period is different from the incubation period, and patency does not necessarily coincide with the beginning or end of clinical symptoms. Schistosomiasis manifests long before eggs appear in the stools or the urine; lymphatic filariae may be eradicated from the host, but the sequelae of the chronic infection (elephantiasis) may continue throughout the patient's life.

Disease

Disease is the reaction of the host to a parasite, which depends on the parasite's degree of virulence, the number of parasites present, the chronicity of the infection, the survival capacity of the parasite, and the immunologic status of the host. Disease does not necessarily correlate with the number of parasites in the host: protozoa are capable of superparasitism, while helminths often occur as a single worm. In either case, host reactions are *disseminated* or are *localized* to the site and surrounding tissues where the parasite is located.

Disseminated Reactions. Disseminated reactions occur most often with parasites that involve many organs (visceral leishmaniasis, *Plasmodium falciparum*) or with parasites located in a given organ but producing systemic toxic reactions, such as *Fasciolopsis buski*. Similarly, *Entamoeba histolytica* and *Trichuris trichiura* produce colitis, sometimes life-threatening with generalized toxemia due to damage of the colonic mucosa. In general terms, disseminated reactions are associated more often with protozoa because they are capable of multiplying in the host. In contrast, helminthic infections, with a few exceptions, do not multiply in the host and do not increase in number. The size of the infective dose limits their number.

Local Reactions. Local reactions are usually necrotic and inflammatory, with formation of microabscesses, abscesses, or granulomas, limited to a small area; examples include *Dirofilaria* infections of the subcutaneous tissues and the lung and *Acanthamoeba* infection of the brain. Local reactions can also involve an entire organ or organ system, usually producing consequences for that organ. *Wuchereria* and *Brugia*, filariids of the lymphatics, damage the lymphatics in the area where they are located, producing difficulties in lymph drainage that result in elephantiasis. *Fasciola hepatica* produces chronic cholangitis. More often, the host has a local reaction to the parasite, a normal response that permits the parasite to survive, such as *Onchocerca volvulus* in fibrous nodules in the subcutaneous tissues. Another example is the inflammatory reaction to a developing unilocular hydatid cyst, which stimulates a fibrous tissue response by the host in an amount necessary to protect the cyst. Local reactions to parasites show infiltration of various cell types: histiocytes and lymphocytes in leishmaniae, predominantly eosinophils in *Anisakis*, neutrophils and lymphocytes in *Toxoplasma*. In some cases, large areas of necrosis occur due to direct action of the parasite on the host's cells, as in *Entamoeba histolytica* in the liver. In other instances, necrosis is due to destruction of the blood vessels, resulting in hemorrhagic infarcts, for example in lesions produced by *Toxoplasma* and *Acanthamoeba* in the brain. In helminthic infections, areas of necrosis usually result from the death of the parasite, for example cysticercus in the brain and other tissues, subcutaneous zoonotic filariids (*Dirofilaria repens*, *Dirofilaria tenuis*), or sparganum larva.

A common reaction to local parasites or their products is a granulomatous inflammation, for example in *Toxocara canis*, producing visceral larva migrans, and *Schistosoma* eggs in the liver, intestine, and other organs. The chronic granulomatous inflammation produced in the liver by schistosomes results in marked fibrosis of the liver that leads to portal hypertension. Another local fibrous reaction in the colon (ameboma) is sometimes produced by *E. histolytica*, a lesion that often simulates a carcinoma.

Peripheral blood eosinophilia is usually associated with helminthic infections in which the parasite has an obligatory phase of migration through the tissues. Peripheral eosinophilia often signifies an abnormal degree of sensitization to parasite antigens, for example when *Ascaris* larvae migrate through the lungs, producing Loeffler's syndrome. In other instances, intense eosinophilia is the result of massive movement of eosinophils from bone marrow to an area where a parasite is dead, for example in *Anisakis* infections. Tissue eosinophilia usually occurs in the area of dead parasites, as in subcutaneous or pulmonary *Dirofilaria* infections. The presence of Charcot-Leyden crystals (the "tombstones" of eosinophils) in tissues signifies that in the past the lesion contained large numbers of eosinophils. In some helminthic infections, peripheral eosinophilia changes throughout the duration of the infection. For example, hookworms produce high peripheral eosinophilia during migration of the worms from the skin through the lungs into the intestine, and this condition continues while the young worms grow and begin to copulate. Soon afterward, the peripheral eosinophilia declines slowly until the eosinophil level becomes normal in spite of continuing local infection. *Toxocara* produces high peripheral eosinophilia during migration of the parasites through the viscera, but the eosinophilia decreases slowly for several months until

the eosinophil level returns to normal when all the larvae become encapsulated in the muscles.

Some parasitic infections evolve rapidly, with a fatal outcome for the host; for example, *Naegleria fowleri* produces amoebic meningoencephalitis in immune-competent hosts. However, most parasites are well adapted to their hosts, where they reside for long periods, sometimes for the life of the host. These chronic infections are often asymptomatic, but sometimes they produce complications. Infections with *Plasmodium malariae*, *Wuchereria bancrofti*, and *Schistosoma* may result in a glomerulonephritis due to the deposition of soluble antigen–antibody complexes in the glomerular membrane. Glomerulonephritis also occurs in infections with *Sarcoptes scabiei* due to secondary infection of the skin lesions with nephritogenic streptococci. *Trypanosoma cruzi* may destroy the effector cells of the parasympathetic nervous system and produce disturbances, or it may produce blocks in the cardiac conduction system. Chronic infection with *Schistosoma haematobium* in certain geographic areas results in higher prevalence of squamous cell carcinoma of the urinary bladder; similarly, infection with the biliary fluke *Clonorchis sinensis* leads to a higher prevalence of cholangiocarcinoma.

Clinically and histologically, parasites sometimes simulate neoplasia. *Dirofilaria immitis* produces coin lesions on chest x-ray films indistinguishable from those of pulmonary carcinoma. *Paragonimus* in the brain often simulates a neoplastic process. *Entamoeba histolytica* produces ulcerating cervicitis in women and ulcerating balanitis in men, lesions that often have been clinically diagnosed as malignant disease. *Echinococcus multilocularis* or alveolar echinococcosis produces metastasis to distant organs, behaving as a malignant disease that often results in death. The hepatic lesion of *Echinococcus multilocularis* has been confused histologically with those of a low-grade sarcoma. *Echinococcus granulosus* usually presents as a mass anywhere in the body, necessitating its distinction from other tissue growths.

The greatest challenge that parasitic infections pose to the clinician examining a patient, and to the pathologist examining tissues, is the diagnosis of parasitic infections encountered outside the known endemic areas of those particular parasites. Because of easy international travel, persons may be infected with *Tunga penetrans*, *Leishmania*, or other organisms that manifest after their return to areas where these parasites do not occur and thus are not commonly known. Similarly, the zoonotic parasites are difficult to suspect and diagnose, by both clinicians and pathologists, because of their infrequent occurrence.

Disease Nomenclature. In recent years the World Association for the Advancement of Veterinary Parasitology has proposed that the names of parasitic diseases be uniformly designated by the suffix *osis* added to the stem of the name of the parasite. The purpose of uniformity in terminology is not only to improve clarity in scientific communication, but also to make the electronic systems of bibliography retrieval more consistent. The new system will result in names such as *endolimacosis* for *Endolimax* infection, *ancylostomosis* for *Ancylostoma* infection, *trypanosomosis* for *Trypanosoma* infection, and so on. This nomenclature system for parasitic diseases has not been widely accepted in the literature of human medicine. Therefore, in this text, the traditional names are retained for the sake of custom: *endolimiasis, ancylostomiasis,* and *trypanosomiasis.*

trast, disseminated diseases with *Entamoeba histolytica* or overwhelming *Giardia lamblia* do not occur in homosexuals with AIDS in spite of their higher prevalence among homosexuals. This fact indicates that their virulence is not enhanced by a CD4$^+$ T-lymphocyte deficiency. Infection with the human T-cell lymphoma/leukemia virus 1 (HTLV-1) correlates with the chronicity and potentiates the virulence of *Strongyloides stercoralis* infections in humans. Homosexual males with AIDS in developed countries often have infections with *Cryptosporidium, Toxoplasma, Encephalitozoon,* and *Enterocytozoon,* while those in developing countries have, in addition to these, infections with *Isospora.* Since the infective stages of *Isospora* require maturation in the environment, infections with *Isospora* correlate better with fecal contamination of the environment than with the fecal-oral route.

Parasitism, Homosexuality, and the Acquired Immune Deficiency Syndrome

The acquired immune deficiency syndrome (AIDS) epidemic has emphasized the need for a better understanding of parasitic infections, better modalities of diagnosis, and constant vigilance for pathogens not normally associated with humans that infect individuals with human immune deficiency virus (HIV). This situation is well illustrated by the recognition of more than ten species of Microspora and Apicomplexa described in immune-compromised and immune-competent humans since the first edition of this text was published.

In immune-competent homosexuals living in developed countries, rates of prevalence of parasites acquired through the fecal-oral route are equal to the rates found in the general population of developing countries. Sexual practices of male homosexuals, for example oral-anal sex, are responsible for the high prevalence of *Entamoeba histolytica, Giardia lamblia, Enterocytozoon bieneusi,* and other nonpathogenic intestinal protozoa. A similar situation is not described in homosexual women.

Individuals with AIDS generally develop parasitic opportunistic infections with organisms that are selectively helped by a CD4$^+$ T-lymphocyte deficiency. In general terms, these organisms belong to the Apicomplexa (*Cryptosporidium, Isospora, Toxoplasma,* and *Cyclospora*), the Microspora (*Enterocytozoon, Encephalitozoon, Vittaforma, Pleistophora, Trachipleistophora,* and others), and related forms. In con-

Diagnosis

The diagnosis of parasitic infection is often difficult clinically. Identification of parasites in the laboratory requires highly trained personnel who are acquainted with the morphologic characteristics of the organisms and, in some instances, with specific methods for their diagnosis. The recognition of given taxonomic groups or species always necessitates morphologic studies of the parasite in question or, in the case of some protists, biochemical analysis. The day when serologic tests can *identify* a given parasite is still far away. Serologic tests indicate to the clinician that antibodies to the parasite in question, or to parasites of related species, are present in the patient's sera, stools, or body fluid. A positive serologic test result may correlate with the clinical symptoms and the history of the patient, but it does not prove that the patient has active infection. There are many case reports in the literature in which specific parasitic agents are "identified," sometimes to the species level, because the patient had a positive serologic test result. These reports are at best spurious because there was no recovery and study of the parasite. The new technologies of DNA analysis are still in their infancy, but their specificity is remarkable. However, identification of the parasite from which the DNA is used as a standard still requires a knowledgeable parasitologist. Clinically, a high degree of suspicion is necessary before a parasitic infection is included among the diagnostic possibilities in a given patient, especially in areas outside the normal endemic range, or in infections occurring in small numbers. The required laboratory samples are then necessary for the pathologist to confirm the clinical suspicion and to identify the parasite.

In recent years, imaging modalities such as compute tomography, nuclear magnetic resonance, ultrasound, and endoscopic retrograde cholangiopancreatography have become the diagnostic methods of choice for hydatid disease, cysticercosis, schistosomiasis, and fascioliasis, respectively. These techniques allow the visualization not only of the lesion and its relationships to other organs and structures, but also sometimes of the parasites themselves, for example *Fasciola* and *Clonorchis-Opistorchis* in bile ducts.

As stated, serologic tests for detection of antibodies are often helpful, but they are rarely diagnostic to the specific level. Detection of circulating antigen (actual parasitic elements or secretions of parasites) and circulating immune complexes is more specific and promising. Diagnosis based on circulating antibodies in scrum or stools in infections with organisms inhabiting the gastrointestinal tract, and easily diagnosed by direct examination of stool samples, is often a futile exercise. The cost is prohibitive, and the interpretation of what constitutes a positive result is still the responsibility of the technologist, who may have a little knowledge of the technique in use or of its limitations. On the other hand, a direct stool examination not only detects the parasite for which the serologic test is set up, it is also excellent for searching for all other organisms potentially present. In addition, the well-trained diagnostician-parasitologist can provide information about the presence of neutrophils, eosinophils, blood, and other important components of the sample, all of which may be helpful to the clinician. Serologic tests are best for infections in which the parasite is in the tissues and either is not accessible or is difficult to recover for direct examination.

Most parasitic infections that shed eggs, larvae, microfilaria, segments of adult worms (tapeworms), or adults are best diagnosed in the clinical laboratory. Different techniques are available for the search, recovery, and identification of these stages. A large number of parasites are generally diagnosed in tissue sections of biopsy specimens taken from patients or in autopsy material; these are the tissue parasites.

cause they are always unusual. Exceptions should be made for organisms associated with AIDS, some of which have become common to most anatomic pathologists. Exceptions should also be made when the parasite is endemic to a given geographic area and pathologists and clinicians are fully familiar with it.

A specimen may reach the cutting room identified as a parasite and grossly identified as a worm or as resembling a worm. In these cases, more often than not, the patient brings the specimen to the physician and reports that he or she passed it in the stools. Less frequently, the worm comes from the tissues of a patient or is coughed up by the individual. If the specimen arrives in saline solution, it should not be placed in formalin; if it is received already fixed, it should remain as such. In either case, the specimen should be referred to the clinical laboratory, where, it is ideally, properly fixed and identified in toto. It is always easier to examine the whole specimen and to identify the parasite based on its gross characteristics since in histologic sections identification is often impossible. Granted, remuneration for the study and for identification of the parasite in the clinical laboratory is small in contrast to what the usual payment if it is sectioned and examined as a surgical sample. However, the patient is poorly served when this procedure is followed.

The second set of circumstances in which an anatomic pathologist encounters a "parasite" is while studying the slides of the day for diagnosis. In the great majority of cases this is an unexpected finding because, if it is a worm, clinicians rarely suspect the patient's true condition. The first step in identifying the parasite is to make sure that it is not an artifact but rather a true organism, often a difficult and frustrating task when one is unfamiliar with the microanatomy of parasites. The purpose of this book is to describe and characterize human parasites in tissues in order to help anatomic pathologists in their daily work. Parasites in sections have characteristics that in most cases allow specific diagnosis, in the same manner that a tumor, on its own, demonstrates that it is a lymphoma, or a squamous cell carcinoma, even if the pathologist knows nothing about the patient's history.

Handling Parasites in the Cutting Room

Tissue pathologists do not usually find parasites in their daily work, and when they do, these parasites are unsuspected and almost invariably pose a problem be-

The Report of Parasites

Reporting to the Clinician. Once the parasite is found and examined, a written report is generated

for the clinician or other interested parties. Specimens referred to the clinical laboratory are reported as clinical specimens. For specimens reported from sections of anatomic specimens, precise language should be used in all written reports, which ideally refers to the genus and species of the parasite, for example "Focal necrosis and abscess formation produced by *Dirofilaria tenuis*, clinically subcutaneous nodule from right forearm," or "Granulomatous inflammation of liver produced by *Toxocara* spp. consistent with clinically visceral larva migrans," or "Cholangitis due to *Clonorchis-Opistorchis*." Note that in these examples the pathologist has seen and identified the filarial worm to the species level, the larvae of *Toxocara* to the generic level, and the trematode in the bile ducts to either one of the two genera found in humans. This is state-of-the-art reporting. If the parasites in question are not found and identified, then none of the above language should be used, regardless of how sure the clinician, the pathologist, or both, are about the cause of the patient's problems. However, if the clinical diagnosis submitted with the specimen is visceral larva migrans, the larvae are not seen in numerous granulomas with eosinophils, and other clinical characteristics of this infection are known, the report should state "Granulomatous inflammation consistent with clinically visceral larva migrans." This example presents a mere suspicion of an infection by *Toxocara*, with clearly defined granulomas in the liver, possibly in a patient with high antibody titers. However, in spite of all this *circumstantial evidence*, the term *Toxocara* (which connotes that a *generic identification* of the worm was made) should not be used in anatomic reports. Nor should such a case be published with the name of a genus or a species, or both, identifying the parasite.

Terms such as *objects*, *fragments of worm*, *foreign bodies*, or *bodies* representing sections of a worm, or consistent with helminthic infection, are at best an indication of the diagnostician's poor judgment. They have no place in a surgical report. To begin with, helminths are living organisms, never objects, foreign bodies, or bodies; they have specific names. In all cases where the nature of the diagnostic sample is in doubt, the help of those familiar with the characteristics of parasites in tissues should be sought. Their guidance usually clarifies an apparently murky case. Fortunately for patients most lesions involving helminths in tissues are obviously not life-threatening, a fact that makes many diagnosticians ignore what could be an important finding academically, biologically, or both.

Reporting in the Literature. Parasites elicit a great deal of interest, curiosity, and often excitement each time they are encountered by a clinician, a pathologist, or other related personnel. This healthy fascination often translates into a desire to share the finding with colleagues at large by means of a literature case report. The report of cases, or clusters of cases, in the surgical pathology, tropical medicine, general and specialty medical, and parasitology literature is a staple for medical parasitologists and physicians interested in these infections. For the basic medical parasitologist, these literature reports are often a fount of information on the basic biology of parasites, which is often not apparent to those who report the case. Well-done reports may help delineate the geographic distribution of parasites, may point to an undescribed species in the fauna of the region from which the reported human case came, or may indicate how long the parasite can live in that host, its rate of growth, and so on. However, the main purpose of case reports is to keep clinicians informed of the diagnostic possibilities in patients with similar clinical presentations and to keep pathologists aware of the diagnostic characteristics of the organisms found.

Unfortunately, incomplete reports of interesting cases are usually the result of these endeavors, making the report suspect, not believable, or at best spurious. Any report of a case, or group of cases, of parasitic infections originating from a study of tissue sections, or of the organisms themselves, should contain a detailed description of the parasite. A description of the morphologic characteristics, with accompanying good-quality photographs and drawings illustrating the diagnostic landmarks used for the identification of the parasite, are essential. The same is true for reports of clinical findings in patients with unusual parasitic diseases. This method of reporting permits future reference for comparison with similar cases, and when a well-known parasite is thought to produce a new or undescribed condition, it provides the only bases that make the findings credible. In reports of series of cases, it is necessary to find the parasite in each patient. Studies with one index case that shows the parasite, together with other cases with similar clinical histories, or serologic test results without the organism, are not justified; they are often inflated reports that delineate imaginary diseases or problems.

Case reports of common parasites published because special stains or esoteric diagnostic technologies were used, often without comparison and correlation with features found in simple hematoxylin and eosin stains, are at best useless. The use of immunofluorescence, transmission, and scanning electron microscopes and molecular technologies in specimens showing obvious known morphologic diagnostic features, easily seen in sections stained with hematoxylin and eosin, are of little importance and constitute overdiagnosis that taxes the health care reimbursement system unnecessarily. Similarly, literature reports in which the species of a parasite is identified on the basis of clinical histories, travel history, serologic reactions, and other similar modalities that constitute circumstantial evidence have little meaning and always lack credibility. Common findings in respected scientific journals are reports with titles such as "Suspected case of (name of parasite) infection in . . ." or "Serologically proven (name of parasite) infection . . .". In all such publications, the field becomes more confused, misinformation grows, and the scientific community is ill served. Well-documented and well-written reports of cases or clusters of cases are the beginning of every scientific advance in human medicine. Examples abound; a classic one is the cluster of cases of young homosexual males with *Pneumocystis* pneumonia, a rare organism at the time, that alerted us to the AIDS epidemic.

Part I

The Protists

Unicellular or *acellular* organisms, those composed of a single cell that carries out all the functions of feeding, locomotion, and reproduction, are referred to in modern classification schemes as the *protists*. The protists are a large group that includes the prokaryotes and eukaryotes, unicellular organisms with the capacity to synthesize carbohydrates from inorganic substances by means of their green plastids, and those that require already formed food. The protists of medical importance are eukaryotes, belonging to the kingdoms Archezoa and Protozoa, both of which require already formed food for their sustenance. Many of the members of these two groups are free-living organisms; some have adapted to a parasitic existence, and the genera and species found in humans are the subject of the following discussion. All generalizations made in this introduction about protists are for didactic purposes to characterize only groups and species found in humans; they should not be construed as applying to all protists found in nature.

Morphology

The morphologic characteristics of the protists are important to the biologist who wishes to classify these organisms, as well as to the pathologist who needs to render an accurate diagnosis in a given sample. Without familiarity with the diverse structures seen under the microscope, it is virtually impossible to recognize the different genera and species of the protists. Moreover, most pathologists are familiar with descriptions of parasites learned in the clinical laboratory, where the organisms are seen in smears (therefore appearing larger) stained with special stains to enhance some organelles. In tissues, organisms are seen in sections; for example, a given protozoon measuring 15 μm in diameter theoretically will appear in two or three sections 5 μm thick. In tissue sections, the size of the organisms is somewhat reduced because of contraction of the tissues during processing for sectioning. The morphologic characteristics of the protists in tissue sections will be discussed in detail for each parasite; here only an overview will be provided as a general guide to how to approach their identification.

Light Microscopy

In tissues, protists are intracellular (Fig. 5–1) or extracellular (Fig. 7–2), the first feature that should be recognized when protists are being identified. The type of cell in which the parasite resides is also of paramount importance: *Leishmania* are found only in histiocytes (Fig. 4–17); *Toxoplasma* and *T. cruzi* are found in all types of cells because they can enter the cell on their own. Protists may be intracellular by necessity, for example the microsporidia, the leishmaniae, some trypanosomes, *Toxoplasma*, and others. However, they appear extracellular because the cell membrane is not readily visible or because they are not seen to be clearly associated with a cell nucleus due to the plane of sectioning; *Toxoplasma* in brain sections is a good example (*color plate* VI *C–D*). In tissue imprints, intracellular protists are often seen outside the cell, but this is due to the artifactual rupture of the cell, resulting in the scattering of the organisms (*color plate* III *A–B*). When one examines tissue imprints, finding one or more intact cells with parasites is sufficient to determine that the parasite in question is intracellular. In general, intracellular protists are smaller than the cell they inhabit, and usually they measure 1 to 5 μm in diameter. Exceptions are certain cysts that have large numbers of organisms, such as *Toxoplasma* and *Sarcocystis* (Fig. 9–1). *Toxoplasma* may measure up to 30 μm in diameter, and *Sarcocystis* may grow large enough to be visible with the naked eye. Some organisms are intracellular but extracytoplasmic, for example *Cryp-*

tosporidium (Figs. 8–3 to 8–6); sometimes extracellular protozoa are found in phagocytic cells.

Extracellular protists are often found in the intestine, such as *Giardia* on the surface of enterocytes, or *Entamoeba histolytica* and *Balantidium coli* on the surface or deep in ulcerations of the colon. In tissues, *E. histolytica* and species of *Acanthamoeba* and *Naegleria* are also extracellular. Sometimes the cysts of *Acanthamoeba* are observed within histiocytes forming giant cells (Fig. 6–21). The size of the amebae in tissues varies roughly from 10 to 30 μm.

In both intracellular and extracellular protists, a few organelles should be recognized for diagnostic purposes. The nuclear characteristics of the amebae are important for the identification of the group to which they belong. *Entamoeba histolytica* has a small central karyosome (Fig. 7–16); *Acanthamoeba* and *Naegleria* have a large one (Figs. 6–3 and 6–11). Intracellular stages of *Leishmania* and *T. cruzi* are identical under the light microscope, recognized by the presence of a kinetoplast, a structure next to the nucleus.

Electron Microscope

With the exception of certain groups of the Microspora, the aid of electron micrographs is rarely necessary for the surgical pathologist's diagnosis of conditions produced by protists. The general ultrastructure of protists is similar to that of eukaryotic cells: a cell membrane composed of three layers limits a cytoplasm that has a nucleus and other organelles, varying in accordance with the group under study. *Entamoeba histolytica* has a nucleus with a defined nuclear membrane and chromatin distributed as small granules attached to the inner surface of the nuclear membrane (Fig. 7–16). In the cytoplasm, numerous digestive vacuoles are present, but *E. histolytica* lacks mitochondria, peroxisomes, rough endoplasmic reticulum, and Golgi dyctiosomes. The trypanosomatids (*Trypanosoma* and *Leishmania*) have a single flagellum arising from a basal body and exiting through a flagellar pocket made by an invagination of the cell membrane (Figs. 4–1 and 5–2). The flagellum arises in the basal body and has the same arrangement of seven plus two microtubules seen in flagella of eukaryotic cells (Fig. 5–2). The trypanosomatids also have a kinetoplast, a single mitochondrion with the largest amount of extranuclear DNA known in any cell. The DNA in the kinetoplast (Fig. 5–2) contains all the information to direct the synthesis of the enzymes needed for aerobic metabolism of carbohydrates. The other flagellates have more than one flagellum arising from different parts of the body; some may have more than one nucleus (*Giardia*) (Fig. 3–1). Most flagellates have an undulating membrane supported by the flagellum (trypanosomatids) or by one of the flagella (trichomonadids) (Fig. 3–9 A). Other structures, such as an axoneme in *Giardia* (Fig. 3–3 B) and an axostyle in the trichomonadids (Fig. 3–9 A), may be seen in some sections. A mouth or cytostome is also present in the trichomonadids and in *Balantidium* (Fig. 11–1 A). The ciliates are characterized by the presence of numerous cilia covering the entire body (Fig. 11–1 A). In electron micrographs, these cilia are similar to those found in ciliated epithelia of vertebrates. In the anterior end of some stages of their life cycles, the members of the Apicomplexa have an apical complex (Figs. 8–1 and 9–4), composed of several organelles such as microtubules, rhopthries, and paired organelles. This complex of organelles permits the entry of the parasites into the cells where they develop. These parasites also have mitochondria, Golgi apparatus, and rough endoplasmic reticulum. Members of the Apicomplexa show various stages of their sexual or asexual development in human tissues. Finally, the presence of a microtubule (Fig. 2–1) and developmental stages in the cell characterize the microsporidians. The microtubule helps to complete their life cycles, which occur in a single host (Fig. 2–2).

Life Cycles

The stage of the protists that performs the functions of motility, feeding, and reproduction is known as the *trophozoite* or *vegetative* stage (Figs. 6–7 *A* and 7–16 *E–G*). The simplest life cycle of parasitic protists consists of a trophozoite that passes unchanged directly to a new host to continue its functions as a trophozoite (*Trichomonas, Entamoeba gingivalis*).

The most common life cycle of protists involves an adaptation to the passage from one host to another by means of a *cyst*, as in *Entamoeba*. Parasitic cysts are stages that usually evolve from a trophozoite by forming a wall on their own, without the intervention of the host. Cysts are forms of reproduction, when the number of nuclei increases as the cyst matures, and of resistance to the adverse environment outside the host (Figs. 7–16 *C–D*). Protists inhabiting the alimentary tract with cysts in their life cycles (*Entamoeba, Endolimax, Iodamoeba, Giardia, and Balantidium*) usually evacuate their cysts into the environment, where they reach the new host by contaminating its food or water. Sometimes cystic stages of protists develop in the tissues, where they remain until the host is ingested by another host, allowing the completion of the cycle (*Toxoplasma, Sarcocystis*). The apicomplexan protists (*Cryptosporidium, Isospora, Sarcocystis,* and *Toxoplasma*) form *oocysts* (*color plate* V *G–H*), the product of their sexual reproduction, and form when the male *microgamete* joins with the female *macrogamete* (see below). Some apicomplexan protists also have sarcocysts (cysts in the skeletal muscles of an intermediate host, for example in *Sarcocystis*) (Figs. 9–1, 9–2, and 9–3). Alternatively, cysts may be formed in many tissues of the intermediate hosts, as in *Toxoplasma* (Figs. 9–8 *D*, 9–13 *B*, 9–15 *D–E*).

Another type of life cycle uses hematophagous arthropods as obligatory intermediate hosts (Fig. 10–1). This type of development is found among the protists inhabiting the blood (*Trypanosoma, Plasmodium*) and tissues of the host (*Leishmania*). The trypanosomes and the leishmaniae are transferred from one host to the next by arthropods in which infective stages develop from the stages taken from the host during a blood meal. In contrast, the plasmodia produce male and female stages, which after ingestion by mosquitoes undergo sexual development that results in the infective stages for the new host (Fig. 10–1). Hematophagous arthropods can transmit the infective stages of protists in different ways. Some hematophagous arthropods inoculate the host with their saliva at the time of feeding (*Plasmodium*, African trypanosomes); others transmit infective stages by their feces, which they excrete at the time of feeding (*T. cruzi*).

Reproduction

The reproduction of protists is varied and sometimes complicated, but in general terms, it is either asexual or sexual. More specifically, the term *multiplication* should be used when speaking of protists without a sexual cycle and *reproduction* when referring to those with a sexual cycle. Protists never undergo *replication*, a term that should be reserved for viruses and prions, as it implies the production of two identical copies. When protists multiply and reproduce, the result is the production of similar but not identical organisms.

Asexual Reproduction

The most common form of reproduction among protists is asexual, which occurs in several ways. (1) *Binary fission*, the division of a trophozoite into two, begins with division of the nucleus, followed by partition of the cytoplasm. Binary fission in the flagellates is longitudinal (Fig. 5–15), and in the ciliates it is transverse. (2) *Schizogony* or *multiple fission*, a process commonly found among the apicomplexan protists, involves division of the nucleus several times before the cytoplasm divides to provide each nucleus with a portion of cytoplasm (Fig. 10–4). The dividing cell is known as a *schizont*. If the resulting cells are *merozoites*, the process is known as *merogony*; if they are *sporozoites*, it is called *sporogony*. Both processes occur in malarial parasites. (3) *External budding* is a process in which a small daughter cell grows and then separates from the surface of the mother cell. Budding of more than two daughter cells at once is known as *ectopolygeny*. (4) *Internal budding* is a process in which the mother cell produces buds internally (*endogeny*) and is destroyed in the process. If two buds are formed, the process is known as *endodyogeny*; if more than two daughter cells differentiate, it is called *endopolygeny*.

Sexual Reproduction

Two forms of sexual reproduction are known in parasitic protists. (1) *Conjugation* involves the temporary fusion of two individuals along some part of their bodies and reciprocal fertilization. (2) *Syngamy* is a type of reproduction seen mainly in the apicomplexan parasites in which special cells produce male and female *gametes* (micro- and macrogametocytes) by a process known as *gamogony*. Gametocytes produce gametes that join (syngamy) to produce a *zygote*. A zygote often divides into many sporozoites, which are the infective stage for a new host.

Geographic Distribution

Protists are widely distributed throughout most areas of the world. Those with a direct form of transmission (intestinal protists) occur in tropical, temperate, and arctic regions because the fecal-oral route is common in all these places. The lower standard of living and poorer hygiene habits frequently found in tropical and subtropical areas play an important role in the higher prevalence of these infections. In developed countries, the same situation is found in institutionalized persons and in small groups of underprivileged individuals; gay males, because of their sexual habits, are exposed to organisms transmitted by contamination in greater proportions. Some of these parasites occur in epidemics due to contamination of drinking water with human (*E. histolytica*, *Giardia lamblia*, *Cyclospora cayetanensis*) or animal (*G. lamblia*, *Cryptosporidium parvum*) excreta.

Protists using arthropods as biologic vectors have a limited distribution that is often restricted to the distribution of their vectors. For example, the African trypanosomes are restricted to tropical Africa (Fig. 5–14) and the *leishmaniae* to tropical and subtropical regions of the world (Figs. 4–3 and 4–15). The leishmaniae as a group produce mostly zoonotic infections. They occur in a wide range of reservoir hosts, and infections in humans result from human interaction with the ecologic niche inhabited by the parasite, the definitive host, and the intermediate host.

This niche is usually the remote, uninhabited regions of tropical countries. In contrast, the plasmodia producing human malaria are more widely distributed because the vectors are domiciliary and peridomiciliary.

Classification

The zoologic classification of the protists is difficult because of the large number of groups that exist both as free-living organisms and as parasites in all animal groups and many plants. Moreover, classically their classification has been based on phenotypic (morphologic) characteristics seen with the light and electron microscopes, methods that have fallen into disfavor, overshadowed by the more glamorous molecular technologies. Unquestionably, this situation represents progress because, with these technologies, more genotypic characteristics are now being used to separate species, resulting in true advances, as in the separation of *E. histolytica* and *E. dispar*, two species phenotypically indistinguishable. This separation has resulted in a clearer understanding of the epidemiology, the biology, and hopefully the true importance of *E. histolytica* as a human pathogen. In contrast, the day when molecular separation of species is a fully mature discipline, at the disposition of most, if not all, laboratories identifying human parasites in the service of patients, has not arrived. Morphology will continue for several decades to be the pivotal discipline dealing with the recognition of human parasitic protists in clinical samples. Molecular classification is a welcome tool for the clinical laboratory, but only if it does not replace the dedicated morphologist.

As stated above, molecular technologies, cell biology studies, and the electron microscope have given us a better understanding of the protists at both the generic and specific levels. However, it is in understanding the relationships of the larger groups (kingdom and phylum) that even greater advances have been made. The modern classification schemes of protists have become more difficult for those whose disciplines are other than the taxonomy and systematics of parasites, basic biology, or zoology, but we need to present the basic principles for those readers who wish to understand the relationships of these parasites. The following approach should suffice for the physician student of medical parasitology.

The protists of medical importance studied in this book are grouped into two kingdoms: the Archezoa (or Archetista) and the Protozoa (or Protista). Two phyla in the Archezoa and six in the Protozoa contain all the species found in humans, as follows:

(A) *Kingdom*: *Archezoa*: The Archezoa are protists lacking mitochondria, plastids, typical Golgi apparatus, peroxisomes, and hydrogenosomes. The ribosomes and their rRNA have prokaryotic features. The Archezoa use anaerobic glycolysis. Some have flagella for locomotion; others use pseudopodia. The majority are parasitic.

Phylum: *Microspora*: Microspora are minute multicellular, intracellular organisms with 70s ribosomes; there are one or two nuclei; no flagella; and possible Golgi apparatus. The Microspora form minute spores that contain an extrusosome with a polar tube and an attachment disc. The spore has a chitinous wall; all are parasitic, and they may be fungi.

Genera: *Encephalitozoon*, *Enterocytozoon*, *Pleistophora*, *Trachipleistophora*, *Vittaforma*, and *Nosema*.

Phylum: *Metamonada*: The Metamonada have two to many flagella; 70s ribosomes; and 16s rRNA. Most are parasitic.

Genera: *Giardia*, *Enteromonas*, *Retortamonas*, and *Chilomastix*.

(B) *Kingdom*: *Protozoa*: The protozoa are protists without walls in the trophozoite stage; most have mitochondria with tubular cristae, Golgi apparatus, and peroxisomes; some may have flagella. Some are free living; others are parasitic.

Phylum: *Parabasala*: The phylum Parabasala has flagellated organisms with three or more flagella. Ribosomes are 70s and lack mitochondria but have hydrogenosomes with a double envelope. The parabasal body is the Golgi apparatus. The Parabasala are parasites of many vertebrates and invertebrates.

Genera: *Trichomonas*, *Pentatrichomonas*, and *Dientamoeba*.

Phylum: *Euglenoida*: The Euglenoida have one to four flagella. Peroxisomes are present, the Golgi apparatus is well developed, and the mitochondria have discoidal cristae. The cytoskeletal cortex is reinforced by microtubules. The nucleus divides, with a persistent nucleolus. Some Euglenoida are free living; others are paraditic.

Genera: *Leishmania* and *Trypanosoma*.

Phylum: *Rhizopoda*: The Rhizopoda have pseudopodia for locomotion and feeding. A Golgi apparatus and mitochondria are present except in Entamoebidae, where mitochondria must have been lost secondarily. Most Rhizopoda are uninucleated; some are free living.

Genera: *Entamoeba*, *Iodamoeba*, and *Endolimax*.

Phylum: *Percolozoa*: The phylum Percolozoa contains primitive organisms lacking a Golgi apparatus. Peroxisomes are present, as well as mitochondria with a discoid or with flat cristae. There are one to four flagella; some species have ameboid and flagellated forms. The Percolozoa are freshwater and marine, with some facultative parasites.

Genera: *Naegleria*, *Acanthamoeba*, *Balamuthia*, *Valh Kanfia*, and *Hartmannella*.

Phylum: *Apicomplexa*: The phylum Apicomplexa has an apical complex in some stage of the life cycle. Parasites are uninucleated or multinucleated; schyzogony is the most common form of multiplication. A cytosome is present, and subpellicular tubes are often found. Sexual reproduction occurs in the form of syngamy and flagella in microgametes. Mitochondria with tubular cristae are found.

Genera: *Cryptosporidium*, *Isospora*, *Cyclospora*, *Caryospora*, *Sarcocystis*, *Toxoplasma*, *Plasmodium* and *Babesia*.

Phylum: *Ciliophora*: The phylum Ciliophora has organisms with numerous cilia, many with complex oral cilia. There are one or more diploid micronuclei and one or more polyploidal macronuclei. Sexual reproduction occurs by conjugation or a related process.

Genus: *Balantidium*.

2

MICROSPORA

Microspora is a large Phylum, containing about 120 genera, that belongs to the kingdom Archetista (Sprague et al. 1992). All the genera of Microspora are obligatory intracellular organisms; most species are parasites of invertebrates, a few of vertebrates, and even fewer of humans. Zoologically, Microspora is characterized by (*1*) the presence of minute spores; (*2*) the existence in the spores of an apparatus to extrude the infective stage into cells; (*3*) the presence of one or two abutted nuclei; (*4*) the presence of 70s ribosomes; and (*5*) at least one chitinous layer of the wall of the spores. It has been suggested that Microspora may belong to the fungi, but there are not sufficient data to support this assumption (Muller, 1997). Microspora is divided into two Classes; one of these, the Microsporea, contains the order Microsporida, which includes all the genera and species affecting humans (Corliss, 1994). Microsporida has two groups: one in which the spores are formed individually in the cell, the Apansporoblastina, the other in which spores develop in packages within vesicles or membranes, the Pansporoblastina. Species belonging to both groups are known to occur in humans.

The study of microsporidians dates back to the first part of the 20th century, but their importance as human parasites has been recognized since the mid-1980s because of the opportunistic infections they produce in individuals with human immune deficiency virus (HIV) infections. The first edition of this book, reflecting what was known at the time of publication, discussed a few cases described in humans, most of which were not well studied and were generally considered oddities. *Enterocytozoon bieneusi* was included, but only the original case and the description of the species were reported at the time. Today we recognize at least six, possibly seven, genera of microsporidians in humans: *Encephalitozoon* (*E. cuniculi, E. hellem, E. intestinalis*), *Enterocytozoon* (*E. bieneusi*), *Vittaforma* (*V. corneae*), *Nosema* (*N. connori*), *Pleistophora*, and *Trachipleistophora* (*T. hominis, T. anthropophthera*). It should be noted that the names, the numbers of genera and species, and the relationships of microsporidia described in humans are changing rapidly.

Morphology and Life Cycle. The general morphology of the spore and the life cycle of microsporidia affecting humans are rather similar in all species and will be dealt with here in detail. The spores vary in size from 1 to 4 μm, are usually oval, and have a relatively thick wall. Inside the spore the most prominent structure is the microtubule, which arises from the attachment disc; the microtubule is up to 24 μm long and is tightly coiled, forming several loops in one or two rows (Fig. 2–1). The sporoplasm is located on the pole opposite the attachment disc, with one or two nuclei, depending on the species. Spores are formed and mature intracellularly. When mature, the spore extrudes its polar tube, which pierces the cell membrane of the host cell, and of a neighboring cell, and enters the cytoplasm to transfer the sporoplasm (a mechanism comparable to a hypodermic needle and a syringe) (Fig. 2–2). Once the sporoplasm is located in the new cell, it becomes a meront and begins growing. In some species, the meront is in direct contact with the cell cytoplasm; in others, it grows inside a vacuole or in an ill-defined cystern (which is not a true vacuole because it lacks a host membrane). The growth and multiplication of the meront is known as *merogony*; it results in the production of sporonts that differentiate into sporoblasts and finally into spores. In some species, the sporonts are large masses of cytoplasm with multiple nuclei, a

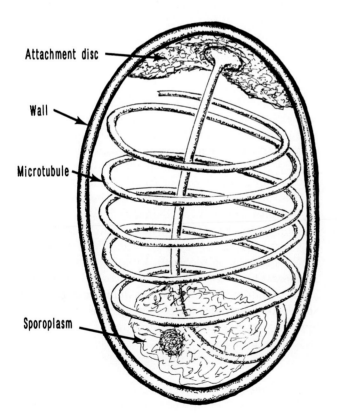

Fig. 2–1. Schematic representation of a spore, as observed in electron micrographs, to demonstrate the arrangement of the internal structures of the parasite.

Attachment disc

Wall

Microtubule

Sporoplasm

stage known as the *plasmodial phase* (Canning, Lom, 1986). Mature spores are eliminated with the feces and other secretions of the host (Fig. 2–2). These spores are then ready to enter another susceptible host via the mouth or respiratory passages or by direct contact with mucosal surfaces.

Encephalitozoon— Encephalitozoonoses

The genus *Encephalitozoon* occurs within vacuoles in the cell, produces two spores from a binucleated sporont, and has spores with a single nucleus. The spores vary from 1 to 1.5 μm 2 to 4 μm, depending on the species, and have five or six coils of the polar tubule arranged in a single row (Cali et al. 1996b). If this definition is applied strictly, the genus should include only the species *cuniculi* and *hellem*. However, if a braoder definition is used, *E. intestinalis* (= *Septata intestinalis*) should also be included (Cali et al. 1996b; Weiss, Cali, 1996). In this text, the most general three-species scheme is adopted. The three species—*cuniculi*, *hellem* and *intestinalis*—are morphologically identical both under the light microscope and on electron micrographs, leaving the molecular technologies as the only methods for distinguishing these species. All three species are pathogenic to humans.

Encephalitozoon cuniculi

Of the microsporidians infecting vertebrates, *E. cuniculi* is probably the best known. The first description of the parasite, and the suggestion that it was a microsporidian, was made in 1923 (Levaditi et al. 1923), though the organism was already known as a producer of encephalitis and nephritis in rabbits and laboratory animals. The true nature of the organism was finally confirmed in 1962 (Nelson, 1962). Previously, the parasite was sometimes grouped with *Toxoplasma*, and often *Toxoplasma* was mistakenly identified as *Encephalitozoon*. In the mid-1960s, *Encephalitozoon* was considered to be synonymous with *Nosema* (Lainson et al. 1964; Weiser, 1964), but later its proper name was reestablished. This is of practical importance because the term *nosematoses* was applied to infections with *Encephalitozoon* creating some confusion (see the discussion of *Nosema* below).

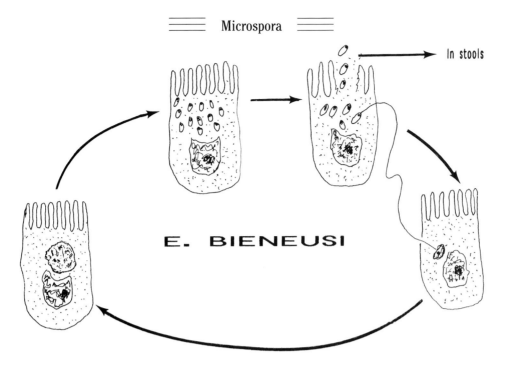

In stools

E. BIENEUSI

Fig. 2–2. Schematic representation of the life cycle of *E. bicncusi* in epithelial cells.

Morphology. Under the light microscope, the spores of *E. cuniculi* are minute intracellular bodies that stain with several histologic stains (*color plate* I *G*). In electron micrographs, the parasites are located inside parasitophorous vacuoles in the cells and show all stages of development. However, the development of the vacuole becomes apparent 24 hours after the parasite has entered the cell (Fig. 2–3) (Pakes et al. 1975). The sporoplasm is a small, uninucleated stage that transforms into a meront that is in close contact with the cell cytoplasm until the vacuole forms. Meronts are larger forms that proliferate and have two, sometimes three nuclei (Fig. 2–4 *A*). Some meronts are elongated, lying close to the vacuole membrane and showing signs of division that gives rise to uninucleated forms (Fig. 2–4 *A*) (Pakes et al. 1975). These uninucleated forms, sporonts, become detached from the vacuole membrane and are free in the vacuole, where they differentiate into sporoblasts (Figs. 2–3 and 2–4 *A–B*), and finally into spores (Figs. 2–4 *A–B*) (Pakes et al. 1975). The maturing sporont develops a thicker cell membrane, and the organelles become more prominent; they become sporoblasts when the cell membrane thickens even more, showing a middle electron-lucent layer. Mature spores have a sporoplasm with a single nucleus, an attachment disc or polar cap, and a microtubule (Figs. 2–1 and 2–5). The spore wall is thick, composed of three layers, of which the middle, translucent one is the thickest (Figs. 2–1 and 2–5). The microtubule, or polar filament, makes up to six coils (Pakes et al. 1975). Most spores of microsporidians have a prominent vacuole, which helps in their recognition in tissue sections for light microscopy (Figs. 2–4 *B* and 2–10 *A–B*).

Life Cycle. The life cycle of *E. cuniculi* is similar to that described above. Both in animals and in humans, the parasite is found in epithelial cells (Fig. 2–2). A great deal of information on natural and experimental infections in animals is available, much of which has relevance to humans. Many species of animals can be infected with *E. cuniculi*, indicating that the parasite has low specificity; it is the only known microsporidian occurring in humans for which natural animal reservoirs are known (Deplazes et al. 1996), making it a zoonotic infection. In animals, the infection may produce encephalitis and nephritis, but the parasite can be found in almost any organ, including the placenta. Spores are eliminated with the urine, feces, and sputum. Once in the environment they move to other hosts, but the exact mode of infection is unknown. The oral route, through ingestion of food contaminated with the feces or urine of infected animals, or by carnivorism, is probably the most important one in animals. Human infections could be acquired in the same manner, but no data are available. Only HIV-positive individuals have been found to be infected, suffering diseases similar to those in animals. The parasite in experimental

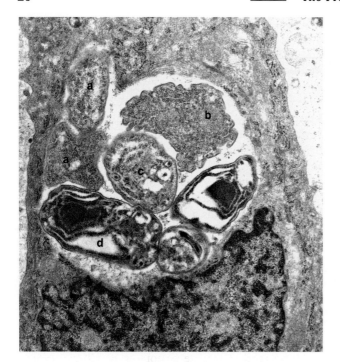

Fig. 2–3. *Encephalitozoon intestinalis*, electron micrograph showing developmental stages in the enterocyte, ×14,170. There are several stages of development, the earliest one with poorly defined organelles (a); another showing early deposition of the spore wall (b); a third, with beginning formation of the microtubule (c); and (d) more advanced stages. Also notable is the apical deformation (cupping) of the cell nucleus. (Courtesy of J. McMahon, Ph.D., Department of Pathology, Cleveland Clinic Educational Foundation, Cleveland, Ohio.)

animals does not cross the placenta (Wilson, 1986); 40% of chick embryos were found to be infected, some of which were dead, indicating that the infection is fatal to chick embryos and that there is a possibility of transmission to humans by ingestion of raw eggs (Reetz, 1994).

How the parasites move from the intestine to the deeper organs is unknown. It has been suggested that in the intestinal wall the parasites are phagocytized by macrophages that transport them to other organs; of importance, in experimental infections by the oral route, the first organ involved is the liver. In intraperitoneal infections, probably mesothelial cells are infected, and ascitis is the main manifestation.

Geographic Distribution and Epidemiology. The geographic distribution of *E. cuniculi* is worldwide in animals; in humans, only a few documented cases are known, most in the United States. Seroprevalence us-

ing an enzyme-linked immunosorbent assay showed that healthy Britons were negative for specific antibodies, but individuals living in the tropics with other parasitic infections were between 6% and 12% positive (Hollister, Canning, 1987). In Orang Asli aborigines of Malaysia, the rate of infection was 43% (Singh et al. 1982). Other investigators have reported similar results in other parts of the world (Hollister et al. 1991; WHO, 1993). In individuals at risk for HIV infection in Britain, 25% of 63 were positive, and of 29 individuals infected with HIV, 6 were positive (Hollister et al. 1991). In homosexual males in Sweden, the positivity rate was 33% (Bergquist et al. 1984). If these

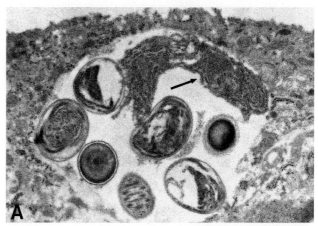

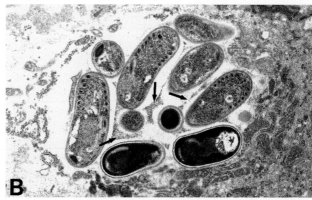

Fig. 2–4. *Encephalitozoon intestinalis*, electron micrographs demonstrating the developmental stages, ×12,000. *A*, Developing parasites within a vacuole or cystern in the cell cytoplasm. The sporont (arrow) is binucleated, dividing many times to produce organisms that develop into spores. *B*, More advanced stages; some are mature spores (bottom). Note that the number and the arrangement of the microtubule loops in a single arrow. The arrows point to the septa, characteristic of this species. (Courtesy of J. McMahon, Ph.D., Department of Pathology, Cleveland Clinic Educational Foundation, Cleveland, Ohio.)

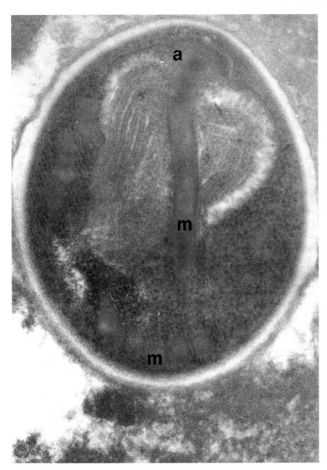

Fig. 2–5. *Encephalitozoon* **spore sectioned longitudinally showing the attachment disc (a) and the microtubule (m), ×93,600. (Courtesy of J. McMahon, Ph.D., Department of Pathology, Cleveland Clinic Educational Foundation, Cleveland, Ohio.)**

positivity rates for antibodies against *E. cuniculi* are accurate, then the infection is widespread in the tropics and in the gay population and suggests that a fecal-oral route is likely the most common mode of transmission in humans. A relationship between trips to or from a tropical place was found to be a factor in developing infections with microsporidians (Cornet et al. 1996).

Pathogenesis. As stated above, the only infections in humans have occurred in immune-suppressed individuals, but how the parasite produces disease is unknown. Destruction of cells is evident from both light and electron microscopic observations. The microsporidians have very low virulence, and all infections occur in immune-suppressed individuals. *Enterocytozoon bieneusi* produces mild infections in immune-competent hosts.

Clinical Findings. Human infections with *Encephalitozoon* described in the past were based mostly on circumstantial evidence and therefore are of questionable validity. In the brain, cases were reported of meningoencephalitis with myositis (Torres, 1927), of granulomatous encephalomyelitis (Wolf, Cowen, 1937), and of encephalitis alone. In another case, a child apparently had parasites in the spinal fluid and urine (Matsubayashi et al. 1959). One case was that of a disseminated carcinoma of the pancreas (Marcus et al. 1973) and the tumor cells were parasitized. Another case featured convulsions without fever (Bergquist et al. 1984), and still another was a disseminated infection in a patient with acquired immune deficiency syndrome (AIDS) (Zender et al. 1989). Some of these cases were *Toxoplasma* infections, others were diagnosed on the basis of serologic tests, and still others were based on light microscopic morphology—none of which are valid criteria for a species identification. Only recently, with the aid of the polymerase chain reaction, was the parasite conclusively identified in humans with AIDS (Croppo et al. 1995; de Groote et al. 1995; Hollister et al. 1995).

The infection, as reported in immune-suppressed individuals, is usually generalized. One patient, a 34-year-old HIV-positive male homosexual, presented with a 4 month history of fever, night sweats, cough, and weight loss. The CD4[+] T-lymphocyte count was 15 cells per cubic milliliter. In addition, the patient complained of poor visual acuity, sinus congestion, paroxysmal cough, and ulcers of the tongue. Rales were heard on both pulmonary bases. Examination of a lung biopsy specimen revealed bronchiolitis and pneumonia, with numerous microsporidians in the epithelial cells of the bronchioles and a polymorphonuclear cell infiltrate. Microsporisians were also present in a biopsy specimen from the nasal sinuses and from an ulcer of the tongue, as well as in the urine and the sputum (de Groote et al. 1995). Treatment with albendazole resulted in clinical improvement and gradual disappearance of the parasites from the sputum and the urine (de Groote et al. 1995). In a second patient with severe renal dysfunction (Fig. 2–6 *A–D* and *color plate* I *G*), the parasites were isolated from urine samples and characterized (Hollister et al. 1995). As more infections with microsporidia are studied at the molecular level, more cases of *E. cuniculi* will be studied clinically and newer syndromes produced by this ubiquitous parasite will be described.

Immunity. Little is known about the immunology of microsporidian infections in humans. Some data from

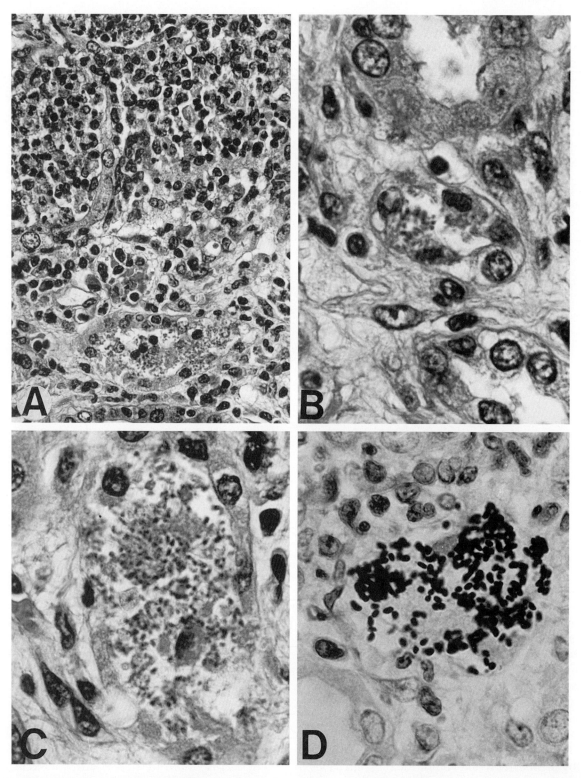

Fig. 2–6. *Encephalitozoon cuniculi* in kidney, *A–C*, sections stained with hematoxylin and eosin. *A,* Low-power view showing the marked infiltration with mononuclear cells and the destruction of the renal parenchyma. At the bottom of the picture, a renal tubule is heavily parasitized and has cells with parasites desquamated in the lumen, ×450. *B* and *C,* Larger magnification shows the parasitized cells, ×1,120. *D,* Section stained with Twort's stain to demonstrate the spores, ×1,120. (Preparations courtesy of D.A. Schwartz, M.D., Department of Pathology, Emory University School of Medicine, Atlanta, Georgia.)

studies of *E. cuniculi* in animals indicate that the tissue response in immune-competent hosts is typically a granulomatous inflammation around a necrotic center and that the lesions persist after the infection has been cleared (Schmidt, Shadduck, 1983). Intact cellular immunity in animals prevents multiplication of the parasites; euthymic mice suffer symptomatic infections, while athymic ones develop a fatal disease (Schmidt, Shadduck, 1984). *Encephalitozoon cuniculi* in immune-intact animals is well tolerated and produces a latent long-lasting infection in spite of an active immune response (Weber, Bryan, 1994). The resistance to infection in mice is related to T cells because T cells harvested from the spleen of resistant animals protect against lethal infections; serum alone does not confer protection (Hermanek et al. 1993; Schmidt, Shadduck, 1984). Mice with severe combined immune deficiency suffer infections with *E. cuniculi* identical to those seen in immune-suppressed humans (Hermanek et al. 1993).

Encephalitozoon hellem

In 1991, *E. hellem* was described on microsporidian isolates from ocular tissue of three patients with AIDS (Didier et al. 1991). The description of the new species was warranted because molecular and immunologic techniques clearly distinguished it from *E. cuniculi*. The electron microscopic appearance of the new parasite was published the same year (Didier et al. 1991). Similar differences between *E. cuniculi* and isolates from the urine of an infected patient were found (Visvesvara et al. 1991). Confirmation of the validity of *E. hellem* as a new species came soon afterward with the development and use of the polymerase chain reaction; *E. cuniculi*, *E. hellem*, and *E. intestinalis* could be differentiated by this technique (Visvesvara et al. 1994; Weiss et al. 1994).

Morphology. The morphologic characteristics of *E. hellem* under the light microscope (*color plate* I C–D) and the electron microscope are very similar to those of *E. cuniculi*. It has been pointed out that the electron-dense coat on the surface of the sporogonic stages (sporont, sporoblast, and spore) in *E. hellem* is deposited as a uniform layer that later thickens. In contrast, in *E. cuniculi*, the deposition begins as discontinuous, narrow bands that later fuse (Baker et al. 1995; Curry, Canning, 1993; Hollister et al. 1993). If this is

a real difference, it would be possible to differentiate these two species on electron micrographs.

Pathogenesis. The mechanism or mechanisms by which *E. hellem* produces disease in humans are unknown. No animal models for study of the disease are available, and as stated, humans immune-suppressed by the HIV infection are the only known hosts capable of sustaining the infection.

Clinical Findings. *Encephalitozoon hellem* has been associated mostly with disseminated disease in HIV-positive individuals, very similar to that produced by *E. cuniculi* and with ocular infections. There are very few reported cases in which speciation of the parasite has been done (Schwartz et al. 1993a, 1993b) because the technology is not widely available. Several reports of keratitis and keratoconjunctivitis produced by an *Encephalitozoon* organism are known (Cali et al. 1991a, 1991b; Desser et al. 1992; Lacey et al. 1992; McCluskey et al. 1993; Metcalfe et al. 1992; Schwartz et al. 1993a; Yee et al. 1991). These conditions have all occurred in HIV-positive individuals, and sometimes the infection has extended to the nasal sinuses, producing sinusitis (Fig. 2–7 B; *color plate* I C–D; Cali et al. 1991b; Metcalfe et al. 1992). The ocular infection is bilateral, characterized by superficial involvement of the epithelial cells of the cornea and the conjunctiva. The patient is usually asymptomatic or may have mild punctate keratopathy, sometimes noted during a routine ophthalmologic examination (Friedberg et al. 1990). The infection is chronic and develops slowly, producing photophobia, blurred vision, and discomfort. Examination reveals conjunctival injection with superficial punctate erosions of the cornea without uveitis. Some patients may have superimposed bacterial infections (Friedberg et al. 1990).

Respiratory infections have been described in patients with disseminated disease (Scaglia et al. 1994), producing mainly a bronchiolitis diagnosed in sputum samples (Schwartz et al. 1993b). Infections of the kidney, ureters, and urinary bladder (Schwartz et al. 1992), of the prostate gland with abscess formation, and of the urethra (Schwartz et al. 1994) have been described. The parasites have been isolated from urine, sputum, conjunctival swabs, and nasal secretions. In one case of disseminated infection in which the parasite was isolated from sputum, urine, and nasal swabs, no systemic symptoms could be attributed to the infection, with the exception of ocular involvement and an asymptomatic microhematuria (Weber et al. 1993).

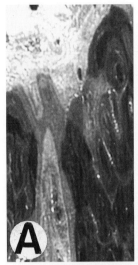
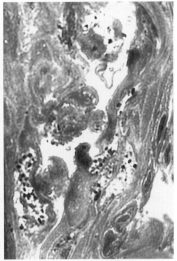

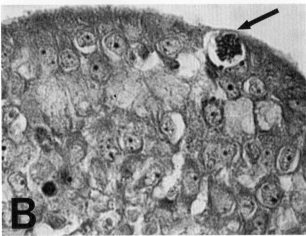

Fig. 2–7. *Encephalitozoon* in cornea and nasal sinuses. *A*, Plastic section of corneal biopsy section, stained with toluidine blue stain, showing the organisms in epithelial cells inside vacuoles, ×756. *B*, Section of a nasal polyp stained with hematoxylin and eosin stain. Note the parasites (arrow), ×756.

Encephalitozoon intestinalis (= *Septata intestinalis*)

In 1991 (Cali et al. 1991c) and in 1992 (Blanshard et al. 1992), reports of HIV patients with chronic diarrhea harboring two different species of microsporidia in the intestine were published. One species was the well-known *E. bieneusi*; the other remained unnamed. The new parasite was described as a new species of a new genus (Septata) related to *Encephalitozoon*, most likely belonging to the same family, Encephalito-

zoonidae (Cali et al. 1993). The reasons for naming a new genus and species were (*1*) the peculiar development of the parasite within vacuoles of enterocytes (Fig. 2–8 *A–C*), macrophages, fibroblasts, and endothelial cells of the lamina propria, in which each stage developed within chambers separated by septae, and (*2*) the development of elongated, binucleated, or tetranucleated cells (Cali et al. 1993).

Based on certain molecular characteristics of the parasite, it was decided that the new genus, *Septata*, was not justified and that it is a synonym of *Encephalitozoon* (Hartskeerl et al. 1995). This decision may be premature, and the genus *Septata* is likely to

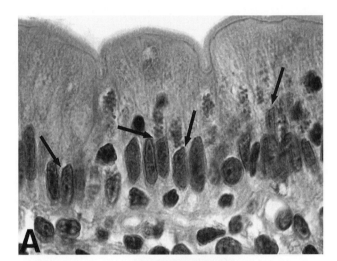

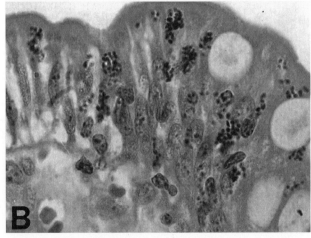

Fig. 2–8. *Encephalitozoon intestinalis* in the small intestine. *A*, Section of a biopsy specimen stained with hematoxylin and eosin. Note the large number of organisms inside the vacuoles. The arrows point to the deformation of the cell nuclei, ×907. *B*, Same specimen stained with Twort's stain, ×907.

be reinstated. *Septata* has enough distinguishing morphologic characteristics to necessitate a redefinition of the genus *Encephalitozoon* in order to accommodate both genera (Cali et al. 1996b). New studies should clarify the true nature of these organisms and their relationships.

Morphology. The morphology of *E. intestinalis* is similar to that described above, except for the presence of septae (Fig. 2–4 *B*), which would permit its separation from *E. cuniculi* and *E. hellem* on electron micrographs (Cali et al. 1993; Orenstein et al. 1992). The mature spores are 2.0 by 1.2 μm and the microtubule has four to seven coils, mostly five. Their development is like that of other members of the genus. *Encephalitozoon hellem* has been found mostly in the United States, with some cases in Europe, probably because of the interest in the parasite and the resources to detect the infection. It will certainly be found to have a worldwide distribution.

Pathogenesis and Clinical Findings. The pathogenicity of *E. intestinalis* is emerging as more cases are studied. It has been isolated in tissue cultures from the stools of patients with *E. bieneusi*, indicating that coinfections with these two microsporidians are common (Blanshard et al. 1992; Orenstein et al. 1992; van Gool et al. 1994). The parasite has been isolated in almost every area of the intestine from AIDS patients with diarrhea and from one without diarrhea (Field et al. 1993a). In human *E. intestinalis* has been found to produce nephritis (Aarons et al. 1994; Case Records of the Massachusetts General Hospital, 1993), keratitis (Lowder et al. 1996), enteritis (Dore et al. 1995; Molina et al. 1995; Orenstein et al. 1992) in one patient with small bowel perforation (Soule et al. 1997), cholangitis (Willson et al. 1995), cystitis (Soule et al. 1997), and disseminated infections (Chu, West, 1996; Dore et al. 1995) similar to those produced by the other two encephalitozoa. Dissemination into the deep organs is probably by infected monocytes traveling in blood vessels from the intestinal wall into the tissues. The clinical manifestations of disseminated disease are variable; asymptomatic cases have been described (Gunnarsson et al. 1995), but unspecific symptoms related to the affected organs may be present. A study of five patients in France revealed that *E. intestinalis* in individuals with AIDS produces chronic diarrhea usually associated with fever, cholangitis, sinusitis, bronchitis, and mild bilateral conjunctivitis (Molina et al. 1995). Most patients with severe disease due to *E. intestinalis* infection have CD4$^+$ T-lymphocyte counts below 100 cells per cubic milliliter (Asmuth et al. 1994; Molina et al. 1995). Infections with all three species of *Encephalitozoon* respond readily to medical therapy, but no treatment is available for infections with the other microsporidians.

Pathology. As the above discussion implies, separation of the clinical manifestations, the organ involvement, and the disease or diseases produced by each species of *Encephalitozoon* is impossible at present, presumably because of the lack of specificity of these species for any tissue or organ system: *E. cuniculi*, *E. hellem*, and *E. intestinalis*. This assumption is supported by the small number of patients from whom the parasites have been isolated and classified to the species level, revealing that the syndromes they produce in humans overlap. Moreover, the pathologic manifestations, the description of the tissue response, the morphologic diagnostic features, and the techniques for diagnosis are essentially identical.

The most important histologic characteristic of *Encephalitozoon* infections in tissue sections studied under the light microscope, is the presence of numerous 1 to 2 μm eosinophilic bodies within cytoplasmic vacuoles of cells that stain relatively well with hematoxylin and eosin stain (Figs. 2–6, 2–7, and 2–8). The cells affected are mostly the epithelial cells of any portion of the intestine, bile ducts, renal tubules, urothelium, pulmonary bronchioles, cornea, and conjunctiva, as well as macrophages and endothelial cells. Destruction of cells without an inflammatory infiltrate sometimes occurs (Chu, West, 1996) unless a concomitant infection is present.

In intestinal infections, the parasites are clustered within vacuoles located in the apical cytoplasm of absorptive enterocytes, particularly those located at the tip of the villi. Careful examination of the parasites under oil immersion shows a birefringent quality produced by the walls of the spores and the vacuole of the spore at one of its poles. The parasites stain well with Giemsa, trichrome, periodic acid–Schiff, Gram, and methenamine silver stains. A peculiar deformation of the apical tip of the nucleus, which becomes cup-like is often present, a feature even more relevant in *Enterocytozoon* (*color plate* I *E–F*; Fig. 2–3; see below). Striking blunting and atrophy of the villi have been described (Orenstein et al. 1992), but these are nonspecific and inconstant characteristics (Bryan et al. 1991a).

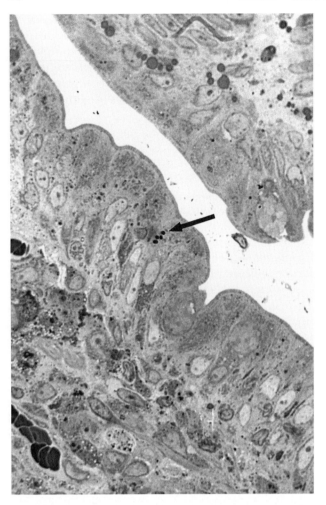

Fig. 2–9. *Enterocytozoon bieneusi* in a plastic section of a biopsy specimen stained with toluidine blue. Note the spores within the cell cytoplasm rather than within a vacuole, ×770.

Enterocytozoon bieneusi

In 1984 an unnamed protozoon was found in an intestinal biopsy specimen of an HIV-positive patient, and was presented at a scientific meeting (Dobbins, Weinstein, 1984). The following year, an electron micrograph of the parasite was published (Dobbins, Weinstein, 1985), and an identical organism, identified as a Microspora, was found in a patient in France (Modigliani et al. 1985). The unnamed microsporidium in these reports was described from the material obtained from the French patient, and a new genus and species were created: *Enterocytozoon bieneusi* (Desportes et al. 1985). Since the time of its recognition as a pathogen that produces diarrhea in patients with

HIV infection, the parasite has been found in one immune-competent adult with acute traveler's diarrhea (Sandfort et al. 1994). The parasite has also been reported in immune-competent African children (1 month to 6 years of age); there was a 1% prevalence in those with diarrhea and a 0.1% prevalence in those without it (Bretagne et al. 1993). *Enterocytozoon* has not been found in animals, and attempts to culture it in the laboratory have been only partially successful (Visvesvara et al. 1995). It is clear that *Enterocytozoon* is a human parasite that was recognized because of the AIDS epidemic (Canning, Hollister, 1990); is well adapted to humans; has low virulence, producing subclinical or asymptomatic infections (Rabeneck et al. 1993); and reactivates in immune-deficient hosts (Weber, Bryan, 1994). As more studies on the epidemiology of the infection are done, the picture should become clearer.

Life Cycle. The life cycle of *E. bieneusi* is similar to that of other microsporidians (Fig. 2–1), except that the way it grows and divides to produce spores is different, making this organism unique. In addition, *E. bieneusi* is not contained within a vacuole, growing in close contact with the cell cytoplasm and its organelles. The spores are oval, about 1.0 × 1.5 μm in their maximum diameter (Figs. 2–3 through 2–9; Fig. 2–10 *A–B*; *color plate* I *E–F*). Once the spore injects the sporo-

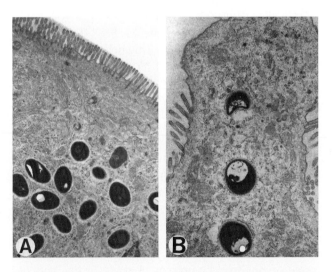

Fig. 2–10. *Enterocytozoon bieneusi*, electron micrographs of sections of a small intestinal biopsy specimen. *A*, ×3,795; *B*, ×6,600. Note the mature spores within the cell cytoplasm; some spores have a vacuole. The enterocyte in *B* appears markedly damaged and is probably desquamating.

plasm into the cell, the parasite begins its sporogonic division, growing considerably to develop a multinucleated form up to 5.0 μm in diameter, known as the *plasmodial phase* or *proliferative stage* (Fig. 2–11 *A–B*). The plasmodial tropozoite is surrounded by the cell mitochondria and is located close to the apical end of the cell nucleus producing a cup-shaped deformation, as described above for the encephalitozoa (Fig. 3–11 *A*). As the division of the nuclei proceeds, electron-lucent clefts appear close to the parasites nuclei, as seen on electron micrographs. As the parasites grow, their cytoplasm develops ribosomes and, later, an endoplasmic reticulum and small amounts of membrane. At the same time, microtubules begin to grow (Fig. 2–11 *B*). As differentiation progresses, the microtubules stack in two rows (Fig. 2–11 *C*) of three coils each. Finally, the parasites separate, becoming individuals that continue to mature into spores (Figs. 2–11 *A* and 2–12) (Cali, Owen, 1990; Orenstein, 1991). Some parasitized enterocytes appear dead and desquamate, to be eliminated with stools, where they are found (*color plate* I *I*). This fact supports the idea that the parasite is transmitted through fecal contamination (Orenstein et al. 1990).

As data were gathered on the importance of the infection in immune-suppressed individuals, surveys carried in many places pointed to a high prevalence in certain human groups. For example, in HIV-positive individuals with chronic diarrhea, the prevalence rates were as follows: the Netherlands, 25% (Eeftinck, van Gool, 1992); Australia, 33% (Field et al. 1993a); France, 16% (Michiels et al. 1993); Canada, 12% (Svenson et al. 1993); the United States, 39% (Kotler, Orenstein, 1994). The parasite has been found in every place where it has been investigated in immune-deficient individuals; and Dutch blood donors and French pregnant women, all immune competent, showed 8% and 5% seropositivity to *Encephalitozoon*, respectively (van Gool et al. 1997). This suggests that among immune-competent individuals, the infection is common. Little more than what has been described above is known about the biology and immunity of the infection because, as mentioned before, no culture method and no animal model for the isolation and study of *Enterocytozoon* are available.

Pathogenesis. The cause-and-effect association between diarrhea and *Enterocytozoon* was taken for granted from the time the first infections were described. Rabeneck and coworkers, who studied two groups of individuals with *Enterocytozoon* in their stools, and with and without diarrhea, found that the groups had similar rates of infection; they concluded that the parasite was not a pathogen (Rabeneck et al. 1993). The opposite conclusion was derived from a similar study using a more refined method, the polymerase chain reaction, for detection of the parasites in stools (Coyle et al. 1996). It should be pointed out that the study of Rabeneck and associates explored the question of virulence, not of pathogenicity, and that their work is important because it suggests that *Enterocytozoon* has very low virulence. This is confirmed by the study of immune-competent African children with and without diarrhea, which showed that infections occurred in both groups (Bretagne et al. 1993), and by other studies reviewed by Wanke et al. (1996).

Clinical Findings. The most important clinical manifestation of enterocytozoonosis is nonspecific chronic diarrhea in HIV-positive individuals that is refractory to treatment. The disease cannot be distinguished from the HIV infection diarrhea or from that produced by other causes. Pulmonary infections (Weber et al. 1992b) have been described as consisting of a chronic cough with scant, nonpurulent sputum and wheezing, symptoms that increase in intensity to dyspnea on exertion. On chest radiographs, small interstitial infiltrates may be present. Infection of the bile ducts and the gallbladder presents with symptoms and signs of chronic cholangitis (Beaugerie et al. 1992; Pol et al. 1993) and sclerosing cholangitis (Pol et al. 1992). Most patients with enterocytozoonosis have a CD4$^+$ T-lymphocyte count below 100 cells per cubic milliliter. Coinfections of *E. bieneusi* and *Cryptosporidium* are relatively common (Garcia et al. 1994). This association is important because it demonstrates the difficulty of attributing symptoms to a given pathogen in HIV-infected individuals shows and that the two organisms have a common route of infection. Patients with organ transplants may also develop chronic diarrhea due to *Enterocytozoon* (Rabodonirina et al. 1996).

Pathology. *Enterocytozoon bieneusi* has been found in all portions of the small intestine (*color plate* I *E–F*; Fig. 2–13 *A–D*; Orenstein, 1991; Peacock et al. 1991), colon (Gourley, Swedo, 1988; Rabeneck et al. 1993), bile ducts (Beaugerie et al. 1992; Pol et al. 1992), gallbladder (Pol et al. 1993), and lung (Weber et al. 1992b). The histologic changes in the duodenum of individuals infected with *Enterocytozoon* consist of blunting of the villi, showing infected cells with obvious damage such as irregular borders with hyperchromatic and vacuolated nuclei. Cupping of the enterocytes is also observed (Fig. 2–13 D). Some cells appear dead; others are in the

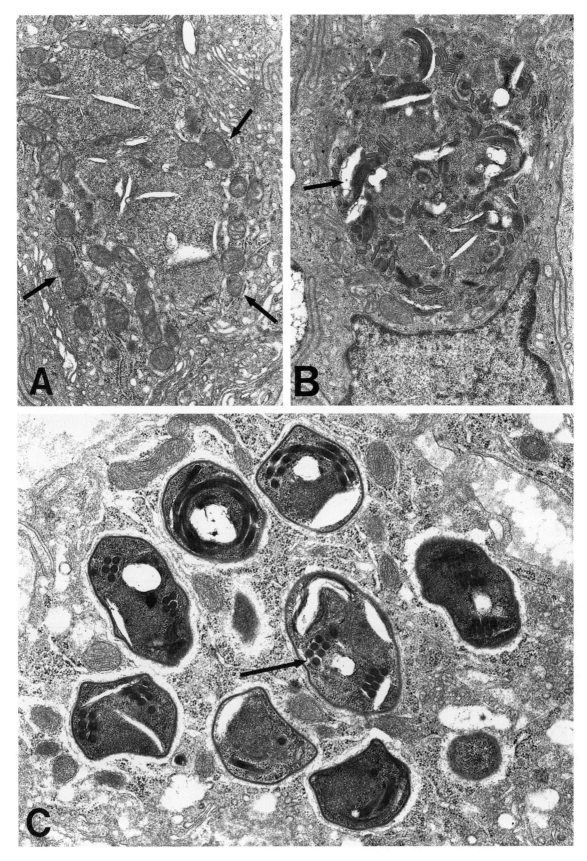

Fig. 2–11.

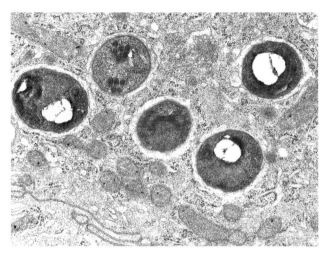

Fig. 2–12. *Enterocytozoon bieneusi,* electron micrographs of sections of a small intestinal biopsy specimen from the same patient in Figure 2–11 showing almost mature spores, ×9,250. (Courtesy of J. McMahon, Ph.D., Department of Pathology, Cleveland Clinic Educational Foundation, Cleveland, Ohio.)

from those produced by the AIDS virus (AIDS enteropathy) is impossible (Greenson et al. 1991).

Infections in sites other than the intestine show similar changes: infected cells with different degrees of degeneration and a nonexistent or scanty cellular infiltrate. In all instances, the diagnosis of the infection is based on the recognition of the parasites, as described below.

Vittaforma corneae
(= Nosema corneum)

The first corneal infection by a microsporidium was found in an 11-year-old boy from Sri Lanka with marked unilateral, deep, granulomatous keratitis, apparently the result of trauma (Ashton, Wirasinha, 1973). A second deep corneal ulceration was discovered in a 26-year-old woman from Africa (Pinnolis et al. 1981) and a third, in a 45-year-old American man with deep stromal keratitis (Davis et al. 1990); all three patients were immune competent (*color plate* I *B*). The parasites were not classified in any of the three reports, but they were isolated in tissue cultures from the third patient and described as *Nosema corneum* (Shadduck et al. 1990). The three parasites are characterized by the size of the spores: 3.5 × 1.5 μm, 5.0 × 3.0 μm, and 4.0 × 1.5 μm, respectively. A fourth case of corneal infection in a patient with clinical characteristics identical to those described above was poorly characterized (Bryan et al. 1991b). Further study of the isolate from the American patient resulted in a full description of the parasite and its placement in a new genus, *Vittaforma corneae* (Silveira, Canning, 1995). Whether the other patients described were infected with the same species seems doubtful based on the size of the spores, but the disease they produced is very similar.

The defining characteristic of *V. corneae* by light microscopy is the size of the spores. This species has been found only in a corneal biopsy specimen from one

process of being desquamated. In areas where the infection is heavier, the changes are more intense, with crowding of the cells, and degenerating cells always contain parasites. Sometimes portions of dead mucosa are seen sloughing off into the lumen, with occasional disruption of the basement membrane and hemorrhages (Orenstein et al. 1990). Changes in the ileum are similar; at low-power magnification, the villus–crypt cell ratio is reduced due to irregular, blunted villi and hyperplastic cryptic cells. Dead cells and macrophages in the villus and the lamina propria are present, with degeneration of the surface epithelium. Higher magnification shows frank disorganization of the epithelium. Parasites are visible in enterocytes located at the tip of the villi but not in those toward the base of the villi or in the crypt (Field et al. 1993a). It is important to keep in mind that these descriptions are from studies in individuals with both HIV and *Enterocytozoon* infections, and that to distinguish the changes produced by these organisms

◀─────────────────────────────────────

Fig. 2–11. *Enterocytozoon bieneusi,* electron micrographs of sections of a small intestinal biopsy specimen demonstrating developmental stages. *A,* Early plasmodial stage surrounded by the cell mitochondria (arrows). The nucleus is not visible in this section, and some electron-lucent clefts are evident, ×13,500. *B,* A more developed plasmodial stage shows early development of the microtubules. Note the cupping of the cell nucleus

and the electron-lucent clefts (arrow), ×14,400. *C,* Spores in a more advanced stage of development. Note that in each electron micrograph only one developmental stage is present at any given time because it is synchronous; also, the arrangement of the microtubule loops in two rows of three each (arrow), ×24,000. (Courtesy of J. McMahon, Ph.D., Department of Pathology, Cleveland Clinic Educational Foundation, Cleveland, Ohio.)

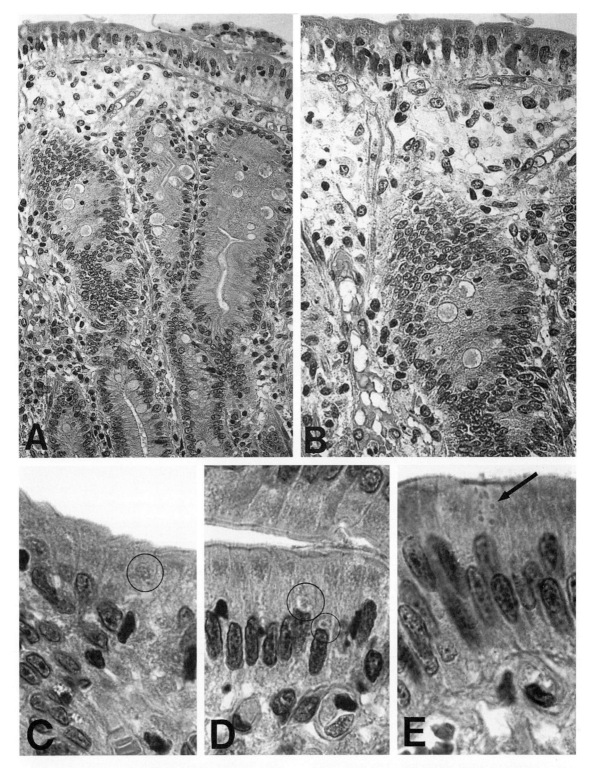

Fig. 2–13. *Enterocytozoon bieneusi* infection of the small intestine, sections stained with hematoxylin and eosin stain. *A*, Low-power view showing the duodenal mucosa, with slight edema of the lamina propria and infiltration by mononuclear cells, ×280. *B*, Higher magnification shows edema and slight infiltration, ×450. *C–E*, Detail of an epithelial cell showing parasites ×1,120. *C*, A few developing spores are seen within the cell cytoplasm (circle); note the lack of a vacuole and the size of the organisms. *D*, Plasmodial stages (circles) growing on top of the nucleus, producing cupping of the apical nuclear pole. The halo surrounding the parasites is a fixation artifact. *E*, Mature spores scattered in the cytoplasm (arrow). These spores are now 1 μm in size. (Preparation courtesy of A. Galian, M.D., Department of Pathology, Hopital Lariivoisiere, Paris, France. Reported by: Modigliani, R., Bories, C., Le Charpentier, Y., et al. 1985. Diarrhoea and malabsorption in acquired immune deficiency syndrome: a study of four cases with special emphasis on opportunistic protozoan infestations. Gut 26:179–187.)

patient, but since under experimental conditions the parasite produced liver infection when injected intraperitoneally into athymic mice (Silveira, Canning, 1995), the possibility of infection in immune-suppressed individuals is real. The electron microscopic characteristics of *V. corneae* are the presence of two abbuted nuclei, all stages of the life cycle growing in a cysterna made by host endoplasmic reticulum, and meronts producing four to eight linearly arranged sporoblasts. The spores have five to seven coils of the microtubule (Fig. 2–14; Silveira, Canning, 1995).

Nosema

Nosema is probably one of the largest genera of Microspora, by some estimates containing over 200 species, parasites of insects. It is characterized by two haploid nuclei in close contact, abutted like a pair of beans that function as a single nucleus throughout the life cycle of the parasite. In addition, the developmental stages are found close to the cell cytoplasm, and division is by binary fission with a disporous pattern (two spores result from each division). The resultant spores are diplokaryotic.

Nosema connori

Only one human infection with *N. connori* is known (Margileth et al. 1973). It occurred in a 4-month-old infant with marked hypogammaglobulinemia, a temperature of 38.5°C, diarrhea, malabsorption, projectile vomiting, and lethargy that waxed and waned for 3 weeks. Rhonchi in the right lung, abdominal distention, and a maculopapular rash were observed. An abdominal x-ray film showed the bowel distended by gas. Exploratory surgery was performed. No obstruction was found, a small bowel biopsy was performed, and the infant died 3 weeks later.

The biopsy specimen and the autopsy showed no gross abnormalities, but microscopically, microsporidial organisms were found, especially in smooth muscle cells of the muscular layers of the in-

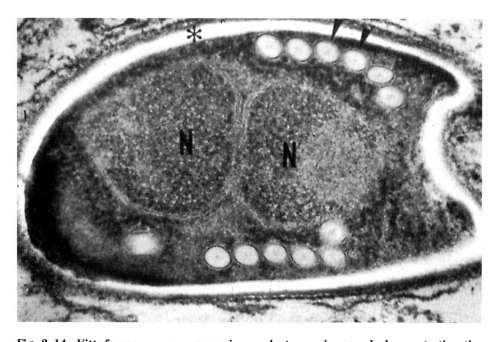

Fig. 2–14. *Vittaforma corneae* spore in an electron micrograph demonstrating the presence of two nuclei (n), the wall of the spore (*), and the microtubule (arrowheads), ×88,800. (Courtesy of R.L. Font, M.D., Cullen Eye Institute, Baylor College of Medicine, Houston, Texas. Reported by: Davies, R.M, Font, R.L., Keisler, M.S., et al. 1990. Corneal microsporidiosis. A case report including ultrastructural observations. Ophthalmology 97:953–957. Reproduced with permission.)

testine and in the arteries of most organs. Skeletal muscles, mostly of the diaphragm, and the epithelial cells of the renal tubules were also parasitized. Other findings at autopsy were an atrophic thymus and a *Pneumocystis* infection.

Further study of the organisms recovered at autopsy resulted in the description of the new species, *N. connori*, based on the size of the spores (4.0 to 4.5 by 2.0 to 2.5 μm) and the presence of two abbuted nuclei (Sprague, 1974). The number of polar tubule coils was later reported as 10 to 12 (Strano et al. 1976). Since other information was impossible to obtain because only formalin-fixed material was available for study, the true nature of the organism remains unknown.

Nosema-like Organism

The other infection with a species of *Nosema* occurred in the skeletal muscles of an HIV-positive patient with severe myositis, but it has not yet been classified (Cali et al. 1996a). The organism inhabits the skeletal muscle cells. It has spores 2.5 to 2.9 by 1.9 to 2.0 μm in size and a wall with a thick, electron-dense exospore coat (the outer layer of the spore wall) and an even thicker, electron-lucent endospore coat. The polar tubule has 7 to 10 coils, usually 9, in one or two rows. On electron micrographs the parasites have all the characteristics of the genus *Nosema* described above (Cali et al. 1996a; Deplazes et al. 1996).

Pleistophora Species

The species of the genus *Pleistophora* are generally parasitic in the muscles of arthropods and vertebrates such as fish, amphibians, and reptiles. The only reports known in mammals concern humans. The multiplication of *Pleistophora* proceeds from the sporoplasm to a sporont-like stage similar to that of all other microsporidia (see above) but then follows a different pathway that characterizes this genus. In *Pleistophora* the sporont, rather than forming one sporoblast, undergoes multiple divisions at the same time that its membrane thickens to form a vesicle where a variable number of sporoblasts mature to spores (Fig. 2–15 A–B). The spores are contained in a sac-like structure known as the *sporoforous vesicle* and generally range

from 3.0 to 4.0 μm, with a single nucleus. *Pleistophora* usually has eight spores in each vesicle. In addition, the early stages of the parasite's development occur in contact with the host cell cytoplasm, with the endoplasmic reticulum overcoating the sporophorous vesicle at the same time that the cisterna forms.

At least three infections with *Pleistophora* are known in immune-suppressed individuals. The first occurred in an immune-impaired, HIV-negative man with generalized muscle weakness and contractures of 7 months' duration. Two biopsy specimens of skeletal muscle revealed an intense inflammatory reaction with plasma cells, lymphocytes, and histiocytes (Fig. 2–16 A–D). Atrophy and degeneration of muscle cells (Fig. 2–15 A and C) accompanied these changes, in some of which numerous spores in sporophorous vesicles were easily seen. The organisms were studied with both the light and electron microscopes and were classified as belonging to the genus *Pleistophora* (Ledford et al. 1985). An electron micrograph accompanying the article indicates that the spores were about 5.0 by 3.0 μm, with 11 coils of the polar filament in two rows. The immunologic status of the patient was studied 4 years later; he was found to be still immune impaired, but HIV negative (Macher et al. 1988).

The second reported *Pleistophora* infection occurred in a 33-year-old HIV-positive Haitian man who presented with symptoms of pain and weakness in the calves that had spread over a 2-month period to the posterior thighs and the upper extremities. Muscle biopsy specimens revealed a marked myositis produced by organisms with the characteristics of a species of *Pleistophora*. The spores in the sporophorous vesicle measured about 4.0 by 2.0 μm (Fig. 2–17 A–C; *color plate* I *H*; Chupp et al. 1993).

The third case also involved an HIV-positive man living in Spain who also presented with a painful, progressive myositis diagnosed in biopsy specimens examined under the electron microscope. A sonogram of the muscles of both legs revealed marked muscle destruction without calcifications (Grau et al. 1996).

Trachipleistophora hominis

A new genus, *Trachipleistophora*, has been created to accommodate microsporidians found in patients with AIDS in Australia (Field et al. 1996b) and Europe (Vavra et al. 1998). These patients presented with a progressive, severe myositis associated with fever and weight loss (Field et al. 1996a) or with generalized dis-

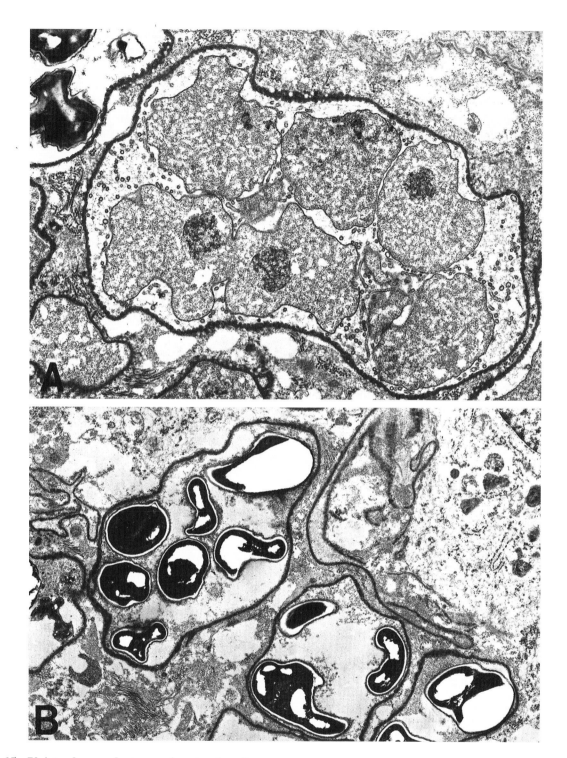

Fig. 2–15. *Pleistophora*, electron micrographs of sections of a muscle biopsy specimen. *A*, The sporont has divided several times at the same time that the surrounding membrane has thickened to form a vesicle that contains the parasites, ×13,000. *B*, Several spores have formed from the sporoblasts, which remain contained in the vesicle. This process is known as *pansporoblastic development*, ×7,500. (The paraffin block from which the preparations for electron microscopy were made is courtesy of M.J. Montana, M.D., Hospital de Figeres, Jirona, Spain. Reported by: Grau, A., Valls, M.E., Williams, J.E., et al. 1996. Miositis por *Pleistophora* en un paciente con sida: Notas clinicas. Med. Clin. 107:779–781.)

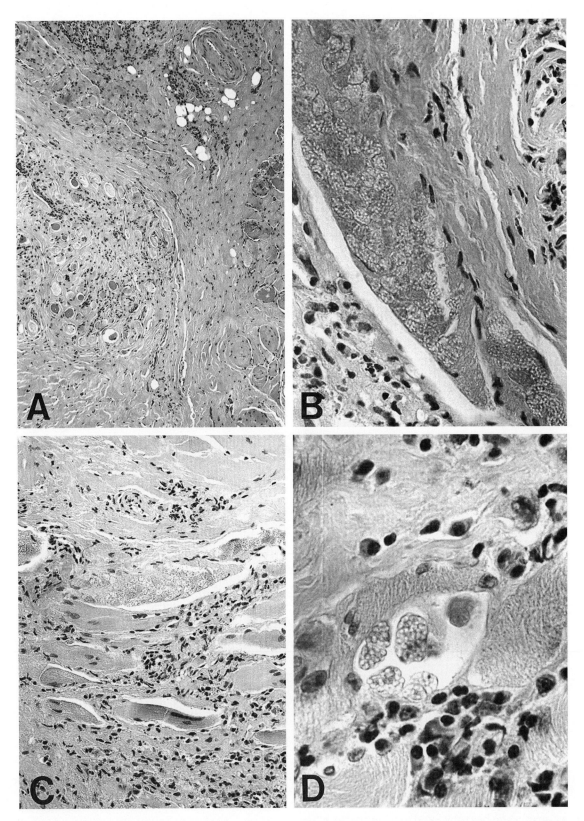

Fig. 2–16. *Pleistophora* in skeletal muscle of a man; sections stained with hematoxylin and eosin stain. *A*, Low-power view showing marked chronic myositis with fibrosis, ×70. *B*, Higher magnification showing the parasites (spores) within a muscle cell. The parasites appear as masses containing birefringent organisms. Note the inflammatory cells, ×450. *C*, Another area with a de-generating muscle cell and inflammation, ×178. *D*, Higher magnification shows spores, ×700. (Preparation courtesy of A. Gonzalvo, M.D., Department of Pathology, Tampa General Hospital, Tampa, Florida. In: Ledford, D.K., Overman, M.D., Gonzalvo, A. et al. 1985. Microsporidosis myositis in a patient with the acquired immunodeficiency syndrome. Ann. Intern. Med. 102:628–630.)

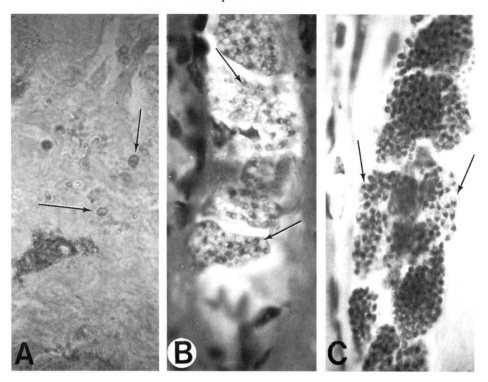

Fig. 2–17. *Pleistophora*, special stains. *A*, Silver methenamine stain showing the spore wall (arrows). *B*, Periodic acid–Schiff stain showing the polar granule, at one end of the spore, staining positively (arrows). *C*, Giemsa stain showing a similar structure staining deep blue (arrows), all ×941. (Preparations courtesy of A. Gonzalvo, M.D., Department of Pathology, Tampa General Hospital, Tampa, Florida. Same patient as in Figure 2–16.)

ease including the brain (Vavra et al. 1998). The characteristics of the new genus in cultures of the parasite are as described for *Pleistophora*, except for the appearance of an electron-dense surface coat surrounding all stages of development (meronts, sporonts, and sporoblasts). This coat, in contrast to that of *Pleistophora*, is rugose ("sun flare-like" projections), thus the name *trachis* (rough). The sporophorous vesicles of *T. hominis* contain 2 to 32 spores. The spores are unenucleated, measure 4.0×2.4 μm, and have an exospore coat that is slightly rugose and a polar tubule with about 11 coils; the extruded polar tubule is about 75 μm in length (Hollister et al. 1996). *Trachipleistophora hominis* is known from a single isolate of a patient with parasites in the cornea, skeletal muscle, and nasal secretions (Field et al. 1996b; Hollister et al. 1996).

Trachipleistophora anthropophthera, in contrast to *T. hominis*, has a dual development, with two kinds of sporophorous vesicles and spores. Type I vesicles have eight spores (2.7×2.0 μm), a thick endospore, and a polar filament with seven thick coils and two thinner

terminal coils. Type II vesicles are smaller, with only two, nearly rounded spores ($2.2–2.5 \times 1.8–2.0$ μm), thin-walled spores, and four or five coils of the polar filament (Vavra et al. 1998). This species was isolated from two patients: one with infection in the brain, the other with infection in the brain, kidneys, pancreas, thyroid, parathyroid, heart, liver, spleen, lymph nodes, and bone marrow (Vavra et al. 1998).

Thelohania-Pleistophora

The genus *Thelohania* is close to *Pleistophora*, sharing most of its diagnostic characteristics. A difference is the number of coils of the polar tubule: 6 or 7 in *Thelohania* and 9 to 11 in *Pleistophora*. In addition, *Thelohania* has two extra thin coils (this is a thinner part of the polar tubule). Another difference is that *Thelohania* has been found in the central nervous system, while

Pleistophora is restricted to the muscles (Yachnis et al. 1996b).

Two cases of infection with a parasite resembling *Thelohania* and *Pleistophora* were described in 1996 in HIV-positive individuals, both with central nervous system involvement, but a decision on the genus or the species of the parasites belong was deferred until more studies were made. It is likely that these organisms are members of *Thelohania*.

The first case involved a 33-year-old man who died 2 months after his illness began. Only the central nervous system was available for examination. The brain, cerebellum, and pons showed multiple areas of necrosis, up to 1.5 cm in diameter, located in the gray matter. Microscopically, the lesions showed necrosis and parasites growing in astrocytes and endothelial cells; spores were being phagocytized and destroyed by macrophages (Yachnis et al. 1996a; Yachnis et al. 1996b). The second case involved in an 8-year-old girl with a congenitally acquired HIV infection and metastatic hemangiopericytoma who presented with episodes of generalized tonic-clonic seizures, poor mental status, and a history of difficulty in walking and breathing. A computed tomography scan of the brain showed lesions similar to those seen in a previous scan, consistent with metastatic tumor, and, in addition, new, smaller lesions in the gray matter. The patient died 1 week after hospitalization. An autopsy revealed disseminated disease heavily involving the brain, heart, kidney, pancreas, and thyroid, as well as other organs to a lesser extent. The organism found was classified as a species of *Pleistophora* based on the morphologic characteristics on light and electron microscopy (Yachnis et al. 1996b).

Diagnosis of Microspora

The diagnosis of Microspora is based on features evident in tissue sections, but the true nature of the spore is best confirmed with the electron microscope. Microsporidians can also be recovered from feces, nasal secretions, sputum, urine, duodenal aspirates, other body fluids, and corneal scrapings. In addition to the hematoxylin and eosin stain, several other special stains are used to stain the spores of microsporidia. Since microsporidiosis is usually diagnosed by the anatomic pathologist, the discussion below is tailored to his or her needs. It also takes into account the fact that the hematoxylin and eosin–stained tissue sections are the first line of work. For convenience, this section will be divided into discussions of intestinal, ocular, and muscle tissues, other tissues, and clinical samples.

Intestinal Microsporidia. Microsporidia in the intestinal tract are frequently overlooked in routine specimens because of the lack of a cellular infiltrate, especially if they are few in number or poorly stained (Case Records of the Massachusetts General Hospital, 1993), or because of lack of familiarity with the parasites. Diagnosticians familiar with these organisms usually detect them under dry objectives, but all suspicious elements should always be investigated with the oil immersion lens (Peacock et al. 1991). Special stains usually do not confirm the diagnosis. They only contrast the organisms with the cytoplasm of the cells, and in most instances they obscure what little morphology is seen under the light microscope. Of help is the diastase periodic acid–Shiff stain to differentiate the organisms (which are negative) from degenerated goblet cells, an often troublesome artifact (Field et al. 1993a). The special stains recommended for staining the parasites in tissues are Giemsa stain (stains the spores and other forms deep blue), Warthin-Starry stain (Field et al. 1993b), calcofluor white (Vavra et al. 1993), Gram stain (the wall of the spore is positive) (Canning, Hollister, 1990), and a "Quick-hot Gram-chromopthrope" (spores stain dark violet) that allows rapid staining of paraffin sections and clinical samples (Moura et al. 1997). Immunofluorescence tests have also been used (van Gool et al. 1993; Zierdt et al. 1993). Each laboratory should become familiar with one or two of these techniques, since performing all of them is too expensive and since no single technique has advantages over the others.

In the hematoxylin and eosin stain, the spores are eosinophilic (*color plate* I *D–F*). Once parasites are recognized, the presence or absence of a vacuole containing the parasites (sometimes difficult to see) should be determined. If a vacuole is present and if the parasites are about 2 μm (*they should be actually measured, not just estimated*), the organism in question is a species of *Encephalitozoon*. In instances where the parasites are scanty, a search for cupping of the apical end of the nucleus should be undertaken, mostly on the cells at the tip of the villi (Fig. 2–8 *A–B*; *color plate* I *E–F*). If cupping is present, the area of the cytoplasm above the nucleus should be studied carefully. Plasmodial stages of *Enterocytozoon* are seen as pale areas containing small gray flecks and faint striations (Fig. 2–13 *D*; Field et al. 1993a), and if measured, they are found to be up to 5 μm in diameter. Any spores found should be measured; if they are about 1 μm, the diagnosis is *Entero-*

cytozoon (Figs. 2–9 and 1–13 C and E). Keep in mind that cupping of the nucleus is also seen in *Encephalitozoon* infections (*color plate* I E; Fig. 2–8 A), but the search for nuclei cupping is more profitable in infections with *Enterocytozoon*, since plasmodial stages are almost invisible in hematoxylin and eosin stains (*color plate* I F).

Once the genus has been identified, the results should be reported, indicating that a species of *Encephalitozoon* or *E. bieneusi* (or both, since double infections have been reported) is present. This report is important because encephalitozoonosis is treatable, with clinical cure and elimination of the parasite, while no therapy is known for enterocytozoonosis.

Electron microscopy, if done, should confirm these findings based on the morphologic description given above for each parasite. Once again, keep in mind that the species of *Encephalitozoon* cannot be separated based on electron micrographs and that all three species have been found in the intestine.

Ocular Microsporidia.

At least three genera of microsporidia have been reported from the eye: *Encephalitozoon*, *Vittaforma*, and *Trachipleistophora*. In biopsy specimens of the cornea and conjunctiva or in smears of the conjunctiva, these genera can be differentiated. The stains used are similar to those used for the intestinal microsporidians. *Encephalitozoon* is seen in vacuoles, and the spores measure 2.0 μm (*color plate* I C) *Vittaforma* has spores measuring 3.8 × 1.2 μm. *Trachipleistophora* has spores measuring 4.0 × 2.4 μm, and the spores are found in groups within the sporophorous sac. All three species of *Encephalitozoon* (*E. cuniculi*, *E. hellem*, and *E. intestinalis*), which produce a benign keratoconjunctivitis, have been recovered from the eye and are treatable. *Vittaforma* produces deep stromal ulcers

Microsporidia of Skeletal Muscles.

At least three genera of microsporidia occur in the skeletal muscles, all in immune-compromised individuals: *Pleistophora*, *Trachipleistophora*, and *Nosema*. The first two belong to the family Pleistophoridae and are characterized by stages forming in polysporophorus vesicles (see above). Further, while the species of *Pleistophora* occurring in humans is undetermined, the species of *Trachipleistophora* is *T. hominis*. *Nosema* is characterized by two abbuted nuclei (see above), and both *N. conori* and a *Nosema* species are found in muscles. The identification of these organisms rests on electron micrographs.

Microsporidia of Other Tissues.

The stains are the same. Parasites are found mostly in epithelial cells of bronchioles, renal tubules, urothelium, the bile duct system, macrophages, and others (*Encephalitozoon*), and in astrocytes and macrophages (*Trachipleistophora*). The size of the spores and the morphologic characteristics described above should help separate these genera.

Microsporidia in Clinical Samples.

In clinical samples, microsporidians have been diagnosed using an array of staining techniques, mainly in stools (*color plate* I I) and duodenal aspirates. Other samples submitted for diagnosis of microsporidiosis are uncommon. The most widely used stain in clinical samples is the Weber's modified trichrome stain, a chromotrope-based stain that stains the spores pale red (Weber et al. 1992a) and is considered the gold standard by some. Also used are the Warthin-Starry (Field et al. 1993b) and Giemsa stains (van Gool et al. 1990). The calcofluor white stain is used in duodenal imprints of biopsy specimens (Vavra et al. 1993) and in fresh stool samples (Luna et al. 1995). A Gram and chromotrope combination stain (Moura et al. 1996) and a trichrome blue stain modification for stool samples (Kokoskin et al. 1994; Ryan et al. 1993) have been proposed. Electron microscopy of pellets of duodenal aspirates (Orenstein et al. 1990) and concentrations of stools also have been recommended. Immunofluorescence (van Gool et al. 1993) and an indirect fluorescent antibody in stool samples (Zierdt et al. 1993) are available.

A polymerase chain reaction and restriction endonuclease in stools (Fedorko et al. 1995), as well as a polymerase chain reaction for stool samples (da Silva et al. 1997), duodenal aspirates, and tissues (Velasquez et al. 1996), have been developed. These techniques allow speciation in tissues if specific parasite primers are used (Fedorko, Hijazi, 1996). Finally, an enzyme-linked immunosorbent assay is also available (Hollister, Canning, 1987).

References

Aarons EJ, Woodrow D, Hollister WS, Canning EU, Francis N, Gazzard BG, 1994. Reversible renal failure caused by a microsporidian infection. AIDS 8:1119–1121

Ashton N, Wirasinha PA, 1973. Encephalitozoonosis (nosematosis) of the cornea. Br. J. Ophthalmol. 57:669–674

Asmuth DM, DeGirolami PC, Federman M, Ezratty CR, Pleskow DK, Desai G, Wanke CA, 1994. Clinical features of microsporidiosis in patients with AIDS. Clin. Infect. Dis. 18:819–825

Baker MD, Vossbrinck CR, Didier ES, Maddox JV, Shadduck JA, 1995. Small subunit ribosomal DNA phylogeny of various microsporidia with emphasis on AIDS related forms. J. Euk. Microbiol. 42:564–570

Beaugerie L, Teilhac MF, Deluol AM, Fritsch J, Girard PM, Rozenbaum W, Le Quintrec Y, Chatelet FP, 1992. Cholangiopathy associated with Microsporidia infection of the common bile duct mucosa in a patient with HIV infection. Ann. Intern. Med. 117:401–402

Bergquist R, Morfeldt Mansson L, Pehrson PO, Petrini B, Wasserman J, 1984. Antibody against *Encephalitozoon cuniculi* in Swedish homosexual men. Scand. J. Infect. Dis. 16:389–391

Blanshard C, Hollister WS, Peacock CS, Tovey DG, Ellis DS, Canning EU, Gazzard BG, 1992. Simultaneous infection with two types of intestinal microsporidia in a patient with AIDS. Gut 33:418–420

Bretagne S, Foulet F, Alkassoum W, Fleury Feith J, Develoux M, 1993. Prevalence des spores d' *Enterocytozoon bieneusi* dans les selles de patients sideens et d'enfants Africains non infectes par le VIH. Bull. Soc. Pathol. Exot. 86:351–357

Bryan RT, Cali A, Owen R, Spencer H, 1991a. Microsporidia: Newly recognized opportunistic pathogens in patients with AIDS. In: Sun T (ed), *Progress in Clinical Parasitology*. New York: W.W. Norton & Co., pp. 1–26

Bryan RT, Cali A, Owen RL, Spencer HC, 1991b. Microsporidia: opportunistic pathogens in patients with AIDS. Prog. Clin. Parasitol. 2:1–26

Cali A, Kotler DP, Orenstein JM, 1993. *Septata intestinalis* n. g., n. sp., an intestinal microsporidian associated with chronic diarrhea and dissemination in AIDS patients. J. Euk. Microbiol. 40:101–112

Cali A, Meisler DM, Lowder CY, Lembach R, Ayers L, Takvorian PM, Rutherford I, Longworth DL, McMahon J, Bryan RT, 1991a. Corneal microsporidioses: characterization and identification. J. Protozool. 38:215S–217S

Cali A, Meisler DM, Rutherford I, Lowder CY, McMahon JT, Longworth DL, Bryan RT, 1991b. Corneal microsporidiosis in a patient with AIDS. Am. J. Trop. Med. Hyg. 44:463–468

Cali A, Orenstein JM, Kotler DP, Owen R, 1991c. A comparison of two microsporidian parasites in enterocytes of AIDS patients with chronic diarrhea. J. Protozool. 38:96S–98S

Cali A, Owen RL, 1990. Intracellular development of *Enterocytozoon*, a unique microsporidian found in the intestine of AIDS patients. J. Protozool. 37:145–155

Cali A, Takvorian PM, Lewin S, Rendel M, Sian C, Wittner M, Weiss L, 1996a. Identification of a new *Nosema*-like microsporidian associated with myositis in an AIDS patient. J. Euk. Microbiol. 43:108S

Cali A, Weiss L, Takvorian P, 1996b. Microsporidian taxonomy: What is a family, genus and species? Joint Meeting of the American Society of Parasitology and Society

of Protozoology. Tucson, Arizona. June 11–15, 1996. Abstracts, pp. 100S–101S.

Canning EU, Hollister WS, 1990. *Enterocytozoon bieneusi* (Microspora): Prevalence and pathogenicity in AIDS patients. Trans. R. Soc. Trop. Med. Hyg. 84:181–186

Canning EU, Lom J, 1986. *The Microsporidia of Vertebrates*. New York: Academic Press

Case Records of the Massachusetts General Hospital, 1993. Weekly clinicopathological exercises. Case 51–1993. A 36-year-old man with AIDS, increase in chronic diarrhea, and intermittent fever and chills. N. Engl. J. Med. 329:1946–1954

Chu P, West AB, 1996. *Encephalitozoon (Septata) intestinalis*. Cytologic, histologic, and electron microscopic features of a systemic intestinal pathogen (Case Report). Am. J. Clin. Pathol. 106:606–614

Chupp GL, Alroy J, Adelman LS, Breen JC, Skolnik PR, 1993. Myositis due to *Pleistophora* (Microsporidia) in a patient with AIDS. Clin. Infect. Dis. 16:15–21

Corliss JO, 1994. An interim utilitarian ("user-friendly") hierarchical classification and characterization of the protists. Acta Protozool. 33:1–51

Cornet M, Romand S, Warszawski J, Bouree P, 1996. Factors associated with microsporidial and cryptosporidial diarrhea in HIV infected patients. Parasite 3:397–401

Coyle CM, Wittner M, Kotler DP, Noyer C, Orenstein JM, Tanowitz HB, Weiss LM, 1996. The association of Microsporidia and AIDS related diarrhea as determined by the polymerase chain reaction (PCR) to ribosomal RNA genes. Joint meeting of the American Society of Parasitology and Society of Protozoology. Tucson, Arizona, June 11–15, 1996. Abstracts, p. 84S

Croppo GP, Visvesvara GS, Leitch GJ, Wallace S, de Groote MA, Reves R, 1995. Antigenic analysis of *Encephalitozoon cuniculi* (CDC:V282) isolated from the urine of a patient with AIDS. Joint meeting of the American Society of Parasitology and American Association of Veterinary Parasitology. Pittsburgh, Pennsylvania, June 1995. Abstracts, p. 104

Curry A, Canning EU, 1993. Human microsporidiosis. J. Infect. 27:229–236

da Silva AJ, Bornay-Llinares FJ, de la Puente CD, Moura H, Mauro P, Sobottka I, Schwartz DA, Visvesvara GS, Slemenda SB, Pieniazek NJ, 1997. Diagnosis of *Enterocytozoon bieneusi* (Microsporidia) infections by polymerase chain reaction in stool samples using primers based on the region coding for small-subunit ribosomal RNA. Arch. Pathol. Lab. Med. 121:874–893

Davis RM, Font RL, Keisler MS, Shadduck JA, 1990. Corneal microsporidiosis. A case report including ultrastructural observations. Ophthalmology 97:953–957

de Groote MA, Visvesvara GS, Wilson ML, Pieniazek NJ, Slemenda SB, Dasilva AJ, Leitch GJ, Bryan RT, Reves R, 1995. Polymerase chain reaction and culture confirmation of disseminated *Encephalitozoon cuniculi* in a patient with AIDS: successful therapy with albendazole. J. Infect. Dis. 171:1375–1378

Deplazes P, Mathis A, Muller C, Weber R, 1996. Molecular epidemiology of *Encephalitozoon cuniculi*, a zoonotic microsporidian infecting HIV-seropositive persons. Joint meeting of the American Society of Parasitology and Society of Protozoology. Tucson, Arizona, June 11–15, 1996. Abstracts, p. 84S

Desportes I, le Charpentier Y, Galian A, Bernard F, Cochand Priollet B, Lavergne A, Ravisse P, Modigliani R, 1985. Occurrence of a new microsporidan: *Enterocytozoon bieneusi* n.g., n. sp., in the enterocytes of a human patient with AIDS. J. Protozool. 32:250–254

Desser SS, Hong H, Yang YJ, 1992. Ultrastructure of the development of a species of *Encephalitozoon* cultured from the eye of an AIDS patient. Parasitol. Res. 78:677–683

Didier ES, Didier PJ, Friedberg DN, Stenson SM, Orenstein JM, Yee RW, Tio FO, Davis RM, Vossbrinck C, Millichamp N, Shadduck JA, 1991. Isolation and characterization of a new human microsporidian, *Encephalitozoon hellem* (n. sp.), from three AIDS patients with keratoconjunctivitis. J. Infect. Dis. 163:617–621

Didier PJ, Didier ES, Orenstein JM, Shadduck JA, 1991. Fine structure of a new human microsporidian, *Encephalitozoon hellem*, in culture. J. Protozool. 38:502–507

Dobbins WO, Weinstein WM, 1984. Electron microscopy of the intestine and rectum in acquired immunodeficiency syndrome. Gastroenterology 86:1063

Dobbins WO, Weinstein WM, 1985. Electron microscopy of the intestine and rectum in acquired immunodeficiency syndrome. Gastroenterology 88:738–749

Dore GJ, Marriott DJ, Hing MC, Harkness JL, Field AS, 1995. Disseminated microsporidiosis due to *Septata intestinalis* in nine patients infected with the human immunodeficiency virus: response to therapy with albendazole. Clin. Infect. Dis. 21:70–76

Eeftinck JKM, van Gool T, 1992. Clinical and microbiological aspects of microsporidiosis. Trop. Geogr. Med. 44:287

Fedorko DP, Hijazi YM, 1996. Application of molecular techniques to the diagnosis of microsporidial infection. Emerg. Infect. Dis. 2:183–191

Fedorko DP, Nelson NA, Cartwright CP, 1995. Identification of microsporidia in stool specimens by using PCR and restriction endonucleases. J. Clin. Microbiol. 33:1739–1741

Field AS, Hing MC, Milliken ST, Marriott DJ, 1993a. Microsporidia in the small intestine of HIV-infected patients. A new diagnostic technique and a new species. Med. J. Aust. 158:390–394

Field AS, Marriott DJ, Hing MC, 1993b. The Warthin-Starry stain in the diagnosis of small intestinal microsporidiosis in HIV-infected patients. Folia Parasitol. 40:261–266

Field AS, Marriott DJ, Milliken ST, Brew BJ, Canning EU, Kench JG, Darveniza P, Harkness JL, 1996a. Myositis associated with a newly described microsporidian, *Trachipleistophora hominis*, in a patient with AIDS. J. Clin. Microbiol. 34:2803–2811

Field AS, Milliken ST, Canning EU, Harkness JL, Brew BJ, Kench JG, Darveniza P, Marriott DJ, 1996b. Clinical presentation and light and electron microscopic findings of a new microsporidian, Trachipleistophora hominis, in a patient with AIDS. Joint meeting of the American Society of Parasitology and Society of Protozoology. Tucson, Arizona, June 11–15, 1996. Abstracts, p. 103S

Friedberg DN, Stenson SM, Orenstein JM, Tierno PM, Charles NC, 1990. Microsporidial keratoconjunctivitis in acquired immunodeficiency syndrome. Arch. Ophthalmol. 108:504–508

Garcia LS, Shimizu RY, Bruckner DA, 1994. Detection of microsporidial spores in fecal specimens from patients diagnosed with cryptosporidiosis. J. Clin. Microbiol. 32:1739–1741

Gourley WK, Swedo JL, 1988. Intestinal infection by microsporidia *Enterocytozoon bieneusi* of patients with AIDS: an ultrastructural study of the use of human mitochondria by a protozoan. U.S. and Canadian Academy of Pathology annual meeting. Washington, D.C., Feb. 28–Mar. 4, 1988. Abstracts, p. 35A

Grau A, Valls ME, Williams JE, Ellis DS, Muntane MJ, Nadal C, 1996. Miositis por *Pleistophora* en un paciente con sida: Notas Clinicas. Med. Clin. (Barcelona) 107:779–781

Greenson JK, Belitsos PC, Yardley JH, Bartlett JG, 1991. AIDS enteropathy: occult enteric infections and duodenal mucosal alterations in chronic diarrhea. Ann. Intern. Med. 114:366–372

Gunnarsson G, Hurlbut D, DeGirolami PC, Federman M, Wanke C, 1995. Multiorgan microsporidiosis: report of five cases and review. Clin. Infect. Dis. 21:37–44

Hartskeerl RA, van Gool T, Schuitema AR, Didier ES, Terpstra WJ, 1995. Genetic and immunological characterization of the microsporidian *Septata intestinalis* Cali, Kotler and Orenstein, 1993: reclassification to *Encephalitozoon intestinalis*. Semin. Respir. Infect. 110:277–285

Hermanek J, Koudela B, Kucerova Z, Ditrich O, Travnicek J, 1993. Prophylactic and therapeutic immune reconstitution of SCID mice infected with *Encephalitozoon cuniculi*. Folia Parasitol. 40:287–291

Hollister WS, Canning EU, 1987. An enzyme-linked immunosorbent assay (ELISA) for detection of antibodies to *Encephalitozoon cuniculi* and its use in determination of infections in man. Semin. Respir. Infect. 94:209–219

Hollister WS, Canning EU, Colbourn NI, Aarons EJ, 1995. *Encephalitozoon cuniculi* isolated from the urine of an AIDS patient, which differs from canine and murine isolates. J. Euk. Microbiol. 42:367–372

Hollister WS, Canning EU, Colbourn NI, Curry A, Lacey CJ, 1993. Characterization of *Encephalitozoon hellem* (Microspora) isolated from the nasal mucosa of a patient with AIDS. Semin. Respir. Infect. 107:351–358

Hollister WS, Canning EU, Weidner E, Field AS, Kench J, Marriott DJ, 1996. Development and ultrastructure of *Trachipleistophora hominis* n.g., n.sp. after in vitro isolation from an AIDS patient and inoculation into athymic mice. Semin. Respir. Infect. 112:143–154

Hollister WS, Canning EU, Willcox A, 1991. Evidence for widespread occurrence of antibodies to *Encephalitozoon cuniculi* (Microspora) in man provided by ELISA and other serological tests. Semin. Respir. Infect. 102:33–43

Kokoskin E, Gyorkos TW, Camus A, Cedilotte L, Purtill T, Ward B, 1994. Modified technique for efficient detection of microsporidia. J. Clin. Microbiol. 32:1074–1075

Kotler DP, Orenstein JM, 1994. Prevalence of intestinal microsporidiosis in HIV-infected individuals referred for gastroenterological evaluation. Am. J. Gastroenterol. 89:1998–2002

Lacey CJ, Clarke AM, Fraser P, Metcalfe T, Bonsor G, Curry A, 1992. Chronic microsporidian infection of the nasal mucosae, sinuses and conjunctivae in HIV disease. Genitourin. Med. 68:179–181

Lainson R, Garnham PCC, Killick-Kendrick R, Bird RG, 1964. Nosematosis, a microsporidial infection of rodents and other animals, including man. Br. Med. J. 470–472

Ledford DK, Overman MD, Gonzalvo A, Cali A, Mester SW, Lockey RF, 1985. Microsporidiosis myositis in a patient with the acquired immunodeficiency syndrome. Ann. Intern. Med. 102:628–630

Levaditi C, Nicolau S, Schoen R, 1923. L'agent etiologique de l'encephalite epizootique du lapin. C. R. Acad. Sci. 89:985–986

Lowder CY, McMahon JT, Meisler DM, Dodds EM, Calabrese LH, Didier ES, Cali A, 1996. Microsporidial keratoconjunctivitis caused by *Septata intestinalis* in a patient with acquired immunodeficiency syndrome. Am. J. Ophthalmol. 121:715–717

Luna VA, Stewart BK, Bergeron DL, Clausen CR, Plorde JJ, Fritsche TR, 1995. Use of the fluorochrome calcofluor white in the screening of stool specimens for spores of Microsporidia. Am. J. Clin. Pathol. 103:656–659

Macher AM, Neafie RC, Angritt P, Athur SM, 1988. Correspondence. Microsporidial myositis and the acquired immunodeficiency syndrome (AIDS): a four-year follow-up. Ann. Intern. Med. 109:343

Marcus PB, Van Der Walt JJ, Burger PJ, 1973. Human tumor microsporidiosis: first reported case. Arch. Pathol. 95:341–95

Margileth AM, Strano AJ, Chandra R, Neafie RC, Blum M, McCully RM, 1973. Disseminated nosematosis in an immunologically compromised infant. Arch. Pathol. 95:145–150

Matsubayashi H, Koike T, Mikata I, Takei H, Hagiwara S, 1959. A case of *Encephalitozoon*-like body infection in man. Arch. Pathol. 67:181–187

McCluskey PJ, Goonan PV, Marriott DJ, Field AS, 1993. Microsporidial keratoconjunctivitis in AIDS. Eye 7:80–83

Metcalfe TW, Doran RM, Rowlands PL, Curry A, Lacey CJ, 1992. Microsporidial keratoconjunctivitis in a patient with AIDS. Br. J. Ophthalmol. 76:177–178

Michiels JF, Hofman P, Saint Paul MC, Loubiere R, Bernard E, LeFichoux Y, 1993. Pathological features of intestinal microsporidiosis in HIV positive patients. A report of 13 new cases. Pathol. Res. Pract. 189:377–383

Modigliani R, Bories C, le Charpentier Y, Salmeron M, Messing B, Galian A, Rambaud JC, Lavergne A, Cochand Priollet B, Desportes I, Cochand-Priollet B, 1985. Diarrhoea and malabsorption in acquired immune deficiency syndrome: a study of four cases with special emphasis on opportunistic protozoan infestations. Gut 26:179–187

Molina JM, Oksenhendler E, Beauvais B, Sarfati C, Jaccard A, Derouin F, Modai J, 1995. Disseminated microsporidiosis due to *Septata intestinalis* in patients with AIDS: clinical features and response to albendazole therapy. J. Infect. Dis. 171:245–249

Moura H, Nunes JL, Sodre FC, Brasil P, Wallmo K, Wahlquist S, Wallace S, Croppo GP, Visvesvara GS, 1996. A combined Gram and chromotrope technique enhances detection of microosporidial spores in clinical samples. Joint meeting of the American Society of Parasitology and Society of Protozoology. Tucson, Arizona, June 11–15, 1996 Abstracts, pp. 84S–85S

Moura H, Schwartz DA, Bornay-Llinares F, Sodre FC, Wallace S, Visvesvara GS, 1997. A new and improved "quick-hot gram-chromotrope" technique that differentially stains microsporidian spores in clinical samples, including paraffin-embedded tissue sections. Arch. Pathol. Lab. Med. 121:888–893

Muller M, 1997. What are the microsporidia? Parasitol. Today 13:455–456

Nelson JB, 1962. An intracellular parasite resembling a microsporidian associated with ascites in Swiss mice. Proc. Soc. Exptl. Biol. 109:714–717

Orenstein JM, 1991. Microsporidiosis in the acquired immunodeficiency syndrome. J. Parasitol. 77:843–864

Orenstein JM, Chiang J, Steinberg W, Smith PD, Rotterdam H, Kotler DP, 1990. Intestinal microsporidiosis as a cause of diarrhea in human immunodeficiency virus–infected patients: a report of 20 cases. Hum. Pathol. 21:475–481

Orenstein JM, Tenner M, Cali A, Kotler DP, 1992. A microsporidian previously undescribed in humans, infecting enterocytes and macrophages, and associated with diarrhea in an acquired immunodeficiency syndrome patient. Hum. Pathol. 23:722–728

Orenstein JM, Zierdt W, Zierdt C, Kotler DP, 1990. Correspondence. Identification of spores of *Enterocytozoon bieneusi* in stool and duodenal fluid from AIDS patients. Lancet 336:1127–1128

Pakes SP, Shadduck JA, Cali A, 1975. Fine structure of *Encephalitozoon cuniculi* from rabbits, mice and hamsters. J. Protozool. 22:481–488

Peacock CS, Blanshard C, Tovey DG, Ellis DS, Gazzard BC, 1991. Histological diagnosis of intestinal microsporidiosis in patients with AIDS. J. Clin. Pathol. 44:558–563

Pinnolis M, Egbert PR, Font RL, Winter FC, 1981. Nosematosis of the cornea. Case report, including electron microscopic studies. Arch. Ophthalmol. 99:1044–1047

Pol S, Romana CA, Richard S, Amouyal P, Desportes Livage I, Carnot F, Pays JF, Berthelot P, 1993. Microsporidia infection in patients with the human immunodeficiency virus and unexplained cholangitis. N. Engl. J. Med. 328:95–99

Pol S, Romana C, Richard S, Carnot F, Dumont JL, Bouche H, Pialoux G, Stern M, Pays JF, Berthelot P, 1992. *En-*

terocytozoon bieneusi infection in acquired immunodeficiency syndrome–related sclerosing cholangitis. Gastroenterology 102:1778–1781

Rabeneck L, Gyorkey F, Genta RM, Gyorkey P, Foote LW, Risser JM, 1993. The role of Microsporidia in the pathogenesis of HIV-related chronic diarrhea. Ann. Intern. Med. 119:895–899

Rabodonirina M, Bertocchi M, Desportes Livage I, Cotte L, Levrey H, Piens MA, Monneret G, Celard M, Mornex JF, Mojon M, 1996. *Enterocytozoon bieneusi* as a cause of chronic diarrhea in a heart-lung transplant recipient who was seronegative for human immunodeficiency virus. Clin. Infect. Dis. 23:114–117

Reetz J, 1994. Naturliche Ubertragung von Mikrosporidien (*Encephalitozoon cuniculi*) uber das Huhnerei. Tierarztl. Prax. 22:147–150

Ryan NJ, Sutherland G, Coughlan K, Globan M, Doultree J, Marshall J, Baird RW, Pedersen J, Dwyer B, 1993. A new trichrome-blue stain for detection of microsporidial species in urine, stool, and nasopharyngeal specimens. J. Clin. Microbiol. 31:3264–3269

Sandfort J, Hannemann A, Gelderblom H, Stark K, Owen RL, Ruf B, 1994. *Enterocytozoon bieneusi* infection in an immunocompetent patient who had acute diarrhea and who was not infected with the human immunodeficiency virus. Clin. Infect. Dis. 19:514–516

Scaglia M, Sacchi L, Gatti S, Bernuzzi AM, Polver PP, Piacentini IC-E, Croppo GP, da Silva AJ, Pieniazek NJ, et al, 1994. Isolation and identification of *Encephalitozoon hellem* from an Italian AIDS patient with disseminated microsporidiosis. APMIS 102:817–827

Schmidt EC, Shadduck JA, 1983. Murine encephalitozoonosis model for studying the host–parasite relationship of a chronic infection. Infect. Immun. 40:936–942

Schmidt EC, Shadduck JA, 1984. Mechanisms of resistance to the intracellular protozoan *Encephalitozoon cuniculi* in mice. J. Immunol. 133:2712–2719

Schwartz DA, Bryan RT, Hewan Lowe KO, Visvesvara GS, Weber R, Cali A, Angritt P, 1992. Disseminated microsporidiosis (*Encephalitozoon hellem*) and acquired immunodeficiency syndrome. Autopsy evidence for respiratory acquisition. Arch. Pathol. Lab. Med. 116: 660–668

Schwartz DA, Visvesvara GS, Diesenhouse MC, Weber R, Font RL, Wilson LA, Corrent G, Serdarevic ON, Rosberger DF, Keenen PC, et al, 1993a. Pathologic features and immunofluorescent antibody demonstration of ocular microsporidiosis (*Encephalitozoon hellem*) in seven patients with acquired immunodeficiency syndrome. Am. J. Ophthalmol. 115:285–292

Schwartz DA, Visvesvara GS, Leitch GJ, Tashjian L, Pollack M, Holden J, Bryan RT, 1993b. Pathology of symptomatic microsporidial (*Encephalitozoon hellem*) bronchiolitis in the acquired immunodeficiency syndrome: a new respiratory pathogen diagnosed from lung biopsy, bronchoalveolar lavage, sputum, and tissue culture. Hum. Pathol. 24:937–943

Schwartz DA, Visvesvara GS, Weber R, Bryan RT, 1994. Male genital tract microsporidiosis and AIDS: prostatic

abscess due to *Encephalitozoon hellem*. J. Euk. Microbiol. 41:61S

Shadduck JA, Meccoli RA, Davis R, Font RL, 1990. Isolation of a microsporidian from a human patient. J. Infect. Dis. 162:773–776

Silveira H, Canning EU, 1995. *Vittaforma corneae* n. comb. for the human microsporidium *Nosema corneum* Shadduck, Meccoli, Davis & Font, 1990, based on its ultrastructure in the liver of experimentally infected athymic mice. J. Euk. Microbiol. 42:158–165

Singh M, Kane GJ, Mackinlay L, Quaki I, Yap EH, Ho BC, Ho LC, Lim KC, 1982. Detection of antibodies to *Nosema cuniculi* (Protozoa: Microsporidia) in human and animal sera by the indirect fluorescent antibody technique. Southeast Asian J. Trop. Med. Public Health 13:110–113

Soule JB, Halverson AL, Becker RB, Pistole MC, Orenstein JM, 1997. A patient with acquired immunodeficiency syndrome and untreated *Encephalitozoon (Septata) intestinalis* microsporidiosis leading to small bowel perforation: response to albendazole. Arch. Pathol. Lab. Med. 121:880–887

Sprague V, 1974. *Nosema connori* n. sp., a microsporidian parasite of man. Trans. Am. Microsc. Soc. 93:400–403

Sprague V, Becnel JJ, Hazard EI, 1992. Taxonomy of phylum Microspora. Crit. Rev. Microbiol. 18:285–395

Strano AJ, Cali A, Neafie RC, 1976. Microsporidiosis. In: Binford CH and Connor DH (eds), *Pathology of Tropical and Extraordinary Diseases*. Vol. 1. Washington, D.C.: Armed Forces Institute of Pathology, pp. 333–339

Svenson J, MacLean JD, Kokoskin Nelson E, Szabo J, Lough J, Gill MJ, 1993. Microsporidiosis in AIDS patients. Can. Communicable Dis. Rep. 19:13–15

Torres CM, 1927. Morphologie d'un nouveau parasite de l'homme, *Encephalitozoon chagasi*, n. sp., observe dans un cas de meningo-encephalo-myelite congenitale avec myosite et myocardite. C.R. Soc. Biol. 97:1787–1790

van Gool T, Canning EU, Gilis H, van den Bergh Weerman MAE-S-J, Dankert J, 1994. *Septata intestinalis* frequently isolated from stool of AIDS patients with a new cultivation method. Semin. Respir. Infect. 109:281–289

van Gool T, Hollister WS, Schattenkerk WE, van den Bergh Weerman MA, Terpstra WJ, van Ketel RJ, Reiss P, Canning EU, 1990. Correspondence. Diagnosis of *Enterocytozoon bieneusi* microsporidiosis in AIDS patients by recovery of spores from faeces. Lancet 336: 697–698

van Gool T, Snijders F, Reiss P, Eeftinck JKM, van den Bergh Weerman MA, Bartelsman JF, Bruins JJ, Canning EU, Dankert J, 1993. Diagnosis of intestinal and disseminated microsporidial infections in patients with HIV by a new rapid fluorescence technique. J. Clin. Pathol. 46: 694–699

van Gool T, Vetter JC, Weinmayr B, Van Dam A, Derouin F, Dankert J, 1997. High seroprevalence of *Encephalitozoon* species in immunocompetent subjects. J. Infect. Dis. 175:1020–1024

Vavra J, Nohynkova E, Machala L, Spala J, 1993. An extremely rapid method for detection of microsporidia in biopsy materials from AIDS patients. Folia Parasitol. 40:273–274

Vavra J, Yachnis AT, Shadduck JA, Orenstein JM, 1998. Microsporidia of the genus *Trachipleistophora*—causative agents of human microsporidiosis: description of *Trachipleistophora anthropophthera* n. sp. (Protozoa: Microsporidia). J. Euk. Microbiol. 45:273–283

Velasquez JN, Carnevale S, Guarnera EA, Labbe JH, Chertcoff A, Cabrera MG, Rodriguez MI, 1996. Detection of the microsporidian parasite *Enterocytozoon bieneusi* in specimens from patients with AIDS by PCR. J. Clin. Microbiol. 34:3230–3232

Visvesvara GS, Leitch GJ, da Silva AJ, Croppo GP, Moura H, Wallace SS-S, Schwartz DA, Moss D, Bryan RT, et al, 1994. Polyclonal and monoclonal antibody and PCR-amplified small-subunit rRNA identification of a microsporidian, *Encephalitozoon hellem*, isolated from man. J. Clin. Microbiol. 32:2760–2768

Visvesvara GS, Leitch GJ, Moura H, Wallace S, Weber R, Bryan RT, 1991. Culture, electron microscopy, and immunoblot studies on a microsporidian parasite isolated from the urine of a patient with AIDS. J. Protozool. 38:105S–111S

Visvesvara GS, Leitch GJ, Pieniazek NJ, da Silva AJ, Wallace S, Slemenda SB, Weber R, Schwartz DA, Gorelkin L, Wilcox CM, et al, 1995. Short-term in vitro culture and molecular analysis of the microsporidian, *Enterocytozoon bieneusi*. J. Euk. Microbiol. 42:506–510

WHO, 1993. Parasitic diseases surveillance. Antibody to *Encephalitozoon cumiculi* in man. Wkly. Epidemiol. Rec. WHO 58:30–32

Wanke CA, DeGirolami P, Federman M, 1996. *Enterocytozoon bieneusi* infection and diarrheal disease in patients who were not infected with human immunodeficiency virus: case report and review. Clin. Infect. Dis. 23:816–818

Weber R, Bryan RT, 1994. Microsporidial infections in immunodeficient and immunocompetent patients. Clin. Infect. Dis. 19:517–521

Weber R, Bryan RT, Owen RL, Wilcox CM, Gorelkin L, Visvesvara GS, 1992a. Improved light-microscopical detection of microsporidia spores in stool and duodenal aspirates. N. Engl. J. Med. 326:161–166

Weber R, Kuster H, Keller R, Bachi T, Spycher MA, Briner J, Russi E, Luthy R, 1992b. Pulmonary and intestinal microsporidiosis in a patient with the acquired immunodeficiency syndrome. Am. Rev. Respir. Dis. 146:1603–1605

Weber R, Kuster H, Visvesvara GS, Bryan RT, Schwartz DA, Luthy R, 1993. Disseminated microsporidiosis due to *Encephalitozoon hellem*: pulmonary colonization, microhematuria, and mild conjunctivitis in a patient with AIDS. Clin. Infect. Dis. 17:415–419

Weiser J, 1964. On the taxonomic position of the genus *Encephalitozoon* Levaditi, Nicolau & Schoen, 1923 (Protozoa: Microsporidia). Semin. Respir. Infect. 54:749– 751

Weiss LM, Cali A, 1996. Microsporidiosis 1996: An overview of the Tucson workshop. J. Euk. Microbiol. 43:111S–112S

Weiss LM, Zhu X, Cali A, Tanowitz HB, Wittner M, 1994. Utility of microsporidian rRNA in diagnosis and phylogeny: a review. Folia Parasitol. 41:81–90

Willson R, Harrington R, Stewart B, Fritsche T, 1995. Human immunodeficiency virus 1–associated necrotizing cholangitis caused by infection with *Septata intestinalis*. Gastroenterology 108:247–251

Wilson JM, 1986. Can *Encephalitozoon cuniculi* cross the placenta? Res. Vet. Sci. 40:138

Wolf A, Cowen D, 1937. Granulomatous encephalomyelitis due to an *Encephalitozoon* (encephalitozoic encephalomyelitis). Bull. Neurol. Inst. N.Y. 6:306–371

Yachnis AT, Bender BS, Martinez-Salazar A, Berg J, Rojiani AM, Eskin TA, Orenstein JM, 1996a. Central nervous system microsporidiosis in acquired immunodeficiency syndrome: A report of two cases. Washington, D.C.: U.S. and Canadian Academy of Pathology annual meeting. Abstracts, p. 133A

Yachnis AT, Berg J, Martinez-Salazar A, Bender BS, Diaz L, Rojiani AM, Eskin TA, Orenstein JM, 1996b. Disseminated microsporidosis especially infecting the brain, heart, and kidneys. Report of a newly recognized pansporoblastic species in two symptomatic AIDS patients. Am. J. Clin. Pathol. 106:535–543

Yee RW, Tio FO, Martinez JA, Held KS, Shadduck JA, Didier ES, 1991. Resolution of microsporidial epithelial keratopathy in a patient with AIDS. Ophthalmology 98:196–201

Zender HO, Arrigoni E, Eckert J, Kapanci Y, 1989. A case of *Encephalitozoon cuniculi* peritonitis in a patient with AIDS. Am. J. Clin. Pathol. 92:352–356

Zierdt CH, Gill VJ, Zierdt WS, 1993. Detection of microsporidian spores in clinical samples by indirect fluorescent-antibody assay using whole-cell antisera to *Encephalitozoon cuniculi* and *Encephalitozoon hellem*. J. Clin. Microbiol. 31:3071–3074

3

INTESTINAL AND UROGENITAL FLAGELLATES

The intestinal and urogenital flagellates of humans were placed in a single taxonomic group, implying a close phylogenetic relationship between the two. However, molecular biology studies indicate the opposite, and modern classifications of the flagellated protists are taking these advances into account (Corliss, 1994). The newest classification indicates that the intestinal and urogenital flagellates actually belong to two Kingdoms, as follows (see also the introduction to Part I):

Kingdom: Archezoa
  Phylum: Metamonada
    Class: Trepomonadea
      Order: Diplomonadida
        Family: Hexamitidae
          Genus: *Giardia*
      Order: Enteromonadida
        Family: Enteromonadidae
          Genus: *Enteromonas*
      Order: Retortamonadida
        Family: Retortamonadidae
          Genus: *Chilomastix, Retortamonas*

Kingdom: Protozoa
  Phylum: Parabasala
    Class: Trichomonadea
      Order: Trichomonadida
        Family: Trichomonadidae
          Genus: *Trichomonas, Pentatrichomonas, and Dientamoeba*

As this classification shows, the protist flagellates of humans are a group of species broadly characterized by having more than one flagellum, but phylogenetically they are very diverse, belonging to two Kingdoms. Only two of these flagellates are unquestionably pathogenic: *Giardia lamblia* in the small intestine and *Trichomonas vaginalis* in the urogenital tract. A third, *Dientamoeba fragilis*, occurs in the large intestine and most likely produces diarrhea, though no definitive proof of its pathogenicity is available (Millet et al. 1983; Shein, Gelb, 1983). The other five species (*Enteromonas hominis, Chilomastix mesnili, Retortamonas intestinalis, Trichomonas tenax,* and *Pentatrichomonas hominis*) exist in the intestinal lumen and the oral cavity of humans. They are commensals and together with *D. fragilis* are diagnosed in the clinical laboratory, where they are often identified in stools and other body fluids. Anatomic pathologists rarely encounter them in their practice.

The intestinal and urogenital flagellates have a worldwide distribution. Their transmission is directly from person to person, which in most species is by the transfer of a cystic stage. In other species, transmission is by the passage of trophozoites, such as in *Diantamoeba* and the trichomonadids. Infections with flagellates involve mouth-to-mouth contact, sexual contact, or fecal contamination for those species inhabiting the mouth, the genitourinary organs, or the intestine, respectively. These infections are usually found in communities and groups of people living in close contact with poor hygienic conditions, such as orphanages and institutions for the mentally retarded. Waterborne epidemics are common with *Giardia* worldwide (Dykes et al. 1980; Lopez et al. 1980), and in the male homosexual community, rates of prevalence are very high (Phillips et al. 1981).

Giardia lamblia—Giardiasis

Giardia lamblia occurs in the small intestine of humans, producing mostly asymptomatic infections and sometimes diarrhea, especially in children, less often in adults. This organism is an important producer of diarrhea in travelers. Several species of animals are naturally infected, and some are implicated as sources of epidemics (Isaac Renton et al., 1993). The parasite is a cosmopolitan organism with a worldwide distribution.

Morphology. *Giardia lamblia* has a trophozoite stage and a cystic stage in its life cycle (Fig. 3–1). Trophozoites are delicate organisms up to 21 μm long by 15 μm wide and 4 μm thick, are rounded anteriorly and pointed posteriorly, and have a symmetric internal organization (Fig. 3–1; *color plate* II *A*). The trophozoites have two nuclei anteriorly and four pairs of flagella: anterior, posterolateral, ventral, and caudal. The flagella are hard to visualize in stained preparations of stool samples and are almost never seen in tissue sections. On the ventral surface, occupying the anterior half of the body, is a suction disc used to attach the parasite to the intestinal mucosa (Figs. 3–2, 3–3 *A–B*, and 3–4). In addition, in the middle line there is a pair

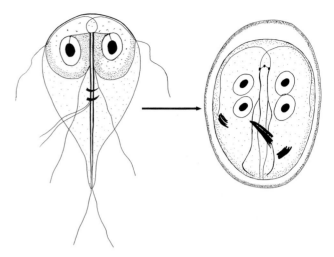

Fig. 3–1. *Giardia lamblia* **life cycle. Trophozoite and cyst.**

of axonemes (the intracytoplasmic portion of the caudal flagella), which exit the body at the posterior end, forming the caudal pair of flagella (Fig 3–3 *B*). Two claw-shaped structures, the median bodies, are easily seen crossing the axonemes at the midportion of the body. The ultrastructure of *Giardia* trophozoites reveals the presence of a Golgi apparatus and an endoplasmic reticulum, but the trophozoites lack mitochondria, peroxisomes, and glycosomes (Farthing

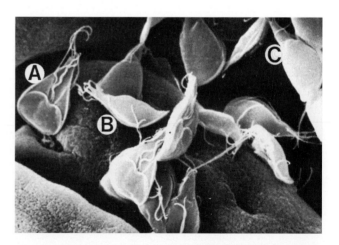

Fig. 3–2. *Giardia lamblia*, **scanning electron micrograph of trophozoites on human duodenal mucosa.** *A*, **Ventral surface of a trophozoite shows the suction disc on the anterior flagella, and the lateral and posterior flagella behind the disc.** *B*, **Lateral view of a trophozoite.** *C*, **Dorsolateral view (In: Owen, R.L. 1980. The ultrastructural basis of *Giardia* infection. Trans. R. Soc. Trop. Med. Hyg. 74:429–433. Reproduced with permission.)**

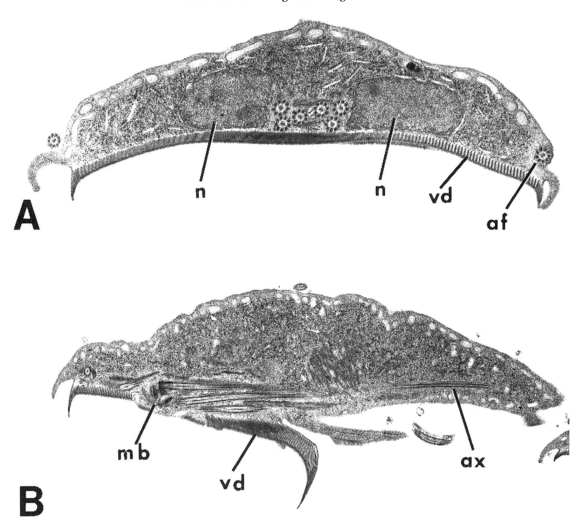

Fig. 3–3. *Giardia lamblia*, transmission electron micrographs of trophozoites. *A*, Transverse section at the level of the two nuclei, ×6,600. *B*, Longitudinal section, ×8,500. Abbreviations: af, anterior flagella; ax, axostyle; mb, medial bodies; n, nucleus; vd, ventral disc. (Courtesy of J. McMahon, Ph.D., Department of Pathology, The Cleveland Clinic Educational Foundation, Cleveland, Ohio.)

1996; Gillin et al. 1996). The interconnections of the flagella and the ultrastructural anatomy of the attachment disc are rather complex (Beaver et al. 1984); for the sake of completion, some landmarks are shown (Fig. 3–3 *A–B*).

The mature cysts are 8 to 12 × 7 to 10 μm, are ovoid with a delicate wall, and have four nuclei similar to those of the trophozoite, plus other organelles and axonemes (*color plate* II *B–D*). Cysts formed in the gastrointestinal tract are evacuated with the feces into the environment and eventually may gain access to a new host with contaminated water or food. In the environment, cysts survive outside the body for about 2 months at 4°C and for 4 days at 37°C.

Life Cycle. Once ingested cysts commence excystation, which in in vitro experiments occurs within 5 to 10 minutes. A break appears at one end of the cyst and flagella appear, moving actively, followed by the posterior end of the parasite, which begins cell division that is completed in about 30 minutes, producing two new individuals (Buchel et al. 1987). Trophozoites must attach immediately to the cell surface (brush border) by their attachment disc, but how attachment occurs is not known. Trophozoites move down in the intestine and secrete a cyst wall, a process completed in 40 to 70 hours. Immature cysts have two nuclei; mature ones have four nuclei and an extra attachment disc so that when they are ingested by a new host, they are ready to divide.

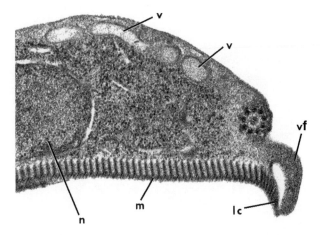

Fig. 3–4. *Giardia lamblia*, **transmission electron micrograph showing the detail of the suction disc. Abbreviations: lc, lateral crest or projecting rim; m, microtubule; n, nucleus; v, vacuole; vf, ventrolateral flange, ×12,230 (Courtesy of J. McMahon, Ph.D., Department of Pathology, The Cleveland Clinic Educational Foundation, Cleveland, Ohio.)**

Epidemiology. *Giardia lamblia* is a cosmopolitan flagellate, mostly of tropical areas where rates of infection are extremely variable in accordance with the population under study. *Giardia* also occurs in temperate zones (Brodsky et al. 1974) and is the only intestinal protozoon among Eskimos of the Canadian Arctic (Cameron, Choquette, 1963). In some populations, prevalence rates of 45% are common (Chunge et al. 1991), and even higher rates are found in children; malnourished children in Bangladesh had a 51% prevalence rate (Gilman et al. 1985). In the United States, *Giardia* is the most commonly diagnosed parasite in the clinical laboratory, and its prevalence is increasing. The parasite was diagnosed in 4% of stool samples across the country in 1976, in 6% in 1981, and in 7% in 1987 (Kappus et al. 1994). Giardiasis in children attending day-care centers is an important problem and one that is growing (Thompson, 1994) in both developed and developing countries. In Brazil, the prevalence in some day-care centers is up to 70% (Guimaraes, Sogayar, 1995). In the male homosexual community the prevalence of *Giardia* and other intestinal protozoa is very high; in a survey in Chicago, 43% of gay males studied were positive for protozoa and 8% had *Giardia* (Peters et al. 1986). In temperate zones, the prevalence in children may be seasonal, with higher rates in the autumn (Rodriguez Hernandez et al. 1996). Many waterborne epidemics due to contaminated drinking water systems also have been reported (Craun, 1979; Kent et al. 1988; Lippy, 1979; Moorehead et al. 1990).

Most of these epidemics are due to the lack of filtration of surface water, the best method for removal of cysts; chlorination alone, in the concentrations recommended for water treatment, does not inactivate the cysts. Under experimental conditions, *Giardia* produced infection in all volunteers ingesting 10 cysts (Rendtorff, 1954). This remarkable rate of infectivity explains why epidemics occur even when only a few cysts are isolated from drinking water. The epidemiologic connection between domestic and wild animals infected with *G. lamblia*, and transmission to humans, was widely believed without convincing evidence. Only recently, have studies addressed this connection in depth. In one report, the transmission from wild animals to humans was proven, based on zymodeme patterns of isolates from humans and animals, during a waterborne outbreak in Canada (Isaac Renton et al. 1993). Another study of transmission of *Giardia* from dogs to humans living together, using the polymerase chain reaction to characterize isolates from both, revealed that the isolates from humans were different from those from dogs. This finding indicates that little or no transmission occurred between dogs and humans (Hopkins et al. 1997).

Pathogenesis. The mechanism by which *Giardia* causes diarrhea and malabsorption in humans is not known. Damage to the brush border and atrophy of the villi likely play a role in the production of diarrhea, but diarrhea also occurs in the absence of brush border and villous alterations, indicating that production of diarrhea must be multifactorial. Marked damage of the villi of the jejunum is often seen in the absence of diarrhea, similar to the condition in celiac disease. In mice with *Giardia*, damage of the brush border results in deficiency of the brush border enzymes, a condition that returns to normal once the infection has been cleared (Buret et al. 1990; Buret et al. 1991). In addition, some patients with selective immunoglobulin A (IgA) deficiency or any other type of hypogammaglobulinemia suffer giardiasis with severe malabsorption symptoms (Ament, Rubin, 1972; Hermans et al. 1966; Hoskins et al. 1967). The role of IgA deficiency in the predisposition to severe giardiasis is controversial because about 10% of the general population have IgA deficiency. Nevertheless, malabsorption does not occur in 10% of cases of giardiasis. Several factors within the mucosa and within the intestinal lumen are proposed as the possible causes for the symptoms produced by *Giardia*. Factors in the mucosa are ultrastructural damage of the villi, reduction of villous height, reduced disaccharidase activity, mucosal inflammation, and immature villous enterocytes due to rapid turnover of ep-ithelial cells. Factors in the lumen are bacterial over-growth, uptake of bile salts by the parasite, and inhi-bition of host hydrolytic enzymes. The role of some of these factors has been tested, with contradictory results; other factors are known to produce diarrhea in infec-tions with agents other than *Giardia*, but their role in *Giardia* infections is untested. Uptake of bile salts by the parasite has been shown in vitro to stimulate growth and encystation of the parasite, but whether this has an effect on the host remains speculative (Far-thing, 1996).

Clinical Findings. The clinical presentation of giar-diasis varies with the host's age, immunologic status, and previous exposure to the parasite. In endemic ar-eas, *Giardia* usually produces symptoms in childhood (Jove et al. 1983; Mason, Patterson, 1987) but rarely in adults, indicating that early exposure confers some protection against the disease. In developed countries, giardiasis occurs in both children and adults, but most cases are found in adults because lack of exposure in childhood results in a large susceptible adult popula-tion.

The incubation period of giardiasis is 12 to 15 days. The acute symptoms are nausea, anorexia, epi-gastric fullness, and malaise, usually followed by sud-den onset of explosive, foul-smelling, watery diarrhea that changes in a few days to bulky, semisolid stools. Abdominal distention associated with increased foul flatulence, foul belching, and epigastric cramps are observed. The acute symptoms usually last for only a few days and may mimic acute viral enteritis, bac-terial enteritis, or other forms of food poisoning en-teritis. Some individuals have mild to moderate weight loss, sometimes up to 30 pounds in cases with malabsorption (Hoskins et al. 1967). Radiographic films of the upper gastrointestinal tract may show changes typical of a duodeno-jejunitis (Fig. 3–5 *A–B*). Chronic infections are characterized by continuous or recurrent, mild to moderate gastrointestinal symp-toms with intestinal cramping, bloating, and bulky stools with fat and undigested food, indicating ab-sorptive alterations of the small intestine (Ament et al. 1973; Wolfe, 1984). Individuals with immune de-ficiency syndromes usually have a more chronic course and develop malabsorption; therefore, all per-sons with chronic giardiasis and malabsorption should be studied to ascertain whether an immune deficiency exists. In a subclinical infection in a 17-year-old male, the presentation was a deficiency of vitamin B_{12} (Springer, Key, 1997). One patient was found to have marked impairment of pancreatic func-tion, which reversed after specific treatment (Carroc-cio et al. 1997). Another patient with a congenital immune deficiency, had a severe hypokalemic my-opathy (Pastorek et al. 1996).

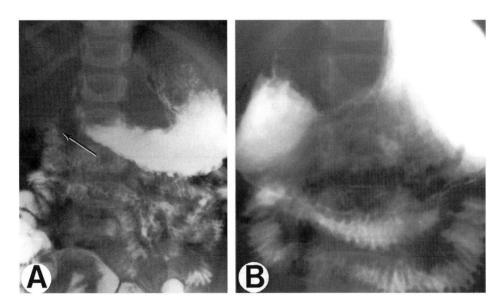

Fig. 3–5. *Giardia lamblia* **enteritis, roentgenogram of the small intestine.** *A,* **Duode-num. Note the characteristic accentuation of the mucosal folds (arrow).** *B,* **Jejunum shows similar mucosal folds. (Courtesy of S. Morrison, M.D., Department of Radiol-ogy, University Hospitals of Cleveland, Cleveland, Ohio.)**

Immunity. It has been known for many years that *Giardia* produces immunity to the disease, which allows spontaneous resolution and reinfection without symptoms. It is also known that the disease occurs mostly in infants and children, the susceptible population in endemic areas, and in those with some forms of immune suppression such as agamma- and hypogammaglobulinemia. This last observation suggests that antibodies play an important role in the defense mechanisms against the parasite.

Since *Giardia* is an intestinal dweller that does not invade the mucosa, it appears that primary stimulation of the immune system occurs at the mucosal surface, mediated by the trophozoites in close contact with the brush border. The role of the cysts is likely minimal because they are formed in the intestinal lumen and are rapidly evacuated with the intestinal contents. The immune response to *Giardia* is then modulated by the lymphoid tissue in the intestinal wall and is closely associated with the type of immune response that this tissue produces, mainly humoral. Cell-mediated responses are also produced by the lymphoid tissues of the intestinal mucosa, but to a much smaller extent (Faubert, 1996). Most studies evaluating the role of antibodies in conferring protection against *Giardia* have been carried out in animal models and in in vitro systems, showing that specific antibodies and complement are capable of lysing the trophozoites. A study of humans demonstrated that in symptomatic and asymptomatic infections, IgE antibodies increase. Moreover, the IgE levels decrease or become normal after eradication of the parasite (Perez et al. 1994). This finding would explain some of the allergic manifestations described in *Giardia* infections. Two other antibody classes, IgA and IgG, were also found to be significantly elevated in infected patients, and titers of IgA were higher in the asymptomatic patients than in the symptomatic ones (Perez et al. 1994).

The cell-mediated immunity to *Giardia* has been studied in mice infected with *G. muris*, with the demonstration that T cells are important in the immune response to the parasite. The CD8$^+$ T cells are increased in infected mice, mainly in the lamina propria and mucosa. As the infection in animals declines, the CD8$^+$ T cells decrease and the CD4$^+$ T cells increase. However, in humans, severe cases of giardiasis invariably occur in those with B-cell defects. Other observations in in vitro systems are more difficult to extrapolate to humans with a natural infection. For example, it has been shown that macrophages from the intestinal Peyer's patches of infected animals, in the presence of specific antibodies, ingest *Giardia* trophozoites in larger numbers. The parasites are killed by the oxidative burst, but whether macrophages also ingest trophozoites in the surface of the intestine is not known.

Pathology. *Giardia* is commonly identified in sections of duodenum and, less frequently, in sections of jejunum (Blenkinsopp et al. 1978; Kociecka et al. 1984; Rosekrans et al. 1981), ileum (Gunasekaran, Hassall, 1996; Oberhuber, Stolte, 1995), and stomach (Quincey et al. 1992). In all these instances, the most common histologic feature of giardiasis is the presence of parasites in scanty, moderate, or large numbers within the crypts and on the surface of the villi (Fig. 3–6 *A–D*). It is generally accepted that *Giardia* does not invade the intestinal mucosa, but studies with light and electron microscopy and with immunoperoxidase stain (Fleck et al. 1985) still report the presence of *Giardia* trophozoites in tissues. In histologic preparations, the parasites are usually detached from the enterocytes, an artifact due to fixation and processing.

The histologic changes of the small intestinal mucosa in giardiasis are variable and do not correlate with the presence or absence of symptoms, the degree of disease, or the number of parasites present (Gillon, Ferguson 1984; Jove et al. 1983; Judd et al. 1983; Oberhuber, Stolte, 1990). Studies of small intestinal biopsy specimens from older children and adults with giardiasis living in hyperendemic areas show a normal mucosa (Fig. 3–6 *A–C*) in spite of the presence of other small intestinal parasitic infections in the majority of cases (Rodriguez Da Silva et al. 1964) or minor nonspecific morphologic changes that persist even after treatment (Jove et al. 1983). In nonendemic areas, studies of adults with symptomatic giardiasis reveal a normal or near-normal mucosa in some patients (Oberhuber, Stolte, 1990). Villous flattening was present in 41% of patients versus 37.5% of subjects, control with intraepithelial lymphocytic infiltrates being similar in both groups (Oberhuber, Stolte, 1990). The changes described are loss of the brush border, damage of epithelial cells, slight flattening of the villi (Fig. 3–7 *A–C*), increased mitotic index and goblet cells, infiltration by polymorphonuclear and mononuclear cells (Fig. 3–7 *C–D*), and absence or diminution of plasma cells in the lamina propria (Ament et al. 1973; Yardley et al. 1964). These histologic changes usually revert to normal in follow-up biopsy specimens after treatment (Ament, Rubin, 1972). In at least one patient, total villus atrophy in the absence of celiac sprue or gastrointestinal immune deficiency syndrome was observed, which reverted to normal after specific treatment (Levinson, Nastro, 1978). The advanced histologic changes seen in some patients with giardiasis resemble those seen in patients with celiac sprue.

An association between bacterial and parasitic infections such as *Giardia* and intestinal nodular lymphoid hyperplasia (Fig. 3–8 *A–B*) is known in individuals with normal immunoglobulin levels (Ward et

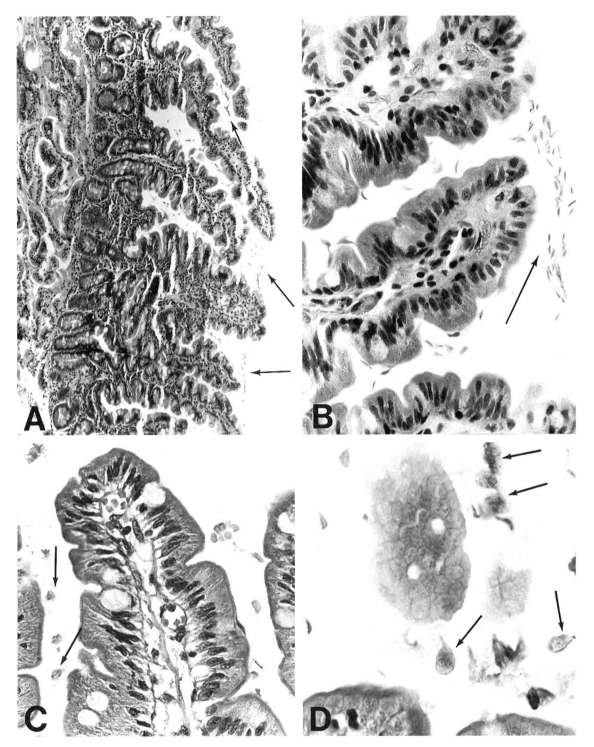

Fig. 3–6. *Giardia lamblia* in a biopsy specimen of duodenum, hematoxylin and eosin stain. *A*, Low-power magnification showing normal villi; note the faint masses of parasite in the lumen (arrows), ×77. *B*, Higher magnification of the same biopsy specimen showing a scanty mononuclear cell infiltrate of the lamina propria and the parasites in the lumen (arrow), ×391. *C*, Another biopsy specimen shows similar features, ×383. *D*, Higher magnification illustrating diagnostic features of the flagellates, sectioned on different planes (arrows), ×600.

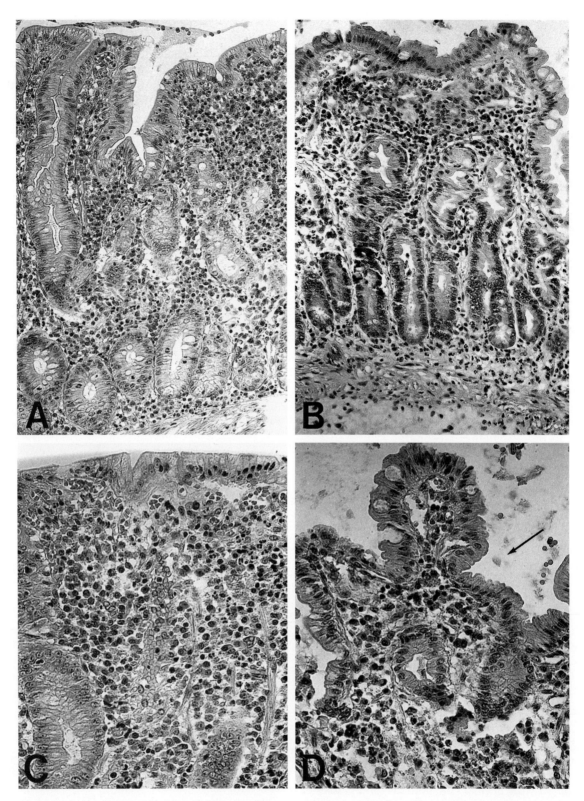

Fig. 3–7. *Giardia lamblia* infection and malabsorption syndrome, duodenal biopsy specimen stained with hematoxylin and eosin stain. *A* and *B*, Low-power view of villi shows flattening and loss of the normal architecture. Note the inflammatory reaction through the thickness of the mucosa, ×180. *C* and *D*, Higher magnification showing the infiltrate, composed mostly of mononuclear cells (plasma and plasmacytoid cells) and a few polymorphonuclear cells. Note the small number of parasites (arrow), ×280. (Preparation courtesy of R.E. Petras, M.D., Department of Pathology, The Cleveland Clinic Foundation, Cleveland, Ohio.)

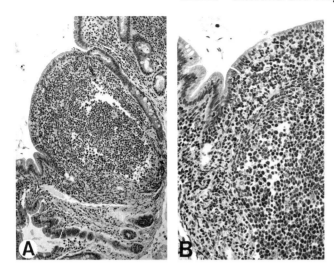

Fig. 3–8. *Giardia lamblia* **and lymphoid nodular hyperplasia, section of duodenal biopsy specimen stained with hematoxylin and eosin stain.** *A,* **Note the lymphoid follicle in the submucosa,** ×76. *B,* **Higher magnification shows detail of the follicle,** ×154.

al. 1983) or with late-onset antibody deficiencies (Ament, 1975). The nature of this association in giardiasis is not well understood (Case Records of the Massachusetts General Hospital, 1997), but a cause–effect relationship has been suggested based on the fact that in individuals without antibody deficiencies, the hyperplasia reversed to normal after treatment (Ward et al. 1983).

Diagnosis. The diagnosis of giardiasis is often made on clinical grounds but requires confirmation by demonstration of the parasite in stools, duodenal aspirates, or small intestinal biopsy specimens (Fig. 3–6 A–D; Isaac Renton, 1991). The method of choice, because of its convenience and low cost, is still the direct examination of fresh or stained smears of fresh or fixed stool samples in the clinical laboratory (Isaac Renton, 1991; Rodriguez Da Silva et al. 1964). It is the general rule that examination of three stool samples collected at 2- to 3-day intervals will detect nearly 100% of infections (Hill, 1993). The low positivity rates sometimes reported for recovery of *Giardia* are usually the result of studies of a single stool sample, poor methodology, or incompetence at the microscope. Elimination of *Giardia* cysts in the stools is somewhat cyclical, with periods of daily positive stools alternating with periods of daily negative stools (Hill, 1993; Rendtorff, 1954). In addition, other data indicate that some individuals continuously excrete large numbers of organisms, oth-

ers only a few (Danciger, Lopez, 1975). If giardiasis is suspected, one stool specimen should be ordered; if it is negative, a second one should follow; and if that is negative, a third. If all three specimens are negative and the patient is not hurt, the collection of a fourth specimen at 7- to 10-day intervals is desirable. A great deal of data on the diagnosis of giardiasis have accumulated in the last ten years, using several technologies. Contradictory rates of recovery of parasites have been reported, making the field very confusing. For example, in one report, imprints of duodenal aspirates were positive in 100% of instances, followed by examination of sections of biopsy specimens and, last, by the stool examination (Kamath, Murugasu 1974). By contrast, another study found that duodenal aspirates are inferior to stool examination for diagnosis of giardiasis (Suzuki et al. 1994). One should always keep in mind that duodenal aspiration and biopsy are costly, invasive techniques, in contrast to the collection of a stool sample. Trophozoites are present in duodenal samples or in loose or liquid stools, and cysts are found in formed stools. Finally, in at least one case, the trophozoites were present in a brush cytology specimen of the stomach (Munoz et al. 1996).

Other sophisticated technologies available for the diagnosis of infectious agents are also applicable for the diagnosis of giardiasis in the clinical laboratory. The basis for these techniques is the detection of parasite antigens in the stools, detection of specific antibodies in stools and serum, and immune staining of parasites in biopsy specimens or stool samples. The enzyme-linked immunosorbent assay seems to be the preferred test for detection of antigen in stools (Hopkins et al. 1993), with data indicating that its cost is comparable to the cost of direct fecal examination (Aldeen et al. 1995). Counterimmunoelectrophoresis of stools for detection of *G. lamblia* antigen, with a sensitivity equal to that of the combined examination of duodenal aspirates and stools, has been described (Craft, Nelson, 1982). A direct immunofluorescence monoclonal antibody test is available for the detection of both *Giardia* and *Cryptosporidium* in stool samples, and in one study it was found to be superior to the direct stool examination (Alles et al. 1995).

In spite of much progress, immune diagnostic techniques are far from routine in the clinical laboratory. Direct microscopy of stool samples is still the gold standard, and in good hands it should detect all cases of giardiasis. When a stool sample is examined, a search for all kinds of parasites is undertaken (not just for one, as serologic tests do). Data on the character of the stool sample, as well as the presence of red blood cells, polymorphonuclear neutrophils, and eosinophils, are collected and reported. A patient with diarrhea returning from an overseas trip may have giardiasis. Direct stool examination may reveal *Giardia*, as suspected by the physician, but it may also show *Cryptosporidium, Enterocytozoon, Clyclospora, Entamoeba histolytica, Aonchoteca philippinensis* (= *Capillaria philippinensis*), and other parasites. These parasites are missed if only antigen or antibody detection techniques for *Giardia* are used. Diarrhea is nonspecific enough to render useless the tests that search for a single pathogen. Immune diagnosis for giardiasis is a useful epidemiologic tool because it is effective in determining rates of prevalence. It is usable during a documented outbreak or epidemic that requires investigation of large numbers of suspected contacts or people at risk in a given community (Aretio et al. 1994) or for testing cures in patients after treatment.

In sections of biopsy specimens, usually taken for reasons other than the diagnosis of giardiasis, the parasites are seen in the crypts and on the surface of the mucosa (Fig. 3–6 *A–D*), showing a variable configuration depending on the plane of sectioning. Only the trophozoites are found. They do not appear as they do in the stools unless a full coronal section of the trophozoite is obtained, usually showing the two nuclei, other organelles, and, rarely, parts of the flagella (Fig. 3–6 *D*). In longitudinal sections the organisms are elongated and slender (Fig. 3–6 *B*), sometimes showing the axonemes of the caudal flagella; in transverse sections they are concave, and the attachment disk may be visible. The important criteria for the identification of the parasites are the recognition of these different shapes and the *presence of organelles*; strands of mucus and other debris are sometimes mistakenly identified as *Giardia*. Special stains are not necessary, but Giemsa stain is better for highlighting the internal structures.

Trichomonas—T. vaginalis and Trichomoniasis

Trichomonas and *Pentatrichomonas* are two genera of the order Trichomonadida (see the introduction to Part I and above), and together they have three species that occur in humans. *Trichomonas tenax* occurs in the oral cavity, in the tartar around the teeth, and is not usually present in the mouths of persons with good oral hygiene. *Trichomonas vaginalis* occurs in the urogenital tract of men and women and *Pentatrichomonas hominis* (= *T. hominis*) in the colon. Several species of *Trichomonas* occur in many animals, including monkeys, birds, and termites. The only species clearly associated with disease in humans is *T. vaginalis*.

Morphology. The trophozoites of *T. vaginalis* are round to oval, sometimes elongated. They have a cytostome (mouth) at the apical end, a single nucleus, three to five flagella on the anterior body, and one posterior flagellum forming the undulating membrane (Figs. 3–9 *A–B*). The undulating membrane has, in addition, a costa (a ribbon-like supporting structure at the base of the undulating membrane). An axostyle (a thick, prominent, rod-like supporting organelle) traverses the body from the anterior to the posterior pole, where it pierces the membrane and protrudes from the body (Fig. 3–9 *A*). The nucleus has uniformly distributed chromatin, and the cytoplasm contains numerous large, siderophilic granules often distributed in larger numbers around the costa and the axostyle (Fig. 3–10). *Trichomonas vaginalis* is morphologically similar to *T. tenax*, except for its larger size (7 to 23 μm, average about 13 μm, vs. 5 to 12 μm, average 7 μm for *T. tenax*) and a shorter undulating membrane. Both species have four flagella on the anterior end. *Pentatrichomonas hominis* has five flagella. In electron micrographs, the organization of the flagella is similar to that of the flagella of other animals. The axostyle is made of a folded membrane with transverse striations, unfolding slightly in the apical aspect, near the nucleus, but more tightly folded at the posterior tip. The costa appears as a ribbon, comb-like structure with clear and dark areas, connected to the undulating membrane by minute fibrils; the posterior flagellum supports the undulating membrane. The cytoplasm has a Golgi apparatus in the form of a parabasal body located next to the nucleus; mitochondria are lacking (Jirovec, Petru, 1968).

Life Cycle. The life cycle of trichomonadids is direct, without a cystic stage; the parasites divide by longitudinal binary fission. Rounded, aflagellar forms of *Trichomonas* are seen in vaginal secretions, in cultures of the parasite (Abonyi, 1995), and more often in secretions of infected males (Jirovec, Petru, 1968). The significance of these forms, which lack a wall, and the role they play in transmission are unknown. Whether they are degenerating parasites is not clearly established. *Trichomonas vaginalis* inhabits the lumen of the vagina, the urethra, and the prostate gland without invading tissues. The duration of the infection in women is about 2 years in prisoners without heterosexual contacts, though other means of transmission have not been

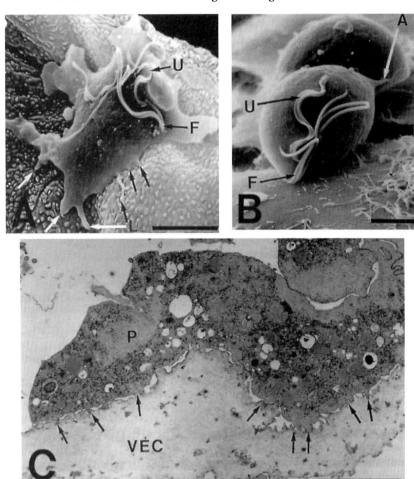

Fig. 3–9. *Trichomonas vaginalis* **and its relationship to cell surfaces shown in electron micrographs.** *A*, *Trichomonas* **trophozoite recently bound to a monolayer culture of HeLa cells shows the typical globose morphology.** *B*, **In contact to vaginal epithelial cells, the parasite transforms rapidly to a "fried egg" appearance, with multiple points of contact to the cell (arrows) and thin lamellopodia.** *C*, **Transmission electron micrograph shows the numerous cytoplasmic projections interdigitating with the epithelial cell surface membrane (arrows). Abbreviations: A, axostyle; F, the four flagella; L, lamellopodia; P, parasite; U, the undulating membrane; VEC, vaginal epithelial cell. Bars = 5 μm. (In: Arroyo R, Gonzales-Robles A, Martinez-Palomo A, et al. 1993. Signaling of** *Trichomonas vaginalis* **for amoeboid transformation and adhesion synthesis follows cytoadherence. Mol. Microbiol. 7:299–309. Reproduced with permission.)**

ruled out. The optimal environment for growth and maintenance of *T. vaginalis* is slightly acid; in general, at a pH below 5.0 or above 7.55 the parasite stops growing (Trussell, 1947). The number of parasites in the vagina of infected women varies with the menstrual cycle phase, being highest in the late luteal and early strogenic phases and lowest toward the end of the cycle and during menstruation (Demes et al. 1988). In menopausal women, the number of parasites is very variable. The parasites survive in the urethra of women and can remain alive for several hours in urine.

Epidemiology. The distribution of *T. vaginalis* is worldwide, and its prevalence varies with the group under study, the geographic location, age, race, number of sexual partners (Zhang, 1996), and other factors (Burch et al. 1959; Cotch et al. 1991). In gen-

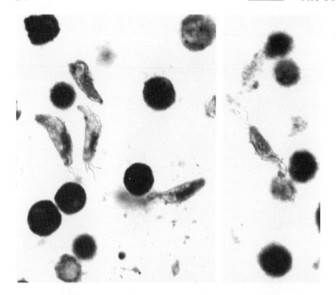

Fig. 3–10. *Trichomonas vaginalis* **in vaginal smear stained with iron-hematoxylin, ×1,342.**

eral, the prevalence is higher in black women (Burch et al. 1959; Cotch et al. 1991; Short et al. 1984) and in prostitutes. In human immune deficiency virus (HIV)-positive women attending a gynecologic clinic in Burkina Faso (Africa), the prevalence was 28% (Meda et al. 1995). In a similar study of HIV-positive women in Los Angeles, the rate of infection was about 17% (Sorvillo et al. 1998). The importance of trichomoniasis in HIV-positive women lies in the possibility that these women are better transmitters and receptor of the virus. The epithelial damage to the cervix and the vagina would allow easier passage of the virus into the vagina for transmission; it would also produce a port of entry for infection. A large study of pregnant women in the United States found that about 13% were infected (Cotch et al. 1991). Rates of prevalence for the general population are not available because no study based on a random sample of women in a given population has been carried out. All studies focus on selective groups, always women or men seeking medical treatment. It is stated that the prevalence of vaginal trichomoniasis in the United States and Scandinavia has declined in part due to the use of metranidozole for therapy (Kent, 1991). The presence of *Trichomonas* in female neonates has been recognized, especially during the first few weeks, acquired in utero from an infected mother; the influence of maternal estrogens makes the vagina of the infant appropriate to sustain the infection (Al-Salihi et al. 1974; Danesh et al. 1995; Trussell, 1947). Trichomoniasis and other sexually transmitted diseases found in very young and adolescent girls should raise the suspicion of sexual abuse (Argent et al. 1995; Robinson, Ridgway, 1994; Siegel et al. 1995), with the caution that methods of transmission other than sexual contact are possible.

The transmission of *T. vaginalis* from host to host is by sexual contact, by fomites, or during delivery. Trichomoniasis is the most common sexually transmitted disease in the developed world and possible worldwide. Transmission to young girls without sexual contact has occasionally been documented: three small children were found to be infected in a family where the mother was also infected and no history of sexual abuse could be elicited (Adu Sarkodie, 1995). Transmission in swimming pools and baths is controversial; however, under experimental conditions, the parasite survived for up to 3 hours in mineral baths (Krieger, Kimmig, 1995). The transmission of *T. tenax* is by mouth-to-mouth contact, saliva droplets, or contaminated dishes and drinking utensils, permitting the passage of trophozoites from person to person. The mode of transmission of *T. hominis* is not clearly established, but it is believed to be by fecal contamination.

Pathogenesis. The concepts of pathogenicity of *T. vaginalis* have changed considerably in recent years as a result of the many studies of its molecular biology (Alderete et al. 1995b). The pathogenic effect of the parasite varies from isolate to isolate: parasites from women with severe cervical abnormalities produced more abscesses when inoculated into experimental mice than those from women with less severe cervical abnormalities (Honigberg et al. 1984). It has also been shown that *Trichomonas* must attach to the epithelial cells of the vagina and cervix (cytoadhesion), and that cytoadhesion is followed by signals to the parasite to change its morphologic appearance (Arroyo et al. 1993). Within 5 minutes after *T. vaginalis* is placed in contact with epithelial cells, it changes from a globose (Fig. 3–9 *A*) to a flattened, ameboid (fried egg) stage (Fig. 3–9 *B*) that begins to attach to the cell by making contact with sites opposite to that of the undulating membrane. In transmission electron micrographs, the parasite shows numerous projections that interdigitate with the microvilli of the vaginal epithelial cells (Fig. 3–9 *C*; Arroyo et al. 1993). The mechanism of cytoadhesion of *T. vaginalis* to cells and surfaces is the subject of numerous in vitro studies (Alderete et al. 1995a). These studies have shown that cytoadhesion is mediated by parasite surface proteins (adhesins) to specific cell surface molecules (receptors) and that the adhesins play a role in the parasite's pathogenicity (Arroyo, Alderete, 1995a). Cytoadhesion is mediated by four specific proteins, and their encoding genes have been characterized (Alderete et al. 1995b; Arroyo et al. 1995b): two of these proteins have been found to be related to cytoadhesion with cytotoxicity in culture cells and the other two to cytoadhesion without cytotoxicity (Arroyo, Alderete, 1995a). Damage of epithelial cells by *T. vaginalis* may also be mediated by the acidic condition created by products resulting from the glycolytic pathway of the parasite (Graves, Gardner, 1993), indicating that the pathogenic effect may be multifactorial. The mechanism of cell damage by the parasite has not been elucidated. Cytoadhesion has not been observed in *T. tenax*, indicating that it is probably an adaptation to the vagina, a constantly changing environment due to the menstrual cycle.

The association between *Trichomonas* infection and complications during pregnancy has been studied, but the results are at best contradictory (Gibbs et al. 1992). One study showed a significant association between *T. vaginalis* infections in pregnant adolescents and the prevalence of low gestational age and birth weight (Hardy et al. 1984). Another study showed a premature rupture of membranes at term (Minkoff et al. 1984). In a larger study, the effect of *Trichomonas* infections on the outcome of pregnancy and its complications could not be fully determined because the factors predisposing to the infection are the same factors associated with adverse pregnancy outcomes (Cotch et al. 1991). The prevalence of trichomoniasis appears to be similar in pregnant and nonpregnant women (Levett, 1995).

Clinical Findings

Females. It is estimated that in general gynecologic practice, between 2% and 3% of healthy women have *Trichomonas* in their vagina; about 50% of this group are asymptomatic (Weinberger, Harger, 1993). Symptoms appear 4 to 28 days after infection and vary from mild to marked acute or chronic vaginitis, sometimes accompanied by vulvitis, which is characterized by erythema often extending down to the inguinal area. The infection is rare in prepuberal girls because the parasite apparently requires an estrogenized epithelium for its survival (Jirovec, Petru, 1968). The main complaint is a greenish, frothy, purulent vaginal discharge, sometimes abundant, accompanied by pruritus and dysuria. These symptoms are characteristic and are usually sufficient for a clinical diagnosis (Wolner Hanssen et al. 1989). Some women have a burning sensation and a feeling of fullness or weight in the pelvis; in others, the only presenting symptom is dysuria. The diagnosis of asymptomatic women without gross abnormalities of the vagina and cervix is often made on routine Papanicolaou smears. The symptoms are usually more pronounced after menstruation, when the number of parasites is highest (Trussell, 1947).

Males. The information on trichomoniasis in males has increased lately because more attention has been devoted to this infection. In the past, the role of *T. vaginalis* as a cause of urethritis in males was controversial, and the predominant belief was that men were mostly asymptomatic carriers, serving as transmitters of the infection to women. A recent well-controlled study defined a more positive role for *T. vaginalis* as the cause of disease in males (Krieger et al. 1993a). The overall prevalence of trichomoniasis in males is unknown. In one study of urethritis in 219 males with and without a discharge, the prevalence of *Trichomonas* was 1% (Janier et al. 1995); in another study of 504 men with a urethral discharge, the rate was 6% (Jackson et al. 1997); and among 147 male partners of women with trichomoniasis, it was 22% (Krieger et al. 1993a). These percentages would be higher if sophisticated techniques such as polymerase chain reaction were used to study men with no pathogens identified by conventional means (Krieger et al. 1996).

The most common complaint is a urethral discharge followed by dysuria, genital or perineal pain, and other symptoms; some patients are asymptomatic (Krieger et al. 1993a). The urethral discharge in male trichomoniasis is usually scanty and clear, resembling that of *Chlamydia trachomatis*, in contrast to the discharge of gonococcal urethritis, which is abundant and purulent (Krieger, 1995; Krieger et al. 1993a). The natural history of the infection in untreated men is resolution in about 33% of cases; some men remain positive and asymptomatic for longer periods (Krieger et al. 1993b). There are rare instances of reports of *T. vaginalis* in histologic sections of patients with prostatitis (Gardner et al. 1986). In another study it was found that a urethral discharge in a male lasting for 4 or more weeks was due to *Trichomonas* because less than 2% of other cases of nongonococcal urethritis last this long (Latif et al. 1987). Examination of the fluid reveals parasites among clumps of epithelial cells and a few polymorphonuclear leukocytes; urinary sediments are also positive. Concurrent infection with *Trichomonas* and *Gonococcus* has not been observed (Latif et al. 1987). In infected men, the parasites are recoverable from urethral discharge, urine, semen, and prepuce.

Infections of the preputial sac producing marked balanitis have been reported, as well as a case of perianal ulcerations from which *T. vaginalis* was cultured (el Sayed, Bazex, 1993). In this instance, the parasite was isolated in culture but was not illustrated or described; the identification was circumstantial, based on infection of the wife. After specific treatment, the patient improved clinically (el Sayed, Bazex, 1993). Cases of urethritis and abscesses in the median raphe of the penis, presenting as a spindle-shaped swelling with a small opening distal to the swelling, are known (Soendjojo, Pindha, 1981; Sowmini et al. 1972); another patient without a coexistent urethritis recovered with specific therapy (Pavithran, 1993).

Immunity. Little is known about the immunologic aspects of *Trichomonas* infections in humans; both cellular and humoral responses have been detected in natural infections, but whether there is protective immunity is not known. Antibodies against *T. vaginalis* found in vaginal secretions and in mucus are against the immunogenic surface proteins of the parasite (Alderete et al. 1991a). An IgG antibody response was present at similar levels, and sometimes at higher levels, in the same women 4 weeks after treatment (Alderete et al. 1991a). Antibodies against *T. vaginalis* were also present in the sera of infected women (Alderete et al. 1991b; Bozner et al. 1992). Patients with cervical neoplasia have a considerably higher prevalence of specific antibodies against *T. vaginalis* in their sera (41% vs. 5% in control subjects). It is suggested that this higher prevalence is due to a possible association between the tumor and the infection (Yap et al. 1995) (see below).

Pathology. No descriptions of prostatic or urethral tissues of men infected with *Trichomonas* are available. Therefore, the following discussion is limited to women. Women with *Trichomonas* vaginitis have a hyperemic and edematous vagina, with minute petechiae and hemorrhages (strawberry cervix). In more advanced cases, there is usually desquamation of the superficial epithelium with granular areas and a frothy, sometimes abundant, discharge. An erythematous reaction may cover the introitus and parts of the vulvar region.

The histologic changes in the vagina and cervix vary from normal to markedly acute, nonspecific inflammation of the mucosa and submucosa (Kessel, Gafford 1935). The surface epithelium is usually covered with coagulated material, mucus, erythrocytes, and white blood cells where the flagellates can be iden-

tified. Focal erosion of the mucosa, usually progressing to necrosis and hemorrhage, with loss of the surface epithelium (Fig. 3–11 *A–B*), and parasites between desquamated cells are commonly seen. Polymorphonuclear leukocytes, lymphocytes, and plasma cells in the epithelial and submucosal layers are often abundant (Fig. 3–11 *B*), but parasites are not seen in the tissues and rarely on the surface. Chronic infection by *Trichomonas* can result in atypia of the squamous mucosa beyond that attributed to inflammation, and the development of cervical neoplasia due to these changes has been postulated several times in the past, without a definitive conclusion about the cause–effect relationship (Ng et al. 1981; Patten, 1978). However, the question has been revived recently in China, using statistical analysis of data collected on nearly 17,000 women followed for 12 years. The conclusion derived from these studies was that an association between *T. vaginalis* infection and the risk of cervical neoplasia is likely, but that the overall increase in cervical carcinomas due to the infection is only about 4% to 5% (Zhang et al. 1995).

Trichomonas outside the urogenital tract, especially in the respiratory tract, is well known. In these cases, infection was ascribed to *T. tenax*, mostly on the basis of circumstantial evidence; only once were the parasites properly identified (Soendjojo, Pindha, 1981). Since the parasite was usually not illustrated and the specific characteristics that allowed its identification as *T. tenax* were not described, the validity of these reports remains doubtful. If the patient is an adult, the parasite is usually referred to as *T. tenax* and is considered a contaminant from the oral cavity, for example, in many cases of pneumonia, lung abscess, bronchiectasis, carcinoma, and other conditions, reviewed by Hersh (1985), or in pleural effusions (Memik, 1968; Ohkura et al. 1985; Radosavljevic Asic et al. 1994) and empyema (Miller et al. 1982; Walzer et al. 1978). One case of mixed bacterial and *Trichomonas* meningitis with repeated recovery of the parasite from the spinal fluid is known (Masur et al. 1976); one case of salivary gland infection was reported recently (Duboucher et al. 1995). In addition, *T. vaginalis* was identified based on specific characteristics on electron micrographs of a pseudodiverticulum of the esophagus producing a stricture (Guccion, Ortega, 1996). If the respiratory tract of an infant is affected, the parasite is called *T. vaginalis* and the idea that it was acquired in the vagina during birth is a forgone conclusion (Hiemstra et al. 1984; McLaren et al. 1983). There is a report of a woman with chronic vulvovaginitis due to

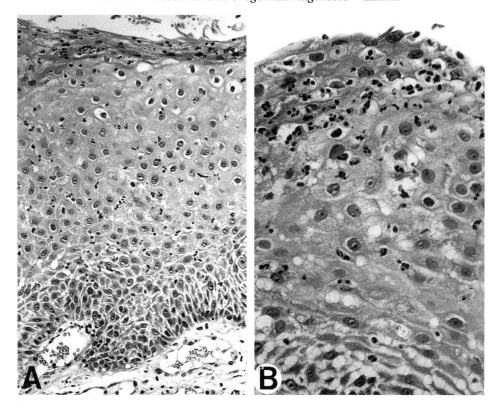

Fig. 3–11. ***Trichomonas vaginalis***, **section of a biopsy specimen of cervix stained with hematoxylin and eosin stain.** *A***, Vaginal epithelium showing scant infiltration and polymorphonuclear cells throughout the entire thickness (exocytosis). The surface of the epithelium is eroded, and it has desquamated cells and an inflammatory infiltrate,** ×187. *B***, Higher magnification shows marked desquamation of superficial layers of the mucosa and an abundant polymorphonuclear cell infiltrate,** ×298.

T. vaginalis who developed a perinephric abscess after trauma, from which *Trichomonas* species were cultured and observed in wet mounts (Suriyanon et al. 1975). This case of an abscess, and those of abscesses in men mentioned above, are not surprising and are akin to the experimental abscesses produced subcutaneously in animals to assess the pathogenicity of *T. vaginalis* (Honigberg et al. 1984).

Diagnosis. The diagnosis of trichomoniasis in women is based on clinical features. It is confirmed by finding the typical flagellates in wet smears of vaginal secretions, sometimes in cultures and more often in preparations stained with Papanicolaou stain. In men the infection is suspected clinically less often, but urethral secretions for *Trichomonas* should be examined in all patients with a nongonococcal urethral discharge, especially if it lasts for 4 weeks or longer. Frequently, the parasites are found during routine ex-

amination of urine sediments in both males and females. These methods have often been evaluated, with contradictory results (Eltabbakh et al. 1995; Krieger et al. 1988; Weinberger, Harger, 1993), but in general, no method used for the diagnosis of trichomoniasis is completely satisfactory because they all miss many infections. The gold standard for over 100 years was the wet preparation, until it was gradually replaced by the smear stained with Papanicolaou stain, because there is no need to examine it immediately and because a permanent record is kept for reexamination at a later day or by other observers. The culture for *Trichomonas* is not widely available in the routine clinical laboratory today, and its adoption requires much more evaluation in spite of its apparent superiority (Beal et al. 1992; Borchardt et al. 1992; Lossick, Kent, 1991; Poch et al. 1996). Monoclonal antibody staining of vaginal specimens is also not generally available and requires further testing (Krieger et al. 1988). A polymerase chain reaction performed

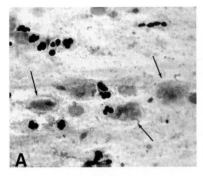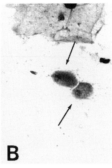

Fig. 3–12. *Trichomonas vaginalis* in a Papanicolaou smear. *A* and *B,* Smears from different women show the appearance of the flagellates with this stain. The morphologic characteristics are mostly lost and appear as an ovoid to round mass of cytoplasm with a poorly staining nucleus (arrows). In some specimens, the siderophilic granules stain pink, ×385.

in a tube with a color indicator for use in vaginal discharges has recently been developed (Shaio et al. 1997). It is doubtful that the diagnosis of trichomoniasis warrants the use of techniques other than a wet mount and a smear stained with Papanicolaou stain in each infected woman.

In preparations stained with Papanicolaou stain, the parasites stain poorly and appear as rounded or oval cytoplasmic masses with no discernible flagella (Fig. 3–12 *A–B*). A faint, elongated nucleus has to be recognized for proper identification; abundant pink siderophilic granules are seen in the cytoplasm, and the faint outline of the axostyle is often evident. Several cellular changes associated with *Trichomonas* infection are seen in smears stained with Papanicolaou stain. These changes include eosinophilia of many cells, numerous naked nuclei due to cytolysis, cytoplasmic alterations such as perinuclear clear zones (always smaller than those produced by the papilloma virus), and an eosinophilic background. Polymorphonuclear cells and red blood cells almost invariably accompany symptomatic *Trichomonas* infections (Patten, 1978). The parasites are not routinely identified in cervical or vaginal biopsy specimens.

References

Abonyi A, 1995. Examination of nonflagellate and flagellate round forms of *Trichomonas vaginalis* by transmission electron microscopy. Appl. Parasitol. 36:303–310

Adu Sarkodie Y, 1995. Correspondence. *Trichomonas vaginalis* transmission in a family. Genitourin. Med. 71: 199–200

Al-Salihi FL, Curran JP, Wang JS, 1974. Neonatal *Trichomonas vaginalis*: Report of three cases and review of the literature. Pediatrics 53:196–200

Aldeen WE, Hale D, Robison AJ, Carroll K, 1995. Evaluation of a commercially available ELISA assay for detection of *Giardia lamblia* in fecal specimens. Diagn. Microbiol. Infect. Dis. 21:77–79

Alderete JF, Arroyo R, Lehker MW, 1995a. Analysis for adhesins and specific cytoadhesion of *Trichomonas vaginalis*. Methods Enzymol. 253:407–414

Alderete JF, Lehker MW, Arroyo R, 1995b. The mechanisms and molecules involved in cytoadherence and pathogenesis of *Trichomonas vaginalis*. Parasitol. Today 11: 70–74

Alderete JF, Newton E, Dennis C, Engbring J, Neale KA, 1991a. Vaginal antibody of patients with trichomoniasis is to a prominent surface immunogen of *Trichomonas vaginalis*. Genitourin. Med. 67:220–225

Alderete JF, Newton E, Dennis C, Neale KA, 1991b. Antibody in sera of patients infected with *Trichomonas vaginalis* is to trichomonad proteinases. Genitourin. Med. 67:331–334

Alderete JF, O'Brien JL, Arroyo R, Engbring JA, Musatovova O, Lopez O, Lauriano C, Nguyen J, 1995c. Cloning and molecular characterization of two genes encoding adhesion proteins involved in *Trichomonas vaginalis* cytoadherence. Mol. Microbiol. 17:69–83

Alles AJ, Waldron MA, Sierra LS, Mattia AR, 1995. Prospective comparison of direct immunofluorescence and conventional staining methods for detection of *Giardia* and *Cryptosporidium* spp. in human fecal specimens. J. Clin. Microbiol. 33:1632–1634

Ament ME, 1975. Immunodeficiency syndrome and gastrointestinal disease. Pediatr. Clin. North Am. 22: 807–825

Ament ME, Ochs HD, Davis SD, 1973. Structure and function of the gastrointestinal tract in primary immunodeficiency syndromes. A study of 39 patients. Medicine 52:227–248

Ament ME, Rubin P, 1972. Relation of giardiasis to abnormal intestinal structure and function in gastrointestinal immunodeficiency syndrome. Gastroenterology 62:216–226

Aretio R, Perez MJ, Martin E, 1994. Evaluacion de dos tecnicas inmunologicas (ELISA, IFD) para el diagnostico de *Giardia lamblia* en heces. Enferm. Infecc. Microbiol. Clin. 12:337–340

Argent AC, Lachman PI, Hanslo D, Bass D, 1995. Sexually transmitted diseases in children and evidence of sexual abuse. Child Abuse Negl. 19:1303–1310

Arroyo R, Alderete JF, 1995a. Two *Trichomonas vaginalis* surface proteinases bind to host epithelial cells and are related to levels of cytoadherence and cytotoxicity. Arch. Med. Res. 26:279–285

Arroyo R, Engbring J, Nguyen J, Musatovova O, Lopez O, Lauriano C, Alderete JF, 1995b. Characterization of cDNAs encoding adhesin proteins involved in *Trichomonas vaginalis* cytoadherence. Arch. Med. Res. 26: 361–369

Arroyo R, Gonzalez-Robles A, Martinez-Palomo A, Alderete JF, 1993. Signalling of *Trichomonas vaginalis* for amoeboid transformation and adhesin [sic] synthesis follows cytoadherence. Mol. Microbiol. 7:299–309

Beal C, Goldsmith R, Kotby M, Sherif M, el Tagi A, Farid A, Zakaria SE-J, 1992. The plastic envelope method, a simplified technique for culture diagnosis of trichomoniasis. J. Clin. Microbiol. 30:2265–2268

Beaver PC, Jung RC, Cupp EW, 1984. *Clinical Parasitology*. Philadelphia: Lea & Febiger

Blenkinsopp WK, Gibson JA, Haffenden GP, 1978. Giardiasis and severe jejunal abnormality. Lancet 1:994

Borchardt KA, Hernandez V, Miller S, Loaiciga K, Cruz L, Naranjo S, Maida N, 1992. A clinical evaluation of trichomoniasis in San Jose, Costa Rica using the In Pouch TV test. Genitourin. Med. 68:328–330

Bozner P, Gombosova A, Valent M, Demes P, Alderete JF, 1992. Proteinases of *Trichomonas vaginalis*: antibody response in patients with urogenital trichomoniasis. Semin. Respir. Infect. 105:387–391

Brodsky RE, Spencer HC, Jr. Schultz MG, 1974. Giardiasis in American travelers to the Soviet Union. J. Infect. Dis. 130:319–323

Buchel LA, Gorenflot A, Chochillon C, Savel J, Gobert JG, 1987. In vitro excystation of *Giardia* from humans: a scanning electron microscopy study. J. Parasitol. 73: 487–493

Burch TA, Rees CW, Reardon LV, 1959. Epidemiological studies on human trichomoniasis. J. Trop. Med. Hyg. 8:312–318

Buret A, Gall DG, Olson ME, 1990. Effects of murine giardiasis on growth, intestinal morphology, and disaccharidase activity. J. Parasitol. 76:403–409

Buret A, Gall DG, Olson ME, 1991. Growth, activities of enzymes in the small intestine, and ultrastructure of microvillous border in gerbils infected with *Giardia duodenalis*. Parasitol. Res. 77:109–114

Cameron T, Choquette L, 1963. Parasitological problems in high northern latitudes, with particular reference to Canada. Polar Rec. 11:567–577

Carroccio A, Montalto G, Iacono G, Ippolito S, Soresi M, Notarbartolo A, 1997. Secondary impairment of pancreatic function as a cause of severe malabsorption in intestinal giardiasis: a case report. Am. J. Trop. Med. Hyg. 56:599–602

Case Records of the Massachusetts General Hospital, 1997. Case 8-1997. N. Engl. J. Med. 336:786–793

Chunge RN, Nagelkerke N, Karumba PN, Kaleli N, Wamwea M, Mutiso N, Andala EO, Gachoya J, Kiarie R, Kinoti SN, 1991. Longitudinal study of young children in Kenya: intestinal parasitic infection with special reference to *Giardia lamblia*, its prevalence, incidence and duration, and its association with diarrhoea and with other parasites. Acta Trop. 50:39–49

Corliss JO, 1994. An interim utilitarian ("user-friendly") hierarchical classification and characterization of the protists. Acta Protozool. 33:1–51

Cotch MF, Pastorek JG II, Nugent RP, Yerg DE, Martin DH,

Eschenback DA, 1991. Demographic and behavioral predictors of *Trichomonas vaginalis* infection among pregnant women. Obstet. Gynecol. 78:1087–1092

Craft JC, Nelson JD, 1982. Diagnosis of giardiasis by counterimmuno-electrophoresis of feces. J. Infect. Dis. 145: 499–504

Craun, CF, 1979. Waterborne outbreaks of giardiasis. In: Jakubowski W and Hoff JC (eds). *Waterborne Transmission of Giardiasis*. Proceedings of a Symposium, Sept. 18–20, 1978. U.S. Environmental Protection Agency, Cincinnati, Ohio. Springfield, Virginia: National Technical Information Service, pp. 127–149.

Danciger M, Lopez M, 1975. Numbers of *Giardia* in the feces of infected children. Am. J. Trop. Med. Hyg. 24: 237–242

Danesh IS, Stephen JM, Gorbach J, 1995. Neonatal *Trichomonas vaginalis* infection. J Emerg. Med 13:51–54

Demes P, Gombosova A, Valent M, Fabusova H, Janoska A, 1988. Fewer *Trichomonas vaginalis* organisms in vaginas of infected women during menstruation. Genitourin. Med. 64:22–24

Duboucher C, Mogenet M, Perie G, 1995. Salivary trichomoniasis. A case report of infestation of a submaxillary gland by *Trichomonas tenax*. Arch. Pathol. Lab. Med. 119:277–279

Dykes AC, Juranek DD, Lorenz RA, Sinclair S, Jakubowski W, Davies R, 1980. Municipal waterborne giardiasis: an epidemiologic investigation. Beavers implicated as a possible reservoir. Ann. Intern. Med. 92:165–170

el Sayed F, Bazex J, 1993. Correspondence. Chronic perianal ulcerations: role of *Trichomonas vaginalis*? Genitourin. Med. 69:483–484

Eltabbakh GH, Eltabbakh GD, Broekhuizen FF, Griner BT, 1995. Value of wet mount and cervical cultures at the time of cervical cytology in asymptomatic women. Obstet. Gynecol. 85:499–503

Farthing MJ, 1996. Giardiasis. Gastroenterol. Clin. North Am 25:493–515

Faubert GM, 1996. The immune response to *Giardia*. Parasitol. Today 12:140–145

Fleck SL, Hames SE, Warhurst DC, 1985. Detection of *Giardia* in human jejunum by the immunoperoxidase method. Specific and non-specific results. Trans. R. Soc. Trop. Med. Hyg. 79:110–113

Gardner WA Jr, Culberson DE, Bennett BD, 1986. *Trichomonas vaginalis* in the prostate gland. Arch. Pathol. Lab. Med. 110:430–432

Gibbs RS, Romero R, Hillier SL, Eschenbach DA, Sweet RL, 1992. A review of premature birth and subclinical infection. Am. J. Obstet. Gynecol. 166:1515–1528

Gillin FD, Reiner DS, McCaffery JM, 1996. Cell biology of the primitive eukaryote *Giardia lamblia*. Annu. Rev. Microbiol. 50:679–705

Gillon J, Ferguson A, 1984. Changes in the small intestinal mucosa in giardiasis. In: Erlandsen SL, Meyer EA (eds), *Giardia and Giardiasis*. New York: Plenum Press, pp. 163–183

Gilman RH, Brown KH, Visvesvara GS, Mondal G, Greenberg

B, Sack RB, Brandt F, Khan MU, 1985. Epidemiology and serology of *Giardia lamblia* in a developing country: Bangladesh. Trans. R. Soc. Trop. Med. Hyg. 79:469–473

Graves A, Gardner WA, 1993. Pathogenicity of *Trichomonas vaginalis*. Clin. Obstet. Gynecol. 36:145–152

Guccion JG, Ortega LG, 1996. Trichomoniasis complicating esophageal intramural pseudodiverticulosis: diagnosis by transmission electron microscopy. Ultrastruct. Pathol. 20:101–107

Guimaraes S, Sogayar MI, 1995. Occurrence of *Giardia lamblia* in children of municipal day-care centers from Botucatu, São Paulo State, Brazil. Rev. Inst. Med. Trop. Sao Paulo 37:501–506

Gunasekaran TS, Hassall E, 1996. Correspondence. Giardiasis diagnosed at colonoscopy with ileoscopy. Am. J. Gastroenterol. 91:407–408

Hardy PH, Nell EE, Spence MR, Hardy JB, Graham DA, Rosenbaum RC, 1984. Prevalence of six sexually transmitted disease agents among pregnant inner-city adolescents and pregnancy outcome. Lancet 2:333–337

Hermans PE, Huizenga KA, Hoffman HN, Brown AL, Markowitz H, 1966. Dysgammaglobulinemia associated with nodular lymphoid hyperplasia of the small intestine. Am. J. Med. 40:78–89

Hersh SM, 1985. Pulmonary trichomoniasis and *Trichomonas tenax*. J. Med. Microbiol. 20:1–10

Hiemstra I, Van Bel F, Berger HM, 1984. Can *Trichomonas vaginalis* cause pneumonia in newborn babies? Br. Med. J. 289:355–356

Hill DR, 1993. Giardiasis. Issues in diagnosis and management. Infect. Dis. Clin. North Am. 7:503–525

Honigberg BM, Gupta PK, Spence MR, Frost JK, Kuczynska K, Choromanski L, Warton A, 1984. Pathogenicity of *Trichomonas vaginalis*: cytopathologic and histopathologic changes of the cervical epithelium. Obstet. Gynecol. 64:179–184

Hopkins RM, Deplazes P, Meloni BP, Reynoldson JA, Thompson RCA, 1993. A field and laboratory evaluation of a commercial ELISA for the detection of *Giardia* coproantigens in humans and dogs. Trans. R. Soc. Trop. Med. Hyg. 87:39–41

Hopkins RM, Meloni BP, Groth DM, Wetherall JD, Reynoldson JA, Thompson RC, 1997. Ribosomal RNA sequencing reveals differences between the genotypes of *Giardia* isolates recovered from humans and dogs living in the same locality. J. Parasitol. 83:44–51

Hoskins LC, Winawer SJ, Broitman SA, Gottlieb LS, Zamcheck N, 1967. Clinical giardiasis and intestinal malabsorption. Gastroenterology 53:265–279

Isaac Renton JL, 1991. Laboratory diagnosis of giardiasis. Clin. Lab. Med. 11:811–827

Isaac Renton JL, Cordeiro C, Sarafis K, Shahriari H, 1993. Characterization of *Giardia duodenalis* isolates from a waterborne outbreak. J. Infect. Dis. 167:431–440

Jackson DJ, Rakwar JP, Chohan B, Mandaliya K, Bwayo JJ, Ndinya Achola JO, Nagelkerke NJ, Kreiss JK, Moses S, 1997. Urethral infection in a workplace population of East African men: evaluation of strategies for screening and management. J. Infect. Dis. 175:833–838

Janier M, Lassau F, Casin I, Grillot P, Scieux C, Zavaro A, Chastang C, Bianchi A, Morel P, 1995. Male urethritis with and without discharge: a clinical and microbiological study. Sex. Transm. Dis. 22:244–252

Jirovec O, Petru M, 1968. *Trichomonas vaginalis* and trichomoniasis. Adv. Parasitol. 6:117–188

Jove S, Fagundes Neto U, Wehba J, Machado NL, Patricio FR, 1983. Giardiasis in childhood and its effects on the small intestine. J. Pediatr. Gastroenterol. Nutr. 2:472–477

Judd R, Deckelbaum RJ, Weizman Z, Granot E, Ron N, Okon E, 1983. Giardiasis in childhood: poor clinical and histological correlations. Isr. J. Med. Sci. 19:818–823

Kamath KR, Murugasu R, 1974. A comparative study of four methods for detecting *Giardia lamblia* in children with diarrheal disease and malabsorption. Gastroenterology 66:16–21

Kappus KD, Lundgren RG Jr, Juranek DD, Roberts JM, Spencer HC, 1994. Intestinal parasitism in the United States: update on a continuing problem. Am. J. Trop. Med. Hyg. 50:705–713

Kent GP, Greenspan JR, Herndon JL, Mofenson LM, Harris JS, Eng TR, Waskin HA, 1988. Epidemic giardiasis caused by a contaminated public water supply. Am. J. Public Health 78:139–143

Kent HL, 1991. Epidemiology of vaginitis. Am. J. Obstet. Gynecol. 165:1168–1176

Kessel JF, Gafford JA Jr, 1935. Pathology of vaginitis due to *Trichomanas*. Arch. Pathol. 20:951

Kociecka W, Gustowska L, Gawronski M, Blotna M, Knapowska M, 1984. Evaluation of jejunal mucosa biopsy in patients with giardiasis. Wiad. Parazytol. 30:311–319

Krieger H, Kimmig P, 1995. Untersuchungen zur Uberlebensfahigkeit von *Trichomonas vaginalis* in Mineralbadern. Gesundheitswesen 57:812–819

Krieger JN, 1995. Trichomoniasis in men: old issues and new data. Sex. Transm. Dis. 22:83–96

Krieger JN, Jenny C, Verdon M, Siegel N, Springwater R, Critchlow CWH-K, 1993a. Clinical manifestations of trichomoniasis in men. Ann. Intern. Med. 118:844–849

Krieger JN, Riley DE, Roberts MC, Berger RE, 1996. Prokaryotic DNA sequences in patients with chronic idiopathic prostatitis. J. Clin. Microbiol. 34:3120–3128

Krieger JN, Tam MR, Stevens CE, Nielsen IO, Hale J, Kiviat NB, Holmes KK, 1988. Diagnosis of trichomoniasis. Comparison of conventional wet-mount examination with cytologic studies, cultures, and monoclonal antibody staining of direct specimens. JAMA 259:1223–1227

Krieger JN, Verdon M, Siegel N, Holmes KK, 1993b. Natural history of urogenital trichomoniasis in men. J. Urol. 149:1455–1458

Latif AS, Mason PR, Marowa E, 1987. Urethral trichomoniasis in men. Sex. Transm. Dis. 14:9–11

Levett PN, 1995. Aetiology of vaginal infections in pregnant and non-pregnant women in Barbados. West. Indian Med. J. 44:96–98

Levinson JD, Nastro LJ, 1978. Giardiasis with total villous atrophy. Gastroenterology 74:271–275

Lippy, E. C. 1979. Water supply problems associated with a waterborne outbreak of giardiasis. In: Jakubowski W, and Hoff JC (eds), Waterborne Transmission of Giardiasis. Proceedings of a Symposium, Sept. 18–20, 1978. U.S. Environmental Protection Agency, Cincinnati, Ohio. Springfield, Virginia: National Technical Information Service, pp. 164–173.

Lopez CE, Dykes AC, Juranek DD, Sinclair SP, Conn JM, Christie RW, Lippy EC, Schultz MG, Mires MH, 1980. Waterborne giardiasis: a communitywide outbreak of disease and a high rate of asymptomatic infection. Am. J. Epidemiol. 112:495–507

Lossick JG, Kent HL, 1991. Trichomoniasis: trends in diagnosis and management. Am J Obstet. Gynecol. 165:1217–1222

Mason PR, Patterson BA, 1987. Epidemiology of Giardia lamblia infection in children: cross-sectional and longitudinal studies in urban and rural communities in Zimbabwe. Am. J. Trop. Med. Hyg. 37:277–282

Masur H, Hook E III, Armstrong D, 1976. A Trichomonas species in a mixed microbial meningitis. JAMA 236:1978–1979

McLaren LC, Davis LE, Healy GR, James CG, 1983. Isolation of Trichomonas vaginalis from the respiratory tract of infants with respiratory disease. Pediatrics 71:888–890

Meda N, Ledru S, Fofana M, Lankoande S, Soula G, Bazie AJ, Chiron JP, 1995. Sexually transmitted diseases and human immunodeficiency virus infection among women with genital infections in Burkina Faso. Int. J. STD. AIDS. 6:273–277

Memik F, 1968. Trichomonads in pleural effusion. JAMA 204:1145–1146

Miller MJ, Leith DE, Brooks JR, Fencl V, 1982. Trichomonas empyema. Thorax 37:384–385

Millet VE, Spencer MJ, Chapin M, Stewart M, Yatabe JA, Brewer T, Garcia LS, 1983. Dientamoeba fragilis, a protozoan parasite in adult members of a semicommunal group. Dig. Dis. Sci. 28:335–339

Minkoff H, Grunebaum AN, Schwarz RH, Feldman J, Cummings M, Crombleholme W, Clark L, Pringle G, McCormack WM, 1984. Risk factors for prematurity and premature rupture of membranes: a prospective study of the vaginal flora in pregnancy. Am. J. Obstet. Gynecol. 150:965–972

Moorehead WP, Guasparini R, Donovan CA, Mathias RG, Cottle R, Baytalan G, 1990. Giardiasis outbreak from a chlorinated community water supply. Can. J Public Health 81:358–362

Munoz E, Carmona T, Chaves F, Paz JI, Bullon A, 1996. Correspondence. Identification of Giardia lamblia by gastric brush cytology. Acta Cytol. 40:1331–1332

Ng HT, Wang KI, Fan PC, Liu HY, 1981. Studies on Trichomonas vaginalis infections in women with carcinoma of the uterine cervix. Proc. Natl. Sci. Counc. Taipei, Taiwan 5:247–251

Oberhuber G, Stolte M, 1990. Giardiasis: analysis of histological changes in biopsy specimens of 80 patients. J. Clin. Pathol. 43:641–643

Oberhuber G, Stolte M, 1995. Histologic detection of trophozoites of Giardia lamblia in the terminal ileum. Scand. J. Gastroenterol. 30:905–908

Ohkura T, Suzuki N, Hashiguchi Y, 1985. Correspondence. Am. J. Trop. Med. Hyg. 34:823–824

Pastorek JG, Cotch MF, Martin DH, Eschenbach DA, 1996. Clinical and microbiological correlates of vaginal trichomoniasis during pregnancy. The Vaginal Infections and Prematurity Study Group. Clin. Infect. Dis. 23:1075–1080

Patten SFJ, 1978. Diagnostic Cytopathology of the Uterine Cervix. New York: S. Karger

Pavithran K, 1993. Trichomonal abscess of the median raphe of the penis. Int. J. Dermatol. 32:820–821

Perez O, Lastre M, Bandera F, Diaz M, Domenech I, Fagundo R, Torres D, Finlay C, Campa C, Sierra G, 1994. Evaluation of the immune response in symptomatic and asymptomatic human giardiasis. Arch. Med. Res. 25: 171–177

Peters CS, Sable R, Janda WM, Chittom AL, Kocka FE, 1986. Prevalence of enteric parasites in homosexual patients attending an outpatient clinic. J. Clin. Microbiol. 24: 684–685

Phillips SC, Mildvan D, William DC, Gelb AM, White MC, 1981. Sexual transmission of enteric protozoa and helminths in a venereal-disease-clinic population. N. Engl. J. Med. 305:603–606

Poch F, Levin D, Levin S, Dan M, 1996. Modified thioglycolate medium: a simple and reliable means for detection of Trichomonas vaginalis. J. Clin. Microbiol. 34:2630–2631

Quincey C, James PD, Steele RJ, 1992. Chronic giardiasis of the stomach. J. Clin. Pathol. 45:1039–1041

Radosavljevic Asic G, Jovanovic D, Radovanovic D, Tucakovic M, 1994. Trichomonas in pleural effusion. Eur. Respir. J. 7:1906–1908

Rendtorff RC, 1954. The experimental transmission of human intestinal protozoan parasites. II. Attempts to transmit Giardia lamblia cysts given in capsules. Am. J. Hyg. 59:202–220

Robinson AJ, Ridgway GL, 1994. Sexually transmitted diseases in children: nonviral including bacterial vaginosis, Gardnerella vaginalis, mycoplasmas, Trichomonas vaginalis, Candida albicans, scabies and pubic lice. Genitourin. Med. 70:208–214

Rodriguez Da Silva J, Coutinho SJ, Dias LB, Figueiredo N, 1964. Histopathologic findings in giardiasis: A biopsy study. Am. J. Digest. Dis. 9:355–365

Rodriguez Hernandez J, Canut Blasco A, Martin Sanchez AM, 1996. Seasonal prevalences of Cryptosporidium and Giardia infections in children attending day care centres in Salamanca (Spain) studied for a period of 15 months. Eur. J. Epidemiol. 12:291–295

Rosekrans PC, Lindeman J, Meijer CJ, 1981. Quantitative

histological and immunohistochemical findings in jejunal biopsy specimens in giardiasis. Virchows Arch. Pathol. Anat. 393:145–151

Shaio MF, Lin PR, Liu JY, 1997. Colorimetric one-tube nested PCR for detection of *Trichomonas vaginalis* in vaginal discharge. J. Clin. Microbiol. 35:132–138

Shein R, Gelb A., 1983. Colitis due to *Dientamoeba fragilis*. Am. J. Gastroenterol. 78:634–636

Short SL, Stockman DL, Wolinsky SM, Trupei MA, Moore J, Reichman RC, 1984. Comparative rates of sexually transmitted diseases among heterosexual men, homosexual men, and heterosexual women. Sex. Transm. Dis. 11:271–274

Siegel RM, Schubert CJ, Myers PA, Shapiro RA, 1995. The prevalence of sexually transmitted diseases in children and adolescents evaluated for sexual abuse in Cincinnati: rationale for limited STD testing in prepubertal girls. Pediatrics 96:1090–1094

Soendjojo A, Pindha S, 1981. *Trichomonas vaginalis* infection of the median raphe of the penis. Sex. Transm. Dis. 8:255–257

Sorvillo F, Kovacs A, Kerndt P, Stek A, Muderspach L, Sanchez-Keeland L, 1998. Risk factors for trichomoniasis among women with human immunodeficiency virus (HIV) infection at a public clinic in Los Angeles County, California: implications for HIV prevention. Am. J. Trop. Med. Hyg. 58:495–500

Sowmini CN, Vijayalakshmi K, Chellamuthiah C, Sundaram SM, 1972. Infections of the median raphe of the penis: report of three cases. Br. J. Vener. Dis. 49:469–474

Springer SC, Key JD, 1997. Vitamin B12 deficiency and subclinical infection with *Giardia lamblia* in an adolescent with agammaglobulinemia of Bruton. J. Adolesc. Health 20:58–61

Suriyanon V, Nelson KE, Ayudhya VCN, 1975. *Trichomonas vaginalis* in a perinephric abscess. A case report. Am. J. Trop. Med. Hyg. 24:776–780

Suzuki HU, de Morais MB, Medeiros EH, do Corral JN, Fagundes Neto U, 1994. Limitacao diagnostica da pesquisa de trofozoitos da *Giardia lamblia* no aspirado duodenal. Arq. Gastroenterol. 31:69–74

Thompson SC, 1994. *Giardia lamblia* in children and the child care setting: a review of the literature. J. Paediatr. Child Health 30:202–209

Trussell RR, 1947. *Trichomonas vaginalis and Trichomoniasis*. Springfield, Illinois: Charles C Thomas

Walzer PD, Rugherford I, East R, 1978. Empyema with *Trichomonas* species. Am. Rev. Respir. Dis. 118:415–418

Ward H, Jalan KN, Mairtra TK, Agarwal SK, Mahalanabis D, 1983. Small intestinal nodular lymphoid hyperplasia in patients with giardiasis and normal serum immunoglobulins. Gut 24:120–126

Weinberger MW, Harger JH, 1993. Accuracy of the Papanicolaou smear in the diagnosis of asymptomatic infection with *Trichomonas vaginalis*. Obstet. Gynecol. 82: 425–429

Wolfe MS, 1984. Symptomatology, diagnosis and treatment. In: Erlandsen SL, Meyer EA (eds), *Giardia and Giardiasis*. New York: Plenum Press, pp. 147–161

Wolner Hanssen P, Krieger JN, Stevens CE, Kiviat NB, Koutsky LC-C, DeRouen T, Hillier S, Holmes KK, 1989. Clinical manifestations of vaginal trichomoniasis. JAMA 261:571–576

Yap EH, Ho TH, Chan YC, Thong TW, Ng GC, Ho LC, Singh M, 1995. Serum antibodies to *Trichomonas vaginalis* in invasive cervical cancer patients. Genitourin. Med. 71:402–404

Yardley JH, Takano J, Hendrix TR, 1964. Epithelial and other mucosal lesions of the jejunum in giardiasis. Jejunal biopsy studies. Bull. Johns Hopkins Hosp. 115: 389–406

Zhang ZF, 1996. Epidemiology of *Trichomonas vaginalis*. A prospective study in China. Sex. Transm. Dis. 23: 415–424

Zhang ZF, Graham S, Yu SZ, Marshall J, Zielezny M, Chen YX, Sun M, Tang SL, Liao CS, Xu JL, et al, 1995. *Trichomonas vaginalis* and cervical cancer. A prospective study in China. Ann. Epidemiol. 5:325–332

4

LEISHMANIAE

The leishmaniae is a group of organisms that inhabit the tissues, specifically the monocyte-macrophage lineage and, to a lesser extent, other phagocytic cells. The leishmaniae and the closely related trypanosomes (see Chapter 5), which inhabit the blood and other tissues, constitute the blood and tissue flagellates. These two groups of organisms are placed in the kingdom Protozoa, phylum Euglenozoa, class Kinetoplastida, order Trypanosomatida, and family Trypanosomatidae. The phylum Euglenozoa is characterized by the presence of one to four flagella, mitochondria with discoidal cristae, a microtubular cytoskeleton, and a well-developed Golgi apparatus. Some species are aquatic, and others are symbiontic (live in other hosts). The Kinetoplastida are defined by having stages in their life cycles with a single flagellum, an undulating membrane, and a kinetoplast, which is a mitochondrion with a core of DNA (Fig. 4–1). The order Trypanosomatida has two genera parasitic in humans: *Trypanosoma* and *Leishmania*, with many species widely distributed in humans and animals.

Members of the genera *Leishmania* and *Trypanosoma* have both invertebrate and vertebrate hosts in their life cycles (Fig. 4–2). The invertebrate hosts are blood-sucking insects where the infective stages develop and are necessary to maintain transmission in any given geographic area. A few exceptions to this general rule of two hosts exist: one species of *Trypanosoma* of horses is transmitted through sexual contact. *Leishmania* and *Trypanosoma* together have about 20 species parasitizing humans, producing some of the most important infectious diseases known. The leishmaniae play a significant role as opportunistic infections in individuals with human immune deficiency virus (HIV) infection, producing a great deal of morbidity and mortality. Most species of trypanosomes and leishmaniae occur in the tropical and subtropical regions of the world, producing diseases of low to high endemicity. However, on occasion they occur in epidemics, the leishmaniae usually following natural disasters such as earthquakes (Dye, Wolpert, 1988), flood, famine, or war (de Beer et al. 1991). In this chapter, we will examine the leishmaniae.

Life Cycle. Species of *Leishmania* have two stages in their life cycle: *amastigotes* (aflagellar forms in histiocytes) and *promastigotes* (flagellar stages in arthropod vectors). Both stages have a prominent kinetoplast; the flagellate has a small, undulating membrane and a sin-

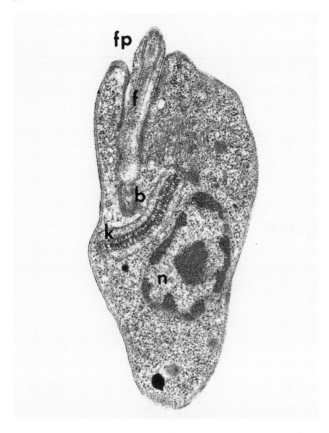

Fig. 4–1. *Trypanosoma cruzi*, electron micrograph of an amastigote illustrating some organelles. Note that the general organization of this stage of *T. cruzi* is similar to that of *Leishmania* amastigotes. Abbreviations: b, basal body; f, flagellum (axoneme); fp, flagellar pocket; k, kinetoplast with central DNA core; n, nucleus, ×22,000. (Courtesy of M. Aikawa, M.D., Institute of Pathology, Case Western Reserve University, Cleveland, Ohio.)

cardiac valve (which separates the esophagus from the thoracic midgut) by digesting a protective layer on the valve composed of chitin fibers. The damaged valve does not operate properly, allowing regurgitation of the promastigotes during the next feeding and passing the parasites into the new host (Schlein, 1993; Schlein et al. 1993). Once the parasite enters the new host, the reverse transformation from promastigote to amastigote occurs within phagocytic cells of the local skin, where the amastigotes may remain, producing skin lesions (cutaneous leishmaniasis). Alternatively, the amastigotes may travel to the tissues to produce a generalized infection (visceral leishmaniasis).

Morphology. Only the morphologic characteristics of the amastigotes are important in this discussion; those of the promastigotes will be omitted. In smears of clinical material or in imprints of biopsy specimens stained with Giemsa stain, the amastigotes appear as 3 to 4 μm oval bodies with a pale blue cytoplasm and a darkly stained nucleus that occupies about one-third to one-half of the parasite. In addition, another structure, also darkly stained, of variable size and shape, the kinetoplast, is located near the nucleus (*color plate* III A–B). The axoneme, that short portion of the flagellum within the body of the parasite, is only occasionally visible because it remains unstained. In these preparations, the amastigotes are seen clearly within a cell (*color plate* II H–J), but more often they are scattered about, an artifact produced during the preparation of the smear or imprint (*color plate* II H–J). Amastigotes are three-dimensional organisms, like an egg, and the location of the nucleus, axoneme, and kinetoplast in the cytoplasm is characteristic. The nucleus is located in the posterior

gle flagellum. The amastigotes are obligatory intracellular parasites of phagocytic cells of vertebrates, because they do not have the ability to enter cells on their own, and multiply asexually by binary fission within the cell. The arthropod vector ingests intracellular amastigotes when it takes its blood meal. Many good natural vectors of the parasite belong to the genus *Phlebotomus*, distributed widely in the Old World, and the genera *Lutzomia* and *Psychodopygus* in the New World, commonly known as *sand flies*.

Once the infected meal is taken by the arthropod, the amastigotes are transformed from a 4 μm organism to an 18 to 20 μm promastigote in the alimentary canal of the vector, where they multiply asexually to produce the infective stages. The flagellates are located in the digestive tube of the sand fly and damage the

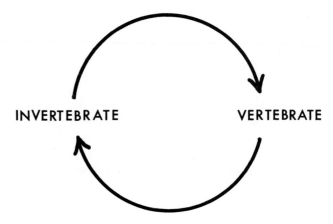

Fig. 4–2. Trypanosomatidae, general life cycle involving a vertebrate definitive host and an invertebrate intermediate host.

half of the body, the kinetoplast anteriorly but toward the dorsal aspect, and the axoneme also in the dorsal aspect anterior to the kinetoplast. This arrangement allows for several morphologic configurations of these structures, depending on the angle of view.

In tissue sections stained with hematoxylin and eosin stain the amastigotes are seen as smaller bodies, less than 2 μm, because of shrinkage of the tissues during processing for sectioning. The organisms are found in clusters. They are often difficult to visualize as individuals because two or three of them may be superimposed on each other (remember that the histologic section is 5 to 6 μm thick). The cytoplasm is so delicate that it is rarely seen stained, but the basophilic nucleus and kinetoplast are darkly stained. In tissue sections, recognition of the nucleus and kinetoplast is the basis for proper identification of these parasites. These structures are closely associated and are seen as large (nucleus) and small (kinetoplast), darkly stained organelles.

In transmission electron micrographs the amastigotes have morphologic characteristics that are similar in all species studied but apparently not identical; minute differences have been found among some species (Gardener et al. 1977). The body is covered by an outer cell membrane under which a row of microtubules is located. These two layers constitute the *periplast* or *pellicle* of the parasite. An invagination of the membrane forms the flagellar pocket, containing the axoneme that later grows to a flagellum in the promastigote. The nucleus is covered with a double-layered membrane and is about 1 μm in diameter, eccentrically located, with one or two nucleoli, and some peripherally located chromatin. The single most characteristic feature of the parasites is the kinetoplast, or mitochondrion, seen as a sausage-shaped structure about 1 μm long. It is covered by a double-layered membrane forming cristae, and at the center it has a tightly coiled mass of DNA (Forteza Bover et al. 1968; Rudzinska et al. 1964). The kinetoplast DNA contains the information for the synthesis of the enzymes necessary for all the steps of aerobic metabolism (Krebs cycle). The kinetoplast enlarges considerably during transformation of the amastigote into the promastigote (Rudzinska et al. 1964). This enlargement occurs when the parasite changes from an intracellular location (amastigotes with anaerobic respiration) to an extracellular location (promastigotes with aerobic respiration). In the cytoplasm, other structures are present, such as the Golgi apparatus, endoplasmic reticulum, and others. The flagellum originates in the cytoplasm, near the kinetoplast, from the basal body, which is identical to other basal bodies: nine peripheral double

fibrils surrounded by a thin sheath, with no central fibrils. As the flagellum exits in the flagellar pocket, the central two fibrils of the flagellum (to form the nine plus two configuration) are present, to run within the flagellar pocket as the axoneme (Molyneux, Killick-Kendrick, 1987). The axoneme, and later the flagellum, are covered by the cell membrane. The ultrastructure of the promastigote has also been reported (Chatterjee, Sen Gupta, 1970; Creemers, Jadin, 1967).

Biology. The biology of the life cycle stages of the leishmaniae, the intracellular amastigote in the vertebrate and the extracellular promastigote in the invertebrate, are being studied intensively. The biologic aspects of the parasites in the arthropod are relevant to the capacity of the vectors to support and transmit the parasites, the manner in which they are transmitted, and their survival and development. These are important aspects of the epidemiology of the disease. The biology of amastigotes is relevant mostly to the disease in the vertebrate, the immunologic mechanisms, the survival of the parasite in phagocytic cells, the mechanism of evasion of the immunologic system, and, to a lesser extent, the therapeutic modalities. Studying the leishmaniae is difficult because there are many species producing different clinical syndromes in humans, which makes generalizations uncertain (Russell, Talamas-Rohana, 1989). Moreover, in most studies of the interaction of the parasites and their host cells, common practice is to use promastigotes because they are easily grown in the laboratory. The amastigotes, which are responsible for infection, are more difficult to obtain because they must be harvested from infected animals or cell cultures. The study of parasites isolated from individuals coinfected with HIV has provided information on the tendency of species of cutaneous leishmaniae to visceralize.

As mentioned before, leishmaniael amastigotes are phagocytized by cells of the monocytic macrophage system and by granulocytes, where they reside and multiply in vacuoles (phagolysosomes). Therefore, the macrophage has a dual role: it acts as the host cell of the parasite and as the antigen-presenting cell of the immune system. In these circumstances, some parasites are killed but others survive, implying that they have developed resistance to the environmental conditions of the vacuole, where they are either loosely or tightly contained (Chang, 1983). The cell lysosomes fuse to the phagolysosome membrane, bursting and discharging their contents, to create an acidic environment that should degrade the parasites; however, some amastigotes survive because they neutralize the lysosomal enzymes (Bogdan et al. 1990; Chang, 1983). The organisms destroyed by the macrophage play a role in conferring immunity to the parasite (see below).

Two biologic forms of *Leishmania* infections are recognized in humans: the dermal and the visceral, defined as such based on the idea that different species of *Leishmania* possess a determined dermal or visceral location. It is now clear that homing of the parasites to the skin or the viscera is not a fixed characteristic of these parasites (Kreutzer et al. 1993; Magill et al. 1993). *Leishmania braziliensis* disseminates to the lymph nodes even before a skin lesion is formed (Barral et al. 1995), as well as to the internal organs in experimental animal infections (Almeida et al. 1996). Cutaneous lesions are well known in natural infections with *L. donovani* (Kumar et al. 1989; Mebrahtu et al. 1993) and *L. infantum* (Ayadi et al. 1992). Visceral disease in humans has been similarly traced to species consider cutaneous in nature (Magill et al. 1993; Ndiaye et al. 1996), as revealed by the molecular classification of *Leishmania* isolates from these patients. Since the lack of homing in *Leishmania* is seen commonly in HIV-positive individuals with low levels of CD4+ T lymphocytes, the leishmaniael tropism to the skin or the viscera must be at least partly determined by the host's immune system (Gradoni, Gramiccia, 1994).

Immunity. The classic view of immunity to leishmaniae was based on the comparison of their different clinical forms, with the spectrum of disease produced by leprosy, supported by histologic and clinical observations. At one end was the tuberculoid type, characterized by skin ulcers that either do not heal or heal and break down again, with no development of immunity to reinfection. At the other end was the lepromatous form, manifesting as disseminated skin nodules that do not ulcerate, with no development of cell-mediated immunity. At the middle of the spectrum was the most common disease, dermal leishmaniasis that heals spontaneously in most cases within months or years, leaving a scar and a strong lifelong cellular immunity to reinfection with the same parasite (Turk, Bryceson, 1971). Dermal leishmaniasis is encountered in endemic areas of cutaneous leishmaniasis throughout the world; the diffuse lepromatous type and the tuberculoid type are seen sporadically. The comparison of cutaneous leishmaniasis with leprosy was helpful in understanding the underlying general immunologic bases for the different clinical presentations of the infection in humans. We now understand how these basic immunologic mechanisms are modulated by the parasite.

Information on immunity to leishmaniae in humans has been difficult to obtain because study populations are not easily available. Most of the work has been done in mice, hamsters, and other animal models for the cutaneous and visceral forms of the disease. The exact mechanism of protective or counterprotective immunity during infections with leishmaniae is not known, but it is clear that in both cases CD4+ T lymphocytes play a fundamental role (Antoine, 1995). The parasites are taken by macrophages, where they supposedly multiply, but when they become activated, the macrophages kill and destroy them. Moreover, macrophages are responsible for presenting antigens to T cells, and they produce cytokines (interleukin-1 [IL-1] tumor necrosis factor [TNF] alpha, and others) that initiate and maintain the specific immune response to the parasite.

In order to survive in the macrophage, leishmaniae avoid activating the infected macrophage, but exactly how this occurs is not known. It has been shown that the parasites can survive in the acidic and proteolytic environment of the parasitophorous vacuole of resting macrophages (Chang, 1983; Chang, Dwyer, 1976) but not in the parasitophorus vacuole of macrophages activated by external stimuli. In the parasitophorous vacuole of activated macrophages, the leishmaniae are killed by toxic nitric oxide (Kemp, 1997). Leishmaniae are also killed and processed in the dendritic cells (Langerhans cells) of the epidermis and by natural killer cells. Dendritic cells, once parasitized, become activated and drain to the regional lymph nodes, presenting leishmaniae antigens to naive parasite-specific T cells. In addition, activated natural killer cells produce cytokines such as interferon gamma, which helps to control the infection.

Degraded parasites in the phagolysosome produce antigens that are processed via the major histocompatibility complex class II molecules (Kemp, 1997), which are responsible for antigen presentation to CD4+ T lymphocytes and thus for their activation. In animal models, activation of CD4+ T lymphocytes produces two types of cells: T helper 1 (Th1) and Th2 cells, distinguished by the cytokines they produce (data suggest that this process also occurs in humans) (Kemp, 1997). In leishmaniae infections these two subsets of CD4+ T lymphocytes act differently, which explains the disease produced by the parasite (Kemp, 1997).

The CD4+ T lymphocytes activated into Th1 lymphocytes produce IL-2 and TNF-gamma, which activate CD8+ T lymphocytes (killer cells), natural killer cells, and macrophages. Activation of these three cells lines results in a self-healing, asymptomatic infection. The CD4+ T lymphocytes activated into Th2 lymphocytes secrete IL-4 and IL-5, which in turn activate B cells to produce antibodies. In this case, no activation of killer cells occurs and the patient suffers the disease with various levels of virulence. The lack of CD4[+] T lymphocytes in individuals with HIV infection makes them highly susceptible to coinfections with *Leishmania* (Alvar, 1994).

Some data obtained in experimental animals and in natural human infections support the concept of immune modulation of leishmaniasis. In experimental *L. donovani* infections in mice, expression of major histocompatibility complex class II molecules, and IL-2 secretion are decreased (Kemp 1997). In addition, macrophages of animals infected with *L. donovani* are refractory to activation by gamma interferon (Reiner et al. 1988). Both of these findings are similar to those in individuals naturally infected with *L. donovani*: these persons have no T-cell response or gamma interferon production (Carvalho et al. 1985; Murray et al. 1987) and no delayed-type hypersensitivity reactions (Sacks et al. 1987). Cells of healthy individuals from endemic areas of *L. infantum* produce high gamma interferon levels when they are challenged with amastigotes (Meller Melloul et al. 1991), and children with *L. chagasi* also show increased gamma interferon production (Bacellar et al. 1991). Isolates of *L. aethiopica* from patients with diffuse cutaneous leishmaniasis and from

patients with localized ulcers modulate production of different cytokines. Promastigotes derived from diffuse cutaneous leishmaniasis, placed in contact with peripheral human monocytes, induce production of IL-10, while those from localized disease induce production of gamma interferon (Akuffo et al. 1997). Since IL-10 is a potent suppressor of natural killer cells, this reaction indicates that the genesis of localized versus diffuse disease is linked to the capacity of a given strain of parasites to modulate the production of cytokines in the host (Akuffo et al. 1997).

The mucocutaneous and visceral leishmaniae infecting humans will be examined separately in the following sections.

Mucocutaneous Leishmaniasis

Skin lesions produced by several species of *Leishmania* are common in some tropical and subtropical areas of the world, where the population at risk is usually the poor, living on minimal or marginal agricultural practices near tropical forests (Fig. 4–3) (WHO 1984;

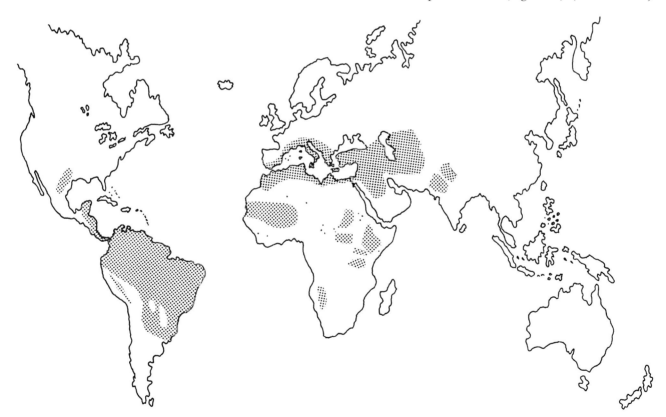

Fig. 4–3. Geographic distribution of cutaneous leishmaniasis. (Redrawn and reproduced by permission. WHO. 1984. The Leishmaniases. Tech. Rep. Ser. No. 701. World Health Organization, Geneva.)

WHO, 1990). A focus of cutaneous leishmaniasis in northern Mexico, the most northern endemic focus on the American continent, extends into the southern portion of Texas (Gustafson et al. 1985; Nelson et al. 1985). Twenty-seven cases of autochthonous leishmaniasis have been identified in this state. All patients lived within the geographic range of a rodent (*Neotoma micropus*), a known reservoir of *L. mexicana* (McHugh et al. 1996).

Geographic Distribution and Epidemiology. The classical concept of two species, *L. tropica* in the Old World and *L. braziliensis* in the New World, as the sole agents of cutaneous leishmaniasis has been revised several times during the last three decades. This revision is due to the necessity to accommodate several species characterized on the basis of their geographic distribution, the clinical picture they produce, and the biologic aspects of the parasites. These classification schemes are applied mostly to the leishmaniae of the New World because of the larger number of species and the need to understand the relationships among them. These classifications are also used for the Old World leishmaniae. Some recent classifications that divide *Leishmania* into two subgenera, *Leishmania* and *Vianna* (Cupolillo et al. 1994; Lainson, Shaw, 1987), have been generally acceptable by specialists in the field. However, for the sake of simplification, we will omit the subgenus name and use only the genus name (*L. Vianna braziliensis* will be referred to as *L. braziliensis*, and so on), similar to the classification proposed earlier by Grimaldi and coworkers (Grimaldi et al. 1989; Grimaldi, McMahon-Pratt, 1996). The dermal leishmaniae, the lesions they produce, and their geographic distribution are as follows (Fig. 4–3):

1. *Cutaneous leishmaniasis of the Old World*

    a. *Leishmania tropica* produces painless, dry ulcerations that heal spontaneously in about 1 year or longer, leading to disfiguring scars. The distribution is usually urban, with a human-vector-human transmission pattern. Endemic countries are Afghanistan, Greece, Iran, Iraq, Israel, Kenya, Syria, Tunisia, Turkey, and Uganda.

    b. *Leishmania major* often produces multiple wet ulcers that heal in 2 to 8 months. In newcomers to the endemic area the lesions may coalesce to form large, painless lesions that are easily infected secondarily. A longer healing period is necessary. The disease is zoonotic and rural in distribution. Endemic countries are Afghanistan, Algeria, Yemen, Djibouti, Egypt,

Guinea, India, Iran, Iraq, Israel, Jordan, Kuwait, Libya, Mali, Mauritania, Morocco, Pakistan, Saudi Arabia, Sudan, Syria, and Turkey.

    c. *Leishmania aethiopica* is responsible for cutaneous ulcers, nasopharyngeal metastasis, and diffuse cutaneous leishmaniasis. The disease develops slowly and lasts for 1 to 3 years. Endemic countries are Ethiopia and Kenya.

2. *Cutaneous leishmaniasis of the New World*

    a. *Leishmania braziliensis* produces chronic, single or multiple ulcers with regional lymph node involvement, which tend to metastasize to naso-oropharyngeal cartilage and cause *espundia*. Endemic countries are Argentina, Belize, Bolivia, Brazil, Colombia, Costa Rica, French Guiana, Guatemala, Honduras, Mexico, Panama, Paraguay, Peru, and Venezuela.

    b. *Leishmania guayanensis* produces painless, dry nodules similar to yaws. In rare cases, it causes mucocutaneous lesions. Endemic countries are Brazil, Colombia, French Guiana, and Surinam.

    c. *Leishmania panamensis* causes wet ulcers with marked lymphatic involvement; lesions are persistent, lasting for several months before spontaneous healing occurs. Mucocutaneous lesions are common. Endemic countries are Colombia, Costa Rica, Ecuador, Honduras, Nicaragua, Panama, and Venezuela.

    d. *Leishmania mexicana* is associated mostly with the *bay sore* or *chiclero's ulcer*, a single ulcer involving the helix of the ear, with destruction of the cartilage, but capable of producing lesions anywhere in the skin. It was once thought to be the sole species responsible for diffuse cutaneous leishmaniasis (see below). Endemic countries are Belize, Colombia, Costa Rica, Guatemala, Honduras, Panama, and the United States (Texas).

    e. *Leishmania liansoni* produces simple, benign ulcerated lesions. Endemic countries are Brazil and Peru.

    f. *Leishmania amazonensis* causes chronic ulcers and mucocutaneous lesions (rarely) that heal spontaneously with difficulty. In addition, it produces diffuse cutaneous leishmaniasis (see below). Endemic countries are Bolivia, Brazil, Colombia, Ecuador, French Guiana, Panama, Peru, and Venezuela.

    g. *Leishmania venezuelensis* produces single nodular lesions and diffuse cutaneous leishmaniasis (Bonfante Garrido et al. 1996). The endemic area is northern Venezuela.

h. *Leishmania colombiensis* has produced only two human cases, both with cutaneous ulcerations. (Kreutzer et al. 1991). The endemic country is Colombia.

Leishmania peruviana was once considered a separate species. It produces *uta*, a disease that occurs in children of the Peruvian Andes and heals spontaneously in 4 months (Davies et al. 1995). Today it is believed to be a variant of *L. braziliensis* (Grimaldi et al. 1989). The species of *Leishmania* found in northern Mexico and the United States is not satisfactorily classified but is likely a variant of *L. mexicana*.

Although there is often an overlap in the distribution of these species, both in the Old and New Worlds, it is apparent that some species predominate in certain geographic areas (Grimaldi et al. 1987, 1989). The epidemiology and clinical characteristics of the cases occurring in Texas have been recently reviewed (McHugh et al. 1996).

Clinical Findings. For practical purposes, the clinical lesions produced by the species of dermal leishmaniae are grossly similar in the New and Old Worlds, but in general, the disease follows a more aggressive course in the New World. The character of the lesion depends on the species of parasite involved and the cellular immunologic status of the host.

Usually, the dermal lesion begins as a small, reddish papule at the site of inoculation, progressing to a larger area of induration and eventually ulceration, starting with a small crust that falls off, exposing the subcutaneous tissues. The lesion expands centrifugally, sometimes rapidly, to form ulcers several centimeters in diameter, taking 3 to 4 weeks to attain a diameter of 6 to 8 cm (Fig. 4–4 A–D). The ulcers commonly have sharp, slightly raised borders, though aggressive ones have irregular, ragged edges with a rim of edema and hyperemia (Fig. 4–4 B). The base of the ulcer is usually clean, with healthy pink granulation tissue with hyperemia and petechiae if the ulcer is not infected secondarily (Fig. 4–4 C). Superimposed infections are the rule, especially in ulcers evolving for some time with little or no medical treatment. Some lesions retain their crusty appearance, producing a dry thickening of the epidermis (Fig. 4–5 A–D). This appearance is common with *L. tropica*, but similar lesions are observed in the New World. The bay sore or chiclero's ulcer is usually limited to the ear, with a clinical evolution and presentation similar to those described above, often resulting in considerable loss of the ear cartilage. These le-

sions are seen throughout Latin America, but they are more commonly associated with *L. mexicana* in Central America (Figs. 4–6 A–B and 4–7 A–D).

Enlargement of satellite lymph nodes, is not uncommon in cutaneous leishmaniasis and is often the first sign of infection with *L. braziliensis* (Barral et al. 1995). In Saudi Arabia *L. tropica* produced lymphadenopathy in 10% of the people studied (Al-Gindan et al. 1989), sometimes in the absence of a clear cutaneous lesion or with only a small, insect bite-like lesion; in some cases, the lymphadenopathy lasted for up to 3 months (Azadeh, 1985), and some patients developed up to 16 satellite lesions (Kubba et al. 1987). In Brazil 67% (Barral et al. 1992) and 77% (Sousa et al. 1995) of patients with *L. braziliensis* had enlarged lymph nodes. Enlargement of lymph nodes often follows the lymph channels, showing a sporotrichoid pattern; sometimes these nodes ulcerate (Kibbi et al. 1987). Enlargement of lymph nodes contralateral to the lesion and recovery of organisms from these lymph nodes have also been described (Ary et al. 1964). Patients with enlarged lymph nodes have enhanced humoral and cellular immune responses compared with those with normal lymph nodes (Barral et al. 1992). In some patients, enlargement of the lymph nodes is the only sign of the infection; in these cases, organisms can be recovered from the nodes, but skin ulcers do not develop (Barral et al. 1995).

Leishmania aethiopica in Africa and members of the *braziliensis* group in the New World metastasize to the naso-oropharyngeal cartilages to produce the mucocutaneous form (*color plate* II *E–F*). This form of the disease is rare in Africa and the Middle East (Farge et al. 1987), but it occurs in up to 80% of untreated primary lesions in the New World, especially in infections with *L. braziliensis* causing espundia. Destruction of the cartilaginous structures of the nose and palate produces marked disfigurement. If the disease is not treated, death results from intercurrent infections or destruction of the pharynx. The pharynx is affected in combination with the nasal cartilages in about 42% of the cases; rarely is the larynx affected alone (Marsden et al. 1985).

Diffuse Cutaneous Leishmaniasis. *Leishmania aethiopica* and *L. tropica* (Abdel-Hameed et al. 1990) in the Old World and several species of cutaneous *Leishmania* in the New World are implicated in diffuse cutaneous leishmaniasis in anergic individuals. The infection starts as a single nodule, usually a small induration, that progresses locally with satellite lesions and soon with distant metastases. Multiple nonulcerating nodules resembling lepromatous leprosy occur

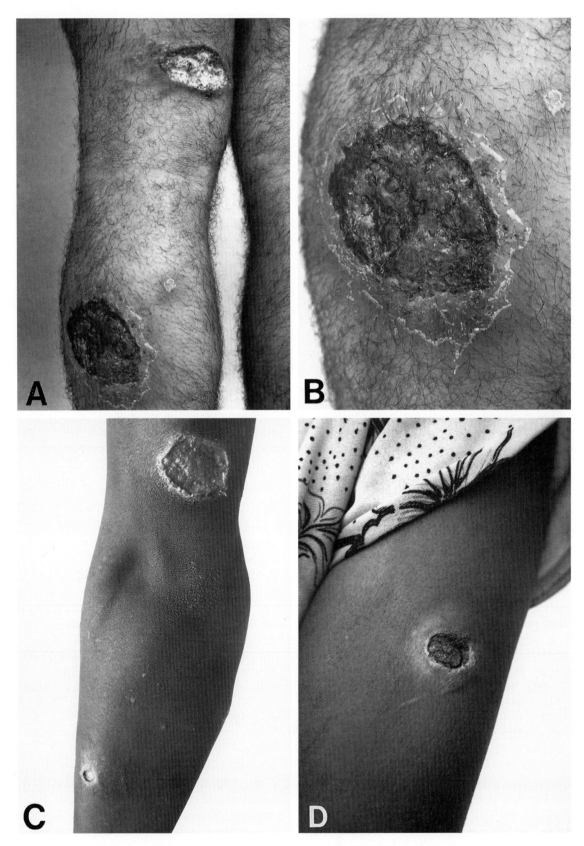

Fig. 4–4. Cutaneous leishmaniasis of approximately 1 month's duration. *A*, A 22-year-old man with leg ulcers; smears were positive, and cultures grew organisms in 5 days. *B*, Close-up view of the bottom ulcer. *C*, Two acute ulcers on a 19-year-old man who also had ulcerations on the forehead, ear, and back; imprints, smear, and cultures were positive. *D*, A 24-year old woman with an acute ulcer. (All patients studied at Tumaco, Colombia. CIDEIM, Cali, Colombia, Tulane University School of Public Health and Tropical Medicine, New Orleans, Louisiana.)

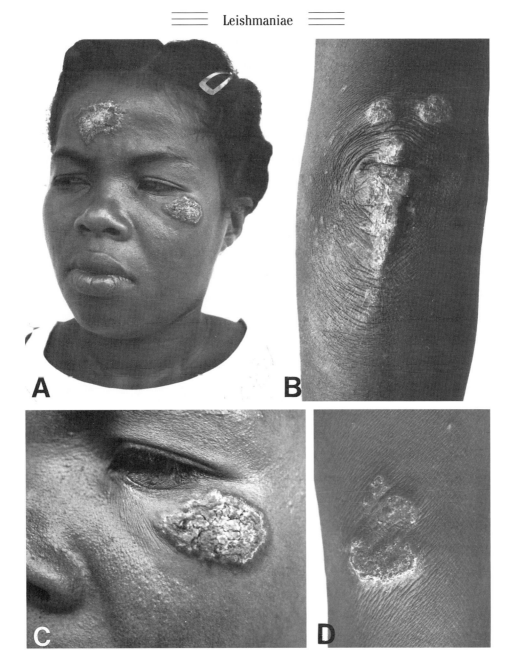

Fig. 4–5. Cutaneous leishmaniasis, crusty lesions. *A* and *C*, that evolves over 2 months, with a crust which sloughs off, exposing the ulcer. *B*. Lesion of 6 years' duration. D, Same person with another ulcer that evolved over 2 years. (Patients studied at Tumaco, Colombia. CIDEIM, Cali, Colombia, Tulane University School of Public Health and Tropical Medicine, New Orleans, Louisiana.)

over the body and face (Figs. 4–8 and 4–9 *A–B*). This lesion was previously attributed to a different species, *L. pifanoi*, described in Venezuela. Now, with the use of molecular speciation of isolates from these patients, it is known that several species on the American continent (if not all species) have the capacity to produce diffuse cutaneous lesions (Grimaldi et al. 1989). Diffuse cutaneous leishmaniasis runs a protracted course but does not ulcerate or visceralize. Also, in contrast to other dermal leishmaniases, antibodies are demonstrable but delayed hypersensitivity to leishmanial antigens is absent.

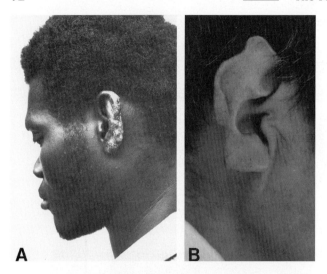

Fig. 4–6. Leishmaniasis of the ear. *A,* Acute ear ulcer (same individual shown in Fig. 4–4 *C*). *B,* Healed leishmaniasis of the ear showing loss of cartilage.

Leishmaniasis Recidivans. The tuberculoid type of cutaneous leishmaniasis, also known as *Leishmania recidivans,* is characterized by a chronic, scarring lesion and a small, advancing, actively ulcerated front. The lesion lasts for months or years and contains a small number of parasites that are difficult to detect (Fig. 4–10 *A–B*). In some cases of leishmaniasis recidivans produced by *L. braziliensis,* the immune response is atypical (Bittencourt et al. 1993).

Finally, cutaneous lesions in HIV-infected individuals are common; these will be discussed below (see *Leishmania* in HIV Infections).

Pathology. The histologic picture of cutaneous leishmaniasis is similar in all species of the New and Old Worlds. The basic lesion is granulomatous, consisting predominantly of a histiocytic infiltrate with a mixture of variable numbers of polymorphonuclear cells, lymphocytes, plasmacytoid cells, and plasma cells.

The early lesions in cutaneous leishmaniasis are aggregates of infected macrophages (histiocytes) resembling poorly formed granulomas with scanty to marked infiltration by lymphocytes and plasma cells. Interface dermatitis develops, extending into the base of the epidermis at first and later to the entire epidermis. This dermatitis is followed by disarray of epidermal cells with eventual necrosis, sloughing off of the epidermis (ulceration), and infiltration by polymorphonuclear cells (Fig. 4–11 *A–B*), usually due to superimposed infections. Dermal involvement develops at the same time, often extending to the deeper layers. A cellular infiltrate and sometimes granulomas are present within dermal collagen bundles and skin adnexa. Lesions with a crust usually have masses of dead epidermal cells on the surface and marked hyperplasia (acanthosis) and papillomatosis at the edge. The inflammatory infiltrate consists of parasitized histiocytes, and mononuclear cells permeate the papillomatous epidermal masses (Figs. 4–11 *C* and 4–12 *D*). Early lesions usually have large numbers of parasites that are easy to find.

The advanced lesion consists of a massive, diffuse histiocytic infiltrate in some areas arranged as poorly formed granulomas, with an abundant lymphoplasmacytic infiltrate (Fig. 4–12 *A–D*). In advanced leishmaniasis, ulceration usually extends from the epidermis into the subcutaneous tissues (Fig. 4–11 *B*), sometimes with mature granulomas and giant cells (Fig. 4–12 *B*). In most cases of cutaneous leishmaniasis there is focal necrosis, often only microscopic, in the dermis, epidermis, or both, with a polymorphonuclear cell infiltrate. In approximately 14% of the biopsy specimens from advanced lesions, intracellular amastigotes are detected in variable numbers, but usually they are scanty and difficult to find (Weigle et al. 1987).

The histologic study of enlarged satellite lymph nodes in cases of cutaneous leishmaniasis shows hyperplasia with focal necrosis, and abundant macrophages with amastigotes are easily found (Berger et al. 1985).

After months or years the ulcer starts to heal, granulation tissue develops, and a scar forms. Completely healed ulcers have some remaining scattered foci of lymphocytic infiltration with a few histiocytes. This process indicates that amastigotes have been controlled and eliminated within the lesion, and it suggests that ulcer formation play a role in the elimination of the parasite (Ridley, Ridley, 1983).

Mucocutaneous Lesions. Mucosal lesions are histologically different from those in the skin. They are characterized by an abundant lymphocytic and plasmacytic infiltrate with a few histiocytes and parasites. Destruction of the cartilaginous structures is evident.

Diffuse Cutaneous Leishmaniasis. Histologically, diffuse cutaneous leishmaniasis is characterized by a histiocytic nodule or *histiocytoma,* with little or no lymphocytic and plasmacytic infiltration (Fig. 4–13 *A–C*). All histiocytes contain loosely packed amastigotes, within large vacuoles (Fig. 4–13 *C–D*). The epidermis overlying the nodule does not ulcerate and appears stretched out, lacking rete pegs (papillae) (Fig. 4–13 *A–B*).

Diagnosis. Histologic proof of cutaneous leishmaniasis is based on finding and identifying the amastigotes

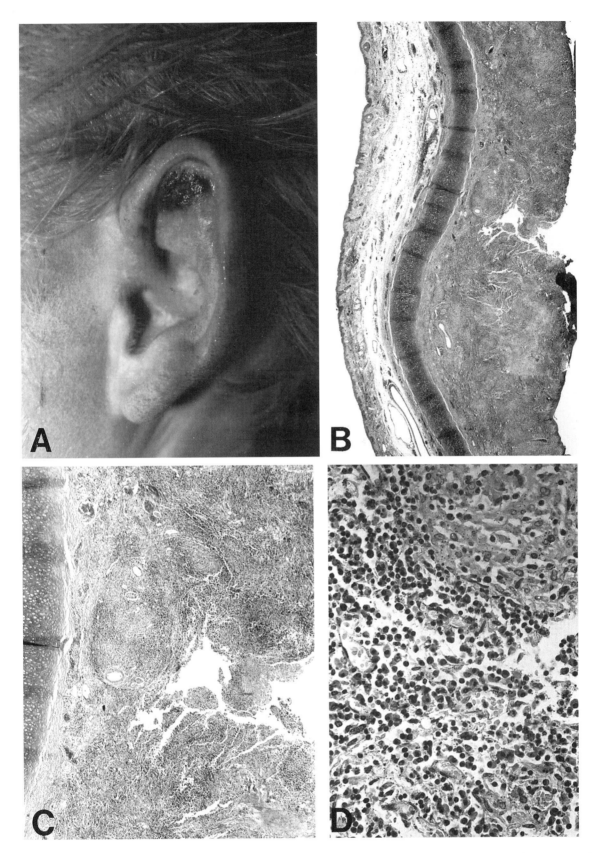

Fig. 4–7. *Leishmania mexicana*, acute ulcer. A 25-year-old archeology student who contracted chiclero's ulcer while excavating in Yucatan, Mexico, and died of a congenital heart condition; an autopsy was performed, and the ear helix was studied. *A*, Gross lesion. *B–D*, Different magnifications showing acute ulceration of the epidermis and dermis, not extending to the cartilage, and the typical histiocytic and mononuclear cell infiltrate; hematoxylin and eosin stain, *B* ×12, *C* ×28, *D* ×280.

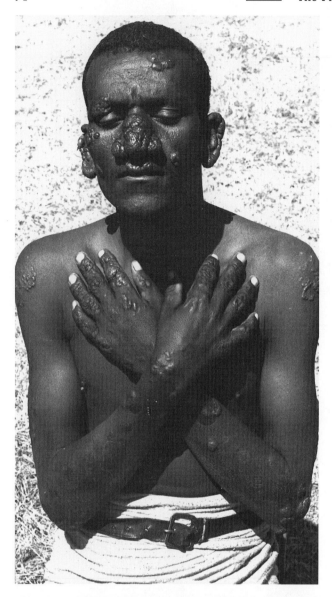

Fig. 4–8. Diffuse cutaneous leishmaniasis. Ethiopian man with multiple nodules over the face and body. (Courtesy of A. Bryceson, M.D., Hospital for Tropical Diseases, London, England.)

in tissues. In the absence of parasites, a histologic picture suggestive of leishmaniasis and a history of travel to endemic areas support the presumptive clinical diagnosis, but they are not proof of infection. Isolation and culture of parasites from the lesion is usually not done in the routine clinical laboratory. However, this procedure should be done if biochemical identification of the species of the parasite is desired, an endeavor undertaken by some specialized or research laboratories. In most cases, diagnosis of human leishmaniasis is based only on the morphologic appearance of the parasite, and clinicians treat their patients based on this information.

The role of the pathologist in the diagnosis of cutaneous leishmaniasis begins with a good understanding of how the lesions are sampled because often the pathologist needs to instruct the clinician (Fig. 4–14 A–C). The first sample should consist of material obtained with a 26-gauge needle on a disposable tuberculin syringe containing 0.1 ml of sterile saline. The needle is inserted intradermally into the border of the ulcer and parallel to it. The saline solution is injected and, without removing the syringe, the area of inoculation is massaged with the finger. The syringe, still in place, is rotated several times to disrupt the tissues, and the tissue fluid is gently aspirated into the needle hub. The syringe is finally withdrawn, hopefully containing a small amount of fluid. If cultures of the parasite are desirable, a drop of the removed fluid should be used to inoculate each of the culture tubes. At least 1 drop of fluid is used to prepare a smear on a slide.

The second sample is taken with a scalpel after anesthetizing a small area at the edge of the ulcer. Perpendicular to the border of the ulcer, a 3 mm long and 3 mm deep cut is made at the border of the ulcer. Tilting the scalpel blade 45° before removal scrapes the wall of the cut. The small amount of material recovered on the edge of the blade is used for a second smear.

The third set of samples consists of a punch biopsy specimen taken at the edge of the ulcer, including both the epidermis and the ulcer, and a tissue imprint of the biopsy specimen before it is fixed. All three slides (two smears, one imprint) should be fixed promptly in 100% alcohol, labeled, and, together with the fixed biopsy specimen, delivered to the laboratory for study (Escobar, Martinez, 1992; Palma, Gutierrez, 1991). Smears should be stained with Giemsa stain and the biopsy specimen processed for hematoxylin and eosin stain.

Smears and imprints are studied by experienced pathologists and technicians familiar with leishmaniae under medium and high dry objectives, and the identity of suspected organisms is confirmed under oil immersion. Sections of biopsy specimens stained with hematoxylin and eosin stain are studied in the usual manner, assessing the characteristics of the lesion first, then searching for the organisms with the high dry objective and using oil immersion for their identification. The typical morphology of the amastigotes should be recognized (see above) before a definitive identification is made. Immunoperoxidase stain is useful because it clearly reveals small numbers of organisms. Other special stains for tissue sections are not recommended unless other organisms need to be excluded. Several studies comparing the relative efficacy of these different

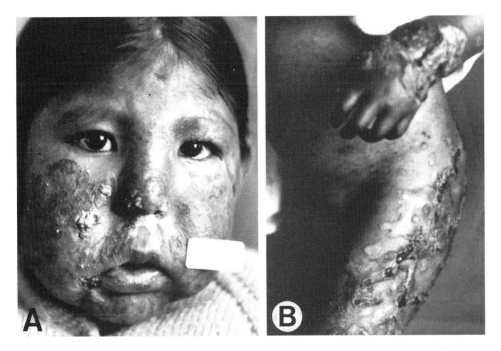

Fig. 4–9. Diffuse cutaneous leishmaniasis. *A* and *B*, Bolivian woman with lesions on the face and trunk. (Courtesy of M. Muños Vera, M.D., Instituto Boliviano de Biologia de las Alturas, Facultad de Medicina, La Paz, Bolivia.)

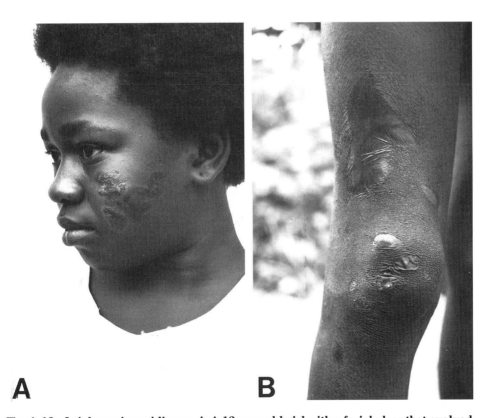

A   B

Fig. 4–10. *Leishmania* recidivans. *A*, A 12-year-old girl with a facial ulcer that evolved over 5 years. Note the scar and the small, active lesion, seen as a white crust. *B*, Young boy with an ulcer on his right leg evolving over several years. Note the upper scars and small, active lesion over the knee.

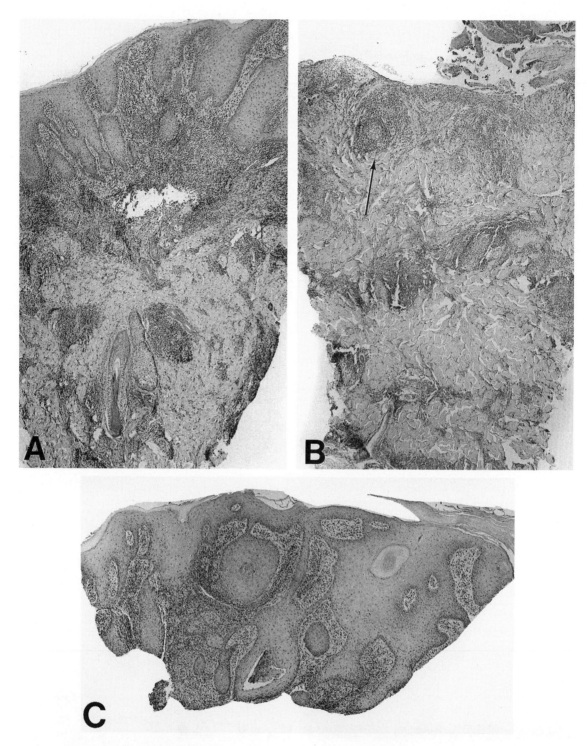

Fig. 4–11. Cutaneous leishmaniasis, low-power view of punch biopsy specimen from three individuals with active American leishmaniasis; hematoxylin and eosin stain. *A*, Section of a biopsy specimen without ulceration, with a marked inflammatory infiltrate of the dermis extending into the skin appendages. Note the interface dermatitis; no parasites were found. ×35. *B*, Section of a biopsy specimen showing a similar infiltrate, pseudogranuloma formation (arrow), and ulceration. Extension of the inflammatory infiltrate goes beyond the skin appendages. Few parasites were found, ×35. *C*, Section of a biopsy specimen from a nonulcerated lesion showing acanthosis and some papillomatosis. No parasites were seen, ×35. (CIDEIM, Cali, Colombia, Tulane University School of Public Health and Tropical Medicine, New Orleans, Louisiana.)

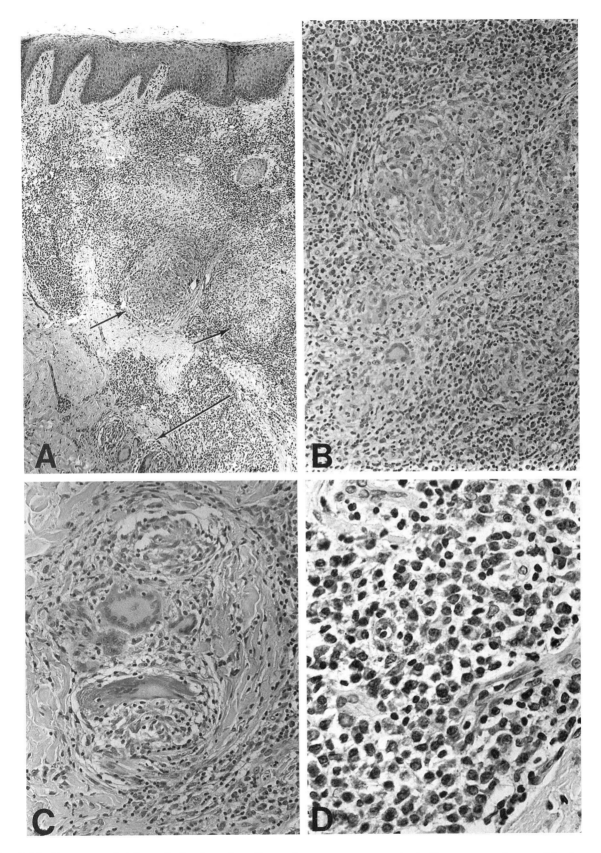

Fig. 4–12. Cutaneous leishmaniasis, hematoxylin and eosin stain. *A*, View of pseudogranulomas (short arrows), mature granulomas (long arrows), and a mononuclear cell infiltrate of the dermis, ×55. *B*. Granulomas and gi-ant cells, ×180. *C*, Mature granuloma with giant cells. No parasites were seen, ×180. *D*, Infiltrate by histiocytes, lymphocytes, plasmacytoid cells, and plasma cells, ×450.

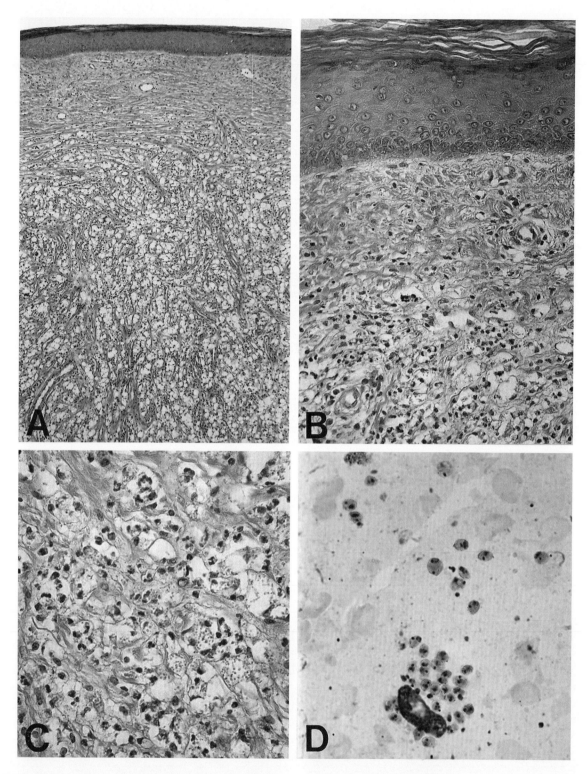

Fig. 4–13. Diffuse cutaneous leishmaniasis, hematoxylin and eosin stain, section of biopsy specimen from a histiocytoma. *A,* Low-power view shows the large number of vacuolated histiocytes infiltrating through the deeper layers of the dermis. Note the absence of rete pegs and the lymphoplasmacytic infiltrate, ×52. *B,* Upper layers of the dermis and epidermis with scanty lymphocytes, ×220. *C.* Higher magnification of the lower dermis showing masses of histiocytes with large vacuoles and numerous parasites, ×350. *D,* Typical imprint of a diffuse cutaneous leishmaniasis nodule showing one histiocyte with amastigotes, ×1120.

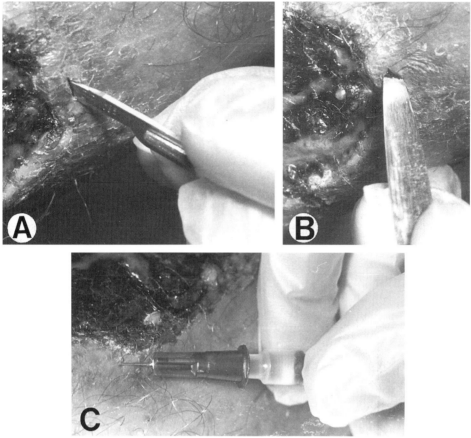

Fig. 4–14. Cutaneous leishmaniae. Methods for collecting necessary samples for diagnosis. See text for detailed explanation. (From Palma, G., and Gutierrez, Y. 1991. Laboratory diagnosis of *Leishmania*. Clin. Lab. Med. 11:909–922. Reproduced with permission.)

methods have been carried out, most of them in endemic areas, where the patient population under study usually presents with ulcers of weeks' to months' duration. In these conditions, recovery of parasites is low. In one study, the biopsy specimens were positive in 14% and the imprints in 19% of the cases (Weigle et al. 1987), both typical results in these kinds of studies. Patients seen in the United States and Europe who travel to endemic areas have much higher rates of positivity because the lesions are usually recently acquired at the time of consultation. The polymerase chain reaction for detection of *Leishmania* has been used on simple scrapings of skin with excellent results, obviating the need for collection of biopsy specimens or other, more invasive techniques (Belli et al. 1998).

The differential diagnosis of *Leishmania* includes *Trypanosoma cruzi*, which is seen in all types of cells (see Chapter 5); *Toxoplasma gondii*, which is also found in all cell types and stains positively with peri-odic acid–Schiff (see Chapter 9); and *Histoplasma*, which is seen in smears and tissue sections exclusively inside macrophages and stains with methenamine silver and periodic acid–Schiff stains.

At the electron microscopic level, differences among some species of *Leishmania* have been found, mainly the relative size of the amastigotes and the number of microtubules in the pellicle (Gardener et al. 1977; Kocan et al. 1983). Similar parameters have been useful in differentiating *Leishmania* from *T. cruzi* (Gardener, 1974).

Visceral Leishmaniasis

Geographic Distribution and Epidemiology. Visceral leishmaniasis is produced by several subspecies of

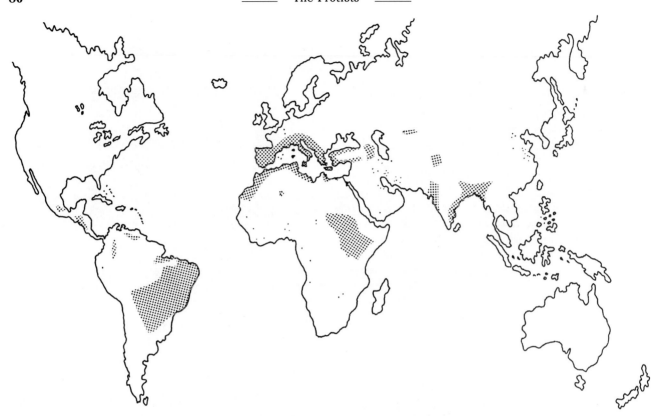

Fig. 4–15. Visceral leishmaniasis, geographic distribution. (Redrawn and reproduced with permission. WHO, 1984. The Leishmaniases. Tech. Rep. Ser. No. 701. World Health Organization, Geneva.)

Leishmania in the tropical and subtropical regions (Fig. 4–15), where the infection may be sporadic, endemic, or sometimes epidemic (WHO, 1984). Visceral leishmaniasis is overwhelmingly a zoonotic infection, and several animal are reservoirs of the infection. Only in a few areas is the infection transmitted in a human-vector-human cycle (Beaver et al. 1984). A focus of visceral leishmaniasis in dogs existing in Oklahoma (Anderson et al. 1989; McVean et al. 1979) is closely related, if not identical, to *L. infantum*, but no human cases in this area are known. Reports of prevalence rates of the infection are available only for limited areas; for example, in the area of Madrid, Spain, 8% of the population is skin test positive (Alvar et al. 1996). The transmission of visceral leishmaniae by blood transfusions (Luz et al. 1997) has been well documented in the past, and transmission due to the use of dirty needles by intravenous drug users has recently been reported (Alvar et al. 1996). In Brazil, a survey of blood donors revealed a prevalence of 9% of antibodies to visceral leishmaniae; in a group of patients with multiple hemodialysis the percentage was 25% (Luz et al. 1997). The species of *Leishmania* produc-

ing visceral leishmaniasis in humans are as follows (Fig. 4–15):

a. *Leishmania donovani* occurs mostly in the Indian continent, producing kala-azar in a human-vector-human cycle without mammalian reservoirs. Endemic countries are East Pakistan, India, Nepal, and China (the north China Plains and east China)

b. *Leishmania infantum*, or Mediterranean visceral leishmaniasis, has dogs as reservoirs in the Mediterranean and Middle East regions. In the Mediterranean basin, it often produces skin lesions. Endemic areas are Europe (Albania, Bosnia, Croatia, France, Greece, Hungary, Italy, Macedonia, Montenegro, Portugal, Romania, Slovenia, Spain, and Yugoslavia); Central Asia (Afghanistan, Armenia, Azerbaijan, Georgia, Kazakhstan, Kirgizia, Tadjikistan, Turkey, Turkmenistan, and Uzbekistan); China (in the northwest); Middle East (Iran, Iraq, Saudi Arabia, South Yemen, and Yemen); and Africa (Algeria, Central African Republic, Chad, Democratic Republic of Congo, Egypt, Gabon, Libya, Malawi, Niger, Nigeria, Tunisia, Upper Volta, and Zambia).

c. *Leishmania archibaldi* in East Africa has wild animals as reservoirs. Endemic countries are Ethiopia (east and south) and probably the Central African Republic, Chad, Democratic Republic of Congo, Djibouti, Niger, Somalia, and Sudan,

d. *Leishmania chagasi*, producing American visceral leishmaniasis, mostly in children, has been conclusively identified in a few places, but the disease is known in many countries of South and Central America. In Honduras *L. chagasi* produces cutaneous lesions, apparently in high numbers (Noyes et al. 1997), and in Brazil at least one case of cutaneous involvement has been described (Oliveira Neto et al. 1986). The parasite has wild and domestic reservoir animals. Endemic countries are Argentina, Bolivia, Brazil, Colombia, Ecuador, El Salvador, Guadeloupe, Guatemala, Honduras, Martinique, Mexico, Paraguay, Surinam, and Venezuela.

Clinical Findings. The clinical picture of visceral leishmaniasis is variable, depending on the species involved and the immunologic status of the host. In endemic visceral leishmaniasis of the Mediterranean area, southwest Asia, China, and Latin America, the 1- to 4-year age group is principally affected, boys twice as often as girls. In Africa and India the peak age is between 5 and 9 years, but the disease also occurs in older children. The incubation period of visceral leishmaniasis can be as short as 10 days or as long as 25 years, indicating that many infections are silent.

The most common symptoms of visceral leishmaniasis are chronic fever, malaise, anorexia, weight loss, and discomfort in the left hypocondrium due to enlargement of the spleen. Diarrhea and cough may be present. The usual sign of the infection is non-tender enlargement of the spleen and liver, sometimes to large proportions (Fig. 4–16). A cutaneous nodule, a skin ulcer, or a mucosal lesion (at the inoculation site) is present in some individuals, especially in the African continent. In India, darkening of the skin of the face, hands, feet, and abdomen is common, hence the name *kala-azar* (black sickness). Hypergammaglobulinemia and leukopenia are common. In a chronic infection in a child that was refractory to treatment, the parasites entered the cerebrospinal fluid and apparently produced meningitis because the disease responded to specific treatment. The exact location of the parasites in the central nervous system remains unknown (Prasad, Sen, 1996).

In sporadic visceral leishmaniasis, the person most commonly affected is the new arrival to the endemic area, a situation in which any person, regardless of age, is susceptible to the infection. In these cases the infec-

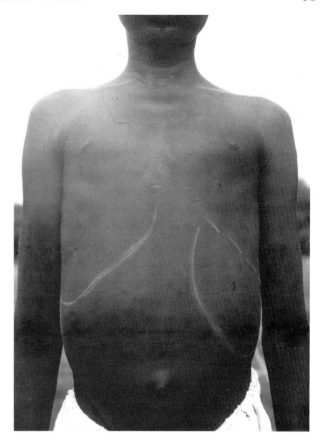

Fig. 4–16. Visceral leishmaniasis. A 14-year-old Sudanese boy with massive hepatosplenomegaly who died of his disease 6 weeks after this photo was taken. (Courtesy of B. Veress, M.D., Ph.D., Karolinska Institutet, Huddinge, Sweden.)

tion begins 3 weeks to 3 years after exposure, with sudden fever and progression of the disease to acute chills and high, undulating fever with two daily peaks. In these patients, the disease runs a more rapid course with wasting, intercurrent infections, severe hemolytic anemia, renal failure, and a hemorrhagic diathesis. In the Indian subcontinent, one to several years after an apparent cure, some individuals develop dermal leishmaniasis after kala-azar. These lesions consist of multiple nodules without ulceration anywhere in the body, sometimes resembling leprosy (Dhar et al. 1995). Hypopigmented macules or erythematous areas may also evolve into nodular lesions.

Leishmaniasis in HIV Infections. The great majority of cases of visceral leishmaniasis in individuals with HIV/acquired immune deficiency syndrome (AIDS) are due to *L. infantum* (Berenguer et al. 1989) in southern Europe (Alvar et al. 1989) and eastern Africa

(Ethiopia). In addition, other countries in the Middle East, Africa, and Latin America have reported visceral leishmaniasis in the AIDS population. It is estimated that in Europe 1.5% to 9.0% of HIV-infected individuals will develop the disease (Alvar, 1994; Anonymous, 1997), and 25% to 70% of cases of visceral leishmaniasis now seen in these areas occur in AIDS patients (Anonymous, 1997). Some believe that transmission of the disease through the use of dirty needles by drug users is common in the area (Alvar et al. 1992; Anonymous, 1997). The lack of reported cases from other endemic areas is probably due to decreased awareness of the infection, lack of diagnostic facilities, or both. The clinical manifestations of visceral leishmaniasis in individuals with HIV/AIDS resemble those described above (Alvar, 1994; Montalban et al. 1989), with fewer patients having splenomegaly, with absent antibody titers, and with many infections refractory to treatment (Alvar et al. 1989; Peters et al. 1990). In addition, other distinct features are seen: the presence of cutaneous lesions, parasites at unusual locations (Del Giudice, 1996), a tendency for the disease to reappear after apparently successful treatment (Alvar, 1994), and relative ease of diagnosis because the lesions contain large numbers of organisms. Mortality is high, about 40% in some series (Montalban et al. 1989), and the disease may develop long before full-blown AIDS (Berenguer et al. 1989).

The cutaneous lesions consist of papules or discrete, asymptomatic infiltrates that develop before or after the appearance of visceral disease. Sometimes the parasites are found in herpes zoster lesions (Barrio et al. 1996; Del Giudice, 1996), or in Kaposi's sarcoma (Perrin et al. 1995; Yebra et al. 1988), or are recovered from a scraping of normal skin (Rab et al. 1992). Recrudescence occurs in about 42% (Montalban et al. 1989) to 50% (Cabie et al. 1992) of the patients. There are two or three repeat infections per patient, but there may be many more, and their number correlates with mortality (Montalban et al. 1989).

The most commonly affected organ in visceral leishmaniasis in AIDS patients is the gastrointestinal tract, with lesions seen from the esophagus to the rectum. In some instances, the infection is limited to ulcerations of the oral cavity and tonsils (Michiels et al. 1994). In the esophagus it produces dysphagia (Datry et al. 1990) or esophagitis (Villanueva et al. 1994), and in the stomach it leads to gastric ulcers (Coppola et al. 1992). The duodenum and jejunum may have severe villous atrophy, with resultant malabsorption (Altes et al. 1991) or duodenitis alone (Datry et al. 1990; Michiels et al. 1992). In some cases, several regions of the intestine are involved (Zimmer et al. 1996). Finally, in the rectum, *Leishmania* produced an enlarging mass that protruded through the anus (Rosenthal et al. 1988).

Outside the intestinal tract, interstitial pneumonitis has been reported (Duarte et al. 1989), as well as pleuritis with effusion (Chenoweth et al. 1993), pleuropulmonary disease (Cabie et al. 1992), and solitary nodules in the larynx (Marsden et al. 1985). In at least one case there was a nodular regenerative hyperplasia of the liver (Fernandez-Miranda et al. 1993), and in another the appearance of polyarthritis, with parasites recovered from the synovial fluid of the wrist (Pearson, Steigbigel, 1981).

Pathology. The most remarkable gross change produced by classic visceral leishmaniasis are the enormous enlargement of the liver, spleen, and lymph nodes. In adult patients, the size of the liver averages 1700 g and, in some instances, more than 4500 g. The cut surface is pale to yellow, with a fatty appearance and a fine, diffuse infiltrate, making the normal lobular pattern difficult to appreciate. The average spleen weighs 880 g; a weight of 4800 g has been recorded. The consistency of the organ is increased due to fibrosis, especially in chronic cases, and infarcts are common. The cut surface is hyperemic, with prominent malpighian corpuscles. The affected lymph nodes appear enlarged, with a whitish, uniform infiltrate on cut section.

Microscopically, the gross change is a massive infiltration of histiocytes containing amastigotes (Fig. 4–17 C). The normal architecture of the liver is disrupted by a large number of parasitized histiocytes (macrophages and Kupffer cells) in the sinusoids (Fig. 4–17 A–B). The parenchymal cells are mostly normal, sometimes with fatty changes. The portal triads have parasitized histiocytes and mononuclear cell infiltrates, often accompanied by bile duct proliferation and slight fibrosis (Fig. 4–17 A). Granulomas in the liver of humans (Andrade, Andrade, 1966) similar to those in experimental animals have been recorded (Fig. 4–17 D; Gutierrez et al. 1984).

The spleen is hyperemic, with large numbers of parasitized histiocytes in the white and red pulp and within the trabeculae. Infiltration by plasma cells is common and polymorphonuclear cells are abundant, especially if intercurrent bacterial infections occur before death. The splenic white pulp is significantly reduced, often with necrosis and fibrosis of the T cell–dependent areas (Veress et al. 1977). Accumulation of dense periodic acid–Schiff–positive material in the interstitium of

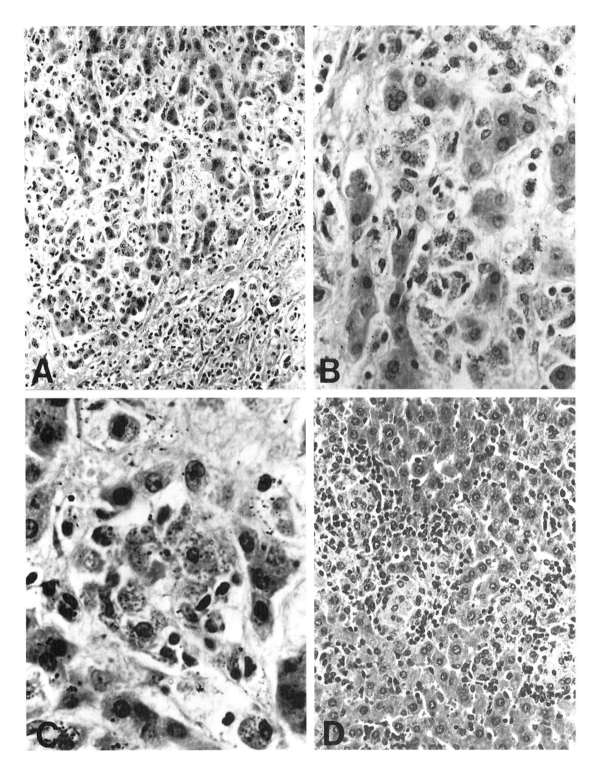

Fig. 4–17. Visceral leishmaniasis in liver, hematoxylin and eosin stain. *A*, Low-power view showing disarrangement of the hepatic architecture by a marked histiocytic infiltrate. Note the normal appearance of the hepatocytes, fibrosis of the portal triad at the lower right, and the scanty lymphocytic infiltrate, ×180. *B* and *C*, Higher magnification showing numerous parasitized histiocytes and a few infiltrating lymphocytes, *B* ×450, *C* ×700. *D*, A 4-week-old experimental infection of BALB/c mice with *L. donovani*. The liver shows several poorly formed granulomas, with histiocytes containing parasites, not appreciable at this magnification, ×240.

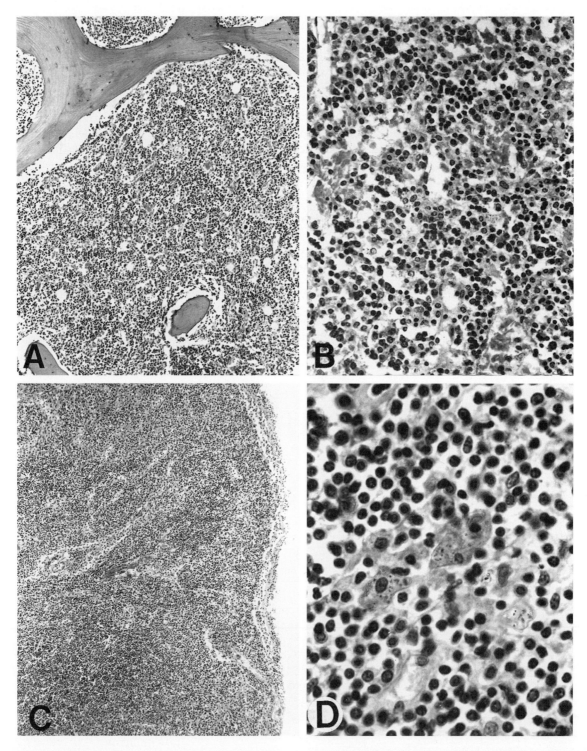

Fig. 4–18. Visceral leishmaniasis in bone marrow and lymph node, hematoxylin and eosin stain. *A*, Bone marrow illustrating hyperplasia of marrow elements with obliteration of fat cells, ×70. *B*, Higher magnification showing both myeloid and erythroid elements with a few parasitized histiocytes, not appreciable at this magnification, ×280. *C*, Lymph node with effacement of lymphoid follicles, ×55. *D*, Higher magnification showing normal lymphocytes with a few histiocytes containing amastigotes, ×705.

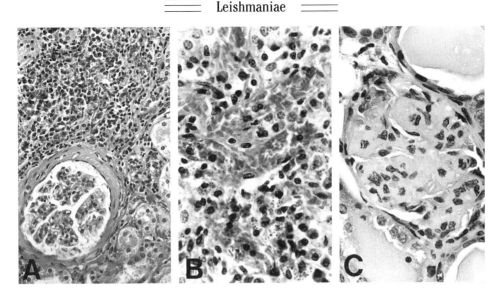

Fig. 4–19. **Visceral leishmaniasis in kidney, hematoxylin and eosin stain.** *A*, Infiltration of renal interstitium by mononuclear cells, ×153. *B*, Higher magnification showing many parasitized histiocytes, ×383. *C*, Guinea pig experimentally infected with *L. donovani*. Marked glomerulonephritis and sclerosis due to amyloid deposition, ×238.

the follicles has been noted. The lymph nodes appear either diffusely infiltrated, with loss of the normal follicular architecture, or hyperplastic, with a normal follicular pattern (Fig. 4–18 *C–D*). The bone marrow has myeloid hyperplasia, decreased numbers of fat cells, and variable numbers of parasitized macrophages (Fig. 4–18 *A–B*). Severely anemic individuals often have extramedullary hemopoiesis, and leukopenia may develop terminally. In treated patients, despite the disappearance of parasites from the liver and spleen, organisms may still be present in the bone marrow.

Finally, small numbers of parasites can be found in almost any tissue in the interstitium, where macrophage infiltrates may occur (Fig. 4–19 *A–B*). In the lungs, an interstitial pneumonitis has been described (Duarte et al. 1989). The kidneys may have an interstitial nephritis (Duarte et al. 1983) or glomerulonephritis with expansion of the mesangium and the basement membrane (Brito et al. 1975) due to accumulation of immune complexes. Guinea pigs infected experimentally develop mesangial proliferative glomerulonephritis with exuberant amyloid deposition (Fig. 4–19 *C*) (Oliveira et al. 1985).

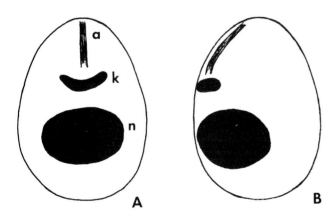

Fig. 4–20. *Leishmania* **amastigote morphology seen in the dorsoventral view** (*A*) **and the lateral view** (*B*). Abbreviations: a, axoneme; k, kinetoplast; n, nucleus.

Diagnosis. The morphologic diagnosis of visceral leishmaniasis is based on the characteristics of cutaneous leishmaniasis (see above) and is made on biopsy material, either from liver, bone marrow, lymph nodes, or other organs. The hallmark of the infection is the presence of macrophages with intracellular amastigotes morphologically indistinguishable from those found in cutaneous leishmaniasis (Figs. 4–20 and 4–21; *color plates* II *H–J* and III *A–B*). Imprints of tissues and bone marrow smears stained with Giemsa stain are best for morphologic identification (*color plate* III *A–B*). Results obtained with Wright stains used in modern automated hematology laboratories comparable to those obtained with Giemsa stains. Cultures in media for leishmaniae usually give positive results in a few days, depending on the number of organisms in the inoculum, and are useful for

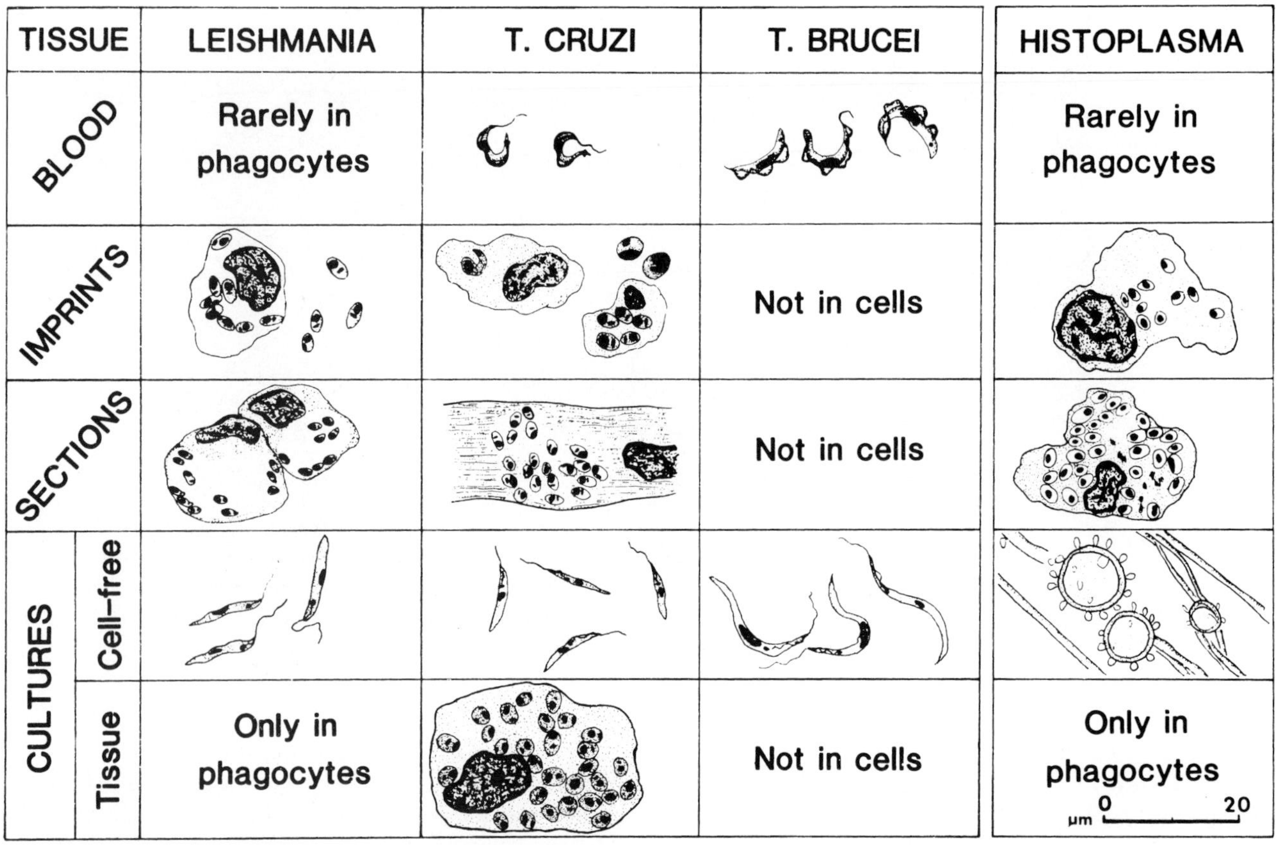

TISSUE	LEISHMANIA	T. CRUZI	T. BRUCEI	HISTOPLASMA
BLOOD	Rarely in phagocytes			Rarely in phagocytes
IMPRINTS			Not in cells	
SECTIONS			Not in cells	
CULTURES — Cell-free				
CULTURES — Tissue	Only in phagocytes		Not in cells	Only in phagocytes

μm 0 — 20

Fig. 4–21. *Leishmania* and *Trypanosoma*, diagnostic stages found in humans and their comparison with *Histoplasma*. All drawings made from photographs identical in magnification. Note that the amastigotes in imprints and tissue cultures appear to be almost twice as large as those in tissue sections.

biochemical identification of the species. Immunoperoxidase is also recommended and gives good results (*color plate* II G).

In the great majority of cases, the diagnosis of leishmaniasis in patients with HIV infection is based on bone marrow or skin biopsy specimens. In bone marrow, the parasites reportedly range from scanty to numerous and easy to detect. In general, biopsy specimens from HIV-infected individuals with leishmanial lesions show abundant organisms. The parasites are usually found in circulating blood, permitting new modalities of diagnosis in the clinical laboratory. Examination of peripheral blood smears shows organisms in one-half of the cases (Fillola et al. 1992; Martinez et al. 1993; Medrano et al. 1993), and smears made from the buffy coat of heparinized blood samples or in leukoconcentrates reveal the parasites (Izri et al. 1993). Bronchoalveolar lavage fluid (Peters et al. 1990) and pleural fluid, made into cell blocks or in smears (Chenoweth et al. 1993), are also used.

The immunodiagnosis of visceral leishmaniasis has been reviewed, with emphasis on visceral leishmaniasis and on visceral lesions produced by *L. tropica* (Reed, 1996). Serologic tests (Delgado et al. 1996; Dye et al. 1993), enzyme-linked immunosorbent assay (El Amin El Roufaie Mohammed et al. 1986; Jensen et al. 1996; Srivastava, Singh, 1988), polymerase chain reaction (Delgado et al. 1996; Piarroux et al. 1994), the indirect fluorescent antibody test, and direct agglutination have been used mostly for diagnosis of visceral leishmaniasis, but these technologies are not yet available in routine clinical laboratories (Nigro et al. 1996; Palma, Gutierrez, 1991). A polymerase chain reaction enzyme-linked immunosorbent assay using bone marrow and blood has been tested for diagnosis in patients infected with HIV (Costa et al. 1996). Detection of amastigote antigens in the urine of patients infected with visceral leishmaniasis, using a Western blot technique, is also a method of diagnosis (de Colmenares et al. 1995).

References

Abdel-Hameed AA, Ahmed BO, Mohamedani AA, El-Harith A, Van Eys G, 1990. A case of diffuse cutaneous leishmaniasis due to *Leishmania major*. Trans. R. Soc. Trop. Med. Hyg. 84:535–536

Akuffo H, Maasho K, Blostedt M, Hojeberg B, Britton S, Bakhiet M, 1997. *Leishmania aethiopica* derived from diffuse leishmaniasis patients preferentially induce mRNA for interleukin-10 while those from localized leishmaniasis patients induce interferon-gamma. J. Infect. Dis. 175:737–741

Al-Gindan Y, Kubba R, El-Hassan AM, Omer AHS, Kutty MK, Saeed MBM, 1989. Dissemination in cutaneous leishmaniasis 3. Lymph node involvement. Int. J. Dermatol. 28:248–254

Almeida MC, Cuba Cuba CA, Moraes MA, Miles MA, 1996. Dissemination of *Leishmania* (*Viannia*) *braziliensis*. J. Comp. Pathol. 115:311–316

Altes J, Salas A, Llomparta A, Obrador A, 1991. Small intestinal involvement in visceral leishmaniasis. Am. J. Gastroenterol. 86:1283

Alvar J, 1994. Leishmaniasis and AIDS co-infection: the Spanish example. Parasitol. Today 10.160–163

Alvar J, Blazquez J, Najera R, 1989. Correspondence. Association of visceral leishmaniasis and human immunodeficiency virus infections. J. Infect. Dis. 160: 560–561

Alvar J, Gutierrez Solar B, Molina R, Lopez Velez R, Garcia Camacho A, Martinez P, Laguna F, Cercenado E, Galmes A, 1992. Correspondence. Prevalence of *Leishmania* infection among AIDS patients. Lancet 339:1427–1427

Alvar J, Gutierrez Solar B, Pachon I, Calbacho E, Ramirez M, Valles R, Guillen JL, Canavate C, Amela C, 1996. AIDS and *Leishmania infantum*. New approaches for a new epidemiological problem. Clin. Dermatol. 14:541–546

Anderson DC, Buckner RG, Glenn BL, MacVean DW, 1989. Endemic canine leishmaniasis. Vet. Pathol. 17:94–96

Andrade ZA, Andrade SG, 1966. Alguns novos aspectos da patologia do calazar (estudo morfologico de 13 casos necropsiados). Rev. Inst. Med. Trop. Sao Paulo 8: 259–266

Anonymous, 1997. *Leishmania*/HIV co-infection. Epidemiological analysis of 692 retrospective cases. Weekly Epidemiol. Rec. WHO 72:49–54

Antoine JC, 1995. Co-stimulatory activity of *Leishmania*-infected macrophages. Parasitol. Today 11:242–243

Ary RA, Zeledon R, Hidalgo W, 1964. Un caso de leishmaniasis verrucosa diseminada por probable intervencion de corticoides curado cn glucantime Un caso de leishmaniasis verrucosa diseminada por probable intervencion de corticoides curado cn glucantime. Acta Med. Costar. 7:105–111

Ayadi A, Loukil M, Lakhoua R, Boubaker S, Debbabi A, Ben Rachid SB, Jedidi H, 1992. A propos d'un cas de manifestations cutanees au cours du kala-azar infantile mediterraneen. Ann. Pediatr. 39:265–267

Azadeh B, 1985. "Localized" *Leishmania* lymphadenitis: a light and electron microscopic study. Am. J. Trop. Med. Hyg. 34:447–455

Bacellar O, Barral Netto M, Badaro R, Carvalho EM, 1991. Gamma interferon production by lymphocytes from children infected with *L. chagasi*. Braz. J. Med. Biol. Res. 24:791–795

Barral A, Barral-Netto M, Almeida R, De Jesus AR, Grimaldi JRG, Netto EM, Santos I, Bacellar O, Carvalho EM, 1992. Lymphadenopathy associated with *Leishmania braziliensis* cutaneous infection. Am. J. Trop. Med. Hyg. 47:587–592

Barral A, Guerreiro J, Bomfim G, Correia D, Barral-Netto M, Carvalho EM, 1995. Lymphadenopathy as the first sign of human cutaneous infection by *Leishmania braziliensis*. Am. J. Trop. Med. Hyg. 53:256–259

Barrio J, Lecona M, Cosin J, Olalquiaga FJ, Hernanz JM, Soto J, 1996. *Leishmania* infection occurring in herpes zoster lesions in an HIV-positive patient. Br. J. Dermatol. 134:164–166

Beaver PC, Jung RC, Cupp EW, 1984. *Clinical Parasitology*. Philadelphia: Lea & Febiger

Belli A, Rodriguez B, Aviles H, Harris E, 1998. Simplified polymerase chain reaction detection of New World *Leishmania* in clinical specimens of cutaneous leishmaniasis. Am. J. Trop. Med. Hyg. 58:102–109

Berenguer J, Moreno S, Cercenado E, Bernaldo de Quiros JC, Garcia de la Fuente A, Bouza E, 1989. Visceral leishmaniasis in patients infected with human immunodeficiency virus (HIV). Ann. Intern. Med. 111:129–132

Berger TG, Meltzer MS, Oster CN, 1985. Lymph node involvement in leishmaniasis. J. Am. Acad. Dermatol. 12: 993–996

Bittencourt AL, Costa JM, Carvalho EM, Barral A, 1993. Leishmaniasis recidiva cutis in American cutaneous leishmaniasis. Int. J. Dermatol. 32:802–805

Bogdan C, Rollinghoff M, Solbach W, 1990. Evasion strategies of *Leishmania* parasites. Parasitol. Today 6:183–187

Bonfante Garrido R, Barroeta S, de Alejos MA, Melendez E, Torrealba J, Valdivia O, Momen H, Grimaldi G Jr, 1996. Disseminated American cutaneous leishmaniasis. Int. J. Dermatol. 35:561–565

Brito TD, Hoshino-Shimizu S, Amato Neto V, Duarte IS, Penna DO, 1975. Glomerular involvement in human kala-azar: a light, immunofluorescent, and electron microscopic study based on kidney biopsies. Am. J. Trop. Med. Hyg. 24:9–18

Cabie A, Matheron S, Lepretre A, Bouchaud O, Deluol AM, Coulaud JP, 1992. Leishmaniose viscerale au cours de l'infection par VIH. Une infection opportuniste a part entiere. Presse Med. 21:1658–1662

Carvalho EM, Badaro R, Reed SG, Jones TC, Johnson WD Jr, 1985. Absence of gamma interferon and interleukin 2 production during active visceral leishmaniasis. J. Clin. Invest. 76:2066–2069

Chang KP, 1983. Cellular and molecular mechanisms of intracellular symbiosis in leishmaniasis. Int. Rev. Cytol. 14 (Suppl):267–305

Chang KP, Dwyer DM, 1976. Multiplication of a human parasite (*Leishmania donovani*) in phagolysosomes of hamster macrophages in vitro. Science 193:678–680

Chatterjee SN, Sen Gupta PC, 1970. Ultrastructure of the promastigote of *Leishmania donovani*. Indian J. Med. Res. 58:70–76

Chenoweth CE, Singal S, Pearson RD, Betts RF, Markovitz DM, 1993. Acquired immunodeficiency syndrome-related visceral leishmaniasis presenting in a pleural effusion. Chest 103:648–649

Coppola F, Recchia S, Ferrari A, Del Sedime L, 1992. Visceral leishmaniasis in AIDS with gastric involvement. Gastrointest. Endosc. 38:76–78

Costa JM, Durand R, Deniau M, Rivollet D, Izri M, Houin R, Vidaud M, Bretagne S, 1996. PCR enzyme-linked immunosorbent assay for diagnosis of leishmaniasis in human immunodeficiency virus–infected patients. J. Clin. Microbiol. 34:1831–1833

Creemers J, Jadin JM, 1967. Etude de l'ultrastructure et de la biologie de *Leishmania mexicana* Biagi, 1953. Bull. Soc. Pathol. Exot. 60:53–58

Cupolillo E, Grimaldi JG, Momen H, 1994. A general classification of new world *Leishmania* using numerical zymotaxonomy. Am. J. Trop. Med. Hyg. 50:296–311

Datry A, Similowski T, Jais P, Rosenheim M, Katlama C, Maheu E, Kazaz S, Fassin D, Danis M, Gentilini M, 1990. AIDS-associated leishmaniasis: an unusual gastro-duodenal presentation. Trans. R. Soc. Trop. Med. Hyg. 84:239–240

Davies CR, Llanos Cuentas EA, Pyke SD, Dye C, 1995. Cutaneous leishmaniasis in the Peruvian Andes: an epidemiological study of infection and immunity. Epidemiol. Infect. 114:297–318

de Beer P, El Harith A, Deng LL, Semiao-Santos SJ, Chantal B, van Grootheest M, 1991. A killing disease epidemic among displaced Sudanese population identified as visceral leishmaniasis. Am. J. Trop. Med. Hyg. 44:283–289

de Colmenares M, Portus M, Riera C, Gallego M, Aisia MJ, Torras S, Munoz C, 1995. Detection of 72–75-kD and 123-kD fractions of *Leishmania* antigen in urine of patients with visceral leishmaniasis. Am. J. Trop. Med. Hyg. 52:427–428

Del Giudice P, 1996. Correspondence. *Leishmania* infection occurring in herpes zoster lesions in an HIV positive patient. Br. J. Dermatol. 135:1005–1006

Delgado O, Guevaara P, Silva S, Belfort E, Ramirez JL, 1996. Follow-up of a human accidental infection by *Leishmania (Viannia) braziliensis* using conventional immunologic techniques and polymerase chain reaction. Am. J. Trop. Med. Hyg. 55:267–272

Dhar S, Kaur I, Dawn G, Sehgal S, Kumar B, 1995. Post-kala-azar dermal leishmaniasis mimicking leprosy: experience with 4 patients, with some unusual features in 1. Lepr. Rev. 66:250–256

Duarte MIS, da Matta VLR, Corbett CEP, Laurenti MD, Chebabo R, Goto H, 1989. Interstitial pneumonitis in human visceral leishmaniasis. Trans. R. Soc. Trop. Med. Hyg. 83:73–76

Duarte MIS, Silva MRR, Goto H, Nicodemo EL, Amato-Neto V, 1983. Interstitial nephritis in human kala-azar. Trans. R. Soc. Trop. Med. Hyg. 77:531–537

Dye C, Vidor E, Dereure J, 1993. Serological diagnosis of leishmaniasis: on detecting infection as well as disease. Epidemiol. Infect. 110:647–656

Dye C, Wolpert DM, 1988. Earthquakes, influenza and cycles of Indian kala-azar. Trans. R. Soc. Trop. Med. Hyg. 82:843–850

El Amin El Roufaie Mohammed, Wright EP, Abdel Rahman AM, Kolk A, Laarman JJ, Pondman KW, 1986. Serodiagnosis of Sudanese visceral and mucosal leishmaniasis: comparison of ELISA-immunofluorescence and indirect haemagglutination. Trans. R. Soc. Trop. Med. Hyg. 80:271–274

Escobar MA, Martinez F, 1992. American cutaneous and mucocutaneous leishmaniasis (tegumentary): a diagnostic challenge. Tropical Doctor 22:69–78

Farge D, Frances C, Vouldoukis I, Wechsler B, Boisnic S, Monjour L, Godeau P, 1987. Chronic destructive ulcerative lesion of the midface and nasal cavity due to leishmaniasis contracted in Djibouti. Clin. Exp. Dermatol. 12:211–213

Fernandez-Miranda C, Colina F, Delgado JM, Lopez-Carreira M, 1993. Diffuse nodular regenerative hyperplasia of the liver associated with human immunodeficiency virus and visceral leishmaniasis. Am. J. Gastroenterol. 88:433–435

Fillola G, Corberand JX, Laharrague PF, Levenes H, Massip P, Recco P, 1992. Peripheral intramonocytic leishmanias in an AIDS patient. J. Clin. Microbiol. 30:3284–3285

Forteza Bover G, Baguena Candela J, Barbera Guillem E, Baguena Candela R, Forteza Vila G, 1968. Estudio con el microscopio electronico de la "*Leishmania donovani*". Sangre 13:9–30

Gardener PJ, 1974. Pellicle-associated structures in the amastigote stage of *Trypanosoma cruzi* and *Leishmania* species. Ann. Trop. Med. Parasitol. 68:167–176

Gardener PJ, Shchory L, Chance ML, 1977. Species differentiation in the genus *Leishmania* by morphometric studies with the electron microscope. Ann. Trop. Med. Parasitol. 71:147–155

Gradoni L, Gramiccia M, 1994. *Leishmania infantum* tropism: strain genotype of host immune status? Parasitol. Today 10:264–267

Grimaldi G Jr, David JR, McMahon-Pratt D, 1987. Identification and distribution of New World *Leishmania* species characterized by serodeme analysis using monoclonal antibodies. Am. J. Trop. Med. Hyg. 36:270–287

Grimaldi G Jr, McMahon-Pratt D, 1996. Monoclonal antibodies for the identification of New World *Leishmania* species. Mem. Inst. Oswaldo Cruz 91:37–42

Grimaldi G Jr, Tesh RB, McMahon-Pratt D, 1989. A review of the geographic distribution and epidemiology of leishmaniasis in the New World. Am. J. Trop. Med. Hyg. 41:687–725

Gustafson TL, Reed CM, McGreery PB, Pappas MG, Fox JC, Lawyer PG, 1985. Human cutaneous leishmaniasis acquired in Texas. Am. J. Trop. Med. Hyg. 34:58–63

Gutierrez Y, Maksem JA, Reiner NE, 1984. Pathologic changes in murine leishmaniasis (*Leishmania donovani*) with special reference to the dynamics of granuloma formation in the liver. Am. J. Pathol. 114:222–230

Izri MA, Robineau M, Petithory JC, Rousset JJ, 1993. Leishmaniose viscerale. Diagnostic parasitologique par leuco-concentration. Presse Med. 22:1010

Jensen AT, Gaafar A, Ismail A, Christensen CB, Kemp M, Hassan AM, Kharazmi A, Theander TG, 1996. Serodiagnosis of cutaneous leishmaniasis: assessment of an enzyme-linked immunosorbent assay using a peptide sequence from gene B protein. Am. J. Trop. Med. Hyg. 55:490–495

Kemp M, 1997. Regulator and effector functions of T-cell subsets in human *Leishmania* infections. APMIS Suppl. 68:1–33

Kibbi A-G, Karam PG, Kurban AK, 1987. Sporotrichoid leishmaniasis in patients from Saudi Arabia: clinical and histologic features. J. Am. Acad. Dermatol. 17:759–764

Kocan KM, MacVean DW, Fox JC, 1983. Ultrastructure of a *Leishmania* sp. isolated from dogs in an endemic focus in Oklahoma. J. Parasitol. 69:624–626

Kreutzer RD, Corredor A, Grimaldi JRG, Grogl M, Rowton ED, Young DG, Morales A, McMahon-Pratt D, Guzman H, Tesh RB, 1991. Characterization of *Leishmania colombiensis* sp. n (kinetoplastida: trypanosomatidae), a new parasite infecting humans, animals, and phlebotomine sand flies in Colombia and Panama. Am. J. Trop. Med. Hyg. 44:662–675

Kreutzer RD, Grogl M, Neva FA, Fryauff DJ, Magill AJ, Aleman-Munoz MM, 1993. Identification and genetic comparison of leishmanial parasites causing viscerotropic and cutaneous disease in soldiers returning from Operation Desert Storm. Am. J. Trop. Med. Hyg. 49:357–363

Kubba R, El-Hassan AM, Al-Gindan Y, Omer AHS, Kutty MK, Saeed MBM, 1987. Dissemination in cutaneous leishmaniasis I. Subcutaneous nodules. Int. J. Dermatol. 26:300–304

Kumar PV, Sadeghi E, Torabi S, 1989. Kala azar with disseminated dermal leishmaniasis. Am. J. Trop. Med. Hyg. 40:150–153

Lainson R, Shaw JJ, 1987. Evolution, classification and geographical distribution. In: Peters W, Killick-Kendrick R (eds), *The Leishmaniases in Biology and Medicine*. London: Academic Press, pp. 1–120

Luz KG, da Silva VO, Gomes EM, Machado FC, Araujo MA, Fonseca HE, Freire TC, D'Almeida JB, Palatnik M, Palatnik-de-Sousa CB, 1997. Prevalence of anti-*Leishmania donovani* antibody among Brazilian blood donors and multiple transfused hemodialysis patients. Am. J. Trop. Med. Hyg. 57:168–171

Magill AH, Grogl M, Gasser RA, Sun W, Oster CN, 1993. Visceral infection caused by *Leishmania tropica* in veterans of operation desert storm. N. Engl. J. Med. 328:1383–1387

Marsden PD, Sampaio RN, Gomes LF, Costa JM, Netto EM, Veiga EP, Llanos-Cuentas EA, 1985. Correspondence. Lone laryngeal leishmaniasis. Trans. R. Soc. Trop. Med. Hyg. 79:424–425

Martinez P, de la Vega E, Laguna F, Soriano V, Puente S, Moreno V, Sentchordi MJ, Garcia Aguado C, Gonzalez Lahoz J, 1993. Diagnosis of visceral leishmaniasis in HIV-infected individuals using peripheral blood smears. AIDS 7:227–230

McHugh CP, Melby PC, LaFon SG, 1996. Leishmaniasis in Texas: epidemiology and clinical aspects of human cases. Am. J. Trop. Med. Hyg. 55:547–555

McVean DW, Buckner RG, Fox JC, Glenn BL, Roberts MA, 1979. Canine leishmaniasis in Oklahoma. C. D. C. Vet. Public Health October:6–7

Mebrahtu YB, Van Eys G, Guizani I, Lawyer PG, Pamba H, Koech D, Roberts C, Perkins PV, Were JB, Hendricks LD, 1993. Human cutaneous leishmaniasis caused by *Leishmania donovani* in Kenya. Trans. R. Soc. Trop. Med. Hyg. 87:598–601

Medrano FJ, Jimenez Mejias E, Calderon E, Regordan C, Leal M, 1993. Correspondence. An easy and quick method for the diagnosis of visceral leishmaniasis in HIV-1-infected individuals. AIDS 7:1399

Meller Melloul C, Farnarier C, Dunan S, Faugere B, Franck J, Mary C, Bongrand P, Quilici M, Kaplanski S, 1991. Evidence of subjects sensitized to *Leishmania infantum* on the French Mediterranean coast: differences in gamma interferon production between this population and visceral leishmaniasis patients. Parasite Immunol. 13:531–536

Michiels JF, Monteil RA, Hofman P, Perrin C, Fuzibet JG, Lel'ichoux Y, Loubiere R, 1994. Oral leishmaniasis and Kaposi's sarcoma in an AIDS patient. J. Oral Pathol. Med. 23:45–46

Michiels JF, Saint Paul MC, Hofman P, Perrin C, Giorsetti V, Bernard E, Montoya ML, Loubiere R, 1992. Aspects histopathologiques des infections opportunistes de l'intestin grele au cours du syndrome d'immunodeficience acquis. Ann. Pathol. 12:165–173

Molyneux DH, Killick-Kendrick R, 1987. Morphology, ultrastructure and life cycles. In: Peters W, Killick-Kendrick R (eds), *The Leishmaniases in Biology and Medicine*. London: Academic Press, pp. 121–176

Montalban C, Martinez Fernandez R, Calleja JL, Garcia Diaz JD, Rubio R, Dronda F, Moreno S, Yebra M, Barros C, Cobo J, 1989. Visceral leishmaniasis (kala-azar) as an opportunistic infection in patients infected with the human immunodeficiency virus in Spain. Rev. Infect. Dis. 11:655–660

Murray HW, Stern JJ, Welte K, Rubin BY, Carriero SM, Nathan CF, 1987. Experimental visceral leishmaniasis: production of interleukin 2 and interferon-gamma, tissue immune reaction, and response to treatment with interleukin 2 and interferon-gamma. J. Immunol. 138:2290–2297

Ndiaye PB, Develoux M, Dieng MT, Huerre M, 1996. Leishmaniose cutanee diffuse au cours du syndrome d'immunodeficience acquise chez un patient senegalais. Bull. Soc. Pathol. Exot. 89:282–286

Nelson DA, Gustafson TL, Spielvogel RL, 1985. Clinical aspects of cutaneous leishmaniasis acquired in Texas. J. Am. Acad. Dermatol. 12:985–992

Nigro L, Vinci C, Romano F, Russo R, 1996. Comparison of the indirect immunofluorescent antibody test and the direct agglutination test for serodiagnosis of visceral leishmaniasis in HIV-infected subjects. Eur. J. Clin. Microbiol. Infect. Dis. 15:832–835

Noyes H, Chance M, Ponce C, Ponce E, Maingon R, 1997. *Leishmania chagasi*: genotypically similar parasites from Honduras cause both visceral and cutaneous leishmaniasis in humans. Exp. Parasitol. 85:264–273

Oliveira AV, Roque-Barreira MC, Sartori J, Campos-Neto A, Rossi MA, 1985. Mesangial proliferative glomerulonephritis associated with progressive amyloid deposition in hamsters experimentally infected with *Leishmania donovani*. Am. J. Pathol. 120:256–262

Oliveira Neto MP, Grimaldi G Jr, Momen H, Pacheco RS, Marzochi MCA, McMahon-Pratt D, 1986. Active cutaneous leishmaniasis in Brazil, induced by *Leishmania donovani chagasi*. Mem. Inst. Oswaldo Cruz 81:303–309

Palma G, Gutierrez Y, 1991. Laboratory diagnosis of *Leishmania*. Clin. Lab. Med. 11:909–922

Pearson RD, Steigbigel RT, 1981. Phagocytosis and killing of the protozoan *Leishmania donovani* by human polymorphonuclear leukocytes. J. Immunol. 127:1438–1443

Perrin C, Taillan B, Hofman P, Mondain V, LeFichoux Y, Michiels JF, 1995. Atypical cutaneous histological features of visceral leishmaniasis in acquired immunodeficiency syndrome. Am. J. Dermatopathol. 17:145–150

Peters BS, Fish D, Golden R, Evans DA, Bryceson AD, Pinching AJ, 1990. Visceral leishmaniasis in HIV infection and AIDS: clinical features and response to therapy. Q. J. Med. 77:1101–1111

Piarroux R, Gambarelli F, Dumon H, Fontes M, Dunan S, Mary C, Toga B, Quilici M, 1994. Comparison of PCR with direct examination of bone marrow aspiration, myeloculture, and serology for diagnosis of visceral leishmaniasis in immunocompromised patients. J. Clin. Microbiol. 32:746–749

Prasad LS, Sen S, 1996. Migration of *Leishmania donovani* amastigotes in the cerebrospinal fluid. Am. J. Trop. Med. Hyg. 55:652–654

Rab MA, Hassan M, Bux D, Mahmood MT, Evans DA, 1992. The isolation and cultivation of *Leishmania infantum* from apparently normal skin of visceral leishmaniasis patients in northern Pakistan. Trans. R. Soc. Trop. Med. Hyg. 86:620–621

Reed SG, 1996. Diagnosis of leishmaniasis. Clin. Dermatol. 14:471–478

Reiner NE, Ng W, Ma T, McMaster WR, 1988. Kinetics of gamma interferon binding and induction of major histocompatibility complex class II mRNA in *Leishmania*-infected macrophages. Proc. Natl. Acad. Sci. USA 85:4330–4334

Ridley DS, Ridley MJ, 1983. The evolution of the lesion in cutaneous leishmaniasis. J. Pathol. 141:83–96

Rosenthal PJ, Chaisson RE, Hadley WK, Leech JH, 1988. Rectal leishmaniasis in a patient with acquired immunodeficiency syndrome. Am. J. Med. 84:307–309

Rudzinska JA, D'alesandro PA, Trager W, 1964. The fine structure of *Leishmania donovani* and the role of the kinetoplast in the Leishmania–Leptomonad transformation. J. Protozool. 11:166–191

Russell DG, Talamas-Rohana P, 1989. *Leishmania* and the macrophage: a marriage of inconvenience. Immunol. Today 10:328–333

Sacks DL, Lal SL, Shrivastava SN, Blackwell J, Neva FA, 1987. An analysis of T cell responsiveness in Indian kala-azar. J. Immunol. 138:908–913

Schlein Y, 1993. *Leishmania* and sandflies: interactions in the life cycle and transmission. Parasitol. Today 9:255–257

Schlein Y, Jacobson RL, Messor G, 1993. *Leishmania* infections damage the feeding mechanism of the sandfly vector and implement parasite transmission by bite. Proc. Natl. Acad. Sci. USA 89:9944–9948

Sousa ADQ, Parise ME, Pompeu MML, Coehlo Filho JM, Vasconcelos IAB, Lima JWO, Oliveira EG, Wilson Vasconcelos A, David JR, Maguire JH, 1995. Bubonic leishmaniasis: a common manifestation of *Leishmania* (*Viannia*) *braziliensis* infection in Ceara, Brazil. Am. J. Trop. Med. Hyg. 53:380–385

Srivastava L, Singh VK, 1988. Diagnosis of Indian kala-azar by dot enzyme-linked immunosorbent assay (dot-ELISA). Ann. Trop. Med. Parasitol. 82:331–334

Turk JL, Bryceson ADM, 1971. Immunological phenomena in leprosy and related diseases. Adv. Immunol. 13: 209–266

Veress B, Omer A, Satir AA, El Hassan AM, 1977. Morphology of the spleen and lymph nodes in fatal visceral leishmaniasis. Immunology 33:605–610

Villanueva JL, Torre Cisneros J, Jurado R, Villar A, Montero M, Lopez F, Sanchez Guijo P, Kindelan JM, 1994. *Leishmania* esophagitis in an AIDS patient: an unusual form of visceral leishmaniasis. Am. J. Gastroenterol. 89:273–275

Weigle KA, Davalos MD, Heredia P, Molineros R, Saravia NG, D'Alessandro A, 1987. Diagnosis of cutaneous and mucocutaneous leishmaniasis in Colombia: a comparison of seven methods. Am. J. Trop. Med. Hyg. 36:489–496

WHO, 1984. The leishmaniases. WHO Technical Report Series No. 701

WHO, 1990. Control of the leishmaniases. WHO Technical Report Series No 793

Yebra M, Segovia J, Manzano L, Vargas JA, Bernaldo de Quiros L, Alvar J, 1988. Disseminated-to-skin kala-azar and the acquired immunodeficiency syndrome. Ann. Intern. Med. 107:490–491

Zimmer G, Guillou L, Gauthier T, Iten A, Saraga EP, 1996. Digestive leishmaniasis in acquired immunodeficiency syndrome: a light and electron microscopic study of two cases. Mod. Pathol. 9:966–969

5

Trypanosomes

As mentioned, the trypanosomes are closely related to the leishmaniae, and their zoologic classification follows the same lines (see Chapter 4; Corliss, 1994). Trypanosomes are known in general as the *blood flagellates*, and under natural conditions they occur in humans and many other species of animals. The important species in humans are the pathogen *Trypanosma cruzi* and the nonpathogen *T. rangeli* in the American continent and two subspecies of *T. brucei brucei*, *T. b. gambiense* and *T. b. rhodesiense*, in Africa. Human infections with trypanosomes have been recorded only within these two continents, where they are responsible for extensive morbidity and mortality, making the trypanosomes of paramount medical interest. Since the basic biologic aspects of the African and American trypanosomes are distinct from each other, they are discussed separately.

Trypanosoma cruzi—American Trypanosomiasis

Trypanosoma cruzi is the agent of Chagas' disease or American trypanosomiasis, an infection widely distributed in humans and wild and domestic animals throughout the Western Hemisphere. The disease is named in honor of the Brazilian physician Carlos Chagas, who discovered it in the early 1900s. Soon after its description, the disease was recognized in many other Latin American countries, where several other unexplained syndromes in some patients were attributed to the infection.

Morphology. *Trypanosoma cruzi* occurs in a vertebrate host and in an arthropod responsible for its transmission. Two stages, or forms of the parasite, are found in the vertebrate host; both stages are relevant for diagnostic purposes and will be studied in detail. One stage is the intracellular amastigote, which for practical purposes is identical, under the light microscope, to the amastigote of leishmaniae (see Chapter 4). The amastigote of *T. cruzi*, in contrast to that of leishmaniae, is found in all kinds of cells, including macrophages, because *T. cruzi* has the capacity to *enter the cell on its own*. The extracellular trypomastigote, or flagellated stage, occurs in peripheral blood. In preparations of blood stained with Giemsa stain, extracellular trypomastigotes slender organism 21 μm in maximum length, with a delicate blue cytoplasm and a dark purplish nucleus at the middle of the body (*color plate* III C). In addition, a large kinetoplast is evident at the posterior end of the body, and a flagellum originating nearby extends anteriorly to form the undulating membrane and terminates as a free flagellum in the anterior end of the body. The flagellum and the undulating membrane usually make two wide undulations, and the trypomastigote usually has the configuration of a wide **C** (Fig. 5–14 *A*).

In electron micrographs, the amastigotes of *T. cruzi* are also similar to leishmaniae amastigotes in the form, shape, and organization of internal organelles (see Chapter 4; Figs. 5–1 *B* and 5–2). One difference is that

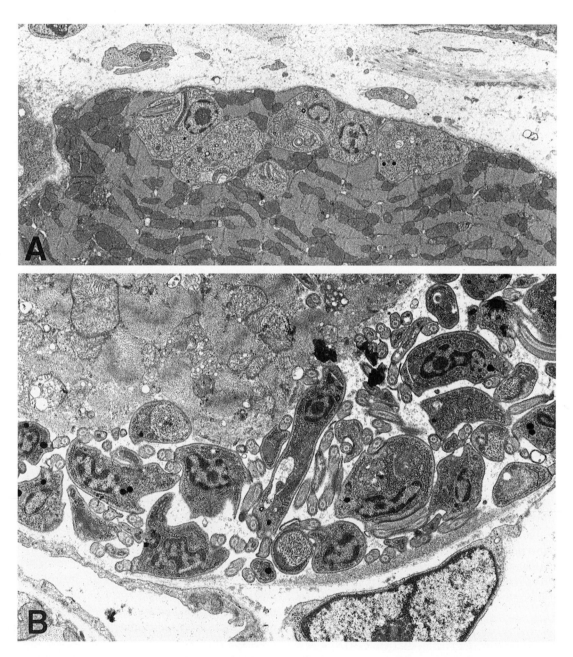

Fig. 5–1. *Trypanosoma cruzi*, **transmission electron micrographs of heart from a mouse infected experimentally.** *A*, **Early nest with amastigotes inside a myocardial cell,** ×6,000. **(Courtesy of M. Aikawa, M.D., Institute of Pathology, Case Western Reserve University, Cleveland,** Ohio.) *B*, **A more advanced nest with many intermediate elongated and flagellated forms. Note the "dissolution" of the cell cytoplasm and the lack of inflammatory infiltrate because the cells are not yet ruptured,** ×10,800.

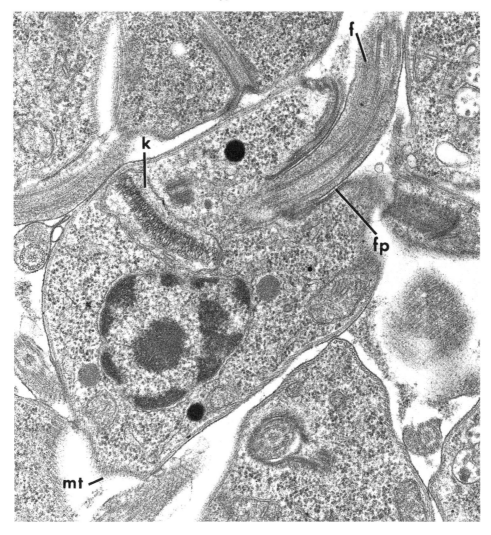

Fig. 5–2. *Trypanosoma cruzi*, transmission electron micrograph of heart from a mouse infected experimentally. High magnification of a flagellated form showing typical structures. Abbreviations: f, flagellum; fp, flagellar pocket; k, kinetoplast showing the DNA arrangement; mt, microtubules, ×20,400.

no parasitophorous vacuole is present and the parasites are in direct contact with the cytoplasm of the cell. Another difference is the presence of intermediate forms since the parasite undergoes the transformation from amastigote to trypomastigote within the cell before entering the bloodstream as well-formed trypomastigotes (Fig. 5–2). In electron micrographs of trypomastigotes, the parasite has a pellicle composed of a cell membrane and microtubules. The nucleus, a mitochondrion filling much of the body, and the kinetoplast and its DNA are other easily recognized organelles. The flagellum originates in the basal body and exits in the flagellar pocket to form the undulating membrane (Fig. 5–2). In addition, the endoplasmic reticulum, ribosomes, and Golgi apparatus, all similar to those described in *Leishmania*, are present (Aikawa, Sterling, 1974).

Life Cycle. The life cycle of *T. cruzi* (Fig. 5–3) begins when the hematophagous arthropod ingests the trypomastigotes with its blood meal. In the arthropod the flagellates multiply in the intestine, and in the posterior intestine they develop into infective (metacyclic) trypomastigotes, which are evacuated in the feces of the insect at the time of its next blood meal. If metacyclic trypomastigotes are deposited on the skin of a susceptible host, they gain access to the tissues through abrasions on the skin or through the normal mucosa

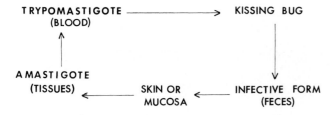

Fig. 5–3. *Trypanosoma cruzi*, **schematic representation of the life cycle.**

of the mouth and conjunctiva (Fig. 5–4). Once in the tissues, the parasites enter the cells (any cell type) on their own, to become amastigotes and to begin multipling as amastigotes. Once the cell is filled with amastigotes, the transformation into trypomastigotes begins, with their eventual release into the bloodstream; parasitized cells die of their parasitism. In the bloodstream the parasites circulate and gain access to distant organs, where they repeat the intracellular cycle (Fig. 5–3; Beaver et al. 1984).

Epidemiology. The distribution of *T. cruzi* in animals on the American continent extends from the northern United States to the northern regions of Argentina (Fig. 5–5). Human infections are restricted mostly to rural

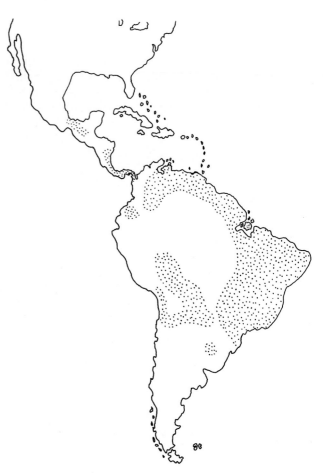

Fig. 5–5. *Trypanosoma cruzi*, **geographic distribution of human infections. The area of enzooticity in wild animals is larger, and comprises much of Latin America and the United States.**

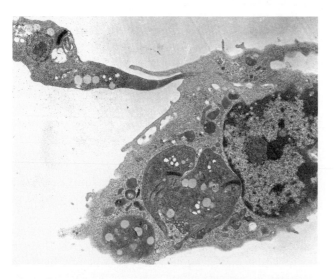

Fig. 5–4. *Trypanosoma cruzi*, **transmission electron micrograph showing the entry of a flagellated epimastigote (?) entering a macrophage in culture. (From: Tanowitz, H., Wittner, M., Kress, Y., et al., 1975. Studies of *in vitro* infection by *Trypanosoma cruzi*. I. Ultrastructural studies on the invasion of macrophages and L cells. Am. J. Trop. Med. Hyg. 24:25–33. Reproduced with permission.)**

areas of Central and South America, where primitive mud huts covered with thatched roofs provide good breeding places for the vectors. At least 100 million people are at risk of contracting the infection in Latin America, and about 16 to 18 million are infected (WHO, 1991). The overall morbidity and mortality produced by *T. cruzi* are unknown. However, it is estimated that in some areas of Brazil more than 13% of all deaths in individuals between the ages of 15 and 74 result from the infection (WHO, 1991). Distribution of the infection is not uniform throughout the continent, with most of the modern cities and the higher altitudes of the Andes, 2000 meters above sea level, being spared. The rate of infection in the population at risk is also variable, but it may reach 100% in focal areas where the conditions for transmission are particularly optimal.

The natural vectors of the parasite are a group of insects of the family Reduviidae, referred to as *reduviids*, commonly known as *kissing bugs* in the United States, and by a different name in each locality studied throughout Latin America. Reduviids have a wide distribution, feeding naturally on wild animals and maintaining the life cycle of the parasite among these animal reservoirs. Some reduviids are adapted to a domiciliary and peridomiciliary habitation, maintaining the parasite among domestic animal reservoirs and humans. Although several genera of the family Reduviidae comprising dozens of species are good natural and experimental intermediate hosts of *T. cruzi*, the most important species belong to the genera *Triatoma*, *Rhodnius*, and *Panstrongylus*. Besides acquisition of the infection through the natural vectors, other modalities of transmission of Chagas' disease are important in humans. Two other methods of transmission are transfusion of contaminated blood and congenital transmission through the placenta. Dirty needles of drug users and transplants of organs from infected individuals are other possible routes of transmission. The most important, modalities, however, are blood transfusions (Grant et al. 1989; Kirchhoff, 1989) and congenital infections (Bittencourt, 1963; Bittencourt, 1976) because of the number of individuals involved. It has been estimated that in different areas of Latin America, between 1% and 11% of mothers suffer from Chagas' disease (Luquetti, 1994).

In the United States *T. cruzi* occurs in wild (Burkholder et al. 1980) and domestic animals (Williams et al. 1977), as well as in the reduviid vectors (Sullivan et al. 1949). However, only a small number of documented human infections naturally acquired in the country have been reported (Schiffler et al. 1984; Woody, 1955; Woody, Woody, 1959). This finding was reinforced by a recent serologic study of samples collected in southern Louisiana, Mississippi, Alabama, and Georgia, areas where the parasite is known to occur. Of 6000 samples examined, only 10 were positive for *T. cruzi* antibodies (Barrett et al. 1997). Infections acquired through contaminated blood (Grant et al. 1989; Nickerson et al. 1989) or found in immigrants from endemic areas (Hagar, Rahimtoola, 1991) have also been few in number. Of 205 Central American immigrants to the Washington, D.C., area, 5% were positive for antibodies to *T. cruzi*, indicating that about 50,000 of these immigrants in the United States are infected (Kirchhoff, 1989; Kirchhoff et al. 1987). It is estimated that in California 1 of every 340 blood donors is at risk of being infected with *T. cruzi* (Galel, Kirchhoff, 1996; Pan, Winkler, 1997).

Pathogenesis and Immunity. *Trypanosoma cruzi* produces a range of manifestations in infected individuals, varying from asymptomatic to fatal. The variations in clinical manifestations are probably due to differences in the parasite, a concept based on animal models that demonstrate differences in virulence among strains of *T. cruzi*. Genotypic differences among strains that produced infections of low and high virulence in humans based on their zymodemes have also been shown (patterns of electrophoretic migration of the enzymes of the glucolytic metabolic pathway) (see *E. histolytica*, Chapter 7) (Montamat et al. 1996). The infection with *T. cruzi* is lifelong, indicating that to some extent the parasite evades the immune response, and that both the lasting infection and active evasion of the immune system modulate the disease process. Thus, in Chagas' disease, pathogenesis and immunity are closely related. Survival of the parasite is due to two general factors: first, the intracellular location within the cytoplasm, without the formation of a parasitophorous vacuole, and the parasitization of cells without killing capabilities such as muscle cells and neurons, and second, the capacity of the parasite to suppress the immune system, such as by decreasing the expression of surface molecules of lymphocytes, especially $CD3^+$, $CD4^+$, and $CD8^+$ lymphocytes.

The course of *T. cruzi* infection has several phases modulated by the immunologic status of the host. Patients with an adequate immune response usually have an *acute* phase, followed by an *undetermined* phase characterized by mild cardiac lesions and symptoms when the heart is challenged during clinical testing. Patients with a hyperergic immune response have an acute phase followed by a *chronic* one that develops over several decades and leads to severe cardiac involvement with or without heart failure. Other patients in the chronic phase may suffer from syndromes due to destruction of the parasympathetic effector cells of the gastrointestinal tract leading to megaesophagus, megacolon, or other conditions.

Examination of tissues from diseased organs of patients with any of the forms of Chagas' disease reveals a common characteristic: marked contrast between the small number of organisms and the large amount of tissue destruction produced. Thus, the question of how *T. cruzi* produces tissue destruction has been investigated almost since the discovery of the disease. At some point, it was established that in Chagas' disease there is a decrease in the number of parasympathetic effector cells of the myoenteric plexuses of Meissner and Auerbach and of the atrioventricular (A-V) node of the heart. This explained elegantly the physiology of the symptoms in megadisease and the abnormalities of the electric impulses in the heart. However, the mechanism by which *T. cruzi* decreases these cell populations, both in humans and in animal models (Caliari et al. 1996), is still under debate. The most plausible explanations proposed at various times were mechanical destruction of cells by the parasite, an allergic reaction, a toxin secreted by the parasite, and an autoimmune reaction (antigens of the parasite are similar to antigens in nerve and myocardial cells). Certain experimental and clinical data support some of these explanations, but most of them have not survived rigorous testing. The two main ideas debated during the last two decades are an autoimmune reaction elicited by antigenic mimicry (Petry, Eisen, 1989) between the parasite and the tissues (Kalil, Cunha-Neto, 1996) or destruction of cells modulated by the immune reaction elicited by persistent parasites in tissues (Higuchi, 1997). A combination of both mechanisms is also suggested in which destruction of tissue is triggered by the immune response to the parasite but is amplified by an autoimmune reaction (DosReis, 1997).

Regarding an autoimmune reaction, parasitic antigens have been isolated and characterized as being similar to antigenic determinants in cardiac muscle and nerve tissue. In addition, antibodies against myocardial cells and other heart structures, and against nerve tissue, have been found in the sera of patients with chagasic cardiomyopathy and gastrointestinal denervation. These two observations support the presence of an autoimmune mechanism, but they do not explain the multifocal nature of the lesions. Nor do these observations explain the period of disease development in chagasic patients, measured in decades, or the development of autoimmunity, measured in weeks or months. In addition, antimyocardial antibodies are commonly found in patients who have had any type of cardiac surgery or cardiac lesion.

Some data strongly support a continuous modulation of cell destruction by the immune system triggered by the persistence of parasites in tissues (Higuchi 1997). The infiltrating lymphocytes in chagasic heart lesions are 96% T cells, and the predominant type is the CD8$^+$ T lymphocyte; CD4$^+$ T lymphocytes are present in small numbers and are poorly stained in comparison to the CD8$^+$ cells. The predominance and superior staining of CD8$^+$ lymphocytes are also found during the acute infection in humans (Voltarelli et al. 1987). This type of infiltrate is the reverse of that seen in the rejection injury of transplanted hearts (D'Avila Reis et al. 1993; Higuchi et al. 1993), indicating that Chagas' cardiomyopathy is not an autoimmune process. The predominance of natural killer CD8$^+$ T lymphocytes in chagasic lesions suggests that these cells are destroying

the cells infected with *T. cruzi*. If the cells killed are parasympathetic ganglion cells or myocardial cells (neither of which divide), a deficit must occur with the production of cardiac disease or megadisease in the intestine. In experimental infections in animals with a deficiency of major histocompatibility complex molecules class I (MHC class I), the tissue parasite load is increased and the animals have a more extensive inflammatory reaction. Because the MHC class I molecule modulates the activation of CD8$^+$ T lymphocytes, a deficiency of these molecules results in a diminution of killer cells and thus a higher parasite load (Tarleton et al. 1996). The presence of parasites, parasite antigens, or both in the tissues of patients with chronic chagasic disease has been demonstrated with the help of immunocytochemistry and the polymerase chain reaction. This is a universal finding and confirms the idea that the parasite is present in the tissue lesions throughout life. In addition, parasites in circulation have been repeatedly demonstrated in patients with chronic infections, albeit with difficulty because of their small number (Monteon Padilla et al. 1996), and reactivation of the infection in immune-suppressed individuals is well known (Lopez-Blanco et al. 1983; Umezawa et al. 1996). At present, it appears that American trypanosomiasis is a progressive inflammatory disease that results in reduction of cell populations and development of fibrosis. In this disease, the inflammatory component plays an important role in the development of myocarditis, dilated cardiomyopathy with heart failure, and probably neuronal injury (Higuchi, 1997). The chronic inflammatory process and the tissue destruction are modulated by the immune system, which is continuously stimulated by parasites that persist in the tissues throughout the patient's life. Chronic inflammation and tissue destruction occur in spite of the fact that demonstration of parasites in damaged tissues under the light microscope is often impossible.

Clinical Findings. Asymptomatic *T. cruzi* infections in endemic areas must occur, as well as infections with mild symptoms, but their frequency is unknown. In individuals with clinical manifestations of Chagas' disease, involvement of many organ systems is often the rule. Frequently, the site of entry of the organism (chagoma) is identified as an area of induration in the skin with enlargement of satellite lymph nodes. Less frequently there is a unilateral inflammation of the conjunctiva and eyelids (Romaña sign), (Fig. 5–6). The acute phase of the infection is present more often in children than in adults. It is characterized by general malaise, fever, irritability, muscle pain, and

The indeterminate phase of the infection manifests as abnormal electrocardiographic responses to pharmacologic overload and positive serology (Andrade, 1983). The chronic phase is lifelong, with symptoms and signs of chronic cardiac tissue damage such as electrocardiographic changes consistent with A-V block, T-wave alterations, and low QRS voltage in some patients (Hagar, Rahimtoola, 1991; Laranja et al. 1956). Other patients have a dilated cardiomyopathy with heart failure and sudden death. Syndromes related to other organs systems such as the gastrointestinal tract may develop in some patients. These syndromes present clinically with symptoms and signs of denervation of the effector cells such as achalasia, megaesophagus, megacolon, or megastomach (Koberle, 1968). Some of these conditions are common in certain endemic areas of South America.

Congenital Infections. The clinical manifestations of congenital Chagas' disease are similar to those seen in acquired infections. Acute symptoms may be observed at birth or months later. The most common manifestations are hepatosplenomegaly, anemia, jaundice, edema, tremors, and convulsions. Central nervous system involvement may occur. The anemia may be profound (sometimes mimicking erythroblastosis), usually requiring blood transfusions, and the edema is of a myxomatous type. Gastrointestinal manifestations may be prominent due to direct involvement by the parasite (Bittencourt, 1976). Megaesophagus may also be a manifestation of the disease in infants (Tafuri et al. 1973). Serology is often negative in the acute phase, and asymptomatic infants of chagasic mothers are often serologically positive; this positivity reverses about 40 days after birth (Bittencourt, 1976). Parasites are undetected for the first 7 to 10 days after delivery (Luquetti, 1994). A congenital pneumonitis, resulting from dissemination of trypomastigotes in amniotic fluid to the respiratory tract, has been observed (Bittencourt et al. 1981).

Chagas' Disease in AIDS Patients. Chagas' disease in individuals with human immune deficiency virus (HIV) infections does not appear to be a problem, judging by the small number of cases reported. Reactivation of an old infection is probably the most common cause of the disease, which usually presents with signs and symptoms of encephalitis (Ferreira et al. 1991; Oddo et al. 1992) or myocarditis (Oddo et al. 1992). The encephalitis may consist of focal necrotic areas, with abundant parasites in the brain lesions (del Castillo, Silva, 1994); in other cases, there is a diffuse encephalitis with areas of microscopic necrosis.

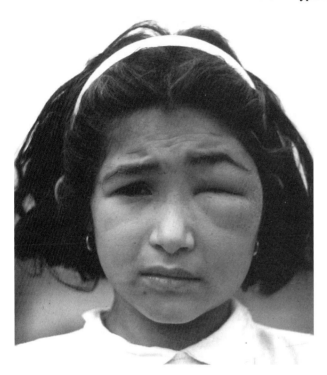

Fig. 5–6. *Trypanosoma cruzi*, Romaña sign. Paraguayan girl with acute Chagas' disease. Note the edema of both the left eyelid and the cheek. Conjunctivitis and preauricular lymph node enlargement are present. (Courtesy of A. D'Alessandro, M.D., School of Public Health and Tropical Medicine, Tulane University, New Orleans, Louisiana. In: Beaver, P.C., Lung, R.C., and Cupp, EW. 1984. *Clinical Parasitology*, 9th ed. Philadelphia: Lea & Febiger. Reproduced with permission.)

sweating; occasionally, vomiting and diarrhea occur (Neto, 1958). Soon after the acute symptoms begin, generalized edema and moderate hepatosplenomegaly often develop. There may be signs of myocardial or central nervous system involvement in severe cases. A myocarditis ranging from mild to severe, with cardiac failure and electrocardiographic changes, especially in children and in new arrivals to endemic areas (immunovirgins), is often fatal. Acute manifestations occur at any age, equally in both sexes. Acute disease is found more commonly in children, the mortality rate in whom is 10% (Laranja et al. 1956). Involvement of the central nervous system is common in acute infections, in spite of the absence of clinical symptoms, as demonstrated by the frequent recovery of parasites in cultures of spinal fluid (Hoff et al. 1978). Spinal fluid abnormalities consist of elevated protein levels and increased numbers of lymphocytes.

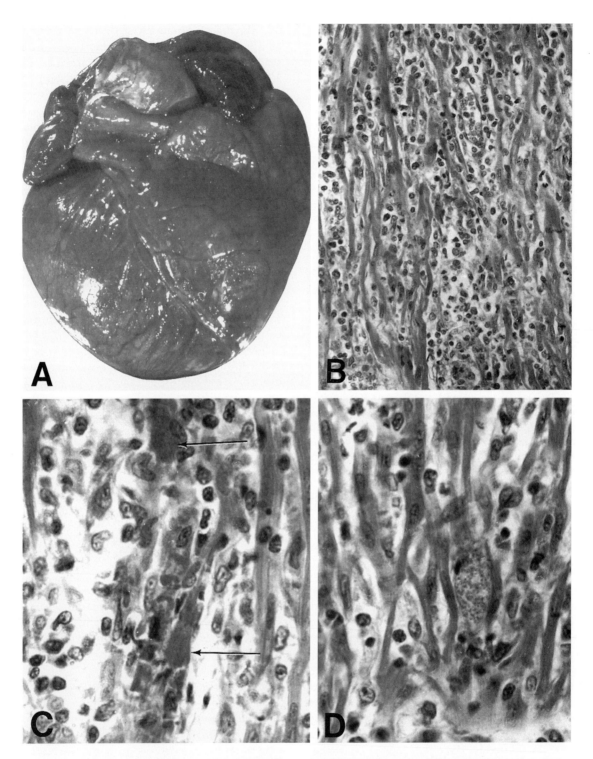

Fig. 5–7. *Trypanosoma cruzi*, acute Chagas' myocarditis. *A*, Gross changes of myocarditis showing enlargement and dilation of the heart. (Courtesy of Z. Andrade, M.D., University of Bahia, School of Medicine, Salvador Bahia, Brazil.) *B–D*, Histologic appearance of a section stained with hematoxylin and eosin stain. *B*, Acute myocarditis showing a mononuclear cell infiltrate and marked disorganization of myocardial fibers, ×280. *C* and *D*, Higher magnification demonstrating individual cell necrosis (arrows), ×705.

Chagas' Disease in Organ Transplant Patients. In patients who are immune suppressed because of an organ transplant, the infection can also be reactivated (Lopez-Blanco et al. 1983; Umezawa et al. 1996). These patients may also acquire the infection with the transplanted organ and suffer acutely because they are more susceptible to the disease (Pizzi et al. 1982). Encephalitis with a focal lesion can also occur (Pizzi et al. 1982). In endemic areas for American trypanosomiasis, heart transplant is a therapeutic modality for patients with chronic chagasic cardiomyopathy, but reactivation of the infection needs monitoring. In Brazil 20% of patients referred for heart transplantation have chagasic cardiomyopathy (Almeida et al. 1996). Many of these patients have reactivation of their infection, manifesting mostly as fever, cutaneous nodules, and myocarditis. It has been stated that fewer chagasic patients suffer from heart transplant rejection than nonchagasic patients (De Carvalho et al. 1996). Skin nodules appear to be common in reactivation of Chagas' disease in transplanted patients; these nodules may become ulcerated (Altclas et al. 1996; Amato et al. 1996).

Pathology. Pathologic descriptions of Chagas' disease have emphasized the lesions produced in the heart and in the myoenteric parasympathetic plexuses because of their clinical importance, but changes occur in most other organ systems as well. As mentioned earlier, heart and parasympathetic ganglionic cells cannot regenerate, and their destruction leads to a deficit.

Heart. Patients dying of acute Chagas' myocarditis with congestive heart failure have a hyperemic, flabby, enlarged heart and pericardial effusion (Fig. 5–7 *A*). In the chronic phase, there is usually cardiac dilation and enlargement of the muscle mass (Koberle, 1968); 60% of autopsied patients have been found to have mural thrombi, one-half with significant embolism (Fig. 5–8 *B*; De Carvalho, 1963). Apical infarcts and apical ventricular aneurysms are found in 50% of cases (Fig. 5–8 *A–B*), but rupture is unusual (Oliveira et al. 1981). However, in 39% of patients dying of Chagas' cardiomyopathy, the cause of death is linked to the aneurysm, either as a source of embolism and thrombosis, or as a source of arrhythmias, or both.

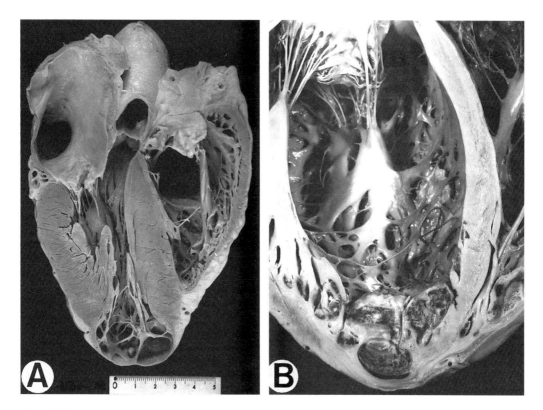

Fig. 5–8. *Trypanosoma cruzi*, gross changes in chronic Chagas' myocarditis. *A*, Apical aneurysm in chronic Chagas' myocarditis. *B*, Chronic dilation of the heart, apical aneurysm, and thrombus formation. (Courtesy of J.S.M. Oliveira, M.D., Faculdade de Medicina de Riberao Preto, São Paulo, Brazil.)

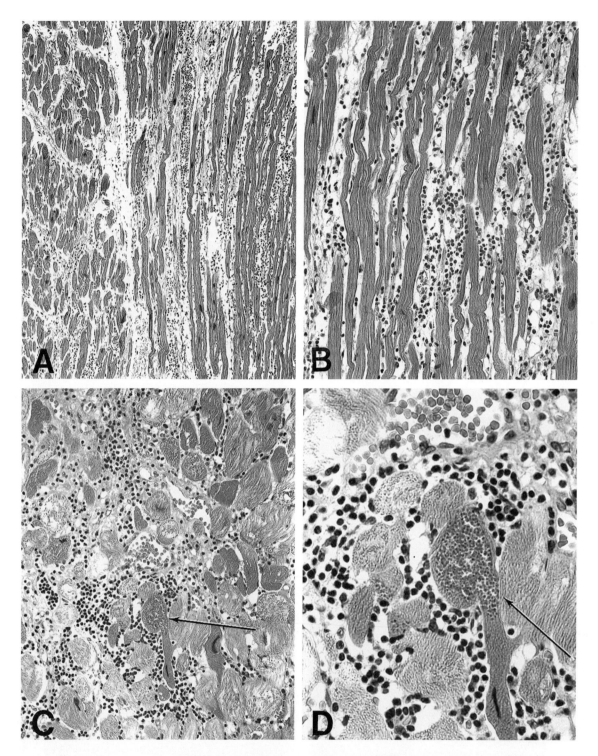

Fig. 5–9. *Trypanosoma cruzi*, microscopic appearance of chronic Chagas' myocarditis, sections stained with hematoxylin and eosin stain. *A* and *B*, Different magnifications showing a diffuse mononuclear cell infiltrate throughout, *A* ×70; *B* ×180. *C* and *D*, Focal area of cellular destruction, more inflammatory changes, and parasites in a muscle cell (arrows), *C* ×180, *D* ×450. (Preparation courtesy of R. Falzoni, M.D., Faculdade de Medicina da Universidade de São Paulo, Brazil.)

The acute phase of Chagas' disease is characterized by a myocarditis with focal destruction of myocytes and massive infiltration by a mixture of mononuclear (lymphocytes, plasma cells, macrophages) and polymorphonuclear leukocytes (Figs. 5–7 *B–D*). Parasites are usually found in small numbers (Fig. 5–7 *D*), somewhat disproportionate to the extent of cell damage; thus the origin of the immunologic explanation for this discrepancy.

Chronic Chagas' myocarditis is characterized by focal inflammatory lesions consisting of degenerated myocytes and a focal mononuclear cell infiltrate throughout the myocardium that lead to fibrosis (Fig. 5–9 *A–D*). Parasites are seldom found in routine examinations of the heart, but if many blocks are prepared and many slides are examined, the parasites may be found in up to 30% of the cases (Fig. 5–9 *D*). However, parasite components are encountered in all cases if molecular techniques are used. The fibrosis is interstitial, focal to diffuse, and in 20% to 30% of infected individuals it leads to chronic Chagas' myocarditis with heart failure (Oliveira et al. 1981). Changes in the fibers of the conduction system during the acute infection consist of hyaline and lytic necrosis, and in the chronic phase of fibrosis, atrophy and fatty infiltration without an inflammatory reaction occur (Andrade et al. 1984). There is also documentation of a progressive decrease in the number of A-V conduction cells as the chronic phase progresses (Koberle, 1968).

Brain. The microscopic changes in the brain are due to direct invasion by the parasites with destruction of cells. In the acute phase, neurons, microglia, and other parasitized cells are surrounded by foci of inflammatory cells. The lesions are located mainly in the brain, cerebellum, basal nuclei, and spinal cord. The arteries have inflammatory changes, and the meninges have a focal inflammatory reaction. The chronic stage of the infection is characterized by a decreased number of neurons and ganglion cells, manifesting as chronic brain syndromes. In HIV-infected individuals necrotic focal lesions (Oddo et al. 1992) and meningoencephalitis (Ferreira et al. 1991) have been found.

Gastrointestinal Tract. The main changes in the gastrointestinal tract are fibrosis and sclerosis of the parasympathetic plexuses of Meissner and Auerbach. These changes begin during the acute phase and persist at a low rate throughout life, with progressive reduction in the number of ganglionic cells. The result is megadisease in the form of megaesophagus or megacolon (Fig. 5–10; Koberle, 1968). The histologic picture of megacolon in Chagas' disease is thus one of aganglionosis similar to that of Hirschsprung's disease.

Placenta. The placenta of mothers with fetuses infected with *T. cruzi* is significantly heavier up to the seventh month of pregnancy and is normal in weight thereafter (Azogue et al. 1985). Placentas of mothers serologically positive for *T. cruzi* show microscopic lesions only in the presence of parasites. Grossly, the placenta is edematous and pale on section. Microscopically, the lesions consist of foci of necrosis, infiltration by lymphocytes and histiocytes, and, in some cases, granuloma formation. Proliferation of Hofbauer cells is usually abundant. Lesions are present in the villi, usually in the stroma but sometimes around and within the wall of the blood vessels. The number of parasites varies from a few to many (Fig. 5–11 *A–B*). There are usually intracellular amastigotes in histiocytes and

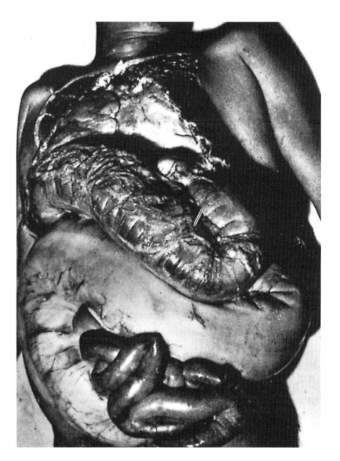

Fig. 5–10. *Trypanosoma cruzi,* **enormous megacolon in chronic Chagas' disease. (From: Koberle, F., 1968. Chagas' disease and Chagas' syndromes: The pathology of American trypanosomiasis. Adv. Parasitol. 6:63–116. Reproduced with permission.)**

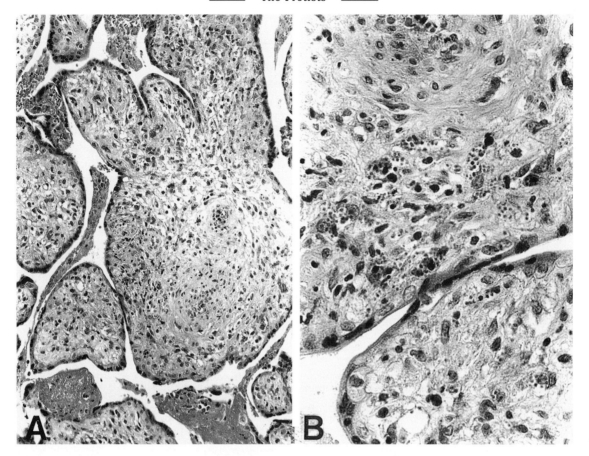

Fig. 5–11. *Trypanosoma cruzi* in congenital Chagas' infection. Sections of placenta stained with hematoxylin and eosin stain. *A*, Low-power view showing the increase in mononuclear cells (villitis), ×119. *B*, Nests of intracellular amastigotes, ×380. **(Preparation courtesy of C. Abramowsky, M.D., Institute of Pathology, Case Western Reserve University, Cleveland, Ohio.)**

other cells, but they are not found in the chorionic epithelium (Bittencourt, 1963, 1976).

Congenital Infection. Lesions in infants with congenital American trypanosomiasis are observed in almost every organ, but the heart, esophagus, intestine, brain, skin, and skeletal muscles are the organs most commonly affected. Intracellular amastigotes are found, and an inflammatory infiltrate of lymphocytes, and less frequently of polymorphonuclear cells, is distributed throughout. Sometimes granulomatous lesions with parasitized giant cells (100 to 120 μm in size) are present. Inflammatory lesions are found only in ruptured amastigote nests. In the brain, microglial nodules, usually perivascular, are common. In the lungs there is a pneumonitis with a nodular pattern, together with many infected cells, granulomas, necrosis, and fibrosis. The gastrointestinal tract and the skin often have many lesions with parasites (Bittencourt, 1976).

Diagnosis. The diagnosis of Chagas' disease is suspected clinically and is confirmed by the laboratory.

Figure 4–21 depicts the morphology of different stages of *T. cruzi* and compares them with the morphology of other members of the group. In the acute phase the trypomastigotes are located in circulating blood, but in certain areas of Latin America, *T. cruzi* must be distinguished from *T. rangeli*, a nonpathogenic species occurring naturally in humans. The trypomastigotes of *T. rangeli* are 31 μm in average length, and have a relatively broad undulating membrane and a small kinetoplast (Fig. 5–12 *A–B*; *color plate* III C).

In cases with low parasitemia, blood cultures in appropriate media or xenodiagnosis (a technique that consists of allowing clean, laboratory-reared reduviids to feed on the patient and examining the insect's intestinal contents several weeks later for the presence of flagellates) are used to demonstrate the organisms. Studies of parasites recovered by any of these methods also need careful assessment and distinction from *T. rangeli*. In reduviids used for xenodiagnosis, *T. rangeli* can also be demonstrated in the hemolymph of the bug. One of the legs of the reduviid is cut, and a small drop of hemolymph that appears at the end of

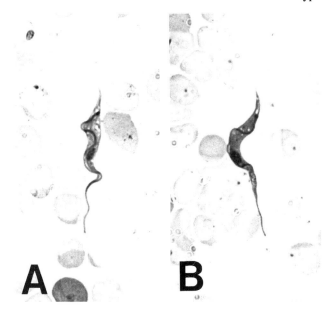

Fig. 5–12. ***Trypanosoma rangeli* in a mouse infected experimentally with parasites from hemolymph of *R. prolixus*, stained with Giemsa stain.** *A* **and** *B*, **Two trypomastigotes illustrating the parasite's size, small kinetoplast, and undulating membrane, both ×1,255. (Preparation courtesy of A. D'Alessandro, M.D., Tulane University School of Public Health and Tropical Medicine, New Orleans, Louisiana.)**

the sectioned leg is collected on a glass slide and examined under the microscope. The presence of the parasites in the hemolymph is characteristic of *T. rangeli* since *T. cruzi* does not invade the hemolymph of the vector (D'Alessandro, 1976; D'Alessandro, del Prado, 1977).

Serologic diagnosis of American trypanosomiasis is one of the most reliable tests of the parasitic infections, but the tests are not widely performed in average laboratories outside endemic areas. The complement fixation test was once used widely for seroepidemiologic studies and for diagnosis; agglutination tests, immunofluorescence tests, and radioimmune precipitation were used mostly for diagnosis. The newer tests include the enzyme-linked immunosorbent assay (Vergara et al. 1992) and the polymerase chain reaction (Silber et al. 1997), both used as research tools and as an immunoblot in clinical samples (Umezawa et al. 1996). Recombinant DNA technology has been used to produce antigens in an attempt to improve the diagnosis (Frasch et al. 1991; Lorca et al. 1995; Vergara et al. 1992). Evaluation of these methods for cross-reactivity with *T. rangeli* has rarely been done. Recent studies have demonstrated that *T. cruzi* antigens react strongly with sera from individuals infected with *T. rangeli*

(Vasquez et al. 1997). Because of these findings, one must be careful in interpreting positive serology for Chagas' disease.

Several tests for detection of parasite antigens in clinical samples are available. Antigens in blood samples have been detected using a dot-immunobinding assay and an enzyme-linked immunosorbent assay in urine from infants with acute or congenital Chagas' disease (Corral et al. 1996).

The anatomic pathologist diagnoses Chagas' disease by properly identifying the organisms in tissue sections or in imprints, based on the morphologic characteristics of the parasites, as described above. Biopsy specimens are seldom taken for the diagnosis of acute Chagas' disease because in the acute phase the parasites are more likely to be recovered in the clinical laboratory. If the clinician wishes to obtain biopsy specimens, he or she should take them from the chagoma, if present, or from satellite lymph nodes. Needle aspirates from the same lesions could be taken for preparations of smears, which should be fixed in alcohol immediately and sent to the laboratory to be stained with Wright or Giemsa stain. Endomyocardial biopsy specimens for diagnosis of the chronic phase of the disease (Pereira-Barretto et al. 1986) have shown nonspecific changes of hypertrophy and fibrosis. These conditions do not contribute to the original clinical diagnosis because parasites are difficult to find. All tissues should be received fresh, and imprints prepared and stained with Wright or Giemsa stain; the remaining tissue is processed and divided into sections, 2 to 3 μm thick to permit better interpretation of the morphologic characteristics of the parasite.

In imprints, the identification of *T. cruzi* follows the same principles outlined for identification of *Leishmania* (see Chapter 4). The parasites are both intracellular (Fig. 5–13 C) and extracellular (Fig. 5–13 B) due to rupture of the cell at the time of imprint preparation. Amastigotes in imprints are as described (Fig. 5–20 A–B), but developmental forms intermediate between amastigotes and trypomastigotes are present. Some appear as large amastigotes (6 to 8 μm) beginning to unfold; others are more elongated, some with an undulating membrane and others with the configuration of trypomastigotes reaching full size (21 μm). Finding and identifying these stages are crucial because they allow the final distinction from *Leishmania* to be made. It should be reemphasized that the intracellular stages of *T. cruzi* are found in all cell types, sometimes in macrophages. *Leishmania* is found only in macrophages (histiocytes) and polymorphonuclear cells (see Fig. 4–21).

In tissue sections, the bases for diagnosis are the morphologic characteristics described for *Leishmania* because the amastigotes of *T. cruzi* are identical to those

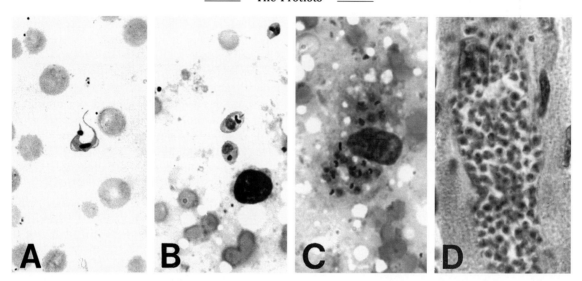

Fig. 5–13. *Trypanosoma cruzi,* **diagnostic stages,** **A–C, stained with Giemsa stain.** *A,* **Trypomastigote in blood.** *B* **and** *C,* **Imprint from spleen of an infected animal showing (artifactually) extracellular amastig-** **otes.** *C,* **Same imprint showing intracellular amastig-** **otes. Compare their size with those in** *B.* *D,* **Parasite nest in muscle cell, hematoxylin and eosin stain, all ×1,120.**

of leishmaniae. It should be remembered that the amastigotes in sections are smaller than those in imprints because of tissue shrinkage during fixation and processing (Fig. 5–13 *D*). Two points must be stressed again: *T. cruzi* is found in all cell types, and developmental forms may be seen in tissue sections, but they are more difficult to determine in tissue sections than in imprints. Differentiation between *T. cruzi* and *Histoplasma* is as discussed for *Leishmania* (see Chapter 4; Fig. 4–21). Differentiation from *Toxoplasma* is based on the presence of a kinetoplast in *T. cruzi* and its absence in *Toxoplasma.* In addition, with periodic acid–Schiff stain, some cytoplasmic granules of *Toxoplasma* are stained positively (see Chapter 7). Polymerase chain reaction using *T. cruzi*–specific DNA sequences is excellent for use both with scrapings of tissue from histologic slides and with tissue sections (Lane et al. 1997).

Trypanosoma brucei rhodesiense and *t. b. gambiense*—African Trypanosomiasis

The African trypanosomes are restricted to tropical Africa, where they produce infections in both humans and animals (WHO, 1986; Fig. 5–14). As mentioned above, the species complex responsible for these infec-

tions is *Trypanosoma brucei brucei,* with three subspecies: *T. b. brucei,* occurring in several animals and often producing a fatal infection, and *T. b. gambiense* and *T. b. rhodesiense* in humans. (The species of African trypanosomes are referred to in this discussion, with the subgenus *brucei* omitted for the sake of brevity.) All three subspecies have similar morphologic characteristics and life cycles, and their classification is based on whether the parasites are found in animals or humans. Those in humans are separated on the basis of their virulence, drug sensitivity, and geographic distribution (Fig. 5–14). *Trypanosoma gambiense* is responsible for a chronic infection in humans with extensive central nervous system involvement, while *T. rhodesiense* produces an acute infection affecting the heart and the central nervous system, with rapid progression to death (WHO, 1979). The human infection is commonly known as *sleeping sickness* or *African trypanosomiasis.*

Morphology. The members of the *T. brucei* group are *polymorphic,* meaning that they occur in circulation in three distinct forms: a long, slender form with a flagellum; a short, stumpy form without a flagellum; and an intermediate form (Fig. 5–15). In preparations of blood stained with Wright or Giemsa stain, the parasites are about 14 to 33 μm long by 1.5 to 3.5 μm wide. The cytoplasm is pale blue, with numerous dark

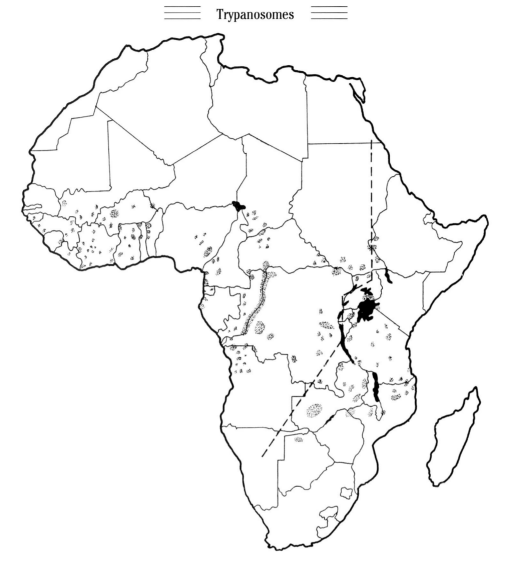

Fig. 5–14. African trypanosomes, geographic distribution. The areas shaded on the left of the broken line correspond to *T. gambiense* and the ones on the right to *T. rhodesiense*. (Redrawn from: WHO. 1986. Epidemiology and Control of African Trypanosomiasis. Tech. Rep. Ser. No. 739. World Health Organization, Geneva. Reproduced with permission.)

blue granules, and at the center of the body is the nucleus, which stains dark reddish or purplish. The undulating membrane originates on the posterior end of the body, is rather broad, and makes several undulations. Also located at the posterior end is the kinetoplast, staining deep red, and nearby is the basal body, from which the flagellum originates. The flagellum runs anteriorly as the support of the undulating membrane and exits at the anterior end as a free flagellum (*color plate* III *D*). Under the electron microscope (Vickerman, 1969), the general morphology and internal organization of the African trypanosomes are similar to those of *T. cruzi*.

Life Cycle. The life cycle of *T. brucei* is complex and starts with the inoculation of the infective stages, known as *metacyclic trypomastigotes*, by the vector. Once in the new host, the parasites enter the bloodstream, where they are found in large numbers (Fig. 5–15). Some enter the interstitium of tissues, especially lymph nodes, brain, and spinal fluid, where they multiply rapidly by binary fission. Intracellular forms (amastigotes) similar to those of *T. cruzi* have been described in the cells of the choroid plexus, and are better demonstrated in stained imprints of the plexus (Mattern et al. 1972; Ormerod, Venkatesan, 1971) but also in electron micrographs (Abolarin et al. 1982).

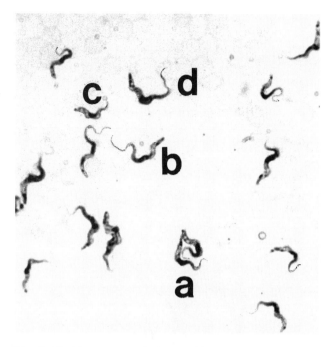

Fig. 5–15. *Trypanosoma b. gambiense* **trypomastigotes in blood of an experimentally infected animal stained with Giemsa stain, ×1,120. Note the dividing forms (a), long slender trypomastigote (b), stumpy trypomastigote (c), and intermediate form (d), ×1,288.**

In the insect vectors, the multiplication of the parasite and the site where it occurs are complicated and outside the scope of this discussion. Flies of the genus *Glossina*, commonly known as *tse-tse* flies, are vectors with several species occurring throughout Africa. The parasites are acquired by the fly while feeding on infected hosts. In the fly's gut the parasites multiply considerably and evolve into metacyclic trypomastigotes. The metacyclic trypomastigotes, the infective stages, migrate to the salivary glands, and during feeding of the fly they are inoculated into the new host with the fly's saliva (Fig. 5–16).

Biology. The African trypanosomes have a distinct capacity to last in the body of the host for long periods by evading the immunologic system with periodic changes of their antigenicity. On entering the host, trypomastigotes cover themselves with a thick coat, visible with the electron microscope, called *variable surface glycoproteins*. In the bloodstream the number of organisms varies cyclically due to changes in the antigenicity of their surface glycoproteins: a scant parasite population increases to reach a high level of parasitemia, from which it decreases to low levels. This cy-

cle lasts for several days and occurs because the parasite population in each cycle has a different antigenic makeup. The inoculated population of trypomastigotes possesses the antigenic determinant A, to which the host mounts a specific antibody response. The anti-A antibodies lyse all trypomastigotes of type A, but a few heterologous trypomastigotes of type B survive to repopulate the bloodstream and eventually become lysed. The cycle is repeated with the appearance of an antigen C population, an antigen D population, and so on (Vickerman, Luckins, 1969). Once the vector is infected with trypomastigotes of any antigenic type, all trypomastigotes lose their coats, but they reacquire the coats as antigenic type A when they become infective metacyclic trypomastigotes. The exact mechanism by which the parasites change their variable surface glycoproteins is not entirely known. It is controlled genetically (Borst et al. 1996), and its importance can be judged by the fact that 5% to 10% of all genes of the parasite are devoted to this mechanism. Morphologically, each cycle begins with slender forms and terminates with a population of stumpy forms.

Humans in Africa are exposed to both their own and animal trypanosomes transmitted by the same insects, but infections with animal trypanosomes do not produce disease because these parasites are lysed effectively in the bloodstream (Rifkin, 1978). Humans lyse animal trypanosomes because of the existence of a *trypanosome lytic factor*, a haptoglobin-related lipoprotein of high density that combines with hemoglobin (Hager, Hajduk, 1997). The parasites internalize hemoglobin with this protein, and in their cytoplasm this compound releases H_2O_2, which the parasites cannot neutralize because they lack the necessary catalases.

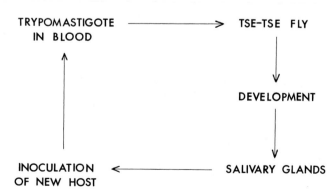

Fig. 5–16. *Trypanosoma brucei* **complex, schematic representation of the life cycle.**

Geographic Distribution and Epidemiology. The exact distribution and prevalence of sleeping sickness are not well known because of the difficulties of obtaining accurate data. In general, the disease exist in the tropical region of the African continent, where *T. gambiense* is limited to the western part of the continent and *T. rhodesiense* to the eastern area (Fig. 5–14). In these areas the disease occurs in restricted foci, with low levels of transmission. It is estimated that about 10 million people are at risk of acquiring the infection (WHO, 1986). The epidemiology of African trypanosomiasis depends on several factors that are distinct for each of the two species. *Trypanosoma gambiense* occurs, in both endemic and epidemic forms, usually in a human-fly-human cycle without animal reservoirs. Humans are the most important reservoirs, especially in the early stages of the infection, because they can have an asymptomatic phase, which lasts for years, with abundant circulating parasites. Animals such as dogs, cattle, sheep, and pigs are naturally infected in endemic areas, as is wild game, but the exact interaction between these different animal reservoirs and humans in maintaining the infections is not clear. Epidemics in endemic areas are produced by parasites of biochemical types different from those prevalent in the area, suggesting that reintroduction from other areas or genetic changes in the parasites occurred (WHO, 1986).

Trypanosoma rhodesiense is more of a zoonotic disease, acquired from species of *Glossina* that naturally feed on wild game. Endemic cases are sporadic (Ormerod, 1961), occurring mostly in adult men who are infected when they enter the wild habitat of the parasite. These men may introduce the parasite into the community, where a human-fly-human cycle is established, to produce an epidemic. In epidemics, men, women, and children become equally infected. The parasites producing human epidemics are biochemically identical to those found in cattle and other animals. The occurrence of African trypanosomiasis is always limited to defined ecologic areas where the disease has persisted for decades because it is impractical to eradicate either the parasite or the vectors. Even in these areas, the true incidence of the infection is unknown because the diagnosis is not always accurate and surveys are limited to small communities.

Clinical Findings. The primary lesion or inoculation chancre, more common with *T. rhodesiense*, develops in 19% to 47% of individuals 2 to 3 days after the infective bite (Duggan, Hutchinson, 1966). This lesion is less frequent among native Africans than among Europeans and Americans. At first, the lesion is a small erythematous, tender swelling that becomes indurated, increases in size to 10 cm or more, and lasts for 2 to 3 weeks. The lesion then subsides, and healing is characterized by desquamation (*color plate* III *F–G*). Sometimes a generalized rash, more common in Europeans and Americans than in native Africans, is the presenting symptom (McGovern et al. 1995). After the inoculation chancre develops, the clinical course is variable in severity and is related to the species involved. In *T. rhodesiense* there is an acute course with a rapidly fatal outcome, while in *T. gambiense* the course is chronic and central nervous system involvement is the rule.

Both infections present with fever, higher with *rhodesiense*, usually coinciding with the crest of the parasitemia. Lymphadenopathy is often generalized, occurring more commonly in the posterolateral triangle of the neck (Winterbottom's sign). A delayed sensation of pain (Kerandel's sign) is sometimes observed. Anemia is a major component of the disease, which in the early phases is due to hemolysis and hemophagocytosis; later, however, other factors are at play. Other organs may be affected, and if the infection is untreated, the outcome is fatal.

Infections with *T. gambiense* are chronic, and half of the patients have central nervous system involvement with encephalitis. This condition is characterized by the presence of trypomastigotes or abnormalities in the spinal fluid, including more than five cells per cubic millimeter and more than 40 mg of protein (Haller et al. 1986). The main symptoms of sleeping sickness encephalitis are lethargy, ataxia, in continence, lack of proprioceptive reflexes, and coma (*color plate* III *E*). Other neurologic symptoms may also occur. Arsenicals (Mel-B), when used for treatment, produce an idiosyncratic reaction encephalopathy in 10% of all patients, a condition that is fatal in one-half of them. Arsenical encephalopathy is characterized by a convulsions with acute brain edema, mental disturbances, without neurologic signs, and coma.

Immunity and Pathogenesis. As mentioned before, *T. gambiense* produces a chronic disease and *T. rhodesiense* an acute one, and each species has strains with different degrees of virulence, which explains in part the differences in the individual clinical manifestations of the disease. It was also mentioned that antibodies capable of lysing trypomastigotes are produced (see Biology above). In the circulation, trypomastigotes either secrete directly or release after their degradation a *trypanosome-derived lymphocyte-triggering factor*, a 185 kDa compound (Olsson et al. 1991). This factor activates CD8$^+$ lymphocytes to secrete gamma interferon and interleukin-2 (Olsson et al. 1991; Pentreath, 1995), which activate macrophages to produce nitrous oxide, tumor necrosis factor alpha, prostaglandins, and other compounds (Dumas, Bouteille, 1996; Okomo-Assoumou et al., 1995). Gamma interferon promotes the growth and multiplication of the parasite, while tumor necrosis factor alpha and nitrous oxide act against it. In addition, these cytokines promote immune suppression of the parasite (Olsson et al. 1991; Pentreath, 1995). The most important cytokine is tumor necrosis factor (Okomo-Assoumou et al. 1995), which acts directly on the membrane of the trypomastigote and indirectly on the production of nitrous oxide. Gamma interferon activates growth of the parasites, which accounts for their large numbers in lymphoid tissues and sensory ganglia because gamma interferon is produced by the dorsal root of the ganglion neurons (Pentreath, 1995).

The cytokines and the nitric oxide produced during the infection modify the endothelial cells of the brain vasculature by damaging their pericytes and breaking down the blood–brain barrier. These processes allow the CD8$^+$ cells and the trypomastigotes to enter the perivascular spaces, where the parasites escape the immunologic system. Proliferation of astrocytes and microglial cells, and further infiltration by lymphocytes and plasma cells around the vessels and the Virchow-Robin spaces follow. The lesions are distributed in the meninges, especially in the pia matter, cerebral cortex, subcortical white matter mostly around the third ventricle, cerebellum, and spinal cord. These lesions consist of focal demyelinization that is never extensive or massive, has no specific character, and spares the fibers of interhemispheric connections (corpus callosum). The distribution of the lesions explains clearly the different symptoms of the disease. Demyelinization of the tuberculo-infundibular and subthalamic areas results in derangement of the internal clock that regulates sleep. The amount of time spent sleeping by individuals with African trypanosomiasis is equal to that of noninfected individuals, but their sleeping pattern is one of small segments distributed throughout the 24 hours of the day, which is interpreted as hypersleepiness. The subthalamic lesions also disrupt the production of cortisol, renin, and prolactine, as well as the circadian rhythm. One explanation suggested for the central nervous system lesions is autoimmunity, and immunoglobulin (IgM) against neurofilaments has been detected (Ayed et al. 1997). However, this mechanism remains speculative.

The antibody response in African trypanosomiasis is prominent and is dominated by production of IgM antibodies that result in a marked hypergammaglobulinemia. The bulk of these antibodies are not directed against the trypanosomes; some are heterophil antibodies, others are autoantibodies against neurofilaments, and some are against DNA autoantibodies. The large amounts of IgM are striking, and the determination of their level is used for diagnosis. In addition, antigen–antibody complexes are in circulation, and they deposit in tissues.

Pathology. The histologic changes in individuals dying of sleeping sickness consist of chronic inflammation, especially in the brain, the lymph nodes, the heart, and, to a lesser degree, other organ systems (Poltera, 1985).

The inoculation site on the skin has marked edema and an intense cellular reaction with mononuclear cells and tissue damage. There usually is a vasculitis with proliferation of endothelial cells, a perivascular mononuclear cell infiltrate, fibroblasts, and trypomastigotes multiplying within the interstitium (Cochran, Rosen, 1983). These trypomastigotes are drained by dermal lymphatics and enter regional lymph nodes, where they proliferate further, or they enter the general circulation. The microscopic changes in the chancre are therefore the beginning of what becomes a generalized vasculitis, interstitial proliferation of parasites, mononuclear cell infiltrates, and tissue damage (Poltera, 1985).

Reports of the histologic appearance of lymph nodes in individuals infected with African trypanosomes are rare. A follicular hyperplasia with sinus histiocytosis and infiltration by plasma cells, numerous lymphocytes, and pale-staining mononuclear cells have been described (Greenwood, Whittle, 1980). Later in the infection the lymph nodes are lymphocyte depleted, and trypomastigotes in the nodes reproduce in larger numbers than in the circulation and develop antigenic characteristics different from those in blood. Multiplication of trypomastigotes in lymph nodes is continuous compared to multiplication in the bloodstream, which occurs in waves (Poltera, 1985).

The heart is affected, especially in infections with *T. rhodesiense*, and in histologic sections there are foci of mononuclear cell infiltrates in the endocardium, myocardium, and pericardium. A pericarditis is often present. Lesions in the conduction system produce electrocardiographic changes and terminal cardiac insufficiency in some cases. Eosinophilia is not present.

The most important findings in African trypanosomiasis occur in the central nervous system, with evidence of meningoencephalitis (Adams et al. 1986). Grossly, the brain is normal or slightly swollen, with expansion of the white matter, decrease in the ventricular spaces, and herniation. Microscopically, the meningoencephalitis (Fig. 5–17 *A–B*) is seen as perivascular (Fig. 5–17 *D*)

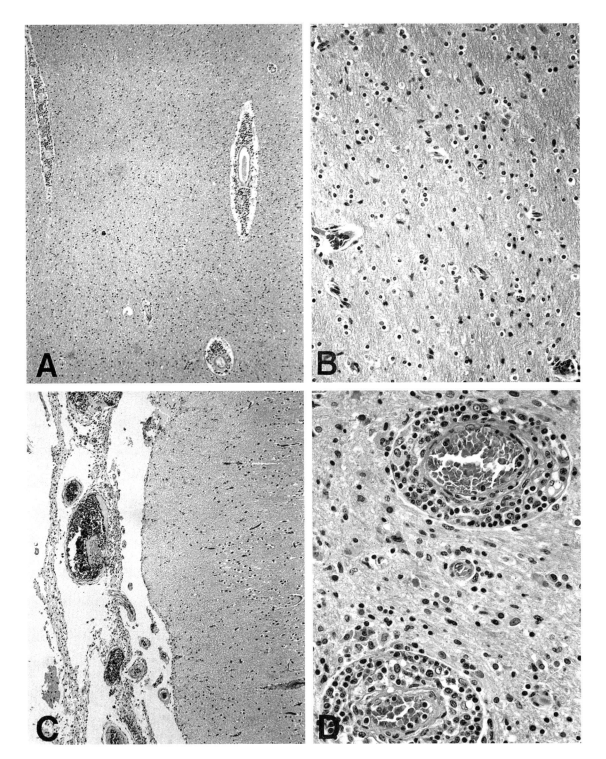

Fig. 5–17. *Trypanosoma b. gambiense* brain lesions, sections of brain stained with hematoxylin and eosin stain. *A*, Low-power view showing an increase in cellular elements and perivascular infiltrates, ×55. *B*, Higher magnification with mononuclear cells evident, ×180. *C*, Meningitis, ×55. *D*, Perivascular infiltrate with lymphocytes and plasma cells, ×280. (Brain tissue samples courtesy of J. Hume Adams, M.D., Department of Neuropathology, Institute of Neurological Sciences, Glasgow, Scotland.)

and meningeal (Fig. 5–17 C) mononuclear cell infiltrates of lymphocytes, macrophages, and plasma cells. Some plasma cells contain large globules of uniform amphophilic material (Russell bodies). These cells, described by Mott, are known as *morular cells*; although not diagnostic, they are highly suggestive of the infection. Both veins and capillaries are affected, sometimes with obliterative changes. Destruction of neurons, a microglial reaction, foci of demyelination with reactive astrocytosis, focal destruction of cellular elements, and hemorrhages are seen in chronic cases. Involvement of choroid plexuses, cranial nerves, and the brain stem has been recorded. The changes are nonspecific, and diagnosis is not possible by gross and microscopic examination of brain tissues alone (Adams et al. 1986; Poltera, 1985). Patients dying of arsenical encephalopathy have a distinct histologic lesion in the brain characterized by acute vasculitis (Haller et al. 1986).

Diagnosis. The clinical diagnosis of African trypanosomiasis is based on the clinical symptoms and a history of having resided in or visited an endemic area. In the clinical laboratory, the diagnosis is established by recovery and identification of trypomastigotes in thin and thick blood smears, in cervical lymph node and bone marrow aspirates, and in smears of cerebrospinal fluid. In any of these preparations the typical polymorphic flagellates can be demonstrated (see Figs. 4–21 and 4–15). Wet preparations of blood and any other fluids may demonstrate motile trypomastigotes if examined directly under the microscope. Cultures in proper media are useful for isolation of the parasite.

The drawback of techniques based on a direct search for the organisms is that the organisms are usually low in number and difficult to detect. Concentration methods have been developed, the simplest of which is centrifugation of the spinal fluid and examination of the sediment. Another method is the hematocrit centrifugation technique, a highly sensitive microscopic examination of the buffy coat zone of centrifuged microhematocrit tubes.

The anatomic pathologist rarely examines biopsy specimens from infected individuals because the parasites are usually not detected in tissue sections, and special histologic stains are not helpful because of the small number of parasites in the interstitium. Imprints of the choroid plexus may reveal intracellular stages. In some studies, aspiration of the inoculation site or from enlarged lymph nodes revealed the parasites, either in fresh (Cohen et al. 1986) or stained preparations in a good number of cases. Other studies showed positivity

of only 3% for lymph node aspirates (Haller et al. 1986). Bone marrow aspirates are often positive in cases where other methods have failed. Autopsy material from patients dying of African trypanosomiasis reveals nonspecific lesions (see above) that are difficult to distinguish from those of a viral encephalitis.

Several tests have been used to determine antibody levels in serum and spinal fluid, such as direct agglutination, indirect hemagglutination, gel precipitation, and immunofluorescence tests. Determination of IgM levels is also recommended, but it is not diagnostic. Increased IgM titers in spinal fluid are considered pathognomonic of central nervous system involvement. The newer tests are the enzyme-linked immunsorbent assay and the polymerase chain reaction (Kanmogne et al. 1996).

References

Abolarin MO, Evans DA, Tovey DG, Ormerod WE, 1982. Cryptic stage of sleeping-sickness trypanosome developing in choroid plexus epithelial cells. Br. Med. J. 285:1379–1382

Adams JH, Haller L, Boa FY, Doua F, Dago A, Konian K, 1986. Human African trypanosomiasis (*T. b. gambiense*): a study of 16 fatal cases of sleeping sickness with some observations on acute reactive arsenical encephalopathy. Neuropathol. Appl. Neurobiol. 12:81–94

Aikawa M, Sterling CR, 1974. *Intracellular Parasitic Protozoa*, New York: Academic Press.

Almeida DR, Carvalho AC, Branco JN, Pereira AP, Correa L, Vianna PV, Buffolo E, Martinez EE, 1996. Chagas' disease reactivation after heart transplantation: efficacy of allopurinol treatment. J. Heart Lung Transplant. 15: 988–992

Altclas J, Jaimovich G, Milovic V, Klein F, Feldman L, 1996. Chagas' disease after bone marrow transplantation. Bone Marrow Transplant. 18:447–448

Amato JG, Amato Neto V, Amato VS, Duarte MI, Uip DE, Boulos M, 1996. Lesoes cutaneas como unicas manifestacoes de reativacao da infeccao pelo *Trypanosoma cruzi* em receptora de rim por transplante. Rev. Soc. Bras. Med. Trop. 30:61–63

Andrade ZA, 1983. Mechanisms of myocardial damage in *Trypanosoma cruzi* infection. In: Ciba Foundation Symposium 99. (ed), *Cytopathology of Parasitic Diseases*. London: Pitman Books, pp. 214–233

Andrade ZA, Andrade SG, Sadigursky M, 1984. Damage and healing in the conducting tissue of the heart (an experimental study in dogs infected with *Trypanosoma cruzi*). J. Pathol. 143:93–101

Ayed Z, Brindel I, Bouteille B, van Meirvenne N, Doua F, Houinato D, Dumas M, Jauberteau MO, 1997. Detection and characterization of autoantibodies directed against neurofilament proteins in human African trypanosomiasis. Am. J. Trop. Med. Hyg. 57:1–6

Azogue E, La Fuente C, Darras C, 1985. Congenital Chagas' disease in Bolivia: epidemiological aspects and pathological findings. Trans. R. Soc. Trop. Med. Hyg. 79: 176–180

Barrett VJ, Leiby DA, Odom JL, Otani MM, Rowe JD, Roote JT, Cox KF, Brown KR, Hoiles JA, Saez-Alquezar A, Turrens JF, 1997. Negligible prevalence of antibodies against *Trypanosoma cruzi* among blood donors in the Southeastern United States. Am. J. Clin. Pathol. 108: 499–503

Beaver PC, Jung RC, Cupp EW, 1984. *Clinical Parasitology*. Philadelphia: Lea & Febiger

Bittencourt AL, 1963. Placentite Chagasica e transmissao congenita da doenca de Chagas. Rev. Inst. Med. Trop. Sao Paulo 5:62–67

Bittencourt AL, 1976. Congenital Chagas' disease. Am. J. Dis. Child. 130:97–103

Bittencourt AL, de Freitas LAR, de Araujo MOG, Jacomo K, 1981. Pneumonitis in congenital Chagas' disease. Am. J. Trop. Med. Hyg. 30:38–42

Borst P, Rudenko G, Taylor MC, Blundell PA, Van Leeuwen F, Bitter W, Cross M, McCulloch R, 1996. Antigenic variation in trypanosomes. Arch. Med. Res. 27:379–388

Burkholder JE, Allison TC, Kelly VP, 1980. *Trypanosoma cruzi* (Chagas) (Protozoa: Kinetoplastida) in invertebrate, reservoir, and human hosts of the lower Rio Grande Valley of Texas. J. Parasitol. 66:305–311

Caliari ER, Caliari MV, de Lana M, Tafuri WL, 1996. Estudo quantitativo e qualitativo dos plexos de Auerbach e Meissner do esofago de caes inoculados com o *Trypanosoma cruzi*. Rev. Soc. Bras. Med. Trop. 29:17–20

Cochran R, Rosen T, 1983. African trypanosomiasis in the United States. Arch. Dermatol. 119:670–674

Cohen MB, Miller TR, Bottles K, 1986. Correspondence. Classics in cytology: note on fine needle aspiration of the lymphatic glands in sleeping sickness. Acta Cytol. 30: 451–452

Corliss JO, 1994. An interim utilitarian ("user-friendly") hierarchical classification and characterization of the protists. Acta Protozool. 33:1–51

Corral RS, Altcheh J, Alexandre SR, Grinstein S, Freilij H, Katzin AM, 1996. Detection and characterization of antigens in urine of patients with acute, congenital, and chronic Chagas' disease. J. Clin. Microbiol. 34:1957–1962

D'Alessandro A, 1976. Biology of *Trypanosoma (Herpetosoma) rangeli* Tejera, 1920. In: Lumsden WHR, Evans DA (eds), *Biology of the Kinetoplastida*. New York: Academic Press, pp. 327–403

D'Alessandro A, del Prado CE, 1977. Search for *Trypanosoma rangeli* in endemic areas of *Trypanosoma cruzi* in Argentina and Brazil. Am. J. Trop. Med. Hyg. 26:623–627

D'Avila Reis D, Jones EM, Tostes S Jr, Reis Lopes E, Gazzinelli G, Colley DG, McCurley TL, 1993. Characterization of inflammatory infiltrates in chronic chagasic myocardial lesions: presence of tumor necrosis factor-alpha cells and dominance of granzyme A+, CD8+ lymphocytes. Am. J. Trop. Med. Hyg. 48:637–644

De Carvalho JA, 1963. Tromboembolismo na doenca de Chagas em Pernambuco-Consideracoes em torno da incidencia em material necroscopico. Rev. Bras. Mal. Doen. Trop. 14:611–616

De Carvalho VB, Sousa EF, Vila JH, da Silva JP, Caiado MR, Araujo SR, Macruz R, Zerbini EJ, 1996. Heart transplantation in Chagas' disease. 10 years after the initial experience. Circulation 94:1815–1817

del Castillo M, Silva M, 1994. Correspondence. Chagas disease: another cause of cerebral mass in AIDS. Am. J. Med. 96:301–302

DosReis GA, 1997. Cell-mediated immunity in experimental *Trypanosoma cruzi* infection. Parasitol. Today 13:335–342

Duggan AJ, Hutchinson MP, 1966. Sleeping sickness in Europeans: a review of 109 cases. J. Trop. Med. Hyg. 69: 124–131

Dumas M, Bouteille B, 1996. Trypanosomose humaine africaine. C.R Seances. Soc Biol. Fil. 190:395–408

Ferreira MS, Nishioka Sde A, Rocha A, Moreira Silva A, Ferreira RG, Olivier W, Tostes S Jr, 1991. Acute fatal *Trypanosoma cruzi* meningoencephalitis in a human immunodeficiency virus-positive hemophiliac patient. Am. J. Trop. Med. Hyg. 45:723–727

Frasch ACC, Cazzulo JJ, Aslund L, Pettersson U, 1991. Comparison of genes encoding *Trypanosoma cruzi* antigens. Parasitol. Today 7:148–151

Galel SA, Kirchhoff LV, 1996. Risk factors for *Trypanosoma cruzi* infection in California blood donors. Transfusion 36:227–231

Grant IH, Gold JWM, Wittner M, Tanowitz HB, Nathan C, Mayer K, Reich L, Wollner N, Steinherz L, Ghavimi F, O'Reily RJ, Armstrong D, 1989. Transfusion-associated acute Chagas disease acquired in the United States. Ann. Intern. Med. 111:849–851

Greenwood BM, Whittle HC, 1980. The pathogenesis of sleeping sickness. Trans. R. Soc. Trop. Med. Hyg. 74: 716–725

Hagar JM, Rahimtoola SH, 1991. Chagas' heart disease in the United States. N. Engl. J. Med. 325:763–768

Hager KM, Hajduk SL, 1997. Mechanism of resistance of African trypanosomes to cytotoxic human HDL. Nature 385:823–826

Haller L, Adamas H, Merouze F, Dago A, 1986. Clinical and pathological aspects of human African trypanosomiasis (*T. b. gambiense*) with particular reference to reactive arsenical encephalopathy. Am. J. Trop. Med. Hyg. 35: 94–99

Higuchi MDL, Morais CF, Pereira B, Lopes EA, Stolf N, Bellotti G, Pileggi F, 1987. The role of active myocarditis in the development of heart failure in chronic Chagas' disease: a study based on endomyocardial biopsies. Clin. Cardiol. 10:665–670

Higuchi MDL, 1997. Invited review: chronic chagasic cardiopathy: the product of a turbulent host–parasite relationship. Rev. Inst. Med. Trop. Sao Paulo 39:53–60

Higuchi MDL, Sampaio Gutierrez P, Demarchi Aiello V, Palomino S, Bocchi E, Kalil J, Bellotti G, Pileggi F, 1993.

Immunohistochemical characterization of infiltrating cells in human chronic chagasic myocarditis: comparison with myocardial rejection process. Virchows Archiv. A. Pathol. Anat. 423:157–160

Hoff R, Teixeira RS, Carvalho JS, Mott KE, 1978. *Trypanosoma cruzi* in the cerebrospinal fluid during the acute stage of Chagas' disease. N. Engl. J. Med. 298: 604–606

Kalil J, Cunha-Neto E, 1996. Autoimmunity in Chagas disease cardiomyopathy: fulfilling the criteria at last? Parasitol. Today 12:396–399

Kanmogne GD, Asonganyi T, Gibson WC, 1996. Detection of *Trypanosoma brucei gambiense*, in serologically positive but aparasitaemic sleeping-sickness suspects in Cameroon, by PCR. Ann. Trop. Med. Parasitol. 90: 475–483

Kirchhoff LV, 1989. Is *Trypanosoma cruzi* a new threat to our blood supply? Ann. Intern. Med. 111:773–775

Kirchhoff LV, Gam AA, Gilliam FC, 1987. American trypanosomiasis (Chagas' disease) in Central American immigrants. Am. J. Med. 82:915–920

Koberle F, 1968. Chagas' disease and Chagas' syndromes: The pathology of American trypanosomiasis. Adv. Parasitol. 6:63–116

Lane JE, Olivares-Villagomez D, Vnencak-Jones CL, McCurley TL, Carter CE, 1997. Detection of *Trypanosoma cruzi* with the polymerase chain reaction and in situ hybridization in infected murine cardiac tissue. Am. J. Trop. Med. Hyg. 56:588–595

Laranja FS, Dias E, Nobrega G, Miranda A, 1956. Chagas' disease. A clinical, epidemiologic, and pathologic study. Circulation 14:1035–1060

Lopez-Blanco OA, Cavalli NH, Jasovich A, Gonzalez-Cappa S, Nadal MA, Boschi A, Arguello EA, Stamboulian D, Favaloro R, Gotlieb D, 1983. Kidney transplantation and Chagas' disease: a two-year follow-up of a patient with parasitemia. Transplantation 36:211–213

Lorca M, Voloso C, Munoz P, Bahamonde MI, Garcia A, 1995. Diagnostic value of detecting specific IgA and IgM with recombinant *Trypanosoma cruzi* antigens in congenital Chagas' disease. Am. J. Trop. Med. Hyg. 52: 512–515

Luquetti AO, 1994. Practical aspects of Chagas disease. Parasitol. Today 10:287–288

Mattern P, Mayer G, Felici M, 1972. Existence de formes amastigotes de *Trypanosoma gambiense* dans le tissu plexuel choroidien de la souris infectee experimentalement. C. R. Acad. Sci. Paris 274:1513–1515

McGovern TW, Williams W, Fitzpatrick JE, Cetron MS, Hepburn BC, Gentry RH, 1995. Cutaneous manifestations of African trypanosomiasis. Arch. Dermatol. 131:1178–1182

Montamat EE, De Luca D-GM, Gallerano RH, Sosa R, Blanco A, 1996. Characterization of *Trypanosoma cruzi* populations by zymodemes: correlation with clinical picture. Am. J. Trop. Med. Hyg. 55:625–628

Monteon Padilla VM, Negrete Garcia C, Reyes Lopez PA, 1996. Chronic chagasic cardiopathy with parasitemic state (preliminary report). Arch. Med. Res. 27:335–337

Neto VA, 1958. Contribuicao ao conhecimento da forma aguda da doenca de Chagas. Thesis, Faculdade de Medicina da Universidade de Sao Paulo.

Nickerson P, Orr P, Schroeder ML, Sekla L, Johnston JB, 1989. Transfusion-associated *Trypanosoma cruzi* infection in a non-endemic area. Ann. Intern. Med. 111:851– 853

Oddo D, Casanova M, Acuna G, Ballesteros J, Morales B, 1992. Acute Chagas' disease (trypanosomiasis americana) in acquired immunodeficiency syndrome: report of two cases. Hum. Pathol. 23:41–44

Okomo-Assoumou MC, Daulouede S, Lesmesre JL, N'Zila-Mouanda A, Vincendeau P, 1995. Correlation of high serum levels of tumor necrosis factor-alpha with disease severity in human African trypanosomiasis. Am. J. Trop. Med. Hyg. 53:539–543

Oliveira JSM, Oliveira JAM, Frederique V Jr, Lima Filho EC, 1981. Apical aneurysm of Chagas' heart disease. Br. Heart J. 46:432–437

Olsson T, Bakhiet M, Edlund C, Hojeberg B, Van der Meide PH, Kristensson K, 1991. Bidirectional activating signals between *Trypanosoma brucei* and CD8+ T cells: a trypanosome-released factor triggers interferon-gamma production that stimulates parasite growth. Eur. J. Immunol. 21:2447–2454

Ormerod WE, 1961. The epidemic spread of Rhodesian sleeping sickness 1908–1960. Trans. R. Soc. Trop. Med. Hyg. 55:525–538

Ormerod WE, Venkatesan S, 1971. An amastigote phase of the sleeping sickness trypanosome. Trans. R. Soc. Trop. Med. Hyg. 65:736–741

Pan AA, Winkler MA, 1997. The threat of Chagas' disease in transfusion medicine. The presence of antibodies to *Trypanosoma cruzi* in the U.S. blood supply. Lab. Med. 28:269–274

Pentreath VW, 1995. Trypanosomiasis and the nervous system. Pathology and immunology. Trans. R. Soc. Trop. Med. Hyg. 89:9–15

Pereira-Barretto AC, Mady C, Arteaga-Fernandez E, Stolf N, Augusto Lopes E, de Lourdes Higuchi M, Bellotti G, Pileggi F, 1986. Right ventricular endomyocardial biopsy in chronic Chagas' disease. Am. Heart J. 111: 307–312

Petry K, Eisen H, 1989. Chagas disease: a model for the study of autoimmune diseases. Parasitol. Today 5:111–116

Pizzi PT, Acosta de Croizet V, Smok G, Diaz AM, 1982. Enfermedad de Chagas en un paciente con trasplante renal y tratamiento immunosupresor. Rev. Med. Chile 110: 1207–1211

Poltera AA, 1985. Pathology of human African trypanosomiasis with reference to experimental African trypanosomiasis and infections of the central nervous system. Br. Med. Bull. 41:169–174

Rifkin MR, 1978. Identification of the trypanocidal factor in normal human serum: high density lipoprotein. Proc. Natl. Acad. Sci. USA 75:3450–3454

Schiffler RJ, Mansur P, Navin TR, Limpakamjanarat K, 1984. Indigenous Chagas' disease (American trypanosomiasis) in California. JAMA 251:2983–2984

Silber AM, Bua J, Porcel BM, Segura EL, Ruiz AM, 1997.

Trypanosoma cruzi: specific detection of parasites by PCR in infected humans and vectors using a set of primers (BP1/BP2) targeted to a nuclear DNA sequence. Exp. Parasitol. 85:225–232

Sullivan TD, McGregor T, Eads RB, Davis DJ, 1949. Incidence of *Trypanosoma cruzi*, Chagas, in Triatoma (Hemiptera, Reduviidae) in Texas. Am. J. Trop. Med. 29:453–458

Tafuri WL, Lopes ER, Nunan B, 1973. Doenca de Chagas congenita. Estudo clinico-patologico de um caso com sobrevida de seis meses. Rev. Inst. Med. Trop. Sao Paulo 15:322–330

Tarleton RL, Grusby MJ, Postan M, Glimcher LH, 1996. *Trypanosoma cruzi* infection in MHC-deficient mice: further evidence for the role of both class I- and class II-restricted T cells in immune resistance and disease. Int. Immunol. 8:13–22

Umezawa ES, Nascimento MS, Kesper N Jr, Coura JR, Borges Pereira J, Junqueira AC, Camargo ME, 1996. Immunoblot assay using excreted-secreted antigens of *Trypanosoma cruzi* in serodiagnosis of congenital, acute, and chronic Chagas' disease. J. Clin. Microbiol. 34:2143–2147

Vasquez JE, Krusnell J, Orn A, Sousa OE, Harris RA, 1997. Serological diagnosis of *Trypanosoma rangeli* infected patients. A comparison of different methods and its implications for the diagnosis of Chagas' disease. Scand. J. Immunol. 45:322–330

Vergara U, Veloso C, Gonzalez A, Lorca M, 1992. Evaluation of an enzyme-linked immunosorbent assay for the diagnosis of Chagas' disease using synthetic peptides. Am. J. Trop. Med. Hyg. 46:39–43

Vickerman K, 1969. On the surface coat and flagellar adhesion in trypanosomes. J. Cell Sci. 5:163–194

Vickerman K, Luckins AG, 1969. Localization of variable antigens in the surface coat of *Trypanosoma brucei* using ferritin conjugated antibody. Nature 1125–1126

Voltarelli JC, Donadi EA, Falcao RP, 1987. Immunosuppression in human acute Chagas disease. Trans. R. Soc. Trop. Med. Hyg. 81:169–170

WHO, 1979. The African trypanosomiases. Report of a WHO Expert Committee. Technical Report Series No. 635. Geneva: WHO

WHO, 1986. Epidemiology and control of African trypanosomiasis. Report of a WHO Expert commitee. Technical Report Series No. 739. Geneva: WHO

WHO, 1991. Control of Chagas disease. Report of a WHO Expert Committee. Technical Report Series No. 811. Geneva: WHO

Williams GD, Adams LG, Yaeger RG, McGrath RK, Read WK, Bilderback WR, 1977. Naturally occurring trypanosomiasis (Chagas' disease) in dogs. JAVMA 171:171–177

Woody NC, 1955. American trypanosomiasis (Chagas' disease). First indigenous case in the United States. JAMA 159:676–677

Woody NC and Woody HB, 1959. Chagas' disease in the United States of North America. Anais do Internacional Doenca de Chagas, Rio de Janeiro, 1959. Rio de Janeiro: pp. 1699–1724.

6

FREE-LIVING AMEBAE

The amebae parasitizing humans belong to two phyla of the kingdom Protozoa. (1) the phylum Percolozoa, comprising primitive organisms some of which may be ameboflagellates that form transitory flagella, lacking a Golgi apparatus, with mitochondria or hydrogenosomes and peroxisomes, and (2) the phylum Rhizopoda, characterized by having pseudopodia for locomotion and feeding, mitochondria generally with tubular cristae, and a free-living existence for most species (Corliss, 1994). Further subdivisions of these two phyla are shown below to illustrate their interrelationships and only because of the importance of these organisms in human medicine.

Phylum: Percolozoa
  Class: Heterolobosea
    Order: Schyzopyrenida
      Family: Vahlkampfiidae
        Genera: *Naegleria* and *Vahlkampfia*

Phylum: Rhizopoda
  Class: Lobosea
    Order: Hartmannellida

      Family: Hartmannellidae
        Genus: *Hartmannella*
      Family: Acanthamoebidae
        Genus: *Acanthamoeba*
    Order: Leptomyxa
      Family: Leptomyxidae
        Genus: *Balamuthia*
  Class: Entamoebidea
    Order: Amoebida
      Family: Entamoebidae
        Genera: *Entamoeba*, *Endolimax*(?), and *Iodamoeba*(?)

Numerous free-living amebae of soil and water exist in nature, but only members of the genera *Naegleria*, *Vahlkampfia*, *Acanthamoeba*, *Balamuthia*, and *Hartmannella* have been recognized in humans. The systematics of the free-living amebae has become complicated because studies of their molecular biology have revealed that their phylogenetic relationships are quite different from those derived from studies with the light and electron microscopes. Thus, the free-living amebae found in humans are placed in the two phyla Percolozoa and Rhizopoda; *Naegleria* and *Vahlkampfia* belong to the former and *Acanthamoeba*, *Balamuthia*, and *Hartmannella* to the latter (Corliss, 1994). *Naegleria* is a very primitive genus of ameba, with organisms that have between one and four temporary flagella at some point in their life cycles and are known as *ameboflagellates*; *Vahlkampfia* organisms do not have temporary flagella.

In this chapter the free-living amebae are discussed, and in Chapter 7 the intestinal amebae are considered. The free-living amebae produce diseases in humans that range from an acute, rapidly fatal disease to chronic tissue invasion with a granulomatous reaction. Infections produced by these organisms in humans and animals have been generally recognized only during the last three decades (Martinez, 1993; Martinez, Janitschke, 1985). Although the number of individuals affected by free-living amebae is small in comparison to the number affected by *Entamoeba histolytica*, the diagnostic problems for the clinician and pathologist are often difficult. The infections produced by the free-living amebae can be separated into the primary amebic meningoencephalitis produced by *Naegleria* and the amebic granulomatous encephalitis produced by the other genera. The free-living amebae have been referred to by other terms frequently encountered in the literature. One term is *limax amebae* from the Latin term for "slug" or "viscous," describing the appearance of the colonies of some groups, which resemble the colonies of molds. Another term, *amphizoic amebae*, indicates that they live both as free-living organisms in the environment (*exozoic*) and as facultative parasites in the bodies of animals and humans (endozoic) (Page, 1974).

Naegleria: Primary Amebic Meningoencephalitis

An infection produced by a free-living ameba causing acute fatal meningitis was recorded for the first time in 1965 in Australia, and the parasite was tentatively identified as a species of *Acanthamoeba* (Fowler, Carter, 1965). The following year, four similar cases were reported in the United States. In three of them the parasite was not named, but it was recognized as different from the known amebae of humans, and the disease produced was named *primary amebic meningoencephalitis* (Butt, 1966) for the first time. In the other

case, it was suggested that a species of *Acanthamoeba* or *Hartmannella* was responsible for the infection (Patras, Andujar, 1966). In 1968, reports from the United States provided, for the first time, the name of the genus *Naegleria* for the ameba producing meningoencephalitis, based on the presence of ameboflagellated stages (Butt et al. 1968; Callicott, 1968). Similar cases were reported the same year from other places, including an outbreak (in retrospect) of 16 cases in Prague (Cerva et al. 1968; Cerva, Novak, 1968). In 1970, the species was named *N. fowleri* based on an isolate from a patient in Australia (Carter, 1970).

The genus *Naegleria* has several species with similar morphologic characteristics. Though some species can be determined on the basis of these characteristics, their speciation is usually based on antigenic and biochemical profiles and on their pathogenicity to animals. All known species of *Naegleria* are free-living organisms that inhabit water and moist soil under natural conditions (Fig. 6–1), and all human infections reported appear to be produced by *N. fowleri* (Beaver et al. 1984). *Naegleria gruberi*, a closely related species, is considered nonpathogenic. One case of keratitis produced by a mixed infection of species of *Vahlkampfia* and *Hartmannella* was described recently in a patient from Scotland (Aitken et al. 1996); two cases of *Vahlkampfia* encephalitis diagnosed on the basis of their morphologic appearance in tissue sections were also reported (Aitken et al. 1996).

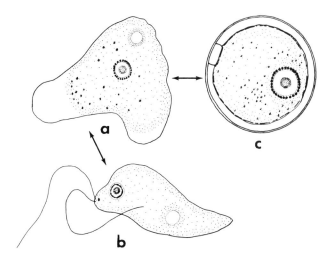

Fig. 6–1. *Naegleria gruberi*, schematic representation of different stages. A trophozoite (a) transforms into an amoeboflagellate (b) or a cyst (c). Not at scale. (Redrawn from: Page, F.C. 1967. Taxonomic criteria for limax amoebae, with descriptions of three new species of *Hartmannella* and three of *Vahlkampfia*. J. Protozool. 14:499–521. Reproduced with permission.)

Morphology. In wet preparations the trophozoites of *Naegleria* are seen as small amebae, with locomotion by small, rounded pseudopods. The trophozoites vary in size and shape from 7 to 15 μm, with a vacuolated cytoplasm, and have a nucleus with a large, rounded, refringent nucleolus, without chromatin, attached to the thin nuclear membrane, making it almost invisible (Figs. 6–1 and 6–2). The cytoplasm has numerous vacuoles aggregated around the nucleus referred to as the *perinuclear vacuoles.* In stained preparations these structures are better appreciated, but no other organelles or structures are discernible. Under certain conditions, for example in water at temperatures between 27°C and 37°C, the trophozoites of species of *Naegleria* grow two temporary flagella in 1 to 20 hours; these flagella last for up to 24 hours under laboratory conditions (Figs. 6–1 and 6–2). Several factors affect both the flagellation and exflagellation of the ameba (Cable, John, 1986). In unstained preparations the cysts are about 7 to 10 μm in diameter and rounded, with a wall about 1 μm thick. Inside the cyst is the ameba, which is seen as a small collection of dark granules with a faint nucleus; the cyst wall has minute pores (*ostyoles*) more readily visible in electron micrographs. In stained preparations, the ameba inside the cyst wall has the morphologic characteristics of a small trophozoite with a well-stained nucleus.

In electron micrographs, the trophozoites of *Naegleria* have the typical elements of a eukaryotic cell (Fig. 6–3). The cellular membrane, composed of three layers surrounding the cytoplasm, contains ribosomes, both free and attached to the endoplasmic reticulum, a primitive Golgi-like complex, smooth endoplasmic reticulum, numerous membrane-bound cytoplasmic organelles, and mitochondria. The mitochondria are discoid or cup-shaped (Fig. 6–3); digestive vacuoles and a contractile vacuole are also seen (Fig. 6–3). The nucleus is prominent, with a delicate membrane and a conspicuous nucleolus or endosome; the space between the nucleolus and the membrane appears to be empty. No centrosomes have been found in *Naegleria*. In scanning electron micrographs the surface of *Naegleria* is seen to possess cup-like structures or *amoebastomes*, used for feeding, formed by outward extensions of the cell surface.

Life Cycle and Biology. The natural history of *Naegleria* involves both a trophozoite stage and a cyst that forms when environmental conditions become adverse and excysts to produce a trophozoite when conditions are suitable (Fig. 6–1). Trophozoites multiply by binary fission and easily colonize cell-free and tissue cell cul-

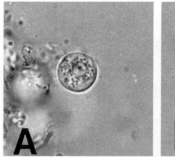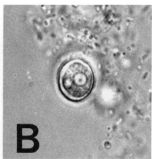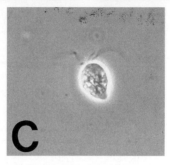

Fig. 6–2. *Naegleria fowleri* in culture. *A,* Trophozoite. *B,* Cyst. *C,* Ameboflagellate. Unstained, ×1,342. (Culture courtesy of G.S. Visvesvara, Ph.D., Centers for Disease Control, Atlanta, Georgia.)

ture media in the laboratory. Cysts are formed in water, soil, and culture media, but not in tissues, and are highly susceptible to desiccation, lasting for less than 5 minutes under dry conditions (Chang, 1978). Airborne cysts are implicated in human infections on circumstantial evidence (Lawande, 1983), but this conclusion seems unlikely given their susceptibility to desiccation (Dorsch et al. 1983).

About a dozen species of *Naegleria* are known. Their classification is based on genetic studies (Adams et al. 1989) or on immunologic characteristics of the isolates; only *N. fowleri* is considered pathogenic for animals and humans. *Naegleria* grows well under natural conditions at environmental temperatures in freshwater lakes, domestic water supplies, soil, air, humidifier systems, and sewage. It also grows in waters with higher than normal temperatures such as thermal springs, thermally polluted water, and chlorinated, heated swimming pools (Visvesvara, Stehr Green, 1990). Strains of *N. fowleri* adapted to higher temperatures (up to 46°C) are thermophilic (Cerva et al. 1982; De Jonckheere, Voorde, 1977) and are virulent to experimental animals, while nonthermophilic strains are avirulent (Cerva et al. 1982). Nevertheless, virulent *Naegleria* has been isolated from water at a temperature of 10°C (De Jonckheere, Voorde, 1977). Infections

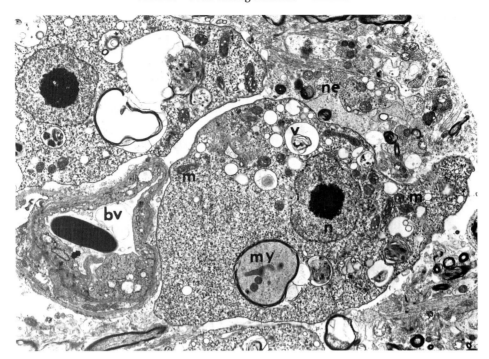

Fig. 6–3. *Naegleria fowleri*, transmission electron micrograph of a section of mouse brain experimentally infected. The parasite has the typical granular cyst with a large nucleolus. In the cytoplasm the mitochondria with tubular cristae, food vacuoles, and a phagocytized myelin sheath are seen. Outside the parasite the neuropil is disrupted. Note the small blood vessel on the lower left and another trophozoite on the upper left. Abbreviations: bv, blood vessel; m, mitochondria; my, myelin; n, nucleus; ne, neuropil; v, vacuole. (Courtesy of A.J. Martinez, M.D., Department of Pathology, University of Pittsburgh School of Medicine, Pittsburgh, Pennsylvania. In: Martinez, A.J., and Visvesvara, G.S. 1991. Laboratory diagnosis of pathogenic free-living amoebas: *Naegleria*, *Acanthamoeba*, and leptomyxid. Clin. Lab. Med. 11:861–872. Reproduced with permission.)

with *N. fowleri* are easily produced in laboratory animals by instillation of trophozoites in the nasal cavity (Martinez et al. 1973), where they attach to the neuro-olfactory epithelium and begin to colonize. Soon thereafter the amebae gain access to the brain, following the olfactory nerve endings that traverse the cribriform plate of the ethmoid bone. Once the amebae reach the brain, colonization of the olfactory bulbs, meninges, and brain tissue takes place rapidly, followed by the appearance of symptoms and death.

Epidemiology and Geographic Distribution. Amebic meningoencephalitis occurs worldwide, with the largest number of cases found in the United States, Australia, and some European countries where interest in the organism is highest. Most known human infections in the United States have occurred in the southeastern half of the country (CDC, 1980, 1992a, 1992b), all of them

during the summer months (Visvesvara, Stehr Green, 1990). The number of cases reported in the literature remains low, estimated at 200 worldwide in 1990 (Visvesvara, Stehr Green, 1990); by now the number of cases is probably about 250, but many remain unreported. Collecting a series of cases for publication in any single institution is difficult; in addition, single case reports have become routine and contribute little to our knowledge.

Naegleria fowleri has been isolated from the nasal mucosa of healthy individuals on several occasions (Cerva et al. 1973). However, how these infections occurred remains speculative. Most known human infections are acquired following swimming in fresh water, especially in thermally polluted streams (Martinez, 1993), natural thermal waters (Cursons et al. 1976), heated swimming pools (Cerva et al. 1968; Cursons et al. 1979), or stagnant water that is heated above normal levels during the summer months. For this reason, it is assumed that trophozoites in water are responsible for the infection in humans, but this has not been firmly established. *Naegleria aerobia*, a species pathogenic for mice, is transmitted more efficiently during the flagellated stage (Das, 1974).

Species of *Naegleria* have been isolated from the nasal passages and upper respiratory tracts of healthy individuals (Abraham, Lawande, 1982; Chang et al. 1975; Lawande et al. 1980; Shumaker et al. 1971). Some of these isolates have been identified only as *Naegleria* or as *N. gruberi*, a nonpathogenic species (Shumaker et al. 1971), but a few have been determined to be the pathogenic *N. fowleri* (Abraham, Lawande, 1982; Chang et al. 1975). The significance of these findings in the epidemiology of the infections remains unclear because passage of the infection from person to person has not been documented and appears unlikely and because reactivation of the infection has not been described.

Pathogenesis. The mechanism of invasion into the brain is not known (Cursons et al. 1978), nor is the mechanism by which *Naegleria* produces disease. Moreover, all information on the pathogenesis of this ameba has been derived from in vitro and animal experiments; how much of this work applies to natural infections in humans is not known. It is well established that virulent strains of *N. fowleri* have a cytopathogenic effect in vitro on cultures of mammalian cells (Culbertson, 1971), a phenomenon either not observed in nonpathogenic species (Cursons et al. 1980) or observed to a lesser degree (Marciano Cabral, 1988). It has been shown that the demyelinization of white matter in *Naegleria* infections, especially adjacent to the inflamed gray matter, is not due to vascular and circulatory alterations with thrombosis, as occurs in other encephalitides. Demyelinization in *Naegleria* is produced by a phospholipolytic effect that works directly on myelin, a pathway shown experimentally in test tubes with solutions of sphingomyelin incubated with the parasites (Chang, 1979). A 30 kDa protease characterized from cultures of *N. fowleri* and *N. gruberi* readily destroys mammalian tissues (Aldape et al. 1994). The enzyme of the nonpathogenic *N. gruberi* is not thermotolerant and does not operate above 30°C (Aldape et al. 1994). Other researchers have shown that destruction of cells is due not only to lysis of cells by enzymes, but also to phagocytosis by the amebae (Visvesvara, Callaway, 1974). In reality, it seems that these two mechanisms operate under different circumstances. Strains of cultured *N. fowleri* ingest cells piecemeal using their amoebastome, and strains serially passed in animals (more virulent) lyse cells (Marciano Cabral, 1988). It has been proposed that either an infectious agent carried by the amebae (Dunnebacke, Schuster, 1974) or a 50 kDa protein isolated from the parasite that acts as an infectious agent (Dunnebacke, Schuster, 1977; Marciano Cabral, 1988) is responsible for cell lysis.

Because the infection with *Naegleria* produces death rapidly, the immune response to the parasite has been little studied. Animal experiments have dealt with production of antibodies in animals infected with low doses of the parasite intraperitoneally and with attempts to elicit a protective immunity. No data on immunity in other animals and humans are available.

Clinical Findings. Primary amebic meningoencephalitis occurs mostly in healthy, immune-competent children and young adults, most of whom report swimming in fresh water just before becoming sick. The incubation period is 3 to 7 days, although in some instances it is up to 2 weeks. The symptoms often begin abruptly, with slight fever and malaise sometimes accompanied by a sore throat and rhinitis. These symptoms progress rapidly, with marked headache and fever, followed by vomiting and neck rigidity, a sign of meningeal irritation. By the end of the third day the patient is severely disoriented, if not comatose. Sometimes mild upper respiratory symptoms occur. At the time of hospital admission the diagnosis is usually pyogenic meningitis. In the hospital, the clinical picture is one of continuing deterioration to confusion, drowsiness, and sometimes convulsions. Spinal taps show a purulent fluid with elevated pressure, consistent with the clinical diagnosis of purulent meningitis. Other neurologic signs and symptoms are absent, and the patient dies of cardiorespiratory failure less than 10 days after the symptoms began (Carter, 1968, 1970, 1972). A few patients have apparently been treated successfully, but the identification of the parasite in some of these cases has been questioned.

Laboratory tests show an increase in peripheral polymorphonuclear leukocytes; the spinal fluid has elevated levels of protein, mononuclear cells, motile amebic trophozoites, and red blood cells. The characteristics of the cerebrospinal fluid and the clinical picture have often been mistaken for viral meningitis; in the absence of a traumatic tap, the presence of blood in the spinal fluid suggests a nonviral etiology. Computed tomography (CT) studies may show the meningeal process, with obliteration of the spaces surrounding the midbrain (Martinez, Janitschke, 1985), or nonspecific diffuse edema alone (Schumacher et al. 1995).

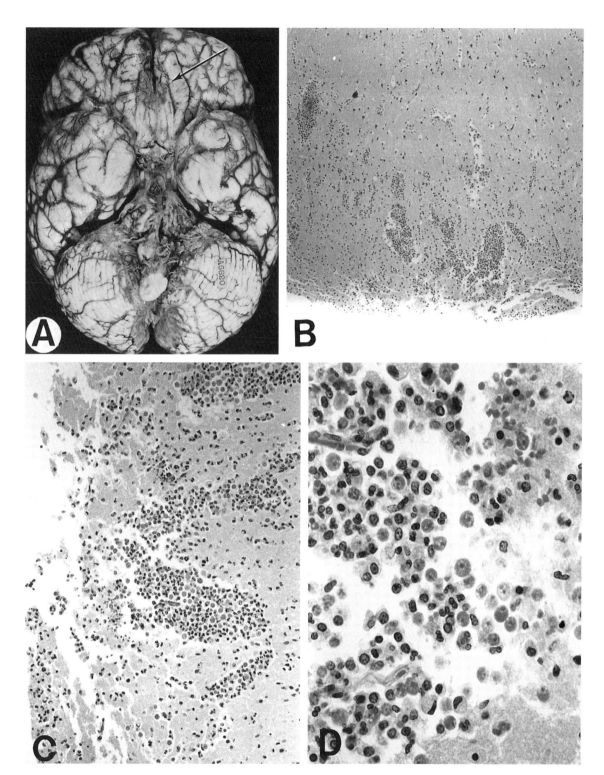

Fig. 6–4. *Naegleria fowleri*, primary meningoencephalitis. *A*, Gross appearance of brain. Note the discrete meningitis with hemorrhages and necrosis of the olfactory bulbs (arrows). (Courtesy of J. Martinez, M.D., Department of Pathology, University of Pittsburgh, School of Medicine, Pittsburgh, Pennsylvania. In: Martinez, J., dos Santos, J.G.N., Nelson, E.C., et al. 1977. Primary amebic meningoencephalitis. Pathol. Annu. 12:225–250. Reproduced with permission.) *B–D* Histologic appearance, sections of brain stained with hema- toxylin and eosin stain. *B*, Cerebral cortex of the right olfactory sulcus, with superficial necrosis and encephalitis represented by large masses of infiltrating cells, ×55. *C*, Higher magnification shows numerous amebae and mild mononuclear and polymorphonuclear cell infiltrates, ×140. *D*, Necrosis, amebic trophozoites, and the typical cellular infiltrate are evident, ×450. (Preparation courtesy of R.F. Carter, M.D., Department of Pathology, Adelaide Children's Hospital, North Adelaide, South Australia.).

Pathology. At necropsy the brain shows congestion with slight to severe swelling. The meninges are diffusely hyperemic, with a scanty purulent exudate, especially at the base of the brain (Fig. 6–4 *A*). The olfactory bulbs are friable and necrotic, with evidence of uncal herniation, and the cerebral cortex has superficial petechiae and areas of hemorrhage, with small areas of necrosis. These changes, variable in distribution, are more often found in the base of the frontal and temporal lobes, as well as in the hypothalamus, midbrain, and pons (Carter, 1968). On coronal sections the brain shows changes related to increased intracranial pressure such as herniation; otherwise, it is normal.

The microscopic changes in primary amebic meningoencephalitis consist of foci of hemorrhage, microscopic necrosis, mononuclear and polymorphonuclear cell infiltrates, and typical amebic trophozoites (Fig. 6–4 *B–D*). Examination of the nasal cavity shows inflammatory changes in the neuro-olfactory epithelium extending into the brain through the cribriform plate, together with marked edema and swelling with a polymorphonuclear cell infiltrate that accounts for the rhinitis seen in some patients (Fig. 6–5 *A–B*; Carter, 1968).

In the cranial cavity the meninges are hyperemic, with moderate to marked infiltration by lymphocytes (Fig. 6–6 *A*). Polymorphonuclear cells are few, and the amebae are seen in this background as discrete, usually poorly stained, rounded structures with a prominent nucleus (Fig. 6–6 *B*). Lesions in the gray matter, sometimes extending into the white matter, consist of foci of microscopic necrosis with inflammatory cells and amebic trophozoites (Fig. 6–4 *C–D*). Often the parasites are found around blood vessels since they enter the brain tissue along the Virchow-Robin spaces (Fig. 6–6 *D*).

Necrosis of small blood vessels with destruction of vessel walls, formation of thrombi (Fig. 6–6 *C*), and

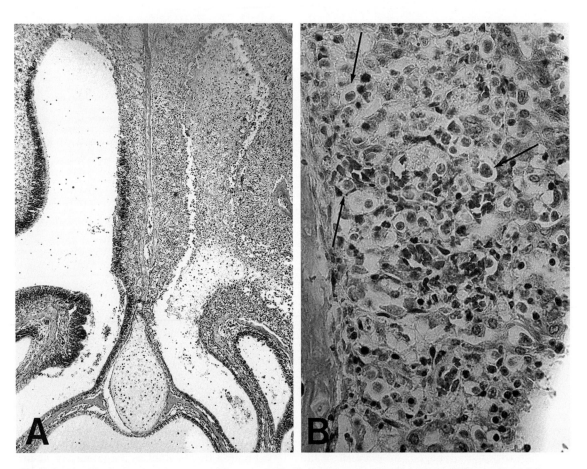

Fig. 6–5. *Naegleria fowleri* in neuro-olfactory epithelium of a mouse infected experimentally, trichrome stain. *A*, Sagittal section of the nasal septum shows destruction of the epithelium and the inflammatory cells, ×55. *B*, Higher magnification shows scanty mononuclear and polymorphonuclear cells and numerous *Naegleria* trophozoites (arrows), ×450. (Preparation courtesy of C.G. Culbertson, Ph.D., Lilly Research Laboratories, Indianapolis, Indiana.)

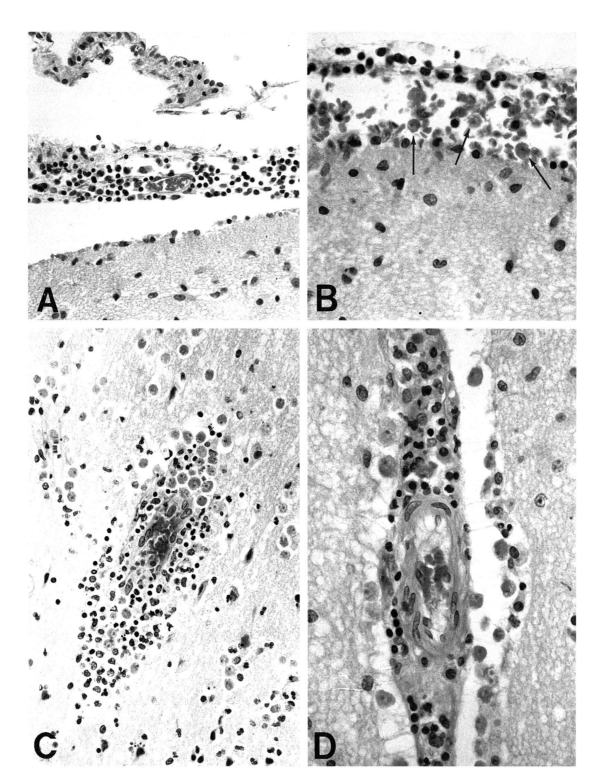

Fig. 6–6. *Naegleria fowleri*, primary amebic meningoencephalitis, hematoxylin and eosin stain. *A*, Meningitis with a mononuclear cell infiltrate, ×280. *B*, Higher magnification showing slight hemorrhage in the meningeal space and a few *Naegleria* trophozoites (arrows), ×280. *C*, Necrosis of small vessel and infiltration by polymorphonuclear and mononuclear cells. Amebae trophozoites are seen throughout the entire field, usually in small groups, ×280. *D*, Deep cerebral sulcus with invasion of the meninges by *Naegleria* trophozoites on the right and the Virchow-Robin space on the left. Note the inflammatory cells, ×448. (Preparation courtesy of R.F. Carter, M.D., Department of Pathology, Adelaide Children's Hospital, North Adelaide, South Australia.)

petechial hemorrhages are common features of primary amebic meningoencephalitis. The organisms circulate in the cerebrospinal fluid to the ventricles and other areas. In no instance, either in tissues or in cerebrospinal fluid, have cysts been identified. The inflammatory response is minimal, probably due to the rapidity with which *Naegleria* multiplies in the tissues and the disease evolves. In foci of necrosis, a few macrophages are present.

A lesion sometimes seen outside the central nervous system is a focal myocarditis consisting of small areas of necrosis with an inflammatory cellular infiltrate (Carter, 1968; Markowitz et al. 1974). Since no parasites have been found, this lesion is believed to be due to a hypoperfusion state (shock).

Diagnosis. The clinical diagnosis of primary amebic meningoencephalitis is difficult, mainly because the small number of reported cases makes it difficult for clinicians to become familiar with the infection. If the clinical diagnosis is suspected, the amebae should be searched for in stained and unstained smears of cerebrospinal fluid.

The amebae in fresh mounts of cerebrospinal fluid sediment are difficult to identify; knowledge of their morphologic characteristics is required. Motile amebae 7 to 15 μm in diameter, with a large nucleolus and a vacuolated cytoplasm, should be found before a diagnosis is made (Fig. 6–2). Lowering the microscope condenser to enhance contrast facilitates visualization of the parasites; phase contrast microscopy may be used. If cerebrospinal fluid is centrifuged and the sediment is resuspended in water, the amebae are transformed into flagellated stages. This characteristic should be kept in mind and explored in the laboratory in all suspected cases of *Naegleria*. Spinal fluid sediment can be stained with Giemsa or trichrome stains; a cytospine preparation of fluid taken postmortem and stained with Papanicolaou stain gave good results in one case (Benson et al. 1985). Stained parasites are recognized more easily than unstained ones.

In tissue sections of autopsy material, where the diagnosis of *Naegleria* is most commonly made, the trophozoites are identical to those in smears (Figs. 6–4 D and 6–7 B–D), except that in tissues the amebae are smaller, with an average size of 7 to 8 μm, and have a nucleus measuring about 2 to 3 μm; in some trophozoites, the nucleus is missing because of the plane of sectioning (Cerva et al. 1968). *Remember, this is a very small ameba.* The trophozoites are found either singly or in groups within the brain tissue, the interstitium of the meninges (pia mater and arachnoid), the brain surface and sulci, and the Virchow-Robin spaces following medium-sized and small blood vessels. The trophozoite membrane is poorly delineated, and the cytoplasm is vacuolated and pale-staining with hematoxylin and eosin stain. The most conspicuous structure is the nucleus, with no apparent nuclear membrane and with a large, darkly stained nucleolus (Figs. 6–4 D and 6–6 D and H). *Naegleria* can be cultured in cell-free media in a manner similar to that of *Acanthamoeba* (see below).

Differentiation of *Naegleria* from other lymax amebae and *E. histolytica* in tissues is aided by measuring the trophozoites. The average diameter of *Naegleria* trophozoites in fixed and processed tissues is 7.5 μm (Cerva et al. 1968). *Naegleria* has not been described outside the neuro-olfactory epithelium and the brain; it does not form cysts in tissues; and it does not produce macroscopic necrosis of brain (Fig. 6–4 A–B).

Acanthamoeba, Balamuthia, and *Hartmannella*—Granulomatous Amebic Encephalitis

The first case of an *acanthamebid* (a term used here to denote any species of the three genera studied) reported in humans occurred in 1948 in a Japanese soldier who died of a disseminated infection. The parasite was identified as closely resembling, if not identical to, *Iodamoeba buetschlii* (Derrick, 1948). Some investigators believe that the parasite in this patient is *Naegleria* (Beaver et al. 1984), but it is now clear that the figures in the report show cysts engulfed by macrophages, a feature of acanthamebids. The second case of human infection occurred in 1960 in Tucson, Arizona, in a 6-year-old girl and was reported as a granuloma of the brain produced by *Iodamoeba* (Kernohan et al. 1960). At this time, Culbertson and coworkers had been conducting experiments with pathogenic free-living amebae in mice (Culbertson, 1961; Culbertson et al. 1958, 1959, 1965) and monkeys (Culbertson et al. 1959), producing lesions similar to those seen in humans. A drawback of this work is that the parasites were referred to as *Hartmannella-Acanthamoeba* because these genera could not be separated at the time. The two genera were defined clearly, and several species belonging to both of them were described in 1967 (Page, 1967a, 1967b). This historic information is provided to explain why the terms *Acanthamoeba* and *Hartmannella*, and sometimes *Naegleria*, were used to refer to human infections with lymax amebae in the literature of the 1960s and 1970s.

Acanthamoeba, Balamuthia, and *Hartmannella,* together with *Entamoeba,* the intestinal amebae, are placed in the phylum Rhizopoda because they have common features (see Chapter 7) (Corliss, 1994). *Acanthamoeba* is characterized by the presence of small, pointed subpseudopodia known as *acanthopodia,* which appear and disappear continuously on the surface of the trophozoite. *Hartmannella* lacks acanthopods but otherwise is very similar to *Acanthamoeba. Balamuthia* also lacks acanthopodia when observed under the light microscope. It is a fastidious ameba that does not grow on bacteria and requires a feeder layer of tissue culture cells for food. It has a uninucleated, plasmodium-like trophic stage that moves by protoplasmic flow into lobose pseudopods (Visvesvara et al. 1993).

Acanthamoeba and *Balamuthia* are the most important of the three genera; several species of *Acanthamoeba* have been isolated from humans, and one species of *Balamuthia, B. mandrillaris,* is responsible for most human infections (Visvesvara et al. 1993). The genus *Hartmannella* is one of the most common in nature, but apparently it has been recovered from humans only in a few instances—once from the brain and identified as *H. rhysodes* (Cleland et al. 1982), from corneal

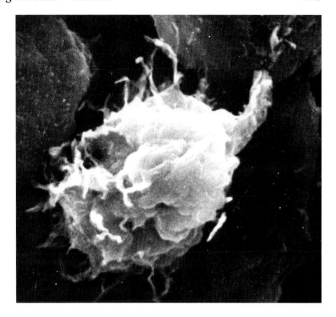

Fig. 6–8. *Acanthamoeba,* **scanning electron micrograph demonstrating the acanthopods, ×3,650. (Courtesy of J. Niederkorn, Ph.D., Department of Ophthalmology, School of Medicine, The University of Texas, Southwestern Medical Center, Dallas, Texas.)**

lesions (Kennedy et al. 1995), and from spinal fluid and identified as *H. vermiformis* (Centeno et al. 1996) or simply as a *Hartmannella* species (Aitken et al. 1996). The morphology and biology of these amebae and the diseases they produce are similar and will be discussed together; if differences exist, they will be pointed out.

Morphology. The trophozoites of species of medically important acanthamebids vary in size and other characteristics (Figs. 6–7 *A* and 6–8). Species of *Acanthamoeba,* as mentioned before, have filamentous projections, the acanthopods (Fig. 6–8). In fresh preparations, the length of actively moving trophic forms of *Acanthamoeba* varies as follows: *A. castellanii,* 21 to 45 μm; *A. astronyxes,* 25 to 60 μm; and *A. polyphaga,* 14 to 41 μm (Page, 1967a). The trophozoites of *B. mandrillaris* are 12 to 60 μm long, with a mean length of 30 μm, and the nucleus is 5 μm in diameter. The cysts are generally 6 to 30 μm in diameter, with a mean of about 25 μm (Fig. 6–7 *B*). The cytoplasm is granular, with numerous food vacuoles distributed around the nucleus; one, and sometimes two, of these food vacuoles are contractile vacuoles that empty their watery content at intervals of 40 to 50 seconds (Page, 1967a). The nucleus is evident as a faint, refractile structure with an even more refractile,

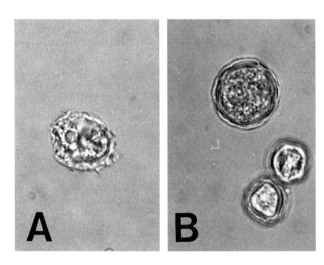

Fig. 6–7. *Acanthamoeba polyphaga* **in culture from human cornea, unstained.** *A,* **Trophozoite shows the nucleus with the large, birefringent nucleolus and minute acanthopodia, ×775.** *B,* **Three cysts illustrate the differences in size. Note the wall with an irregular ectocyst and the smoother endocyst containing the ameba, ×775. (Culture courtesy of I. Rutheford, M.D., Department of Pathology, The Cleveland Clinic Educational Foundation, Cleveland, Ohio.)**

rounded karyosome (Fig. 6–7 B). The cysts vary in size from 10 to 20 μm and have a wall composed of an ectocyst or outer wall, which is irregular, polyhedral, somewhat wrinkled, and very refractile, and an endocyst or inner wall, which is smoother. The inner content is the parasite itself, which also is polyhedral, containing numerous dark granules and a nucleus similar to that of the trophozoite. In preparations well stained with iron hematoxylin or trichrome stain these characteristics are better appreciated. In tissue sections stained with hematoxylin and eosin stain the acanthopods do not stain, the nucleolus stains dark red, and the cytoplasm stains eosinophilically. The nuclear membrane is delicate and is often outlined only by the perinuclear vacuoles.

In electron micrographs, the acanthamebids are similar to those of *Naegleria* and other amebae (Figs. 6–9 and 6–10 A). A cytoplasmic membrane with the characteristic two electron-dense layers and an electron-lucent layer in the middle surrounds the trophozoite; the acanthopods are seen projecting from the membrane (Fig. 6–10 A). The cytoplasm has numerous mitochondria, usually with tubular cristae (Fig. 6–9); in contrast, *Entamoeba* lacks mitochondria, probably due to an evolutionary secondary loss. The cytoplasm also has an abundant endoplasmic reticulum, mostly of the rough variant, free ribosomes, and granules of glycogen. The Golgi apparatus has a paranuclear position. The food vacuoles are numerous, and in some sections endocytotic vesicles are seen. The con-

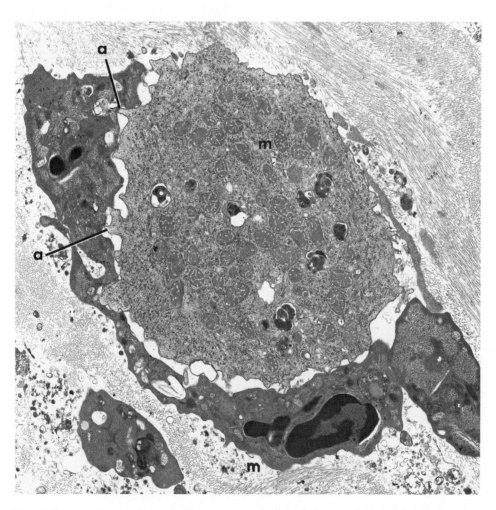

Fig. 6–9. *Acanthamoeba polyphaga*, transmission electron micrograph of a section from a corneal biopsy specimen. Note the trophozoite being engulfed by a macrophage, ×8,465. Abbreviation: a, acanthopods. (Courtesy of J. McMahon, Ph.D., Department of Pathology, The Cleveland Clinic Educational Foundation, Cleveland, Ohio.)

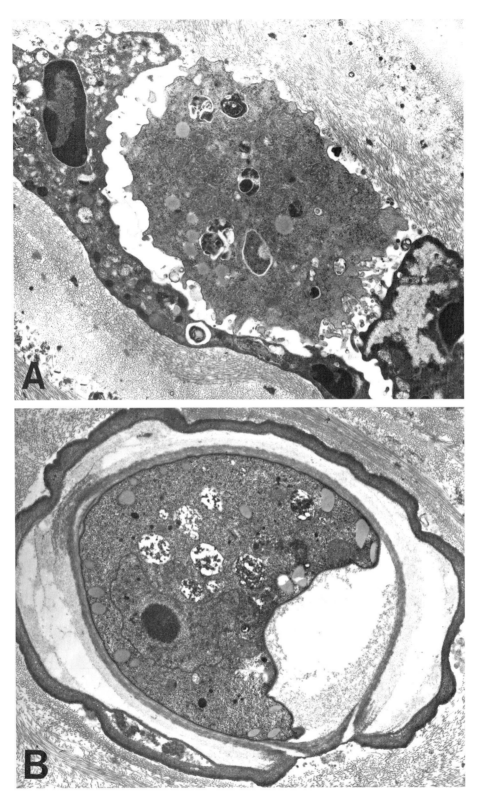

Fig. 6–10. *Acanthamoeba polyphaga*, transmission electron micrographs of a section from a corneal biopsy specimen. *A*, Trophozoite, ×5,000. *B*, Cyst. Note the wall with a ostyole and the parasite with a single nucleus, ×5,000. (Courtesy of J. McMahon, Ph.D., Department of Pathology, The Cleveland Clinic Educational Foundation, Cleveland, Ohio.)

tractile vacuole is surrounded by a spongioma consisting of numerous canaliculi, and the vacuolar membrane, when full, appears distended. The nuclear membrane is delicate, with numerous nuclear pores, and the large karyosome at the center shows clumps of heterochromatin (Proca-Ciobanu et al. 1975). The cysts have a thick, irregular wall with numerous pores or ostyoles (Fig. 6–10 B). In tissues, both immature (Fig. 6–11) and mature cysts are often seen phagocytized and being destroyed by the macrophages (Fig. 6–12 A–B). Species of *Balamuthia* lack acanthopods under the light microscope, but in electron micrographs a few small ones are seen (Fig. 6–13 A). The cysts are mostly round, with a wall composed of three layers (Fig. 6–13 B) (Visvesvara et al. 1993).

Life Cycle and Biology. For practical purposes, the life cycles of all the free-living amebae are similar, involv-ing a trophozoite and a cystic stage (Fig. 6–7). The trophozoites require a liquid or highly humid environment with plentiful bacteria for their subsistence; in the case of *Balamuthia*, the trophozoites need other living protozoa to feed on. Under adverse conditions, the trophozoites form cysts that revert to trophozoites under suitable conditions. The cysts of *Acanthamoeba* and *Hartmannella* are transported in dust by the wind and have been isolated from air in every place where they have been sought. The cysts of acanthamebids are found in the tissues, a characteristic that helps to distinguish them from *Naegleria*. However, their significance in maintaining the parasite in nature or in transmitting the infection to other hosts is not known.

For our purposes, the most important biologic characteristic of the acanthamebids is their capacity to cause infections in immune-competent hosts and to become opportunistic infections in immune-deficient ones (Martinez, 1980). Some species of *Acanthamoeba* pos-

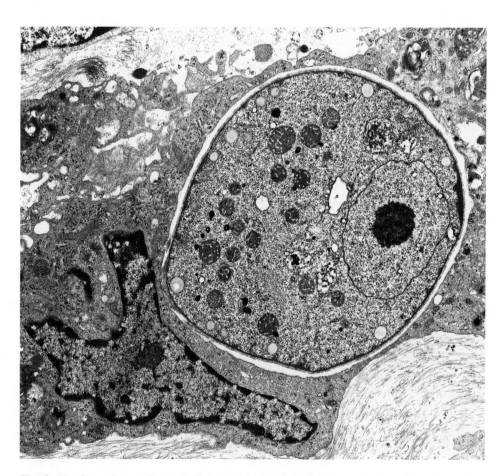

Fig. 6–11. *Acanthamoeba polyphaga*, transmission electron micrographs of a section from a corneal biopsy specimen, showing an immature cyst within a macrophage, ×8,755. (Courtesy of J. McMahon, Ph.D., Department of Pathology, The Cleveland Clinic Educational Foundation, Cleveland, Ohio.)

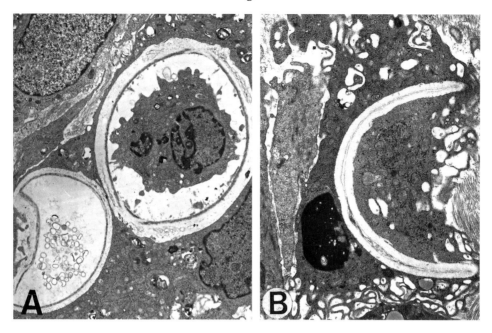

Fig. 6–12. *Acanthamoeba polyphaga*, transmission electron micrographs of a section from a corneal biopsy specimen. *A* and *B*, Cysts within macrophages in different stages of disintegration, ×4,250 (Courtesy of J. McMahon, Ph.D., Department of Pathology, The Cleveland Clinic Educational Foundation, Cleveland, Ohio.)

sess distinct morphologic and biologic characteristics, but in general these are not sufficient to allow their separation. Immunoperoxidase, immunofluorescence stains, and the polymerase chain reaction (Vodkin et al. 1992) are used for this purpose.

One biologic characteristic of *Acanthamoeba* and *Hartmannella* is that they are commonly parasitized by *Legionella*-like amebal pathogens (LLAP). These pathogens are adapted to survive in digestive vacuoles of the amebae in the same manner that *Legionella pneumophila* does in human alveolar macrophages (Abu, 1996). The relevance of these *Legionella*-like organisms in clinical medicine has been studied recently, "suggesting that they may be an unrecognized and possible significant cause of respiratory disease" (Adeleke et al. 1996). A strain of LLAP was isolated from a patient with pneumonia (using cultures of *Acanthamoeba* as the isolating media) in whom *L. pneumophila* was not demonstrated by conventional means. After successful treatment for *Legionella*, the patient showed specific antibodies to the LLAP isolate. Cultures of amebae have been used to isolate *L. pneumophila* from clinical samples from patients with respiratory disease (Adeleke et al. 1996).

Epidemiology. The free-living amebae occur worldwide, and human cases have been found in every

place where physicians and diagnosticians have become aware of their existence. Human infections with these amebae have probably occurred since the dawn of humankind. Their recognition during the last few decades is the result of the enormous advances in infectious disease treatment in the antibiotic era. The acquired immune deficiency syndrome (AIDS) epidemic highlighted the importance of the acanthamebids because of their capacity to become opportunistic and produce significant morbidity and mortality.

Because the cysts of acanthamebids are found in air, infections in humans must occur through the upper respiratory airways and by contact with exposed mucosa such as the conjunctiva. *Acanthamoeba* and *Hartmannella* have been isolated in cultures of swabs taken from the nose and upper respiratory tract of normal individuals (Cerva et al. 1973; Wang, Feldman, 1961), but the most common isolates from the respiratory tract are species of *Hartmannella* (Wang, Feldman, 1967). Human-to-human transmission has not been demonstrated. Thus, all infections are acquired from the environment, and the term *econozes* (from the Greek *oikos*, "house," + *nosos*, "disease") is proposed here to refer to the diseases caused by organisms that are free-living but occasionally facultative parasites.

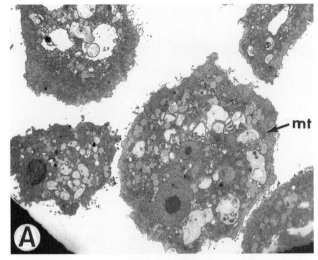

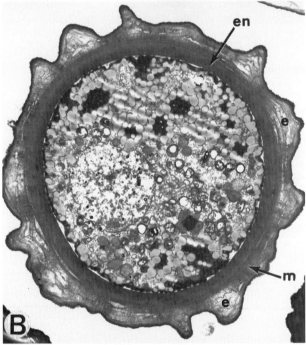

Fig. 6–13. *Balamuthia mandrillaris*, transmission electron micrograph of trophozoites and a cyst. *A,* Trophozoite. Note the general lack of acanthopods and the cytoplasm with numerous small, elongated, oval mitochondria (mt). There are numerous vacuoles, most of which are empty, others with electron-dense nuclear material. The nucleus has dense, compacted chromatin, ×6,000. *B,* The cyst is spherical, with a wall consisting of three layers: the highly irregular ectocyst (e), the thicker endocyst (en) with a smooth inner surface, and a middle one of variable thickness filled with reticulate material (m). The cyst is filled with numerous lipid droplets, ×12,920. (Courtesy of A.J. Martinez, M.D., Department of Pathology, University of Pittsburgh School of Medicine, Pittsburgh, Pennsylvania.)

Pathogenesis. The pathogenicity of species of *Acanthamoeba*, *Balamuthia*, and *Hartmannella* is unquestionable. That some of these species are highly virulent is also evident given time sequence of symptom development and the degree of disease seen in some human infections. However, these amebae need hosts who are immune suppressed or at least immune deficient to become facultative parasites. *Balamuthia* infections found in young adults and children with no known immune deficit (Riestra-Castaneda et al. 1997; Taratuto et al. 1991) suggest that this genus may be more virulent than *Acanthamoeba* and *Hartmannella*. The mechanism by which the parasites invade tissues and produce lesions is not known. The only work done on interaction of the amebae with tissue cells has focused on the cornea because of the interest in ocular lesions. *Acanthamoeba* in the cornea produces a progressive necrotizing keratitis. In in vitro studies, this keratitis has been shown to occur only in human, pig, and hamster corneas, other animals being refractory. In the corneas of susceptible animals the parasites attach firmly to the corneal epithelium, producing deep pits and exfoliation of the epithelium (Niederkorn et al. 1992). In in vivo studies the parasites attach only to previously damaged corneal epithelium, never to intact epithelium, and the presence of Langerhans cells in the cornea prevents the development of lesions (Klink et al. 1994). Macrophages appear to act as the first line of defense by ingesting the parasites (Klink et al. 1996). How the parasites attach to either damaged or intact cornea and how the lesions are produced are not known. The role of collagenase isolated from the supernatant of an *A. castellanii* culture seems to play a role in lesion production because it is active both in vivo and in vitro against corneal tissue (He et al. 1990).

Disease. Infections with acanthamebids have been described in immune-competent individuals and in those who are debilitated, have an underlying disease, or are immune suppressed. In immune-competent hosts the infections usually occur in the cornea, skin, ear, and bone. The main predisposing factors to the disease are skin ulcers or skin trauma, diabetes mellitus, cirrhosis of the liver, pneumonia, Hodgkin's disease, glucose-6-phosphate dehydrogenase deficiency, broad-spectrum antibiotic use, steroid therapy, antineoplastic agent use, radiation therapy, alcoholism, and human immune deficiency virus (HIV) infection (Martinez, 1980). During the last two decades, the great majority of cases have occurred in patients with AIDS (Gordon et al. 1992; Gregorio et al. 1992; Murakawa et al. 1995), who sometimes develop disseminated disease. Infections with *B. mandrillaris* in immune-competent individuals, especially children, have also been identified (Riestra-Castaneda et al. 1997; Taratuto et al. 1991).

The ports of entry used by the free-living amebae are damaged skin, the upper respiratory tract, and the conjunctiva. There the parasites produce dermal lesions, nasal sinus infections, and keratitis. Radial keratotomy has been complicated by *Acanthamoeba* infection (Friedman et al. 1997). As noted earlier, infections in the upper respiratory tract may be asymptomatic. Depending on the immunologic condition of the host, the parasites may disseminate to secondary loci, mainly in the brain and the lungs. The species implicated in human infections are *A. culbertsoni*, *A. polyphaga*, *A. castellanii*, *A. astronyxes*, *A. griffini*, *B. mandrillaris*, *H. rhysodes*, and *H. vermiformis*. Since the clinical and histologic characteristics of each syndrome produced by these acanthamebids are distinct, we will consider them separately in order of importance.

Central Nervous System. As stated, infection of the central nervous system with acanthamebids usually occurs in immune-impaired individuals (see above), in whom it produces a granulomatous amebic encephalitis (Martinez et al. 1980). The amebae reach the brain from a primary locus somewhere in the body; probably the most common locus is the upper respiratory tract, followed by the skin. Dissemination from the cornea has not been demonstrated. The parasites probably travel via the circulatory system, since arteritis with thrombosis and infarction is commonly seen in the brain and other sites.

Clinical findings. Involvement of the brain by acanthamebids occurs at all ages, equally in both sexes and with no racial predilection. The clinical manifestations are variable, but most patients present with focal or diffuse encephalopathy and meningeal irritation. Sometimes the main manifestations consist of a space-occupying lesion with signs of increased intracranial pressure (Martinez et al. 1980). The most common symptoms are mental status abnormalities, seizures, headache, hemiparesis, and meningism. Fever is present in about one-half of the cases, and nausea, vomiting, anorexia, ataxia, and aphasia are present to a lesser degree. The course of the disease is subacute or chronic and lasts for 7 to 120 days (Martinez, 1980). Some patients have concurrent skin ulcerations.

The most significant laboratory abnormalities in the cerebrospinal fluid are pleocytosis of 20% to 100% lymphocytes, a borderline normal glucose level, an elevated protein level, and few or no polymorphonuclear cells. The borderline normal glucose level and the sub-

normal polymorphonuclear cell count, help to distinguish the infection from a bacterial meningoencephalitis. Imaging techniques (CT scans, cerebral angiograms, and gallium scans) usually demonstrate several avascular lesions located anywhere in the brain, commonly in the cerebellum or midbrain. In some patients, CT scanograms reveal large arterial occlusions and magnetic resonance imaging (MRI) demonstrates lesions in the spinal cord (Schumacher et al. 1995). A shift of the ventricular spaces may be demonstrated. In a 7-year-old girl, the presentation was that of a tumor mass in the left parietal area, with incoordination of the right upper extremity and unsteady gait progressing to left-sided weakness, increased deep tendon reflexes, and a positive Babinski sign on the right side (Ofori-Kwakye et al. 1986). An infection with *Balamuthia* presented as a brain stem glioma (Lowichik et al. 1995). The great majority of patients deteriorate progressively into coma and death.

Pathology. Gross examination of the brain in granulomatous amebic encephalitis shows swollen, edematous cerebral hemispheres, with evidence of increased intracranial pressure: uncal and cerebellar tonsillar herniation or lateral deviation of one of the hemispheres. The superficial cortex has areas of softening, with focal areas of inflammatory exudate on the meninges. On cut section the areas of softening appear hemorrhagic and necrotic, extending into the white and gray matter (Fig. 6–14); these areas are more common in the cerebellum, brain stem, and basal ganglia (Martinez et al. 1980). Cortical lesions filled with dark brown, friable debris extend several centimeters from the cortex into the white matter; some of these lesions are indistinguishable from hemorrhagic infarcts.

The microscopic tissue changes consist of extensive necrosis with hemorrhage and mononuclear and polymorphonuclear cell infiltrates in varying amounts, but the amebae are the hallmark of the lesion (Figs. 6–15 A–B). In viable tissues, a granulomatous inflammation is the characteristic finding in these patients. Recent granulomas have the ameba at their center (Fig. 6–16 A). Older granulomas consist of many histiocytes, with both cysts and trophozoites engulfed by giant cells (Fig. 6–16 B). The cysts are found in different stages of disintegration and are finally destroyed by the macrophages (Fig. 6–16 B; see also Fig. 6–12 A–B). Parasites are seen throughout the necrotic tissue; in viable brain tissue they are more numerous, usually following the Virchow-Robin spaces, and occurring around and within the walls of medium-sized and large blood vessels. Both trophozoites and cysts are recognized (Fig. 6–15 D). Many blood vessels show changes of vasculitis and necrosis of the wall with thrombosis,

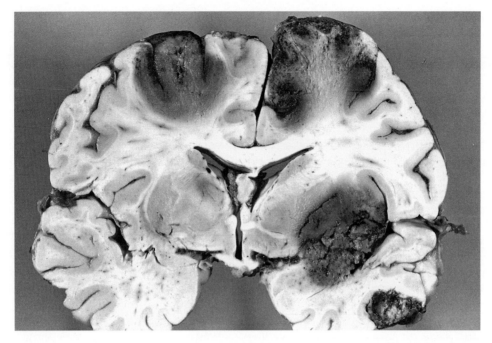

Fig. 6–14. *Acanthamoeba castellanii.* **Gross appearance of brain lesions. Note the multiple foci of hemorrhagic necrosis involving cortex and white matter. (Courtesy of J. Martinez, M.D., Department of Pathology, University of Pittsburgh, School of Medicine, Pittsburgh, Pennsylvania. In: Martinez, J. 1982. Acanthamoebiasis and immunosuppression. Case report. J. Neuropathol. Exp. Neurol. 41:548–557. Reproduced with permission.)**

a mechanism responsible for the large amount of tissue necrosis and thus the infarct-like appearance of these lesions. Smaller vessels have fibrinoid necrosis (Fig. 6–15 C). The cellular infiltrate is variable: some patients with intact bone marrow have lymphocytes and abundant polymorphonuclear cells; others, with low or absent lymphoid and myeloid elements, have no inflammatory reaction (Fig. 6–15 D). The presence of macrophages is variable. Sometimes the macrophages contain phagocytized amebae, especially cysts, in various stages of degradation. Cysts in multinucleated giant cells have a smooth ectocyst due to the digestive capacity of the macrophages. Plasma cells may be present, especially if the lesion has been evolving for some time.

Amebic Keratitis and Keratoconjunctivitis. Amebic keratitis has become an important infection, especially in individuals who wear soft contact lenses (Stehr-Green et al. 1989). In the United States, 208 cases of amebic keratitis were reported up to mid-July 1988, but this figure does not represent the true number of cases because only those reported in the literature or to the Centers for Disease Control were available. This is a minuscule number if we consider that about 25 million Americans use contact lenses. About 85% of the infected patients used daily-wear or extended-wear soft lenses; the type of solution used for cleaning the lenses was known in 138 patients, 64% of whom used saline prepared by dissolving salt tablets in water (Stehr-Green et al. 1989). The prevalence of amebic

Fig. 6–15. *Acanthamoeba,* **histologic appearance of lesions in brain sections stained with hematoxylin and eosin stain. *A,* Low-power view of cerebellar lesion showing marked necrosis and hemorrhage, ×9. *B,* Higher magnification shows amebic trophozoites within the granular layer of the cerebellum, ×220. *C,* Section of brain from another patient showing necrosis of a small vessel; numerous trophozoites and necrosis with scanty** polymorphonuclear and mononuclear cells are present, ×750. *D,* **Blood vessel showing numerous *Acanthamoeba* cysts in the wall. Note the lack of inflammatory reaction due to marked leukopenia, ×450. (Preparations from autopsies in *A, B,* and *D* courtesy of A.J. Martinez, M.D., Department of Pathology, University of Pittsburgh, School of Medicine, Pittsburgh, Pennsylvania).**

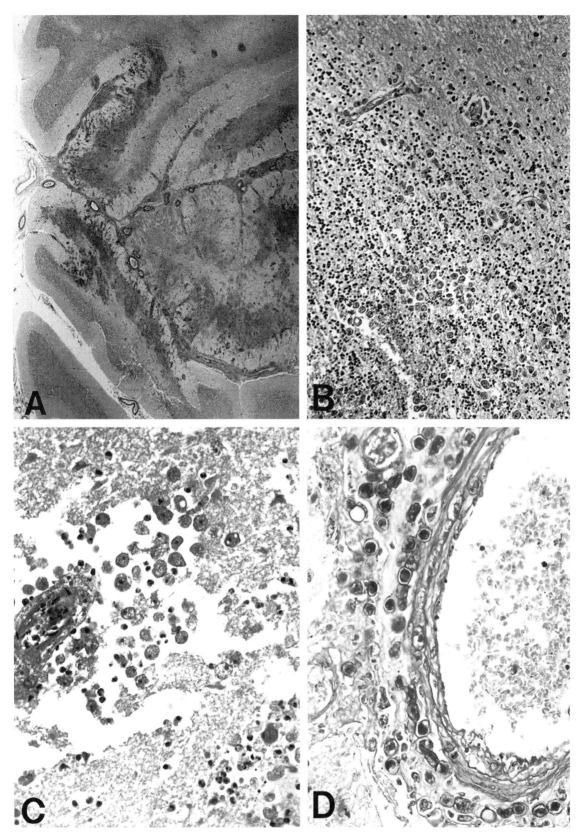

Fig. 6–15.

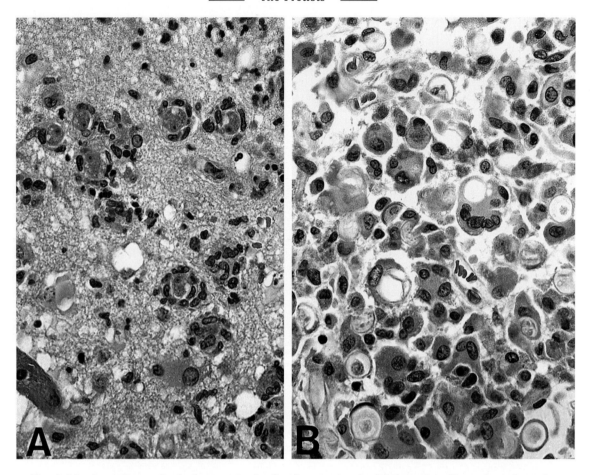

Fig. 6–16. *Acanthamoeba* in human brain. Sections stained with hematoxylin and eosin stain. *A*, Section of viable tissue shows the early granulomas, consisting of histiocytes surrounding amebae trophozoites, ×350. *B*, Area showing an older reaction consisting of numerous histiocytes with phagocytized cysts in different stages of disintegration, ×450.

keratitis appears to be decreasing among users of soft contact lenses in the United States (Cohen et al. 1996). Identification of a few amebic isolates from cases of keratitis has shown *A. polyphaga* to be the causal agent in some instances (Visvesvara et al. 1975). However, this finding is probably due to the fact that *A. polyphaga* survives more often when exposed to some of the recommended soft contact lens disinfection agents (Ludwig et al. 1986). In other patients *A. castellanii* has been cultured and identified (Florakis et al. 1988; Jones et al. 1975), and *A. griffini* has been characterized on molecular bases (Ledee et al. 1996). *Acanthamoeba polyphaga* has been described as having a broad hyaline lobopodium, with numerous acanthopods formed in the direction of movement, but these characteristics do not permit identification (Fig. 6–7 *A*). Recently, a species of *Hartmannella* was isolated from the cornea in a coinfection with *Vahlkampfia* (Kennedy et al. 1995).

Clinical findings. The presenting symptoms of amebic keratitis usually consist of a corneal ulcer or abrasion that often resembles adenoviral keratitis (*color plate* III *H*; Goodall et al. 1996). Persons without contact lenses often have a history of a foreign body in the eye, minor ocular trauma, or washing their eyes with dirty water. The wearer of contact lenses, especially soft ones, complains of sudden discomfort and irritation. The symptoms become worse, with increasing pain, tearing, and photophobia. Examination of the eye usually shows redness and often a corneal epithelial defect, which may become recurrent or persistent (Cohen et al. 1985; Moore et al. 1986). Other patients show superficial punctate keratitis (Samples et al. 1984), scattered epithelial and subepithelial opacities (Nagington et al. 1974), epithelial infiltrates (Mannis et al. 1986), irregularities (Jones, 1986), stippling (Key et al. 1980), roughened epithelium (Watson, 1975), epithelial irregularities (Hanssens et al. 1985), or elevated corneal ep-

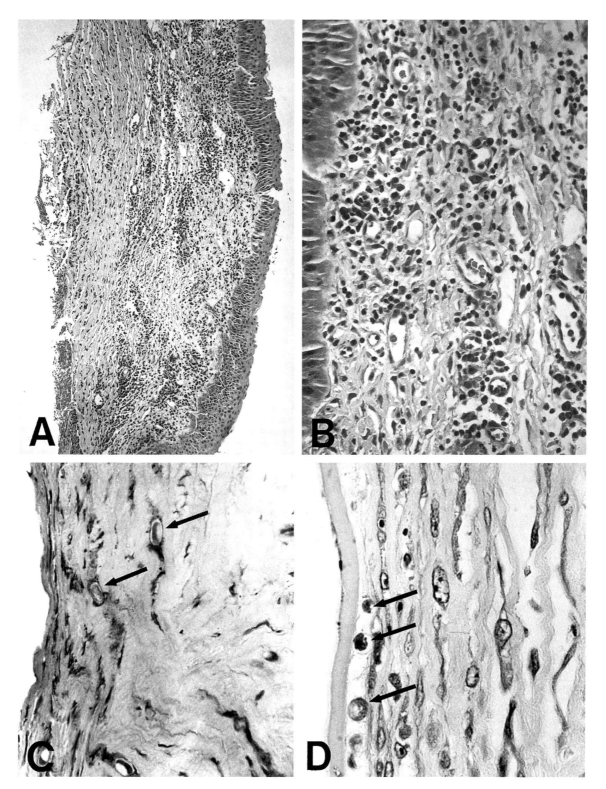

Fig. 6–17. *Acanthamoeba* keratitis. Sections of cornea stained with hematoxylin and eosin stain. *A*, Low-power view shows the marked inflammatory reaction, ×70. *B*, Higher magnification; amebae are not present in this field, ×220. Section of cornea from another case, showing fibrosis, a scant inflammatory reaction, and amebae. *C*, Cysts (arrows), ×450. *D*. Higher magnification of the posterior cornea shows Descemet's membrane with amebic trophozoites below it (arrows), fibroblasts, and a few mononuclear cells. The nuclei of the corneal stroma appear abnormally ballooned, ×450. (*C* and *D* from a preparation courtesy of H.S. Levine, M.D., Department of Pathology, The Cleveland Clinic Foundation, Cleveland, Ohio.)

ithelial lines (Florakis et al. 1988). If the diagnosis is not suspected, conventional treatment results in further deterioration over several months, with periods of quiescence and recrudescence, especially if steroid therapy is given. The keratitis progresses relentlessly, and conjunctivitis and iritis can develop; marked deterioration of visual acuity with destruction of the cornea follows (*color plate* III *H*), necessitating vigorous therapy and keratoplasty. A ring stromal infiltrate develops in over two-thirds of affected individuals, manifesting as a paracentral annular corneal infiltrate or abscess (Theodore et al. 1985); if this condition is recognized by the clinician, it can lead to an early diagnosis. Rarely does *Acanthamoeba* keratitis extend beyond the cornea to produce uveitis (Jones et al. 1975). In AIDS patients with *Acanthamoeba* encephalitis, uveitis without corneal involvement has been described (Jones et al. 1975; Sotelo-Avila et al. 1974), as well as isolated anterior uveitis and retinitis (Heffler et al. 1996).

Pathology. Examination of a corneal biopsy specimen, or of the entire cornea if transplantation is performed, reveals a slight to marked granulomatous inflammatory reaction composed of mononuclear and polymorphonuclear cells (Figs. 6–17 *A–B*). The corneal stroma has increased fibroblasts and proliferation of small blood vessels throughout. Both trophozoites and cysts of *Acanthamoeba* are recognized in variable numbers (Fig. 6–17 *C–D*). No amebic isolates from cornea have been identified as *Balamuthia*, but it is not unlikely that this genus is responsible for some infections, especially in cases where amebae are not cultured in the usual nonnutrient agar plates. Since *Balamuthia* must feed on living cells, keratitis is more likely to be produced by this group.

Skin. Skin lesions produced by acanthamebids have been described in patients with and without factors that contribute to the infection. However, the great majority of dermal acanthamoebiases have been recorded in individuals with AIDS (Chandrasekar et al. 1997; Murakawa et al. 1995; Park et al. 1994; Tan et al. 1993).

Clinical findings. Some individuals with chronic skin lesions negative for bacteria, fungi, and other common pathogens have *Acanthamoeba*, with subsequent central nervous system dissemination. The lesion in one woman began 1 year earlier, with a bruise attributed to a bite by her son (Gullett et al. 1979). In 6 months a pruritic pustule developed that ruptured, ulcerated, and increased in size. The lesion became indurated and painful during the following months. A skin biopsy specimen showed a granulomatous inflammation, but no organisms were recognized or isolated in cultures. Death occurred after central nervous system symptoms developed. Autopsy revealed *Acanthamoeba* in both the central nervous system and the skin lesion (Gullett et al. 1979). The skin lesion (Fig. 6–18 *A*) was a large, nodular mass of indurated tissue with superficial ulceration having irregular, violaceous borders; the rest of the lesion was red-pink. Small, dry fragments of epidermis covered some areas, and the lesion was painful on manipulation. In individuals with AIDS, the skin lesions are usually ulcerated (Fig. 6–19 *A*). They may begin as single or multiple subcutaneous nodules (Chandrasekar et al. 1997; Deluol et al. 1996) that evolve to necrosis, with drainage of pus, or as pruritic papules that ulcerate. The lesions are usually multiple and painless, and the patient is afebrile. As stated before, these ulcerations are often the port of entry by which the parasite reaches the central nervous system (Murakawa et al. 1995; Park et al. 1994; Tan et al. 1993).

Pathology. The microscopic picture consists of granulomatous inflammation with marked histiocytic infiltration, as well as poorly formed and mature granulomas, some with multinucleated giant cells of foreign bodies (Fig. 6–18 *B–C*). A mononuclear cell infiltrate consisting of lymphocytes, lymphocytoid cells, and plasma cells is abundant, with a few polymorphonuclear cells in microscopic areas of necrosis. The inflammatory cells are seen infiltrating from the epidermis through the

Fig. 6–18. *Acanthamoeba astronyxis* in the skin. *A*, Skin lesion that evolved over 1 year in a 24-year-old woman, illustrating the nodular verrucous character. (Courtesy of J. Gullett, M.D., San Francisco General Hospital Medical Center, San Francisco, California. In: Gullett, J., Mills, J., Hadley, K., et al. 1979. Disseminated granulomatous *Acanthamoeba* infection presenting as an unusual skin lesion. Am. J. Med. 67:891–896. Reprinted with permission.) *B–D* Histologic appearance, hematoxylin and eosin stain. *B*, Biopsy specimen of the skin lesion shows the marked inflammatory reaction involving the dermis, ×55. *C*, Higher magnification shows the histiocytic nature of the infiltrate in subcutaneous tissues and the mature granulomas with multinucleated foreign body giant cells, ×180. *D*, Granuloma composed of numerous histiocytes, a few mononuclear cells, and one *Acanthamoeba* trophozoite at the center, ×1,120. (Preparation courtesy of W. Margaretten, M.D., Department of Pathology, San Francisco General Hospital, University of California, San Francisco.)

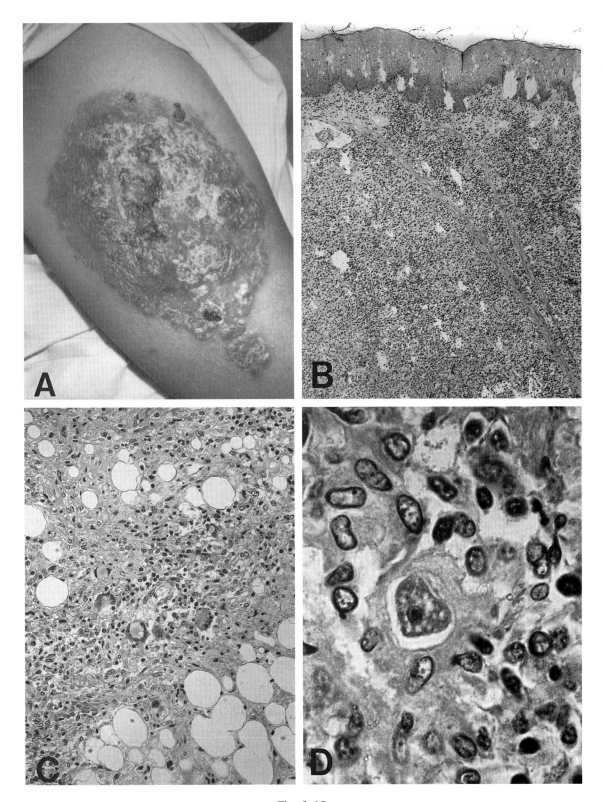

Fig. 6–18.

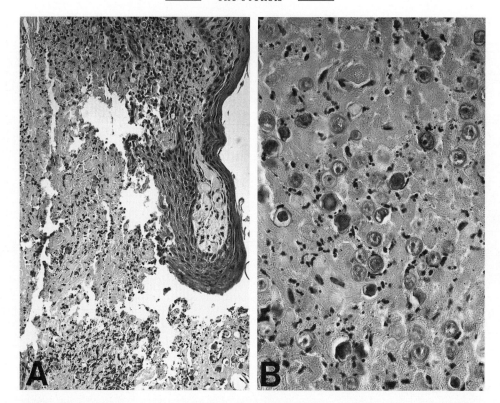

Fig. 6–19. *Acanthamoeba* **in sections of a skin ulcer in a patient with AIDS stained with hematoxylin and eosin stain.** *A,* **Low-power view of the ulcer,** ×119. *B,* **Higher magnification shows necrotic tissue and numerous cysts,** ×298.

dermis and subcutaneous tissues. Parasites may be few in number and difficult to find (Fig. 6–18 *D*), or abundant, with numerous cysts associated with the granulomas (Figs. 6–19 *A–B*).

Other Tissues. *Acanthamoeba* was recovered from bone in osteomyelitis of the mandible (Borochovitz et al. 1981), from the ear in otitis media (Jakovljevich, Talis, 1969; Lengy et al. 1971), from the lung in pneumonic consolidation (Fig. 6–20 *A–B*; Derrick, 1948), from the nasal cavity in a case of sinusitis in a Haitian man with HIV infection (Gonzalez et al. 1986; Helton et al. 1993), and from other tissues in disseminated infections (Figs. 6–21 *A–D*; Murakawa et al. 1995; Ringsted et al. 1976; Tan et al. 1993).

Immunity. No information on the immunologic aspects of infections with acanthamebids in humans or animals is available.

Diagnosis. The diagnosis of *Acanthamoeba* is suspected clinically based on the patient's history and symptoms, but demonstration and identification of the

amebae in tissues or fluids is required for confirmation (Martinez, Visvesvara, 1991). Recently, it has been suggested that examination of patients by tandem scanning confocal microscopy results in a larger number of clinical diagnoses of keratitis (Mathers et al. 1996). Isolation of the parasite in cultures is necessary for biochemical and immunologic identification of the species. The specimens should be collected in sterile Page's amebae saline for transport to the laboratory (Gradus et al. 1989). *Acanthamoeba* and *Hartmannella* can be cultured in cell-free media composed of nonnutrient agar. Plates are prepared, cooled, and seeded with *Escherichia coli* suspended in 0.5 ml of sterile saline to make a light milk-colored solution. Then the plates are refrigerated and are ready to use at any time. The sample, cerebrospinal fluid, pus from an ulcer, abscess, or another source, or teased biopsy tissue fragments are placed on the plates and incubated at room temperature. Filtering the sample through a sterile cellulose filter and lying the filter on the agar plate has also been recommended (Gradus et al. 1989). The trophozoites multiply and feed on the bacteria (which do not multiply because the agar is nonnutrient). The plates are examined with low-power microscopy, searching for small, circular spaces devoid of bacteria with active

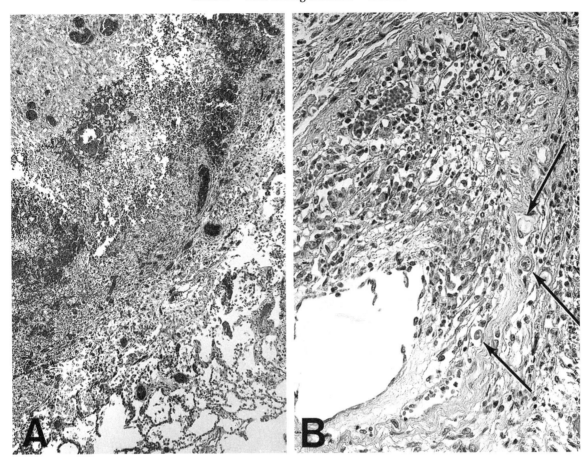

Fig. 6–20. *Acanthamoeba* **in sections of lung from a patient with AIDS, stained with hematoxylin and eosin stain.** *A,* **Low-power view shows marked consolidation, ×45.** *B,* **Higher magnification demonstrates the inflammatory reaction. The amebae are not seen well at this magnification (arrows), ×182.**

trophozoites at the margins. Cultures can be examined daily starting 2 days after seeding and continuing for 8 to 10 days at which time the plates can be discarded. *Balamuthia* requires culture cells for isolation; in case of doubt, clinical samples should be cultured both in agar plates and in tissue culture cells. If the parasite grows in agar, it is *Acanthamoeba* or *Hartmannella*; if it grows only in culture cells, it is *Balamuthia.* From the cultures, preparations in saline for observation of the amebae or smears for stain preparations should be made. If amebic keratitis is proven in tissue sections and cultures are negative, other soil amebae such as *Balamuthia,* should be consider (Aitken et al. 1996).

Acanthamoeba can be identified in wet preparations of cerebrospinal fluid based on the size of the amebae, characteristic lobopodia with acanthopodia, a nucleus with a large nucleolus, and a vacuolated cytoplasm (see Morphology above; Fig. 6–7 *A*). *Hartmannella* and *Balamuthia* have some of the same characteristics as *Acanthamoeba* but lack acanthopods. The size, the presence

of cysts (Fig. 6–1 *B*), the acanthopods, and the lack of flagellated organisms are features that distinguish the acanthamebids from *Naegleria* (see below).

Scrapings from cornea (Epstein et al. 1986) or skin ulcerations, aspirates from osteomyelitic lesions, or abscesses from infected individuals should be smeared on a glass slide and fixed in absolute alcohol. Stains reveal amebae with the characteristics described above. Stains of corneal scrapings with Giemsa stain have been recommended for demonstration of trophozoites and cysts (Margo et al. 1986); indirect fluorescent antibody staining is also useful (Epstein et al. 1986). Calcofluor white, a chemofluorescent dye with affinity for the polysaccharide of the amebic cyst wall, has been used for rapid diagnosis of cysts (Wilhelmus et al. 1986). In preparations of bronchoalveolar lavage fluid made with cytocentrifugation, stained with hematoxylin and eosin, trichrome, and Papanicolaou stains, the amebae were easily identified. The best stain was hematoxylin and eosin stain, followed by the trichrome and Papa-

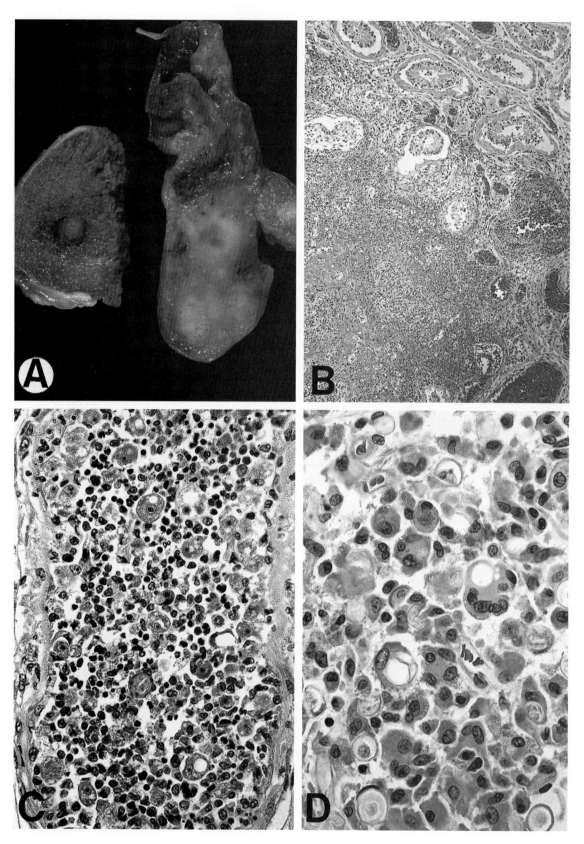

Fig. 6–21. *Acanthamoeba* in testis and epididymis of a patient with AIDS stained with hematoxylin and eosin stain. *A*, Gross picture of sections of testis and epididymis demonstrating the lesions. *B–C*, sections of epididymis stained with hematoxylin and eosin stain. *A*, Low-power view shows the necrotic area, ×55. *B*, Higher magnification demonstrates trophozoites within the inflammatory infiltrate, ×350. *D*, Area where the infection has evolved for a longer period showing numerous cysts in different stages of disintegration, within macrophages, ×450.

nicolaou stains (Newsome et al. 1992). It should be emphasized that amebae in smears of body fluids are larger than those seen in tissue sections (due to shrinkage during tissue processing).

In tissue sections, both trophozoites and cysts of *Acanthamoeba*, *Hartmannella*, and *Balamuthia* are present in variable numbers, probably depending on the duration of the infection. The trophozoites in tissues measure, on average, 22 μm in diameter and have the characteristic nucleus with a large nucleolus that stains darkly with hematoxylin and eosin. The cytoplasm is vacuolated, and the acanthopodia, seen easily in smears, are not recognizable in tissue sections unless iron hematoxylin stain is used (Fig. 6–18 *D*). The cysts are also easily identified by their thick, irregular ectocyst with ostyoles containing the ameba, often shrunken and represented by a dark mass with a nucleus similar to that of the trophozoite (*color plate* III *I*). The wall does not stain with hematoxylin and eosin. It appears refringent, with greater variability in size than that seen in the trophozoites (*color plate* III *I*).

Distinction between *Acanthamoeba*, *Hartmannella*, *Vahlkampfia*, and *Balamuthia* under the light microscope is not possible. In electron micrographs, *B. mandrillaris* generally lacks acanthopods, the cyst is more rounded, and the wall is thicker, with three layers (Fig. 6–13 *A–B*). Distinction between these genera and *E. histolytica* in tissue sections is based on their nuclear morphology and is relatively easy; moreover, the presence of cysts in tissues completely rules out *Entamoeba*. The histologic pattern of lesions produced by *Naegleria* (meningoencephalitis) and the acanthamebids (granulomas and extensive necrosis) should help to distinguish the two infections in most cases.

References

Abraham SN, Lawande RV, 1982. Incidence of free-living amoebae in the nasal passages of local population in Zaria, Nigeria. J. Trop. Med. Hyg. 85:217–222

Abu KY, 1996. The phagosome containing *Legionella pneumophila* within the protozoan *Hartmannella vermiformis* is surrounded by the rough endoplasmic reticulum. Appl. Environ. Microbiol. 62:2022–2028

Adams M, Andrews RH, Robinson B, Christy P, Baverstock PR, Dobson PJ, Blackler SJ, 1989. A genetic approach to species criteria in the amoeba genus *Naegleria* using allozyme electrophoresis. Int. J. Parasitol. 19:823–834

Adeleke A, Pruckler J, Benson R, Rowbotham T, Halablab M, Fields B, 1996. *Legionella*-like amebal pathogens—phylogenetic status and possible role in respiratory disease. Emerging Infect. Dis. 2:225–230

Aitken D, Hay J, Kinnear FB, Kirkness CM, Lee WR, Seal

DV, 1996. Amebic keratitis in a wearer of disposable contact lenses due to a mixed *Vahlkampfia* and *Hartmannella* infection. Ophthalmology 103:485–494

Aldape K, Huizinga H, Bouvier J, McKerrow J, 1994. *Naegleria fowleri*: characterization of a secreted histolytic cysteine protease. Exp. Parasitol. 78:230–241

Beaver PC, Jung RC, Cupp EW, 1984. *Clinical Parasitology*. Philadelphia: Lea & Febiger

Benson RL, Ansbacher L, Hutchison RE, Rogers W, 1985. Cerebrospinal fluid centrifuge analysis in primary amebic meningoencephalitis due to *Naegleria fowleri*. Arch. Pathol. Lab. Med. 109:668–671

Borochovitz D, Martinez AJ, Patterson GT, 1981. Osteomyelitis of a bone graft of the mandible with *Acanthamoeba castellani* infection. Hum. Pathol. 12:573–576

Butt CG, 1966. Primary amoebic meningoencephalitis. N. Engl. J. Med. 274:1473–1476

Butt CG, Baro C, Knorr RW, 1968. *Naegleria* (sp.) identified in amebic encephalitis. Am. J. Clin. Pathol. 50:568–574

Cable BL, John DT, 1986. Conditions for maximum enflagellation in *Naegleria fowleri*. J. Protozool. 33:467–472

Callicott JHJ, 1968. Amebic meningoencephalitis due to free-living amebas of the *Hartmannella (Acanthamoeba)-Naegleria* group. Am. J. Clin. Pathol. 49:84–91

Carter RF, 1968. Primary amoebic meningo-encephalitis: clinical, pathological, and epidemiological features of six fatal cases. J. Pathol. Bacteriol. 96:1–25

Carter RF, 1970. Description of a *Naegleria* sp. isolated from two cases of primary amoebic meningo-encephalitis, and of the experimental pathological changes induced by it. J. Pathol. 100:217–244

Carter RF, 1972. Primary amoebic meningo-encephalitis. An appraisal of present knowledge. Trans. R. Soc. Trop. Med. Hyg. 66:193–208

CDC, 1980. Primary amebic meningoencephalitis—United States. Morb. Mort. Weekly Rep. 29:405–407

CDC, 1992a. Primary amebic meningoencephalitis—North Carolina, 1991. JAMA 268:862–863

CDC, 1992b. Primary amebic meningoencephalitis—North Carolina, 1991. Morb. Mort. Weekly Rep. 41:437–440

Centeno M, Rivera F, Cerva L, Tsutsumi V, Gallegos E, Calderon A, Ortiz R, Bonilla P, Ramirez E, Suarez G, 1996. *Hartmannella vermiformis* isolated from the cerebrospinal fluid of a young male patient with meningoencephalitis and bronchopneumonia. Arch. Med. Res. 27:579–586

Cerva L, Kasprzak W, Mazur T, 1982. *Naegleria fowleri* in cooling waters of power plants. J. Hyg. Epidemiol. Microbiol. Immunol. 26:152–161

Cerva L, Novak K, 1968. Amoebic meningoencephalitis: sixteen fatalities. Science. 160:92

Cerva L, Novak K, Culbertson CG, 1968. An outbreak of acute, fatal amebic meningoencephalitis. Am. J. Epidemiol. 88:436–444

Cerva L, Servus C, Skocil V, 1973. Isolation of limax amoebae from the nasal mucosa of man. Folia Parasitol. 20:97–103

Chandrasekar PH, Nandi PS, Fairfax MR, Crane LR, 1997. Cutaneous infections due to *Acanthamoeba* in patients with acquired immunodeficiency syndrome. Arch. Intern. Med. 157:569–572

Chang SL, 1978. Resistance of pathogenic *Naegleria* to some common physical and chemical agents. Appl. Environ. Microbiol. 35:368–375

Chang SL, 1979. Pathogenesis of pathogenic *Naegleria* amoeba. Folia Parasitol. 26:195–200

Chang SL, Healy GR, McCabe L, Shumaker JB, Schultz MG, 1975. A strain of pathogenic *Naegleria* isolated from a human nasal swab. Health Lab. Sci. 12:1–7

Cleland PG, Lawande RV, Onyemelukwe G, Whittle HC, 1982. Chronic amebic meningoencephalitis. Arch. Neurol. 39:56–57

Cohen EJ, Buchanan HJW, Laughrea PA, Adams CP, Galentine PG, Visvesvara GS, Folbero R, Arentsen JJ, Laibson PR, 1985. Diagnosis and management of *Acanthamoeba* keratitis. Am. J. Ophthalmol. 100:389–395

Cohen EJ, Fulton JC, Hoffman CJ, Rapuano CJ, Laibson PR, 1996. Trends in contact lens–associated corneal ulcers. Cornea 15:566–570

Corliss JO, 1994. An interim utilitarian ("user-friendly") hierarchical classification and characterization of the protists. Acta Protozool. 33:1–51

Culbertson CG, 1961. Pathogenic *Acanthamoeba* (*Hartmanella*). Am. J. Clin. Pathol. 35:195–202

Culbertson CG, 1971. The pathogenicity of soil amebas. Annu. Rev. Microbiol. 25:231–254

Culbertson CG, Ensminger PW, Overton WM, 1965. The isolation of additional strains of pathogenic *Hartmanella*. sp.(*Acanthamoeba*). Am. J. Clin. Pathol. 35:383–387

Culbertson CG, Smith JW, Cohen HK, Minner JR, 1959. Experimental infection of mice and monkeys by *Acanthamoeba*. Am. J. Pathol. 35:185–197

Culbertson CG, Smith JW, Minner JR, 1958. *Acanthamoeba*: Observations on animal pathogenicity. Science 127:1506

Cursons RTM, Brown TJ, Bruns BJ, Taylor DE, 1976. Primary amoebic mengingoencephalitis (sic) contracted in a thermal tributary of the Waikato River—Taupo: a case report. NZ Med. J. 84:479–481

Cursons RTM, Brown TJ, Keys EA, Moriarty KM, Till D, 1980. Immunity to pathogenic free-living amoebae: role of cell-mediated immunity. Infect. Immun. 29:408–410

Cursons RTM, Brown TJ, Keys EA, 1978. Virulence of Pathogenic Free-living amebae. J. Parasitol. 64:744–745

Cursons RTM, Brown TJ, Keys EA, Gordon EH, Leng RH, Havill JH, Hyne BE, 1979. Primary amoebic meningo-encephalitis in an indoor heat-exchange swimming pool. NZ Med. J. 89:330–331

Das SR, 1974. Pathogenicity of flagellate stage of *Naegleria aerobia* and its bearing on the epidemiology of exogenous amoebiasis. Ann. Soc. Belge Med. Trop. 54:327–332

De Jonckheere J, Voorde H, 1977. The distribution of *Naegleria fowleri* in man-made thermal waters. Am. J. Trop. Med. Hyg. 26:10–15

Deluol AM, Teilhac MF, Poirot JL, Maslo C, Luboinski J, Rozenbaum W, Chatelet FP, 1996. Cutaneous lesions due to *Acanthamoeba* sp in a patient with AIDS. J. Euk. Microbiol. 43:130S–131S

Derrick EH, 1948. A fatal case of generalized amoebiasis due to a protozoon closely resembling, if not identical with, *Iodamoeba buetschlii*. Trans. R. Soc. Trop. Med. Hyg. 42:191–198

Dorsch MM, Cameron AS, Robinson BS, 1983. The epidemiology and control of primary amoebic meningoencephalitis with particular reference to South Australia. Trans. R. Soc. Trop. Med. Hyg. 77:372–377

Dunnebacke TH, Schuster FL, 1974. An infectious agent associated with amebas of the genus *Naegleria*. J. Protozool. 21:327–329

Dunnebacke TH, Schuster FL, 1977. The nature of a cytopathogenic material present in amebae of the genus *Naegleria*. Am. J. Trop. Med. Hyg. 26:412–421

Epstein RJ, Wilson LA, Visvesvara GS, Plourde EG Jr, 1986. Rapid diagnosis of *Acanthamoeba* keratitis from corneal scrapings using indirect fluorescent antibody staining. Arch. Ophthalmol. 104:1318–1321

Florakis GJ, Folbero R, Krachmer JH, Tse DT, Roussel TJ, Vrabec MP, 1988. Elevated corneal epithelial lines in *Acanthamoeba* keratitis. Arch. Ophthalmol. 106:1202–1206

Fowler M, Carter RF, 1965. Acute pyogenic meningitis probably due to *Acanthamoeba* sp: a preliminary report. Br. Med. J. 2:740–742

Friedman RF, Wolf TC, Chodosh J, 1997. *Acanthamoeba* infection after radial keratotomy. Am. J. Ophthalmol. 123:409–410

Gonzalez MM, Gould E, Dickinson G, Martinez AJ, Visvesvara GS, Cleary TJ, Hensley GT, 1986. Acquired immunodeficiency syndrome associated with *Acanthamoeba* infection and other opportunistic organisms. Arch. Pathol. Lab. Med. 110:749–751

Goodall K, Brahma A, Ridgway A, 1996. Correspondence. *Acanthamoeba* keratitis: masquerading as adenoviral keratitis. Eye 10:643–644

Gordon SM, Steinberg JP, DuPuis MH, Kozarsky PE, Nickerson JF, Visvesvara GS, 1992. Culture isolation of *Acanthamoeba* species and leptomyxid amebas from patients with amebic meningoencephalitis, including two patients with AIDS. Clin. Infect. Dis. 15:1024–1030

Gradus MS, Koenig SB, Hynduik RA, DeCarlo J, 1989. Filter-culture technique using amoeba saline transport medium for the noninvasive diagnosis of *Acanthamoeba* keratitis. Am. J. Clin. Pathol. 92:682–685

Gregorio CD, Rivasi F, Mongiardo N, Rienzo BD, Wallace S, Visvesvara GS, 1992. *Acanthamoeba* meningoencephalitis in a patient with acquired immunodeficiency syndrome. Arch. Pathol. Lab. Med. 116:1363–1365

Gullett J, Mills J, Hadley K, Podemski B, Pitts L, Gelber R, 1979. Disseminated granulomatous *Acanthamoeba* infection presenting as an unusual skin lesion. Am. J. Med. 67:891–896

Hanssens M, De Jonckheere JFM, De Meunynck C, 1985. *Acanthamoeba* keratitis. A clinicopathological case report. Int. Ophthalmol. 7:203–213

He Y, Niederkorn JY, McCulley JP, Stewart GL, Meyer DR, Silvany R, Daugherty J, 1990. *In vivo* and *in vitro* collagenolytic activity of *Acanthamoeba castellani*. Invest. Ophthalmol. Vis. Sci. 31:2235–2240

Heffler KF, Eckhardt TJ, Reboli AC, Stieritz D, 1996. *Acanthamoeba* endophthalmitis in acquired immunodeficiency syndrome. Am. J. Ophthalmol. 122:584–586

Helton J, Loveless M, White CRJ, 1993. Cutaneous acanthamoeba infection associated with leukocytoclastic vasculitis in an AIDS patient. Am. J. Dermatopathol. 15:146–149

Jakovljevich R, Talis B, 1969. Recovery of a hartmannelloid amoeba in the purulent discharge from a human ear. J. Protozool. 16:36

Jones BR, McGill JI, Steele ADM, 1975. Recurrent suppurative keratouveitis with loss of eye due to infection by *Acanthamoeba castellani*. Trans. Ophthalmol. Soc. UK 95:210–213

Jones DB, 1986. *Acanthamoeba*—the ultimate opportunist? Am. J. Ophthalmol. 102:527–530

Jones DB, Visvesvara GS, Robinson NM, 1975. *Acanthamoeba polyphaga* keratitis and *Acanthamoeba* uveitis associated with fatal meningoencephalitis. Trans. Ophthalmol. Soc. UK 95:221–232

Kennedy SM, Devine P, Hurley C, Ooi YS, Collum LM, 1995. Correspondence. Corneal infection associated with *Hartmannella vermiformis* in contact-lens wearer. Lancet 346:637–638

Kernohan JW, Magath TB, Schloss GT, 1960. Granuloma of brain probably due to *Endolimax williamsi* (*Iodamoeba butschlii*). Arch. Pathol. 70:576–580

Key SN III, Green WR, Willaert E, Steven AR, Key SN Jr, 1980. Keratitis due to *Acanthamoeba castellani*. A clinicopathologic case report. Arch. Ophthalmol. 98:475–479

Klink F van, Alizadeh H, He Y, Mellon JA, Silvany RE, McCulley JP, Niederkorn JY, 1994. The role of contact lenses, trauma, and Langerhans cells in a Chinese hamster model of *Acanthamoeba* keratitis. Invest. Ophthalmol. Vis. Sci. 34:1937–1944

Klink, F van, Taylor WM, Alizadeh H, Jager MJ, van RN, Niederkorn JY, 1996. The role of macrophages in *Acanthamoeba* keratitis. Invest. Ophthalmol. Vis. Sci. 37:1271–1281

Lawande RV, 1983. Recovery of soil amoebae from the air during the harmattan in Zaria, Nigeria. Ann. Trop. Med. Parasitol. 77:45–49

Lawande RV, Macfarlane JT, Weir WR, Awunor Renner C, 1980. A case of primary amebic meningoencephalitis in a Nigerian farmer. Am. J. Trop. Med. Hyg. 29:21–25

Ledee DR, Hay J, Byers TJ, Seal DV, Kirkness CM, 1996. *Acanthamoeba griffini*. Molecular characterization of a new corneal pathogen. Invest. Ophthalmol. Vis. Sci. 37:544–550

Lengy J, Jakovljevich R, Talis B, 1971. Recovery of a hartmanelloid amoeba from a purulent ear discharge. Harefuah 80:23–24

Lowichik A, Rollins N, Delgado R, Visvesvara GS, Burns DK, 1995. Leptomyxid amebic meningoencephalitis mimicking brain stem glioma. A. J. Neuroradiol. 16:926–929

Ludwig IH, Meisler DM, Rutherford I, Bicon FE, Langston RHS, Visvesvara GS, 1986. Susceptibility of Acanthamoeba to soft contact lens disinfection systems. Invest. Ophthalmol. Vis. Sci. 27:626–628

Mannis MJ, Tamaru R, Roth AM, Burns M, Thirkill C, 1986. *Acanthamoeba* sclerokeratitis. Determining diagnostic criteria. Arch. Ophthalmol. 104:1313–1317

Marciano Cabral F, 1988. Biology of *Naegleria* spp. Microbiol. Rev. 52:114–133

Margo CE, Brinser JH, Groden L, 1986. Exfoliated cytopathology of *Acanthamoeba* keratitis. JAMA 255:2216

Markowitz SM, Martinez AJ, Duma RJ, Shiel FO, 1974. Myocarditis associated with primary amebic (*Naegleria*) meningoencephalitis. Am. J. Clin. Pathol. 62:619–628

Martinez AJ, 1980. Is *Acanthamoeba* encephalitis an opportunistic infection? Neurology 30:567–574

Martinez AJ, 1993. Free-living amebas: infection of the central nervous system. Mt. Sinai J. Med. 60:271–278

Martinez AJ, Garcia CA, Halks-Miller M, Arce-Vela R, 1980. Granulomatous amebic encephalitis presenting as a cerebral mass lesion. Acta Neuropathol. 51:85–91

Martinez AJ, Janitschke K, 1985. *Acanthamoeba*, an opportunistic microorganism: a review. Infection 13:251–256

Martinez AJ, Nelson EC, Duma RJ, 1973. Animal model of human disease. Primary amebic meningoencephalitis, *Naegleria* meningoencephalitis, CNS protozoal infection. Am. J. Pathol. 73:545–548

Martinez AJ, Visvesvara GS, 1991. Laboratory diagnosis of pathogenic free-living amoebas: *Naegleria*, *Acanthamoeba*, and Leptomyxid. Clin. Lab. Med. 11:861–872

Mathers WD, Sutphin JE, Folberg R, Meier PA, Wenzel RP, Elgin RG, 1996. Outbreak of keratitis presumed to be caused by *Acanthamoeba*. Am. J. Ophthalmol. 121:129–142

Moore MB, McCulley JP, Kaufman HE, Robin JB, 1986. Radial kerato-neuritis as a presenting sign in *Acanthamoeba* keratitis. Ophthalmology 93:1310–1315

Murakawa GJ, McCalmont T, Altman J, Telang GH, Hoffman MD, Kantor GR, Berger TG, 1995. Disseminated acanthamebiasis in patients with AIDS. A report of five cases and a review of the literature. Arch. Dermatol. 131:1291–1296

Nagington J, Watson PG, Playfair TJ, McGill J, Jones BR, Steele ADMC, 1974. Amoebic infection of the eye. Lancet 2:1537–1540

Newsome AL, Curtis FT, Culbertson CG, Allen SD, 1992. Identification of *Acanthamoeba* in bronchoalveolar lavage specimens. Diagn. Cytopathol. 8:231–234

Niederkorn JY, Ubelaker JE, McCulley JP, Stewart GL, Meyer DR, Mellon JA, Silvany RE, He Y, Pidherney M, Martin JH, Alizadeh H, 1992. Susceptibility of corneas from various animal species to in vitro binding and invasion by *Acanthamoeba castellani*. Invest. Ophthalmol. Vis. Sci. 33:104–112

Ofori-Kwakye SK, Sidebottom DG, Herbert J, Fischer EG, Visvesvara GS, 1986. Granulomatous brain tumor caused by *Acanthamoeba*. J. Neurosurg. 64:505–509

Page FC, 1967a. Re-definition of the genus *Acanthamoeba* with descriptions of three species. J. Protozool. 14:709–724

Page FC, 1967b. Taxonomic criteria for limax amoeba, with descriptions of 3 new species of *Hartmannella* and 3 of *Vahlkampfia*. J. Protozool. 14:499–521

Page FC, 1974. *Rosculus ithacus* Hawes, 1963 (Amoebida, Flabelluidae) and the amphizoic tendency in amoebae. Acta Protozool. 13:143–154

Park CH, Iyengar V, Hefner L, Pestaner JP, Vandel NM, 1994. Cutaneous *Acanthamoeba* infection associated with acquired immunodeficiency syndrome. Lab. Med. 25:386–388

Patras D, Andujar JJ, 1966. Meningoencephalitis due to *Hartmannella* (*Acanthamoeba*). Am. J. Clin. Pathol. 46:226–233

Proca-Ciobanu M, Lupascu G, Petrovici A, Ionescu MD, 1975. Electron microscopic study of a pathogenic *Acanthamoeba castellani* strain: the presence of bacterial endosymbionts. Int. J. Parasitol. 5:49–56

Riestra-Castaneda JMA, Riestra-Castaneda R, Gonzalez-Garrido AA, Pena Moreno P, Martinez AJ, Visvesvara GS, Jardon Careaga F, Oropeza de Alba JL, Gonzalez Cornejo S, 1997. Granulomatous amebic encephalitis due to *Balamuthia mandrillaris* (Leptomyxiidae): report of four cases from Mexico. Am. J. Trop. Med. Hyg. 56:603–607

Ringsted J, Jager BV, Suk D, Visvesvara GS, 1976. Probable *Acanthamoeba* meningoencephalitis in a korean child. Am. J. Clin. Pathol. 66:723–730

Samples JR, Binder PS, Luibel FJ, Font RL, Visvesvara GS, Peter CR, 1984. *Acanthamoeba* keratitis possibly acquired from a hot tub. Arch. Ophthalmol. 102:707–710

Schumacher DJ, Tien RD, Lane K, 1995. Neuroimaging findings in rare amebic infections of the central nervous system. Am. J. Neuroradiol. 16:930–935

Shumaker JB, Healy GR, English D, Schultz M, Page FC, 1971. *Naegleria gruberi*: isolation from nasal swab of a healthy individual. Lancet 2:602–603

Sotelo-Avila C, Taylor FM, Ewing CW, 1974. Primary amebic meningoencephalitis in a healthy 7-year-old boy. J. Pediatr. 85:131–136

Stehr-Green JK, Bailey TM, Visvesvara GS, 1989. The epidemiology of *Acanthamoeba* keratitis in the United States. Am. J. Ophthalmol. 107:331–336

Tan B, Weldon Linne CM, Rhone DP, Penning CL, Visvesvara GS, 1993. *Acanthamoeba* infection presenting as skin lesions in patients with the acquired immunodeficiency syndrome. Arch. Pathol. Lab. Med. 117:1043–1046

Taratuto AL, Monges J, Acefe JC, Meli F, Paredes FA, Martinez AJ, 1991. Leptomyxid amoeba encephalitis: report of the first case in Argentina. Trans. R. Soc. Trop. Med. Hyg. 85:77

Theodore FH, Jakobiec FA, Juechter KB, Ma P, Troutman RC, Pang PM, Iwamoto T, 1985. The diagnostic value of a ring infiltrate in acanthamoebic keratitis. Ophthalmology 92:1471–1479

Visvesvara GS, Callaway CS, 1974. Light and electron microscopic observations on the pathogenesis of *Naegleria fowleri* in mouse brain and tissue culture. J. Protozool. 21:239–250

Visvesvara GS, Jones DB, Robinson NM, 1975. Isolation, identification, and biological characterization of *Acanthamoeba polyphaga* from a human eye. Am. J. Trop. Med. Hyg. 24:784–790

Visvesvara GS, Schuster FL, Martinez AJ, 1993. *Balamuthia mandrillaris*, n. g., n. sp., agent of amebic meningoencephalitis in humans and other animals. J. Euk. Microbiol. 40:504–514

Visvesvara GS, Stehr Green JK, 1990. Epidemiology of free-living ameba infections. J. Protozool. 37:25S–33S

Vodkin MH, Howe DK, Visvesvara GS, McLaughlin GL, 1992. Identification of *Acanthamoeba* at the generic and specific levels using the polymerase chain reaction. J. Protozool. 39:378–385

Wang SS, Feldman HA, 1961. Occurrence of *Acanthamoeba* in tissue cultures inoculated with human pharyngeal swabs. Antimicrob. Agents Chemother. 1:50–53

Wang SS, Feldman HA, 1967. Isolation of *Hartmannella* species from human throats. N. Engl. J. Med. 277:1174–1179

Watson PG, 1975. Amoebic infection of the eye. Trans. Ophthalmol. Soc. UK 95:204–206

Wilhelmus KR, Osato MS, Font RL, Robinson NM, Jones DB, 1986. Rapid diagnosis of *Acanthamoeba* keratitis using calcofluor white. Arch. Ophthalmol. 104:1309–1312

7

INTESTINAL AMEBAE

In this chapter, we will study members of the class Entamoebidae, containing the order Amoebida, which includes many parasitic and free-living amebae with naked protoplasts (see Chapter 6). Most parasitic genera and species of the Amoebidae inhabit the alimentary canal of most known vertebrates and of some invertebrates. Of the three genera found in humans, *Entamoeba* definitely belongs in this family, while *Endolimax* and *Iodamoeba* are assigned to it provisionally (Corliss, 1994). These genera have several species living in the colon and one species living in the mouth, and they are still separated on the basis of the morphologic characteristics of the nucleus. The separation of some species of *Entamoeba* important to humans on the basis of their morphology is no longer possible; molecular analysis is required.

The genera *Endolimax* and *Iodamoeba* have one species each in humans, *E. nana* and *I. buetschlii*. The genus *Entamoeba* has six: *E. histolytica*, *E. dispar*, *E. hartmanni*, *E. coli*, *E. polecki*, and *E. gingivalis*; the last inhabits the mouth, the others the large intestine. For clinical diagnostic purposes, these amebae are identified in the clinical laboratory in stool samples. Since only *E. histolytica* is pathogenic to humans and to some animals, and since it is found in tissues, the anatomic pathologist needs to diagnose the infection in biopsy specimens, autopsy material, and other samples. For these reasons, the following discussion will deal only with this organism.

Entamoeba histolytica—Amebiasis

Amebiasis is an infection of the colon that has the potential to disseminate to other organs, producing morbidity and mortality. The infection occurs with higher frequency in the tropical areas of the world and to a lesser extent in temperate areas. Since the discovery of *E. histolytica* in 1875 and its definitive association with disease during the last decade of the 19th century, the parasite has been the subject of intensive study. Most investigations have focused on the pathogenicity of the parasite since most infected individuals do not develop disease. Some workers suspected that *E. histolytica* actually consisted of more than one species. Early in the 20th century, *E. hartmanni* was described as a nonpathogenic ameba, different from *E. histolytica*, because its cysts are smaller, but *E. hartmanni* fell into disfavor and its existence was not generally accepted until the early 1960s. The existence of two almost identical species not recognized until then rendered most of the work done on the epidemiology of the disease, and some of the experimental work, either invalid or difficult to interpret.

Throughout the 1980s, work by Sargeaunt (Sargeaunt et al. 1987; Sargeaunt, Williams, 1979; Sargeaunt, Williams, 1982) showed that *E. histolytica* isolated from patients could be separated into pathogenic and nonpathogenic forms based on their zymodemes. A *zymodeme*, as previously noted, is the pattern produced by certain enzymes, extracted from parasites grown in cultures, when submitted to gel electrophoresis. The glucolytic enzymes of the Krebs cycle are frequently used. Their zymodemes are constant, reproducible, and reliable features that separate pathogenic from nonpathogenic isolates. At the same time, genetic and immunologic parameters that also allowed distinction between pathogenic and nonpathogenic *E. histolytica* were found. Based on all of this information Diamond and Clark described *E. dispar* as a nonpathogenic species morphologically identical to *E. histolytica* but distinguishable on the basis of its molecular characteristics (Diamond, Clark, 1993).

Morphology and Life Cycle. In fresh preparations of stool specimens the trophozoites of *E. histolytica* are seen as delicate, refringent organisms with ameboid movements measuring 10 to 60 μm in diameter. Trophozoites in dysenteric stools tend to be larger than those found in formed stools. The movement of trophozoites is rapid and capricious, sometimes unidirectional but changing course often; movement is by the formation of finger-like, hyaline pseudopods consisting of extensions of the ectoplasm to the endoplasm. The cytoplasm has a distinct clear ectoplasm and an endoplasm. The endoplasm contains numerous granules, digestive vacuoles, and a round nucleus about 5 μm in diameter with a small, highly refringent karyosome. The cysts are rounded and measure 10 to 20 μm in diameter, averaging 12 to 13 μm. In fresh preparations the mature cysts are birefringent, with four nuclei identical to those in the trophozoite, though slightly smaller. The cytoplasm often contains elongated structures with rounded ends, the chromatoidal bodies. Less mature cysts may have one to three nuclei and sometimes a large glycogen mass that stains golden yellow with iodine (Beaver et al. 1984).

In well-fixed, well-stained preparations of stool samples, the morphology of the organisms is better appreciated (Fig. 7–16). The digestive vacuoles may contain food and sometimes red blood cells, especially in dysenteric stools. The nucleus has small granules of chromatin, sometimes seen as irregular plaques, arranged against the inner surface of the nuclear membrane. The nucleolus or karyosome is small and excentric, but depending on the angle of view, it may be seen as centrally located. Preparations of cysts stained with iron hematoxylin stain show their nuclei, identical to the nucleus of the trophozoite, and the chromatoidal bodies as dark structures (Beaver et al. 1984).

Under the electron microscope, trophozoites of *E. histolytica* have a smooth outer membrane composed of three layers (Osada, 1959); no mitochondria or Golgi complex have been observed, and the endoplasmic reticulum is poorly developed (Byrd, 1937). In addition, the cytoplasm has glycogen particles; small, cylindrical, electron-dense bodies; and some crystalline structures. Studies of cultured amebae with the electron microscope have revealed that some trophozoites have dead trophozoites in their digestive vacuoles (El-Hashimi, Pittman, 1970). Recently, it has been found that *E. histolytica* also lack perixosomes and Golgi dictiosomes (Clark, Roger, 1995).

The life cycle of *E. histolytica* has the following stages: trophozoite, precyst, cyst, metacyst, and metacystic trophozoite. In studies with *E. muris*, the natural habitat of the trophozoites has been found to be the crypts and mucous layer of the cecum and large intestine. The trophozoites are located in an area termed the *biotic zone* of the parasite, where they live in colonies of variable size (Lin, 1971). In monkeys naturally infected with *E. histolytica,* the parasite is found in the crypts between the epithelium and the basement membrane, causing no damage or only minor necrosis (Beaver et al. 1988). In the colon the trophozoite develops into a cyst under conditions that are not entirely known; at first, the trophozoite becomes round and nonmotile and stops feeding; some of its digestive vacuoles disappear to become a *precyst*, with a single nucleus. Secretion of a thin wall and further condensation of the cytoplasm continue, with formation of a glycogen mass and chromatoidal bodies. The cyst is completely formed and mature after two divisions of the nuclei and is ready to survive in the adverse environment outside the host. Ingestion of mature cysts by an appropriate host results in infection. In the stomach the cysts survive the acidic conditions, but lower in the small intestine where the pH becomes neutral or slightly alkaline, the cysts open and release the multinucleated *metacysts*, which begin to divide into four *metacystic trophozoites*. In the colon, the parasites begin forming colonies (Beaver et al. 1984).

Epidemiology. *Entamoeba histolytica* has a cosmopolitan distribution and, as mentioned earlier, its prevalence is greater in the tropical areas of the world than in the temperate zones. This preponderance of the parasite in the tropics probably is related less to climatic conditions than to socioeconomic ones. Contamination of the environment with fecal excreta, and as a consequence contamination of food and water, are ideal conditions for transmission of the infection. Amebiasis is generally more common in poorly developed areas, orphanages, and mental institutions. In homosexual men living in the developed areas of the world, rates of infection approach those found in the general population of endemic areas (Allason-Jones et al. 1986; Bocket et al. 1992; Phillips et al. 1981). Although monkeys, dogs, and cats are sometimes infected under natural and experimental conditions, their significance in the maintenance of human infection is unknown. Epidemics produced by contaminated water have been reported on many occasions; in one instance, an outbreak was produced by the use of contaminated devices for colonic irrigation (CDC, 1981). Amebiasis occurs sporadically throughout the United States (Krogstad et al. 1978), more commonly in the southern region of the country; its overall prevalence is unknown (Healy, 1986). The average number of cases of amebiasis reported to the Centers for Disease Control for more than 20 years has been approximately 3500 per year. Overdiagnosis of amebiasis in clinical practice is common, more so than underdiagnosis, but a false-negative diagnosis is more serious because it can result in fatal disease (Krogstad et al. 1978).

Rates of prevalence of *E. histolytica* sensu stricto are not known because the data collected during the last three decades on prevalence rates of *E. histolytica* include *E. dispar*. For example, in 1981 it was estimated that 480 million people were infected with *E. histolytica* worldwide, of whom 36 million developed amebic abscess or colitis each year and at least 40,000 died (Walsh, 1986). However, these data include both species, inflating the numbers considerably. A few studies have been carried out to determine the actual prevalence of *E. histolytica* and *E. dispar* in endemic communities. A survey of 633 individuals in Brazil living in three different places showed prevalence rates of 18%, 31%, and 36% of *Entamoeba* in the stools; 108 strains of amebae were isolated and submitted to electrophoresis, but there was no single strain with a pathogenic zymodeme (Aca et al. 1994). In another study in South Africa, it was found that only 1% of healthy individuals carried amebae with a pathogenic zymodeme (*E. histolytica*) (Gathiram, Jackson, 1985). It is also suggested that travelers to endemic areas become infected far more often with *E. histolytica* than with *E. dispar* (Walderich et al. 1997), but this idea needs confirmation. If true, it would suggest a marked difference in infectivity between the two species. Taken together, these reports of prevalence rates of pathogenic amebae (*E. histolytica*) indicate that the problem of amebiasis is overestimated worldwide.

Pathogenesis. The mechanism by which *E. histolytica* produces disease in humans and animals has been debated for over 100 years. Since the name *histolytica* was given in the belief that the parasite produces lysis of the tissues, lytic products released by the parasite, either actively or passively after its death in tissues, have been intensively studied, mostly with negative results. Moreover, the clinical observation that many people were infected with the parasite but very few suffered disease defied most explanations. Further, much confusion was added because, when amebiasis was discussed, the terms *pathogenicity* and *virulence* were used synonymously. *Pathogenicity* is the capacity to produce disease; it is a yes-or-no phenomenon. *Virulence* refers to the degree of disease produced by a pathogen in an individual or a given population (Clark, Diamond, 1994). We know that *E. histolytica* is a pathogen and that, at least in some places, it has very low virulence. In a longitudinal study in South Africa, individuals harboring amebae with pathogenic zymodemes (*E. histolytica*) were largely asymptomatic carriers, and only 10% developed symptoms; moreover, within a year, most carriers had lost their infections spontaneously (Gathiram, Jackson, 1987).

The separation of *E. dispar* from *E. histolytica*, and the new data on how the ameba interacts with cells, have opened new avenues of understanding regarding its pathogenicity. *Entamoeba histolytica* produces tissue damage in certain individuals, but why these individuals suffer disease is not entirely known. In persons in whom tissue damage occurs, the damage is modulated by (*1*) adhesion of the parasite to cells (cytoadhesion) and (*2*) killing of the cells (by pore-forming proteins or amebapores).

Cytoadhesion. It has been shown that *E. histolytica* possesses an adhesive molecule on its cell membrane. The function of this molecule can be inhibited by the terminal oligosaccharides of *N*-acetyl-D-galactosamine; thus, it has been termed the *inhibitable GalNac molecule* (Ravdin et al. 1985b; Ravdin, Guerrant, 1981). Adhesion of *E. histolytica* by means of this molecule has been shown in vitro on different culture cells, on polymorphonuclear cells (Ravdin et al. 1985b), and on fixed and unfixed rat colonic epithelial cells (Ravdin et al. 1985a). Colonic mucins act as powerful ligands for the adhesion molecule and inhibit the parasite from making contact with rat colonic cells (Chadee et al. 1987). The native amebic adhesion protein has been isolated and characterized as a 260 kDa heterodimer of glycoprotein composed of 170 kDa heavy and 31–35 kDa light subunits (Petri et al. 1987). The heavy subunit is antigenic and is recognized by 90% of human immune sera (Petri et al. 1987). It stimulates T lymphocytes in vitro to produce gamma interferon (Schain et al. 1992); it is immunogenic, preventing 67% of gerbils from acquiring experimental amebic liver abscess (Petri, Ravdin, 1991); and patients with intestinal amebiasis have immunoglobulin A (IgA) in their saliva that reacts against the adhesin molecule (Carrero et al. 1994). In spite of this information, however, the role of the adhesin molecule in developing immunity remains unknown. Adhesion of E. histolytica to any cell studied resulted in swelling of the target cell followed by its death, indicating that cytoadhesion is the first step in the pathogenicity of the parasite.

Amebapores. In the 1980s it was discovered that E. histolytica produces a protein capable of destroying cells by forming ion channels that make the target cell membrane permeable to K, Ca, and Na ions (Lynch et al. 1982; Rosenberg, Gitler, 1985). This protein, known as the *ameba pore forming protein*, or *amebapore*, is released by the parasite into the intercellular space between the parasite and the target cell soon after the parasite makes contact with the cell (Leippe, 1997). The amebapore has been isolated and characterized; it is composed of 77 amino acid residues arranged in four alpha domains. These peptides have been synthesized and studied in detail (Leippe et al. 1994). Four residues, labeled H1 through H4, have been tested separately; H1 and H3 have been found to have pore-forming activity. Amebapores have certain characteristics in common with other natural pore-forming peptides occurring on cells from many phylogenetically diverse organisms; they are soluble, but they can change into a membrane-inserted state to form ion channels on contact with target cells. Thus, the amebapore is related to NK-lysine, the effector molecule of mammalian natural killer cells (Leippe, 1997)

Other amebic toxic factors have also been found in E. histolytica trophozoites. These toxic factors include (1) a cytotoxin/enterotoxin with protease activity (Lushbaugh et al. 1981); (2) a collagenase active against collagens I and III (Munoz et al. 1982); (3) serotonin that in vitro actively alters electrolyte transport across the intestinal mucosa (McGowan et al. 1983);

(4) neutral proteinases, the amount of which is directly proportional to the virulence of the parasite (Lushbaugh et al. 1984); (5) cathepsin B, a cysteine protease more potent than the cytotoxin (Lushbaugh et al. 1985); and others. The role of these toxic factors in pathogenicity has not been demonstrated in natural or experimental infections in animals, much less in humans.

The capacity of some strains of E. histolytica to make contact with tissue cells and produce lysis appears to be unique among the intestinal amebae (no data are available on E. invadens, the pathogenic species in snakes and other cold-blooded animals). In the colon the amebae may start to destroy the epithelium, invade into the mucosa and intestinal wall, and travel via the bloodstream to other organs, producing the infection known as *amebiasis*. The role of neutrophils in the genesis of amebic lesions is also important because E. histolytica has powerful chemoattractants for neutrophils, which degranulate on making contact with the parasite (Guerrant et al. 1981). Degranulation of neutrophils contributes to the lysis of tissues, but probably not in large amounts, since mechanisms are available to check their enzymes (Weiss, 1989). It has long been observed that tissues with amebic lesions have a small number of infiltrating polymorphonuclear cells (Beaver, 1958; Councilman, LaFleur, 1891).

Immunity. Little is known about immunity to amebiasis, probably because no good animal model for the disease is available (Denis, Chadee, 1988). The presence of circulating antibodies in patients suffering from intestinal or extraintestinal amebiasis is well known. The presence of IgA in the saliva of patients with colitis has also been demonstrated (Carrero et al. 1994). The presence of antibodies is of little help in making a diagnosis because antibody titers do not distinguish between present and past invasive disease (Ximenez et al. 1993). Recently, it has also been shown that infections with the nonpathogenic E. dispar do not elicit an antibody response. In contrast, even in asymptomatic individuals, the infection with E. histolytica results in passage of amebic antigens or soluble amebic products through the intestinal wall to elicit a humoral response (Denis, Chadee, 1988). In animals with luminal infection but without disease, peripheral blood lymphocytes are unresponsive to amebic antigens (Denis, Chadee, 1988). The role of antibodies in protecting against the infection or the disease remains unknown.

Regarding knowledge of cellular immunity, most progress has been made in the area of in vitro interaction between parasites and cells of the immune system. Survival of the amebae in the host may be aided by the development of a transient immune suppression. Some studies indicate that patients with amebiasis have a serum component that suppresses T-cell proliferation and production of interferon gamma, effects in which the adhesin molecule is involved. The parasite may also suppress the interaction between macrophages and T lymphocytes, decreasing the host's defenses against the ameba. Other mechanisms not entirely determined have been outlined on the basis of incomplete experimental data (Campbell, Chadee, 1997).

Intestinal Amebiasis

Clinical Findings. The clinical manifestations of intestinal amebiasis vary with the susceptibility of the individual and the virulence of the parasite. Most infec-

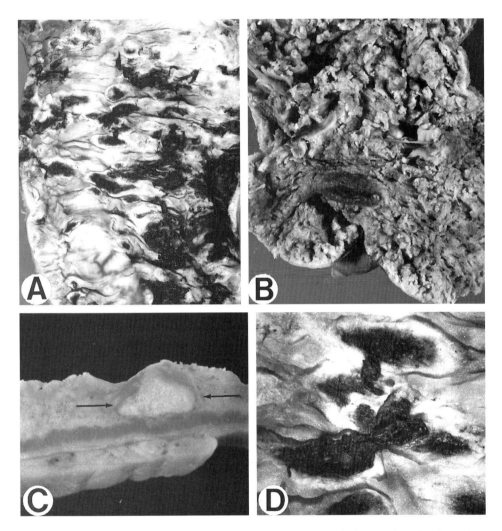

Fig. 7–1. *Entamoeba histolytica*, gross intestinal lesions. *A*, Ulcerations in the colon of a 58-year-old man who died of acute intestinal amebiasis, peritonitis, and amebic liver abscess. *B*, Generalized mucosal necrosis in a 2-year-old boy with a 2-week history of dysentery and amebic trophozoites in his stools. *C*, Cross section of colon showing an area of necrosis extending down to the muscle layers (arrows), with a flask-shape configuration ×4. *D*, Higher magnification of *A* with several ulcers showing the elongated shape. Note that these ulcers are grossly indistinguishable from those of ulcerative colitis. (Courtesy of H. Estrada, M.D., Facultad de Medicina, Universidad de Caldas, Manizales, Colombia.)

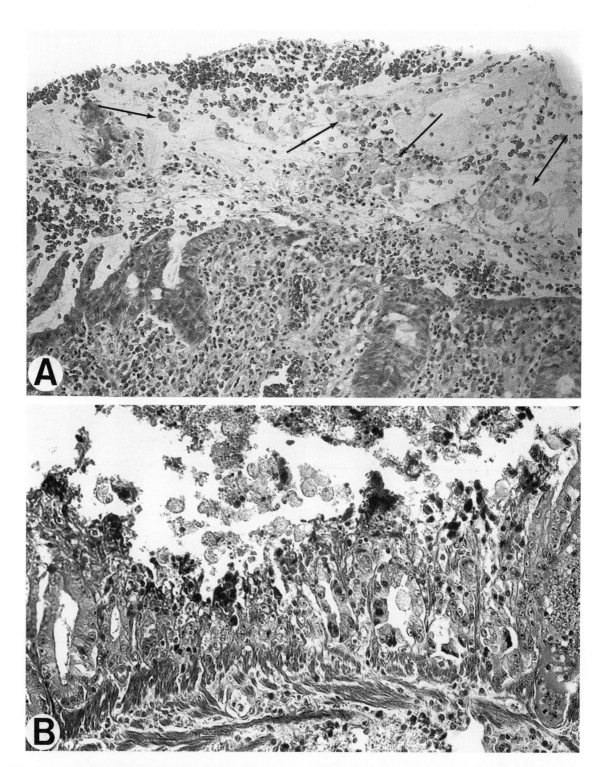

Fig. 7–2. *Entamoeba histolytica*, sequence of lesions in sections of colon stained with hematoxylin and eosin stain. *A*, Early contact of the parasite with the mucosa produces chronic damage of superficial epithelium, distortion of the crypts, and flattening of the mucosa. Note the large colony of parasites (arrows) on the surface and the large number of inflammatory cells, ×180. *B*, Lesion comprising half of the thickness of the mucosa; cat experimentally infected, ×250.

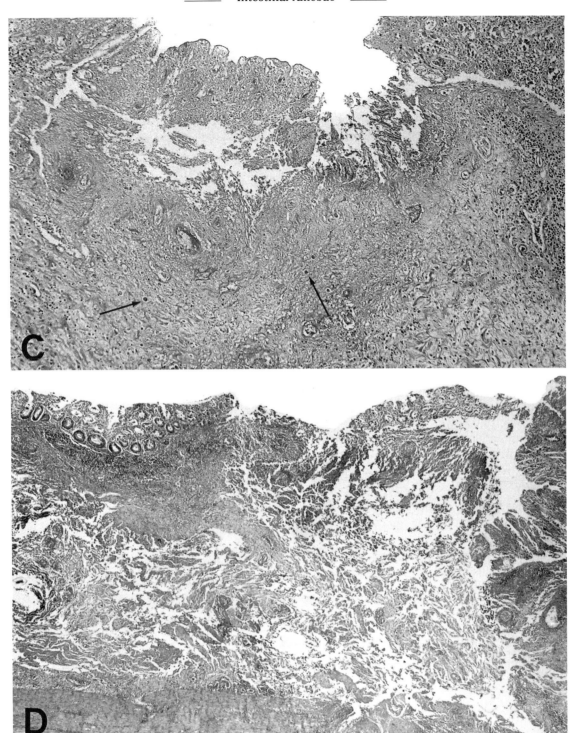

Fig. 7–2. *(continued). C*, Ulceration involving part of the submucosa. Note the necrosis, the slight inflammatory reaction, and, barely seen at this magnification, a few amebic trophozoites (arrows), ×63. *D*, Ulcer extending laterally to the left in the submucosa and down to the muscle layers, ×26.

tions are clinically silent, resulting from colonization of the intestinal lumen alone or from minimal superficial invasion of the mucosa, with a physiologic equilibrium between the host and the parasite. Generalizations about susceptibility to infection among persons of any particular age, sex, or race are difficult because comparison of data from different sources is not possible. It appears that the highest incidence of both infection and disease occurs in the third to fifth decades; in this age group, infection is more common in women but disease is more prevalent in men (Wilmot, 1962).

The incubation period of amebiasis varies between 1 and 3 weeks. Symptoms develop either slowly or suddenly, a common feature during epidemics. The gradual onset of disease with abdominal symptoms and slight diarrhea often precedes frank dysentery by days or weeks. General malaise, loss of appetite and weight, and diffuse abdominal pain, often more intense in the lower abdomen, are common symptoms. If the involvement is primarily cecal or purely appendiceal, the symptoms may mimic those of acute appendicitis; if it is sigmoidal, a dysenteric picture may predominate. The number of daily stools increases, sometimes with mucus and blood. The symptoms progress until full-blown dysentery develops, with numerous bowel movements per day containing blood and mucus. On physical examination, the individual appears chronically ill without dehydration, with a temperature of 37°C to 38.5°C, abdominal tenderness especially in the right iliac fossa, and a slightly enlarged liver. In some individuals with severe amebic dysentery, a more pronounced clinical picture may develop. The patient appears toxic, with a temperature of 39°C to 40°C, dehydration, low blood pressure, and marked abdominal tenderness. Severe ulceration of the colon is always observed. In some patients, this condition may lead to perforation, peritonitis, and death. In endemic areas, the diagnosis is often not made clinically by physicians familiar with the disease; the outcome of severe amebic dysentery is high mortality, regardless of medical or surgical treatment (Wilmot, 1962).

Pathology. The gross appearance of the colon in amebiasis ranges from small (1 to 2 mm), superficial ulcerations scattered throughout the mucosa, more numerous in the cecum, to larger ulcerations with necrosis (Fig. 7–1 A–D; color plate IV A). In some cases, peritonitis is indicative of microscopic or inapparent perforation. In dysenteric colitis the ulcerations vary in size from 2 to 3 cm in diameter and often appear shallow, with hemorrhagic, necrotic material. When numerous ulcers are present, they are usually elongated, arranged perpendicular to the axis of the colon. In most instances, the mucosal surface between the ulcers appears normal (Fig. 7–1 A and D). In advanced cases, necrosis of the entire colonic mucosa is evident (Fig. 7–1 B). Gross perforation may be seen but often it is not appreciated, even though leakage of intestinal contents into the peritoneal cavity with peritonitis is observed. On cross section the intestinal

wall may be thin and appear friable, or more often thickened and edematous (Fig. 7–1 C), with necrosis extending downward and laterally from the opening of the ulcer, showing the typical flask-shaped ulcer. The overlying mucosa appears normal on the surface, but it is often undermined and sloughs off easily. In most cases of amebic colitis, the appearance of the colon is indistinguishable grossly from that of advanced ulcerative colitis or advanced inflammatory bowel disease produced by other microorganisms. Finally, colitis and amebae in the stools may not be indicative of colonization or of a cause–effect relationship between the parasite and the lesion.

Microscopically, the lesion produced by E. histolytica in the colon begins when one ameba on the mucosal surface cytoadheres to one epithelial cell and destroys it (see above). If more cells and more amebae are involved, the lesion progresses down into the mucosa (Fig. 7–2 A–B). As soon as the initial necrosis begins, an inflammatory reaction composed of polymorphonuclear cells occurs; the leukocytes degranulate and release their enzymes, which contribute to the tissue destruction (Takeuchi et al. 1977). Necrosis of the mucosa (Fig. 7–2 C) continues into the submucosa, extending laterally to form the flask-shaped ulcer, with its bottom composed of the intestinal muscle layer. The ulcer is filled with amorphous necrotic debris; degenerated polymorphonuclear, epithelial, and other host cells; and fibrin. The amebae are seen at the edge of the lesion in the interface between dead and viable tissues, either singly or in groups. The inflammatory infiltrate around the necrotic lesion consists of scanty polymorphonuclear cells and lymphocytes interspersed among abundant nuclear dust, especially in ulcers not secondarily infected with bacteria. In most cases of uncomplicated amebiasis, the ulcers are limited to the mucosa and submucosa and do not extend beyond the muscle layers (Fig. 7–2 D).

In transmural lesions, various degrees of invasion and tissue destruction are observed. Trophozoites follow the plane of less resistance between muscle bundles until they reach the peritoneal surface (Fig. 7–3 A–D), producing necrosis of muscles and other tissues. Blood vessels are usually compromised early by lysis of the wall. Small thrombi composed of fibrin red blood cells and amebae form; these thrombi may embolize to the liver or, less frequently, to distant organs (Carrera, 1950). The walls of larger vessels show invasion by the parasites, often reaching the endothelial layer (Fig. 7–3 D). Edema, hyperemia, and necrosis of large areas of tissue due to ischemia are seen at this time. The vascular lesions, especially of large vessels, may explain the extent of tissue necrosis in some cases (Luvuno et

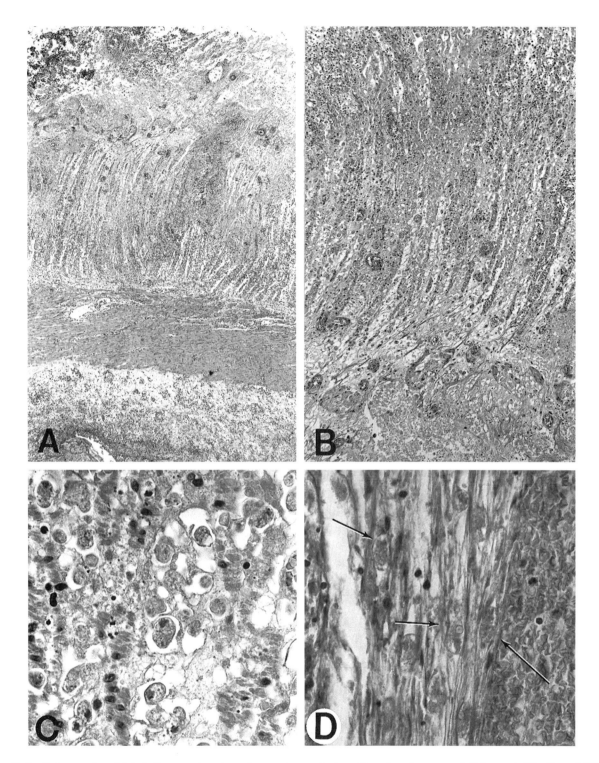

Fig. 7–3. *Entamoeba histolytica*, extension to peritoneum, hematoxylin and eosin stain. *A*, Total destruction of the mucosa and submucosa, with a marked inflammatory reaction and necrosis of muscle layers. Note the serositis at the bottom, ×28. *B*, Higher magnification showing numerous amebae invading through the muscle bundles, barely seen at this magnification, ×70. *C*, Parasites between necrotic muscle bundles, ×450. *D*, Large vein with parasitic invasion of its wall (large arrows). Note the parasites reaching the endothelial layer (long arrow) and the lumen of the blood vessel filled with red blood cells at the right, ×450.

al. 1985). Fibrinopurulent peritonitis is usually the rule in transmural infection (Fig. 7–3 A).

In 1% or 2% of persons with amebiasis, a palpable mass simulating a tumor may develop in the colon. This complication, which may occur in combination with other symptoms of acute amebiasis or which may develop after an episode of clinical disease with spontaneous or therapeutic remission, is known as *amebic granuloma* or *ameboma* (Fig. 7–4 A–D). Ameboma develops in an area of ulceration as a hard, uniform thickening of the colonic wall that reduces the lumen of the colon; it is easily demonstrated on x-rays (Fig. 7–4 A). Amebomas may be a few centimeters in size or may occupy a portion of the colon up to 25 cm in length. They develop most often in the cecum (50%), followed by the rectum and anal canal (27%), transverse colon (9%), sigmoid colon (5%), and to a lesser degree at other sites (Adams, MacLeod, 1977; Radke, 1955; Spicknall, Peirce, 1954). In a study of 214 patients with amebiasis, 4% developed amebomas (Spicknall, Peirce, 1954).

Microscopically, amebomas are composed of three distinct zones: the inner one, of necrosis; the middle one, of granulation; and the outer one, of fibrous tissue (Fig. 7–4 B). Parasites are seen close to the necrotic material and infiltrating in small numbers down into the granulation tissue (Fig. 7–4 C–D). This lesion develops as necrosis with repair and scar formation. Sometimes the lesion is circumferential, producing a thickening of the wall varying from 1 to 3 cm (Bravo, Duque, 1965). If not treated, amebomas may progress to further scarring with stenosis (Spicknall, Peirce, 1954).

Extraintestinal Amebiasis

Disease. From the primary intestinal foci, *E. histolytica* trophozoites find their way to secondary locations in the internal organs, where they produce extraintestinal lesions. Parasites traveling from the intestine through the portal vein lodge in the liver. Those traveling from the sigmoid colon and rectum through some of the communicating plexuses between the portal system and the inferior vena cava lodge in the lungs, brain, and other organs. Parasites that leak into the peritoneal cavity because of intestinal perforation seed the peritoneum and the peritoneal surface of abdominal organs.

Liver. In intestinal amebiasis, the liver is often involved due to mucosal damage that allows absorption of toxic substances, bacteria, and amebic trophozoites. The clinical symptoms of hepatic tenderness, mild enlargement, and sometimes slightly altered liver function tests are nonspecific; they are seen equally in inflammatory bowel disease due to other causes. This condition, sometimes referred to inaccurately as *amebic hepatitis*, was attributed to amebae arriving in the liver in large numbers and producing inflammation (Powell et al. 1959). If amebic hepatitis occurs, it still needs to be demonstrated histologically; however, cultures of portions of liver from experimentally infected guinea pigs with intestinal disease were positive in 50% of cases (Rees et al. 1954). On the other hand, it is known that in a few cases of either symptomatic or asymptomatic amebiasis, an amebic liver abscess develops.

Clinical Findings. Amebic liver abscess has a male preponderance. In most cases the disease presents with pain in the right hypochondrium; sometimes the pain affects the right side of the chest or the epigastrium (Adams, MacLeod, 1977). In 20% of cases a previous history of dysentery is discovered, and in 14% of cases diarrhea or dysentery or both are present concurrently. Tenderness of the right hypochondrium with a tender, palpable liver is present in over 80% of patients; 75% have fever, and 47% have signs in the right lung base. The patient appears acutely ill and dehydrated, with a rapid pulse, and sometimes is mildly icteric, though liver function tests are rarely abnormal. In a series of 100 patients with amebic liver abscesses, 69% had elevated alkaline phosphatase in the presence of normal serum glutamic-oxaloacetic transaminase and serum glutamic-pyruvic transaminase (Gupta, 1984). Jaundice per se does not exclude the diagnosis (it is present in 9% of cases), but its presence makes amebic liver abscess less likely; biliary obstruction rarely occurs. X-ray films and other imaging techniques such as ultrasound and computed tomography (CT) scans demonstrate the abscess(es), its size, its location, and its extension to adjacent structures (Fig. 7–5 A–C). Often a simple chest x-ray film shows elevation of the hemidiaphragm, with fluid in one of the pleural cavities. Laboratory tests demonstrate leukocytosis and anemia due to chronic infection. Serologic tests using amebic antigens are positive in 94% of the patients; thus, negative results make the diagnosis of hepatic amebiasis unlikely. Amebic liver abscesses in children occur equally in both sexes and produce a mortality of 67% (Scragg, 1960). If the abscess is aspirated, the "anchovy paste" consistency and color of the aspirated contents may facilitate the clinical diagnosis. However, this appearance is not often seen, and lack of this characteristic does not rule amebic liver abscess (Krogstad et al. 1978). In the laboratory, the amebae can be identified in aspirates from

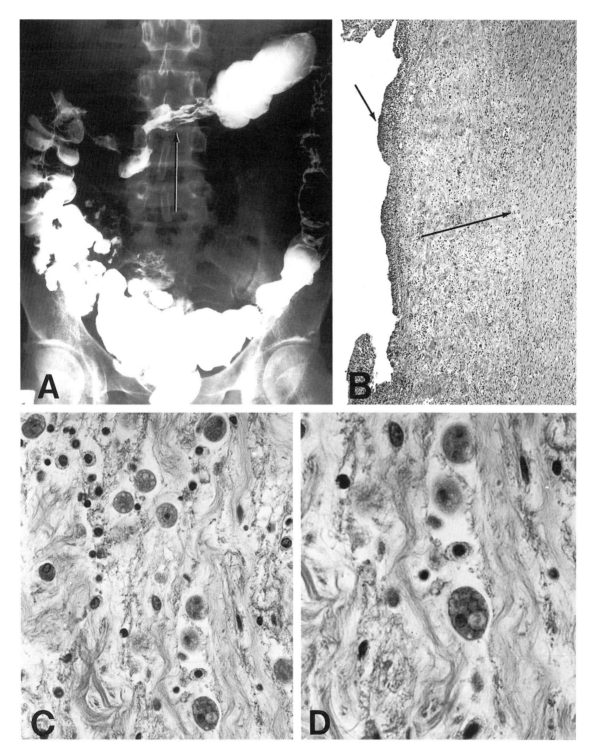

Fig. 7–4. *Entamoeba histolytica*, ameboma. *A*, X-ray film of barium enema showing an area of constriction (arrow). (Courtesy of F. Abdul-Karim, M.D., Department of Pathology, American University of Beirut, Beirut, Lebanon.) *B*, Low-power view of the lesion showing necrosis (short arrow), granulation tissue, and fibrosis (long arrow), ×45. *C* and *D*, Higher magnification of amebae within the granulation and fibrous tissue showing the scanty mononuclear cell infiltrate, *C* ×450, *D* ×705.

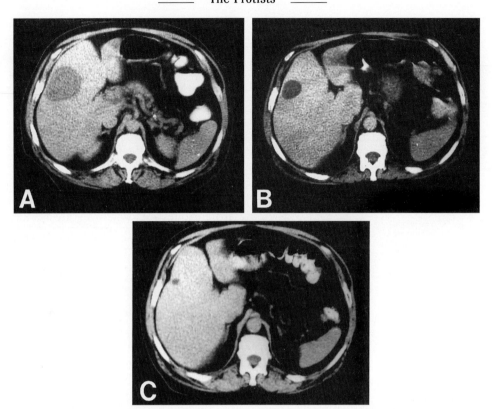

Fig. 7–5. *Entamoeba histolytica*, CT scans of amebic liver abscess. *A*, Lesion at the time of admission. *B*, Three weeks after drainage and specific therapy. *C*, Nine months later (Courtesy of K.V. Gopalakrishna, M.D., Infectious Diseases Service, Fairview General Hospital, Cleveland, Ohio.)

the abscess in 68% of cases (Biagi, Navarrete, 1958); bacteriologic cultures are usually negative unless the abscess is infected. Resolution of amebic and pyogenic liver abscess was studied longitudinally for 6 months with a monthly ultrasonogram in patients treated successfully with a medical regimen. At 6 months, only 30% of amebic abscesses had resolved compared with 94% of pyogenic ones (Sheen et al. 1989).

Pathology. The liver is often enlarged and may show the abscess if it is located on or near the surface. If the abscess has ruptured the capsule of Glisson or has extended into other adjacent organs, the full size of the abscess cavity is appreciated. In most cases there is a single abscess (Fig. 7–6 *A*; *color plate* IV *B*) located in the right lobe, where it occurs six times more often than in the left lobe. Less often, multiple abscesses are scattered randomly throughout the parenchyma (Fig. 7–6 *B*).

Recent amebic abscesses have irregular edges with no clear demarcation between the abscess and the normal parenchyma. The cavity is filled with dark brown necrotic material with a sweet odor corresponding to liquefied liver parenchyma. Sometimes the abscess fluid has the consistency and color of anchovy paste. A white fibrous wall of irregular thickness delineates older abscesses more clearly. The contents of these abscesses are variable in consistency and color, depending on the stage of evolution. After treatment and parasitologic cure, the organizing sterile abscess may have whitish debris or sometimes only clear fluid. Abscesses may persist after parasitologic cure (Watt et al. 1986), and some may calcify (D'Alessandro et al. 1966).

The early histologic events in the development of amebic liver abscess in humans have been described in a few cases. Amebic trophozoites originating in colonic lesions travel through the portal system within small thrombi composed of fibrin, red blood cells, and amebae. In the interlobular region, these trophozoites lodge in the smaller branches of the portal vein. At first, the lesion formed resembles a microinfarct. It extends toward the center of the lobule, with proliferation of the parasite and an early polymorphonuclear cell infiltrate (Palmer, 1938). This early sequence of events has been duplicated in experimental amebiasis complicated by amebic liver abscess in cats (Carrera, 1950).

The sequence of experimental amebic liver abscess formation in hamsters (Tsutsumi et al. 1984) and gerbils (Chadee, Meerovitch, 1984) has been described. In these animal models the early liver lesion was granulomatous, followed by necrosis produced by the rupture of infiltrating polymorphonuclear cells and liberation of their lysosomal enzymes. In these models, the rupture of polymorphonuclear cells was due to some form of active interaction with the parasite (see above); it did not occur with fixed (dead) amebae. Although

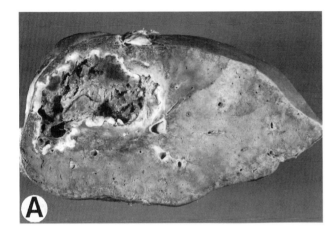

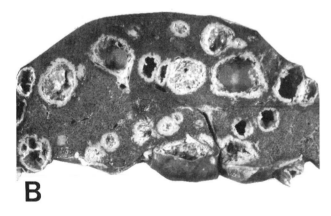

Fig. 7–6. *Entamoeba histolytica*, liver abscess. *A*, Liver from the patient described in Figure 7–1 showing a single large, amebic abscess of the right lobe. Note the irregular, thick white wall indicating organization and fibrosis. *B*, Multiple liver abscesses in a child. Note that some abscesses appear empty because of recent necrosis and liquefaction, while others are filled with thick material indicating a longer period of evolution. (Courtesy of P. Valencia Mayoral, M.D., Department of Pathology, Hospital Infantil de Mexico Dr-Marquez–Dr-Jimenez, Mexico City, Mexico.)

this sequence of events may be similar in humans and animals, such a conclusion appears unwarranted at present because in the experimental hamster and gerbil models, an inordinately large number of parasites was used to produce the lesions (Chadee, Meerovitch, 1984; Tsutsumi et al. 1984).

The initial stages of a human amebic abscess show dissolution of the parenchyma, with necrosis and a relatively scant infiltrate composed of polymorphonuclear cells and lymphocytes (Fig. 7–7 *A–B*). Most leukocytes arriving at the lesion are lysed in contact with the parasite (see above), hence their low number. The amebic trophozoites are few and are always located at the edge (wall) of the abscess (Fig. 7–7 *C–D*). In older abscesses there is usually a variable amount of collagenous, fibrous tissue separating the lesion from the liver parenchyma (Fig. 7–8 *A*). If the lesion is active, trophozoites are present between the fibrocytes (Fig. 7–8 *B*); in parasitologically cured abscesses, trophozoites are absent.

Lungs. Invasion of the pleural cavity or the lung parenchyma is most commonly due to extension from a liver abscess. This invasion occurs in less than 1% of patients with amebic dysentery, in 3% of all patients dying of amebiasis, and in 15% of patients with liver abscess (Anderson et al. 1953; Blyth, Pirie, 1978). Solitary amebic abscesses of lung due to hematogenous metastasis from the intestine occur in 14% of all patients with pleuropulmonary amebiasis. Similar solitary lung lesions are found in 10% of patients with concurrent hepatic abscesses. Extension into the pulmonary parenchyma from a liver abscess occurs in about 37% of patients and rupture into a major bronchus (bronchohepatic fistula), with expectoration of abscess contents and little pulmonary involvement, in 20%. Perforation of a hepatic abscess into the pleural cavity (empyema) has been observed in approximately 18% of cases (Fig. 7–9; Ochsner, De Bakey, 1936).

Clinical Findings. The clinical manifestations of pleuropulmonary amebiasis vary with the mode of extension into the lung. In disease extending from the liver, the first clinical symptoms are liver abscess followed by severe pain in the lower chest, often referred to the right shoulder. A nonproductive cough (pleural involvement), expectoration of large amounts of dark brown material with a sweet odor ("anchovy sauce"; bronchohepatic fistula, or dyspnea are possible presenting symptoms. In solitary metastatic abscess, the symptoms are similar to those of any bacterial abscess of the lung. X-ray films show the characteristic consolidation or cavitation, and other imaging techniques may delineate the relationship between the pulmonary

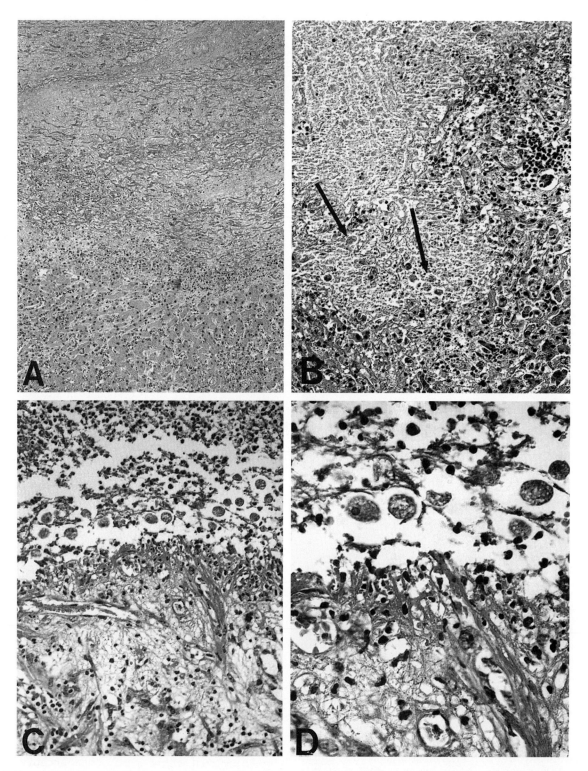

Fig. 7–7. *Entamoeba histolytica*, sections of liver abscess stained with hematoxylin and eosin stain. *A*, Low-power view of an early abscess showing necrosis (top), normal liver (bottom), and a few inflammatory cells at the interface, ×70. *B*, Higher magnification showing necrosis, a few necrotic trophozoites (arrows), inflammation, and liver parenchymal cells, ×140. *C* and *D*, Amebic abscess from another patient with early granulation tissue in the wall. Note the amebic trophozoites next to the wall of the abscess, *C* ×280, *D* ×450.

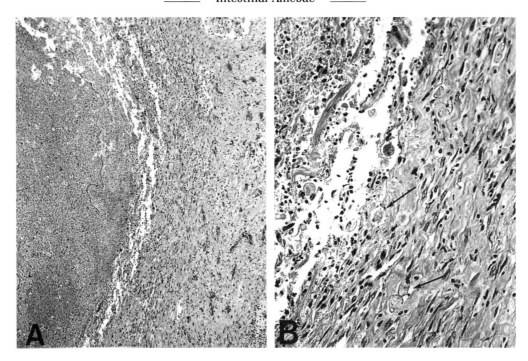

Fig. 7–8. *Entamoeba histolytica*, **sections of old liver abscess stained with hematoxylin and eosin stain.** *A*, **Fibrous wall with scanty infiltrate on the right and necrotic** content of the abscess on the left, ×58. *B*, **Amebic trophozoites are still present at the interface between the abscess and the fibrous wall (arrows),** ×230.

and liver lesions. Other general symptoms of infection are similar to those found in hepatic abscesses; mortality is high (Kubitschek et al. 1985).

    Pathology. The gross appearance of amebic lung abscesses is similar to that of abscesses produced by other infectious agents. The main feature is rapidly extending necrosis, with poorly defined, irregular borders and remnants of pulmonary fibrous septa across the lesion. Pulmonary abscesses usually do not develop a good wall because of the speed of spread. Superimposed bacterial infections are common. Amebic abscesses of the lung are often located in the right lower lobe. The content is variable in color and composition. Abscesses communicating with the liver are filled with the anchovy paste type of material; all others are filled with uncharacteristic debris or fluid.

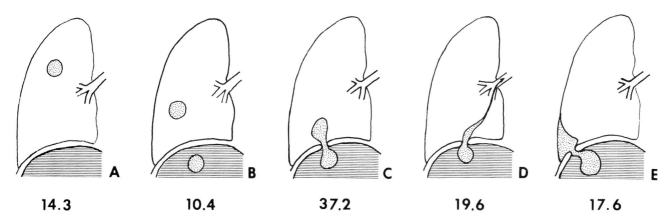

| 14.3 | 10.4 | 37.2 | 19.6 | 17.6 |

Fig. 7–9. *Entamoeba histolytica*, **routes of dissemination into the lung, with percentages of occurrence. (Adapted from: Ochsner, A., and DeBakey, M. 1936. Pleu-** ropulmonary complications of amebiasis. An analysis of 153 collected and 15 personal cases. J. Thorac. Surg. 5:225–258.)

The early amebic lesion in the lung consists of consolidation due to edema, as well as infiltration of the alveoli by polymorphonuclear leukocytes and lymphocytes (Fig. 7–10 A). Soon afterward the alveolar septae become necrotic, with extravasation of blood, fibrin, and other debris. As the lesion enlarges, the inflammation spreads irregularly throughout the lung parenchyma. Alveolar macrophages are often mistaken for *E. histolytica* trophozoites, which usually occur in small numbers at the edges of the abscess (Fig. 7–10 B).

Heart. Involvement of the heart by *E. histolytica* is a rare complication (MacLeod et al. 1966). With few exceptions, it is a pericardial infection that occurs in less than 1% of all patients with amebic liver abscesses, especially those of the left lobe. Involvement of the pericardial sac occurs as a sympathetic reaction, with accumulation of fluid and symptoms of pericarditis in response to an abscess of the left lobe of the liver. The liver abscess may rupture into the pericardial cavity, with colonization of the pericardium by the amebae. Mortality may be as high as 30%, and the clinical diagnosis is difficult to make (MacLeod et al. 1966).

Clinical Findings. The clinical symptoms suggest an amebic liver abscess of the left lobe associated with pericarditis; retrosternal, epigastric, or left shoulder pain accompanied by dyspnea and cough are early symptoms. On examination, pericardial effusion, low-grade fever, signs and symptoms of chronic disease, high jugular venous pressure, pulsus paradoxus, and a muffled heart apex beat are found. Leukocytosis, pericardial effusion, and electrocardiographic changes suggestive of pericarditis are positive laboratory test results. In addition, emaciation and anemia are common (MacLeod et al. 1966). Communication between the pericardium and the liver abscess can be demonstrated

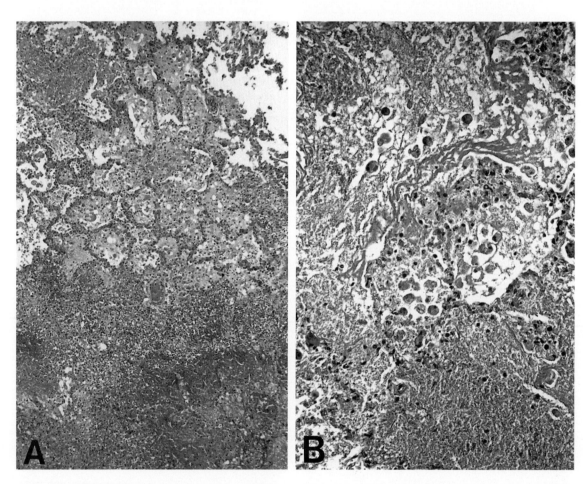

Fig. 7–10. *Entamoeba histolytica* in sections of lung stained with hematoxylin and eosin stain. *A*, Low-power view of an area of consolidation and necrosis in a Vietnam veteran who died with disseminated amebiasis, ×70. *B*, Higher magnification showing the dissolution of the pulmonary parenchyma and amebic trophozoites, ×180. (Preparation courtesy of M. Gravanis, M.D., Department of Pathology, Emory University School of Medicine, Atlanta, Georgia.)

radiologically (Ganesan, Kandaswamy, 1975); pneumopericardium has been described as a rare occurrence (Freeman, Bhoola, 1976).

Pathology. Fluid is a characteristic finding in amebic pericarditis. If the fluid is clear, the amebae have not reach the pericardium. However, all cases of true amebic pericarditis (due to rupture from the liver) have pus with characteristics similar to those of hepatic abscess (Fig. 7–11 A; *color plate* IV D). The parietal pericardium, often friable, can rupture, with extension into the mediastinum and pleural cavity. Aspirated fluid may reveal the amebic trophozoites or liver material, indicative of perforation. Microscopically, the visceral and parietal pericardia have marked necrosis (Fig. 7–11 B) and amebic trophozoites; the visceral pericardium is covered with fibrin, polymorphonuclear cells, and parasites.

Brain. Amebic brain abscesses are rare complications of amebiasis and occur as metastasis from an abscess in the liver, the lung, or, less frequently, the intestine (Lombardo et al. 1964; Powell, Neame, 1960); primary brain abscesses may occur without intestinal or other organ involvement (Kchouk et al. 1993). Amebic brain abscesses are usually multiple and go unrecognized clinically. The diagnosis is often made at postmortem examination, since these abscesses are usually fatal and have rarely been treated successfully (Kchouk et al. 1993; Ohnishi et al. 1994). The symptoms depend on the location of the abscess in the brain and are similar to those of any other destructive, rapidly evolving brain lesion. Plain radiographs and other imaging techniques demonstrate the exact location and size of the abscess, which appears grossly

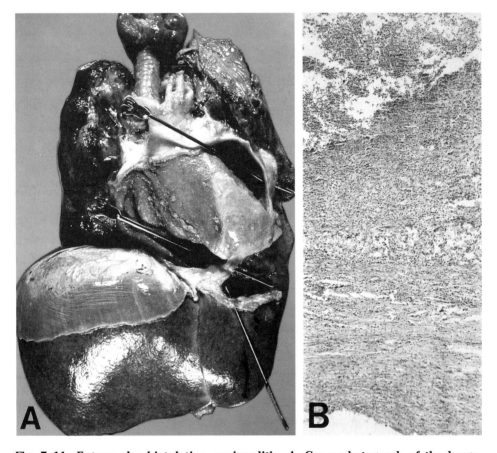

Fig. 7–11. *Entamoeba histolytica,* pericarditis. *A,* Gross photograph of the lungs, heart, and liver showing several perforations between a left lobe liver abscess and the pericardial sac. (Courtesy of P. Valencia Mayoral, M.D., Department of Pathology, Hospital Infantil de Mexico, Dr-Marquez–Dr-Jimenez, Mexico City, Mexico.) *B,* Microscopic low-power view of a section of parietal pericardium showing necrosis and infiltration throughout the thickness. The purulent content of the pericardial sac is seen above. Amebae were scanty and mostly appear vacuolated, hematoxylin and eosin stain, ×10. (Same case as shown in *color plate* IV D. Preparation courtesy of N. Gispert, M.D., Mexico City, Mexico.)

as an area of necrosis involving the white and gray matter (Fig. 7–12 A).

Microscopically, the lesion is a typical necrotic area with a scant infiltrate of polymorphonuclear leukocytes and lymphocytes. Amebic trophozoites should be recognized to make the diagnosis (Fig. 7–12 B).

Skin. Cutaneous amebiasis is a rare disease seen mostly in children and occurs in four distinct situations: first, from perforation of a liver or pulmonary abscess into the skin to form a sinus tract or from intestinal perforation into the skin to form a fistula; second, in surgical wounds infected secondarily from an internal amebic lesion; third, as a primary focus in the ocular orbit, the face, and other sites (Baez-Mendoza, Ramirez-Barba, 1986; Beaver et al. 1978; Brandt, Perez Tamayo, 1956); and fourth, in the perineal (*color plate* V A) and genital areas (*color plate* IV C; Magana-Garcia, Arista-Viveros, 1993; Poltera, 1973; Wynne, 1980), the most common sites for cutaneous amebiasis. These lesions usually occur in patients with intestinal disease and are due to extension from the rectum, or they result from contamination with fecal material (Magana-Garcia, Arista-Viveros, 1993). The common presentation is a slow ulceration (*color plate* IV C) involving first the epidermis and later the dermis. The ulcer is usually clean, with well-demarcated borders and a fundus containing granulation tissue. Secondary infections may occur with formation of pus and other necrotic debris. Microscopically, the parasites are seen in smears or biopsy specimens from the ulcer, which show a marked, nonspecific necrosis with mononuclear and polymorphonuclear leukocyte infiltration.

Pseudocondylomatous Lesions. In some instances, an inflammatory, slow-growing, condyloma-like lesion (pseudocondyloma) develops (*color plate* V A). Grossly, these lesions appear as firm growths or as verrucous lesions of different sizes in the perineal area, with or without ulceration and up to 2 cm or more in thickness. In one report, a lesion in the clitoris resembled a carcinoma (Majmudar et al. 1976). Microscopically, these lesions are large tissue masses with squamous epithelium (Fig. 7–13 A–B) showing changes varying from marked acanthosis to pseudoepitheliomatous hyperplasia and various degrees of spongiosis. The dermal papillae are elongated and, together with the upper corion, have edema, capillary proliferation, and a marked mononuclear cell infiltrate (Fig. 7–13 C). Parasites are recognizable in many areas, especially among groups of histiocytes and inflammatory cells (Fig. 7–13 D).

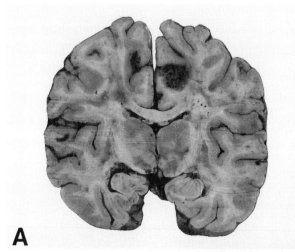

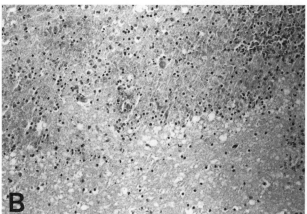

Fig. 7–12. *Entamoeba histolytica*, **brain abscess. A, Gross appearance of an amebic brain abscess showing two symmetrical necrotic areas. (Courtesy of P. Valencia Mayoral, M.D., Department of Pathology, Hospital Infantil de Mexico, Dr-Marquez–Dr-Jimenez, Mexico City, Mexico.) B, Microscopic section of a small metastatic lesion in the brain from the same autopsy material shown in Figure 7–10, with marked necrosis and inflammatory cells, hematoxylin and eosin stain, ×575. (Preparation courtesy of M. Gravanis, M.D., Department of Pathology, Emory University School of Medicine, Atlanta, Georgia.)**

Genitalia. Since the 1950s, genital amebiasis has been recognized in the gynecologic and urologic literature as an important infection because of the morbidity it produces. In women, the lesion may occur as a cervicitis with marked ulceration (Balasubrahmanyan, Cheriyan, 1949), as cervicovaginitis with destruction of the adjacent vaginal wall (Bhoumik, 1951), as a vulvar infection (Eyles et al. 1953), or as an endometrial lesion (Munguia et al. 1966; Othman, Ismail, 1993). Clinically, the cervical, cervicovaginal, and endometrial le-

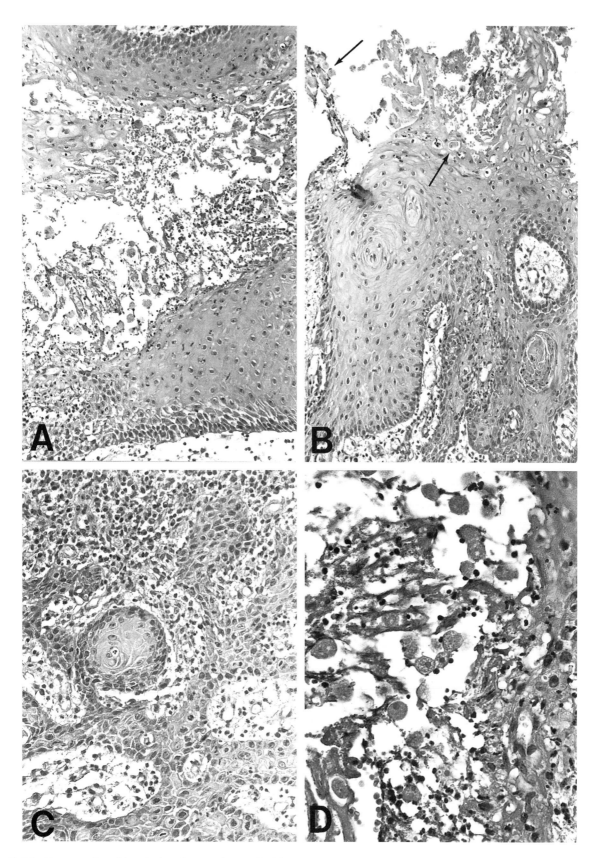

Fig. 7–13. *Entamoeba histolytica* in sections of skin stained with hematoxylin and eosin stain. *A–D*, Histologic appearance of the lesion. *A*, Low-power view, ×140. *B*, Section of a biopsy specimen showing sloughing of the superficial epidermis and amebic trophozoites (arrows), ×140. *C*, Higher magnification showing a mononuclear cell infiltrate, ×220. *D*, Even higher magnification showing the parasites, ×350.

sions often resemble a carcinoma, but biopsy specimens or Papanicolaou smears may reveal the parasites (Fig. 7–14 A–B; Munguia et al. 1966). If the clinical diagnosis is carcinoma and only necrotic tissue with amebae are found, the surgical report should include a warning that biopsies need to be repeated after specific antiamebic treatment. The carcinoma and the amebal infection may coexist (Acevedo Olvera et al. 1962, 1963; Mhlanga et al. 1992). In men, the parasites colonize the prepuce (Fig. 7–15 A) or the glans penis and may simulate ulcerated squamous cell carcinomas (*color plate* V *C*). Histologically, all of these lesions have a similar picture of necrosis, leukocytic infiltration, and parasites (Fig. 7–15 B; Mylius, Seldam, 1962).

Riboprinting techniques to characterize isolates of amebae colonizing the cervix of women using an intrauterine device have shown that the parasite is *E. gingivalis*, which is morphologically indistinguishable from *E. histolytica*. In addition, these patients have a concomitant infection with *Actinomyces* without cervical or vaginal ulcerations (Clark, Diamond, 1992). Removal of the intrauterine device rapidly cured one patient (McNeill, Moraes-Ruehsen, 1978).

Other Organs. Metastatic lesions of *E. histolytica* affect almost every organ system in the body. The gross appearance and histologic characteristics of these lesions are nonspecific, with necrosis and an inflammatory reaction. The presence of trophozoites is necessary for the etiological diagnosis. In one report, *E. histolytica* was isolated from a knee joint from a patient with arthritis, who responded to specific antiameba treatment (Than-Saw et al. 1992).

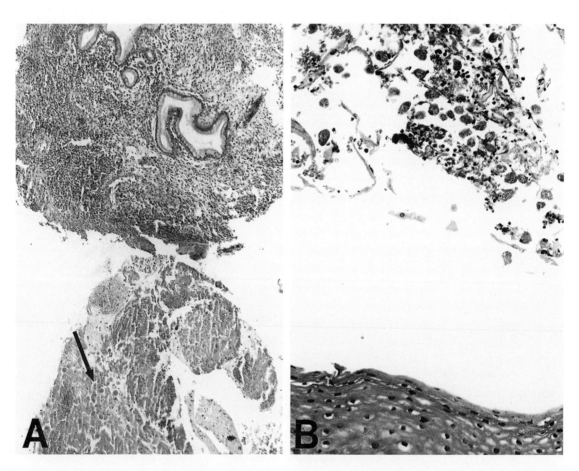

Fig. 7–14. *Entamoeba histolytica* **in sections of cervix stained with hematoxylin and eosin stain.** *A,* **Biopsy specimen of cervix from a patient with amebiasis. Note the necrotic debris (lower half), with the parasites (arrow) barely discernible at this magnification, ×70. (Preparation courtesy of H. Estrada, M.D., Facultad de** Medicina, Universidad de Caldas, Manizales, Colombia.) *B,* **Biopsy specimen with a similar lesion. Note the amebae in the exudate above, ×220. Biopsy was performed again 1 month after specific treatment. The patient was found to have an invasive squamous cell carcinoma of the cervix.**

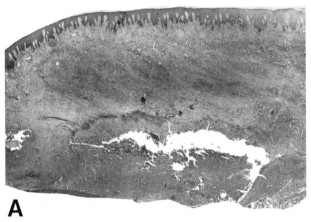

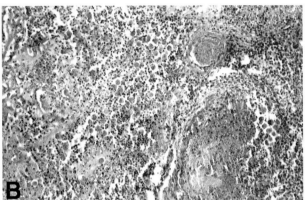

Fig. 7–15. *Entamoeba histolytica* in sections of skin stained with hematoxylin and eosin stain. *A*, Low-power view of prepuce from a man with an ulcerating lesion of the penis and prepuce clinically simulating a malignancy, ×12. *B*, Higher magnification showing necrosis, inflammatory cells, and numerous amebic trophozoites, ×100. (Preparation courtesy of H. Estrada, M.D., Facultad de Medicina, Universidad de Caldas, Manizales, Colombia.)

Diagnosis. Amebiasis is usually suspected clinically but requires laboratory confirmation, which involves finding the typical amebic trophozoites and cysts in various samples. *Entamoeba histolytica* and *E. dispar* cannot be distinguished morphologically. Correct identification of the parasite, if desired, must be based on isolation of the parasite in cultures, and the species must be determined using molecular techniques (see above). Since these methods are not used in the routine clinical laboratory, amebae found with morphologic characteristics of *E. histolytica* in stool samples should be reported as *E. histolytica*-like. Parasites found in tissues, in lesions, or in other body fluids may be reported as consistent with *E. histolytica* infection on the assumption that if the parasite is found in tis-

sues, it must be pathogenic and thus, *E. histolytica*. When amebae with morphologic characteristics identical to those of *E. histolytica* are found in a vaginal smear, in the absence of lesions, in women using an intrauterine device, the possibility of *E. gingivalis* should be considered. Distinction between *E. histolytica* and *E. gingivalis* has been made based on the presence of red blood cells in *histolytica* and their absence in *gingivalis* (Rachman, Rosenberg, 1986). However, this is not a valid criterion because all amebae ingest red blood cells if they are present (Montfort, Perez-Tamayo, 1994).

Serology. Many serologic tests are available and are useful for the diagnosis of cases in which parasites are not easily recoverable (Healy, 1986), for example in extraintestinal amebiasis. These tests, such as direct and indirect immunoagglutination tests, immunodiffusion tests, and others are still used to detect circulating antibodies. However, all serologic tests can only demonstrate past or present infection; on their own, they are not diagnostic. In recent years, the emphasis has been on the use of tests that allow differentiation between *E. histolytica* and *E. dispar*, either in serum or in stool samples. An enzyme-linked immunosorbent assay for stool samples is considered highly specific and sensitive (Haque et al. 1994). Direct DNA extraction and amplification from stools, without the need for culture, has been described as capable of detecting one trophozoite of *E. histolytica* per milligram of feces (Katzwinkel Wladarsch et al. 1994). The cytoadhesion protein of the trophozoites of *E. histolytica* (see above) has been used as an antigen to detect antibodies in both stools and serum samples (Ravdin, 1994). The immunoblot has been applied to distinguish *E. histolytica* from *E. dispar* in cyst passers (Lee, Hong, 1996). As mentioned earlier, these tests are still experimental. When they become routine in every clinical laboratory, the era of morphologic diagnosis of *E. histolytica* will have ended—not sooner, as some have claimed (Ravdin, 1994). Pathologists and other diagnosticians will continue using the morphologic characteristics of the amebae several decades into the next century to make diagnoses and influence clinical decisions.

Stools. In stools the parasite can be recovered and identified in wet preparations and in those stained with iron-hematoxylin or trichrome stains (Proctor, 1991). Trophozoites without ingested red blood cells (Fig. 7–16 A–B) and cysts (Fig. 7–16 C–D) are found mostly in asymptomatic carriers. Hematophagous amebae (Fig. 7–16 E–G) with ingested red blood cells in dysenteric or diarrheic stools occur in patients suffering from

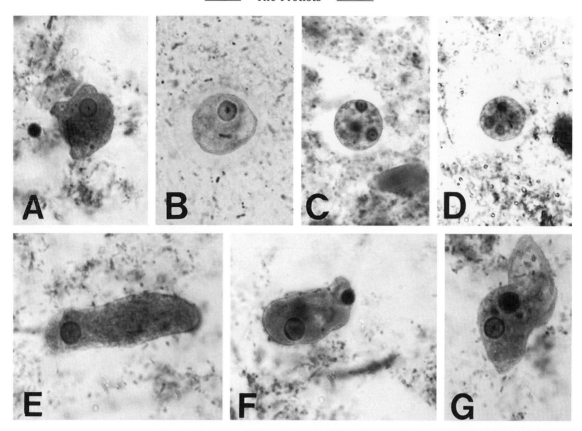

Fig. 7–16. *Entamoeba histolytica*-like diagnostic stages in human stools. *A* and *B*, Trophozoites without red blood cells, iron-hematoxylin stain. *C* and *D*, Mature cysts, trichrome stain. *E–G*, Hematophagous trophozoites of *E. histolytica* from diarrheic stools, iron-hematoxylin stain, all ×1,120.

invasive amebiasis. The morphologic characteristics of these stages are as described above.

Body Fluids. In smears of body fluids, as well as in aspirates from abscesses, skin ulcers, and genital lesions, only the trophozoites are found in either wet or stained preparations (*color plate* IV *G*) because *E. histolytica* does not form cysts in tissues.

Tissue Sections. Amebic trophozoites in tissue sections of any organ appear considerably smaller than those in wet mounts or smears due to shrinkage during fixation and processing (*color plate* IV *E–F*). The trophozoites vary between 15 and 25 μm, sometimes occurring with recognizable ingested red blood cells and often with only uniformly vacuolated cytoplasm (Fig. 7–16 *A–B*, and *E–G*). In abscesses, the trophozoites are usually found in the interface between healthy and necrotic tissue. The trophozoites are often found within clear spaces, an artifact produced by shrinkage of both the tissues and the parasite during fixation and processing. Amebic trophozoites in tissues are best

studied after being stained with hematoxylin and eosin stain (*color plate* IV *E–F*). The cytoplasm appears finely granular, with amphophilic tinctorial properties and sometimes containing phagocytized red blood cells; the cell membrane is smooth and sharply delineated. If the nucleus is present in the histologic section studied, the morphologic characteristics described above are easily recognizable. These characteristics—nuclear chromatin in small, uniform granules against the inner surface of the nuclear membrane and a small karyosome—are diagnostic of the genus *Entamoeba*. Obvious as it may seem, it must be emphasized that in tissues one deals with sections of the ameba and that the nucleus appears in only one or two of the possible four or five sections that each parasite yields.

Distinguishing the organism from histiocytes is usually not difficult if the nuclear structures of both cells are compared. The nucleus of histiocytes is more convoluted, with a different chromatin pattern. In addition, because of its larger size, the nucleus appears in almost all sections of the histiocyte, while the nucleus of the ameba does not.

The use of periodic acid–Schiff and immunoperoxidase stains (*color plate* V *B*) for the identification of *E. histolytica* in tissues is often recommended because the amebae stain positively and are easy to find under low-power magnification. However, this stain is not specific, macrophages stain equally positive, and the morphologic characteristics of the parasite are obscured. Periodic acid–Schiff should be used to *locate* the area where the parasites reside in the tissue section, making it easier to find them in the hematoxylin and eosin stain for exact morphologic identification. In our present state of knowledge, it is safe to assume that an ameba with a typical *Entamoeba* nucleus, if found in tissues, is probably *E. histolytica*. Specific identification is not possible until the parasite is studied with molecular, biochemical, and immunologic tests that determine the species.

References

Aca I-S, Kobayashi S, Carvalho LB Jr, Tateno S, Takeuchi T, 1994. Prevalence and pathogenicity of *Entamoeba histolytica* in three different regions of Pernambuco, northeast Brazil. Rev. Inst. Med. Trop. Sao Paulo 36:519–524

Acevedo Olvera A, Biagi FF, Santoyo J, 1963. Tres casos de amibiasis cervicouterina. Rev. Med. Hosp. Gen. (Mexico) 26:185–193

Acevedo Olvera A, Santoyo IJ, Biagi FF, 1962. Amibiasis cervico-uterina. Rev. Inst. Med. Trop. Sao Paulo 4:338–340

Adams EB, MacLeod IN, 1977. Invasive amebiasis. II. Amebic liver abscess and its complications. Medicine 56:325–334

Allason-Jones E, Mindel A, Sargeaunt P, Williams P, 1986. *Entamoeba histolytica* as a commensal intestinal parasite in homosexual men. N. Engl. J. Med. 315:353–356

Anderson HH, Bostick WL, Johnstone MG, 1953. Pulmonary amebiasis and abscess. In: Anderson HH, Bostick WL, Johnstone MG (eds), *Amoebiasis. Pathology, Diagnosis and Chemotherapy*. Springfield, Illinois: Charles C Thomas, pp. 142–147

Baez-Mendoza J, Ramirez-Barba EJ, 1986. Cutaneous amebiasis of the face: a case report. Am. J. Trop. Med. Hyg. 35:69–71

Balasubrahmanyan M, Cheriyan O, 1949. A case of amoebic vaginitis. Indian Med. Gaz. 85:501–502

Beaver PC, 1958. The exudates in amebic colitis. Proceedings of the Sixth International Congresses on Tropical Medicine and Malaria 6:419–434

Beaver PC, Blanchard JL, Seibold HR, 1988. Invasive amebiasis in naturally infected New World and Old World monkeys with and without clinical disease. Am. J. Trop. Med. Hyg. 39:343–352

Beaver PC, Jung RC, Cupp EW, 1984. *Clinical Parasitology*. Philadelphia: Lea & Febiger

Beaver PC, Lopez-Villegas A, Cuello C, D'Alessandro A, 1978. Cutaneous amebiasis of the eyelid with extension into the orbit. Am. J. Trop. Med. Hyg. 27:1133–1136

Bhoumik A, 1951. Amoebic infection of the female genital organs with report of a case. Indian Med. Gaz. 86:355–357

Biagi FF, Navarrete F, 1958. Busqueda de amibas en abscesos hepaticos. Rev. Latinoam. Microbiol. 1:243–248

Blyth DF, Pirie D, 1978. Haematogenous amoebic lung abscess. A case report. S. Afr. Med. J. 53:147–148

Bocket L, Marquette CH, Dewilde A, Hober D, Wattre P, 1992. Isolation and replication in human fibroblast cells (MRC-5) of a microsporidian from an AIDS patient. Microbiol. Pathol. 12:187–191

Brandt H, Perez Tamayo R, 1956. Amibiasis cutanea. Presentacion de un caso. Prensa Med. Mexicana 21:1–6

Bravo C, Duque O, 1965. Ameboma. Presentacion de 26 casos. Antioquia Med. 15:39–52

Byrd EE, 1937. The intestinal parasites observed in fecal samples from 729 college freshmen. J. Parasitol. 23:213–215

Campbell D, Chadee K, 1997. Survival strategies of *Entamoeba histolytica*: modulation of cell mediated immune responses. Parasitol. Today 13:184–190

Carrera GM, 1950. Pathology of early amebic hepatitis. An experimental study. Arch. Pathol. 50:440–449

Carrero JC, Diaz MY, Viveros M, Espinoza B, Acosta E, Ortiz Ortiz L, 1994. Human secretory immunoglobulin A anti–*Entamoeba histolytica* antibodies inhibit adherence of amebae to MDCK cells. Infect. Immun. 62:764–767

CDC, 1981. Amebiasis associated with colonic irrigation—Colorado. Morb. Mort. Weekly Rep. 30:101–102

Chadee K, Meerovitch E, 1984. The pathogenesis of experimentally induced amebic liver abscess in the gerbil (*Meriones unguiculatus*). Am. J. Pathol. 117:71–80

Chadee K, Petri JA Jr, Innes DJ, Ravdin JI, 1987. Rat and human colonic mucins bind to and inhibit adherence lectin of *Entamoeba histolytica*. J. Clin. Invest. 80:1245–1254

Clark CG, Diamond LS, 1992. Colonization of the uterus by the oral protozoan *Entamoeba gingivalis*. Am. J. Trop. Med. Hyg. 46:158–160

Clark CG, Diamond LS, 1994. Pathogenicity, virulence and *Entamoeba histolytica*. Parasitol. Today 10:46

Clark CG, Roger AJ, 1995. Direct evidence for secondary loss of mitochondria in *Entamoeba histolytica*. Proc. Natl. Acad. Sci. USA 92:6518–6521

Corliss JO, 1994. An interim utilitarian ("user-friendly") hierarchical classification and characterization of the protists. Acta Protozool. 33:1–51

Councilman WT, LaFleur HA, 1891. Amoebic dysentery. Johns Hopkins Hosp. Rep. 2:395–548

D'Alessandro A, Lega J, Vera MA, 1966. Cystic calcifications of the liver in Colombia. Echinococcosis or calcified abscesses? Am. J. Trop. Med. Hyg. 15:908–913

Denis M, Chadee K, 1988. Immunopathology of *Entamoeba histolytica* infections. Parasitol. Today 4:247–252

Diamond LS, Clark CG, 1993. A redescription of *Entamoeba histolytica* Schaudinn, 1903 (Emended Walker, 1911) separating it from *Entamoeba dispar* Brumpt, 1925. J. Euk. Microbiol. 40:340–344

El-Hashimi W, Pittman F, 1970. Ultrastructure of *Entamoeba histolytica* trophozoites obtained from the colon and from in vitro cultures. Am. J. Trop. Med. Hyg. 19:215–226

Eyles DE, Jones FE, Smith CS, 1953. A study of *Entamoeba histolytica* and other intestinal parasites in a rural west Tennessee community. Am. J. Trop. Med. Hyg. 2:173–190

Freeman AL, Bhoola KD, 1976. Pneumopericardium complicating amoebic liver abscess. A case report. S. Afr. Med. J. 50:551–553

Ganesan TK, Kandaswamy S, 1975. Amebic pericarditis. Chest 67:112–113

Gathiram V, Jackson TFHG, 1985. Frequency distribution of *Entamoeba histolytica* zymodemes in a rural South African population. Lancet 1:719–721

Gathiram V, Jackson TFHG, 1987. A longitudinal study of asymptomatic carriers of pathogenic zymodemes of *Entamoeba histolytica*. S. Afr. Med. J. 72:669–672

Guerrant RL, Brush J, Ravdin JI, Sullivan JA, Mandell GL, 1981. Interaction between *Entamoeba histolytica* and human polymorphonuclear neutrophils. J. Infect. Dis. 143:83–93

Gupta RK, 1984. Amebic liver abscess: a report of 100 cases. Int. Surg. 69:261–264

Haque R, Neville LM, Wood S, Petri WA Jr, 1994. Short report: detection of *Entamoeba histolytica* and *E. dispar* directly in stool. Am. J. Trop. Med. Hyg. 50:595–596

Healy GR, 1986. Immunologic tools in the diagnosis of amebiasis: epidemiology in the United States. Rev. Infect. Dis. 8:239–246

Katzwinkel Wladarsch S, Loscher T, Rinder H, 1994. Direct amplification and differentiation of pathogenic and non-pathogenic *Entamoeba histolytica* DNA from stool specimens. Am. J. Trop. Med. Hyg. 51:115–118

Kchouk M, Ghedas K, Bouhaouala MH, Larnaout A, Touibi S, Khaldi M, Ben Rachid MS, 1993. Abces cerebral amibien. A propos d'un cas. Ann. Radiol. Paris. 36:332–335

Krogstad DJ, Spencer HC Jr, Healy GR, Gleason NN, Sexton DJ, Herron CA, 1978. Amebiasis: epidemiologic studies in the United States, 1971–1974. Ann. Intern. Med. 88:89–97

Kubitschek KR, Peters J, Nickeson D, Musher DM, 1985. Amebiasis presenting as pleuropulmonary disease. West. J. Med. 142:203–207

Lee M, Hong ST, 1996. Differentiation of *Entamoeba histolytica* and *Entamoeba dispar* in cyst-passers by immunoblot. Korean J. Parasitol. 34:247–254

Leippe M, 1997. Amoebapores. Parasitol. Today 13:178–183

Leippe M, Andra J, Muller Eberhard HJ, 1994. Cytolytic and antibacterial activity of synthetic peptides derived from amoebapore, the pore-forming peptide of *Entamoeba histolytica*. Proc. Natl. Acad. Sci. USA 91:2602–2606

Lin TM, 1971. Colonization and encystation of *Entamoeba muris* in the rat and the mouse. J. Parasitol. 57:375–382

Lombardo L, Alonso P, Saenz A, Brandt H, Humberto M, 1964. Cerebral amebiasis. Report of 17 cases. J. Neurosurg. 21:704–709

Lushbaugh WB, Hofbauer AF, Kairalla AA, Cantey JR, Pittman FE, 1984. Relationship of cytotoxins of axenically cultivated *Entamoeba histolytica* to virulence. Gastroenterology 86:1488–1495

Lushbaugh WB, Hofbauer AF, Pittman FE, 1985. *Entamoeba histolytica*: purification of cathepsin B. Exp. Parasitol. 59:328–336

Lushbaugh WB, Kairalla AB, Hofbauer AF, Arnaud P, Cantey JR, Pittman FE, 1981. Inhibition of *Entamoeba histolytica* cytotoxin by alpha 1 antiprotease and alpha 2 macroglobulin. Am. J. Trop. Med. Hyg. 30:575–585

Luvuno FM, Mtschali Z, Baker LW, 1985. Vascular occlusion in the pathogenesis of complicated amebic colitis: evidence for a hypothesis. Br. J. Surg. 72:123–127

Lynch EC, Rosenberg IM, Gitler C, 1982. An ion-channel forming protein produced by *Entamoeba histolytica*. EMBO J. 1:801–804

MacLeod IN, Wilmot AJ, Powell SJ, 1966. Amoebic pericarditis. Q. J. Med. 35:293–311

Magana-Garcia M, Arista-Viveros A, 1993. Cutaneous amebiasis in children. Pediatr. Dermatol. 10:352–355

Majmudar B, Chaiken ML, Lee KU, 1976. Amebiasis of clitoris mimicking carcinoma. JAMA 236:1145–1146

McGowan K, Kane A, Asarkof N, Wicks J, Guerina V, Kellum J, Baron S, Gintzler AR, Donowitz M, 1983. *Entamoeba histolytica* causes intestinal secretion: role of serotonin. Science 221:762–764

McNeill RE, Moraes-Ruehsen MD, 1978. Ameba trophozoites in cervico-vaginal smear of a patient using an intrauterine device. A case report. Acta Cytol. 22:91–92

Mhlanga BR, Lanoie LO, Norris HJ, Lack EE, Connor DH, 1992. Amebiasis complicating carcinomas: a diagnostic dilemma. Am. J. Trop. Med. Hyg. 46:759–764

Montfort I, Perez-Tamayo R, 1994. Is phagocytosis related to virulence in *Entamoeba histolytica* Schawdinn, 1903. Parasitol. Today 10:271–275

Munguia H, Franco E, Valenzuela P, 1966. Diagnosis of genital amebiasis in women by the standard Papanicolaou technique. Am. J. Obstet. Gynecol. 94:181–188

Munoz MDL, Calderon J, Rojkind M, 1982. The collagenase of *Entamoeba histolytica*. J. Exp. Med. 155:42–51

Mylius RE, Seldam REJT, 1962. Venereal infection by *Entamoeba histolytica* in a New Guinea native couple. Trop. Geogr. Med. 14:20–26

Ochsner A, De Bakey M, 1936. Pleuropulmonary complications of amebiasis. An analysis of 153 collected and 15 personal cases. J. Thorac. Surg. 5:225–258

Ohnishi K, Murata M, Kojima H, Takemura N, Tsuchida T, Tachibana H, 1994. Brain abscess due to infection with *Entamoeba histolytica*. Am. J. Trop. Med. Hyg. 51:180–182

Osada M, 1959. Electron-microscopic studies on protozoa I. Fine structure of *Entamoeba histolytica*. Keio J. Med. 8:99–103

Othman NH, Ismail AN, 1993. Endometrial amoebiasis. Eur. J. Obstet. Gynecol. Reprod. Biol. 52:135–137

Palmer RB, 1938. Changes in the liver in amebic dysentery. With special reference to the origin of amebic abscess. Arch. Pathol. 25:327–335

Petri WA Jr, Joyce MP, Broman J, Smith RD, Murphy CF, Ravdin JI, 1987. Recognition of the galactose- or N-acetyl-galactosamine-binding lectin of *Entamoeba histolytica* by human immune sera. Infect. Immun. 55:2327–2331

Petri WA Jr, Ravdin JI, 1991. Protection of gerbils from amebic liver abscess by immunization with the galactose-specific adherence lectin of *Entamoeba histolytica*. Infect. Immun. 59:97–101

Petri WA Jr, Smith RD, Schlesinger PH, Murphy CF, Ravdin JI, 1987. Isolation of the galactose-binding lectin that mediates the in vitro adherence of *Entamoeba histolytica*. J. Clin. Invest. 80:1238–1244

Phillips SC, Mildvan D, William DC, Gelb AM, White MC, 1981. Sexual transmission of enteric protozoa and helminths in a venereal-disease-clinic population. N. Engl. J. Med. 305:603–606

Poltera AA, 1973. Pseudomalignant cutaneous amoebiasis in Uganda. Trop. Geogr. Med. 25:139–146

Powell SJ, Neame PB, 1960. A case of amoebic brain abscess. Br. Med. J. 2:1136–1137

Powell SJ, Wilmot AJ, Elsdon-Dew R, 1959. Hepatic amoebiasis. Trans. R. Soc. Trop. Med. Hyg. 53:190–195

Proctor EM, 1991. Laboratory diagnosis of amebiasis. Clin. Lab. Med. 11:829–859

Rachman R, Rosenberg M, 1986. Correspondence. Distinction between *Entamoeba gingivalis* and *Entamoeba histolytica*, revisited. Acta Cytol. 30:82

Radke RA, 1955. Ameboma of the intestine: an analysis of the disease as presented in 78 collected and 41 previously unreported cases. Ann. Intern. Med. 43:1048–1065

Ravdin JI, 1994. Diagnosis of invasive amoebiasis—time to end the morphology era. Gut 35:1018–1021

Ravdin JI, Guerrant RL, 1981. Role of adherence in cytopathogenic mechanisms of *Entamoeba histolytica*: study with mammalian tissue culture cells and human erythrocytes. J. Clin. Invest. 68:1305–1313

Ravdin JI, John JE, Johnston LI, Innes DJ, Guerrant RL, 1985a. Adherence of *Entamoeba histolytica* trophozoites to rat and human colonic mucosa. Infect. Immun. 48:292–297

Ravdin JI, Murphy CF, Salata RA, Guerrant RL, Hewlett EL, 1985b. N-acetyl-D-galactosamine-inhibitable adherence lectin of *Entamoeba histolytica*. I. Partial purification and relation to amoebic virulence in vitro. J. Infect. Dis. 151:804–815

Rees CW, Taylor DJ, Reardon LV, 1954. The presence of *Entamoeba histolytica* in the liver of guinea pigs with experimental intestinal amebiasis. J. Parasitol. 40:1–2

Rosenberg I, Gitler C, 1985. Subcellular fractionation of amoebapore and plasma membrane components of *Entamoeba histolytica* using self-generating percoll gradients. Mol. Biochem. Parasitol. 14:231–248

Sargeaunt PG, Jackson TFHG, Wiffen S, Bhojnani R, Williams JE, Felmingham D, Goldmeir D, Allason-Jones E, Mindel A, Phillips E, 1987. The reliability of *Entamoeba histolytica* zymodemes in clinical laboratory diagnosis. Arch. Invest. Med Mex. 18:69–74

Sargeaunt PG, Williams JE, 1979. Electrophoretic isoenzyme patterns of the pathogenic and non-pathogenic intestinal amoebae of man. Trans. R. Soc. Trop. Med. Hyg. 73:225–227

Sargeaunt PG, Williams JE, 1982. A study of intestinal protozoa including non-pathogenic *Entamoeba histolytica* from patients in a group of mental hospitals. Am. J. Public Health 72:178–180

Schain DC, Salata RA, Ravdin JI, 1992. Human T-lymphocyte proliferation, lymphokine production, and amebicidal activity elicited by the galactose-inhibitable adherence protein of *Entamoeba histolytica*. Infect. Immun. 60:2134–2146

Scragg J, 1960. Amoebic liver abscess in African children. Arch. Dis. Child. 35:171–176

Sheen IS, Chang-Chien CS, Lin DY, Liaw YF, 1989. Resolution of liver abscesses: comparison of pyogenic and amebic liver abscesses. Am. J. Trop. Med. Hyg. 40:384–389

Spicknall CG, Peirce EC II, 1954. Amebic granuloma. Report of four cases and review of the literature. N. Engl. J. Med. 250:1055–1062

Takeuchi A, Jervis HR, Phillips BP, 1977. Electron microscope studies of experimental *Entamoeba histolytica* infection in the guinea pig: III. Histolysis of the cecum. Virchows Arch. Cell. Pathol. 24:263–277

Than-Saw, Mar-Mar-Nyein, Oo MM, Tin-Tin-Aye, Myint-Lwin, Win KM, Naing KM, Kaneda Y, Tanaka T, 1992. Isolation of *Entamoeba histolytica* from arthritic knee joint. Trop. Geogr. Med. 44:355–358

Tsutsumi V, Mena-Lopez R, Anaya-Velazquez F, Martinez-Palomo A, 1984. Cellular bases of experimental amebic liver abscess formation. Am. J. Pathol. 117:81–91

Walderich B, Weber A, Knobloch J, 1997. Differentiation of *Entamoeba histolytica* and *Entamoeba dispar* from German travelers and residents of endemic areas. Am. J. Trop. Med. Hyg. 57:70–74

Walsh JA, 1986. Problems in recognition and diagnosis of amebiasis: estimation of the global magnitude of morbidity and mortality. Rev. Infect. Dis. 8:228–238

Watt G, Padre LP, Adapon B, Cross JH, 1986. Nonresolution of an amebic liver abscess after parasitologic cure. Am. J. Trop. Med. Hyg. 35:501–504

Weiss SJ, 1989. Tissue destruction by neutrophils. N. Engl. J. Med. 320:365–376

Wilmot AJ, 1962. *Clinical Amoebiasis*. London: Billing and Sons Ltd.

Wynne JM, 1980. Perineal amoebiasis. Arch. Dis. Child. 55:234–236

Ximenez C, Leyva O, Moran P, Ramos F, Melendro EI, Ramiro M, Martinez MC, Munoz O, Kretschmer R, Arellano J, 1993. *Entamoeba histolytica*: antibody response to recent and past invasive events. Ann. Trop. Med. Parasitol. 87:31–39

8

INTESTINAL APICOMPLEXA

A large number of organisms previously placed in different zoologic groups were found to have a set of organelles seen in electron micrographs and called the *apical complex*. The apical complex is located in the anterior part of the body and is present in one or more stages of the life cycle of these parasites. Its main function is to attach to and enter the host cell (Fig. 8–1). The presence of the apical complex is the basis for classifying all organisms that possess it in a separate phylum, the Apicomplexa. All organisms placed in the Apicomplexa are intracellular parasites at some point in their life cycles.

The classification of the Apicomplexa is better defined than that of other groups of the Protozoa; following is a simplified version showing the relationships of the genera and species important in human medicine (Beaver et al. 1984; Corliss, 1994). For didactic purposes, we will divide this phylum into three groups in accordance with the organ systems where they occur: the intestinal, tissue, and blood Apicomplexa. Each group will be studied in separate chapters.

A glance at this list of species demonstrates the importance of the Apicomplexa as human parasites, their wide distribution among animals and humans, and the morbidity and mortality they produce worldwide. The

Phylum: Apicomplexa
  Class: Coccidia
    Order: Eucoccidia
      Family: Cryptosporidiidae
        Genus: *Cryptosporidium*
      Family: Eimeriidae
        Genus: *Isospora* and *Cylospora*
      Family: Sarcocystidae
        Genus: *Sarcocystis* and *Toxoplasma*
      Family: Plasmodiidae
        Genus: *Plasmodium*
    Order: Piroplasmodia
      Family: Babesiidae
        Genus: *Babesia* and *Entopolypoides*

following paragraph presents a general statement on the biology and life cycles of the Apicomplexa. More detailed information will be found in the discussion of each species.

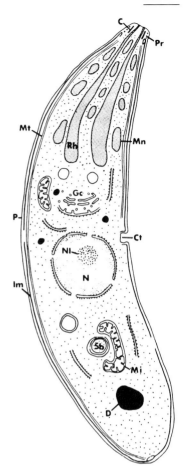

Fig. 8–1. Apicomplexan organism, schematic representation. Abbreviations: C, conoid; Ct, cytostome or micropore; D, dense body; Gc, Golgi complex; Im, inner membrane; Mi, mitochondria; Mn, micronemes; Mt, microtubules; N, nucleus; Ni, nucleolus; P, pellicle; Pr, polar ring; Rh, rhoptries; Sb, spherical body. (From: Aikawa, M., and Sterling, C.R. 1974. *Intracellular Parasitic Protozoa*. New York: Academic Press. Reproduced with permission.)

All apicomplexans have male and female sexual stages and reproduce both sexually and asexually as alternating generations in one or two hosts. *Asexual* reproduction is known as *schizogony*, a process by which the nucleus of the intracellular trophozoite divides a certain number of times, after which each nucleus acquires a small portion of cytoplasm to form an independent organism, the merozoite. The merozoites are freed after the cell ruptures and enter other cells to repeat the asexual cycle. *Sexual* development or *sporogony* involves the production of two sexual forms that develop from merozoites, known as the *microgametocytes* and *macrogametocytes*, or male and female, respectively. These sexual forms join to produce a zygote

that develops into an oocyst and, finally, into the infective stages, the sporozoites (Beaver et al. 1984). The sporozoites may remain in the oocysts, as in most intestinal species, or they may be freed from the oocysts to be inoculated by a biologic vector into the next host, as in malarial parasites.

This sketch of the life cycles of the apicomplexan parasites has variations that apply to each species. These variations include the number and kinds of hosts where the species occur, the type of cell where they develop, and the absence or presence of some stages in their life cycles. For example, *Cryptosporidium* has only one host where asexual and sexual development occurs. *Toxoplasma* also has one host, the cat, where both asexual and sexual reproduction occurs, but it has many alternate (intermediate) hosts where asexual reproduction occurs in the tissues. *Plasmodium* has two obligatory hosts: humans, where asexual development occurs, and mosquitoes, where sexual reproduction takes place.

Cryptosporidium—Cryptosporidiasis

The first cases of *Cryptosporidium* infection in humans were reported in 1976 (Meisel et al. 1976; Nime et al. 1976) in two immune-suppressed individuals suffering from overwhelming watery diarrhea. These cases were followed by reports of the disease in patients with hypogammaglobulinemia (Clinicopathological conference, 1980; Lasser et al. 1979), with a renal transplant (Weisburger et al. 1979), and with other conditions (Stemmerman et al. 1980). Soon afterward, a report of a self-limited, severe acute infection in an immune-competent man appeared in the literature (Anderson et al. 1982). At about this time, the acquired immune deficiency syndrome (AIDS) was identified, and cryptosporidiasis was recognized as a producer of untreatable diarrhea in this population. The first cases of cryptosporidiasis were thought to be zoonotic because the infection was known to occur in domestic animals, cows, horses, and other animals, but soon it was realized that *Cryptosporidium* is a human parasite previously unrecognized. Human cases occur worldwide, especially in the pediatric population, and the parasite has become another common pathogen, a producer of diarrhea.

Cryptosporidium has several species, classified on the basis of their morphologic characteristics and the species of animal they infect (Levine, 1984; Upton, Current, 1985). *Cryptosporidium parvum* occurs in several animals, including humans, and together with *C. muris* of rats and mice is the only species found in mammals. The total number of species of *Cryptosporidium* is not known. Other species will certainly be described, some of which are probably capable of infecting humans. One species of veterinary importance, *C. baileyi*, is responsible for cryptosporidiasis in chickens and other birds, producing a disease of the upper respiratory tract.

Life Cycle and Biology. The habitat of *Cryptosporidium* is the brush border of the epithelial cells of the gastrointestinal, respiratory, biliary, and pancreatic tracts (Fig. 8–2). The infection is acquired by the ingestion of water or food contaminated with mature oocysts passed in the feces. Once in the intestine, the oocysts release four sporozoites, which attach to the cell membrane of the enterocytes by means of their apical complex and enter the cell to become intracellular trophozoites. Inside the cell, the parasites are located in the area of the brush border; thus, we refer to *Cryptosporidium* as being intracellular but extracytoplasmic. Once the parasites are inside the cell, asexual development (schizogony) commences, terminating with several nuclear divisions that produce a certain number of merozoites. Once they mature, the merozoites are freed to enter the lumen of the intestine; in turn, the merozoites invade other cells to repeat the asexual cycle. At some point, some trophozoites differentiate into male and female gametes that unite to form the oocyst, of which two morphologic and biologic forms are known: thick- and thin-walled oocysts. The thick-walled oocysts are evacuated with the feces, at which time they are already infective, to transmit the infection to other hosts. The thin walled oocysts release their four sporozoites within the intestine to infect other cells, producing a form of autoinfection (Fig. 8–2). The four sporozoites in the oocyst of *Cryptosporidium* are free within the oocyst (not contained within a membrane), a feature not found in most coccidia. This membrane is called the *sporocyst*; therefore, we say that the oocysts of *Cryptosporidium* lack a sporocyst.

Morphology. For the purpose of diagnosis, the most important stage is the oocyst found in the feces of infected hosts (*color plate* V G). In fresh preparations of stool in saline solution, oocysts are seen as delicate, translucent, spherical structures measuring 4 μm in diameter. The wall of oocysts is birefringent and is thick relative to the size of the parasite; if the condenser of

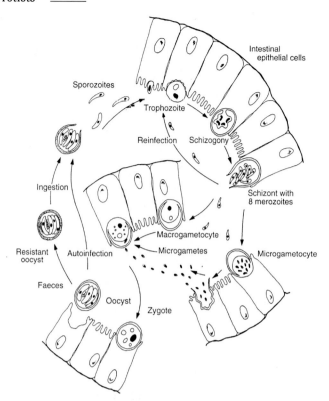

Fig. 8–2. *Cryptosporidium*, schematic representation of the life cycle. After ingestion of oocysts, the sporozoites are released in the intestine and in the brush border of the epithelial cells and begin asexual reproduction (schizogony). Some merozoites become gametocytes (male and female), which couple to form zygotes that evolve into oocysts. Oocysts are either thin-walled, rupturing in the intestine to produce autoinfection, or thick-walled and evacuated with the feces. Oocysts are infectious at the time they leave the body. (From: Smith, H.V., and Rose, J.V. 1990. Waterborne cryptosporidiosis. Parasitol. Today 6:8–12. Reproduced with permission.)

the microscope is lowered, four elongated structures may be seen inside the oocyst: these are the four sporozoites. In stained preparations with modified acid-fast stain (see below), the sporozoites stain red. In tissue sections of epithelia with brush borders, all stages of the sexual and asexual cycles are present. The organisms within the brush border of the cell appear as rounded structures no larger than the size of the oocysts in stools (*color plate* V D). The different developmental stages of the cycle are separated with difficulty with light microscopy but relatively easily with electron microscopy.

Scanning electron micrographs of the mucosa show the parasites firmly attached and protruding into the lumen as small spheres (Fig. 8–3). In transmission electron micrographs of *Cryptosporidium* in the intestinal

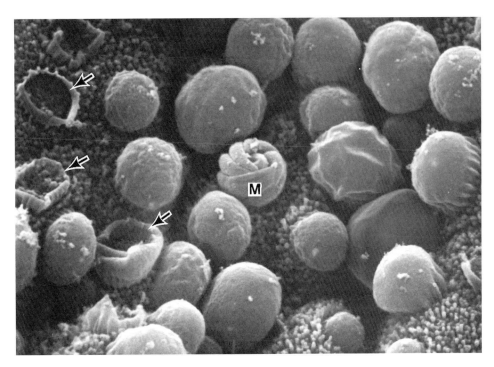

Fig. 8–3. *Cryptosporidium parvum*, scanning electron micrograph of the intestinal mucosa showing numerous developmental stages. Because of rupture of the cell membrane during processing, some merozoites are exposed (M). The arrows point to craters left by released parasites. (In: Current, W.L. and Garcia, L. 1991. Cryptosporidiosis. Clin. Lab. Med. 11:873–897. Reproduced by permission.)

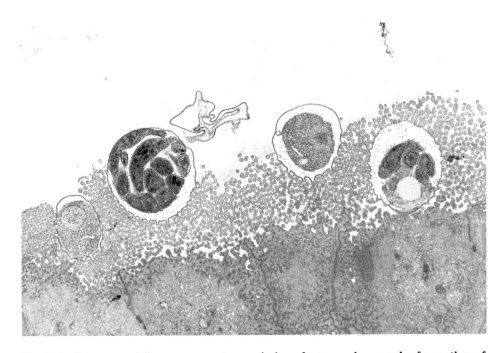

Fig. 8–4. *Cryptosporidium parvum*, transmission electron micrograph of a section of an intestinal biopsy specimen from a patient with AIDS. Note the mature schizont on the left with well-formed merozoites; at the middle is a gametocyte, and at the right a maturing schizont, ×6,630.

mucosa the sporozoites are rarely seen between the microvilli as elongated stages (a point at which they are motile) with the nucleus, endoplasmic reticulum, and Golgi apparatus. Often they are seen making contact with the host cell membrane by means of the apical complex, which consists of rhoptries, micronemes, a polar ring, and preconidial rings (Figs. 8–4 and 8–5). Once inside the cell, the sporozoites become rounded forms, with their nucleus and other organelles in evidence. However, the most striking feature is the change in the host cell at the point where the parasite makes contact with the cytoplasm (Figs. 8–5 and 8–6). A thick electron area, the filamentous zone, fuses the parasite to the cell cytoplasm, and some believe that the parasite derives its food through this area (Fig. 8–6). The parasite is covered by a double layer of the host cell membrane, derived from the membrane of the microvilli (Fig. 8–6). Intermediate stages from trophozoite to mature merozoite have marked cytoplasmic proliferation and up to eight nuclei. Mature merozoites are elongated and covered by a triple membrane; in their cytoplasm, the nucleus, the endoplasmic reticulum with

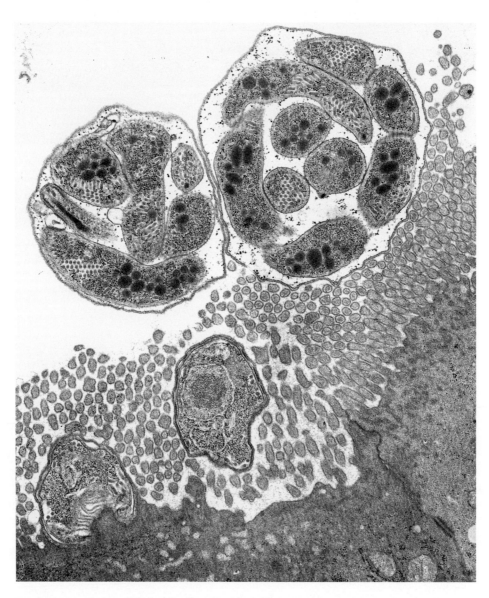

Fig. 8–5. *Cryptosporidium parvum*, transmission electron micrograph of sections of a biopsy specimen from the patient in Figure 8–4. Showing larger magnification of two mature schizonts with merozoites. Note the apical complex organelles; at the bottom are two other developmental forms, ×17,300.

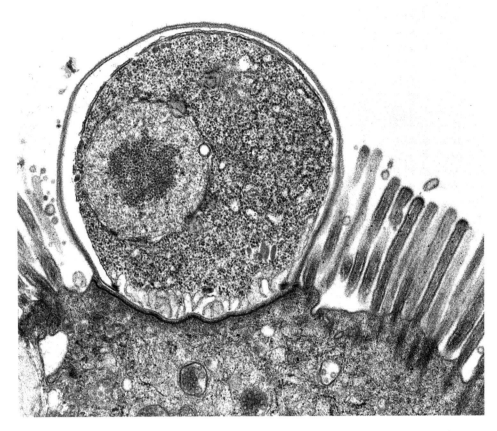

Fig. 8–6. *Cryptosporidium parvum*, transmission electron micrograph of sections of the biopsy specimen from the patient in Figure 8–4. Showing larger magnification of the gametocyte. Note the area of attachment to the cell cytoplasm and the host cell membrane covering the parasite, forming a vacuole for the parasite, ×26,200.

attached ribosomes, the Golgi apparatus, and the apical complex are the most prominent structures. The mature merozoite leaves the cell through a split in the cell membrane to parasitize other cells. The macrogametocyte is similar in size to the early merozoite but lacks cellular division (Fig. 8–6). The microgametocyte is characterized by the presence of microgametes, budding at the periphery, with minute, compact nuclei. The oocyst is distinguished by its thick wall and by the four sporozoites inside (Bird, Smith, 1980; da Costa-Ribeiro et al. 1989; Lumb et al. 1988).

Geographic Distribution and Epidemiology. Human infections with *Cryptosporidium* are worldwide, with prevalences related to the socioeconomic and hygienic conditions of the group under study. These infections are more common in places where groups of individuals live close together, for example in institutions or day-care centers (CDC, 1984). The oocysts of *Cryp-*

tosporidium are infectious at the time of evacuation with feces; thus, transmission from person to person follows the fecal-oral route. Waterborne epidemics and outbreaks due to contamination of drinking water with either human or animal excreta are important sources of large numbers of infections (Kramer et al. 1996). Molecular analysis of *Cryptosporidium* isolates from humans and bovines shows that the human phenotypes are similar and are different from those of bovines. However, isolates of *Cryptosporidium* from humans in contact with bovines show the bovine phenotype (Peng et al. 1997). The epidemiologies of *Cryptosporidium* and *Giardia* (see Chapter 3) are intimately related. The same factors are responsible for their prevalence, incidence, and transmission (Kramer et al. 1996; Rodriguez Hernandez et al. 1996). However, the prevalence of *Giardia* increased in children attending a day-care center throughout a five-season study period, while that of *Cryptosporidium* remained relatively constant (Rodriguez Hernandez et al. 1996). Several species of domestic and wild animals are naturally infected, and they serve as reservoirs of the parasite; *Cryptosporidium* has low host specificity.

More than 200 surveys carried out in many countries, targeting groups of individuals living under different conditions, are now available. The data from these surveys are sometimes difficult to interpret because the methodologies used to collect the data are not uniform. However, as a whole these surveys show that cryptosporidiasis is an infection more common in tropical than in temperate regions and that the infection is predominant in infants less than 1 year of age. In areas with wet and dry seasons, disease prevalence is highest during the rainy season (Enriquez et al. 1997). Disease prevalence is also higher in individuals with diarrhea, and in areas of high transmission, seropositivity in the general population is extremely high—95% in one study (Newman et al. 1994).

In the United States, of 216,000 stool specimens from persons of all ages examined by state diagnostic laboratories in 1987, only 0.2% were positive for *Cryptosporidium* (Kappus et al. 1991). In addition, a survey in a day-care center showed a prevalence of less than 1% (Addiss et al. 1991). In contrast, in 202 individuals of all ages studied in Venezuela, the prevalence was 10%; six children (28% of the children in the study) had diarrhea, four of whom were infants (Chacin Bonilla et al. 1993). In Bedouin children in Israel, only 1% were positive (el On et al. 1994). In Australia, of about 7000 patients studied, 100, or 1.4%, were positive. Of the 100 patients who tested positive, 29 were less than 1 year old, 50 were 1 to 2 years of age, and the other 21 were older (Assadamongkol et al. 1992). In Venezuela, the positivity among children with diarrhea was 11% (Chacin-Bonilla et al. 1997). In Bolivia, 32% of healthy Aymara children from the Altiplano examined were positive (Esteban et al. 1998). Studies of prevalence in Europe have shown a situation similar to that of the United States. Seroepidemiologic studies of the infection have revealed high rates of seropositivity in random samples of individuals from different countries. Rates of prevalence of immunoglobulin G (IgG) antibodies have varied from 25% to 95%, with the highest rates found in tropical countries (Garcia, Current, 1989). Seroepidemiologic studies of IgM (to determine the presence of recent or active infection) in developing countries show up to 20% positivity (Ungar et al. 1988). This finding indicates that many individuals come in contact with the infection and may have had symptoms at least once.

The prevalence of *Cryptosporidium* in the male homosexual communities of advanced countries varies from none (Jokipii et al. 1985; Laughon et al. 1988) to relatively high. In a group of human immune deficiency virus (HIV)-positive homosexual men in Los Angeles, 6% were positive for *Cryptosporidium*, and the prevalence in this group correlated with anal-penile sex practices (Esfandiari et al. 1995). In the same area, the prevalence of cryptosporidiasis in all HIV-positive individuals (about 17,000) was less than 4%; whites and Latinos had similar rates, and blacks had a much lower rate (Sorvillo et al. 1994). In Malaysia, asymptomatic drug users who were HIV positive without symptoms of AIDS showed a prevalence of 23% (Kamel et al. 1994).

Several outbreaks of cryptosporidiasis produced by contaminated drinking water have been studied, most of them in the United States (Hayes et al. 1989; MacKenzie et al. 1994) and Europe (Casemore et al. 1994; Smith, Rose, 1998). In the United States, 30 outbreaks of waterborne diarrhea occurred during 1993–1994 in which 405,366 people became ill. Ten of these outbreaks were produced by *Cryptosporidium* and *Giardia*. One outbreak caused by *Cryptosporidium* in Milwaukee, by far the largest reported in the world, was responsible for 403,000 of the 405,366 cases of illness (Kramer et al. 1996; MacKenzie et al. 1994; Widmer et al. 1996). The Milwaukee outbreak was due to contamination of drinking water with cattle excreta. Cattle have a high prevalence of the infection (more than 90% of dairy herds in the United States are positive) (Widmer et al. 1996), and oocysts of *Cryptosporidium* are very resistant to chlorine. In a hospital setting, about a dozen nurses who took care of a patient with *Cryptosporidium* contracted the infection (Gardner, 1994).

Some of the risk factors for the infection have been investigated in Africa, where the presence of pigs and dogs in the household was found to correlate with infections in children; breast-feeding appeared to protect infants (Molbak et al. 1994). In Brazil, a serologically positive child less than 3 years of age (index case) in a household was responsible for a secondary case in 58% of the households studied, indicating a transmissibility rate of 19% (Newman et al. 1994). Studies of dairy farmers in Wisconsin, in the United States, showed positive serology in 44% compared with 24% in the control group (Lengerich et al. 1993).

Pathogenesis. Little is known about the mechanism by which *Cryptosporidium* produces disease, mainly because of the lack of a suitable model. Neonatal piglets used in experimental work are not ideal. From limited experiments, the diarrhea in cryptosporidiasis appears to be secretory, a fact supported by some clinical observations (Clark, Sears, 1996). The mechanism proposed for this hypersecretion is based on the damage to the enterocytes caused by the multiplying parasites, which results in hyperplasia of the crypt cells. The destruction of absorptive cells at the tips of the villi and the hyperplasia of the secreting crypt cells together are enough to tilt the balance toward secretion of fluid and ions by the intestinal mucosa. This response may be amplified by the cytokine response of the enterocytes to damage of the inflammatory cells resulting from the immunologic response to the parasites (Clark, Sears, 1996). However, this scenario remains speculative.

Clinical Findings. Cryptosporidiasis is a disease affecting equally individuals of both sexes and all ages, but most illnesses occur in infants. Clinically, cryptosporidiasis presents as gastroenteritis. The severity of the symptoms depends on the immunologic status of the host (Pitlik et al. 1983). In immune-competent hosts, clinically silent infections occur. However, the majority of patients have self-limited, watery diarrhea with cramps, loss of appetite, and loss of weight that last for periods ranging from a few days to 2 weeks (Jokipii, Jokipii, 1986; Reese et al. 1982). Some patients may have severe cramps and vomiting (Tzipori et al. 1980). The mean incubation period is approximately 7 days, and the mean duration of illness is about 12 days (range, 2 to 26 days). In some individuals, oocysts are recovered from stools between 7 and 28 days of infection; in many, between 1 and 15 days after cessation of symptoms; and in a few, beyond 2 months (Jokipii, Jokipii, 1986; Shepherd et al. 1988). The clinical picture of cryptosporidiasis in immune-competent hosts is similar to that of traveler's diarrhea, in which *Cryptosporidium* plays an important role (Gatti, 1993; Jokipii, 1983). Infection of the colon in immune-competent hosts may produce symptoms of colitis (Hart et al. 1989).

In immune-suppressed individuals, cryptosporidiasis presents with a clinical picture similar to that of immune-competent hosts, but it is more pronounced and lasts for months or years (Current et al. 1983; Meisel et al. 1976; Nime et al. 1976; Soave et al. 1984). The most severe symptoms, with malabsorption and poor D-xylose absorption, are found in patients with small bowel infection. Less severe symptoms and reduced morbidity are found in patients with colon infection (Clayton et al. 1994). The conditions associated with intractable cryptosporidiasis are AIDS, low IgA level, congenital hypogammaglobulinemia, and cyclophosphamide and prednisolone therapy. Some malignancies, especially lymphomas (Gentile et al. 1991), are also as-

sociated with the infection and, in one case, with insulin-dependent diabetes mellitus (Chan et al. 1989). In individuals with AIDS, cryptosporidiasis usually occurs in those with 150 or fewer CD4$^+$ T lymphocytes per cubic millimeter; those with higher T-lymphocyte counts are able to clear the infection (Flanigan et al. 1992).

Lung. Bronchopulmonary cryptosporidiasis is usually found in persons with AIDS who have very low CD4$^+$ T lymphocyte levels (Brea Hernando et al. 1993a; Goodstein et al. 1989; Moore, Frenkel, 1991; Poirot et al. 1996), though one case occurred in a patient with lymphoma (Travis et al. 1990) and another in an infant with combined immune deficiency (Kocoshis et al. 1984). The symptoms of pulmonary cryptosporidiasis are nonspecific and consist of chronic cough, dyspnea, fever, and chest pain. The cough sometimes occurs with profuse mucus production. Other patients may have symptoms of bronchiolitis or pneumonia. Some chest x-ray films are normal; others show diffuse infiltrates, or areas of consolidation. Death is due to respiratory failure, but whether *Cryptosporidium* is the cause of death is not known because most affected individuals have other pathogens in the lung, including cytomegalovirus and *Pneumocystis*. In an asymptomatic patient infected with HIV and with intestinal cryptosporidiasis, shedding of oocysts in the sputum was demonstrated (Miller et al. 1984). In one child, a severe laryngotracheitis with ulceration was the main presentation of the infection (Harari et al. 1986). One case of pulmonary, gastrointestinal, hepatic, and urinary cryptosporidiasis was caused by *C. baileyi* (Ditrich et al. 1991).

Biliary Tract and Pancreas. Involvement of the biliary tract by *Cryptosporidium*, producing symptoms and histologic abnormalities consistent with sclerosing cholangitis, has been documented repeatedly in patients with advanced AIDS (stage IV of the Centers for Disease Control classification) and extremely low CD4$^+$ T-lymphocyte counts (Brea Hernando et al. 1993b; Teixidor et al. 1991). The disease has also been documented in a child with a congenital immune deficiency (Davis et al. 1987). The main clinical symptoms are pain in the right upper quadrant, diarrhea, fever, and cholestasis. Radiographs of the bile ducts show stenosis of the distal portion of the common bile duct with dilation; in other patients, the obstruction and dilation are accompanied by distortion of the intrahepatic bile ducts (Benhamou et al. 1993; Dolmatch et al. 1987). In persons with HIV infection this syndrome is called *AIDS-related cholangitis*. Because other organisms are often found in association with *Cryptosporidium* in the biliary tract, the role of *Cryptosporidium* in producing the syndrome is not known. The distal obstruction of the common bile duct, with dilation and distortion of the intrahepatic bile ducts, correlates significantly with infections with cytomegalovirus and *Cryptosporidium*, while obstruction and dilation without distortion of the intrahepatic bile ducts do not (Benhamou et al. 1993). The obstruction of the common bile duct is caused by stenosis of the ampulla due to an inflammatory reaction, sometimes with papillary proliferation of the epithelium (Gremse et al. 1989). An acalculous cholecystitis has also been attributed to *Cryptosporidium* (Gould et al. 1989), and in one case, together with cytomegalovirus, it produced a gangrenous cholecystitis (Blumberg et al. 1984).

Symptoms of pancreatitis in the pancreatic ducts have also been reported in patients with AIDS (Cappell, Hassan, 1993) and in those with congenital immune suppression syndromes (Kocoshis et al. 1984). The number of cases is very small (Cappell, Hassan, 1993), and in one immune-competent patient the diagnosis was circumstantial (Hawkins et al. 1987). The parasite was found in pancreatic sections in cases of disseminated cryptosporidiasis (Gross et al. 1986; Kocoshis et al. 1984).

Other Organs. There are reports of *Cryptosporidium* involvement of the esophagus (Kazlow et al. 1986) and the gastric mucosa, with resulting pyloric obstruction (Cersosimo et al. 1992; Garone et al. 1986). Whether the cases of gastric cryptosporidiasis were produced by *C. muris* (the species parasitizing the stomach of mice) has not been explored. *Cryptosporidium muris* is distinguished from *C. parvum* by its larger size: of 5×7 μm; a report of *C. muris* in the stools of a patient turned out to be an infection with *Cyclospora* (Narango et al. 1989). A urinary bladder infection has also been reported (Ditrich et al. 1991).

Immunity. The immune mechanism that limits *Cryptosporidium* infections in the immune-competent host to a self-limited disease is not known. It is also not known whether the host is protected against reinfection or against the disease after the first infection occurs. The presence of infected individuals without symptoms suggests that the immunity is to the infection, not to reinfection with the parasite. The protective role of specific IgG and IgM antibodies present in large numbers of individuals is also not known, as is the role of secretory IgA antibodies present in the saliva and serum of chronically infected individuals (Cozon et al. 1994). However, since the infection is chronic in

patients with several kinds of congenital agammaglobulinemias, the antibodies must play an important role in establishing immunity to the infection. In addition, the CD4$^+$ T lymphocytes must play an important function in controlling both the infection and the disease because, in patients with low levels of these cells, the symptoms and the parasites are not cleared from the intestine. Athymic mice infected with *Cryptosporidium* have a disease course similar to that of humans with low CD4$^+$ T-lymphocyte counts. It seems that both humoral and cellular immunity need to be intact to control *Cryptosporidium* infections. In infants, secretory antibodies in milk provide some protection (Sterling et al. 1991).

Pathology. The gross and microscopic picture of cryptosporidiasis in immune-competent patients is seldom reported. In one case, the intestinal mucosa of immune-competent children showed mild to moderate enteropathy, with evidence of brush border effacement in areas where the parasites were located; reduced villous height and increased levels of intraepithelial lymphocytes were also found (Phillips et al. 1992). Gross and microscopic lesions in immune-suppressed individuals have been described in autopsy and biopsy specimens (Clayton et al. 1994; Genta et al. 1993). However, caution is needed in interpreting this information because the presence of other organisms has been documented in about one-half of these cases (Clayton et al. 1994). Further, in patients with no other organisms, HIV enteropathy has to be kept in mind.

Cryptosporidium in the intestinal tract is often distributed predominantly in the small intestine, where the parasites are concentrated at the tips of the villi or deep in the crypts; alternatively, *Cryptosporidium* may be located mainly in the colon. The clinical manifestations are different with each of these distribution patterns (Clayton et al. 1994). Involvement of the small intestine produces more severe symptoms with malabsorption, while colon involvement results in less morbidity (Clayton et al. 1994). The intestinal mucosa in some *Cryptosporidium* infections is grossly normal (Gross et al. 1986); in others it is hyperemics, with signs of acute inflammation and petechial hemorrhages without ulcerations. In a few studies of the microscopic appearance of the intestinal mucosa in cryptosporidiasis, changes ranged from minimal in up to 70% of patients (Genta et al. 1993) to marked structural abnormalities (Chiampi et al. 1983; Lefkowitch et al. 1984; Meisel et al. 1976). In some cases of chronic cryptosporidiasis, the small intestine has pronounced mucosal damage (Fig. 8–7 *A*), with blunting, shortening, villous atrophy, and metaplastic changes with increased mitosis.

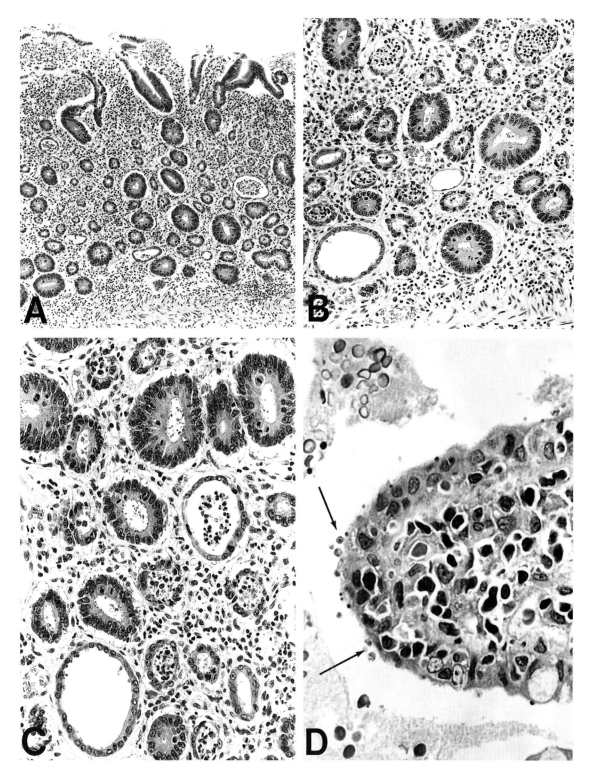

Fig. 8–7. *Cryptosporidium* infection in a patient with AIDS. Histologic appearance of small intestine in sections stained with hematoxylin and eosin stain. *A*, Low-power view showing marked distortion of the mucosa and inflammatory cells, indicating chronic damage, ×70. *B* and *C*, Higher magnification; note the crypt abscesses, the glands with low cuboidal epithelium, the rapid turnover (mitosis) of the epithelium, the inflammatory cells, and the parasites on the brush border, *B* ×140, *C* ×220. *D*, Higher magnification illustrating the parasites (arrows), ×705.

Inflammation with crypt abscess may be due to other coinfecting organisms (Fig. 8–7 *B*). The damaged epithelial cells have a cuboidal rather than a columnar appearance, with decreased mucin production (Fig. 8–7 *C*). The infiltrating cells are plasma cells, lymphocytes, and polymorphonuclear leukocytes filling the interstitium of the mucosal glands, lamina propria, and submucosa; sometimes they occur in small numbers down in the muscular layers (Figs. 8–7 *C–D*). In cases with flattening of the mucosa, polymorphonuclear cells are predominant (Genta et al. 1993). Within the brush border of the epithelial cells, the presence of parasites is the most striking feature and the hallmark of the infection (Fig. 8–7 *D*). One case of pulmonary cryptosporidiasis showed moderate metaplasia of the epithelium (Fig. 8–8; Kocoshis et al. 1984). Another case of infection of the gallbladder and intrahepatic ducts showed inflammatory changes, but in addition to *Cryptosporidium*, cytomegalovirus was present, probably with a superimposed bacterial infection (Fig. 8–9 *A–B*; Kahn et al. 1987). Electron microscopic studies have revealed the different stages of the life cycle of the parasite; otherwise, the changes correlate well with those seen with light microscopy (Figs. 8–4, 8–5, and 8–6).

Diagnosis. In the clinical laboratory, *Cryptosporidium* is identified by the study of recovered typical oocysts in

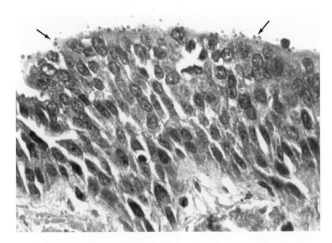

Fig. 8–8. ***Cryptosporidium* in sections of respiratory epithelium stained with hematoxylin and eosin stain. Respiratory epithelium of a medium-sized bronchus with moderate metaplastic changes and *Cryptosporidium* parasites on the brush border (arrows), ×500. (Preparation courtesy of M.L. Cibull, Department of Pathology, University of Kentucky, Lexington, Kentucky Reported by: Kocoshis, S.A., Cibull, M.L., Davis, T.E., et al. 1984. Intestinal pulmonary cryptosporidiasis in an infant with severe combined immune deficiency. J. Pediatr. Gastroenterol. Nutr. 3:149–157.)**

the stools, duodenal aspirates, and sputum in both fresh (*color plate* V *G*) and stained smears (Current, Garcia, 1991). Modified Kinyoun Acid Fast (MKA) or Ziehl-Nielsen carbolfuchsin, Giemsa, safranin-methylene blue (malachite green), methylene blue eosin, and other stains are good for easy screening and identification of oocysts (Ma, Soave, 1983). The routine trichrome stain used for diagnosis of parasites in stools, the Gram stain, and the silver methenamine stain poorly stain the oocysts of *Cryptosporidium* (Garcia, Current, 1989). Sheather's sugar and zinc sulfate concentration are excellent for recovering organisms when they are present in small numbers. A comparison of positive yields using small intestinal biopsy specimens and other laboratory methods showed that studying stools stained with Ziehl-Nielsen carbolfuchsin and preserved in 10% formalin is a satisfactory method for diagnosis of cryptosporidiasis (Garcia et al. 1983).

In addition to the stains mentioned above, several other immunologic methods for diagnosis using stool samples have been employed, such as direct immunofluorescence using fluorescein-conjugated monoclonal antibodies and several modifications of indirect immunofluorescence. The auramine-rhodamine stain and indirect immunofluorescence using antibody labeled with biotin hydrazide were found to be the best methods for staining cysts in experimental conditions (Arrowood, Sterling, 1989). Serologic tests are not available commercially in the routine laboratory; they have been used mostly in seroepidemiologic surveys. Commercial kits for an enzyme immunoassay and for an immunofluorescent antibody for detection of *Cryptosporidium* oocysts and *Giardia* cysts in stool samples are now available (Graczyk et al. 1996). Finally, enzyme-linked immunoassays for *Cryptosporidium* antigens in stools have been described (Ungar, 1990).

In tissue sections, the diagnosis is made by recognizing *Cryptosporidium* in the brush border of the intestinal mucosa or on the surface of other mucosae, for example the esophagus. The parasites are small, basophilic, spherical structures 3 to 4 μm in diameter arranged in rows or clusters. The different stages of the life cycle are usually unrecognizable, though 1 to 2 μm sections of paraffin- or plastic-embedded tissues show more details. Special stains in tissue are not necessary for identification, although Ziehl-Nielsen carbolfuchsin facilitates the screening of sections. Immunoperoxidase with monoclonal antibodies is used for staining paraffin-embedded tissues and for easy detection of parasites (*color plate* V *E*; Bonnin et al. 1990; Loose et al. 1989). A polymerase chain reaction technique for detection of parasite DNA in paraffin-embedded tissues is also available (Laxer et al. 1992).

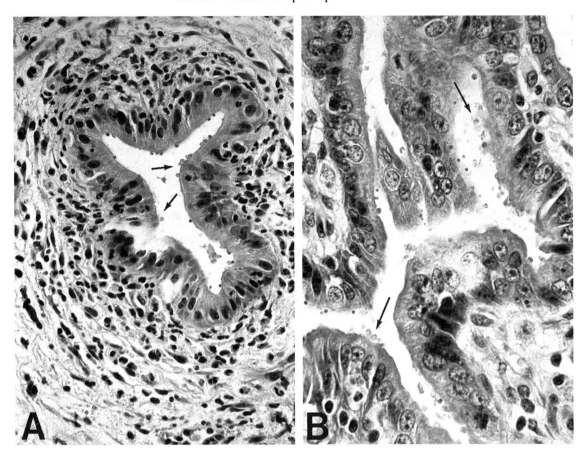

Fig. 8–9. *Cryptosporidium* in bile epithelium of a patient with AIDS. Sections stained with hematoxylin and eosin. *A*, In liver bile duct (arrows), ×298. *B*, In gallbladder (arrows), ×470. (Preparation courtesy of Douglas G. Kahn, M.D., Sherman Oaks Community Hospital, Sherman Oaks, California. Reported by: Kahn, D.C., Garfinkle, J.M., Klonoff, D.C., et al. 1987. Arch. Pathol. Lab. Med. 111:879–881.)

Isospora belli—Human Coccidiosis or Isosporiasis

The characteristic of the genus *Isospora* is that the oocysts have two sporocysts, each with four sporozoites. This genus has over 200 species, most of them in vertebrates. It is believed that only one species, *I. belli*, is parasitic in humans. Infections with *Isospora* have been known since the 1860s. Until recently, it was believed that two species, *I. belli* and *I. hominis*, were human parasites, distinguished on the basis of the morphology of the oocysts in feces. In 1972 the life cycle of *I. hominis* was described and was found to be similar to the life cycles of species of *Sarcocystis*. The parasite was then transferred to this genus (see *Sarcocystis* below) (Rommel, Heydorn, 1972).

Morphology and Life Cycle. The habitat of *I. belli* is the epithelial cells of the small intestine. After mature oocysts are ingested with food or water, the four sporozoites contained in the two sporocysts are released in the intestinal lumen and enter the epithelial cell. There they develop in the cytoplasm in a manner similar to that of other intestinal coccidia (Fig. 8–10). All stages—trophozoites, schizonts, merozoites, gametocytes, and oocysts—are found, developing as described above for *Cryptosporidium*. The differences between *Isospora* and *Cryptosporidium* are several. (*1*) *Isospora* develops in the cell cytoplasm, and because it is larger, it distends and deforms the cell. (*2*) *Isospora* is located above, below, or next to the nucleus. (*3*) The oocyst of *Isospora* is unsporulated (not infective) at the time of evacuation with feces. (*4*) *Isospora* requires a phase of development in the environment to become infective.

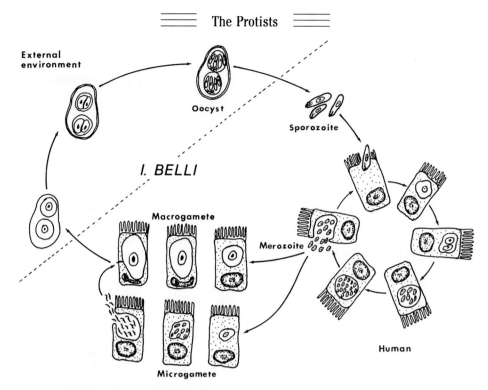

External
environment

Oocyst

Sporozoite

I. BELLI

Macrogamete

Merozoite

Microgamete

Human

Fig. 8–10. *Isospora belli,* **schematic representation of the life cycle. After ingestion of oocysts, the sporozoites penetrate the epithelial cells of the small intestine, where asexual reproduction produces merozoites. Merozoites repeat the cycle; some become male and female gametocytes, which produce gametes. Gametes join to produce the oocyst, which is evacuated with the stools and continues developing (sporulation) in the environment to become infective.**

(5) Finally, *Isospora* oocysts measure up to 33 μm, or up to seven times the size of *Cryptosporidium* (Beaver et al. 1984). At the time of evacuation with the feces, *I. belli* oocysts have a single sporoblast, the cell that develops into two sporocysts in about a week at environmental temperatures.

The stages of *Isospora* in the tissues are larger than those of *Cryptosporidium,* and the morphology of the different stages of development is easier to determine. Merozoites are sometimes single organisms in the cell cytoplasm, measuring about 2×5 μm, with a prominent nucleus. The stages from sporozoite to mature schizont and from merozoite to mature schizont are identical morphologically. Some merozoites developing into gametocytes are difficult to distinguish from developing schizonts until they are fully mature, with a prominent single nucleus. During schizogony, the organism grows to a relatively large size before it begins nuclear division, and in mature schizonts the merozoites are clearly delineated as elongated structures with single nuclei. The microgametocyte contains numerous nuclei, with each nucleus corresponding to a microgamete. Identification of one or more of these stages is neces-

sary for diagnosis. Electron microscopic studies of tissues from patients with isosporiasis have been done recently (Boldorini et al. 1996; Comin, Santucci, 1994).

Geographic Distribution and Epidemiology. Infections with *Isospora* are reported worldwide, usually as sporadic cases or as small clusters of cases in parasitologic surveys. Prevalence data are rarely collected because interest in the infection is low due to its benign nature. A review of all cases up to 1935 found over 200 cases (Magath, 1935). Another review in 1960 for the Western Hemisphere disclosed over 800 credibly reported cases, 43 of which occurred in the United States, mostly in the southern states (Faust et al. 1961). Since that time many more cases have been reported, some in outbreaks in an orphanage (12 cases; Campos et al. 1969) and in a town in Chile (90 cases; Sagua et al. 1978). In contrast to *Cryptosporidium,* which uses the fecal-oral route, *Isospora* is acquired from the environment by ingestion of dirt or food contaminated with dirt containing the oocysts. Water may play a role, but epidemics of isosporiasis due to contaminated drinking water have not been reported. *Isospora* is more common in the tropics and in poor areas where contamination of the environment with human excreta is more common than in the temperate zone.

The prevalence of *Isospora* in large numbers of stools submitted for parasitologic examination is reportedly over 3% in Chile (Jarpa et al. 1960), 0.3% in Brazil (de Oliveira et al. 1973), and 0.2% in the aboriginal population of Queensland, Australia (Prociv et al. 1992). One of the highest reported prevalence rates was in an institution for medically handicapped children in the United States (Jeffery, 1958). *Isospora* is difficult to detect in stool samples because of its delicate, translucent nature. Its detection requires subdued illumination of the microscopic field, which is not often used during regular diagnostic work (Elsdon-Dew, Freedman, 1950). For this reason, the parasite is not reported in most surveys of intestinal parasites; it requires special interest and a specific search before it is recognized.

The interest in *Isospora* today is due to its prevalence among individuals infected with HIV, in whom it causes chronic gastroenteritis (DeHovitz et al. 1986). The number of infections in the HIV/AIDS population is lower than that of *Cryptosporidium* in developing countries, and it is minuscule in developed countries, where infections are found mostly in immigrants from tropical countries. In developing countries, 3% to 19% prevalence rates have been reported (DeHovitz et al. 1986; Henry et al. 1986; Pape et al. 1989); in the United States, rates as low as 0.2% in New York City (Soave, Johnson, 1988) to 1% to 3% (Esfandiari et al. 1995; Sorvillo et al. 1995) in Los Angeles have been reported. The 3% prevalence rate in Los Angeles corresponded to ten cases equally divided between blacks and Latinos (Esfandiari et al. 1995). Because transmission does not occur through fresh feces, dissemination of the organism among the male gay population does not occur; when it occurs, it is acquired from the environment (Forthal, Guest, 1984). In contrast to *Cryptosporidium*, *I. belli* is highly host specific and is not found in the intestine of animals.

Clinical Findings. The clinical symptoms of human coccidiosis in immune-competent hosts are relatively unknown. Many infected individuals are asymptomatic; others have manifestations consisting mainly of self-limited mild diarrhea, abdominal discomfort, and low-grade fever of about 1 week's duration. This is the clinical picture found in immune-competent hosts after an accidental laboratory infection (McCracken, 1972) and in experimental infections (Matsubayashi, Nozawa, 1948).

In these cases, the oocysts were found in the stools 20 days after all symptoms disappeared.

In immune-suppressed hosts, *Isospora* is an opportunistic infection clinically indistinguishable from cryptosporidiasis. It produces a chronic illness consisting of diarrhea lasting for 1 month or more, diffuse crampy abdominal pain, nausea, and loss of at least 10% of body weight during the 2 months preceding diagnosis (DeHovitz et al. 1986; Felez et al. 1990). The number of stools is between 5 and 15 per day, and some patients become dehydrated. Signs of malabsorption are found in some patients if investigated. Steatorrhea, similar to that of tropical sprue, enterocolitis, and nonspecific jejunitis, with weight loss of 36 kg has been reported (Brandborg et al. 1970; French et al. 1964). Most patients have peripheral eosinophilia, sometimes up to 25% (one of the rare instances in which a protozoon produces eosinophilia). In some patients the illness lasts for up to 20 years, with an intermittent character (Ravenel et al. 1976; Trier et al. 1974). A case of acalculous cholecystitis in a patient with AIDS was attributed to *Isospora* because the parasites were seen in the gallbladder epithelium (Benator et al. 1994). In individuals with AIDS coinfected with *Isospora*, specific treatment results in rapid disappearance of symptoms, but they often recur after cessation of therapy (DeHovitz et al. 1986). Isosporiasis has also been identified as a chronic infection in individuals with the human T-cell leukemia virus type I (Greenberg et al. 1988).

Immunity and Pathogenesis. No information on either the immunology or the mechanism of pathogenicity of isosporiasis in animals or humans is available.

Pathology. The histologic changes produced by *I. belli* are described in biopsy specimens from patients with clinical disease (Brandborg et al. 1970; Liebman et al. 1980; Trier et al. 1974). The small intestinal mucosa (duodenum and upper jejunum) has villi with "clubbed" tips progressing to flattening or complete atrophy in severe cases (Fig. 8–11 *A–D*). The epithelial cells appear normal; some have intracytoplasmic stages of the parasite (Fig. 8–11 *D*). Minimal to moderate infiltration by lymphocytes and polymorphonuclear leukocytes is observed in the lamina propria and around the capillaries (Fig. 8–11 *A–B*). Eosinophils are increased in the lamina propria, sometimes occurring in large numbers, as in eosinophilic enteritis. Submucosal edema, abundant inflammation with tissue

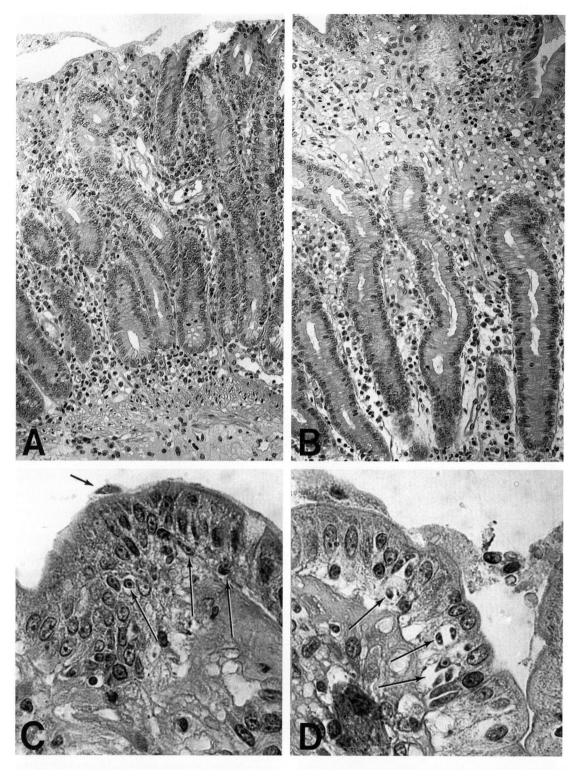

Fig. 8–11. *Isospora belli* in small intestine in a patient with AIDS, sections stained with hematoxylin and eosin stain. *A* and *B*, Medium-power view showing flattening of the villi and a mononuclear cell infiltrate, ×180. *C*, Higher magnification showing a parasite on top of the brush border, ready to enter the epithelial cell (short arrow) and other early stages within the cells (long arrows), ×700. *D*, Another area showing other parasites within the cells (arrows), ×700. (Preparation courtesy of A. Galian, M.D., Department of Pathology, Hospital Larivoisiere, Paris, France. Reported by: Modigliani, R., Bories, C., LeCharpentier, Y., et al. 1985. Diarrhea and malabsorption in acquired immune deficiency syndrome: a study of four cases with special emphasis on opportunistic protozoan infestations. Gut 26:179–187.)

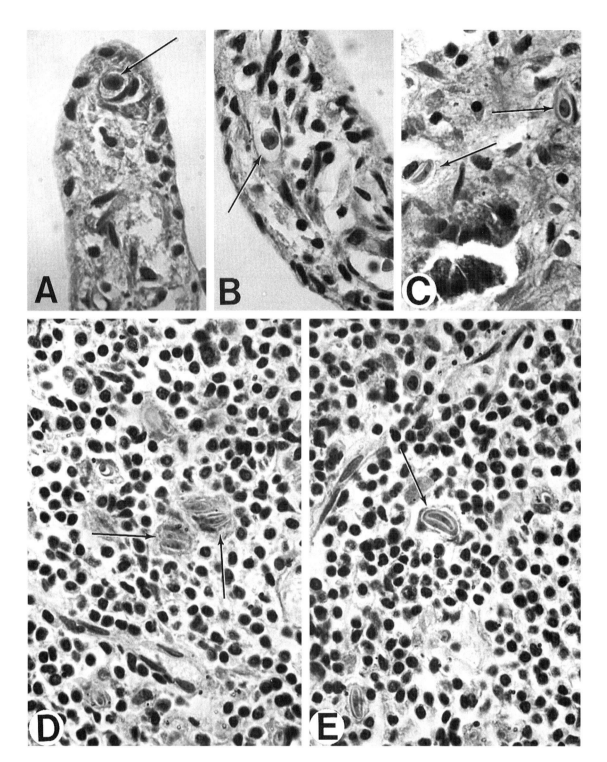

Fig. 8–12. *Isospora belli* disseminated infection in a patient with AIDS, sections stained with hematoxylin and eosin stain. *A–C*. Small intestine. *A*, Villus showing marked lysis and a poorly preserved stage of *I. belli* (arrow), ×700. *B*, Another stage (arrow), ×700. *C*, Tissue stages within the submucosa of the small intestine (arrows), ×700. *D* and *E*, Lymph node with tissue stages (arrows), ×700. (Preparation for *A–D* courtesy of M.J. Merino, M.D., Laboratory of Pathology, National Institutes of Health, Bethesda, Maryland. *D* and *E* courtesy of C. Restrepo, M.D., Department of Pathology, Louisiana State University, School of Medicine, New Orleans, Louisiana. Reported by: Restrepo, C., Macher, A.M., and Radany, E.H. 1987. Disseminated extraintestinal isosporiasis in a patient with acquired immune deficiency syndrome. Am. J. Clin. Pathol. 87:536–542.)

eosinophilia, and flattening of villi are present in some patients with a histologic picture of eosinophilic enteritis (Brandborg et al. 1970). The gallbladder may also be parasitized (Benator et al. 1994).

The striking and common histologic feature of all cases of *Isospora* is the presence of parasites in the cytoplasm of epithelial cells in variable numbers and different stages of development. Parasites vary from small bodies 3 to 4 μm (Fig. 8–11 *C–D*) to 15 to 20 μm in diameter (Fig. 8–12 *A–B*), often bearing down on the nucleus of the epithelial cell (Fig. 8–12 *A*) and sometimes growing below or next to the cell nucleus. Mature schizonts and oocysts distend and deform the cell considerably, a feature that helps to distinguish *Isospora* from *Cyclospora* and the intestinal microsporidia (see Chapter 1).

In autopsy material from individuals dying of AIDS and coinfection with *Isospora*, tissue stages of the parasite have been found in mesenteric lymph nodes and in the interstitium of the small and large intestines (Fig. 8–12 *A–D*). These stages are located within the histiocytes and appear as elongated 10 to 30 μm $\times$ 5 to 8 μm organisms. They are surrounded by a thick wall and occur either singly (Fig. 8–12 *E*) or in pairs (Fig. 8–12 *D*). These stages are *cysts* with a wall consisting of an amorphous material that does not stain with hematoxylin and eosin stain or with periodic acid–Schiff hematoxylin stain. Inside the cyst is a single zoite with one nucleus that stains basophilically (Michiels et al. 1994; Restrepo et al. 1987). The ultrastructure of the cysts of *I. belli* from a patient (Michiels et al. 1994) was described recently (Lindsay et al. 1996; Lindsay et al. 1997). These cysts are similar to those found in *I. rivolta* and *I. felis* of cats (Frenkel, Dubey, 1972; Fig. 8–12 *C–E*) and *I. canis* of dogs (Markus, 1983). They are responsible for transmission of the parasite through carnivorism. The question is whether *I. belli* uses the same form of transmission or if the infection in these patients was with an *Isospora* of animals.

Diagnosis. *Isospora belli* infection is diagnosed by examination of stool samples or duodenal aspirates (Elsdon-Dew et al. 1953; Elsdon-Dew, Freedman, 1950; Orrego et al. 1959). The presence of typical unsporulated oocysts (*color plate* V *I*) in preparations of stool samples, either directly or by concentration, is sufficient for diagnosis. The oocysts measure 20 to 33 μm $\times$ 10 to 9 μm and at the time of evacuation contain a single sporoblast, seen as a rounded granular mass, at the center. Oocysts in stool samples stain with acid-fast stain, allowing easy identification. The sporoblast

stains deep red, and the wall is outlined by precipitated stain around it (DeHovitz et al. 1986; Ng et al. 1984). The presence of Charcot-Leyden crystals in the stools is a common finding in these patients.

In biopsy specimens of small intestine or in autopsy material, the alterations in the villi may be present or absent, but the different stages of the life cycle should be recognized in the epithelial cells for proper diagnosis. The cysts in the interstitium of the small intestine have not been reported in biopsy specimens but only in autopsy material (Fig. 8–12 *D*). Special stains are not necessarily helpful in the identification of *Isospora*. To reemphasize, the following organisms should be considered in the differential diagnosis of *Isospora*: *Cryptosporidium* (in the brush border), *Cyclospora* (in the cytoplasm of the enterocytes, probably in a parasitophorous vacuole; it is smaller than *Isospora*—see below), *Sarcocystis* (only oocysts in the lamina propria; see below), *Enterocytozoon* and *Encephalitozoon* (less than 2 μm in the enterocyte cytoplasm; see Chapter 2). One should also keep in mind *Toxoplasma* (in any type of cell in mucosa and submucosa; see Chapter 9) and *Leishmania* (in macrophages in the submucosa; see Chapter 4).

Cyclospora cayetanensis— Cyclosporiasis

Cyclospora was recognized as a human parasite during the 1980s. Apparently, the parasite was first mentioned in 1979 in three patients seen in Papua, New Guinea, with "an undescribed coccidian" in their stools (Ashford, 1979). The second report appeared in 1986 (Soave et al. 1986) and described large, coccidia-like bodies found in the stools of four persons who had traveled to Haiti and Mexico. These individuals were immune competent, with complaints of explosive diarrhea, nausea, vomiting, anorexia, and weight loss (Soave et al. 1986). In 1990 two reports, one dealing with similar cases reported to the Centers for Disease Control, suggested that the organism in question was an alga (Long et al. 1990). The other report, concerning an HIV-positive patient seen in Chicago, stated that the parasite was different from the known organisms infecting humans (Hart et al. 1990). At various times, the unknown organism was called an *unsporulated coccidian*, an *alga-like* (Shlim et al. 1991), *cyanobacterium-like body* (Kaminsky, 1991; Long et al. 1991), a *coccidian-like body* (Hoge et al. 1993), *atypical Cryptosporidium* (Baxby, Blundell, 1988), and *Cryptosporidium muris-*

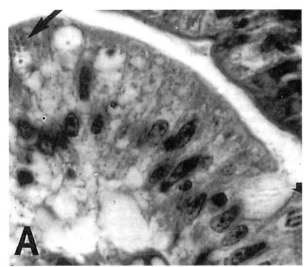
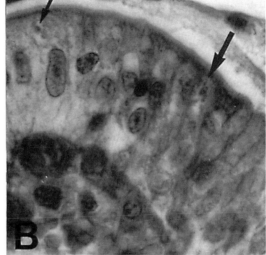

Fig. 8–13. *Cyclospora* in a duodenal biopsy specimen from a patient with AIDS, section stained with hematoxylin and eosin stain. *A*, A probable maturing schizont (thick arrow) and a probable immature one (thin arrow) are seen in the area between the nucleus and the brush border, ×420. *B*, A maturing schizont (long arrow) and a mature one showing merozoites (short arrow), ×420. Note that the parasites appear to be located in parasitophorous vacuoles. (In Nhieu, J.T.V., Nin, F., Fleury-Feith, J., et al. 1996. Identification of intracellular stages of *Cyclospora* species by light microscopy of thick sections using hematoxylin. Hum. Pathol. 27:1107–1109. Reproduced with permission.)

like (Narango et al. 1989). The parasite was referred to as *Cyclospora cayetanensis* for the first time in an abstract to the meeting of the American Society of Tropical Medicine and Hygiene in 1992 (Ortega et al. 1992). The reasons for classifying the organism as a *Cyclospora* were given in 1993 (Ortega et al. 1993) and were fully described in 1994 (Ortega et al. 1994).

The genus *Cyclospora* has about ten known species characterized by having oocysts with two sporocysts, each giving rise to two sporozoites. The entire life cycle of *Cyclospora* is not known, but what is known of its development in the enterocytes appears similar to that of *Cryptosporidium* and *Isospora* (Fig. 8–13 A–B). The oocysts of *C. cayetanensis* are immature at the time of evacuation with the feces (Fig. 8–14), and complete sporulation takes place in about 5 days at 25°C to 32°C under laboratory conditions (Ortega et al. 1992). Ingestion of mature oocysts about 8 to 10 μm in size produces the infection in the duodenum (and possibly, in other parts of the small intestine not known at present). *Cyclospora* is located in the cytoplasm of enterocytes, usually above the nucleus and within parasitophorous vacuoles (Fig. 8–13 A–B; Bendall et al. 1993; Deluol et al. 1996; Nhieu et al. 1996; Sun et al. 1996). Only its asexual development is known from the study of biopsy specimens. The merozoites measure 1 to 2 × 6 μm and the trophozoites measure 2 × 4 μm; the schizonts were said to have 10 to 16 merozoites in one study (Sun et

al. 1996) and 6 to 8 in another (Deluol et al. 1996). The typical structures of an apicomplexan organism were present in the merozoites. The presence and development of the sexual stages have not been described.

Cyclospora has become an important pathogen easily transmitted through food and water; it is found in every place where it is investigated. In the United

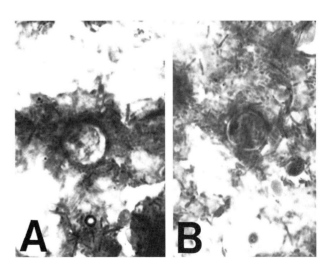

Fig. 8–14. *Cyclospora* oocysts in stools of a patient with AIDS. *A* and *B*, Preparation stained with modified acid-fast stain, ×1,340.

States, the infections seen until 1996 were in international travelers (CDC, 1997c), but since then, many outbreaks in different parts of the country have been studied (CDC, 1996, 1997a, 1997b, 1997d), including two due to pseudoinfections (laboratory error because of unfamiliarity with the parasite; CDC, 1997c). Outbreaks among foreigners living in developing countries have also been reported (Shlim et al. 1991; Taylor et al. 1988). In HIV-positive patients in Haiti presenting with diarrhea the prevalence of *Cyclospora* was 11%, similar to that of *Isospora* but only one-third of the rate of *Cryptosporidium* infection (Pape et al. 1994).

Cyclospora produces diarrhea in both immunocompetent and immune-compromised individuals. The incubation period of the disease is 1 to 7 days after exposure to contaminated water (Chiodini, 1994). The clinical presentation consists of abrupt onset of watery diarrhea in 68% of the cases and gradual onset in the rest (Shlim et al. 1991), with anorexia, fatigue, and abdominal cramps similar to those in patients with *Cryptosporidium* and *Isospora* infections. Other symptoms such as muscle pain and nausea may also occur, but vomiting is uncommon; flatulence and bloating have also been reported. The diarrhea is prolonged, with remissions and relapses lasting for several weeks. The median duration of the illness in immune-competent hosts has been estimated to be 7 weeks (Hoge et al. 1993), and in HIV-positive individuals the duration of diarrhea has varied from days to months (Wurtz, 1994). Some patients can be asymptomatic while excreting cysts (Pollock et al. 1992). Laboratory tests are not helpful except for the stool examination, which reveals the typical oocysts. Jejunal aspirates reveal the oocysts in wet preparations (Pollock et al. 1992). Absorption tests for xylose are abnormal (Shlim et al. 1991). As stated above, cyclosporiasis is an important cause of traveler's diarrhea (Bendall et al. 1993; Deluol et al. 1994; Hoge et al. 1993).

Histologically, the jejunum in cyclosporiasis shows villous blunting and fusion, with a mononuclear cell infiltrate of the lamina propria; the mitotic index is increased (Connor et al. 1993; Pollock et al. 1992). At this time, tissue diagnosis is difficult because not enough information is available. Cyclosporiasis should be part of the differential diagnosis of other parasites in enterocytes (see *Isospora* above), and confirmation with electron microscopic studies seems desirable.

The diagnosis of cyclosporiasis is made in the clinical laboratory based on stool samples, using concentration methods such as the standard formalin-ethyl acetate sedimentation, flotation methods such as zinc sulfate, and sugar flotation methods similar to those used for *Cryptosporidium*. Stained smears with acid-fast stain, as recommended for all coccidial oocysts, give variable results that are sometimes difficult to interpret if small numbers of organisms are present. Fluorescence microscopy is helpful because the oocysts of *Cyclospora* autofluoresce (Berlin et al. 1998; Eberhard et al. 1997). A polymerase chain reaction of high specificity but low sensitivity has also been used (Pieniazek et al. 1996).

Sarcocystis hominis and *S. suihominis*— Intestinal Sarcocystosis

Sarcocystis and *Toxoplasma* are two genera of coccidia that belong to the family Sarcocystidae and are characterized by two hosts in their life cycle. The genus *Sarcocystis* was created to include organisms found in the skeletal muscles of animals that form large cysts (sarcocysts) containing many zoites. Some sporadic cases of parasitism in humans with *Sarcocystis* (sarcosporidiosis) in the muscle were described under the name *S. lindenmani*. Little was known about the nature and life cycle of *Sarcocystis* until the 1960s, when it was established that the sarcocysts in muscles were one stage of the life cycle of some species of intestinal coccidia. In the 1970s it was recognized that *I. hominis* of humans belongs to the genus *Sarcocystis*, with two species in humans: *S. hominis* (Heydorn et al. 1975) and *S. suihominis* (Heydorn, 1977). Here we will study the species of *Sarcocystis* found in the small intestine of humans; in the next chapter we will consider the *Sarcocystis* in muscles.

Life Cycle. The life cycle of *Sarcocystis* requires two hosts: the definitive final host (carnivore), in which sexual reproduction takes place in the intestinal wall, and the intermediate host (prey), in which asexual reproduction occurs in the tissues, resulting in the formation of infective sarcocysts in the muscles (Fig. 8–15).

In humans, infection with *Sarcocystis* occurs by ingestion of uncooked pork with infective stages of *S. suihominis* and uncooked beef with *S. hominis*. The ingested sarcocysts contain thousands of sporozoites, which are freed in the small intestine to enter the mucosa and parasitize *nonepithelial* cells located in the lamina propria; the nature of the cells is not known. The zoites develop directly into macro- and microgametocytes (no other stages are formed), and they join to produce a cygote that matures within the intestinal

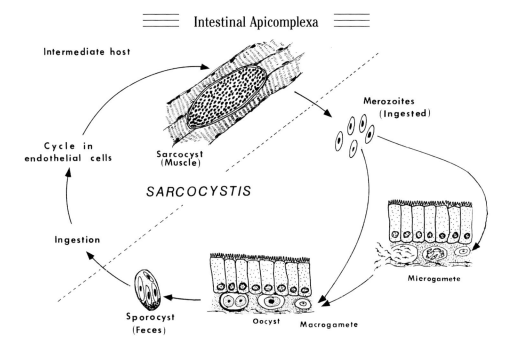

Fig. 8–15. *Sarcocystis*, **schematic representation of the life cycle. Two hosts are required for the development of *Sarcocystis*; the definitive host is infected by ingestion of sarcocysts containing merozoites in muscles of animals. The merozoites are released in the intestine, and within cells located in the lamina propria of the small intestine, they develop directly into male and female gametocytes. The gametocytes join and produce the oocysts (sporogony), which become infective within the tissues and is excreted by sporocysts with the feces. After sporocysts are ingested, the oocyst develop in the intermediate host, first in the endothelial cells and finally in the skeletal muscles or heart, where they form sarcocysts.**

wall into an oocyst. The oocyst has two sporoblasts, each of which develops four sporozoites. The oocysts release the two sporulated (infective) sporocysts, which are excreted with the feces (*color plate* V *H*).

The intermediate host ingests the fully mature sporocysts passed with the feces of the definitive host, and in the intestinal tract the sporozoites are released. The sporozoites enter the blood vessels of the intestinal mucosa and are distributed via the bloodstream throughout the body, entering the endothelial cells of medium-sized and small blood vessels of many organs. In the endothelial cells asexual reproduction of the parasite occurs. Two or three cycles usually take place, considerably increasing the number of parasites. The zoites produced in the last of these cycles enter the striated muscles of the heart, the skeletal muscles, or both and develop to sarcocysts containing thousands of zoites (Figs. 8–15 and 9–1 to 9–3; Beaver et al. 1984). In the endothelial cells of some animals, *Sarcocystis* produces a significant arteritis that is sometimes fatal.

Morphology. Four stages of the parasite theoretically occur in humans with intestinal sarcocytosis: male and female gametocytes and sporocysts in tissues and stools. The gametocytes stained with hematoxylin and eosin stain are about 10 μm in size, with a red cytoplasm and a nucleus at the center. The sporocysts in tissues are about 10 to 15 μm in diameter and show two to four sporozoites, depending on the plane of sectioning. In stools, the sporocysts of *S. hominis* are 15 $\times$ 9 μm and those of *S. suihominis* are 13 $\times$ 10 μm. In unstained preparations the sporocysts are delicate and translucent; with subdued illumination of the microscope, the four sporozoites and the residual body can be seen. The electron microscopic appearance of the tissue stages has been described only in culture cells (Mehlhorn, Heydorn, 1979).

Distribution. Human intestinal *Sarcocystis* has a worldwide distribution in the intermediate hosts (pigs and cattle) and in humans; infections are probably more

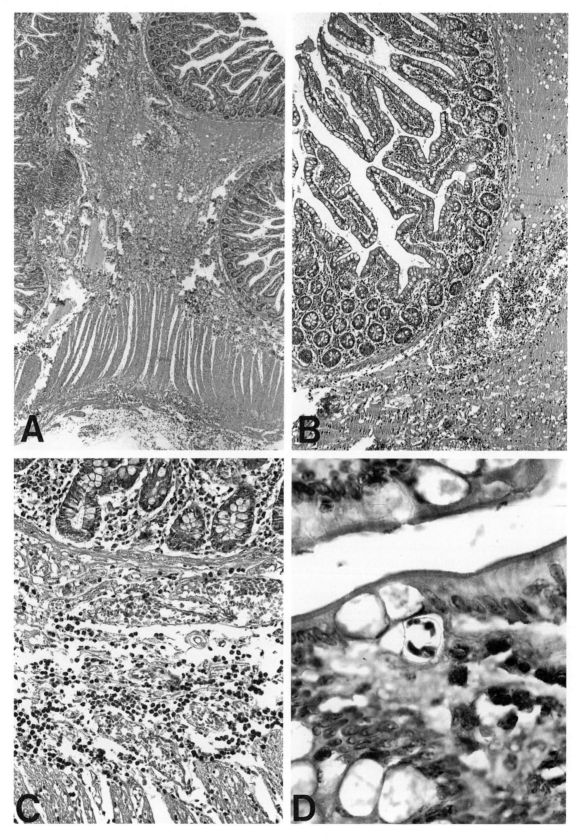

Fig. 8–16.

common than is generally recognized. However, since, as stated above, *S. hominis* and *S. suihominis* were known as *I. hominis* until the 1970s, reports on the distribution and prevalence of these two species are accurate. Surveys in cattle to determine the prevalence of sarcocysts in muscles (the infective stages to humans) in southern Germany have shown that almost 100% of the slaughtered cattle are positive (Boch et al. 1978).

Clinical Findings.

Sarcocystis hominis. Reports before 1972 of clinical symptoms produced by *Sarcocystis* (called *I. hominis*) in humans are uninterpretable because two different species were grouped under *I. hominis*. Experimental infection of two volunteers (Rommel, Heydorn, 1972) and later of five volunteers (Aryeetey, Piekarski, 1976) produced asymptomatic infections.

In Thailand a series of six patients presented with acute symptoms consisting of fever, acute abdominal pain, vomiting, diarrhea, leukocytosis, and mild to moderate distention of the small intestine on x-ray films. All six individuals required surgical resection of a portion of the jejunum or ileum due to marked inflammation (Bunyaratvej et al. 1982). Since the time of the original report, other cases have been diagnosed; the total number of patients is now 22 (Bunyaratvej et al. 1992; Bunyaratvej, Unpunyo, 1992). In all surgical specimens, a *Sarcocystis* organism was found microscopically, considered *S. hominis* on epidemiologic grounds (Bunyaratvej et al. 1982, 1992; Bunyaratvej, Unpunyo, 1992).

Sarcocystis suihominis. In experimental infections of human volunteers with *S. suihominis*, only mild symptoms occurred, consisting of acute diarrhea, vomiting, chills, slight fever, and perspiration 6 to 24 hours after ingestion of the infective stages in pork (Rommel, Heydorn, 1972). The sporocysts were found in the feces for at least 40 days; the prepatent period was 10 days in one case. In 55 natural infections diagnosed by finding the sporocysts in stools, the symptoms were similar to those in the volunteers,

but in addition, anemia and eosinophilia occurred (Wentai et al. 1986).

Pathology. Histologic studies of the small intestinal mucosa of individuals with *Sarcocystis* infections and few or no symptoms are lacking. The report of Bunyaratvej et al. (1982) presents a complete description of their cases of segmental eosinophilic enteritis or segmental necrotizing enteritis. The segment of resected ileum measured 2 to 20 cm in length; one patient had a right hemicolectomy. The ileum was thickened and edematous, with discoloration ranging from grayish-white to dark brown; in extreme cases, its appearance was gangrenous. On section, there was infiltration and edema of all layers of the viscus.

Six pieces of bowel were resected; histologically, all of them showed eosinophilic ileitis with necrotizing features (Fig. 8–16 *A–B*). In some cases the mucosa appeared normal, with intact villi; in others, ulcerations were found. An abundant polymorphonuclear cell infiltrate with many eosinophils, a few mononuclear cells, and edema occurred in all layers (Fig. 8–16 *C*), more extensive in some areas than in others. The parasites, which were sometimes difficult to find, were developmental gametes and sporulating or mature oocysts in the lamina propria (Fig. 8–16 *D*) with no inflammatory infiltrate or cell damage around them. The type of cell in which the parasites were located was not discernible with light microscopy.

Diagnosis. *Sarcocystis* is usually identified in the clinical laboratory by finding the typical sporocysts, with four sporozoites (*color plate V H*), in wet or stain smears made directly from stools or from concentrated stools. The sporocysts are infective at the time of evacuation and are usually seen singly, though sometimes in pairs, surrounded by the thin oocyst wall.

In tissues, sarcocystosis is diagnosed by finding the typical forms of gamogony, i.e., male and female gametocytes, and mature sporocysts located below the epithelial cells in the lamina propria. In all cases of seg-

Fig. 8–16. *Sarcocystis* infection of the small intestine, segmental necrotizing enteritis, hematoxylin and eosin stain. *A*, Low-power view of a section of small intestine showing necrosis and inflammatory infiltration of the submucosa. Peritonitis is seen at the bottom, ×28. *B* and *C*, Higher magnification showing detail of the necrosis and inflammatory reaction composed of mononuclear and polymorphonuclear cells; eosinophils are present in large numbers (*B* ×70, *C* ×180). *D*, Higher magnification showing the parasite (sporocyst) under the epithelial cell within the lamina propria, ×800. (Preparation courtesy of S. Bunyaratvej, M.D., Department of Pathology, Ramathibody Hospital, Bangkok, Thailand. Reported by: Bunyaratvej, S., Bunyawongwiroj, P., and Nitiyanant, P. 1982. Human intestinal sarcosporidiosis: report of six cases. Am. J. Trop. Med. Hyg. 31:3641.)

mental eosinophilic ileitis, with or without necrosis and with no known cause, a search for *Sarcocystis* in the intestinal tissues and stools should be undertaken.

References

Addiss DG, Stewart JM, Finton RJ, Wahlquist SP, Williams RM, Dickerson JW, Spencer HC, Juranek DD, 1991. *Giardia lamblia* and *Cryptosporidium* infections in child day-care centers in Fulton County, Georgia. Pediatr. Infect. Dis. J. 10:907–911

Anderson BC, Donndelinger T, Wilkins RM, Smith J, 1982. Cryptosporidiosis in a veterinary student. JAVMA 180:408–409

Arrowood MJ, Sterling CR, 1989. Comparison of conventional staining methods and monoclonal antibody-based methods for *Cryptosporidium* oocyst detection. J. Clin. Microbiol. 27:1490–1495

Aryeetey ME, Piekarski G, 1976. Serologicsche *Sarcocystis*-Studien an Menschen und Ratten. Z. Parasitenk. 50:109–124

Ashford RW, 1979. Occurrence of an undescribed coccidian in man in Papua New Guinea. Ann. Trop. Med. Parasitol. 73:497–500

Assadamongkol K, Gracey M, Forbes D, Varavithya W, 1992. *Cryptosporidium* in 100 Australian children. Southeast Asian J. Trop. Med. Public Health 23:132–137

Baxby D, Blundell N, 1988. Recognition and laboratory characteristics of an atypical oocyst of *Cryptosporidium*. J. Infect. Dis. 158:1038–1045

Beaver PC, Jung RC, Cupp EW, 1984. *Clinical Parasitology*. Philadelphia: Lea & Febiger

Benator DA, French AL, Beaudet LM, Levy CS, Orenstein JM, 1994. *Isospora belli* infection associated with acalculous cholecystitis in a patient with AIDS. Ann. Intern. Med. 121:663–664

Bendall RP, Lucas S, Moody A, Tovey G, Chiodini PL, 1993. Diarrhoea associated with cyanobacterium-like bodies: a new coccidian enteritis of man. Lancet 341:590–592

Benhamou Y, Caumes E, Gerosa Y, Cadranel JF, Dohin E, Katlama C, Amouyal P, Canard JM, Azar N, Hoang C, et al, 1993. AIDS-related cholangiopathy. Critical analysis of a prospective series of 26 patients. Dig. Dis. Sci. 38:1113–1118

Berlin OG, Peter JB, Gagne C, Conteas CN, Ash LR, 1998. Autofluorescence and the detection of *Cyclospora* oocysts. Emerg. Infect. Dis. 4:127–128

Bird RG, Smith MD, 1980. Cryptosporidiosis in man: parasite life cycle and fine structural pathology. J. Pathol. 132:217–233

Blumberg RS, Kelsey P, Perrone T, Dickersin R, Laquaglia M, Ferruci J, 1984. Cytomegalovirus- and *Cryptosporidium*-associated acalculous gangrenous cholecystitis. Am. J. Med. 76:1118–1123

Boch VJ, Laupheimer KE, Erber M, 1978. Drei Sarkospori-

dienarten bei schlachtrindern in Suddeutschland. Berl. Munch. Tierarztl. Wschr. 91:426–431

Boldorini R, Tosoni A, Mazzucco G, Cernuschi M, Caramello P, Maran E, Costanzi G, Monga G, 1996. Intracellular protozoan infection in small intestinal biopsies of patients with AIDS. Light and electron microscopic evaluation. Pathol. Res. Pract. 192:249–259

Bonnin A, Petrella T, Dubremetz JF, Michiels JF, Puygauthier Toubas D, Camerlynck P, 1990. Histopathological method for diagnosis of cryptosporidiosis using monoclonal antibodies. Eur. J. Clin. Microbiol. Infect. Dis. 9:664–666

Brandborg LL, Goldberg SB, Breidenbach WC, 1970. Human coccidiosis—a possible cause of malabsorption. The life cycle in small-bowel mucosal biopsies as a diagnostic feature. N. Engl. J. Med. 283:1306–1313

Brea Hernando AJ, Bandres Franco E, Mosquera Lozano JD, Lantero Benedito M, Ezquerra Lezcano M, 1993a. Criptosporidiasis pulmonar y SIDA. Presentacion de un caso y revision de la literatura. Ann. Med. Interne 10:232–236

Brea Hernando AJ, Sacristan Terroba B, Bandres Franco E, Mosquera Lozano JD, Garcia Moreno V, Yanguela Terroba J, 1993b. Colangitis esclerosante en un paciente con sindrome de inmunodeficiencia adquirida. Rev. Esp. Enferm. Dig. 83:205–208

Bunyaratvej S, Bunyawongwiroj P, Nitiyanant P, 1982. Human intestinal sarcosporidiosis: report of six cases. Am. J. Trop. Med. Hyg. 31:36–41

Bunyaratvej S, Unpunyo P, 1992. Combined *Sarcocystis* and gram-positive bacterial infections. A possible cause of segmental enterocolitis in Thailand. J. Med. Assoc. Thailand 75 Suppl 1:38–44

Bunyaratvej S, Visalsawadi P, Likitarunrat S, 1992. *Sarcocystis* infection and actinomycosis in tumorous eosinophilic enterocolitis. J. Med. Assoc. Thailand 75 Suppl 1:71–75

Campos R, Amato Neto V, Lacerda Campos L, 1969. Brote de isosporosis en ninos de un orfelinato. Bol. Chil. Parasitol. 24:127–129

Cappell MS, Hassan T, 1993. Pancreatic disease in AIDS—a review. J. Clin. Gastroenterol. 17:254–263

Casemore DP, Gardner CA, O'Mahony C, 1994. Cryptosporidial infection, with special reference to nosocomial transmission of *Cryptosporidium parvum*: a review. Folia Parasitol. 41:17–21

CDC, 1984. Cryptosporidiosis among children attending day-care centers—Georgia, Pennsylvania, Michigan, California, New Mexico. Morb. Mort. Weekly Rep. 33:599–601

CDC, 1996. Update: outbreaks of *Cyclospora cayetanensis* infection—United States and Canada, 1996. Morb. Mort. Weekly Rep. 45:611–612

CDC, 1997a. Outbreak of cyclosporiasis—Northern Virginia—Washington, D.C.—Baltimore, Maryland, metropolitan area, 1997. Morb. Mort. Weekly Rep. 46:689–691

CDC, 1997b. Outbreaks of cyclosporiasis—United States, 1997. Morb. Mort. Weekly Rep. 46:451–452

CDC, 1997c. Outbreaks of pseudo-infection with *Cyclospora* and *Cryptosporidium*—Florida and New York City, 1995. Morb. Mort. Weekly Rep. 46:354–358

CDC, 1997d. Update: outbreaks of cyclosporiasis—1997. Morb. Mort. Weekly Rep. 46:521–523

Cersosimo E, Wilkowske CJ, Rosenblatt JE, Ludwig J, 1992. Isolated antral narrowing associated with gastrointestinal cryptosporidiosis in acquired immunodeficiency syndrome. Mayo Clin. Proc. 67:553–556

Chacin-Bonilla L, Bonilla MC, Soto-Torres L, Rios-Candida Y, Sardina M, Enmanuels C, Parra AM, Sanchez-Chavez Y, 1997. *Cryptosporidium parvum* in children with diarrhea in Zulia State, Venezuela. Am. J. Trop. Med. Hyg. 56:365–369

Chacin Bonilla L, Mejia De Young M, Cano G, Guanipa N, Estevez J, Bonilla E, 1993. *Cryptosporidium* infections in a suburban community in Maracaibo, Venezuela. Am. J. Trop. Med. Hyg. 49:63–67

Chan AW, MacFarlane IA, Rhodes JM, 1989. Correspondence. Cryptosporidiosis as a cause of chronic diarrhoea in a patient with insulin-dependent diabetes mellitus. J. Infect. 19:293

Chiampi NP, Sundberg RD, Klompus JP, Wilson AJ, 1983. Cryptosporidial enteritis and *Pneumocystis* pneumonia in a homosexual man. Hum. Pathol. 14:734–737

Chiodini PL, 1994. A "new" parasite: human infection with *Cyclospora cayetanensis*. Trans. R. Soc. Trop. Med. Hyg. 88:369–371

Clark DP, Sears CL, 1996. The pathogenesis of cryptosporidiosis. Parasitol. Today 12:221–225

Clayton F, Heller T, Kotler DP, 1994. Variation in the enteric distribution of Cryptosporidia in acquired immunodeficiency syndrome. Am. J. Clin. Pathol. 102:420–425

Clinicopathological conference, 1980. Immunodeficiency and cryptosporidiosis. Br. Med. J. 281:1123–1127

Comin CE, Santucci M, 1994. Submicroscopic profile of *Isospora belli* enteritis in a patient with acquired immune deficiency syndrome. Ultrastruct. Pathol. 18:473–482

Connor BA, Shlim DR, Scholes JV, Rayburn JL, Reidy J, Rajah R, 1993. Pathologic changes in the small bowel in nine patients with diarrhea associated with a coccidia-like body. Ann. Intern. Med. 119:377–382

Corliss JO, 1994. An interim utilitarian ("user-friendly") hierarchical classification and characterization of the protists. Acta Protozool. 33:1–51

Cozon G, Biron F, Jeannin M, Cannella D, Revillard JP, 1994. Secretory IgA antibodies to *Cryptosporidium parvum* in AIDS patients with chronic cryptosporidiosis. J. Infect. Dis. 169:696–699

Current WL, Garcia LS, 1991. Cryptosporidiosis. Clin. Lab. Med. 11:873–897

Current WL, Reese NC, Ernst JV, Bailey WS, Heyman MB, Weinstein WM, 1983. Human cryptosporidiosis in immunocompetent and immunodeficient persons. Studies of an outbreak and experimental transmission. N. Engl. J. Med. 308:1252–1257

da Costa-Ribeiro H Jr, Teichberg S, Sun T, Fagundes Neto U, Lifshitz F, 1989. Ultrastructure of human cryptosporidial infection: a review. Prog. Clin. Parasitol. 1:143–158

Davis JJ, Heyman MB, Ferrell L, Kerner J, Kerlan R Jr, Thaler MM, 1987. Sclerosing cholangitis associated with chronic cryptosporidiosis in a child with a congenital immunodeficiency disorder. Am. J. Gastroenterol. 82: 1196–1202

de Oliveira GS, Barbosa W, da Silva AL, 1973. Isosporose humana em Goias I. Dados epidemiologicos, clinicos e imunologicos. Rev. Pat. Trop. 2:387–395

DeHovitz JA, Pape JW, Boncy M, Johnson WDJ, 1986. Clinical manifestations and therapy of *Isospora belli* infection in patients with the acquired immunodeficiency syndrome. N. Engl. J. Med. 315:87–90

Deluol AM, Junod C, Poirot JL, Heyer F, N'Go N, Cosnes J, 1994. Travellers diarrhea associated with *Cyclospora* sp. J. Euk. Microbiol. 41:32S

Deluol AM, Theillac MG, Poirot JL, Heyer F, Beaugerie L, Chatelet FP, 1996. *Cyclospora* sp.: life cycle by electron microscopy examination in HIV infected patients. Joint meeting of the American Society of Parasitology and Society of Protozoology, Tucson, Arizona, Nov. 11–15, 1996, p. 180

Ditrich O, Palkovic L, Sterba J, Prokopic J, Loudova J, Giboda M, 1991. The first finding of *Cryptosporidium baileyi* in man. Parasitol. Res. 77:44–47

Dolmatch BL, Laing FC, Ferderle MP, Jeffrey RB, Cello J, 1987. AIDS-related cholangitis: radiographic findings in nine patients. Radiology 163:313–316

Eberhard ML, Pieniazek NJ, Arrowood MJ, 1997. Laboratory diagnosis of *Cyclospora* infections. Arch. Pathol. Lab. Med. 121:792–797

el On J, Dagan R, Fraser D, Deckelbaum RJ, 1994. Detection of *Cryptosporidium* and *Giardia intestinalis* in Bedouin children from southern Israel. Intern. J. Parasitol. 24:409–411

Elsdon-Dew R, Freedman L, 1950. Coccidiosis in Natal. Infections with *Isospora hominis* (Rivolta). S. Afr. J. Clin. Sci. 1:185–195

Elson-Dew R, Roach GG, Freedman L, 1953. Correspondence. *Isospora belli* (Wenyon) from duodenal intubation. Lancet 1:348

Enriquez FJ, Avila CR, Santos JI, Tanaka-Kido J, Vallejo O, Sterling CR, 1997. Cryptosporidium infections in Mexican children: clinical, nutritional, enteropathogenic, and diagnostic evaluations. Am. J. Trop. Med. Hyg. 56: 254–257

Esfandiari A, Jordan WC, Brown CP, 1995. Prevalence of enteric parasitic infection among HIV-infected attendees of an inner city AIDS clinic. Cell Mol. Biol. 41 Suppl 1:S19–S23

Esteban JG, Aguirre C, Flores A, Strauss W, Angles R, Mas-Coma S, 1998. High *Cryptosporidium* prevalences in healthy Aymara children from the northern Bolivian Altiplano. Am. J. Trop. Med. Hyg. 58:50–55

Faust EC, Giraldo LE, Caicedo G, Bonfante R, 1961. Human isosporiasis in the Western Hemisphere. Am. J. Trop. Med. Hyg. 10:343–349

Felez MA, Miro JM, Mallolas J, Valls ME, Moreno A, Gatell

JM, Soriano E, 1990. Enteritis por *Isospora belli* en pacientes con sindrome de immunodeficiencia adquirida. Descripcion de 9 casos. Med. Clin. Barcelona 95:84–88

Flanigan T, Whalen C, Turner J, Soave R, Toerner J, Havlir D, Kotler D, 1992. *Cryptosporidium* infection and CD4 counts. Ann. Intern. Med. 116:840–842

Forthal DN, Guest SS, 1984. *Isospora belli* enteritis in three homosexual men. Am. J. Trop. Med. Hyg. 33:1060–1064

French JM, Whitby JL, Whitfield AGW, 1964. Steatorrhea in a man infected with coccidiosis (*Isospora belli*). Gastroenterology 47:642

Frenkel JK, Dubey JP, 1972. Rodents as vectors for feline coccidia, *Isospora felis* and *Isospora rivolta*. J. Infect. Dis. 125:69–72

Garcia LS, Bruckner DA, Brewer TC, Shimizu RY, 1983. Techniques for the recovery and identification of *Cryptosporidium* oocysts from stool specimens. J. Clin. Microbiol. 18:185–190

Garcia LS, Current WL, 1989. Cryptosporidiosis: clinical features and diagnosis. Crit. Rev. Clin. Lab. Sci. 27: 439–460

Gardner C, 1994. An outbreak of hospital-acquired cryptosporidiosis. Br. J. Nurs. 3:152, 154–158

Garone MA, Winston BJ, Lewis JA, 1986. Cryptosporidiosis of the stomach. Am. J. Gastroenterol. 81:465–470

Gatti S, 1993. Cryptosporidiosis in tourists returning from Egypt and the Island of Mauritius. Clin. Infect. Dis. 16:344–345

Genta RM, Chappell CL, White AC Jr, Kimball KT, Goodgame RW, 1993. Duodenal morphology and intensity of infection in AIDS-related intestinal cryptosporidiosis. Gastroenterology 105:1769–1775

Gentile G, Venditti M, Micozzi A, Caprioli A, Donelli G, Tirindelli C, Meloni G, Arcese W, Martino P, 1991. Cryptosporidiosis in patients with hematologic malignancies. Rev. Infect. Dis. 13:842–846

Goodstein RS, Colombo CS, Illfelder MA, Skaggs RE, 1989. Bronchial and gastrointestinal cryptosporidiosis in AIDS. J. Am. Osteopath. Assoc. 89:195–197

Gould E, Angeles-Angeles A, Albores-Saavedra J, 1989. Cytomegalovirus and *Cryptosporidium*-associated acalculous cholecystitis in the acquired immunodeficiency syndrome (AIDS). Patologia 27:143–146

Graczyk TK, Cranfield MR, Fayer R, 1996. Evaluation of commercial enzyme immunoassay (EIA) and immunofluorescent antibody (IFA) test kits for detection of *Cryptosporidium* oocysts of species other than *Cryptosporidium parvum*. Am. J. Trop. Med. Hyg. 54: 274–279

Greenberg SJ, Davey MP, Zierdt WS, Waldmann TA, 1988. *Isospora belli* enteric infection in patients with human T-cell leukemia virus type I-associated adult T-cell leukemia. Am. J. Med. 85:435–438

Gremse DA, Bucuvalas JC, Bongiovanni GL, 1989. Papillary stenosis and sclerosing cholangitis in an immunodeficient child. Gastroenterology 96:1600–1603

Gross TL, Wheat J, Bartlett M, O'Connor KW, 1986. AIDS and multiple system involvement with *Cryptosporidium*. Am. J. Gastroenterol. 81:456–458

Harari MD, West B, Dwyer B, 1986. Correspondence. *Cryptosporidium* as cause of laryngotracheitis in an infant. Lancet 1:1207

Hart AS, Ridinger MT, Soundarajan R, Peters CS, Swiatlo AL, Kocka FE, 1990. Correspondence. Novel organism associated with chronic diarrhea in AIDS. Lancet 335:169–170

Hart MH, Kruger R, Nielsen S, Kaufman S, 1989. Acute self-limited colitis associated with *Cryptosporidium* in an immunocompetent patient. J. Pediatr. Gastroenterol. Nutr. 8:401–403

Hawkins SP, Thomas RP, Teasdale C, 1987. Acute pancreatitis: a new finding in *Cryptosporidium* enteritis. Br. Med. J. Clin. Res. Ed. 294:483–484

Hayes EB, Matte TD, O'Brien TR, McKinley TW, Logsdon GS, Rose JB, Ungar BL, Word DM, Pinsky PF, Cummings ML, Wilson MA, Long EG, Hurwitz ES, Juranek DD, 1989. Large community outbreak of cryptosporidiosis due to contamination of a filtered public water supply. N. Engl. J. Med. 320:1372–1376

Henry MC, De Clercq D, Lokombe B, Kayembe K, Kapita B, Mamba K, Mbendi N, Mazebo P, 1986. Parasitological observations of chronic diarrhoea in suspected AIDS adult patients in Kinshasa (Zaire). Trans. R. Soc. Trop. Med. Hyg. 80:309–310

Heydorn AO, 1977. Beitrage zum Lebenzyklus der Sarkosporidien. IX. Entwicklungszyklus von *Sarcocystis suihominis* n. spec. Berl. Munch. Tierarztl. Wschr. 90: 218–224

Heydorn AO, Gestrich R, Mehlhorn H, Rommel M, 1975. Proposal for a new nomenclature of the Sarcosporidia. Z. Parasitenk. 48:73–82

Hoge CW, Shlim DR, Rajah R, Triplett J, Shear M, Rabold JH, Echeverria P, 1993. Epidemiology of diarrheal illness associated with coccidian-like organism among travellers and foreign residents in Nepal. N. Engl. J. Med. 341:1175–1179

Jarpa A, Montero E, Navarro C, Mayerholz M, Vasquez A, Zuloaga M, 1960. Isosporosis humana. Bol. Chil. Parasitol. 15:50–54

Jeffery GM, 1958. Epidemiologic considerations of isosporiasis in a school for mental defectives. Am. J. Hyg. 67: 251–255

Jokipii L, 1983. *Cryptosporidium*: a frequent finding in patients with gastrointestinal symptoms. Lancet. 2:358–361

Jokipii L, Jokipii AM, 1986. Timing of symptoms and oocyst excretion in human cryptosporidiosis. N. Engl. J. Med. 315:1643–1647

Jokipii L, Pohjola S, Valle SL, Jokipii AM, 1985. Frequency, multiplicity and repertoire of intestinal protozoa in healthy homosexual men and in patients with gastrointestinal symptoms. Ann. Clin. Res. 17:57–59

Kahn DG, Garfinkle JM, Klonoff DC, Pembrook LJ, Morrow DJ, 1987. Cryptosporidial and cytomegaloviral hepatitis and cholecystitis. Arch. Pathol. Lab. Med. 111: 879–881

Kamel AGM, Maning N, Arulmainathan S, Murad S, Nasuruddin A, Lai KPF, 1994. Cryptosporidiosis among HIV positive intravenous drug users in Malaysia. Southeast Asian J. Trop. Med. Public Health 25:650–653

Kaminsky RG, 1991. Cuerpos Semejantes a *Cyanobacteria* Asociados con Diarrea en Honduras. Rev. Med. Hondur. 59:179–182

Kappus KK, Juranek DD, Roberts JM, 1991. Results of testing for intestinal parasites by state diagnostic laboratories, United States, 1987. MMWR CDC Surveill. Summ. 40:25–45

Kazlow PG, Shah K, Benkov KJ, Dische R, LeLeiko NS, 1986. Esophageal cryptosporidiosis in a child with acquired immune deficiency syndrome. Gastroenterology 91:1301–1303

Kocoshis SA, Cibull ML, Davis TE, Hinton JT, Seip M, Banwell JG, 1984. Intestinal and pulmonary cryptosporidiosis in an infant with severe combined immune deficiency. J. Pediatr. Gastroenterol. Nutr. 3:149–157

Kramer MH, Herwaldt BL, Craun GF, Calderon RL, Juranek DD, 1996. Surveillance for waterborne-disease outbreaks—United States, 1993–1994. MMWR CDC Surveill. Summ. 45:1–33

Lasser KH, Lewin KJ, Ryning FW, 1979. Cryptosporidial enteritis in a patient with congenital hypogammaglobulinemia. Hum. Pathol. 10:234–240

Laughon BE, Druckman DA, Vernon A, Quinn TC, Polk BF, Modlin JF, Yolken RH, Bartlett JG, 1988. Prevalence of enteric pathogens in homosexual men with and without acquired immunodeficiency syndrome. Gastroenterology 94:984–993

Laxer MA, D'Nicuola ME, Patel RJ, 1992. Detection of *Cryptosporidium parvum* DNA in fixed, paraffin-embedded tissue by the polymerase chain reaction. Am. J. Trop. Med. Hyg. 47:450–455

Lefkowitch JH, Krumholz S, Feng Chen KC, Griffin P, Despommier D, Brasitus TA, 1984. Cryptosporidiosis of the human small intestine: a light and electron microscopic study. Hum. Pathol. 15:746–752

Lengerich EJ, Addiss DG, Marx JJ, Ungar BL, Juranek DD, 1993. Increased exposure to cryptosporidia among dairy farmers in Wisconsin. J. Infect. Dis. 167:1252–1255

Levine ND, 1984. Taxonomy and review of the coccidian genus *Cryptosporidium* (Protozoa, Apicomplexa). J. Protozool. 31:94–98

Liebman WM, Thaler MM, De Lorimier A, Brandborg LL, Goodman J, 1980. Intractable diarrhea of infancy due to intestinal coccidiosis. Gastroenterology 78:579–584

Lindsay DS, Dubey JP, Toivio-Kinnucan MA, Michiels JF, Blagburn BL, 1997. Examination of extraintestinal tissue cysts of *Isospora belli*. J. Parasitol. 83:620–625

Lindsay DS, Toivio-Kinnucan MA, Dubey JP, Michiels JF, Blagburn BL, 1996. Examination of the tissue cyst of *Isospora belli* in an AIDS patient. J. Protozool. 44:20a

Long EG, Ebrahimzadeh A, White EH, Swisher B, Callaway CS, 1990. Alga associated with diarrhea in patients with acquired immunodeficiency syndrome and in travelers. J. Clin. Microbiol. 28:1101–1104

Long EG, White EH, Carmichael WW, Quinlisk PM, Raja R, Swisher BL, Daugharty H, Cohen MT, 1991. Morphologic and staining characteristics of a *Cyanobacterium*-like organism associated with diarrhea. J. Infect. Dis. 164:199–202

Loose JH, Sedergran DJ, Cooper HS, 1989. Identification of *Cryptosporidium* in paraffin-embedded tissue sections with the use of a monoclonal antibody. Am. J. Clin. Pathol. 91:206–209

Lumb R, Smith K, O'Donoghue PJ, Lanser JA, 1988. Ultrastructure of the attachment of *Cryptosporidium* sporozoites to tissue culture cells. Parasitol. Res. 74:531–536

Ma P, Soave R, 1983. Three-step stool examination for cryptosporidiosis in 10 homosexual men with protracted watery diarrhea. J. Infect. Dis. 147:824–828

MacKenzie WR, Hoxie NJ, Proctor ME, Gradus MS, Blair KA, Peterson DE, Kazmierczak JJ, Addiss DG, Fox KR, Rose JB, Davis JP, 1994. A massive outbreak in Milwaukee of *Cryptosporidium* infection transmitted through the public water supply. N. Engl. J. Med. 331:161–167

Magath TB, 1935. The coccidia of man. Am. J. Trop. Med. Hyg. 15:91–129

Markus MB, 1983. The hypnozoite of *Isospora canis*. S. Afr. J. Sci. 79:273

Matsubayashi H, Nozawa T, 1948. Experimental infection of *Isospora hominis* in man. Am. J. Trop. Med. 28:633–637

McCracken AW, 1972. Natural and laboratory-acquired infection by *Isospora belli*. South. Med. J. 65:800, 818

Mehlhorn H, Heydorn AO, 1979. Electron microscopical study on gamogony of *Sarcocystis suihominis* in human tissue cultures. Z. Parasitenk. 58:97–113

Meisel JL, Perera DR, Meligro C, Rubin CE, 1976. Overwhelming watery diarrhea associated with a *Cryptosporidium* in a immunosuppressed patient. Gastroenterology. 70:1156–1160

Michiels JF, Hofman P, Bernard E, Saint PM, Boissy C, Mondain V, LeFichoux Y, Loubiere R, 1994. Intestinal and extraintestinal *Isospora belli* infection in an AIDS patient. A second case report. Pathol. Res. Pract. 190:1089–1093

Miller RA, Wasserheit JN, Kirihara J, Coyle MB, 1984. Detection of *Cryptosporidium* oocysts in sputum during screening for mycobacteria. J. Clin. Microbiol. 20:1192–1193

Molbak K, Aaby P, Hojlyng N, da Silva AP, 1994. Risk factors for *Cryptosporidium* diarrhea in early childhood: a case-control study from Guinea-Bissau, West Africa. Am. J. Epidemiol. 139:734–740

Moore JA, Frenkel JK, 1991. Respiratory and enteric cryptosporidiosis in humans. Arch. Pathol. Lab. Med. 115:1160–1162

Narango J, Sterling C, Gilman R, Miranda E, Diaz F, Cho M, Benel A, 1989. *Cryptosporidium muris*-like objects from fecal samples of Peruvians. Honolulu, Hawaii. Abstracts, 38th annual meeting of the American Society for Tropical Medicine and Hygiene, Abstract No. 324.

Newman RD, Zu SX, Wuhib T, Lima AA, Guerrant RL, Sears CL, 1994. Household epidemiology of *Cryptosporidium parvum* infection in an urban community in northeast Brazil [see comments]. Ann. Intern. Med. 120:500–505

Ng E, Markell EK, Fleming RL, Fried M, 1984. Demonstration of *Isospora belli* by acid-fast stain in a patient with acquired immune deficiency syndrome. J. Clin. Microbiol. 20:384–386

Nhieu JTV, Nin F, Fleury-Feith J, Chaumette MT, Schaeffer A, Bretagne S, 1996. Identification of intracelluar stages of *Cyclospora* species by light microscopy of thick sections using hematoxylin. Hum. Pathol. 27: 1107–1109

Nime FA, Burek JD, Page DL, Holscher MA, Yardley JH, 1976. Acute enterocolitis in a human being infected with the protozoan *Cryptosporidium*. Gastroenterology. 70: 592–598

Orrego F, Faiguenbaum J, Apablaza A, 1959. Hallazgo de *Isospora belli* en jugo duodenal. Bol. Chil. Parasitol. 14:55–56

Ortega YR, Gilman RH, Sterling CR, 1994. A new coccidian parasite (Apicomplexa: Eimeriidae) from humans. J. Parasitol. 80:625–629

Ortega YR, Sterling CR, Gilman RH, Cama VA, Diaz F, 1992. *Cyclospora cayetanensis*: a new protozoan pathogen of humans. Program and Abstracts, 41st annual meeting of the American Society for Tropical Medicine and Hygiene, Seattle, Nov. 15–19, 1992.

Ortega YR, Sterling CR, Gilman RH, Cama VA, Diaz F, 1993. *Cyclospora* species—a new protozoan pathogen of humans. N. Engl. J. Med. 328:1308–1312

Pape JW, Verdier RI, Boncy M, Boncy J, Johnson WD Jr, 1994. *Cyclospora* infection in adults infected with HIV. Clinical manifestations, treatment and prophylaxis. Ann. Intern. Med. 121:654–657

Pape JW, Verdier RI, Johnson WDJ, 1989. Treatment and prophylaxis of *Isospora belli* infection in patients with the acquired immunodeficiency syndrome. N. Engl. J. Med. 320:1044–1047

Peng MM, Xiao L, Freeman AR, Arrowood MJ, Escalante AA, Weltman AC, Ong CS, MacKenzie WR, Lal A, Beard CB, 1997. Genetic polymorphism among *Cryptosporidium parvum* isolates: evidence of two distinct human transmission cycles. Emerg. Infect. Dis. 3:567– 573

Phillips AD, Thomas AG, Walker-Smith JA, 1992. *Cryptosporidium*, chronic diarrhoea and the proximal small intestinal mucosa. Gut 33:1057–1061

Pieniazek NJ, Slemenda SB, da Silva AJ, Alfano EM, Arrowood MJ, 1996. PCR confirmation of infection with *Cyclospora cayetanensis*. Emerging Infect. Dis. 2:357–358

Pitlik SD, Fainstein V, Garza D, Guarda L, Bolivar R, Rios A, Hopfer RL, Mansell PA, 1983. Human cryptosporidiosis: spectrum of disease. Report of six cases and review of the literature. Arch. Intern. Med. 143:2269–2275

Poirot JL, Deluol AM, Antoine M, Heyer F, Cadranel J, Meynard JL, Meyohas MC, Girard PM, Roux P, 1996. Broncho-pulmonary cryptosporidiosis in four HIV-infected patients. J. Euk. Microbiol. 43:78S–79S

Pollock RC, Bendall RP, Moody A, Chiodini PL, Churchill DR, 1992. Traveller's diarrhoea associated with *Cyanobacterium*-like bodies. Lancet 340:556–557

Prociv P, Luke R, Quayle P, 1992. Isosporiasis in the aboriginal population of Queensland. Med. J. Aust. 156:115–117

Ravenel JM, Suggs JL, Legerton CW Jr, 1976. Human coccidiosis: recurrent diarrhea of 26 years duration due to *Isaspora* (sic) *belli*: A case report. J. South. Carolina Med. Assoc. 72:217–219

Reesc NC, Current WL, Ernst JV, Bailey WS, 1982. Cryptosporidiosis of man and calf: a case report and results of experimental infections in mice and rats. Am. J. Trop. Med. Hyg. 31:226–229

Restrepo C, Macher AM, Radany EH, 1987. Disseminated extraintestinal isosporiasis in a patient with acquired immune deficiency syndrome. Am. J. Clin. Pathol. 87: 536–542

Rodriguez Hernandez J, Canut Blasco A, Martin Sanchez AM, 1996. Seasonal prevalences of *Cryptosporidium* and *Giardia* infections in children attending day care centres in Salamanca (Spain) studied for a period of 15 months. Eur. J. Epidemiol. 12:291–295

Rommel VM, Heydorn AO, 1972. Beitrage zum Lebenszyklus der Sarkosporidien III. *Isospora hominis* (Railliet und Lucet, 1891) Wenyon, 1923, eine Dauerform der Sarkosporidien des Rindes und des Schweins. Berl. Munch. Teirarztl. Wsch. 85:143–145

Sagua H, Soto J, Delano B, Fuentes A, Becker P, 1978. Brote epidemico de isosporosis por *Isospora belli* en la ciudad de Antofagasta, Chile. Consideraciones sobre 90 casos diagnosticados en 3 meses. Bol. Chil. Parasitol. 33:8–12

Shepherd RC, Reed CL, Sinha GP, 1988. Shedding of oocysts of *Cryptosporidium* in immunocompetent patients. J. Clin. Pathol. 41:1104–1106

Shlim DR, Cohen MT, Eaton M, Rajah R, Long EG, Ungar BL, Ungar BLP, 1991. An alga-like organism associated with an outbreak of prolonged diarrhea among foreigners in Nepal. Am. J. Trop. Med. Hyg. 45:383–389

Smith HV, Rose JB, 1998. Waterborne cryptosporidiosis: current status. Parasitol. Today 14:14–22

Soave R, Danner RL, Honig CL, Ma P, Hart CC, Nash T, Roberts RB, 1984. Cryptosporidiosis in homosexual men. Ann. Intern. Med. 100:504–511

Soave R, Dubey JP, Ramos LJ, Tumings M, 1986. A new intestinal pathogen? Clin. Res. 34:533A

Soave R, Johnson WD Jr, 1988. *Cryptosporidium* and *Isospora belli* infections. J. Infect. Dis. 157:225–229

Sorvillo FJ, Lieb LE, Kerndt PR, Ash LR, 1994. Epidemiology of cryptosporidiosis among persons with acquired immunodeficiency syndrome in Los Angeles County. Am. J. Trop. Med. Hyg. 51:326–331

Sorvillo FJ, Lieb LE, Seidel J, Kerndt P, Turner J, Ash LR, 1995. Epidemiology of isosporiasis among persons with acquired immunodeficiency syndrome in Los Angeles County. Am. J. Trop. Med. Hyg. 53:656–659

Stemmerman GN, Hayashi T, Glober GA, Oishi N, Frankel RI, 1980. Cryptosporidiosis. Report of a fatal case complicated by disseminated toxoplasmosis. Am. J. Med. 69:637–642

Sterling CR, Gilman RH, Sinclair NA, Cama V, Castillo R,

Diaz F, 1991. The role of breast milk in protecting urban Peruvian children against cryptosporidiosis. J. Protozool. 38:23S–25S

Sun T, Ilardi CF, Asnis D, Bresciani AR, Goldenberg S, Roberts B, Teichberg S, 1996. Light and electron microscopic identification of *Cyclospora* species in the small intestine. Evidence of the presence of asexual life cycle in human host. Am. J. Clin. Pathol. 105:216–220

Taylor DN, Houston R, Shlim DR, Bhaibulaya M, Ungar BL, Echeverria P, 1988. Etiology of diarrhea among travelers and foreign residents in Nepal. JAMA 260:1245–1248

Teixidor HS, Godwin TA, Ramirez EA, 1991. Cryptosporidiosis of the biliary tract in AIDS. Radiology 180:51–56

Travis WD, Schmidt K, MacLowry JD, Masur H, Condron KS, Fojo AT, 1990. Respiratory cryptosporidiosis in a patient with malignant lymphoma. Report of a case and review of the literature. Arch. Pathol. Lab. Med. 114:519–522

Trier JS, Moxey PC, Schimmel EM, Robles E, 1974. Chronic intestinal coccidiosis in man: intestinal morphology and response to treatment. Gastroenterology 66:923–935

Tzipori S, Angus KW, Gray EW, Campbell I, 1980. Vomiting and diarrhea associated with cryptosporidial infection. N. Engl. J. Med. 303:818

Ungar BLP, 1990. Enzyme-linked immunoassay for detection of *Cryptosporidium* antigens in fecal specimens. J. Clin. Microbiol. 28:2491–2495

Ungar BLP, Gilman RH, Lanata CF, Perez-Schael I, 1988. Seroepidemiology of *Cryptosporidium* infection in two Latin American populations. J. Infect. Dis. 157:551–556

Upton SJ, Current WL, 1985. The species of *Cryptosporidium* (Apicomplexa: Cryptosporidiidae) infecting mammals. J. Parasitol. 71:625–629

Weisburger WR, Hutcheon DF, Yardley JH, Roche JC, Hillis WD, Charache P, 1979. Cryptosporidiosis in an immunosuppressed renal-transplant recipient with IgA deficiency. Am. J. Clin. Pathol. 72:473–478

Wentai L, Zhenbing Z, Ziqiang L, Congen X, Yangxian Z, Fuqiang C, 1986. Clinical analysis and treatment of 55 cases of intestinal sarcosporidiosis. Chinese J. Parasitol. Parasit. Dis. 4:49

Widmer G, Carraway M, Tzipori S, 1996. Water-borne *Cryptosporidium*: a perspective from the USA. Parasitol. Today 12:286–290

Wurtz R, 1994. *Cyclospora*: a newly identified pathogen of humans. Clin. Infect. Dis. 18:620–623

9

TISSUE APICOMPLEXA

Members of the Apicomplexa in human tissues other than the intestine and blood belong to the genera *Sarcocystis* and *Toxoplasma* of the family Sarcocystidae, characterized, as already stated, by two hosts in their life cycles. The *Sarcocystis* organisms occurring in the intestine of humans were studied in Chapter 8. The *Sarcocystis* organism parasitizing skeletal muscles and myocardium will be discussed here under the generic name *S. lindemanni* to denote several species not determined at present. Although the importance of *S. lindemanni* in human medicine is not as great as that of *Toxoplasma*, it is discussed in some detail because of the diagnostic problems it may pose for pathologists.

Sarcocystis lindemanni— Sarcocystosis or Sarcosporidiosis

Humans are the accidental intermediate hosts of several species of *Sarcocystis* of animals, which produce sarcocystosis or sarcosporidiosis. These infections are acquired by the ingestion of sporocysts passed in the feces of a animal, the definitive host, with intestinal *Sarcocystis*. The animal is a carnivore, either a domestic or wild dog or cat, or possibly a hawk, owl, or reptile (see Chapter 8, and Fig. 6–9; Beaver et al. 1984). Up to now, fewer than 70 such cases have been reported in the world's literature. Disease has been found in the heart, skeletal muscles, and tongue, usually incidental findings in autopsy material or in muscle biopsy specimens. A survey in Denmark of 112 human autopsies from which 50 g of diaphragmatic muscles recovered from autopsied bodies were artificially digested found four cases of sarcosporidiosis (Greve, 1985). This suggests that the infection may be more common in the general population than the number of cases described indicates. In a histologic study of tongues and diaphragms from 50 autopsied patients in Ireland, no evidence of infection was found (Wong et al. 1993). Although it is assumed that the development of *Sarcocystis* in humans follows the same pattern of generation in the endothelial cells of blood vessels before reaching the muscles, neither these stages nor lesions associated with them have been found (Beaver et al. 1984). All cases of sarcosporidiosis were once thought to belong to a single species, *S. lindemanni*. Then, in 1979, Beaver and coworkers reviewed all reported cases, added five more, and classified them into at least seven morphologic types, each presumably corresponding to a different species (Beaver et al. 1979). At least 40 cases of cardiac sarcosporidiosis and 29 cases of skeletal sarcosporidiosis had been described up to 1979; since then, others have been added (Kan, 1985; Kouyoumdhian, Tognola, 1985; Lele et al. 1986; Pamphlett, O'Donoghue, 1990; Troedsen et al. 1992; Wong, Pathmanathan, 1992, 1994). Features common to all cases of sarcosporidiosis in humans are their higher frequency in the tropics, except for a few in Europe, and their zoonotic nature. The life cycle of *Sarcocystis* was studied in Chapter 8.

Morphology. In some ways, the morphology of a sarcocyst resembles that of a cyst of *Toxoplasma*, and sometimes it is difficult to distinguish between the two. Once the merozoites are freed from the endothelial cells (see Life Cycle, Chapter 8), they reach the muscles and enter the myocytes. The earlier stages occur within parasitophorous vacuoles, and as growth progresses, the cyst wall begins to form around the membrane of the vacuole (Entzeroth, 1982). The cyst membrane becomes strengthened by deposited osmiophilic material to constitute the *primary cyst wall*. This membrane is common to all species of *Sarcocystis* and *Toxoplasma*, but in *Sarcocystis* it continues to differentiate becoming the much thicker wall of the mature sarcocyst (Entzeroth, 1982).

In mature sarcocysts, the appearance of the wall differs in accordance with the species. Most sarcocysts have a thick wall; in others, the wall is relatively thin for the size of the cyst. Villosities may form part of the wall, giving the appearance of striations, which are helpful in distinguishing different types of cysts. Cyst growth begins with two types of cells, the round metrocytes and the elongated, banana-shaped merozoites. Metrocytes are temporary cells located at the periphery of the cyst against the cyst wall; they are not found in mature cysts. Division by endodyogeny (a form of asexual reproduction in which two daughter cells form within the parent cell) of both metrocytes and merozoites occurs as the cyst grows. At the same time septae form, dividing the sarcocyst into several compartments. Well-defined septae with clearly marked eosinophilic bands of tissue are present in most species; in some, they are difficult to see and may appear as empty spaces. The zoites in mature cysts are elongated and banana-shaped, with a single nucleus, and stain basophilically with hematoxylin and eosin stain; the cyst wall is eosinophilic. The zoites are several times larger than those of *Toxoplasma* and are easily seen under the light microscope. The size of the mature sarcocyst

varies with the species; sometimes this structure is seen in the muscles of animals with the naked eye. The elongated sarcocyst follows the shape of the myocyte but enlarges it considerably. In general, in most known species of *Sarcocystis*, the mature sarcocyst is several times larger than the cyst of *Toxoplasma*. The metrocytes, when present, are an important feature distinguishing between the two genera. The cysts grow in muscle cells without eliciting an inflammatory response; therefore, the muscle phase of the infection is clinically silent.

The morphologic characteristics of the seven types of *Sarcocystis* found parasitizing humans are summarized here, closely following the findings of Beaver and coworkers (Beaver et al. 1979).

Type 1. Four cases of type 1 *Sarcocystis* in the skeletal muscles are known, two in France and one each in China and Uganda. The cysts are characterized by a thick, radially striated wall, multiple microvilli (Fig. 9–1 B), large zoites, and clearly visible metrocytes. In the case from Uganda the cysts were up to 2.25×200 μm, the wall had microvilli (cytophaneres) up to 12 μm, and the primary membrane was about 0.5 μm, extending inside the cyst to form numerous compartments. The zoites were falciform, measuring 10 to 12 $\times$ 2 μm. The parasite in this cases resembles one observed in *Cercopithecus talopian*, a primate from west and central Africa (Fig. 9–1 A–B).

Type 2. Type 2 corresponds to cases of *Sarcocystis* in the skeletal muscles observed once in Sudan, five times in India, and once in Angola. The sarcocysts are usually large, with a thin, smooth cyst wall. The zoites are medium-sized, located in compartments formed by well-defined septae (Fig. 9–2 C) some of which appeared empty, especially at the center of the cyst. These cases resemble *Sarcocystis nesbitti* described in *Macaca mulatta* (Fig. 9–2 A–D).

Type 3. Type 3 *Sarcocystis* occurred in the skeletal muscles of three individuals from India, one from Southeast Asia, and one from Sudan. Morphologically, the parasites closely resemble those of type 2 *Sarcocystis*. They have small and medium-sized sarcocysts with a thin wall, medium-sized zoites, and septae apparent only by the manner in which the zoites are grouped (they appear as clefts). In one case from India, the cyst ranged from 60 to 70 μm in diameter and from 65 to 90 μm in length. The wall, 0.5 μm in thickness, and the parasitized skeletal muscle cell, 80 μm in diameter, were twice as big as those of the normal adjacent cells. The zoites were relatively slender,

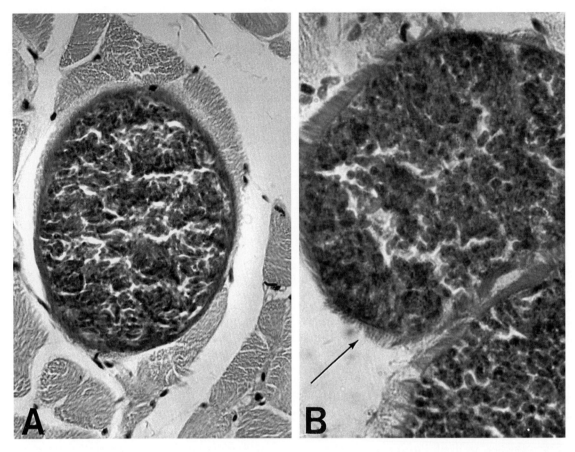

Fig. 9–1. *Sarcocystis* in sections of skeletal muscle of *Cercopithecus talopian*, identical to the human type 1, stained with hematoxylin and eosin stain. *A*, Cross section of a sarcocyst showing the thick wall. The geographic arrangement of the zoites indicates the presence of compartments. Note the enormous enlargement of the muscle cells, ×450. *B*, Higher magnification showing the large zoites and the cytophaneres (arrow), ×550. (Preparation courtesy of P.C. Beaver, Ph.D., School of Public Health and Tropical Medicine, Tulane University, New Orleans, Louisiana.)

1.5 μm in diameter by approximately 6 to 8 μm in length.

Type 4. Type 4 *Sarcocystis* was reported in the skeletal muscles of six individuals from Malaysia, two from Indonesia, two from Singapore, one from Southeast Asia, one from Asia, and one from an unspecified location. The sarcocysts are large to medium-sized, with a thin wall, small zoites not distinctly grouped, and septae visible only in the central portion where the zoites are sparse. Two of those cases studied (by Beaver et al. 1979) showed sarcocysts up to 400 μm in length by 130 μm in width. The cyst wall was smooth and less than 1.0 μm thick, surrounded by a thin layer of sarcoplasm. The six cases reported from Malaysia, plus five new ones, were reviewed recently, and it was con-

Fig. 9–2. *Sarcocystis nesbitti* in sections of skeletal muscle of *Macaca mulatta*, identical to the human type 2. *A–C.* Stained with hematoxylin and eosin stain. *A*, Longitudinal section of the sarcocyst, ×280. *B*, Higher magnification showing the arrangement of zoites, with a suggestion of compartments. The membrane is thin and smooth, ×550. *C*, Cross section of the cyst showing compartments and a smooth membrane, ×350. *D*, Stained with periodic acid–Schiff hematoxylin stain. Low magnification showing slightly oblique sections of the cyst. The zoites have small periodic acid–Schiff–positive elements. (Preparation courtesy of P.C. Beaver, Ph.D., School of Public Health and Tropical Medicine, Tulane University, New Orleans, Louisiana.)

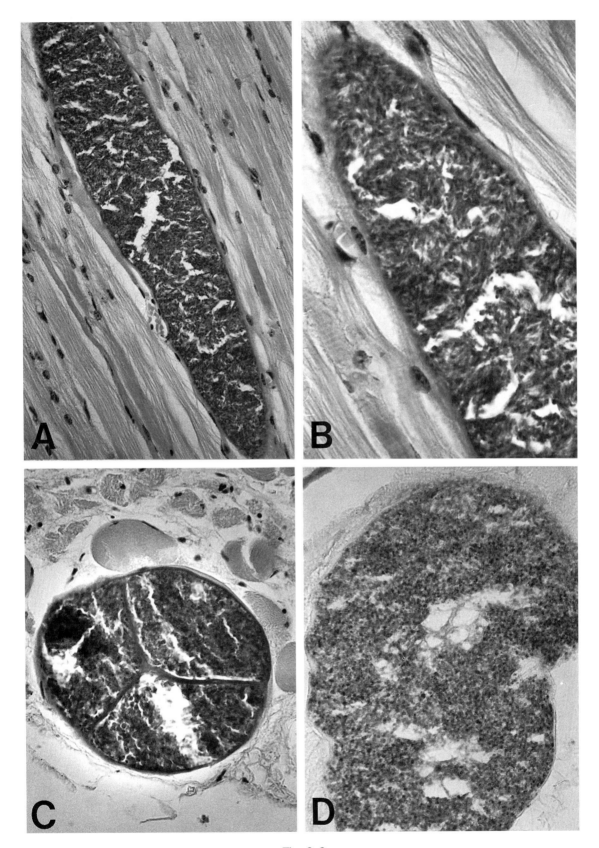

Fig. 9–2.

cluded that the new ones best fit type 4 (Pathmanathan, Kan, 1981, 1992; Wong et al. 1994; Wong, Yusoff, 1995).

Type 5. Type 5 *Sarcocystis* occurred in the myocardium of one person from Italy and another from England; it is characterized by small sarcocysts with a thin wall and medium-sized zoites. Since the descriptions and the illustrations in both of these cases are insufficient, no statements can be made about their morphologic characteristics.

Type 6. Type 6 *Sarcocystis* occurred in the myocardium of three persons, one each from Britain, Brazil, and Costa Rica. The sarcocysts are small to medium-sized, with a thin wall and large, basophilic zoites (Fig. 9–3 A–C). The cyst is 30 μm in diameter, with a maximum length of 110 μm. The cyst wall is 0.5 μm thick, with no cytophaneres or septa; the

zoites measure 2.5 to 3.0 μm in diameter by 12 μm in length. The parasitized myocardial cell is enlarged. The distribution of the zoites suggests a compartment for each zoite. Morphologically, the organism resembles *S. bovicanis*, a parasite occurring in the tropics and subtropics, with wild and domestic dogs as the final hosts and cattle as the intermediate host. Although this type may represent one or more species, it is appropriate to refer to it as *S. bovicanis*-like (Fig. 9–3 A–C).

Type 7. Type 7 *Sarcocystis* corresponds to sarcocysts in the myocardium. It has been reported twice from Panama, once from Brazil, and three times in immigrants from the West Indies, Germany, and Puerto Rico residing in New York. The parasites found in the heart consist of small cysts with a thin wall and small zoites. The cysts vary from 21 to 51 μm in diameter; the wall is 1.5 to 3.0 μm thick; and the zoites are 7 to 10 μm

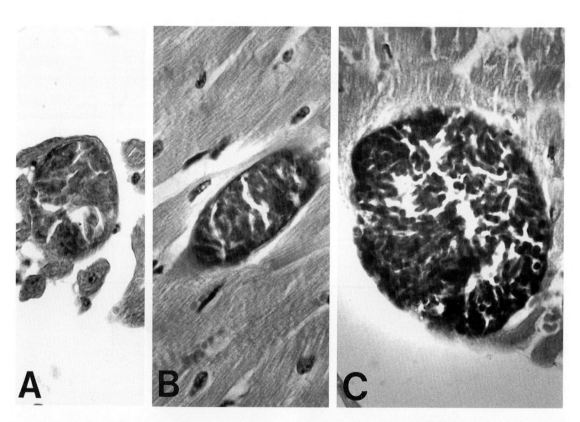

Fig. 9–3. *Sarcocystis* **in sections of cardiac muscle of humans and sheep, human type 6, stained with hematoxylin and eosin stain.** *A,* **Slightly oblique section in muscle of a child from Costa Rica showing enlargement of the cardiac muscle cell, the thin smooth cyst wall, and the large zoites. The septae are evident only because of the arrangement of the zoites, ×705.** *B* **and** *C,* **Identical cysts found** in sheep. Note the similarity to the characteristics described in *A,* ×550. (Preparations courtesy of P.C. Beaver, Ph.D., School of Public Health and Tropical Medicine, Tulane University, New Orleans, Louisiana. Human slide is from case No. 5 in: Beaver, P.C., Gadgil, R.K., and Morera, P. 1979. Sarcocystis in man: a review and report of five cases. Am. Trop. Med. Hyg. 29:819–844.)

long by 2.0 to 2.5 μm wide. The cardiac fiber containing the sarcocysts is enlarged three to five times its normal size. The cyst resembles *Toxoplasma* and must be carefully differentiated from it based on the increased size of the myocyte.

Disease. As mentioned earlier, sarcosporidiosis in humans is mostly an asymptomatic infection, usually found incidentally. A few reported cases have been associated with symptoms that apparently occurred during development of the parasites in the tissues before they became mature sarcocysts. Although the identity of the parasite is doubtful, one author reported a chronic illness consisting of general weakness and muscular soreness with peripheral eosinophilia of 20% (Price, 1933). Two other patients presented with eosinophilia and progressive weakness of the muscles, for which muscle biopsies were performed (Jeffrey, 1974; Mandour, 1965), and one presented with fever, chronic myositis, and peripheral eosinophilia (Van-den et al. 1995). In addition, one patient was diagnosed with periarteritis nodosa (McGill, Goodbody, 1957) and another with necrotizing vasculitis (McLeod et al. 1980).

Diagnosis. *Sarcocystis* is diagnosed in biopsy specimens or in autopsy material from skeletal muscle and myocardium. Biopsy specimens are usually taken for reasons other than the *Sarcocystis* infection since at present no specific symptoms are associated with the parasite in humans. Moreover, the mature muscle sarcocysts are asymptomatic. Thus the finding of *Sarcocystis* is usually incidental, and recognition and identification should be based on the morphologic characteristics described above (Figs. 9–1 to 9–3). The infection is commonly misdiagnosed. In earlier years, cases of toxoplasmosis were mistakenly identified as sarcosporidiosis; in others, artifacts have been the culprits (Cone, 1922). A case of pulmonary infection should be disregarded because it does not conform to the biology of the parasite, i.e., *Sarcocystis* does not occur in the lung (Lancastre et al. 1989). *Sarcocystis* species found in humans should be differentiated from *Toxoplasma* (see below) based on their size, thickness of the cyst wall, presence of compartments (Fig. 9–2 *C*), metrocytes, microvilli in the wall of some species (Fig. 9–1 *B*), and the relative size of the zoites. Some species, especially those with small cysts (Fig. 9–3), are difficult to distinguish from *Toxoplasma*. The earlier developmental stages of *Sarcocystis* have not been described. They may be indistinguishable from the mature cysts of *Toxoplasma*.

Toxoplasma gondii—Toxoplasmosis

The other genus of the family Sarcocystidae important in human medicine is *Toxoplasma*, an intestinal coc-

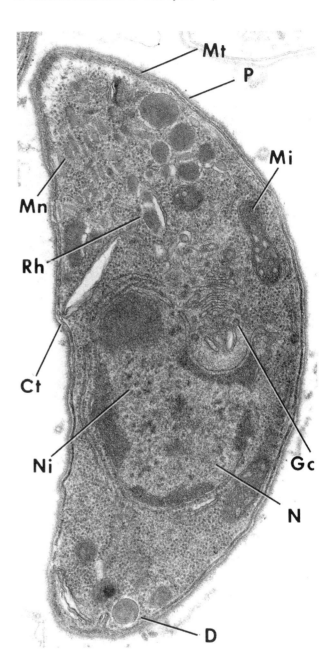

Fig. 9–4. *Toxoplasma gondii* **trophozoite in experimental animal, electron micrograph. Slightly oblique section. Ct, cytosome; D, dense bodies; Gc, Golgi complex; Mi, mitochondria; Mn, micronemes; Mt, microtubules; N, nucleus; Ni, nucleolus; P, pellicle; Rh, rhoptries, ×42,900. (Courtesy of M. Aikawa, M.D., Institute of Pathology, Case Western Reserve University, Cleveland, Ohio.)**

cidian of cats. In cats, the definitive hosts of *Toxoplasma*, the life cycle can be direct (similar to that of *Isospora*), but many species of animals, including humans, can become infected with *Toxoplasma* in their tissues and serve as intermediate hosts in an indirect life cycle. This dual form of development helps make *Toxoplasma* one of the most ubiquitous parasites in nature. Other genera of apicomplexan parasites closely related to *Toxoplasma*, such as *Neospora*, *Hammondia*, and *Frenkelia*, are known in animals and produce infections very similar to that of toxoplasmosis.

Toxoplasma has long been known as a parasite of humans and animals. It produces disease sporadically in the general population, sometimes in the unborn, who became infected in utero. The mode of transmission, and the high rates of positivity to *Toxoplasma*

antibodies in almost every population studied, remained puzzling for decades. In the late 1960s, the discovery that the *Toxoplasma* of humans was a stage in the life cycle of an intestinal coccidian of cats (Frenkel et al. 1969) opened the field for a more comprehensive study of the infection. In the early 1980s, the acquired immune deficiency syndrome (AIDS) epidemic increased awareness of the parasite because of its capacity to produce opportunistic infections in these patients.

Morphology. The stages of the life cycle of *Toxoplasma* in humans that are important for the understanding and diagnosis of the disease are the trophozoites, pseudocysts, and cysts, all of which are intracellular. In *tissue imprints, tissue culture cells*, and

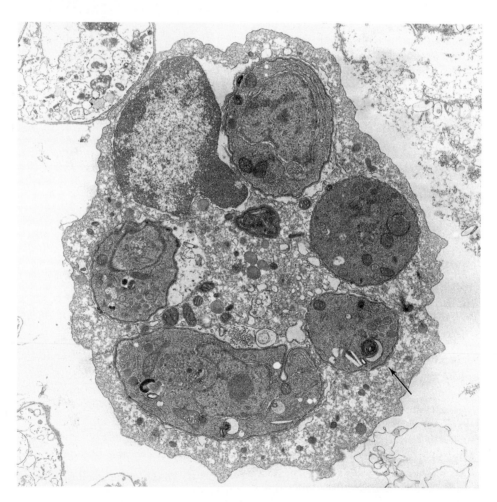

Fig. 9–5. *Toxoplasma gondii*, **electron micrograph of a macrophage with several trophozoites (tachyzoites). Note the parasites contained within parasitophorous vacuoles, sometimes appreciated only as a double cell membrane (arrow), ×14,250. (Courtesy of M. Aikawa, M.D., Institute of Pathology, Case Western Reserve University, Cleveland, Ohio.)**

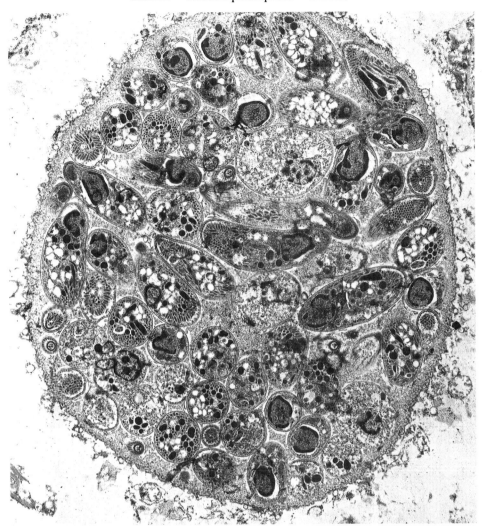

Fig. 9–6. *Toxoplasma gondii*, transmission electron micrograph of a cyst. Note the numerous zoites with all the characteristics of an apicomplexan parasite. (Courtesy of J. Filo, M.D., Department of Pathology, Cleveland Clinic Educational Foundation, Cleveland, Ohio.)

smears of fluids stained with Giemsa stain, the tropho- zoites (or tachyzoites) are crescent-shaped organisms about 4 to 8 μm in length by 2 to 3 μm in width, with one end slightly broader than the other (Fig. 9–24 A–B; *color plate* VI A–B). The cytoplasm stains blue and the nucleus, located near the broader end of the parasite, dark red (*color plate* VI A–B). The pseudocysts are cells containing from a few to numerous tachyzoites in their cytoplasm (Fig. 9–25 A; *color plate* VI C). The cysts (or bradyzoites) are up to 40 μm in diameter, have a delicate cyst wall, and contain numerous organisms in- distinguishable from the trophozoites described above (Fig. 9–25 C; *color plate* VI B). In electron micrographs, the tachyzoites and zoites in the bradyzoite have all the

characteristics of an apicomplexan organism (Figs. 9–4 and 9–6).

In *tissue sections* stained with hematoxylin and eosin stain, all stages are morphologically identical to that described above, but their size is much smaller due to shrinkage during fixation and processing for sec- tioning. Moreover, the organisms themselves may be sectioned. The tachyzoites are small bodies with a dark nucleus and scanty eosinophilic cytoplasm measuring no more than 4 μm in length. The pseudocysts are col- lections of intracellular parasites with no cyst wall. The cysts are rounded except in muscle cells, where they may be elongated; they measure about 30 μm in di- ameter (also because of shrinkage), and the cyst wall, about 1 μm thick, is clearly seen. In electron micrographs, the tachyzoites are located within parasitophorous vacuoles in the cell cytoplasm (Fig. 9–5), where they multiply by endodyogeny. They have all the organelles of an apicomplexan organism (see Chapter 8). The bradyzoites are characterized by their wall and by the presence of hundreds of organisms.

Life Cycle and Biology. As stated above, the life cycle of *Toxoplasma* (Fig. 9–7) resembles that of *Sarcocystis* in the sense that two hosts may be involved. The biologic differences between the two organisms are great and must be known to understand some aspects of the infection in humans. In the final hosts *Toxoplasma* develops asexually in the epithelial cells of the small intestine, producing merozoites and gametes, and sexually, producing oocysts in a manner similar to that of other coccidial organisms (Frenkel et al. 1970). The oocysts excreted with the feces of cats require a period of maturation (sporogony) outside the host, which results in the formation of two sporocysts, each with four sporozoites (identical to those of *Isospora*). Both cats (final hosts) and other animals, including humans (intermediate hosts), may become infected by ingestion of sporulated oocysts found in the environment. Infected cats develop an intestinal infection. Other hosts, including humans, do not support the parasite in the intestine; the parasite enters the mucosal vessels to disseminate into the tissues. Once the parasites enter the cell (any type of cell), they began developing as tachyzoites, fill the cell, and escape to parasitize other cells and repeat the cycle. Some tachyzoites, on entering the cell, began forming bradyzoites, a slow process that

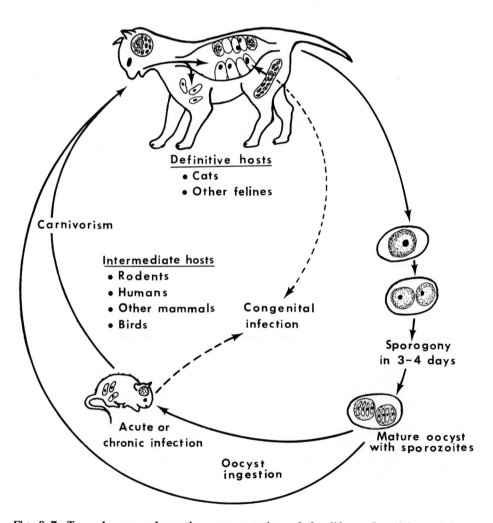

Fig. 9–7. *Toxoplasma*, schematic representation of the life cycle. (Adapted from: Frenkel, J. 1988. Pathophysiology of toxoplasmosis. Parasitol. Today 4:273–278. Reproduced with permission.)

starts with secretion of the membrane. Eventually, after the cell dies, mature bradyzoites rest in the interstitium, where they remain for the life of the host.

The function of tissue bradyzoites in the life cycle of the parasite is to transmit the infection to other hosts, which may ingest flesh and organs with the bradyzoites. Cats ingesting bradyzoites develop an intestinal infection, other animals a tissue infection. Therefore, both bradyzoites and oocysts are infective stages of the parasite, but their later development and the type of infection they produce depend on the hosts: cats or all other animals (Frenkel, 1988).

Geographic Distribution and Epidemiology.

Toxoplasmosis is a worldwide infection with high prevalence in the general population, as countless seroepidemiologic surveys demonstrate. In these surveys, the percentage of individuals with antibodies against *Toxoplasma* always increases with age, indicating that infections occur at all ages. Since clinical disease is extremely rare in immune-competent individuals, asymptomatic toxoplasmosis must be considered the rule. The infection is acquired by consumption of raw meat containing bradyzoites or by ingestion of soil, water, or food contaminated with oocysts shed by cats (Benenson et al. 1982; Stagno et al. 1980). Other routes of infection are in utero, transmission, blood transfusions, organ transplants, and leukocyte transfusions (Siegel et al. 1971).

Serologic surveys of college students in the United States revealed a 20% positivity rate for *Toxoplasma* antibodies (Remington et al. 1963), and it is estimated that one-half of the entire U.S. population is seropositive for *Toxoplasma* (Krick, Remington, 1978). The prevalence of seropositivity for *Toxoplasma* in the U.S. population appears to have fallen by at least one-third in the last three decades (Smith et al. 1996). Surveys in other countries have shown even higher prevalence rates of seropositivity, due in some cases to contamination of the environment with cat feces and in others to consumption of raw or undercooked beef. Seropositivity of 100% for *Toxoplasma* antibodies in adults was found in the Marshall Islands (Adams et al. 1987). In Panama City, Panama, follow-up of over 571 children for 5 years showed seroconversion in 72, a rate of almost 13%. The only significant risk factor was owning a dog (Frenkel et al. 1995). Thus, dogs pose a more important risk than cats, probably due to the practice of xenosmophilia by dogs (rolling over soil contaminated with cat feces and other odoriferous matter) and getting the mature oocysts on their hair (Frenkel et al. 1996).

Studies of farm animals in the United States showed that swine are infected in percentages varying from less than 3% (Dubey et al. 1995) to 34% (Patton et al. 1966). In addition, cats and other domestic and wild animals on these farms were found to have a high prevalence of antibodies to *Toxoplasma*, helping to maintain the infection in nature (Dubey et al. 1995). In spite of these data, it is estimated that the role of pork in the transmission of the infection is negligible (Patton et al. 1966). Epidemics of toxoplasmosis in humans due to consumption of beef have been reported, but these reports are based more on circumstantial evidence than on scientific facts (Kean et al. 1969). An outbreak due to ingestion of oocysts from an infected cat that contaminated a riding stable in Atlanta, in which 37 persons became ill, is well documented. This episode revealed that the symptoms of toxoplasmosis are more common than was previously believed (Teutsch et al. 1979).

Regarding the prevalence of specific anti-*Toxoplasma* antibodies among the human immune deficiency virus (HIV)/AIDS population, several studies show that the rates are similar in groups with AIDS and in those at risk for AIDS. This finding indicates that the disease in AIDS is usually due to reactivation (Derouin et al. 1986). Serology for *Toxoplasma* in 411 patients with AIDS was positive in 130 (32%), of whom 31, or (24%), developed toxoplasmosis, indicating a 28% probability of developing the disease; 26% will develop it in less than 2 years (Grant et al. 1990). Similar studies in Europe showed that in patients who had AIDS and positive *Toxoplasma* serology, 47% developed *Toxoplasma* encephalitis (Zangerle, Allerberger, 1994; Zangerle et al. 1991). An autopsy series of 135 patients dying of AIDS in Switzerland revealed toxoplasmic encephalitis in 26% (Lang et al. 1989). The risk of acquiring the infection by HIV-positive individuals owing a cat has been estimated as nil (Wallace et al. 1993).

The oocysts of *Toxoplasma* survive for more than 1 year in soil under optimal conditions (Frenkel et al. 1975). The cysts in pork meat survive for 10 minutes at 52°C; temperatures of 61°C or higher kill all cysts in less than 4 minutes (Dubey et al. 1990).

Immunity and Pathogenesis.

Toxoplasma gondii is a pathogen for humans with an extremely low virulence in immune-competent hosts and requires strong immune suppression to express significant virulence; in these hosts, marked virulence is universal. The mechanism by which *Toxoplasma* damages cells is not known, other than the observation that mechanical destruction of the parasitized cell occurs together with death of neighboring cells, resulting in microscopic areas of necrosis. This process is observed in tissues of patients with early lesions; arteritis with thrombosis and destruction of blood vessels mainly in the brain, produces infarcts in larger areas of brain tissue. *Toxoplasma* parasitizes all kinds of cells, including macrophages. In the macrophages the parasite is located within parasitophorous vacuoles and may survive the killing mechanisms of the macrophages by neutralizing the enzymes released by the lysosomes. Macrophages activated by interferon gamma kill phagocytized *Toxoplasma*, which provides some protection to animals against reinfection. The presence of interferon gamma is necessary for mice to develop immunity to the infection (Deckert et al. 1996).

Humoral and cellular immunity to *Toxoplasma* has been investigated for many years because the parasite is easy to keep in infected laboratory animals and tissue cell cultures. It has long been known that specific anti-*Toxoplasma* antibodies lyse extracellular organisms, but no amount of specific antibodies given to an animal can prevent the infection. Moreover, immunity to the infection develops in animals with a genetic defect that prevents production of antibodies. The role of T lymphocytes in the immunopathology of toxoplasmosis was demonstrated over three decades ago in experimental animals by irradiation and destruction of their immune cells and by selective replacement of T cells and B cells. These experimental data from animals were proven correct later in humans infected by HIV. The immune response to toxoplasmosis resembles the response to *T. cruzi*, another species that parasitizes all kinds of cells. The organisms invade the body and somehow activate macrophages that destroy the parasites in acidic vacuoles, releasing peptides that bind to major histocompatibility complex molecules type II, to be expressed on the surface of the macrophage. Presentation of the antigen to CD4+ T lymphocytes activates them, causing them to differentiate into T helper 1 (Th1) cells that secrete interleukin-2 (IL-2) and interferon gamma, cytokines that activate more macrophages, natural killer cells, and the killer CD8+ T lymphocytes. Thus primed, the immune system controls the parasite and results in an asymptomatic infection. This process is demonstrated in experimental animals, in which innate immunity to the infection is related to their different levels in interferon gamma and IL-12 (Walker et al. 1997). The difference between the immune response to *Toxoplasma* and to *T. cruzi* is that in *T. cruzi*, modulation of the immune response allows controlled multiplication of the parasite, producing a

lifelong silent infection with clinical manifestations decades later.

In individuals with immune deficiencies, especially HIV infection, a decrease in CD4+ T lymphocytes and a gradual shift from a Th1 cell population to a Th2 cell population (Clerici, Shearer, 1993) permit uncontrolled multiplication of the parasite and expression of its virulence until it kills the host.

Disease. Prior to the AIDS epidemic, toxoplasmosis was an infection sporadically seen in aborted fetuses and premature infants; in other patients, benign lymphadenitis and chorioretinitis were the only two diseases observed. Rare opportunistic infections were also seen in individuals with organ transplants, malignancies, and other forms of immune impairment. Today the overwhelming majority of cases of toxoplasmosis occur in HIV-positive individuals, and most pathologists have become acquainted with a disease that was once extremely unusual and difficult to diagnose. In general, three forms of toxoplasmosis are recognized in humans: (*1*) acquired in immune-competent hosts, (*2*) acquired (or reactivated) in immune-deficient hosts, and (*3*) acquired congenitally.

Acquired Toxoplasmosis in Immune-Competent Hosts. As stated before, toxoplasmosis is a common infection in the general population acquired by ingestion of mature oocysts or cysts (bradyzoites) in animal meat. It is universally believed that only a few infected individuals may have transitory symptoms, but evidence from a study of a toxoplasmosis epidemic due to ingestion of oocysts indicates otherwise. Of 37 patients detected in the epidemic, 35 were symptomatic, and of 25 symptomatic patients who consulted a physician, only 3 were diagnosed correctly as having toxoplasmosis (Teutsch et al. 1979). Thus, it appears that most infected persons have symptoms consisting of malaise, fever, enlarged lymph nodes, myalgia, stiff neck, anorexia, arthralgia, skin rash, confusion (associated with fever), and hepatitis. These symptoms are self-limited, are seen in different degrees and combinations, and are not specific. A small number of infected individuals may have a chronic lymphadenitis; others have eye lesions. These two diseases are discussed here.

Lymph nodes. Toxoplasmic lymphadenitis is said to be common in immune-competent children and young adults, mostly women. In England and Wales, the peak age for the disease is between 25 and 34 years of age, with a few cases in persons 65 years of age and older (Jackson, Hutchison, 1989). The clinical features range from asymptomatic lymphadenopathy to lymphaditis of varying severity, in extreme cases producing a chronic debilitating illness with fever, malaise, and progressive swelling of lymph nodes. The swollen nodes are painful, nonsuppurative, and bilateral, with a cervical distribution. Swelling of the nodes begins 2 to 4 weeks after infection and may last for several weeks, a clinical picture that often suggests a malignant lymphoma. In most patients with unusually prolonged clinical toxoplasmic lymphadenitis, removal of an affected lymph node is often necessary for diagnosis. Exception for demonstration of an elevated white blood cell count, and especially lymphocytosis with atypical lymphocytes, the usual laboratory tests are not helpful.

The gross appearance of the removed lymph node is unremarkable except for its enlarged size; it is firm, and the cut surface is slightly pale. The microscopic changes associated with lymphatic toxoplasmosis are marked follicular hyperplasia with relatively well-preserved architecture and prominent epithelioid histiocytic infiltration of the cortical and paracortical regions (Fig. 9–8 *A*). Clusters of epithelioid cells appear to be encroaching on the margins of the follicles, with effacement of their borders. Sometimes epithelioid cells are found within the germinal center. The subcapsular sinuses have abundant mononuclear cells producing marked distention (Fig. 9–8 *B*). In some areas the histiocytic elements are grouped as poorly formed granulomas (Fig. 9–8 *C*) with rare Langhans-type giant cells, and other histiocytic elements have focal areas of necrosis with polymorphonuclear cells. Parasites are rarely found in histologic sections or in lymph node imprints (Fig. 9–8 *D*; Aisner et al. 1983; Fernandez-Rivero, Ramirez, 1984), but if experimental animals (Siim, 1956) or tissue culture cells are inoculated with lymph node tissues, the parasite can often be recovered. The polymerase chain reaction failed to identify *Toxoplasma* DNA in a series of cases diagnosed histologically as toxoplasmic lymphadenitis. It was suggested that the lymph node reaction we have become accustomed to labeling toxoplasmic lymphadenitis may not be due entirely to the parasite (Weiss et al. 1992). Serologic tests are helpful, especially if rising titers are demonstrated. The diagnosis of lymphatic toxoplasmosis is usually based on the microscopic appearance of the lymph node; however, it is not known whether this histologic picture is specific for *Toxoplasma* or if other infectious agents can elicit similar changes.

Eye. Acquired *toxoplasmic retinochoroiditis*, as the disease is known in immune-competent hosts, is probably the most common form of toxoplasmosis. In addition, *Toxoplasma* is the most common cause of retinochoroiditis in the United States (Montoya, Remington, 1996). The disease was misdiagnosed as tuberculosis for many years by clinicians and pathologists alike until it was conclusively demonstrated to be due to *Toxoplasma* in 1952 (Wilder, 1952). It is believed that the disease results from reactivation of a dormant *Toxoplasma* cyst formed during a past active infection in the retina or choroid (Frenkel, Jacobs, 1958). It has also been stated that the active infection responsible for the cyst in the eye is always acquired in utero (Dutton, 1986), but observations of patients with serologic profiles of an acute toxoplasmic infection have shown that some of them can develop chorioretinitis (Montoya, Remington, 1996). Reactivation of a retinal cyst can occur in the presence of corticosteroid therapy (Morhun et al. 1996). Ocular toxoplasmosis is very unusual in patients less than 5 years of age; the majority of cases occur between 15 and 64 years of age (Jacobs et al. 1960). In the Marshall Islands, with 100% *Toxoplasma* seropositivity in adults, the prevalence of retinal lesions is 4% and the incidence of the disease is 273 cases per year per 100,000 seropositive persons (Adams et al. 1987).

Clinically, ocular toxoplasmosis in immune-competent adults manifests as a unilateral, focal, or multifocal retinochoroiditis at the border of an inactive scar, or as a focal necrotizing retinochoroiditis accompanied by various degrees of vitreitis (Fig. 9–9). The primary lesion is acute or subacute, followed by recrudescences that sometimes last for many years. The typical acute lesion is a white, elevated focus of necrotizing retinochoroiditis near an old pigmented scar known as the *satellite lesion* (Pavesio, Lightman, 1996). Other lesions, such as papillitis, have also been described. The lesion usually occurs in the inner retinal layers and is associated with a vitreous reaction; sometimes the outer retinal layers are compromised, causing macular detachment (Doft, Gass, 1985). Outer retinal lesions are seen as multifocal gray-white, discrete patches (Doft, Gass, 1985); the disease appears to be more aggressive in elderly patients (Johnson et al. 1997). In the past, the infection was frequently progressive and led to enucleation after the eye had become phthisic (Frenkel, Jacobs, 1958).

The histologic changes due to ocular toxoplasmosis are known only from descriptions of the final stage of the disease; the manner in which the lesions begin and progress in humans is not known. Lesions occur principally in the retina, the only place where proliferative stages of the parasite are found; sometimes an inflammatory reaction occurs in the choroid, but in spite of its intensity, no organisms are found. The histologic

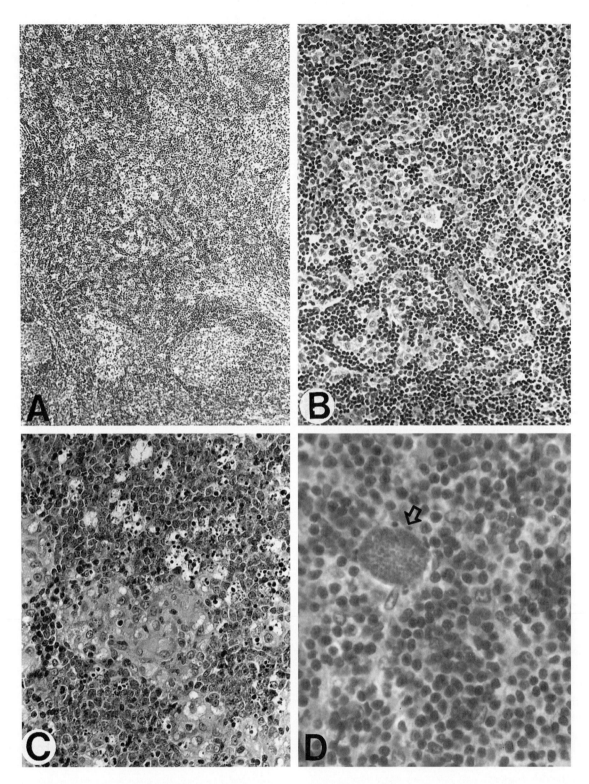

Fig. 9–8. *Toxoplasma gondii.* Microscopic lesions of an acquired lymph node infection in immune-competent hosts, sections stained with hematoxylin and eosin stain. *A*, Low-power view of a lymph node showing hyperplastic changes. The sinusoids are filled with histiocytes, ×70. *B*, Higher magnification showing the infiltration by histiocytes, ×180. *C*, Masses of histiocytes forming pseudogranulomas; microscopic foci of necrosis are seen, ×220. *D*, Cyst (arrow), ×600 (Photograph of cyst courtesy of D. Hood, M.D., Department of Pathology, Cleveland Clinic Foundation, Cleveland, Ohio.)

picture is that of a granulomatous inflammation in the retina sometimes involving the choroid (Fig. 9–10 A–B). Under low-power magnification, expansion and disorganization of the retina due to the granulomas can be seen, with destruction of the retina and cellular infiltration. The granulomas consist of histiocytic cells, and the inflammatory reaction is composed of lymphocytes and plasma cells (Fig. 9–10 B). In active lesions, necrosis and proliferative forms of *Toxoplasma* are present; otherwise, only granulomas are seen and parasites are difficult to find (Fig. 9–10 B). Completely healed lesions have well-formed granulomas with epithelioid and giant cells. Cases of toxoplasmic iridocyclitis have rarely been reported (Frenkel, Jacobs, 1958). The polymerase chain reaction has been used in aqueous humor for specific diagnosis of ocular toxoplasmosis (Brezin et al. 1991).

Other lesions allegedly produced by *Toxoplasma* in immune-competent patients have been described, such as chronic cardiomyopathy (Niedmann et al. 1959; Niedmann et al. 1962). In these cases, demonstration and description of the parasite have been unsatisfactory. Skin lesions (Binazzi, Papini, 1980) and dermatomyositis (Lapetina, 1989) have also been attributed to *Toxoplasma*, based mostly on positive serology. In some cases, organisms in skin biopsy specimens were "demonstrated" (i.e., shown in accompanying photographs) (Binazzi, 1986). However, in none of these cases were the identifying characteristics of the organisms described, casting doubt on the role of *Toxoplasma* in cardiac, hepatic, and dermal lesions in immune-competent individuals.

Acquired (or reactivated) Toxoplasmosis in Immune-Suppressed Hosts. It has already been stated that the great majority of cases of acquired toxoplasmosis in immune-deficient hosts are seen in individuals in the HIV/AIDS group. In these individuals, the disease is similar in many respects to that seen in persons immune-suppressed for other reasons. However, in the HIV/AIDS group the infection tends to be more disseminated, sometimes targets organs other than the central nervous system, and is often easier to diagnose microscopically because of the large number of organisms.

Clinical disease in immune-suppressed individuals results from reactivation of a latent infection, though seldom from a newly acquired one. The mechanism of reactivation is unknown. Reactivation occurs when a cyst in the tissues ruptures, freeing zoites that infect other cells (Frenkel, Escajadillo, 1987). The infection may be localized to the area where the cyst ruptures, producing encephalitis, orchitis, pancreatitis, pneu-

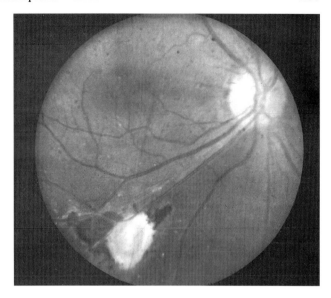

Fig. 9–9. *Toxoplasma gondii* in the eye. Area of chorioretinitis showing an inactive lesion with gliosis and inflammation (white area at the bottom) of the retina and an active lesion consisting of hypertrophy and hyperplasia of retinal pigment epithelium (dark area at the bottom). (Courtesy of H. Grossniklaus, M.D., Department of Ophthalmology and Pathology, University Hospitals of Cleveland, Cleveland, Ohio.)

monitis, myocarditis, gastroenteritis, colitis, cystitis, or any combination of these diseases. Often the infection becomes generalized. Encephalitis is the most commonly diagnosed condition because it is life-threatening and is in the minds of clinicians every time symptoms occur in the central nervous system. It is estimated that in the United States, 5% to 10% of individuals with AIDS will develop toxoplasmic encephalitis (McCabe, Remington, 1988). A study in Norway showed that of 238 HIV-infected patients, 40 (18%) were positive for *Toxoplasma*, 20 (8%) of whom developed the disease (Dunlop et al. 1996). These estimates will probably decrease in some countries due to advances in the treatment of HIV infection. In the following sections, we will consider the clinical aspects and morphologic changes in each organ affected by the parasite in this group of patients.

Central nervous system. Clinically, acquired central nervous system toxoplasmosis usually presents as an acute illness with fever, headache, focal neurologic deficit, and seizures (Porter, Sande, 1992). With computed tomography (CT) scans and magnetic resonance imaging (MRI), contrast-enhancing lesions can be found facilitating the diagnosis. Diffuse meningoencephalitis with headache, disorientation, and drowsi-

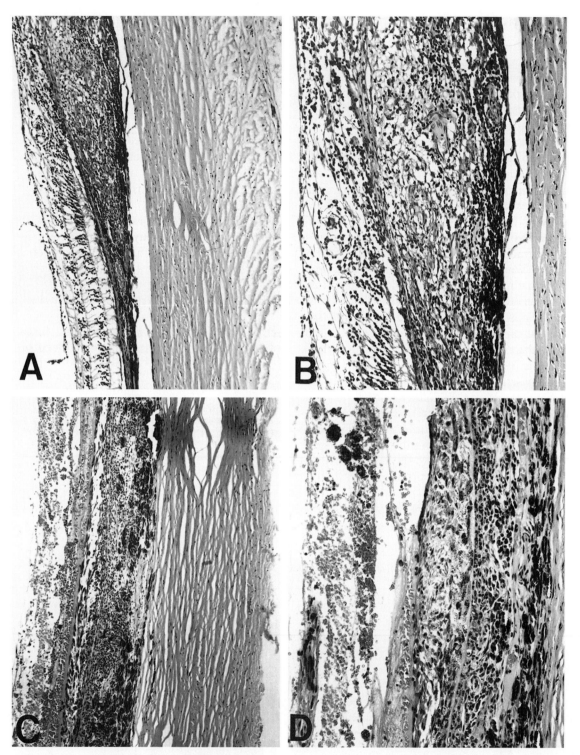

Fig. 9–10. *Toxoplasma gondii*, microscopic lesions of ocular infections; sections stained with hematoxylin and eosin stain. *A* and *B*, immune-competent host. *A*, Low-power view showing marked expansion of the choroid layer and destruction of the retina, ×70 (normal retina at bottom). *B*, Higher magnification showing the granulomatous nature of the inflammatory reaction in the choroid; there are many histiocytes and poorly formed granulomas. Lymphocytes and plasma cells are abundant. Parasites (not shown) are few in number, ×140. *C* and *D*, immune-suppressed host. *C*, Low-power view showing massive necrosis of the retina and hemorrhage. The choroid has an abundant inflammatory reaction, ×70. *D*, Higher magnification showing the inflammatory reaction. Clinically, the picture is identical to that of acute retinal necrosis syndrome, ×140. (Preparations for *C* and *D* courtesy of R.L. Font, M.D., Department of Pathology, Cullen Eye Institute, Baylor College of Medicine, Houston, Texas. Reported by: Parke, D.W. II, and Font, R.L. 1986. Diffuse toxoplasmic retinochoroiditis in a patient with AIDS. Arch. Ophthalmol. 104:571–575.)

ness, rapidly progressing to coma and death, is the presentation in some patients (Caramello et al. 1993). If brain damage is extensive, symptoms of a space-occupying lesion may be observed. If damage is confined to the cortical motor zones, hemiparesis or seizures can be the presenting symptoms. Other neurologic signs include decreased mental status, coma, papilledema, involvement of cranial nerves, and cord lesions. Psychotic symptoms were not described in *Toxoplasma* encephalitis before the AIDS epidemic began. When present, they may be a manifestation of the HIV infection rather than of the parasite. In addition, HIV encephalopathy can produce symptoms similar to those of central nervous system toxoplasmosis (Navia et al. 1986; Wanke et al. 1987). Cases of toxoplasmosis manifesting as outright dementia, with no radiologic lesions and no demonstrable HIV virus in the brain, have been reported (Arendt et al. 1991). Another clinical presentation, which appears to be rare, is that of a thalamic syndrome (Dejerine-Roussy) with pain due to a lesion in the thalamus (Gonzales et al. 1992). Symptoms and signs of myelities such as motor loss, usually paraparesis, bilateral sensory loss, urinary bladder dysfunction, and local pain are seen in patients with spinal cord lesions (Vyas, Ebright, 1996). The most relevant laboratory findings are the lesions found with CT (Fig. 9–11 *A*), MRI (Fig. 9–11 *B*), and other imaging techniques. The lesions seen in CT scans are either single or multiple and are located anywhere in the brain. Contrast studies show most lesions with contrast uptake, some focally, others as single rings.

Edema is usually marked, hydrocephalus is moderate to marked (Nolla Salas et al. 1987), and a mass effect is present in most patients (Donovan Post et al. 1983). In some cases, CT scans have shown only hydrocephalus and a prominent choroid plexus (Bourgouin et al. 1992). MRI is useful to detect spinal cord lesions (Poon et al. 1992). Based on radiographic studies and spinal fluid examination alone, distinction between central nervous system lymphoma and *Toxoplasmosis* in patients with AIDS is almost impossible (Edwards, Pendlebury, 1987).

The standard laboratory tests are not specific; the cerebrospinal fluid may be normal or may have increased glucose, protein, and polymorphonuclear cells. In 90% of patients CD4+ T lymphocyte counts are less than 200 cells per cubic millimeter, and in two-thirds of the patients they are less than 100 (Porter, Sande, 1992). Serology is positive in most patients, but up to 16% are negative. Spinal fluid immunoglobulin G (IgG) titers are positive in the majority of patients (Porter, Sande, 1992). Negative serologic tests may signify a newly acquired infection. Smears of spinal fluid sediment stained with Wright or Giemsa stain (Threlkeld et al. 1987), as well as cytocentrifuge smears (DeMent et al. 1987), should be examined. Culture of spinal fluid in tissue culture cells may reveal the parasites (Caramello et al. 1993). Finally, the polymerase chain reaction can detect parasite DNA (Parmley et al. 1992; Schoondermark van de Ven et al. 1993).

The gross appearance of central nervous system toxoplasmosis is that of a swollen, edematous brain

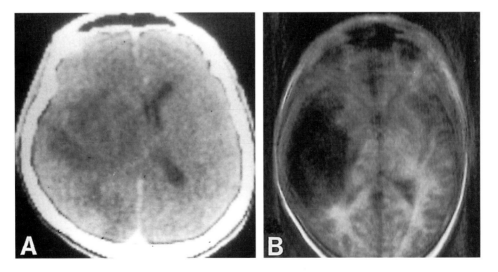

Fig. 9–11. *Toxoplasma gondii*. Radiographs of central nervous system infection in AIDS. *A*, CT scan showing a large lesion on the right cerebral hemisphere. *B*, MRI scan of the brain of a young hemophiliac who was treated successfully for *Toxoplasma* infection and died 18 months later of other complications.

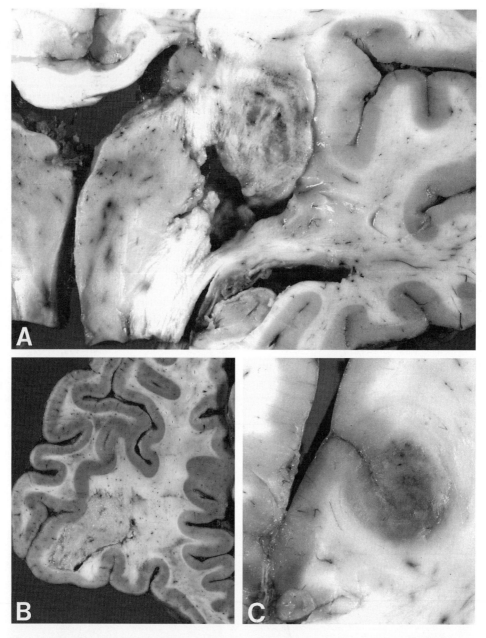

Fig. 9–12. *Toxoplasma gondii.* Gross lesions of central nervous system infection in three patients with AIDS. *A,* Coronal section of brain, same patient as in Figure 9–11 *A,* showing extensive necrosis on the right basal ganglia. *B* and *C,* Coronal brain sections from two other patients showing necrotic lesions.

Fig. 9–13. *Toxoplasma gondii.* Microscopic lesions of central nervous system infection in a patient with AIDS, sections stained with hematoxylin and eosin stain. *A,* Focal necrosis with a minimal inflammatory infiltrate around a capillary. Parasitized cells are present (arrows), ×350. *B,* Larger area of necrosis with many infiltrating cells (mononuclear and polymorphonuclear) and abundant parasites. Some stages appear to be cysts, but often this is difficult to determine, ×180. *C,* Medium-sized vessel with arteritis. All layers of the wall show infiltration by lymphocytes and plasma cells, ×350. *D,* Low-power view of the area between necrotic tissue (top) and less involved tissue (bottom). The center shows walling off of the lesion, with marked hyperemia, macrophages, a leukocytic infiltrate, and earlier granulation tissue, ×55.

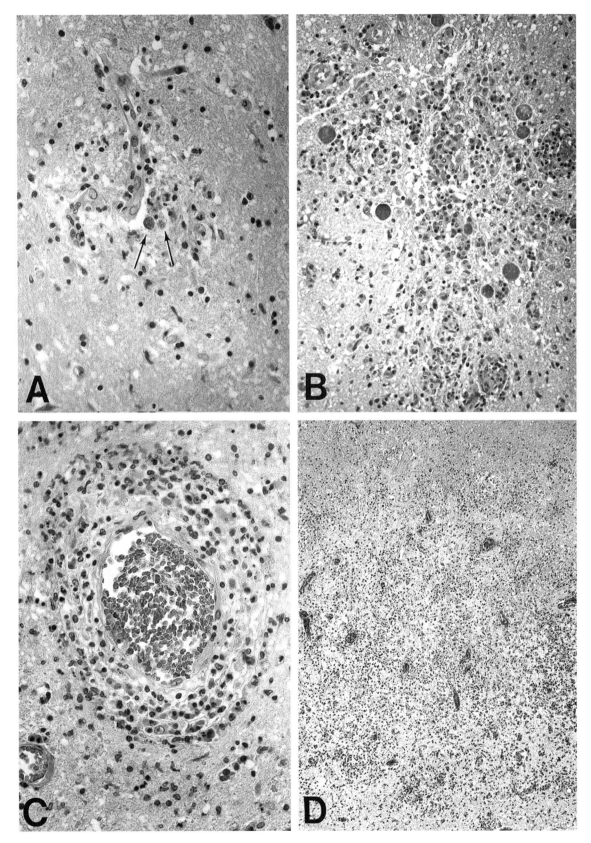

Fig. 9–13.

with signs of uncal, tonsillar, or transtentorial herniation. Lesions on the surface of the brain may not be appreciated. However, coronal sections show multiple necrotic, sometimes hemorrhagic, areas (Fig. 9–12 A–C), varying from a few millimeters to 5 cm in diameter, in the basal ganglia and other central areas of the brain, cerebellum, and spinal cord.

The most important microscopic features of central nervous system toxoplasmosis are the extensive necrosis in various stages of organization (Fig. 9–13 D) and a prominent vasculitis involving small, medium-sized, and large vessels (Fig. 9–13 C). The vasculitis is responsible for thrombosis, which produces the extensive infarct-like necrosis (Frenkel, 1971; Huang, Chou, 1988). At the periphery, the lesions have variable amounts of acute and chronic inflammation, and often contain proliferative forms (tachyzoites) and cysts (bradyzoites; Fig. 9–13 B). The amount of infiltration depends on the clinical stage of the HIV infection (Falangola et al. 1994). Patients in whom toxoplasmosis manifests early in the HIV in-

fection have moderate cell infiltration, while those in whom the infection manifests later have little or none (Falangola et al. 1994). The surrounding brain tissue has microscopic areas of necrosis with parasites (Fig. 9–13 A) or glial nodules (granulomas) and scanty inflammation (Fig. 9–13 A–B). In successfully treated patients who die months later from other complications of AIDS, the healed lesions in the brain are indistinguishable from healed, cavitated infarcts (Fig. 9–14 A–B). In some patients presenting with dementia, the histologic picture consists of diffuse involvement of the brain without gross lesions, with numerous parasites producing glial nodules (Arendt et al. 1991). In patients with hydrocephalus alone, diffuse destruction (necrosis) of the ependymal lining of the ventricles with a marked inflammatory reaction of the periventricular brain tissue is seen (Bourgouin et al. 1992). The choroid plexus is involved in half of the patients and in about three-fourths of those with acute necrotizing encephalitis. Abscesses of the choroid plexus are found in some cases; rarely is the choroid

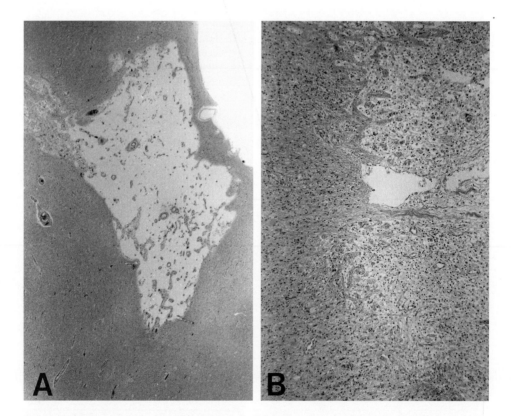

Fig. 9–14. *Toxoplasma gondii*, healed brain lesion in a patient with AIDS, sections stained with hematoxylin and eosin stain. Same individual described in Figure 9–11 *A*, 18 months after successful treatment for *Toxoplasma* infection. *A* and *B*, The lesion appears as a healed, cavitated infarct with abundant granulation tissue and macrophages at the edge of the lesion, *A* ×10, *B* ×47.

plexus the only structure involved by *Toxoplasma* (Falangola, Petito, 1993).

Heart. The heart is the second most common organ involved by *Toxoplasma* in the immune-suppressed patient (Hofman et al. 1993a; Jautzke et al. 1993). In a few cases the cardiac disease is an isolated infection; more commonly, it occurs together with disease in other viscera (Hofman et al. 1993b). The disease is important both in individuals with AIDS and in those with heart transplants. In transplant patients the disease has received much attention because *Toxoplasma* myocarditis, or any other organ involvement, is the source of unwarranted morbidity and mortality in this group. In England, 35% of heart transplant recipients had negative serology, whereas 26% of donors were positive, resulting in an approximately 17% chance that a heart from a seropositive donor went to a seronegative recipient (Nagington, Martin, 1983). In the United States, the figure is about 7% (Luft et al. 1983). Between 2% and 5% of individuals with a heart transplant develop toxoplasmic encephalitis, more often acquired from the infected transplanted heart than from other sources (Luft et al. 1986). Reactivation of an old *Toxoplasma* infection in the recipient due to the use of immune-suppressive therapy is important (Wreghitt et al. 1989), but to a lesser extent (Gallino et al. 1996). Seropositive recipients who receive a heart from a seropositive donor have an increase in antibody titers, sometimes of IgM, but they do not develop disease (Luft et al. 1983). Prophylaxis in all transplant patients who are seronegative for *Toxoplasma* antibodies before surgery is recommended (Wreghitt et al. 1989).

The clinical findings in *Toxoplasma* myocarditis are similar to those in any other type of myocarditis. The gross appearance of the heart is often unremarkable, but in some cases it is flabby and moderately to markedly dilated; on cut sections it may have a discolored appearance or show multiple punctate hemorrhages. The microscopic findings are variable. In some cases, areas of dropout myocytes with an inflammatory infiltrate or areas of microscopic necrosis with a more marked infiltration by mononuclear and polymorphonuclear cells are seen (Fig. 9–15 A–B). In some areas, only myocytes containing nests of proliferative forms of *Toxoplasma* (pseudocysts) without inflammation or necrosis are found (Fig. 9–15 C). Cysts are rare in acute infections (Fig. 9–15 D–E), and in some cases, the histologic demonstration of parasites is difficult because of their small number. In cases where only a lymphocytic infiltration is present, anti-*Toxoplasma* immunolabeling demonstrates the parasites (Hofman et al. 1993b). *Toxoplasma* organisms in myocardial sections of autopsy material or in sections of myocardial biopsy specimens are usually unexpected because the infection is usually not suspected on clinical grounds. In autopsy material from patients without clinical myocarditis, the finding may consist of a few organisms with little or no inflammatory reaction. In these patients, the presence of the parasites should be interpreted cautiously: the patient had an infection that did not have time to develop fully; this is *Toxoplasma* infection without toxoplasmosis. On cardiac biopsy specimens, the finding of one or two nests of parasites is more difficult to interpret because these specimens often are obtained for diagnosis in patients with heart transplants and signs of rejection. The histologic lesion produced by rejection and the lesion produced by *Toxoplasma* in the heart are indistinguishable, making either diagnosis impossible unless abundant parasites and the myocarditis are found. Further, the question that often arises is whether the parasites were present in the transplanted heart or whether they are the product of reactivation of an infection in the recipient. The serologic status for *Toxoplasma* of the donor and the recipient may clarify the situation in some cases (Ryning et al. 1979).

In a clinical myocarditis without microscopic demonstration of *Toxoplasma* in tissue sections, the parasite was recovered with animal inoculations (Potts, Williams, 1956). This finding should remain doubtful because circulating *Toxoplasma* in individuals with HIV is common (Asensi et al. 1993; Tirard et al. 1991), and inoculating cultures or animals with tissue fragments may produce positive results. To determine the toxoplasmic nature of these cases of myocarditis, organisms should be demonstrated with immune staining or with the polymerase chain. In rare cases, both myocarditis and pericarditis attributed to *Toxoplasma* have been reported (Hakkila et al. 1958).

Lung. The lungs are the third most common organ involved by toxoplasmosis (Hofman et al. 1993a; Jautzke et al. 1993; Rabaud et al. 1996). This condition occurs either alone (Schnapp et al. 1992) or accompanied by cerebral or disseminated infection (Bergin et al. 1992; Garcia et al. 1991). The percentage of cases of toxoplasmic pneumonitis remains low in comparison to that of encephalitis; it was estimated at 5% in a prospective study based on bronchoalveolar lavage samples (Derouin et al. 1990). Pulmonary toxoplasmosis is found in individuals with malignancies (Bendelac et al. 1984) and bone marrow transplants (Saad et al. 1996), but it is more common in those with HIV infections (Prosmanne et al. 1984).

The clinical manifestations vary, depending on the stage of the infection, from asymptomatic (Catterall et al. 1986) to rapidly progressive respiratory failure re-

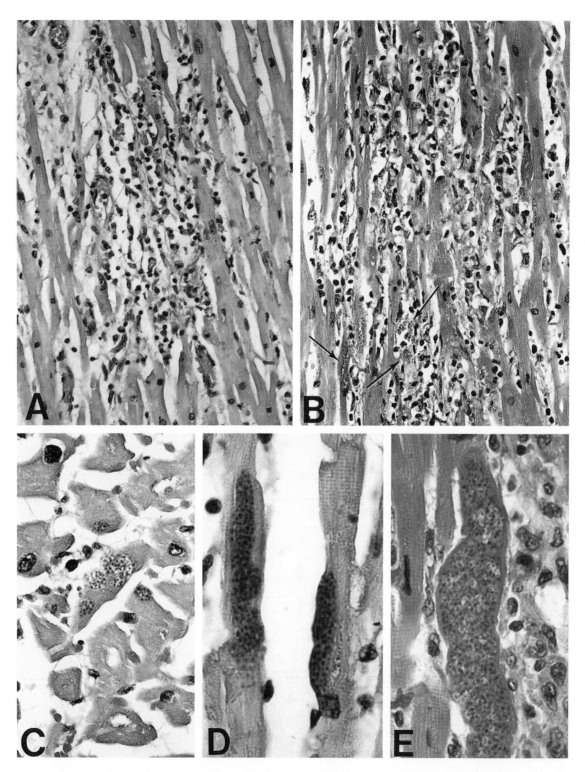

Fig. 9–15. *Toxoplasma gondii* myocarditis, sections stained with hematoxylin and eosin stain. *A*, Microscopic areas of myocarditis without parasites, ×220. *B*, Section from another patient with generalized toxoplasmosis. The changes are identical to those seen in the previous picture; numerous parasites are present, but they are difficult to see at this magnification (arrows), ×280. *C* and *D*, Higher magnification of another area of the heart from the autopsy material in A. Note that the colonies (pseudocysts) in cells cut on cross sections do not enlarge the parasitized muscle cells (*C*), and the colonies in cells cut longitudinally illustrate their elongated shape (*D*), *C* ×450, *D* ×700. *E*, Section of another patient's heart showing a *Toxoplasma* cyst in a muscle cell. Note the thin wall, the tightly packed minute zoites, the lack of compartments (compared with *Sarcocystis*), and the normal width of the muscle cell, ×700.

sembling *Pneumocystis* pneumonia (Bonilla, Rosa, 1994). The clinical diagnosis remains elusive, and the condition is often recognized at autopsy (Knani et al. 1990; Touboul et al. 1986). The presenting symptoms and signs and the radiologic appearance of the disease are nonspecific (Oksenhendler et al. 1990). The main symptoms are cough and shortness of breath, and the signs are high fever and rales (Pomeroy, Filice, 1992). On x-ray films a conspicuous diffuse, small nodular or reticulonodular infiltrate of both lungs is apparent, especially during the earlier stages of the infection (Bergin et al. 1992; Prosmanne et al. 1984). However, this infiltrate changes rapidly as the infection evolves (Bonilla, Rosa, 1994). Laboratory tests not helpful; biopsy specimens (Derouin et al. 1989) or bronchoalveolar lavage samples should be taken to demonstrate the organisms (Bonilla, Rosa, 1994). The extreme elevation of serum lactic dehydrogenase seen in toxoplasmic pneumonitis appears useful in distinguishing this disease from *Pneumocystis* pneumonia (Pugin et al. 1992).

The gross appearance of the lungs in *Toxoplasma* pneumonitis is similar to that seen in other pneumonitides. The microscopic changes consist of hyperemia and an alveolar exudate consisting mostly of macrophages, other mononuclear and polymorphonuclear cells, and often abundant proliferative forms of *Toxoplasma* parasites in both interstitial and alveolar cells (Fig. 9–16 A–D; Bergin et al. 1992; Nash et al. 1994). In some patients, there are widespread foci of microscopic necrosis (Fig. 9–16 C) that correlate with the x-ray picture of small nodular infiltrates (Prosmanne et al. 1984). Larger areas of parenchymal necrosis may also be present (Nash et al. 1994). The lesions can be diffuse, confined to one lung, or have a lobar pattern.

Pancreas. A single case of involvement of the pancreas by *Toxoplasma*, with a histologic picture of pancreatitis, is known (Ahuja et al. 1993). However, the most frequent finding is that of pancreatic disease in disseminated toxoplasmosis (Hofman et al. 1993a; Jautzke et al. 1993).

Eye. The clinical and histologic pictures of *Toxoplasma* retinitis in immune-suppressed patients vary greatly from those seen in immune-competent hosts. Retinitis in immune-suppressed patients is due mainly to cytomegalovirus, but herpes simplex virus, herpes zoster virus, and *Toxoplasma* also play a role. Clinical distinction between these forms of retinitis is not possible, and most cases often require invasive techniques for etiologic diagnosis. Clinically, the infection may be acute, sometimes bilateral (Holland et al. 1988), progressing in a confluent manner, with lesions that are larger than those seen in immune-competent hosts. The

lesions are sometimes multiple, in others more diffuse; in some cases, optic nerve involvement with severe loss of vision has been documented (Berger et al. 1993; Grossniklaus et al. 1990). A miliary-type presentation consisting of numerous regularly spaced lesions (Berger et al. 1993) and rapid necrosis of the retina and the choroid, similar to that produced by some viruses, are also forms of the infection (Bottoni et al. 1990; Parke, Font, 1986).

Grossly, the enucleated eye has only a hazy brown lesion, or lesions at the posterior pole and a friable, necrotic retina (Grossniklaus et al. 1990). Histologically, the retinal necrosis is marked, and mononuclear cells, hemorrhage, and thrombosis of blood vessels are evident (Fig. 9–10 C–D). Within the necrotic retina and pigment epithelium, few or no inflammatory cells are present (Holland et al. 1988). Free melanin pigment and proliferative *Toxoplasma* forms are seen, as well as mononuclear cell infiltration of the choroid. Macrophages containing pigment are also present within a proteinaceous eosinophilic matrix (Parke, Font, 1986).

Skin. Skin lesions produced by *Toxoplasma* have been described, especially in disseminated infections; clinically, they manifest as a rash, sometimes with small nodules. In an immune-suppressed individual with multiple purpuric skin nodules up to 1 cm in diameter, parasites with some characteristics of *Toxoplasma* in electron micrographs were found (Leyva, Santa Cruz, 1986).

Gastrointestinal Tract. In the gastrointestinal tract, *Toxoplasma* in immune-suppressed individuals produces some important syndromes. It has been found in the stomach (Falcone et al. 1991), sometimes producing narrowing of the antrum (Smart et al. 1990). It has also appeared in the small intestine (Jautzke et al. 1993) in patients with marked necrosis of the mucosa and gastrointestinal symptoms (Fig. 9–18 A–D). In the colon, it produces colitis (Pauwels et al. 1992). It should be kept in mind that these cases may not represent reactivation of an old infection, especially if no other organs are involved, but may instead be an acquired infection. The lesions are mostly necrotic mucosa because the parasite invades most cells, including enterocytes, where it develops asexually, as in all other tissues (Fig. 9–18 A–D). These patients may be seronegative for *Toxoplasma* antigens because of the recently acquired infection.

Other organs. Invasion of almost every organ system by *Toxoplasma* is well documented in the literature. The histologic picture is similar to that described above: nests of organisms with no cellular infiltrate, or focal necrosis with organisms and inflammatory cells in variable numbers, or larger necrotic areas. The fol-

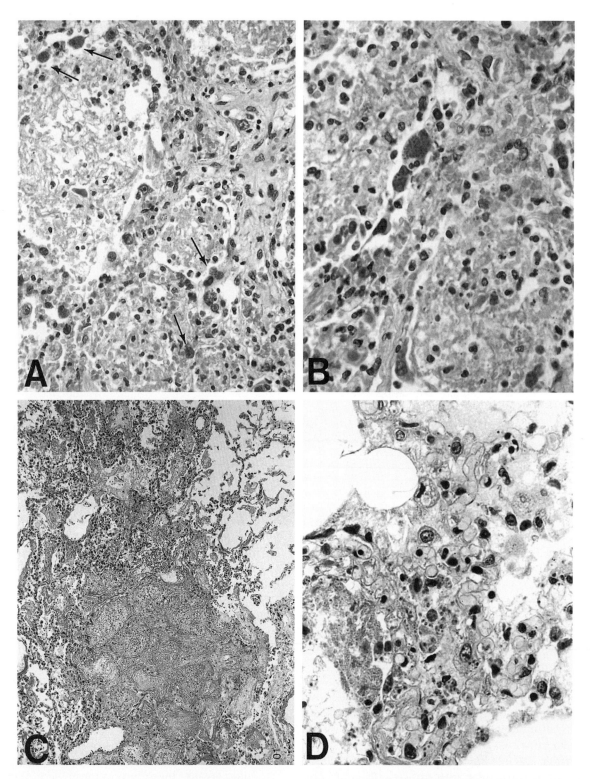

Fig. 9–16. *Toxoplasma gondii*. Microscopic lesions of a pulmonary infection in immune-suppressed hosts, sections stained with hematoxylin and eosin stain. *A* and *B*, Medium-power magnification showing expansion of the septa, with a small lymphocytic infiltrate. Alveoli contain desquamated necrotic cells, fibrin, and a few infiltrating cells. Parasitized cells are seen throughout the septa and alveoli, most with tachyzoites, ×450. *C*, Low-power view of lung section from another patient showing focal microscopic areas of necrosis, ×70. *D*, Higher magnification of lung section from another patient showing abundant tachyzoites in the septa, ×450.

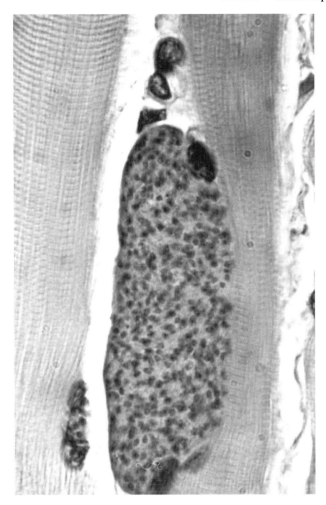

Fig. 9–17. *Toxoplasma gondii* in skeletal muscle from a patient with AIDS, sections stained with hematoxylin and eosin stain. *Toxoplasma* cyst in section of skeletal muscle. The parasite appears to be located in the skeletal muscle, but it is in an unidentified interstitial cell. Note the lack of septae, the small zoites, the thin cyst wall, and the cell nucleus (top), ×1,340.

Congenital Toxoplasmosis. Toxoplasma is transmitted to the fetus only if the mother acquires the infection during pregnancy, regardless of the presence or absence of symptoms in the mother. Only during the acute infection do the trophozoites of *Toxoplasma* circulate in blood and enter the placenta and the fetus. Thus, in any given woman, only one pregnancy can result in congenital toxoplasmosis (Desmonts, Couvreur, 1974; Dische, Gooch, 1981). This view, once considered firmly established, has been shaken by the description of cases in which the infection was transmitted by mothers known to be immune before conception (Vogel et al. 1996). The situation in women who are HIV positive is clearly different. Women supposedly immune (with circulating antibodies to *Toxoplasma*) often have circulating parasites and may pass the infection to the fetus at any time (Mitchell et al. 1990). Yet, the infection is rarely acquired by the fetus (Dunn et al. 1996; Minkoff et al. 1997). The prevalence of toxoplasmosis in women of childbearing age is relatively low in the United States (38%) and Great Britain and is high in France (84%) and the Central American countries. These data indicate that in the United States 62% and in France 16% of women of childbearing age are at risk of contracting the infection during pregnancy. However, only a small fraction do so, and transmission to the fetus occurs in less than 50% of this group (Dische, Gooch, 1981). These prevalence data also indicate that congenital toxoplasmosis is more common in France than in the United States and England because transmission is more active in France. Several studies show that the incidence of congenital toxoplasmosis in various countries varies from 0.5 to 8.7 per 1000 people (Jackson, Hutchison, 1989). Toxoplasmosis in the fetus differs from acquired toxoplasmosis in that the fetus has an immature immunologic system, and although it receives circulating antibodies from the mother, it has no cell-mediated immunity. In many respects, congenital toxoplasmosis parallels acquired toxoplasmosis in immune-suppressed individuals.

Clinical findings. The clinical manifestations of congenital toxoplasmosis are multiple and variable, and the disease should be included in the differential diagnosis of every obscure illness of fetuses and infants. The severity of the manifestations in the fetus varies according to when during pregnancy the infection is acquired; they are more severe during the first two trimesters. The role of the parasite as a cause of abortion appears minimal (Desmonts, Couvreur, 1974). Infants born with toxoplasmosis have abnormalities such as hydrocephalus and microphthalmia of different de-

lowing organ systems can be affected: testis (Crider et al. 1988; Haskell et al. 1989; Hofman et al. 1993a; Jautzke et al. 1993); skeletal muscles (Fig. 9–17; Gherardi et al. 1992); urinary bladder, where it has presented as an intravesical mass (Gluckman, Werboff, 1994), or as thickening of the wall (Hofman et al. 1993c), or as a cystitis (Welker et al. 1994); lymph nodes (Hofman et al. 1993a; Jautzke et al. 1993); peritoneum (Israelski et al. 1988); and pituitary gland, with manifestations of panhypopituitarism (Milligan et al. 1984).

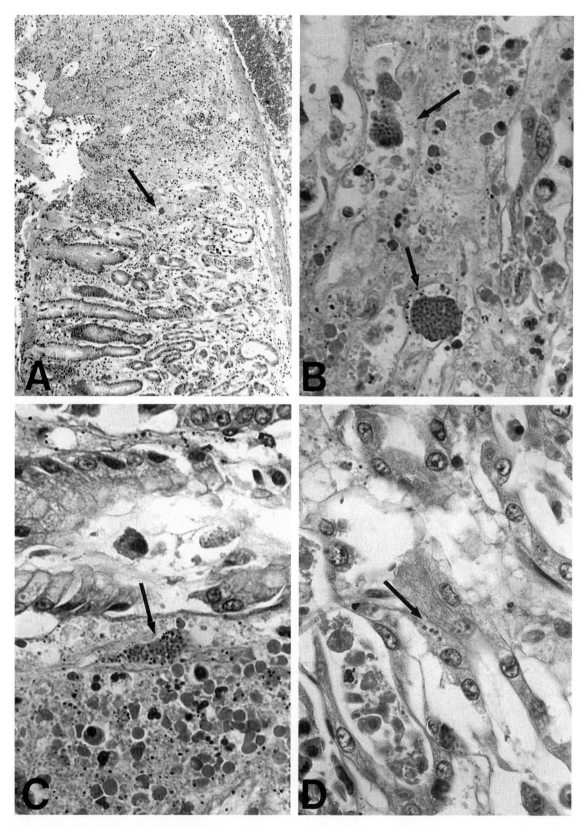

Fig. 9–18. *Toxoplasma gondii* in small intestine of a patient with AIDS, sections stained with hematoxylin and eosin stain. *A*, Low-power view showing necrosis of the intestinal mucosa. A pseudocyst is visible at the center of the picture (arrow), ×70. *B–D*, Higher magnification showing the lesion and the parasites in several cells (arrows), ×570. Note the damage and distortion of the architecture of the glandular epithelium in *A* and *D*.

grees, depending on the severity of the infection. Other symptoms and neurologic deficits manifest as the infant grows, sometimes beginning as early at 3 weeks of age (Dutton, 1986).

In aborted fetuses, the manifestations of congenital toxoplasmosis are severe hydrocephalus, microphthalmia, brain calcifications, generalized icterus, and enlarged liver. In newborn infants, the symptoms vary from subclinical to mild or fulminant. In subclinical cases, the disease is frequently undiagnosed. Sequelae such as mental retardation, convulsive seizures (Eichenwald, 1960), cerebral calcifications, chorioretinitis, and other central nervous system symptoms appear later in infancy or in childhood.

Acute or fulminant *Toxoplasma* infection of the neonatal period is commonly associated with the tetrad of chorioretinitis, hydrocephalus, intracerebral calcifications, and convulsions. In other organ systems there are symptoms of heart failure, anemia, hepatomegaly, petechial hemorrhages, and jaundice, similar to those seen in other congenital infections. The chronic course of these infections may continue, with progressive weight loss, failure to thrive, and death.

Placenta. The gross appearance of the placenta does not parallel the severity of fetal disease and often is unimpressive; however, in one case, placental hydrops and a history of cerebral calcification suggested the diagnosis of *Toxoplasma* (Altshuler, 1973). Microscopically, there usually are changes of mild to florid infection in the villi (Fig. 9–19 *A–B*), in the membranes, the villous plate, and the umbilical cord (Fig. 9–19 *C–D*), with variable numbers of lymphocytes, plasma cells, and a few polymorphonuclear cells (Fig. 9–19 *C*). Areas of microscopic necrosis, calcification (Fig. 9–19 *C*), and vasculitis may be present (Garcia et al. 1983). The parasites (tachyzoites and bradyzoites) are usually difficult to demonstrate in the placenta (Fig. 9–19 *D*).

Central nervous system. The most impressive changes in congenital toxoplasmosis occur in the central nervous system. Grossly, the brain is small in some cases, but an increase in size due to hydrocephalus is more common (Fig. 9–20 *B*). The external brain surface varies from marked attenuation of the gyri (*color plate* V *E*) to lysencephaly, and some patients have subarachnoid hemorrhage; areas of microgyra and polygyra are common. The cut surface shows variable changes; the most impressive one is enormous dilation of the ventricles due to hydrocephalus. In microcephalic brains and in brain remnants from hydrocephalic children, gross necrotic lesions are randomly distributed throughout the tissue. Calcifications are present in the cortex and around the ventricles, appearing as white, chalky, gritty material (Fig. 9–20 *A*). Areas of necrosis

of variable size, confluent and sometimes resembling a tumor, are prominently distributed throughout the white and gray matter (Fig. 9–20 *B*; Dische, Gooch, 1981). The dilation of the ventricles in small brains is due to loss of tissue. Ependymitis resulting in obstruction of the aqueduct of Sylvius is present in all cases of hydrocephalus. Cystic spaces are found in brain tissue.

Microscopically, the lesion in the central nervous system is a chronic meningoencephalitis in various stages of evolution from microscopic areas of necrosis (Fig. 9–21 *A*) with a mononuclear cell infiltrate (Fig. 9–21 *B*) to calcification. These lesions indicate a continuous process of brain tissue destruction. The microscopic nodules of the cellular infiltrate are the earliest reaction to *Toxoplasma* in the central nervous system. These nodules consist of aggregations of microglial cells 80 to 140 μm in diameter (Fig. 9–21 *B*). In the center of the nodules the brain elements are distorted and swollen, and nearby neurons show signs of degeneration. These nodules tend to undergo central necrosis and coalesce to form larger areas of tissue destruction. The small and medium-sized blood vessels show evidence of inflammation. Larger areas of necrosis, when present, have the characteristics of liquefaction necrosis (Fig. 9–21 *D*) and result either from the coalescence of smaller areas, or from occlusion of blood vessels due to arteritis. The edge and the central portion of the necrotic lesions have different stages of organization, depending on their age, and eventually they organize into small cystic spaces. The inflammatory reaction is mainly mononuclear, with abundant lymphocytes, polymorphonuclear cells, and macrophages (Fig. 9–21 *C*). The ependymal lining is also markedly inflamed, especially in the area of the choroid plexus (Fig. 9–21 *C*). *Toxoplasma* bradyzoites and tachyzoites within the tissues are not difficult to find. Parasites are present in 10% to 20% of the cellular nodules examined (Frenkel, Friedlander, 1951).

Eye. The great majority of patients with congenital toxoplasmosis have ocular disease of variable intensity. Often the ocular lesion is the only manifestation of infection at birth, but equally often it may develop later in infancy or childhood to produce blindness as the sole sequela of congenital toxoplasmosis. On gross examination the eyes are markedly deformed, often microphthalmic, with complete disorganization of the choroid and retina, mostly in the posterior pole, beginning at the macula and extending peripherally to involve all structures of the eye (Fig. 9–22 *A–D*).

Microscopically, marked destruction of the ocular tissues with inflammation and edema of all layers and disorganization of the retina, is observed (Fig. 9–22 *B–C*). The chronic damage manifests as an intense

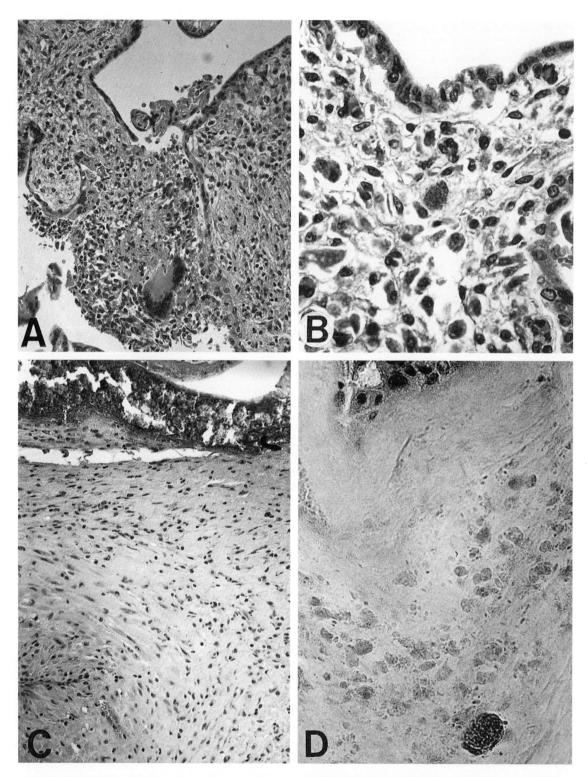

Fig. 9–19. *Toxoplasma gondii* in placenta, sections stained with hematoxylin and eosin stain. *A*, Villitis showing an area of microscopic necrosis, inflammatory cells, and a giant cell, ×180. *B*, Higher magnification of a cell with parasites, ×450. *C* and *D*, Funisitis showing calcification (*C*, top) and a *Toxoplasma* cyst (*D*, bottom), *C* ×180, and *D* ×450. (Preparations courtesy of C.H. Sander, M.D., Department of Pathology, Michigan State University, East Lansing, Michigan.)

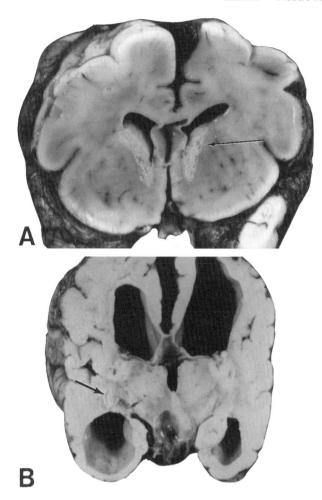

A

B

Fig. 9–20. *Toxoplasma gondii*, coronal brain sections from an infant with congenital infection. *A*, Section showing marked periventricular calcification (arrow). *B*, Coronal section illustrating the hydrocephalus; note the necrosis of the basal ganglia (arrow). (Courtesy of C. Abramowsky, M.D., Institute of Pathology, Case Western Reserve University, Cleveland, Ohio.)

appears flabby and dilated. Microscopically, myocarditis with focal necrosis, inflammatory lymphocytes, histiocytes, and polymorphonuclear leukocytes are found. Proliferative stages of the parasite are usually found in myocardial cells. Microscopically, this lesion is similar to *Toxoplasma* myocarditis of the adult (Fig. 9–15 A–D).

Other tissues. In congenital toxoplasmosis, almost every tissue examined shows microscopic evidence of the disease. Sometimes cysts are found with no inflammatory reaction (Fig. 9–23 A), but more often there is microscopic necrosis and inflammation, with or without proliferative stages of the parasite (Fig. 9–23 B).

Diagnosis. In toxoplasmosis of the immune-competent patient, laboratory diagnosis (i.e., demonstration of the parasite) remains difficult; often serologic tests, interpreted correctly, are most helpful. Specific treatment for toxoplasmosis, with a dramatic response, is also good circumstantial evidence of the infection. In patients who are immune suppressed, the diagnosis is easier because of the large number of parasites in the tissues and in circulation. In patients with AIDS, *Toxoplasma* should be considered in the differential diagnosis of every illness with central nervous system manifestations, as well as in every case of pneumonitis, retinitis, and any form of carditis. *Toxoplasma* infection of other organs is harder to find; only biopsy specimens or other samples may reveal the organisms. It addition, in every newborn who has symptoms of unclear significance, toxoplasmosis should figure in the differential diagnosis. In the diagnosis of congenital toxoplasmosis, the clinician should attempt to isolate *Toxoplasma* from the placenta, umbilical cord, and white blood cells (buffy coat) of cord blood. *Toxoplasma* is identified in body fluids, cell cultures, tissue imprints, and tissue sections.

Body Fluids. Body fluids can be used for direct recovery and visualization of *Toxoplasma* and for inoculation into tissue culture cells (Fig. 9–24 A–B). The fluid samples most commonly submitted to the laboratory are bronchoalveolar lavage fluid (Bendelac et al. 1984; Bonilla, Rosa, 1994) and cerebrospinal fluid (Threlkeld et al. 1987) for preparation of smears, staining, and diagnosis under the microscope. In addition, blood (Tirard et al. 1991), tissue fragments, and other samples may be submitted for culture in tissue cells. Tissue imprints of biopsy specimens and autopsy material for staining and diagnosis also can be received; potentially, *Toxoplasma* can be found and visualized

mononuclear cell infiltrate with organization and calcification (Fig. 9–22 C–D). Persistence of fetal pupillary vessels indicates intrauterine onset of the lesion. The damage of the retina and choroid extends to the vitreous humor, often massively, clinically stimulating a tumor in older children (Fig. 9–22 A–B). Parasites are usually few, but both trophozoites and cysts may be demonstrated.

Heart. The myocardium is involved in many children dying of congenital toxoplasmosis, but the condition is often undiagnosed clinically. The gross appearance of the heart varies with the intensity of the infection; if marked myocarditis is present, the heart

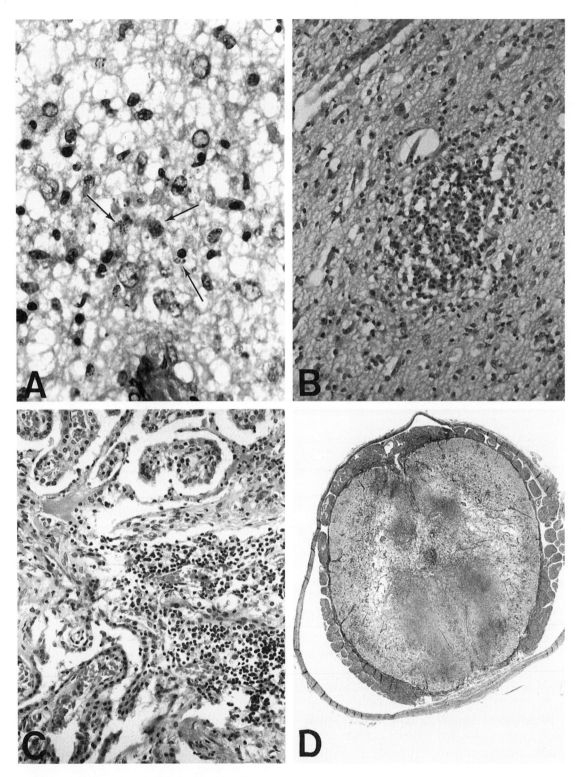

Fig. 9–21. *Toxoplasma gondii*, congenital infection, sections stained with hematoxylin and eosin stain. *A*, Low-power view of early necrosis in white matter showing a small mononuclear cell infiltrate and a few cells with organisms (arrows), ×350. *B*, The cellular nodule composed mostly of mononuclear cells. No parasites are seen in this field, but they are found in 10% to 20% of the nodules studied, ×180. *C*, Marked choroiditis showing a mononuclear cell infiltrate, ×180. *D*, Cross section of spinal cord with marked necrosis. At higher magnification, many organisms were found to be present, ×12. (Tissues courtesy of A. Gutierrez-Hoyos, M.D., Servicio de Patologia, Hospital Aranzazu, San Sebastian, Universidad del Pais Vasco, Spain.)

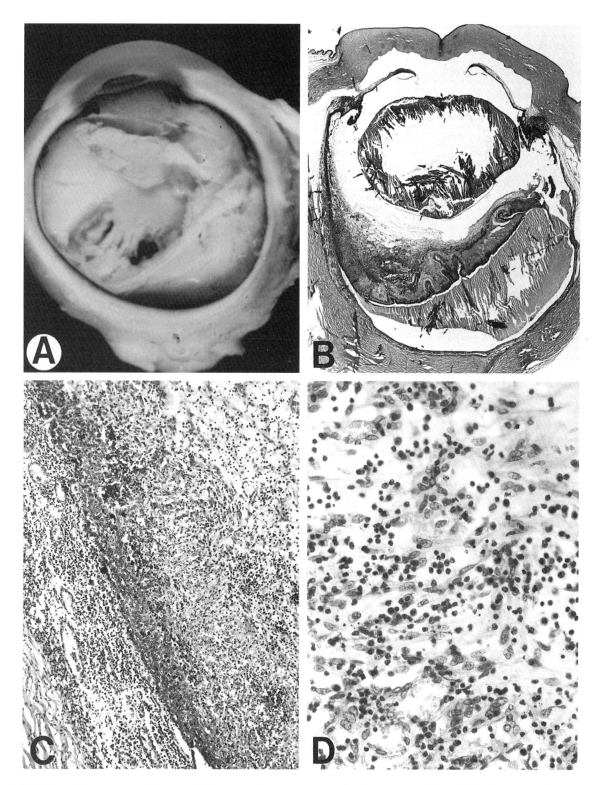

Fig. 9–22. *Toxoplasma gondii*, congenital ocular infection. *A,* Gross picture of a cross section of eye showing marked chorioretinitis. The posterior chamber is filled with blood, granulation tissue, and necrotic debris. *B–C.* Microscopic pictures, sections stained with hematoxylin and eosin stain. *B,* Low-power view showing detachment of the retina due to hemorrhage; florid chorioretinitis with destruction of the retina and choroid with abundant granulation tissue, ×8.7. *C,* Higher magnification showing the inflammatory exudate and destruction of the choroid and retina, ×70. *D,* Higher magnification illustrating fibrosis (repair) and the nature of the infiltrate, consisting of lymphocytes, plasma cells, and polymorphonuclear cells, ×280. (Tissues courtesy of A. Gutierrez-Hoyos, M.D., Servicio de Patologia, Hospital Aranzazu, San Sebastian, Universidad del Pais Vasco, Spain.)

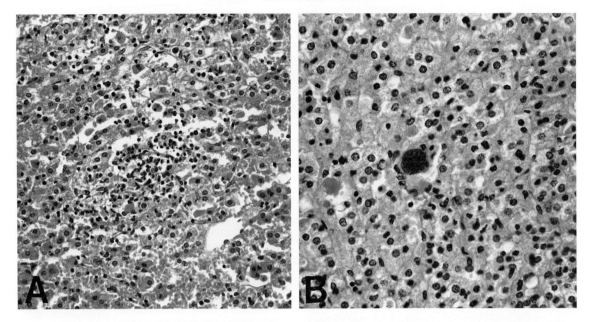

Fig. 9–23. *Toxoplasma gondii*, congenital infection, sections of adrenal gland stained with hematoxylin and eosin stain. *A*, Low-power view of focal necrosis with a mononuclear cell infiltrate, ×180. *B*, Higher magnification of the cyst. Note the lack of inflammatory cells, ×280. (Tissues courtesy of A. Gutierrez-Hoyos, M.D., Servicio de Patologia, Hospital Aranzazu, San Sebastian, Universidad del Pais Vasco, Spain.)

with proper stains in any sample from any other organ. In infants with congenital toxoplasmosis, the polymerase chain reaction in urine samples detects the infection (Fuentes et al. 1996).

Smears. Smears of fluids or tissue imprints are best if stained with Giemsa or Wright-Giemsa stains. The Papanicolaou stain is also used for cytospine preparations, smears of fluids, fine needle aspiration samples, and

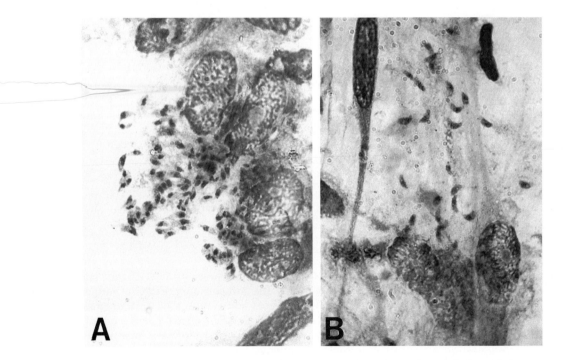

Fig. 9–24. *Toxoplasma gondii* in culture cells, Giemsa stain. *A* and *B*, Two different fields showing the typical morphology of trophozoites, ×950.

others. All stained preparations should be examined under the microscope using oil immersion. Tissue imprints are best for rapid demonstration of organisms and are especially efficient when biopsy specimens are submitted for frozen sections. Imprints are air-dried and stained directly with Wright stain, or they can be fixed in absolute methyl alcohol and stained with Giemsa stain. *Toxoplasma* organisms recovered in body fluids and tissue imprints have identical morphologic characteristics. Tachyzoites, *pseudocysts*, or *terminal colonies* (collection of tachyzoites within a cell without a cyst wall, usually pushing the cell nucleus to the side) (*color plate* VI A), and bradyzoites (true cysts with a thin membrane) (*color plate* VI B) can be observed. In cell cultures, tachyzoites are the predominant stage seen (Fig. 9–24 A–B). The morphologic characteristics of the parasite described above have to be recognized for proper identification.

Cell Cultures. *Toxoplasma* grows well in any of the standard cell culture lines used for viral isolation, a method employed for experimental work but now recommended for recovery of the organisms in cases of active infection (Hofflin, Remington, 1985; Shepp et al. 1985) (Fig. 9–24 A–B). Cultures of blood from patients with AIDS and toxoplasmic encephalitis are positive 50% of the time, as well as in other forms of the infection in both immune-competent and immune-suppressed individuals (Asensi et al. 1993). Separating white blood cells from 10 ml of peripheral blood and using these cells as an inoculum for culture tissue cells has been proposed as a good method for detecting the parasites (Tirard et al. 1991).

Tissue Sections. In tissue sections stained with hematoxylin and eosin stain, the same forms are seen, i.e., tachyzoites, pseudocysts, and cysts. Their size is smaller due to shrinkage during fixation and processing. The morphologic characteristics of the organisms stained with hematoxylin and eosin stain are greatly attenuated (*color plate* VI C–D). Trophozoites (tachyzoites) are found in the cytoplasm of any cell (Fig. 9–25 A), an important diagnostic characteristic. They occur in small numbers, especially in areas of necrosis, where they often appear artifactually as extracellular organisms. If the tissue is well preserved and the sections are thin enough, the cytoplasm and the nucleus of individual trophozoites can be seen (Fig. 9–25 A). The lack of a kinetoplast distinguishes *Toxoplasma* from *T. cruzi* and *Leishmania* (see Chapter 4). In terminal colonies (pseudocysts), the morphology of the individual organisms is difficult to determine (Fig. 9–25 A–B). The colony is definitively intracellular, even if it does not appear as such, but sometimes the cell nucleus is pushed to one side. It generally appears as a collection of small, dark bodies within a thin membrane. The size of the colony varies from 8 to 10 μm up to 25 to 30 μm and the shape of the organism is sometimes irregular, accommodating to the parasitized cell.

Cysts in tissues are mostly spherical (Fig. 9–25 C); in muscle cells, they are elongated (Figs. 9–15 D–E and 9–25 F). Their diameter is up to 30 μm; their length in muscles is up to five times the diameter of the cyst. *Toxoplasma* cysts contain hundreds of tightly packed organisms, seen as small, dark nuclei with no evident cytoplasm; the cyst membrane, 0.5 to 1.0 μm thick, is eosinophilic, weakly positive with periodic acid–Schiff stain (Fig. 9–25 C), and argyrophilic (Fig. 9–25 F). The zoites within the cysts are strongly periodic acid–Schiff positive (Fig. 9–25 C), and diastase resistant, as are the intracellular tachyzoites (Fig. 9–25 A–B). The pseudocysts are recognized because they do not have a wall when stained with argentaffin stain (Fig. 9–25 D–E). *Toxoplasma* cysts in striated muscle need careful differentiation from *Sarcocystis* (see above) and other members of the Apicomplexa. The polymerase chain reaction in paraffin-embedded tissue detects most proven (parasites are present in tissues) cases, as well as a few that are histologically negative but suggestive of toxoplasmosis (Tsai, O'Leary, 1993). The immunoperoxidase stain is very specific and sensitive.

Serology. Serology should be part of the workup in all HIV-positive patients to provide a baseline of antibody titers for future clinical evaluations (Grant et al. 1990). The main serologic tests for diagnosis of toxoplasmosis are the methylene blue dye test, complement fixation, indirect hemagglutination, direct agglutination, latex agglutination, indirect fluorescence, enzyme-linked immunosorbent assay, and tests for detecting specific IgM antibodies. For diagnosis of acute infection, a negative test essentially excludes the diagnosis. Seroconversion from negative to positive, with more than a fourfold rise of titers in specimens drawn several weeks apart, confirms the diagnosis. Care should be taken to use the same test and the same laboratory used previously (Wilson, McAuley, 1991).

Serologic diagnosis of congenital infection begins by establishing the serologic status of the mother before or soon after conception. A positive diagnosis indicates that the mother is immune to reinfection and is probably not at risk of transmitting the infection to her unborn child (see above). All testing for IgG after conception should follow testing for IgM to determine if the woman is suffering from acute infection. A positive IgM test requires treatment of the mother and follow-up testing of the fetus for congenitally acquired infec-

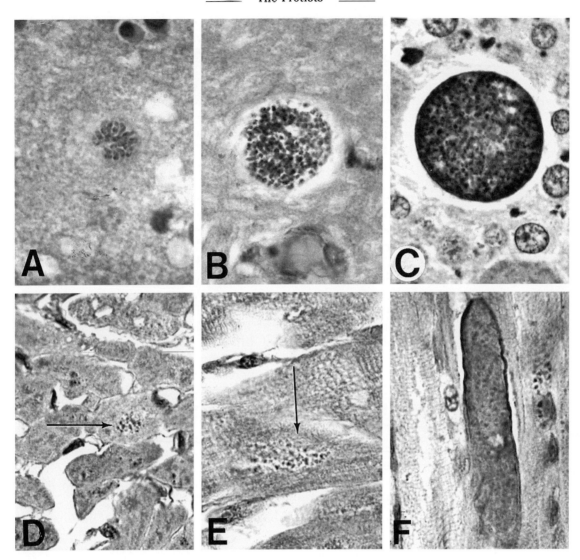

Fig. 9–25. *Toxoplasma gondii*. Diagnostic stages, special stains of tissue sections. *A–C.* Periodic acid–Schiff hematoxylin stain of human brain. *A*, Trophozoites. *B*, Pseudocyst showing some zoites with periodic acid–Schiff–positive material. *C*, Cyst with weakly periodic acid–Schiff–positive wall and intensely positive zoites, obscuring their morphology. *D–F.* Argentaffin stain of human heart. *D*, Very faint, almost indistinguishable trophozoites (arrow). *E*, Very faint, almost indistinguishable pseudocyst (arrow) with no stainable wall. *F*, Cyst with argentaffin-positive wall; zoites are faint, all ×1,120.

tion. Diagnosis in the newborn requires examination of tissues including the placenta, cord, and umbilical cord for the presence of the parasite; serologic tests for different species of antibodies and radiologic examination of the central nervous system are also recommended (Wilson, McAuley, 1991).

Other Methods. Detection of circulating specific antigens by enzyme-linked immunosorbent assay (Acebes et al. 1994) and analysis of genomic DNA (Blanco et al. 1992) have been tested experimentally for detection of parasites in fluids. The polymerase chain reaction is used in brain biopsy specimens, amniotic fluid, aqueous humor (Norose et al. 1996), and spinal fluid. In spinal fluid of patients with *Toxoplasma* encephalitis, detection of parasite DNA gave very low positivity (Cingolani et al. 1996). Similar results were obtained using venous blood (Dupouy Camet et al. 1993; Filice et al. 1993; Parmley et al. 1992; Schoondermark van de Ven et al. 1993). These studies are difficult to interpret because it was not known whether all the patients used had toxoplasmosis. The small number of infected patients detected with these tests and their unavailability in most laboratories make their clinical use limited at best.

References

Acebes MV, Diez B, Garcia-Rodriguez JA, Viens P, Cisterna R, 1994. Detection of circulating antigens in the diagnosis of acute toxoplasmosis. Am. J. Trop. Med. Hyg. 51:506–511

Adams WH, Kindermann WR, Walls KW, Heotis PM, 1987. *Toxoplasma* antibodies and retinochoroiditis in the Marshall Islands and their association with exposure to radioactive fallout. Am. J. Trop. Med. Hyg. 36:315–320

Ahuja SK, Ahuja SS, Thelmo W, Seymour A, Phelps KR, 1993. Necrotizing pancreatitis and multisystem organ failure associated with toxoplasmosis in a patient with AIDS. Clin. Infect. Dis. 16:432–434

Aisner SC, Aisner J, Moravec C, Arnett EN, 1983. Acquired toxoplasmic lymphadenitis with demonstration of the cyst form. Am. J. Clin. Pathol. 79:125–127

Altshuler G, 1973. Toxoplasmosis as a cause of hydranencephaly. Am. J. Dis. Child. 125:251–252

Arendt G, Hefter H, Figge C, Neuen Jakob E, Nelles HW, Elsing C, Freund HJ, 1991. Two cases of cerebral toxoplasmosis in AIDS patients mimicking HIV-related dementia. J Neurol. 238:439–442

Asensi V, Carton JA, Maradona JA, de Ona M, Melon S, Martinez A, Asensi JM, Villar H, Mendcz FJ, Arribas JM, 1993. Significado clinico del cultivo de *Toxoplasma gondii* en sangre y otros medios organicos. Med. Clin. Barcelona 100:651–654

Beaver PC, Gadgil RK, Morera P, 1979. *Sarcocystis* in man: a review and report of five cases. Am. J. Trop. Med. Hyg. 28:819–844

Beaver PC, Jung RC, Cupp EW, 1984. *Clinical Parasitology*. Philadelphia: Lea & Febiger

Bendelac A, Laporte JP, Marteau M, Mougeot G, Najman A, Poirot JL, Roux P, 1984. Decouverte d'une localisation pulmonaire de *Toxoplasma gondii* chez une malade immunodeprimee. Presse Med. 13:1213–1214

Benenson MW, Takafuji ET, Lemon SM, 1982. Oocyst-transmitted toxoplasmosis associated with ingestion of contaminated water. N. Engl. J. Med. 307:666–669

Berger BB, Egwuagu CE, Freeman WR, Wiley CA, 1993. Miliary toxoplasmic retinitis in acquired immunodeficiency syndrome. Arch. Ophthalmol. 111:373–376

Bergin C, Murphy M, Lyons D, Gaffney E, Mulcahy FM, 1992. *Toxoplasma* pneumonitis: fatal presentation of disseminated toxoplasmosis in a patient with AIDS. Eur. Respir. J. 5:1018–1020

Binazzi M, 1986. Profile of cutaneous toxoplasmosis. Int. J. Dermatol. 25:357–363

Binazzi M, Papini M, 1980. Cutaneous toxoplasmosis. Int. J. Dermatol. 19:332–335

Blanco JC, Angel SO, Maero E, Pszenny V, Serpente P, Garberi JC, 1992. Cloning of repetitive DNA sequences from *Toxoplasma gondii* and their usefulness for parasite detection. Am. J. Trop. Med. Hyg. 46:350–357

Bonilla CA, Rosa UW, 1994. *Toxoplasma gondii* pneumonia in patients with the acquired immunodeficiency syndrome: diagnosis by bronchoalveolar lavage. South. Med. J. 87:659–663

Bottoni F, Gonnella P, Autelitano A, Orzalesi N, 1990. Diffuse necrotizing retinochoroiditis in a child with AIDS and toxoplasmic encephalitis. Graefes. Arch. Clin. Exp. Ophthalmol. 228:36–39

Bourgouin PM, Melancon D, Carpenter S, Tampieri D, Ethier R, 1992. Hydrocephalus and prominence of the choroid plexus: an unusual computed tomographic presentation of cerebral toxoplasmosis in AIDS. Can. Assoc. Radiol. J. 43:55–59

Brezin AP, Eqwuagu CE, Silveira C, Thulliez P, Martins MC, Mahdi RM, Belfort JR, Nussenblatt RB, 1991. Analysis of aqueous humor in ocular toxoplasmosis. N. Engl. J. Med. 324:699

Caramello P, Forno B, Lucchini A, Pollono AM, Sinicco A, Gioannini P, 1993. Meningoencephalitis caused by *Toxoplasma gondii* diagnosed by isolation from cerebrospinal fluid in an HIV-positive patient. Scand. J. Infect. Dis. 25:663–666

Catterall JR, Hofflin JM, Remington JS, 1986. Pulmonary toxoplasmosis. Am. Rev. Respir. Dis. 133:704–705

Cingolani A, de Luca A, Ammassari A, Murri R, Linzalone A, Grillo R, Giancola ML, Antinori A, 1996. Detection of *T. gondii*-DNA by PCR in AIDS-related toxoplasmic encephalitis. J. Euk. Microbiol. 43:118S–119S

Clerici M, Shearer GM, 1993. A TH1 to TH2 switch is a critical step in the etiology of HIV infection. Immunol. Today 14:107–111

Cone SM, 1922. Sarcosporidiosis involving the bone. Surg. Gynecol. Obstet. 34:247–251

Crider SR, Horstman WG, Massey GS, 1988. *Toxoplasma* orchitis: report of a case and a review of the literature. Am. J. Med. 85:421–424

Deckert SM, Rang A, Weiner D, Huang S, Wiestler OD, Hof H, Schluter D, 1996. Interferon-gamma receptor-deficiency renders mice highly susceptible to toxoplasmosis by decreased macrophage activation. Lab. Invest. 75:827–841

DeMent SH, Cox MC, Gupta PK, 1987. Diagnosis of central nervous system *Toxoplasma gondii* from the cerebrospinal fluid in a patient with acquired immunodeficiency syndrome. Diagn. Cytopathol. 3:148–151

Derouin F, Beauvais B, Lariviere M, 1986. Serological study of the prevalence of toxoplasmosis in 167 patients with acquired immunodeficiency syndrome (AIDS) or chronic lymphadenopathy syndrome (LAS). Biomed. Pharmacother. 40:231–232

Derouin F, Sarfati C, Beauvais B, Garin YJ, Lariviere M, 1990. Prevalence of pulmonary toxoplasmosis in HIV-infected patients. AIDS 4:1036

Derouin F, Sarfati C, Beauvais B, Iliou MC, Dehen L, Lariviere M, 1989. Laboratory diagnosis of pulmonary toxoplasmosis in patients with acquired immunodeficiency syndrome. J. Clin. Microbiol. 27:1661–1663

Desmonts G, Couvreur J, 1974. Congenital toxoplasmosis. A prospective study of 378 pregnancies. N. Engl. J. Med. 290:1110–1116

Dische MR, Gooch WMI, 1981. Congenital toxoplasmosis. In: Rosenberg HS, Bernstein J (eds), *Perspectives in Pediatric Pathology*. New York: Masson Publishing, Inc. pp. 83–113

Doft BH, Gass JDM, 1985. Punctate outer retinal toxoplasmosis. Arch. Ophthalmol. 103:1332–1336

Donovan Post MJ, Chan JC, Hensley GT, Hoffman TA, Moskowitz LB, Lippmann S, 1983. *Toxoplasma* encephalitis in Haitian adults with acquired immunodeficiency syndrome: a clinical–pathologic–CT correlation. Am. J. Roentgenol. 140:861–868

Dubey JP, Kotula AW, Sharar A, Andrews CD, Lindsay DS, 1990. Effect of high temperature on infectivity of *Toxoplasma gondii* tissue cysts in pork. J. Parasitol. 76:201–204

Dubey JP, Weigel RM, Siegel AM, Thulliez P, Kitron UD, Mitchell MA, Manelli A, Mateus-Pinilla NE, Shen SK, Kwok OCH, Todd KS, 1995. Sources and reservoirs of *Toxoplasma gondii* infection on 47 swine farms in Illinois. J. Parasitol. 81:723–729

Dunlop O, Rootwelt V, Sannes M, Goplen AK, Abdelnoor M, Skaug K, Baklien K, Skar A, Melby K, Myrvang B, Bruun JN, 1996. Risk of toxoplasmic encephalitis in AIDS patients: indications for prophylaxis. Scand. J. Infect. Dis. 28:71–73

Dunn D, Newell M-L, Gilbert R, Mok J, Petersen E, Peckham C, 1996. Low incidence of congenital toxoplasmosis in children born to women infected with human immunodeficiency virus. European Collaborative Study and Research Network on Congenital Toxoplasmosis. Eur. J. Obstet. Gynecol. Reprod. Biol. 68:93–96

Dupouy Camet J, de Souza SL, Maslo C, Paugam A, Saimot AG, Benarous R, Tourte Schaefer C, Derouin F, 1993. Detection of *Toxoplasma gondii* in venous blood from AIDS patients by polymerase chain reaction. J. Clin. Microbiol. 31:1866–1869

Dutton GN, 1986. The causes of tissue damage in toxoplasmic retinochoroiditis. Trans. Ophthalmol. Soc. UK 105:404–412

Edwards KR, Pendlebury WW, 1987. Correspondence. Central nervous system lymphomas versus toxoplasmosis in a patient with AIDS. N. Engl. J. Med. 317:1540

Eichenwald HF, 1960. A study of congenital toxoplasmosis. In: Siim JC (ed), *Human Toxoplasmosis*. Baltimore: Williams & Wilkins, pp. 41–51

Entzeroth R, 1982. A comparative light and electron microscope study of the cysts of *Sarcocystis* species of roe deer (*Capreolus capreolus*). A. Parasitenkd. 66:281–292

Falangola MF, Petito CK, 1993. Choroid plexus infection in cerebral toxoplasmosis in AIDS patients. Neurology 43:2035–2040

Falangola MF, Reichler BS, Petito CK, 1994. Histopathology of cerebral toxoplasmosis in human immunodeficiency virus infection: a comparison between patients with early-onset and late-onset acquired immunodeficiency syndrome. Hum. Pathol. 25:1091–1097

Falcone S, Murphy BJ, Weinfeld A, 1991. Gastric manifestations of AIDS: radiographic findings on upper gastrointestinal examination. Gastrointest. Radiol. 16:95–98

Fernandez-Rivero CS, Ramirez C, 1984. Correspondence. Acquired toxoplasmic lymphadenitis with demonstration of the cyst in imprints. Am. J. Clin. Pathol. 82:751–752

Filice GA, Hitt JA, Mitchell CD, Blackstad M, Sorensen SW, 1993. Diagnosis of *Toxoplasma* parasitemia in patients with AIDS by gene detection after amplification with polymerase chain reaction. J. Clin. Microbiol. 31:2327–2331

Frenkel JK, 1971. Toxoplasmosis, mechanisms of infection, laboratory diagnosis and management. Curr. Top. Pathol. 54:28–75

Frenkel JK, 1988. Pathophysiology of toxoplasmosis. Parasitol. Today 4:273–278

Frenkel JK, Dobesh M, Parker BB, Lindsay DS, 1996. Xenosmophilia of dogs: a habit favoring the mechanical transmission of *Toxoplasma gondii* and other fecal microbes. Abstracts of the Joint Meeting of the American Society of Parasitology and Society of Protozoologists, Tuczon, Arizona, June 11–12, 1996, p. 110

Frenkel JK, Dubey JP, Miller NL, 1969. *Toxoplasma gondii*: fecal forms separated from eggs of the nematode *Toxocara cati*. Science 164:432–433

Frenkel JK, Dubey JP, Miller NL, 1970. *Toxoplasma gondii* in cats: fecal stages identified as coccidian oocysts. Science 167:893–896

Frenkel JK, Escajadillo A, 1987. Cyst rupture as a pathogenic mechanism of toxoplasmic encephalitis. Am. J. Trop. Med. Hyg. 36:517–522

Frenkel JK, Friedlander S, 1951. *Toxoplasmosis*. Washington, D.C.: U.S. Public Health Service

Frenkel JK, Hassanein KM, Hassanein RS, Brown E, Thulliez P, Quintero-Nunez R, 1995. Transmission of *Toxoplasma gondii* in Panama City, Panama: A five-year prospective cohort study of children, cats, rodents, birds, and soil. Am. J. Trop. Med. Hyg. 53:458–468

Frenkel JK, Jacobs L, 1958. Ocular toxoplasmosis. Pathogenesis, diagnosis, and treatment. Arch. Ophthalmol. 59:260–279

Frenkel JK, Ruiz A, Chincilla M, 1975. Soil survival of *Toxoplasma* oocysts in Kansas and Costa Rica. Am. J. Trop. Med. Hyg. 24:439–443

Fuentes I, Rodriguez M, Domingo CJ, del Castillo F, Juncosa T, Alvar J, 1996. Urine sample used for congenital toxoplasmosis diagnosis by PCR. J. Clin. Microbiol. 34:2368–2371

Gallino A, Maggiorini M, Kiowski W, Martin X, Wunderli W, Schneider J, Turina M, Follath F, 1996. Toxoplasmosis in heart transplant recipients. Eur. J. Clin. Microbiol. Infect. Dis. 15:389–393

Garcia AGP, Coutinho SG, Amendoeira MR, Assumpcao MR, Albano N, 1983. Placental morphology of newborns at risk for congenital toxoplasmosis. J. Trop. Pediatr. 29:95–103

Garcia LW, Hemphill RB, Marasco WA, Ciano PS, 1991. Acquired immunodeficiency syndrome with disseminated toxoplasmosis presenting as an acute pulmonary and gastrointestinal illness. Arch. Pathol. Lab. Med. 115:459–463

Gherardi R, Baudrimont M, Lionnet F, Salord JM, Duvivier C, Michon C, Wolff M, Marche C, 1992. Skeletal muscle toxoplasmosis in patients with acquired immunodeficiency syndrome: a clinical and pathological study. Ann. Neurol. 32:535–542

Gluckman GR, Werboff LH, 1994. Toxoplasmosis of the bladder: case report and review of the literature. J. Urol. 151:1629–1630

Gonzales GR, Herskovitz S, Rosenblum M, Foley KM, Kanner R, Brown A, Portenoy RK, 1992. Central pain from cerebral abscess: thalamic syndrome in AIDS patients with toxoplasmosis. Neurology 42:1107–1109

Grant IH, Gold JW, Rosenblum M, Niedzwiecki D, Armstrong D, 1990. Toxoplasma gondii serology in HIV-infected patients: the development of central nervous system toxoplasmosis in AIDS. AIDS 4:519–521

Greve E, 1985. Sarcosporidiosis—an overlooked zoonosis. Man as intermediate and final host. Danish Med. Bulletin 32:228–230

Grossniklaus HE, Specht CS, Allaire G, Leavitt JA, 1990. Toxoplasma gondii retinochoroiditis and optic neuritis in acquired immune deficiency syndrome. Report of a case. Ophthalmology. 97:1342–1346

Hakkila J, Frick HM, Halonen PI, 1958. Pericarditis and myocarditis caused by Toxoplasma: report of a case and review of the literature. Am. Heart J. 55:758–765

Haskell L, Fusco MJ, Ares L, Sublay B, 1989. Case report: disseminated toxoplasmosis presenting as symptomatic orchitis and nephrotic syndrome. Am. Med. Sci. 298:185–190

Hofflin JM, Remington JS, 1985. Tissue culture isolation of Toxoplasma from blood of a patient with AIDS. Arch. Intern. Med. 145:925–926

Hofman P, Bernard E, Michiels JF, Thyss A, Le Fichoux Y, Loubiere R, 1993a. Extracerebral toxoplasmosis in the acquired immunodeficiency syndrome (AIDS). Pathol. Res. Pract. 189:894–901

Hofman P, Drici MD, Gibelin P, Michiels JF, Thyss A, 1993b. Prevalence of Toxoplasma myocarditis in patients with the acquired immunodeficiency syndrome. Br. Heart J. 70:376–381

Hofman P, Quintens H, Michiels JF, Taillan B, Thyss A, 1993c. Toxoplasma cystitis associated with acquired immunodeficiency syndrome. Urology 42:589–592

Holland GN, Engstrom RE Jr, Glasgow BJ, Berger BB, Daniels SA, Sidikaro Y, Harmon JA, Fischer DH, Boyer DS, Rao NA, Eagle RCJ, Kreiger AE, Foos RY, 1988. Ocular toxoplasmosis in patients with the acquired immunodeficiency syndrome. Am. J. Ophthalmol. 106:653–667

Huang TE, Chou SM, 1988. Occlusive hypertrophic arteritis as the cause of discrete necrosis in CNS toxoplasmosis in the acquired immunodeficiency syndrome. Hum. Pathol. 19:1210–1214

Israelski DM, Skowron G, Leventhal JP, Long I, Blankenship CF, Barrio GW, Prince JB, Araujo FG, Remington JS, 1988. Toxoplasma peritonitis in a patient with acquired immunodeficiency syndrome. Arch. Intern. Med. 148:1655–1657

Jackson MH, Hutchison WM, 1989. The prevalence and source of Toxoplasma infection in the environment. Adv. Parasitol. 28:55–105

Jacobs L, Remington JS, Melton ML, 1960. The resistance of the encysted form of Toxoplasma gondii. J. Parasitol. 46:11–21

Jautzke G, Sell M, Thalmann U, Janitschke K, Gottschalk J, Schurmann D, Ruf B, 1993. Extracerebral toxoplasmosis in AIDS. Histological and immunohistological findings based on 80 autopsy cases. Pathol. Res. Pract. 189:428–436

Jeffrey HC, 1974. Sarcosporidiosis in man. Trans. R. Soc. Trop. Med. Hyg. 68:17–29

Johnson MW, Greven GM, Jaffe GJ, Sudhalkar H, Vine AK, 1997. Atypical, severe toxoplasmic retinochoroiditis in elderly patients. Ophthalmology 104:48–57

Kan SP, 1985. A review of sarcocystosis with special reference to human infection in Malaysia. Trop. Biomed. 2:167–175

Kean BH, Kimball AC, Christenson WN, 1969. An epidemic of acute toxoplasmosis. JAMA 208:1002–1004

Knani L, Bouslama K, Varette C, Gonzalez Canali G, Cabane J, Lebas J, Imbert JC, 1990. Toxoplasmose pulmonaire au cours du SIDA. A propos de 3 cas. Ann. Med. Interne 141:469–471

Kouyoumdhian JA, Tognola WA, 1985. Muscular sarcosporidiosis: report of a case. Arq. Neuropsiquiatr. 43:269–302

Krick JA, Remington JS, 1978. Toxoplasmosis in the adult—an overview. N. Engl. J. Med. 298:550–554

Lancastre F, Delalande A, Deluol AM, Matrat C, Georges E, Roux P, 1989. Sarcosporidiosis revealed in sputum. Lancet 1:791

Lang W, Miklossy J, Deruaz JP, Pizzolato GP, Probst A, Schaffner T, Gessaga E, Kleihues P, 1989. Neuropathology of the acquired immune deficiency syndrome (AIDS): a report of 135 consecutive autopsy cases from Switzerland. Acta Neuropathol. 77:379–390

Lapetina F, 1989. Toxoplasmosi e dermatomiositi: nesso causale o casuale? Pediatr. Med. Chir. 11:197–203

Lele VB, Dhopavkar PV, Kher A, 1986. Sarcocystis infection in man (a case report). Ind. J. Pathol. Microbiol. 29:87–90

Leyva WH, Santa Cruz DJ, 1986. Cutaneous toxoplasmosis. J. Am. Acad. Dermatol. 14:600–605

Luft BJ, Billingham M, Remington JS, 1986. Endomyocardial biopsy in the diagnosis of toxoplasmic myocarditis. Transplant. Proc. 18:1871–1873

Luft BJ, Naot Y, Araujo FG, Stinson EB, Remington JS, 1983. Primary and reactivated Toxoplasma infection in patients with cardiac transplant. Ann. Intern. Med. 99:27–31

Mandour AM, 1965. Pathology and symptomatology of *Sarcocystis* infection in man. Trans. R. Soc. Trop. Med. Hyg. 59:432–435

McCabe R, Remington JS, 1988. Toxoplasmosis: the time has come. N. Engl. J. Med. 318:313–315

McGill RJ, Goodbody RA, 1957. Sarcosporidiosis in man with periarteritis nodosa. Br. Med. J. 2:333–334

McLeod R, Hirabayashi RN, Rothman W, Remington JS, 1980. Necrotizing vasculitis and *Sarcocystis*: a cause and effect relationship. South. Med. J. 73:1380–1382

Milligan SA, Katz MS, Craven PC, Strandberg DA, Russell IJ, Becker RA, 1984. Toxoplasmosis presenting as panhypopituitarism in a patient with the acquired immune deficiency syndrome. Am. J. Med. 77:760–764

Minkoff H, Remington JS, Holman S, Ramirez R, Goodwin S, Landesman S, 1997. Vertical transmission of *Toxoplasma* by human immunodeficiency virus–infected women. Am J Obstet. Gynecol. 176:555–559

Mitchell CD, Erlich SS, Mastrucci MT, Hutto SC, Parks WP, Scott GB, 1990. Congenital toxoplasmosis occurring in infants perinatally infected with human immunodeficiency virus 1. Pediatr. Infect. Dis. J. 9:512–518

Montoya JG, Remington JS, 1996. Toxoplasmic chorioretinitis in the setting of acute acquired toxoplasmosis. Clin. Infect. Dis. 23:277–282

Morhun PJ, Weisz JM, Elias SJ, Holland GN, 1996. Recurrent ocular toxoplasmosis in patients treated with systemic corticosteroids. Retina 16:383–387

Nagington J, Martin AL, 1983. Correspondence. Toxoplasmosis and heart transplantation. Lancet 2:679

Nash G, Kerschmann RL, Herndier B, Dubey JP, 1994. The pathological manifestations of pulmonary toxoplasmosis in the acquired immunodeficiency syndrome. Hum. Pathol. 25:652–658

Navia BA, Petito CK, Gold JWM, Cho ES, Jordan BD, Price NG, 1986. Cerebral toxoplasmosis complicating the acquired immune deficiency syndrome: clinical and neuropathological findings in 27 patients. Ann. Neurol. 18:224–238

Niedmann G, Del Campo E, Thiermann E, Sanchez J, Levy M, 1962. Miocarditis de probable etiologia toxoplasmosica. Bol. Chil. Parasitol. 17:58–63

Niedmann G, Thiermann E, Campo ED, 1959. Un caso de miocarditis cronica toxoplasmosica. Bol. Chil. Parasitol. 14:59–61

Nolla Salas J, Ricart C, D'Olhaberriague L, Gali F, Lamarca J, 1987. Hydrocephalus: an unusual CT presentation of cerebral toxoplasmosis in a patient with acquired immunodeficiency syndrome. Eur. Neurol. 27:130–132

Norose K, Tokushima T, Yano A, 1996. Quantitative polymerase chain reaction in diagnosing ocular toxoplasmosis. Am. J. Ophthalmol. 121:441–442

Oksenhendler E, Cadranel J, Sarfati C, Katlama C, Datry A, Marche C, Wolf M, Roux P, Derouin F, Clauvel JP, 1990. *Toxoplasma gondii* pneumonia in patients with the acquired immunodeficiency syndrome. Am. J. Med. 88:18N–21N

Pamphlett R, O'Donoghue P, 1990. *Sarcocystis* infection of human muscle. Aust. NZ J. Med. 20:705–707

Parke DW, Font RL, 1986. Diffuse toxoplasmic retinochoroiditis in a patient with AIDS. Arch. Ophthalmol. 104:571–575

Parmley SF, Goebel FD, Remington JS, 1992. Detection of *Toxoplasma gondii* in cerebrospinal fluid from AIDS patients by polymerase chain reaction. J. Clin. Microbiol. 30:3000–3002

Pathmanathan P, Kan SP, 1981. Human *Sarcocystis* infection in Malaysia. Southeast Asian J. Trop. Med. Public Health 12:247–250

Pathmanathan R, Kan SP, 1992. Three cases of human *Sarcocystis* infection with a review of human muscular sarcocystosis in Malaysia. Trop. Geogr. Med. 44:102–108

Patton S, Zimmerman J, Roberts T, Faulkner C, Diderrich V, Assadi-Rad A, Davies P, Kliebenstein J, 1966. Seroprevalence of *Toxoplasma gondii* in hogs in the National Animal Health Monitoring System (NAHMS). J. Euk. Microbiol. 43:121S

Pauwels A, Meyohas MC, Eliaszewicz M, Legendre C, Mougeot G, Frottier J, 1992. *Toxoplasma* colitis in the acquired immunodeficiency syndrome. Am. J. Gastroenterol. 87:518–519

Pavesio CE, Lightman S, 1996. *Toxoplasma gondii* and ocular toxoplasmosis: pathogenesis. Br. J. Ophthalmol. 80:1099–1107

Pomeroy C, Filice GA, 1992. Pulmonary toxoplasmosis: a review. Clin. Infect. Dis. 14:863–870

Poon TP, Tchertkoff V, Pares GF, Masangkay AV, Daras M, Marc J, 1992. Spinal cord *Toxoplasma* lesion in AIDS: MR findings. J. Comput. Assist. Tomogr. 16:817–819

Porter SB, Sande MA, 1992. Toxoplasmosis of the central nervous system in the acquired immunodeficiency syndrome. N. Engl. J. Med. 327:1643–1648

Potts RE, Williams AA, 1956. Acute myocardial toxoplasmosis. Lancet 2:483–484

Price RM, 1933. Human sarcosporidiosis—case report. J. Kans. Med. Soc. 34:132–135

Prosmanne O, Chalaoui J, Sylvestre J, Lefebvre R, 1984. Small nodular pattern in the lungs due to opportunistic toxoplasmosis. J. Can. Assoc. Radiol. 35:186–188

Pugin J, Vanhems P, Hirschel B, Chave JP, Flepp M, 1992. Extreme elevations of serum lactic dehydrogenase differentiating pulmonary toxoplasmosis from pneumocystis pneumonia. N. Engl. J. Med. 326:1226

Rabaud C, May T, Lucet JC, Leport C, Ambroise TP, Canton P, 1996. Pulmonary toxoplasmosis in patients infected with human immunodeficiency virus: a French National Survey. Clin. Infect. Dis. 23:1249–1254

Remington JS, Dalrymple W, Jacobs L, Finland M, 1963. *Toxoplasma* antibodies among college students. N. Engl. J. Med. 269:1394–1398

Ryning FW, McLeod R, Maddox JC, Hunt S, Remington JS,

1979. Probable transmission of *Toxoplasma gondii* by organ transplantation. Ann. Intern. Med. 90:47–49

Saad R, Vincent JF, Cimon B, de Gentile L, Francois S, Bouachour G, Ifrah N, 1996. Pulmonary toxoplasmosis after allogeneic bone marrow transplantation: case report and review. Bone Marrow Transplant. 18:211–212

Schnapp LM, Geaghan SM, Campagna A, Fahy J, Steiger D, Ng V, Hadley WK, Hopewell PC, Stansell JD, 1992. *Toxoplasma gondii* pneumonitis in patients infected with the human immunodeficiency virus. Arch. Intern. Med. 152:1073–1077

Schoondermark van de Ven E, Galama J, Kraaijeveld C, van Druten J, Meuwissen J, Melchers W, 1993. Value of the polymerase chain reaction for the detection of *Toxoplasma gondii* in cerebrospinal fluid from patients with AIDS. Clin. Infect. Dis. 16:661–666

Shepp DH, Hackman RC, Conley FK, Anderson JB, Meyers JB, 1985. *Toxoplasma gondii* reactivation identified by detection of parasitemia in tissue culture. Ann. Intern. Med. 103:218–221

Siegel SE, Lunde MN, Gelderman AH, Halterman RH, Brown JA, Levine AS, Graw RG Jr, 1971. Transmission of toxoplasmosis by leukocyte transfusion. Blood 37:388–394

Siim JC, 1956. Toxoplasmosis acquisita lymphonodosa: clinical and pathological aspects. Ann. N.Y. Acad. Sci. 64:185–206

Smart PE, Weinfeld A, Thompson NE, Defortuna SM, 1990. Toxoplasmosis of the stomach: a cause of antral narrowing. Radiology 174:369–370

Smith KL, Wilson M, Hightower AW, Kelley PW, Struewing JP, Juranek DD, McAuley JB, 1996. Prevalence of *Toxoplasma gondii* antibodies in US military recruits in 1989: comparison with data published in 1965. Clin. Infect. Dis. 23:1182–1183

Stagno S, Dykes AC, Amos CS, Head RA, Juranek DD, Walls K, 1980. An outbreak of toxoplasmosis linked to cats. Pediatrics 65:706–712

Teutsch SM, Juranek DD, Sulzer A, Dubey JP, Sikes RK, 1979. Epidemic toxoplasmosis associated with infected cats. N. Engl. J. Med. 300:695–699

Threlkeld MG, Graves AH, Cobbs CG, 1987. Cerebrospinal fluid staining for the diagnosis of toxoplasmosis in patients with the acquired immune deficiency syndrome. Am. J. Med. 83:599–600

Tirard V, Niel G, Rosenheim M, Katlama C, Ciceron L, Ogunkolade W, Danis M, Gentilini M, 1991. Correspondence. Diagnosis of toxoplasmosis in patients with AIDS by isolation of the parasite from the blood. N. Engl. J. Med. 324:634

Touboul JL, Salmon D, Lancastre F, Mayaud C, Fermand JP, Fouret P, Akoun G, 1986. Pneumopathie a *Toxoplasma gondii* chez un a patient atteint de syndrome d'immunodepression acquis: mis en evidence du parasite par lavage bronchiolo-alveolaire. Rev. Pneumol. Clin. 42:150–152

Troedsen C, Pamphlett R, Collins H, 1992. Correspondence. Is sarcocystosis common in Sydney? Med. J. Aust. 156:136

Tsai MM, O'Leary T, 1993. Methods in pathology: identification of *Toxoplasma gondii* in formalin-fixed, paraffin-embedded tissue by polymerase chain reaction. Mod. Pathol. 6:185–188

Van-den EE, Praet M, Joos R, Van GA, Gigasse P, 1995. Eosinophilic myositis resulting from sarcocystosis. J. Trop. Med. Hyg. 98:273–276

Vogel N, Kirisits M, Michael E, Bach H, Hostetter M, Boyer K, Simpson R, Holfels E, Hopkins J, Mack D, Mets MB, Swisher CN, Patel D, Roizen N, Stein L, Stein M, Withers S, Mui E, Egwuagu C, Remington J, Dorfman R, McLeod R, 1996. Congenital toxoplasmosis transmitted from an immunologically competent mother infected before conception. Clin. Infect. Dis. 23:1055–1060

Vyas R, Ebright JR, 1996. Toxoplasmosis of the spinal cord in a patient with AIDS: case report and review. Clin. Infect. Dis. 23:1061–1065

Walker W, Roberts CW, Ferguson DJ, Jebbari H, Alexander J, 1997. Innate immunity to *Toxoplasma gondii* is influenced by gender and is associated with differences in interleukin-12 and gamma interferon production. Infect. Immun. 65:1119–1121

Wallace MR, Rossetti RJ, Olson PE, 1993. Cats and toxoplasmosis risk in HIV-infected adults. JAMA 269:76–77

Wanke C, Tuazon CU, Kovacs A, Dina T, Davis DO, Barton N, Katz D, Lunde M, Levy C, Conley FK, Lane HC, Fauci AS, Masur H, 1987. *Toxoplasma* encephalitis in patients with acquired immune deficiency syndrome. diagnosis and response to therapy. Am. J. Trop. Med. Hyg. 36:509–516

Weiss LM, Chen YY, Berry GJ, Strickler JG, Dorfman RF, Warnke RA, 1992. Infrequent detection of *Toxoplasma gondii* genome in toxoplasmic lymphadenitis: a polymerase chain reaction study. Hum. Pathol. 23:154–158

Welker Y, Geissmann F, Benali A, Bron J, Molina JM, Decazes JM, 1994. *Toxoplasma*-induced cystitis in a patient with AIDS. Clin. Infect. Dis. 18:453–454

Wilder HC, 1952. *Toxoplasma* chorioretinitis in adults. Arch. Ophthalmol. 48:127–136

Wilson M, McAuley JB, 1991. Laboratory diagnosis of toxoplasmosis. Clin. Lab. Med. 11:923–939

Wong KT, Clarke G, Pathmanathan R, Hamilton PW, 1994. Light microscopic and three-dimensional morphology of the human muscular sarcocyst. Parasitol. Res. 80:138–140

Wong KT, Leggett PF, Heatley M, 1993. Correspondence. Apparent absence of *Sarcocystis* infection in human tongue and diaphragm in Northern Ireland. Trans. R. Soc. Trop. Med. Hyg. 87:496

Wong KT, Pathmanathan R, 1992. High prevalence of human skeletal muscle sarcocystosis in south-east Asia. Trans. R. Soc. Trop. Med. Hyg. 86:631–632

Wong KT, Pathmanathan R, 1994. Ultrastructure of the human skeletal muscle sarcocyst. J. Parasitol. 80:327–330

Wong KT, Yusoff M, 1995. Scanning electron microscopy of the human muscular sarcocyst. Parasitol. Res. 81:359–360

Wreghitt TG, Hakim M, Gray JJ, Balfour AH, Stovin PG, Stewart S, Scott J, English TA, Wallwork J, 1989. Toxoplasmosis in heart and heart and lung transplant recipients. J. Clin. Pathol. 42:194–199

Zangerle R, Allerberger F, 1994. Correspondence. High risk of developing toxoplasmic encephalitis in AIDS patients seropositive to *Toxoplasma gondii*. J. Acq. Immun. Defic. Syndrome 7:207–208

Zangerle R, Allerberger F, Pohl P, Fritsch P, Dierich MP, 1991. High risk of developing toxoplasmic encephalitis in AIDS patients seropositive to *Toxoplasma gondii*. Med. Microbiol. Immunol. 180:59–66

10

APICOMPLEXA OF THE BLOOD

The Apicomplexa of blood belong to the class Haematozoea, which has two orders: Haemosporida and Piroplasmida. Haemosporida has the family Plasmodiidae, with the genus *Plasmodium*. Piroplasmida has the family Babesiidae, with the genera *Babesia* and *Entopolypoides* (Corliss, 1994). These three genera have species parasitic in humans, all of which are intraerythrocytic, with complicated life cycles necessitating two hosts, a vertebrate and an invertebrate. *Plasmodium* produces malaria, and *Babesia* and *Entopolypoides* produce piroplasmosis; both diseases are well known in both humans and animals. The zoologic distinction between these two groups of organisms is that all species of *Plasmodium* produce pigment from the metabolism of hemoglobin of the parasitized erythrocyte, while *Babesia* and *Entopolypoides* do not. Malaria is a disease of animals and humans produced by many species of *Plasmodium*. Piroplasmosis is a disease exclusively of animals, also produced by many species of *Babesia* and by one known species of *Entopolypoides*. In humans piroplasmosis occurs as an occasional zoonotic infection. Both malaria and piroplasmosis have a worldwide distribution (Beaver et al. 1984).

Plasmodium—Malaria

The plasmodia causing malaria in humans belong to four species, three of which—*P. vivax*, *P. malariae*, and *P. ovale*—are characterized biologically by having rounded gametocytes and medically by producing a rather benign, nonfatal infection. The fourth species, *P. falciparum*, has elongated gametocytes and causes a great deal of morbidity and mortality (WHO, 1987).

Life Cycle. The life cycle of human plasmodia has many similarities to the cycles of other apicomplexans, already studied (Chapters 8 and 9). Plasmodia have two hosts in their life cycle: the vertebrate host, where intrinsic or intermediate asexual development (schizogony) occurs in the red blood cells, and mosquitoes, the invertebrate hosts, where extrinsic or definitive development (sporogony) takes place (Fig. 10–1). Development begins with ingestion of gametocytes by mosquitoes during their blood meal on infected individuals. In the stomach of the mosquito the male and female gametocytes mature rapidly to form gametes, which

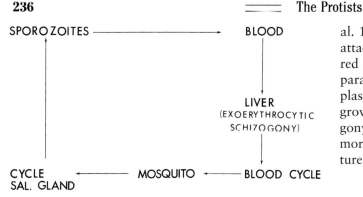

SPOROZOITES ──────────────▶ BLOOD

LIVER
(EXOERYTHROCYTIC
SCHIZOGONY)

CYCLE ◀──── MOSQUITO ◀──── BLOOD CYCLE
SAL. GLAND

Fig. 10–1. *Plasmodium*, schematic representation of the general life cycle.

join to become a fertilized stage (oocyte) that undergoes a series of cellular divisions. These cellular divisions culminate in the production of infective stages, the sporozoites. Sporozoites are set free in the general cavity of the mosquito and migrate to the salivary glands, where they are inoculated into the next host with the saliva of the mosquito. Inoculated sporozoites are in circulation no longer than 30 minutes. They rapidly enter the parenchymatous liver cells, where they undergo a phase of asexual development known as primary *exoerythrocytic* schizogony or *preerythrocytic* schizogony. In the liver, *all inoculated* sporozoites of *P. falciparum* and *P. malariae* develop in approximately 10 days to produce merozoites, which invade the circulating red blood cells. In contrast, only *a portion* of the inoculated sporozoites of *P. vivax* and *P. ovale* develop in 10 days; the rest remain in the hepatocytes as dormant stages, the hypnozoites. If infections with *P. vivax* and *P. ovale* are untreated, the liver stages of these species remain dormant for up to $3^1/_2$ years. These liver stages produce *relapses* (reappearance of disease after complete absence of circulating parasites) at any time during this $3^1/_2$ year period. Untreated *P. falciparum* lasts $1^1/_2$ years in its host, and *P. malariae* lasts for several decades. Since both of these species lack hypnozoites in the liver, they do not produce relapses; instead, they produce *recrudescences* (reappearance of disease due to undetectable circulating parasites). Genetic studies of *P. falciparum* isolates from children have demonstrated that recrudescences are due to the same isolate (Al-Yaman et al. 1997); thus, they are not reinfections, as some have suggested.

Merozoites formed in the liver leave the parenchymal cell and, in the sinusoid, make contact with specific molecules on the red blood cell membrane, entering the corpuscle in less than 1 minute (Figs. 10–2 and 10–3; Aikawa et al. 1978). The Duffy blood group antigen is the attachment molecule for *P. vivax* (Miller et

al. 1977a; Miller et al. 1977b), and glycophorin is the attachment molecule for *falciparum*. Once inside the red blood cell, the young trophozoite locates within a parasitophorous vacuole and begins feeding on cytoplasmic material of the host cell. At the same time, growth and division of its nucleus (erythrocytic schizogony) occur, with formation of schizonts (forms with more than one nucleus). The schizonts continue to mature and finally evolve into independent forms, the

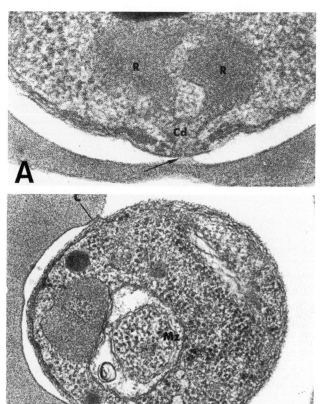

Fig. 10–2. *Plasmodium*, entry into red blood cells. *A* and *B*, Transmission electron micrographs demonstrate the morphologic mechanism of penetration into red blood cells. *A*, Attachment of the parasite by means of its apical complex to a red blood cell (arrow), ×90,000. *B*, The parasite with one-third of its body inside the red blood cell. Note that attachment is still occurring, forming a ring around the parasite; the parasitophorous vacuole is also beginning to form, ×40,500. Abbreviations: cd, common duct; c, junctional attachment; mz, merozoite; r, rhophtries. (In: Aikawa, M. Miller, L.H., Johnson, J., and Rabbege, J. 1978. Erythrocyte entry by malarial parasites. A moving junction between erythrocyte and parasite. J. Cell Biol. 77: 72–82. Reproduced with permission.)

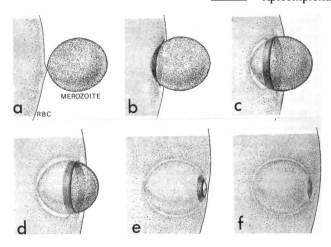

Fig. 10–3. Diagram depicting the moving circumferential junction between merozoite and erythrocyte. (In Aikawa, M., Miller, L.H., Johnson, J., and Rabbege, J. 1978. Erythrocyte entry by malarial parasites. A moving junction between erythrocyte and parasite. J. Cell Biol. 77: 72–82. Reproduced with permission.)

merozoites. Completion of erythrocytic schizogony requires 48 hours for *P. falciparum*, *P. vivax*, and *P. ovale* and 72 hours for *P. malariae*. Erythrocytic schizogony terminates with rupture of the parasitized red blood cell, freeing the newly formed merozoites, which enter other erythrocytes to start the cycle again (Fig. 10–4). Rupture of parasitized red blood cells produces the clinical manifestations of malaria. Some merozoites transform into sexual forms, micro- and macrogametes, which, if ingested by mosquitoes, reinitiate the sexual life cycle (Fig. 10–4; Beaver et al. 1984).

Morphology. The morphology of malaria parasites in the erythrocytes is very well known. It is illustrated in every textbook of parasitology and every manual dealing with the diagnosis of malaria because it is the basis for diagnosis of the infection. The plasmodia observed in erythrocytes correspond to the different stages of schizogony, which in good preparations of blood stained with Giemsa stain are seen as pale blue structures with one or more dark red nuclei. Once inside the red blood cell, the merozoites become trophozoites; they measure less than 2 μm and have a small nucleus. Trophozoites at this stage are identical in all four human species; thus, *based on the presence of small trophozoites alone, identification of the species is not possible*. Trophozoites grow and acquire a pseudovacuole at the center that gives them the appearance of a ring, a name used to characterize these stages. The parasite continues to grow, and movement of the trophozoite is inferred by the strands of delicate cytoplasm extending out from the body of the parasite. At this stage, about 24 hours after initiation of schizogony, some of the morphologic characteristics of the parasites and the red blood cell they inhabit allow identification of the species. Morphologically, the parasitized red blood cell in *P. falciparum* and *P. malariae* is normal in both size and shape, as determined by comparison with adjacent, nonparasitized red blood cells. The parasitized red blood cell in *P. vivax* and *P. ovale* is enlarged and deformed.

In *P. falciparum* the trophozoite is about one-third to one-half the diameter of the red blood cell. It does not have prominent pseudopods, appearing instead as a slightly deformed, resting organism with a prominent

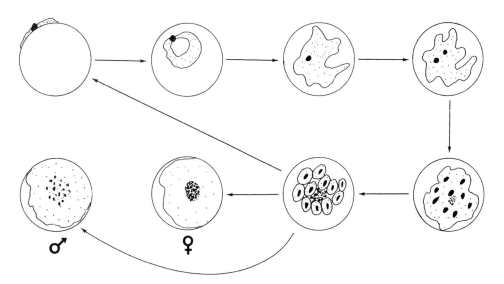

Fig. 10–4. *Plasmodium*, schematic representation of erythrocytic schizogony.

pseudovacuole. Granules of malarial pigment begin forming as small clumps of refractile dark yellow or greenish material next to the parasite. These clumps grow as the parasite matures and are freed from the erythrocyte when the merozoites are released. Under polarized light, the malaria pigment crystals polarize strongly. Further growth of the parasite is accompanied by nuclear division resulting in schizonts; young schizonts have two to six nuclei, and mature ones have 21 to 24 nuclei. Toward the end of schizogony, 48 or 72 hours after beginning to develop, each nucleus claims a small portion of the cytoplasm to become a merozoite. Merozoites are soon released into the circulation to enter other erythrocytes and repeat the asexual cycle. Some merozoites began differentiating into gametocytes, but they disappear into the spleen and bone marrow until full development is completed, and they reappear in the circulation as full-grown gametocytes. Mature gametocytes have the characteristic shape of a banana extending across the red blood cell, protruding from it at either end. *Plasmodium malariae* and *P. falciparum* have some similarities. However, the trophozoites of *P. malariae* are slightly larger and sometimes appear stretched across the red blood cell, forming a band of variable width; they are also slow moving (no pseudopods) and the gametocytes are round, filling most of the red blood cell.

In *P. vivax* the development is as described above, but the trophozoite grows to a much larger size and has numerous pseudopods, seen as irregular strings of cytoplasm that give the parasite bizarre shapes. In addition, the red blood cells are pale, enlarged, and deformed. The young schizonts are also larger, with prominent extensions of the cytoplasm. The mature schizonts have a variable number of merozoites, usually 12 to 18, but as few as 8 or as many as 24 are not uncommon. The gametocytes are rounded and large, occupying most of the red blood cell. *Plasmodium ovale* has characteristics similar to those of *P. vivax*, but the deformation of the red blood cell is oval, hence the name of the species.

The parasitized red blood cells of *P. vivax* and *P. ovale* develop Schüfner's stippling of the cytoplasm, seen as multiple small, eosinophilic dots; in *P. falciparum* the erythrocytes have coarser Maurer's stippling, and *P. malariae* has Ziemann's stippling. These changes are seen only in excellent preparations stained with Giemsa stain and rinsed with buffer solutions at a pH of 7.2. In most clinical laboratories these stains are not done as carefully, or the automated Wright-Giemsa stain is used, so the stippling is not demonstrated. Note that the absence of stippling does not facilitate identification of the species, but its presence is helpful.

The electron microscopic appearance of plasmodia has been studied intensely, and all the stages of both human and animal malarial parasites have been examined. The account given here is a composite of observations made mostly on animal plasmodia, with the understanding that minor differences may exist in species found in humans; the discussion is also limited to the stages in the erythrocytes. Merozoites freed from hepatocytes or from red blood cells are oval, about 1.5 by 1.0 μm in size, with a well-develop apical complex, a nucleus, mitochondria, a cytostome, ribosomes, and an endoplasmic reticulum. The wall of the merozoite, known as the *pellicular complex*, consists of a thin outer membrane, a thick interrupted inner membrane, and a system of microtubules forming the cytoskeleton of the parasite. Merozoites rapidly attach by means of their apical end to other erythrocytes, forming a slight depression on the membrane of the erythrocyte. The attachment site on the red blood cell thickens and forms a junction with the merozoite's membrane, rapidly extending to form a ring around the moving merozoite. As the merozoite moves inward, the red cell–merozoite attachment ring moves back on the merozoite until the parasite is inside a parasitophorous vacuole formed by the red cell membrane (Aikawa et al. 1978).

Once the merozoite is inside the red blood cell, the cytoskeleton (microtubules and the inner membrane) and the apical complex organelles break down, and the merozoite becomes a rounded trophozoite with a single cell membrane. The most interesting organelle in the trophozoite is the cytostome for ingestion of red blood cell cytoplasm; in addition, mitochondria, the endoplasmic reticulum, ribosomes, and a nucleus are present. The ameboid movements of the parasites are inferred from the tortuous extensions and invaginations of their cytoplasm. These ameboid movements are also responsible for the pseudovacuole that gives the appearance of a ring. Schizonts are characterized by the presence of more than one nucleus and by the relatively larger size of the trophozoite (Aikawa, 1971). The changes in the parasitized red blood cells are discussed in the section on Biology and Pathogenesis (see below).

Geographic Distribution and Epidemiology. Human plasmodia are widely distributed in tropical and most subtropical regions, where they produce one of the most important parasitic infections in the world (Fig. 10–5). Malaria has been endemic in latitudes as northerly as the location of Moscow and as southerly as the northern third of Argentina. The control and eradication campaigns of most countries have altered the geographic range and prevalence of malaria, but

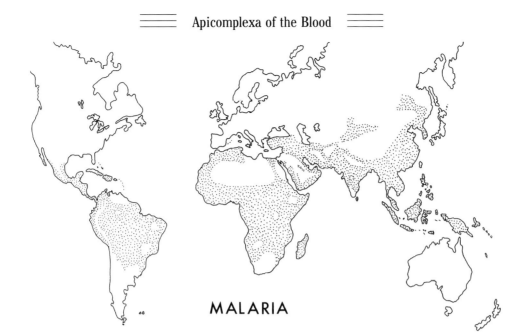

MALARIA

Fig. 10–5. *Plasmodium*, geographic distribution of human malaria.

the number of cases is still large, though no reliable estimates are available. The most commonly quoted figure is 200 million cases worldwide per year, with 1% mortality. The World Health Organization estimated that in 1986, 100 million cases occurred worldwide, a figure challenged based on the calculation of populations living in malarious areas and the risk of contracting the infection. The result is a staggering 489 million clinical cases, 234 million of which are due to *P. falciparum*, with a mortality of 2.3 million (Sturchler, 1989). In some highly endemic areas, the year-round prevalence is between one-third and one-half of the population. In an island in the southwestern Pacific, the prevalence in children is 30% year around, with *P. falciparum* infections predominating during the rainy season and *P. vivax* during the dry season (Maitland et al. 1996). Epidemics of malaria in the past were relatively common and resulted in deaths counted in the tens of thousands, but they have steadily decreased. However, it is estimated that in recent years in Venezuela there has been an increase in malaria cases the year after the El Niño phenomenon (Bouoma, Dye, 1997). *Plasmodium vivax* has the largest geographic range, comprising most of the tropical and subtropical regions of the world. *Plasmodium falciparum* is restricted to the tropical areas but can also occur in subtropical locations. *Plasmodium malariae* has a patchy distribution in the same range as *P. falciparum* (Beaver et al. 1984), and *P. ovale* occurs in tropical Africa and sporadically in the western Pacific (Alves et al. 1969; Baird et al. 1990).

The lowest number of cases of malaria worldwide occurred in the early 1970s, but since then there has been a resurgence in many places, especially in Southeast Asia and Africa. It has been said that the oil embargo of the mid-1970s, which resulted in a considerable increase in oil prices, forced many countries to stop or reduce considerably their malaria eradication programs. Their money was used not to purchase insecticides, but rather oil to run their economies. This has created a situation in which malaria needs to be considered as a reemerging disease (Krogstad, 1996). Malaria was endemic in the continental United States until several control projects eradicated the infection, and in the early 1950s the country was malaria free. Europe was also an indigenous zone, but it is now free of malaria. Today, most malaria infections in Europe and North America are imported (Lobel et al. 1985); their number has increased considerably. In 1991 in Canada 674 cases of malaria were diagnosed, 5 of which were fatal (Carsley, MacLean, 1997). Outbreaks with small clusters of cases occurred in the United States due to reintroduced malaria (CDC, 1986a, 1986b, 1997; Maldonado et al. 1990). The increased number of resistant strains of *P. falciparum* and possibly of *P. vivax* (Collins, Jeffery, 1996), as well as international travel, could lead to reintroduction of malaria in the United States (Zucker, 1996).

The endemicity of malaria is determined by the presence of humans infected in an area where the vectors can breed and multiply in sufficient numbers to allow transmission from human to human. There are no known animal reservoirs for any of the species of human plasmodia. The vectors of malaria are female mosquitoes belonging to the genus *Anopheles*, containing about 400 species, 60 of which are considered good vectors of the parasite. These different species occur in distinct geographic locations to which they are adapted, and in any given endemic area for malaria, two or three species are the vectors of importance (Gilles, Warrell, 1993). Good mosquito malaria vectors feed preferentially, if not exclusively, on humans. These vectors have a life span long enough to permit development of the parasite, and they are adapted to temperature and humidity conditions that are consistent with the needs of the parasite.

One method of transmission of malaria in humans is through blood transfusions (Dover, Schultz, 1971). The most important species in this form of malaria is *P. malariae* because it lacks liver stages (hypnozoites; see above), and its long-lasting infection is due to persistence of stages in the blood. In African children, anemia due to several causes, including *falciparum* malaria produced by resistant strains, is responsible for a high percentage of hospital admissions. Anemia in these children is treated mainly with blood transfusions, which has increased the number of human immune deficiency virus (HIV) cases in this patient group (Hedberg et al. 1993). In Saudi Arabia, the sequential use of single syringes in patients receiving heparin blocks resulted in a number of infections with *P. falciparum* (Abulrahi et al. 1997). Transfusion malaria (Taylor, 1996) and its counterpart, malaria caused by dirty needles used by drug addicts, has resulted in outbreaks; one of the most remarkable outbreaks occurred in New York City in one of the winters of the 1930s. Malaria has also been acquired from bone marrow (Lefrere et al. 1996) and organ transplants (Holzer et al. 1985), a problem more acute in endemic areas or in transplanted patients with organs from endemic areas (Turkmen et al. 1996).

Biology and Pathogenesis. The pathogenesis of human malaria is related to the erythrocytic life cycle of the parasite. The symptoms occur when the infected erythrocytes rupture, releasing the newly formed merozoites. The symptoms of fever, muscle pain, headache, and nausea are related to the parasitemia; nonimmune patients develop symptoms at lower levels of parasitemia than semi-immune ones. It is almost certain that the fever in malaria is modulated by endogenous pyrogens released by monocytes and macrophages responding to the rupture and release of merozoites by infected red blood cells. Endogenous pyrogens are cytokines that affect the thermoregulatory center in the

hypothalamus and induce synthesis of prostaglandin E_2, which initiates the physiologic responses that produce fever, shivering, vasoconstriction, and other clinical manifestations (Kwiatkowski, 1995). However, tumor necrosis factor alpha appears to be the most important cytokine responsible for both fever and cerebral malaria. There is an increase in circulating tumor necrosis factor alpha at the end of schizogony of *P. vivax* (Karunaweera et al. 1992) and in children infected with *P. falciparum* (Kwiatkowski, 1995). Moreover, *P. falciparum* cultured in the presence of monocytes induces the production of tumor necrosis factor alpha, which increases sharply when merozoites are released from red blood cells (Kwiatkowski, 1995). The amount of tumor necrosis factor alpha produced during infection by a given isolate of *P. falciparum* varies with the strain of the parasite, which may explain why some patients in endemic areas develop cerebral malaria and others do not (Allan et al. 1993; see below). Wild isolates of *P. falciparum* from patients with severe malaria produce, on average, more tumor necrosis factor alpha than isolates from mild cerebral malaria; however, there is overlap between individual patients from the two groups (Allan et al. 1995).

Other important biologic aspects of plasmodia necessary for understanding the disease in humans involve the relationship between the parasite and its host cell, the erythrocyte. Changes induced by the parasites on infected red blood cells modulate the interaction of the red blood cells with endothelial cells and cells of the immune system. For example, erythrocytes infected with the asexual stages of *P. falciparum* form electron-dense, cone-shaped excrescences (knobs) on the plasma membrane (Figs. 10–6 and 10–7; Miller, 1972). These excrescences extend over the entire membrane and serve as the focal points for attachment (cytoadhesion) to the endothelial cells. This adhesion results in sequestration of the parasites to the capillary and postcapillary venous endothelium during their asexual multiplication (Aikawa et al. 1972). The electron-dense material composing the knobs is produced and secreted by the parasite in the parasitophorous vacuole. Once this material is secreted, it is incorporated into the vacuole membrane and transported on fragments of that membrane to the surface membrane of the red blood cell, where it is expressed as knobs (Fig. 10–6; Aikawa, 1988a).

The mechanism of cytoadhesion of *P. falciparum* to endothelial cells by means of knobs is difficult to study in vivo (Grau, Kossodo, 1994); most studies have been done in in vitro systems with different kinds of cells, including endothelial cells. Several molecules are thought to be the cell receptors for cytoadhesion of *P.*

falciparum to endothelial cells. Among them are the cell adhesion molecule 1 (VCAM-1), intracellular molecule 1 (ICAM-1), endothelial adhesion molecule 1 (ELAM-1) or E-selectin, and, to a lesser extent, CD36 (platelet glycoprotein IIIb or IV, OKM5 antigen) and thrombospodin (Berendt et al. 1990; Cooke, Coppel, 1995; Fujioka, Aikawa, 1996; Mendis, Carter, 1995; Ockenhouse et al. 1992; Roberts et al. 1985). A variety of cells, including endothelial cells, express these molecules, but their exact distribution in the endothelia of capillary beds in humans is not known. Nor is it known whether different levels of expression of these molecules are responsible for different levels of parasite sequestration (and thus different clinical pictures of the infection) (Berendt et al. 1990). The level of ICAM-1 molecule expression in the microcirculation of

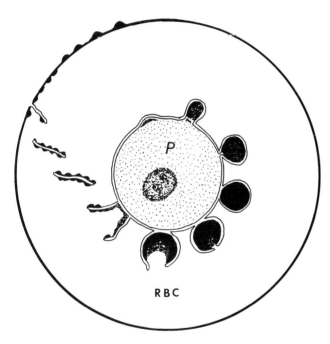

Fig. 10–6. *Plasmodium*, **schematic representation of a parasitized red blood cell showing the morphologic events that lead to the formation of knobs on the cell membrane. Note that the electron-dense material originates in the parasite, is excreted, and then in small fragments of the vacuole membrane is transported to the surface of the erythrocyte. (In: Howard, J.R., Uni, S., Lyon, J.A., et al. 1987. Export of *Plasmodium falciparum* protein to the host erythrocyte membrane: Special problems of protein trafficking and topogenesis. In: Chang, K.P., and Snary, D. (eds.) Host-Parasite Cellular and Molecular Interactions in Protozoal Infections. New York: Springer-Verlag, 281–296. Reproduced with permission.)**

the brain has been found to correlate with the amount of sequestration of parasitized red blood cells (Fujioka, Aikawa, 1996).

Sequestration of *P. falciparum*–infected erythrocytes in the brain is responsible for cerebral malaria, one of the major manifestations of severe malaria (Grau, Kossodo, 1994). Based on morphologic observations, a correlation between the severity of the disease and the amount of parasites sequestered in the microcirculation of the brain has long been known. The logical postulate derived from this observation is mechanistic: the masses of infected red blood cells in the capillaries decrease the microcirculation, followed by hypoxia, brain edema, coma, and death. The mechanical blockage of small blood vessels in the brain also explains the microscopic hemorrhages in individuals dying of cerebral malaria, a finding that cannot be accounted for solely on the basis of a cytokine-mediated mechanism of cerebral malaria (Grau, Kossodo, 1994). Blockage of blood vessels, hemorrhage, and tissue damage produce irreversible changes that manifest with a neurologic deficit in patients who recover from cerebral malaria (Newton et al. 1996). Because of these observations, the most accurate account of the physiopathology of cerebral malaria should include the morphologic observations together with a local and generalized release of metabolically active substances. These substances are lactic acid, locally induced cytokines, and substances with neurotransmitter or vasomotor activity such as tumor necrosis factor alpha (see above) and nitric oxide (Berendt et al. 1994; Clark et al. 1991). It is thought, but unproven, that the cytokines interleukin 1, tumor necrosis factor alpha, and lymphotoxin stimulate the release of nitric oxide by many cells, including endothelial cells (Mendis, Carter, 1995). Increased levels of nitrous oxide, which regulates the maintenance of vascular tone and neurotransmission, produce vasodilation that results in systemic hypotension and intracranial hypertension (Newton et al. 1996); these conditions are responsible for the manifestations of cerebral malaria (Clark et al. 1991; Clark et al. 1994; Clark, Rockett, 1994). The exact mechanism of cerebral malaria will probably be elucidated in the future (Mendis, Carter, 1995).

Other abnormalities found in the cell membranes of infected erythrocytes are the caveola–vesicle complexes in *P. vivax*, consisting of a caveola surrounded by vesicles in a fashion reminiscent of the arrangement of a terminal bronchiole and its alveoli. These caveola–vesicle complexes correspond to the Schüfner's stippling seen with the light microscope (Aikawa et al. 1975). In *P. malariae*, infected erythrocytes have the clefts and caveola–vesicle complexes that correspond to

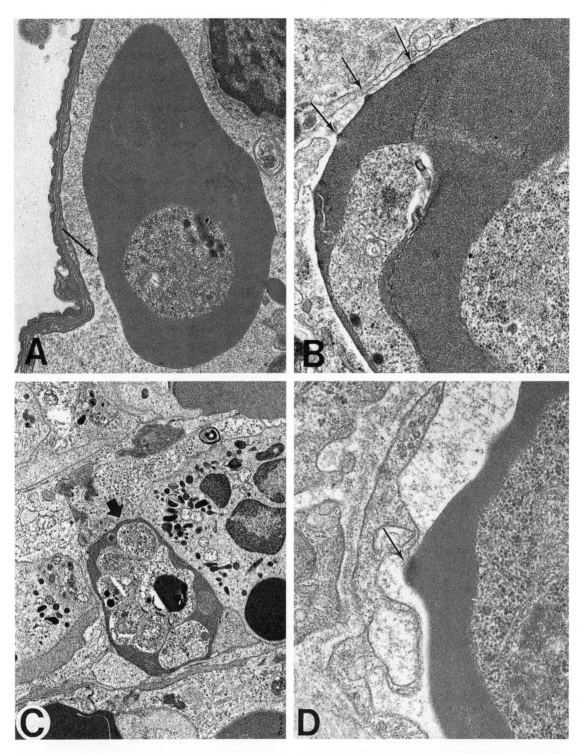

Fig. 10–7. *Plasmodium falciparum*, transmission electron micrographs of different organs from *Aotus trivirgatus* infected experimentally. *A*, Pulmonary capillary showing an erythrocyte with an advanced trophozoite; note that excrescences (knobs) are beginning to form on the parasitized red blood (arrow), ×5,000. *B*, Sequestered, parasitized red blood cell in a capillary of spleen showing the excrescences on the membrane, seen as electron-dense knobs (arrows), ×7,800. *C*, Spleen sinusoid with sequestered red blood cells with a mature schizont (arrow) containing six merozoites and a residual body with electron-dense material corresponding to malarial pigment, ×2,400. *D*, Higher magnification showing the red blood cells excrescence (arrow), ×12,000.

the Ziemann's dots and knobs similar to those of *P. falciparum* (Aikawa, 1988b).

Immunity. Exposure to malarial parasites confers specific immunity; thus, in endemic areas, individuals with the infection do not necessarily become ill or die. This acquired immunity is observed in young children and adults, leaving infants as the population most likely to suffer from serious illness and die of the infection. In addition to this acquired specific immunity, other innate factors are responsible for the immunity, or resistance to the infection, seen in some individuals and population groups. The best-known forms of innate immunity occur in persons with the genetic trait to produce hemoglobin S, which in the homozygote produces sickle cell anemia, a disease that is often fatal. In the heterozygote, however, there is no sickle cell disease, but rather a resistance to *falciparum* malaria. The mechanism that produces the resistance to the infection in the heterozygote is not known, but it may be related to sickling of infected red blood cells, which allows them to be rapidly cleared by the macrophage-monocyte system. Another well-known cause of innate resistance is lack of the Duffy antigen on the red blood cells, which occurs almost universally in the black population. The Duffy antigen is the molecule that allows merozoites of *P. vivax* to attach to and enter red blood cells. If this antigen is not present, this step in the cycle does not occur and infection cannot take place. The glucose-6-phosphate dehydrogenase deficiency seen in large numbers of persons living in areas endemic for malaria appears to be a selected trait that protects these individuals from malaria. The genetic defect is in chromosome X, so only in males and in female homozygotes is the deficiency fully expressed. The mechanism by which this genetic defect works is probably related to malarial parasites' use of the host pathway for the hexose-monophosphate shunt; any alteration in this pathway affects the parasites adversely. Although these individuals have the infection, they are protected against higher levels of parasitemia. Other innate factors providing some protection against malaria are hemoglobin E, some of the thalassemias, and some cytoskeletal abnormalities of the red blood cells.

The acquired immunity to malaria is seen under natural conditions in newborn infants with immune mothers; these newborns are refractory to the disease for about 6 months after birth. During this period infection can occur, but it is mild and almost never fatal. After this period, the children become increasingly susceptible to the disease and may die of profound anemia or cerebral malaria. Children usually acquire a protective immunity by the age of 5 years if they survive the infection; after this age, death due to the disease is rare. This acquired immunity requires continued reexposure to the infection to be maintained. Immunity is acquired when the individual is infected with all the prevailing strains of the parasite that occur in the endemic area. Thus, immunity to malaria is strain specific and takes a long time to develop. In the adult population, the prevalence of the infection is often 100%.

The malarial parasites spend most of their lives inside cells, where they are generally protected from the immune system. The sporozoites inoculated directly by the mosquito into the bloodstream are exposed to immune cells and antibodies. Antibodies directed against surface antigens, in conjunction with complement, may lyse the parasites or may prevent their entry into the hepatocyte. This action is the basis for the development of vaccine against malaria, and work in this area has had some success in experimental systems. However, one should remember that the circulation of sporozoites is short-lived and that some sporozoites gain access to the hepatocyte 3 minutes after their inoculation. The response to the infected hepatocyte seems nil since no symptoms, signs, inflammatory response to the parasites occur. Merozoites leaving the hepatocytes, or the red blood cells after completion of schizogony, rapidly enter the red blood cells to multiply asexually. Within the red blood cells, the parasites are also protected from the action of antibodies. In addition, because the erythrocyte does not interact with other cells of the immune system, no cell-mediated response is elicited by these cells. In animal models and in in vitro systems T cell–mediated immunity is evident, but how it operates in human infections is not known.

The alterations produced by the parasite on the red blood cells render these cells susceptible to clearance by the macrophage-monocyte system, especially in the spleen. This form of protection keeps the parasitemia at low levels but it also destroys the erythrocytes, resulting in anemia. The high levels of parasitemia seen in *P. falciparum* infections are not only the result of the higher rate of parasite multiplication, but are also due to the fact that by sequestering in the capillary bed during schizogony, the parasites avoid passage through the spleen. In this context, sequestration in *P. falciparum* is a parasite defense mechanism.

The anatomic pathologist regards malaria infections as belonging to one of two groups. One group is the infections produced by *P. falciparum*. In some individuals these infections produce fatal cerebral malaria, a disease diagnosed in the clinical laboratory in blood films and sometimes by the anatomic pathologist in tissues often obtained at autopsy. The other group is the infections produced by *P. vivax*, *P. malariae*, and *P. ovale*. These species produce a clinical infection that that is usually not fatal and is diagnosed exclusively in the clinical laboratory.

Plasmodium falciparum

Plasmodium falciparum is the most important species producing human malaria. It is sometimes referred to as *tertian malignant* because the malarial attack occurs every third day. This species is responsible for almost all the deaths attributed to the infection, with perhaps a few due to *P. malariae* nephrosis in children (see below). Death due to *falciparum* malaria occurs in nonimmune individuals traveling or residing in the endemic area; the former group consists mostly of children. This fact indicates that in endemic areas the infection confers a form of resistance or protection to the disease since in these areas up to 40% of the population usually have moderate parasitemia without symptoms.

To reemphasize, the main morphologic and biologic characteristics of *P. falciparum* that distinguish it from the other species are as follows: (*1*) The gametocytes have a falciform shape. (*2*) Parasite development in the liver occurs once at the beginning of the infection; no residual stages remain in the liver. (*3*) Erythrocytic schizogony occurs in red blood cells attached to the endothelial cells of the capillary vasculature. (*4*) Some strains of *P. falciparum* develop abnormal responses and resistance to some chemotherapeutic agents (Lobel et al. 1985; WHO, 1987). (*5*) In nonimmune hosts, infection with *P. falciparum* is potentially fatal even in large medical centers (Gilles, Warrell, 1993; Miller, 1984; WHO, 1987).

Clinical Findings. The incubation period of *falciparum* malaria depends largely on the number of sporozoites received from the mosquito; it is usually 1 to 2 weeks, but on some occasions it has been measured in months. The prodromal symptoms consist of bone aches, headache, chills, nausea, and sometimes vomiting and diarrhea. The onset of the disease may be delayed in persons with partial immunity, in whom the prodromal symptoms may last longer. Parasites may be detected in blood before the full-blown infection develops.

At the beginning of the disease the fever is irregular, without periodicity, sometimes occurring daily because different parasite broods complete erythrocytic schizogony at different times. However, the fever tends to become more synchronous as the disease progresses with its every-third-day pattern. In one-third of the patients, the fever becomes periodic after a few days; in the rest, the fever is remittent, intermittent, or even continuous. The typical *falciparum* malarial attack begins with low-grade fever, headache, bone and muscle pains, malaise, anxiety, and mental confusion, followed by a fever lasting for several hours and then by sweating, which is sometimes profuse. If no clear-cut paroxysms occur, the fever and sweating may persist. If the malarial attack is well defined, the individual becomes asymptomatic after the sweating subsides, only to have symptoms recur 48 hours later (on the third day, i.e., tertian malaria); however, this presentation is rare in *falciparum* malaria. The infection follows a course of similar episodes that continuously diminish in intensity. Uncomplicated disease lasts for 2 to 3 weeks.

In complicated *P. falciparum* malaria (pernicious or malignant malaria), different clinical syndromes are observed, depending on the organ system involved. Gastrointestinal involvement, sometimes fatal, usually occurs with nausea, vomiting, and profuse diarrhea that is often dysenteric. Pulmonary edema (Deaton, 1970) and insufficiency are sometimes fatal (Marsh et al. 1996; Punyagupta et al. 1974); anemia, hypoglycemia, jaundice, hepatic dysfunction, and other symptoms are also observed. Glomerulonephritis in the acute phase of *falciparum* malaria, with proteinuria, cylindruria, and mild urinary sediment abnormalities, has been found in up to 50% of cases. A large proportion of these patients develop renal failure associated with acute intravascular hemolysis or with a heavy parasitic load. Hemolysis is often the result of antimalarial therapy and should be distinguished from blackwater fever (see below). The most important complications of *falciparum* malaria are cerebral malaria and severe anemia (Imbert et al. 1997).

Cerebral Malaria. For practical purposes, cerebral malaria is defined as any impairment of consciousness or development of convulsions in a patient exposed to malaria (Gilles, Warrell, 1993). The prodromal symptoms are variable and nonspecific, the most common one being fever. The fever is followed by central nervous system symptoms such as drowsiness, headache, and rapid development of coma, often followed by death. Otherwise, the major clinical manifestations are meningismus, paresias, mental changes, and, in children, epileptiform attacks (seizures) such as status epilepticus, partial motor convulsions, or generalized tonic-clonic convulsions (Crawley et al. 1996). Since these manifestations are nonspecific, other causes for their occurrence should be ruled out even in patients with circulating *falciparum* parasites. More commonly, the presentation of cerebral malaria consists of convulsions, either generalized tonic-clonic, focal clonic, or bilateral. In addition, ocular symptoms and intracranial hypertension are commonly seen. In the youngest patients, intracranial hypertension manifests with tense, bulging fontanels. In children, as in adults, it is also important to rule out other causes for the clinical manifestations before making the diagnosis of cerebral malaria. The mortality in children with cerebral malaria in a university hospital was about 15% with most deaths occurring within the first 48 hours of admission. In children who survived, neurologic sequelae at discharge were found in 9% (Carme et al. 1993). A 2-year follow-up of these children revealed that the neurologic sequelae were responsible for death in some of them; in others, the sequelae were still present at the end of the study. However, the long-term outcome of the neurologic deficit in these children is unknown (Carme et al. 1993). In contrast, children surviving the disease without major neurologic sequelae show no neuropsychologic sequelae (Muntendam et al. 1996).

Congenital Malaria. Congenital malaria is diagnosed in an infant within 7 days of birth, later in nonendemic areas. The disease is acquired at birth, when rupture of blood vessels allows maternal and infant blood to be mixed. Clinically, the disease usually presents as fever; other symptoms are variable and nonspecific. All four species of plasmodia produce congenital or neonatal malaria, but *P. malariae* produces a larger number of infections (as in transfusion malaria; see above). In endemic areas, congenital malaria occurs less often than expected, judging by the number of infected mothers, and is more often seen in children born to nonimmune mothers. Primigravid women in endemic areas suffer the heaviest infections, and parity seems to influence susceptibility to the infection (Cot et al. 1993). Malaria in the pregnant woman increases the risk of delivering a low-birth-weight baby (Foster, 1996; Leopardi et al. 1996; Matteelli et al. 1996). Neonatal malaria increases the rate of perinatal death. Chemoprophylaxis for malaria in pregnant women provides some protection against infection of the infant (Bouvier et al. 1997a; Nyirjesy et al. 1993). Malaria is also the major cause of moderate to severe anemia in pregnant women living in endemic areas (Shulman et al. 1996); routine chemoprophylaxis has been recommended (Bouvier et al. 1997b).

The placenta of malarious mothers has gross and microscopic changes that are seen more commonly in primigravids infected with *P. falciparum*. The average weight of the placenta is significantly lower (by 46 g), and histologic changes are similar to those found in other tissues, with large numbers of parasitized red blood cells and malaria pigment in the maternal circulation (Walter et al. 1982). Increased fibrin deposition and many lymphocytes in the intervillous spaces of women with both active and previous malaria are found in the placenta (Leopardi et al. 1996). The effect of *P. falciparum* parasitization of the placenta is responsible for prematurity (Archibald, 1956). However, infection of the placenta does not correlate with perinatal mortality (McDermott et al. 1997). In congenital malaria, transfusion malaria (Dover, Schultz, 1971), and malaria acquired with organ transplants (Holzer et al. 1985), there are no developmental stages in the liver and these patients do not require therapy for these stages.

Blackwater Fever. Blackwater fever is a loose translation of the French term *fièvre bilieuse mélanurique* during the last part of the 19th century. The disease is seen in areas where *falciparum* malaria is endemic, and it is associated with a concurrent or recent malaria infection. The main characteristics of the disease are massive erythrocytic hemolysis, usually in patients who used quinine for treatment in the past. The symptoms begin with the usual malarial attack, but in a few days the patient develops abdominal pain, vomiting, diarrhea, and oliguria with mahogany brown urine that progresses to renal failure. Hypertension, renal failure, and coma are common, often with low parasitemia; mortality is 20% to 30%. The cause of blackwater fever is not known; it appears to be due to an autoimmune response to red blood cells altered by quinine in some patients. In other patients with a deficiency of the red blood cell enzyme glucose-6-phosphate dehydrogenase, development of blackwater fever is due to primaquine and other oxidant drugs, and may occur even in the absence of the infection. The syndrome produced by both of these mechanisms is identical (Tran et al. 1996).

Malaria and HIV Infection. The distribution of HIV infection in Africa and other tropical areas overlaps the distribution of malaria. An interaction between *Plasmodium*, an apicomplexan parasite, and the HIV virus was expected, but it did not occur (Butcher, 1992). In longitudinal studies of children with perinatally acquired HIV infection, there was no increase in the number of cases or the severity of *P. falciparum* (Greenberg et al. 1991). Studies in adults showed similar findings; in addition, there were no differences in the therapeutic response to malaria between HIV-positive and HIV-negative patients (Muller, Moser, 1990). Some explanations for this lack of enhanced morbidity due to malaria in HIV infections are presented above (see Immunity).

Pathology. The morphologic changes produced by *P. falciparum* result from its sequestration in small blood vessels and the capillary bed. Accumulation of malarial pigment in histiocytes is the gross and histologic hallmark of the infection. The pigment is the end product of the parasite's digestion of the erythrocyte's hemoglobin. The pigment consists of a ferric ion containing porphyrin conjugated with a protein moiety derived from partial proteolysis of the globin portion of hemoglobin. The metabolism of malarial pigment by macrophages is slow, and eventually the pigment reverts to its basic components, which are reused as building blocks for hemoglobin. Hemosiderin, another hemoglobin pigment found in infections with malaria, results from red blood cell lysis.

Central Nervous System. Grossly, the brains of patients dying of *falciparum* infection have flattened gyri due to marked swelling. The blood vessels are congested, and the cut surface of the fresh organ is pink with a dark gray cortex due to pigment deposition (Fig. 10–8). Microscopically, the distended capillaries have masses of erythrocytes filling the lumen (Fig. 10–9 *A–B*). In slightly larger blood vessels, the parasitized erythrocytes are clearly seen lying against the endothelial surface, with the parasites' nuclei stained darkly with hematoxylin and eosin stain. Malarial pigment in parasitized red blood cells, in macrophages, and sometimes free in the circulation is abundant. Some vessels contain thrombi.

In cerebral malaria lasting for more than 10 days, small, hemorrhagic areas known as *ring hemorrhages* may be observed around blood vessels (Fig. 10–9 *C–D*). These hemorrhages are due to endothelial damage and thrombosis of medium-sized blood vessels, which produce blood leakage in the tissue. In individuals who survive an episode of cerebral malaria, the damaged hemorrhagic areas heal and form small areas of fibrosis known as *Durck's granulomas.*

Spleen. The spleen shows changes early in the infection, such as hyperemia and slight enlargement. Later, during the chronic phase, spleen enlargement becomes clinically apparent, a change known as *tropical splenomegaly syndrome* (Pitney, 1968). Gross evaluation of splenomegaly in patients was used to assess the prevalence of malaria in endemic areas. It is well known that

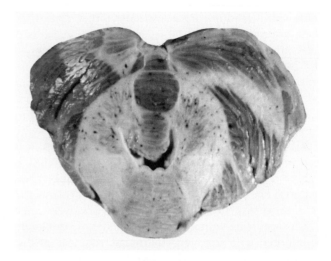

Fig. 10–8. *Plasmodium falciparum*, section of pons and cerebellum from a patient with fatal acute falciparum malaria. Note the marked hyperemia and petechial hemorrhages. (Courtesy of D.H. Connor, M.D., Division of Geographic Medicine, Armed Forces Institute of Pathology, Washington, D.C., AFIP No. 70-11647.)

populations receiving massive antimalaria chemotherapy have lower levels of splenomegaly syndrome. In Uganda, 45% of individuals with tropical splenomegaly syndrome had *P. malariae* (Marsden et al. 1965); however, in New Guinea this correlation was absent (Marsden et al. 1967). The slight splenomegaly found in individuals with acute *P. falciparum* infection plays a role in the accelerated clearance of abnormal erythrocytes from the circulation (Looareesuwan et al. 1987). Splenic rupture is a complication of infections with all forms of malaria, but it is more common in *P. vivax* infections.

The spleen in acute *falciparum* infections is friable, dark red to dark brown, due to congestion and accumulation of pigment; in chronic infections it is black, with a firm consistency (Fig. 10–10 *A*). The white pulp is prominent against the dark background in acute infections but is usually indistinguishable in chronic ones.

Microscopically, both the white and red pulp are distended due to massive hyperemia. Numerous parasitized red cells and macrophages with large, amorphous clumps of dark pigment are scattered throughout the organ; polymorphonuclear cells increase, some with phagocytized pigment (Fig. 10–10 *B*). In chronic infections, the hyperemia is less severe and the white pulp becomes depleted; fibrosis may be prominent. The macrophages with pigment increase, as does the fibrous tissue of the trabeculae, follicles, and capsule. Accumulation of pigment in the spleen and other organs depends on the intensity and duration of the infection. After treatment, metabolism of the pigment is slow;

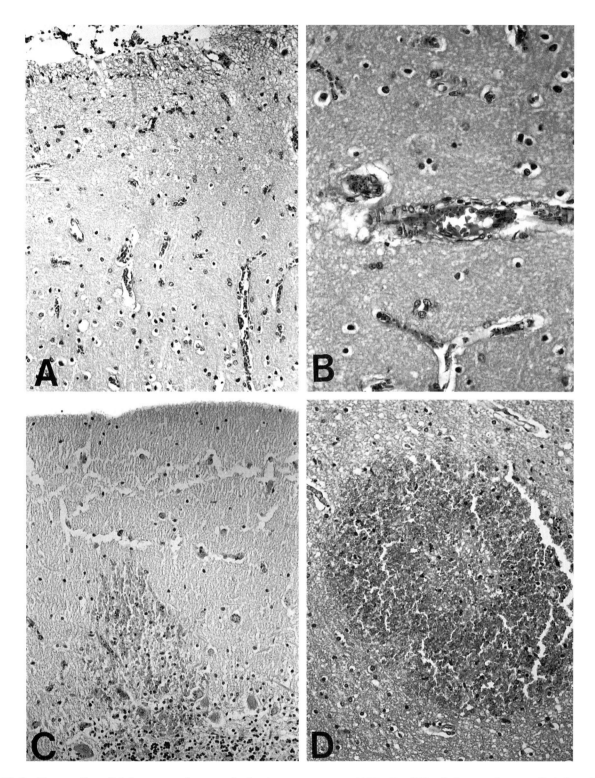

Fig. 10–9. *Plasmodium falciparum*, microscopic changes in the central nervous system, sections stained with hematoxylin and eosin stain. *A*, Low-power view of a brain section showing marked hyperemia, ×140. *B*, Higher magnification showing capillaries and a small blood vessel filled with parasitized red blood cells, ×280. *C*, Early microscopic hemorrhage in the cerebellar cortex, ×40. *D*, "Ring" hemorrhage, slightly older than the previous one, in a brain from another patient. Note the central necrosis, ×280. (Preparation for *A–C* courtesy of K.T. Tham, M.D., Hong Kong. Preparation for *D* courtesy of M. Aikawa, M.D., Institute of Pathology, University Hospitals of Cleveland, Cleveland, Ohio.)

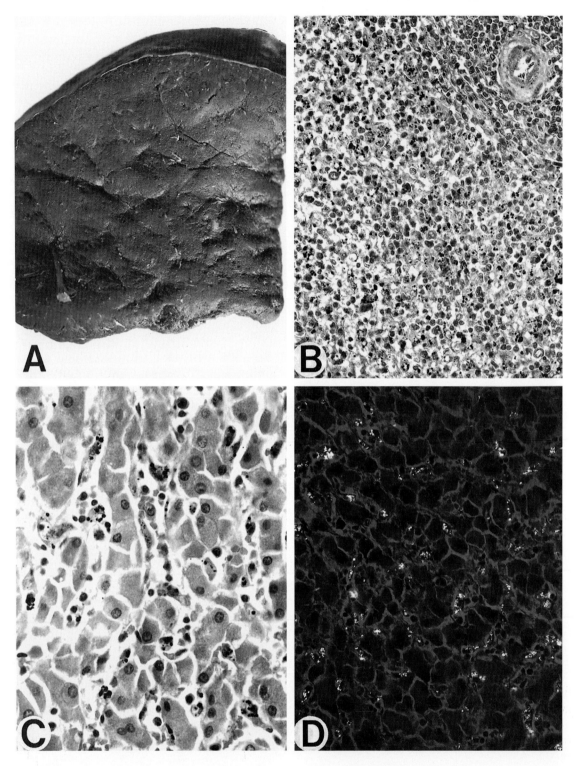

Fig. 10–10. *Plasmodium falciparum* infection in spleen and liver. *A*, Gross photograph of a slice of spleen; note the black slate color produced by accumulation of malarial pigment. *B*, Low-power view of a histologic section of spleen showing marked accumulation of pigment in phagocytic cells, stained with hematoxylin and eosin stain, ×280. *C–D*, Liver sections stained with hematoxylin and eosin stain. *C*, Medium-power view of liver showing congested sinusoids containing Kupffer cells with pigment and parasitized red blood cells, ×280. *D*, Same section under polarized light, ×280 (Tissues courtesy of K.T. Tham, M.D., Hong Kong.)

sometimes pigment is present after 1 year. Small, hemorrhagic infarcts of the spleen due to thrombosis in the sinusoids are common, and in long-lasting infections with profound anemia, there are foci of extramedullary hemopoiesis.

Liver. The liver is an important organ in the life cycle of *Plasmodium.* Invasion of hepatocytes by mosquito sporozoites and further development of the sporozoites produce no detectable histologic changes on light or electron microscopy (Hollingdale, 1985). The changes in the liver occur during the clinical infection.

Grossly, the liver is moderately enlarged due to fluid overload; in experimental animals the wet weight was increased, while the dry weight remained constant (Jervis et al. 1972). The most dramatic abnormality is the color change from dark brown in acute infections to black in chronic ones due to accumulation of pigment. Microscopically, there is distention of the sinusoids, an increased number of macrophages with pigment, and a few polymorphonuclear cells (Fig. 10–10 C). At first, the Kupffer cells hypertrophy and begin to phagocytize pigment, but circulating monocytes soon infiltrate the sinusoids. Early in the infection, pigment is deposited in the perilobular zone. Then it spreads to the midlobular zone and later to the central vein portion, correlating with the portal blood flow. Large numbers of parasitized red blood cells attach to the sinusoidal endothelial cells, which have alterations in their ultrastructure (Gutierrez et al. 1976). The macrophages with pigment change as the infection progresses, becoming round and more compact, with masses of clumped pigment in older infections. Under polarized light the pigment polarizes, producing a bright yellowish color (Fig. 10–10 D). Changes in the hepatocytes are evident only on electron micrographs. They consist of mitochondrial damage, swelling, and loss of microvilli in the space of Disse and the bile canaliculi. These changes may contribute to the hyperbilirubinimia in some cases of malaria (Bhamarapravati et al. 1973; Brito et al. 1962).

Kidneys. In the kidneys, the gross abnormalities are mainly hyperemia and darkening due to pigment deposition. Microscopically, the changes are subtler, sometimes evident only on electron micrographs or with immunofluorescence. These microscopic changes are responsible for glomerulonephritis, especially in individuals with chronic infections.

Individuals with *P. falciparum* infections and renal involvement have hypercellularity and scant infiltration by inflammatory cells in the glomeruli. Electron micrographs show thickening of the basement membrane and electron-dense deposits in the subendothelial and paramesangial areas. Immunofluorescent stains that show these deposits contain immunoglobulin G (IgG), IgM, beta-1-C globulin, and C3 (Boonpucknavig, Sitprija, 1979). A few individuals with *P. falciparum* infection develop nephrotic syndrome, but in certain geographic areas this condition is more common in children infected with *P. malariae* (see below).

Other Organs. All other organ systems and tissues are affected by *falciparum* malaria. Also, patients dying of the infection have gross changes caused by congestion due to accumulation of sequestered parasites. Under the microscope, abundant parasitized red blood cells are found within the dilated vessels, and pigment is seen if polarized light is used (Fig. 10–11 A–B). In placentas from infected mothers, parasitized red blood cells and pigment are observed in the maternal circulation (intervillous spaces); they are almost never seen in the fetal circulation (Fig. 10–12 A–B).

Plasmodium vivax, P. malarie, and *P. ovale*

As stated before, *P. vivax*, *P. ovale*, and *P. malariae* produce an infection that is not fatal and if untreated, in the absence of reinfection, is self-limited. The liver stages of *P. vivax* and *P. ovale* produce relapses of progressively lower intensity and duration for a period of no more than 4 years. In *P. malariae*, recrudescences occur even several decades later, but the infection becomes asymptomatic soon after the acute episode and remains so for many years. The symptoms are similar to those described above for *P. falciparum*, but none of its complications occur. There are no descriptions of gross or microscopic lesions in tissues from patients infected with these three species.

An association between *P. malariae* and nephrotic syndrome in children was established more than three decades ago (Gigioli, 1962a, 1962b; Gilles, Hendrickse, 1960, 1963), and the pathophysiology of the disease was determined soon thereafter (Allison et al. 1969; Soothill, Hendrickse, 1967). The average age of children with nephrotic syndrome produced by *P. malariae* is about 8 years, older than the average age of children with this condition in nonendemic areas. The peak number of hospital admissions for patients with nephrotic syndrome in endemic areas coincides with the peak incidence of malaria. Since most glomerulopathies in malaria occur in individuals with *P. malariae*, the term given to this syndrome is *quartan malarial nephropathy.*

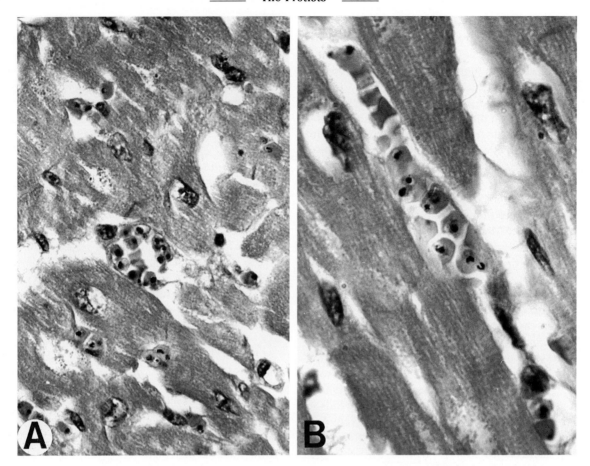

Fig. 10–11. *Plasmodium falciparum*, microscopic changes in heart; sections stained with hematoxylin and eosin. *A*, Cross section of small vessel showing parasitized red blood cells attached to endothelium; parasites, pigment, or both are seen as dark-staining dots, ×1,400. *B*, Higher magnification of a capillary vessel with similar features, ×1,400.

Quartan malarial nephropathy is clinically similar to the nephropathy produced by other conditions, but the histologic, electron microscopic, and immunofluorescence features are different (Allison et al. 1969; Hendrickse, Adeniyi, 1979). Histologically, the lesion of malarial nephrotic syndrome in Ugandan children consists of a proliferative glomerulonephritis produced by circulating soluble antigen–antibody complexes that deposit on the epithelial side of the basement membrane (Allison et al. 1969). Morphologically, the lesions in the glomeruli are grouped into five categories: (*1*) diffuse changes throughout the glomerulus; (*2*) lobular lesions; (*3*) focal glomerular changes; (*4*) chronic changes with capsular lesions and fibrosis; and (*5*) minimal lesions (Kibukamusoke, Hutt, 1967). Immunofluorescence studies of kidney sections demonstrate bound immunoglobulins and complement C3 in the base membrane deposits, and antibodies eluted from the kidney react against antigens of *P. malariae* (Allison et al. 1969). The gammaglobulins in the glomerulus are IgM, associated mostly with a granular pattern of deposits, and IgG, associated with either a continuous or a granular pattern (Houba et al. 1971). In children who respond to therapy, the basement membrane deposits resolve. However, in those who do not respond, the antigen–antibody complexes persist, indicating that the *P. malariae* nephritis is damaging the glomerulus, liberating antigens that react with autoantibodies and perpetuating the lesion (Houba et al. 1971). In a study of Nigerian children, the glomerular lesions were quantified and graded as grade I if 30% of glomeruli were affected; grade II if 30 to 75% were affected, and grade III if over 75% were affected. The patients who responded to treatment were all in group I. Those who did not respond were in groups II and III, and the disease progressed to hypertension and renal failure within 3 to 5 years (Hendrickse, Adeniyi, 1979).

Diagnosis. Clinical suspicion of malaria should arise when the epidemiologic circumstances (living in or having been in an endemic area) and the symptoms suggest the infection. The clinical diagnosis is usually confirmed in the laboratory using good, well-stained blood smears. The blood smear, if read by a well-trained technician, is a cheap, reliable, and fast method. In spite of progress in the development of other technologies for diagnosis, the morphologic study of blood smears is still the gold standard and apparently will not be replaced soon. The development of a rapid, cost-effective method for detection and identification of malarial parasites in blood is desirable and should eliminate the use of the microscope. Meanwhile, careful examination of all parasites found in thin or thick blood smears is necessary to identify the organism in question. Morphologic diagnosis of malaria and identification of the parasites are widely discussed in textbooks on clinical pathology (Woods, Gutierrez, 1993).

Several other techniques are used for the diagnosis of malaria. The *ParaSight f test* is based on a capture assay of a histidine-rich protein of *P. falciparum* in peripheral blood. The *ICT Malaria Pf test* is similar but uses a monoclonal antibody against the histidine-rich protein. The *OptiMAL test* is based on the detection of lactate dehydrogenase produced by the parasites; it distinguishes the species based on differences between the lactate dehydrogenase isoforms. This test uses whole blood and a dipstick with reagents. The *QBC system* uses acridine orange stain for staining malaria parasites in blood contained in a capillary tube. The blood and the stain are mixed in the tube and read with a microscope illuminated with blue-violet light, under which the parasites fluoresce. The technique has given good results for both *Plasmodium* and *Babesia* (Mattia et al. 1993). A polymerase chain reaction has very low sensitivity and the results vary greatly, depending on the geographic area where it is used (Jelinek et al. 1996). Serologic methods such as the enzyme-linked immunosorbent assay and the immunofluorescence antibody test detect antibodies against blood stages of the parasites. Most of these newer tests are best for epidemiologic work in which large numbers of samples are available for examination. Although most of these

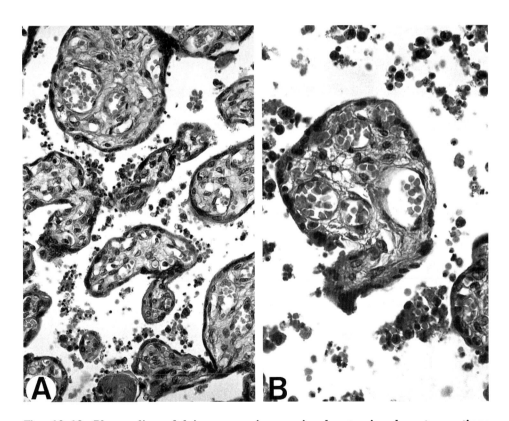

Fig. 10–12. *Plasmodium falciparum*, **microscopic changes in placenta, sections stained with hematoxylin and eosin stain.** *A* **and** *B*, **Different magnifications showing the maternal side with abundant parasitized red blood cells and malarial pigment. Note that the erythrocytes in capillaries within the villi are parasite free and have no pigment,** *A* **×240,** *B* **×380.**

tests are available commercially, the routine clinical laboratory is hard pressed to justify their cost for the few samples examined. In the following paragraphs, we will discuss only the diagnosis of tissue sections.

Only *P. falciparum* occurs in tissue sections. In hematoxylin and eosin–stained preparations of autopsy material from patients dying of malaria (almost never seen in biopsy specimens because they are not submitted for diagnosis) there is a marked hyperemia. Examination of engorged capillaries under oil immersion reveals masses of erythrocytes with small, dark dots (parasite nuclei) and clumps of refractile dark or dark greenish malarial pigment. Arterioles and venules show clearly that the infected erythrocytes are located against the endothelium. Visualization of individual parasites in tissue sections generally is not difficult in hematoxylin and eosin–stained specimens because the cytoplasm does not stain. Preparations stained with Giemsa stain may be helpful, but this or other special stains are not necessary for diagnosis because the changes are characteristic of *P. falciparum* infection. The pigment in the red blood cells and macrophages polarizes if viewed under polarized light, a feature common to all malarial pigments. The use of polarized light has also been recommended for screening of blood smears (Field et al. 1963; Field, Shute, 1956). The malaria pigment occurs in infected red blood cells, especially after prolonged parasite evolution, in peripheral monocytes, and in tissue macrophages. On treatment, clearance of pigment begins. Pigment disappears first from red blood cells, followed by peripheral monocytes (median period, 216 hours) and finally from tissue macrophages (median period, 12 days) (Day et al. 1996). This fact is mentioned here because polarization of pigment can be used as the basis for diagnosis of *P. falciparum* in patients living in endemic areas who have the disease but are parasite free. This condition occurs when these patients receive empirical therapy (administered by themselves, by pharmacies, or by primary care clinics), which clears the parasites rapidly from circulation, but later they develop signs and symptoms of cerebral malaria. Assessment of the presence of pigment in the three compartments—infected red blood cells, monocytes, and tissue macrophages—may provide a diagnosis and the approximate time elapsed after treatment (Day et al. 1996). To obtain tissue macrophages easily, intradermal pricks are made with a needle in a small area of the volar surface. Then the skin is gently squeezed to produce a small amount of serosanguinous fluid that is applied to a slide; the slide is then stained and examined (Day et al. 1996).

In some instances, when an autopsy is not possible in individuals dying of suspected malaria, transeth-moidal needle biopsy is desirable. The brain tissue obtained with a needle is smeared on slides stained with Giemsa stain to demonstrate the parasitized red blood cells (Ranque, 1986). However, a sample from almost any tissue in the body will serve the same purpose.

Babesia and *Entopolypoides*— Babesiosis or Piroplasmosis

Organisms resembling *Plasmodium* have been described in individuals suffering from an acute febrile illnes that is sometimes fatal. These organisms belong to the family Babesiidae, in which two genera have species that infect humans: *Babesia* and *Entopolypoides*. The diseases produced by these organisms are known as *piroplasmosis*, which is characterized by a massive hemolytic syndrome that is sometimes fatal. Since many species of mammals suffer from this disease, it is of veterinary importance in many regions of the world. *Babesia*, like *Plasmodium*, has a two-host cycle; the invertebrate hosts are ticks (Beaver et al. 1984).

Babesia

Babesia species are intraerythrocytic organisms of different shapes, commonly pyriform, and arranged within the cell as pairs or tetrads, sometimes with a characteristic arrangement resembling a Maltese cross (Fig. 10–15 D). Although many species of *Babesia* occur in animals, only four or five are known to infect humans. These are *B. divergens* and *B. bovis* (= *B. caucasica*) in Europe; *B. microti* in the New England area and the eastern United States; *B. equi* in California; and possibly *B. canis* in Mexico and France (Marsaudon et al. 1995). Two general areas where the infection is recognized are Europe (Brasseur, Gorenflot, 1992), with about two dozen cases, and the United States, where over 200 cases have been reported (Fernandez Villar et al. 1991).

Life Cycle. The life cycle of *Babesia* involves a vertebrate host, where asexual multiplication occurs in the erythrocytes, producing four merozoites, and an invertebrate host, a tick, where sexual development occurs. The vertebrate host acquires the infection when the tick inoculates the infective stages in its salivary glands. The infective stages have an apical complex and a pellicle (cytoskeleton) similar to that of the sporozoites of plasmodia. The inoculated forms enter the erythrocytes, where they lose their pellicles and transform into trophozoites that begin feeding on the hemoglobin of the host cell. Before division occurs the trophozoite forms all of its organelles, including the apical complex. Then the trophozoite divides into two organisms, one of which retains the apical complex and the other of which forms its own. Sexual stages do not form in the vertebrate host.

In the tick, the ingested parasites undergo development that is not completely understood. Sexual reproduction takes place, with formation of an intracellular stage in the gut cells of the arthropod. This stage enlarges and divides its nucleus and cytoplasm several times, finally producing numerous *vermicules*. The vermicules pass from the gut epithelial cells to the cavity of the tick (filled with hemolymph), where they distribute and invade hemocytes, the cells of the Malpighian tubules (the urinary system of arthropods), and, in female ticks, the oocytes. In the oocytes the parasites develop throughout the process of oviposition of the tick and continue to develop to merozoites in the ticks's eggs. The merozoites enter the gut epithelium of the tick's larva (vertical transmission). When the larva begins to feed, the parasite forms vermicules that are distributed throughout the body of the tick, including the salivary glands. Vertical transmission occurs in one or more generations, depending on the tick species, maintaining the parasite in nature. Both humans and animals acquire the disease by the bite of the infected tick.

Geographic Distribution and Epidemiology. The extent of *Babesia* infections in humans is not known; judging by the fragmentary data available, it may be an extensive zoonosis. In Nigeria, a serologic study of 173 males revealed antibodies to *Babesia* in 54% (Leeflang et al. 1976). In Mexico, of 101 persons studied, 38 reacted to antigen from *B. canis*; from 3 of these subjects, *Babesia* isolates were obtained with inoculations in animals (Osorno et al. 1976). In North Carolina, of 186 serum samples from children on an Indian reservation, 6 were positive for *B. microti* (Chisholm et al. 1986). In the United States, the first case of *Babesia* was reported in 1904 in Montana. The parasite was described as *Piroplasma hominis* and was thought to cause Rocky Mountain spotted fever (Wilson, Chowning, 1904). More recently, the first case identified as *Babesia* occurred in 1976 (Grunwaldt, 1977) in New York State. Other cases followed, demonstrating that the infection occurs mainly on the northeastern seashore and its offshore islands (Ruebush et al. 1981a). Isolated cases have been reported from California, (Bredt et al. 1981; Scholtens et al. 1968), Wisconsin (Steketee et al. 1985), and Georgia (Healy et al. 1976). The species infecting humans on the northeastern seashore is *B. microti*; the vector is *Ixodes dammini* (Ruebush et al. 1981b; Spielman, 1976), which is also the vector of *Borrelia burgdorferi*, the agent of Lyme disease. However, it appears that *I. dammini* is a synonym of *I. scapularis*, which is known in the part of the country south of Maryland (Sanders, 1998; Telford, 1998). The correct name probably will be determined in the near future. Sixty percent of patients with Lyme disease are seropositive for *B. microti*, and one-half of the patients with babesioses have antibodies for *B. burgdorferi* (Benach et al. 1985), closely linking these two infections epidemiologically.

Since *I. dammini* is a tick with a 2-year cycle, with mice (*Peromyscus leucopus*) (Spielman et al. 1981) and white-tail deer (*Odocoileus virginianus*) as its obligatory hosts, the prevalence of these infections depends on the populations of these animals (Healy, 1989). The prevalence of both Lyme disease and babesiois is increasing because the white-tail deer population in the United States is exploding (Dammin et al. 1981). Reports of coinfections with both diseases are known (Grundwalt et al. 1983; Marcus et al. 1985). Careful study of patients with Lyme disease has shown that 10% of them have babesiosis, and that these patients have more symptoms and longer disease duration than patients with Lyme disease alone (Krause et al. 1996). Transmission of both *B. microti* and *B. burgdorferi* in the northeastern United States is higher during the months of May and June, the peak period for the vector seeking a host to feed on (Piesman et al. 1987). *Babesia* infection is also transmitted through blood transfusions (Gerber et al. 1994; Gordon et al. 1984; Grabowski et al. 1982; Jacoby et al. 1980; Wittner et al. 1982). Only one instance of infection in a pregnant woman is known, with no transmission to the fetus (Raucher et al. 1984). Serologic surveys of blood donors in Massachusetts have shown a seropositivity of about 4% (Popovsky et al. 1988). In healthy individuals living under endemic conditions in Shelter Island, New York, seropositivity was 4.4% in June and almost 7% in October (Filstein et al. 1980). This increase, and the increase in titers in persons who tested positive in June, represented an almost 6% incidence for the season (Filstein et al. 1980). In Europe, *Ixodes ricinus* and *Dermacentor marginatus* (Oteo, Estrada, 1992) transmit *B. divergens* and *B. bovis*, both parasites of cattle. *Babesia divergens* is widely distributed in Europe and is considered the main agent of babesiosis, while *B. bovis* occurs mostly in southern Europe (Brasseur, Gorenflot, 1996). Prevention of the infection must be stressed, especially to splenectomized patients. Prevention involves the use of insect repellents every time exposure is likely (walking in the woods) and, upon returning home, close inspection of the entire body to remove any ticks promptly. Transmission of babesiosis starts 48 hours after attachment of the tick.

In recent years, a *Babesia*-like organism called WA1 has been found in patients in the states of California and Washington (Persing et al. 1995). Genetic sequence analysis showed that the parasite is closer to *B. gibsoni* from dogs and to species of *Theileria* than to other species of *Babesia* (Persing et al. 1995; Quick et al. 1993; Thomford et al. 1994). Experimental infections in hamsters with WA1 and with *B. microti* have shown that WA1 in animals produces more morbidity and mortality (Wozniak et al. 1996). In another patient from Missouri, a *Babesia* (MO1) distinct from *B. microti* and WA1, and reacting strongly against *B. divergens*, was also isolated (Herwaldt et al. 1996). The patient was seronegative to *B. microti*, which should arise concern about relying on serologic testing for diagnosis; negative results do not rule out babesiosis produced by other species (Herwaldt et al. 1996). In Taiwan, a strain (TW1) with characteristics of *B. microti* has been studied (Shih CM, Lien JC, 1994; Shih et al. 1997). At the time of this writing, no definite species determination is available for any of these three isolates.

Immunity. Little information available on immunity to babesiosis in humans. The disease tends to occur more often in patients with some form of immune impairment, as well as in older and asplenic individuals (see below). Patients with acute babesiosis have a peripheral lymphocytosis, due to an increase in B lymphocytes and a decrease in T lymphocytes, in a manner similar to that observed in malarial infections. However, the T-cell subpopulation bearing an IgG receptor is relatively increased. The response to nonspecific mitogens decreases, and the level of circulating immune complexes is ele-

vated in these patients. The elevation of circulating immune complexes in animals has resulted in glomerulonephritis, but whether this occurs in humans has not been established (Benach et al. 1982).

Clinical Findings. Babesiosis occurs at all ages, but the elderly are the group most commonly affected (Benach et al. 1982). The clinical manifestations of *Babesia* infections are variable. Some patients are asymptomatic (Healy et al. 1976); others have mild symptoms and often are not diagnosed (Krause et al. 1992). The infection tends to develop more readily in individuals who have an altered immune system (Benach et al. 1982). Some conditions, such as old age (Benach, Habicht, 1981), lymphoma, IgA deficiency (Cahill et al. 1981), Waldenström's macroglobulinemia (Bruckner et al. 1985), and especially splenectomy (see below) are predisposing factors. Babesiosis has developed in individuals with acquired immune deficiency virus (AIDS) (Benezra et al. 1987), presenting in one individual with prolonged fever of unknown origin (Falagas, Klempner, 1996) and in another, who was also spenectomized, with a high parasitemia (Ong et al. 1990). Babesiosis manifests with a gradual onset of malaise, anorexia, and fatigue, followed by fever of up to 1 week's duration, with profound sweating and muscle and joint pains. Some individuals experience nausea, vomiting, and shaking chills; the temperature at the time of examination has ranged from 37.6°C to 40.0°C. Another physical finding is mild splenomegaly (Ruebush et al. 1977a; Ruebush et al. 1977b). Some patients have infarcts in the retina (Ortiz, Eagle, 1982) or acute respiratory distress syndrome (Gordon et al. 1984). Laboratory tests show anemia with a progressive decrease in red blood cells due to hemolysis, sometimes necessitating blood transfusions. Elevated bilirubin, elevated alkaline phosphatase, and thrombocytopenia are frequent (Gombert et al. 1982; Ruebush et al. 1977b). White blood cell counts are normal, but reticulocyte levels are increased. Serologic tests for *Babesia* are positive. The diagnosis is often missed by the clinical laboratory or the disease is mistakenly diagnosed as malaria (Ruebush et al. 1977a).

Fig. 10–13. *Babesia divergens*, **kidney lesions in human infection, sections stained with hematoxylin and eosin stain.** *A*, **Low-power view showing many renal tubules filled with granular casts, ×55.** *B*, **Two glomeruli, mostly intact, and renal tubules with granular casts, ×180.** *C*, Higher magnification showing renal capillaries; some red blood cells with parasites are seen as very faint dots (arrows), ×705. *D*, **Higher magnification of tubular casts, ×705. (Preparation courtesy of C.C. Kennedy, M.D., Consultant Pathologist, Belfast City Hospital, Belfast, Ireland.)**

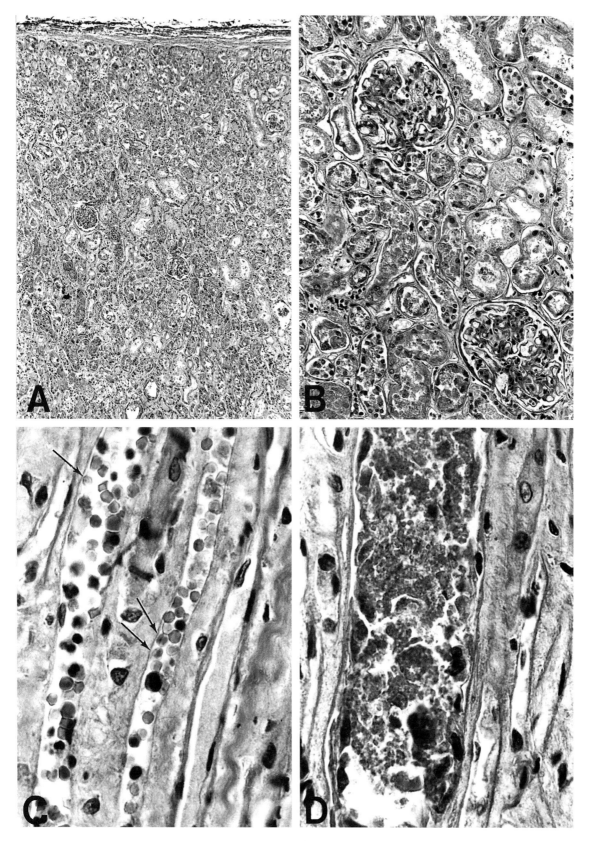

Fig. 10–13.

Babesia in Splenectomized Individuals. In splenectomized and older individuals, *Babesia* infection follows a more severe course characterized by high fever, massive hemolysis, hemoglobulinemia, and hemoglobinuria sometimes diagnosed as Weil's disease. The outcome has been fatal in some cases in which profound shock with brain anoxia, bilirubinemia, and acute renal tubular necrosis developed. Fatality in splenectomized patients occurs more often in Europe (Belgium, France, Russia, Spain, Sweden, Switzerland, the United Kingdom, and Yugoslavia) (Brasseur, Gorenflot, 1996; Etrican et al. 1979; Fitzpatrick et al. 1969; Harambasic et al. 1976; Skrabalo, Deanovic, 1957), mostly produced by *B. divergens*, the most pathogenic species. *Babesia bovis*, *B. caucasica*, and possibly *B. equi* (Rosner et al. 1984) also infect individuals in Europe. One patient who died in the United States was infected with *Entopolypoides*, a closely related organism (see below). Most splenectomized patients surviving the infection have been found in the United States; the species responsible for these infections was *B. microti* (Mathewson et al. 1984; Rosner et al. 1984; Scholtens et al. 1968). A splenectomized elderly woman in France also survived the infection (Bazin et al. 1976). A presentation with pancytopenia due to hemophagocytosis is observed in splenectomized patients with severe disease (Gupta et al. 1995; Slovut et al. 1996).

Pathology. The usual infection with *Babesia* produces no known histologic changes other than the presence of the parasites in the red blood cells. In splenectomized persons with fatal infections, the organs have gross changes related to massive hemolysis and acute tubular necrosis. Microscopically, the kidneys have tubular necrosis, edema (Fig. 10–13 *A–B*), massive amounts of hemoglobin, casts in the tubules filling the lower collecting system (Fig. 10–13 *D*), and debris in the capil-

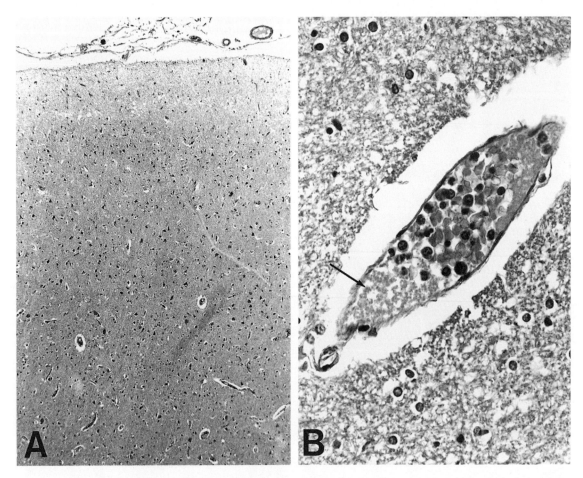

Fig. 10–14. ***Babesia divergens*, brain lesions in fatal human infection, hematoxylin and eosin stain. *A*, Low-power view of cerebral cortex illustrates the lack of hyperemia, ×47. *B*, Higher magnification of a medium-sized vessel showing the lack of margination of parasitized red blood cells. Note the granular material from hemolyzed red blood cells (arrow), ×380. (Preparation courtesy of C.C. Kennedy, M.D., Consultant Pathologist, Belfast City Hospital, Belfast, Ireland.)**

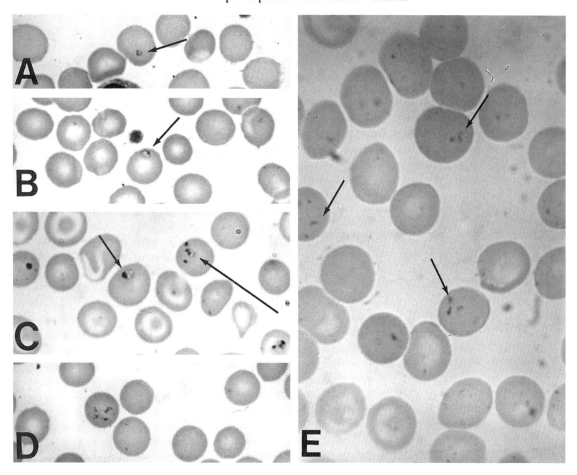

Fig. 10–15. *Babesia microti* and *Entopolypoides* in humans. *A–D. Babesia microti* from a case in New England, preparation stained with Giemsa stain. *A* and *B*, Small rings (arrows). *C*, One (short arrow) and four trophozoites (long arrow) are represented by faint cytoplasm and small chromatin granules. *D*, Characteristic arrangements of a tetrad, ×1,700. *E*, Blood smear from a patient with *Entopolypoides* (arrows), ×2,000. (Photographs courtesy of G.R. Healy, Ph.D., Centers for Disease Control, Atlanta, Georgia. The photo in *B* corresponds to case no. 2 reported by: Wolf, R.E., Gleason, N.N., Schoenbaum, S.C., et al. 1978. Intraerythrocytic parasitosis in humans with *Entopolypoides* species (Family Babesiidae): Association with hepatic dysfunction and serum factors inhibiting lymphocyte response to phytohemagglutinin. Ann. Intern. Med. 88:769–773.)

laries debris corresponding to lysed red blood cells. The brain has mild hyperemia (Fig. 10–14 *A–B*), but no parasitized red blood cells are attached to the endothelium of blood vessels, an important difference from *P. falciparum* (see above). The parasites in hematoxylin and eosin stains appear as faintly visualized structures in the red blood cells that are difficult to recognize (Fig. 10–13 *C* and 10–14 *B*).

Diagnosis. The diagnosis of *Babesia* is made on peripheral blood films (Fig. 10–15 *A–E*; Healy, Ruebush, 1980) or films of the buffy coat (see malaria, Diagnosis) (Mattia et al. 1993). In patients who are negative, reexamination of the blood in 1 or 2 weeks may give positive results. It is necessary to recognize the typical *Babesia*

organisms based on their morphology (Healy, Ruebush, 1980) and, if possible, to identify the species. Polarization of blood smears gives negative results, which is helpful in distinguishing *Babesia* from *Plasmodium* (see above). Serologic tests such as indirect immunofluorescence (Chisholm et al. 1978; Krause et al. 1994; Ruebush et al. 1977b) and enzyme-linked immunosorbent assay are available (Reiter, Weiland, 1989). The polymerase chain reaction for determination of *Babesia* DNA in circulating blood yielded positive results 53 days after the parasites were cleared (Pruthi et al. 1995).

Entopolypoides

The genus *Entopolypoides* has only one species, *E. macaci*, which is parasitic in primates. Some authors regard it as synonymous with *Babesia* (Hoare, 1981). *Entopolypoides* is characterized by the presence of minute areas of intraerythrocytic nuclear material, with delicate strands of cytoplasm that lack pigment production.

At least two patients infected with organisms thought to be *Entopolypoides* are known, both in the United States (Wolf et al. 1978). One patient was a native of Turkey who, soon after arriving in the United States, was found to have hepatosplenomegaly with hypersplenism, esophageal varices, and other medical problems. The patient underwent splenectomy; a liver biopsy specimen taken at the time showed periportal fibrosis. The second patient had hepatic failure. The parasites in these two patients were identified as *Entopolypoides* based on the morphologic characteristics of the intraerythrocytic stages found in peripheral blood smears (Fig. 10–15 *E*). The epidemiologic circumstances did not indicate that infection with this species was possible. Whether *Entopolypoides* is synonymous with *Babesia* awaits clarification.

References

Abulrahi HA, Bohlega EA, Fontaine RE, Seghayer S, 1997. *Plasmodium falciparum* malaria transmitted in hospital through heparin locks. Lancet 349:23–25

Aikawa M, 1971. *Plasmodium*: the fine structure of malarial parasites. Exp. Parasitol. 30:284–320

Aikawa M, 1988a. Human cerebral malaria. Am. J. Trop. Med. Hyg. 39:3–10

Aikawa M, 1988b. Morphological changes in erythrocytes induced by malarial parasites. Biol. Cell 64:173–181

Aikawa M, Miller LH, Johnson J, Rabbege J, 1978. Erythrocyte entry by malarial parasites: a moving junction between erythrocyte and parasite. J. Cell Biol. 77:72–82

Aikawa M, Miller LH, Rabbege J, 1975. Caveola–vesicle complexes in the plasmalemma of erythrocytes infected by *Plasmodium vivax* and *P. cynomolgy*. Am. J. Pathol. 79:285–294

Aikawa M, Rabbege JR, Wellde BT, 1972. Junctional apparatus in erythrocytes infected with malarial parasites. Z. Zellforsch. 124:72–75

Al-Yaman F, Genton B, Reeder JC, Anders RF, Alpers MP, 1997. Evidence that recurrent *Plasmodium falciparum* infection is caused by recrudescence of resistant parasites. Am. J. Trop. Med. Hyg. 56:436–439

Allan RJ, Beattie P, Bate C, Hensbroek MB, Morris-Jones S, Greenwood BM, Kwiatkowski D, 1995. Strain variation in tumor necrosis factor induction by parasites from children with acute *falciparum* malaria. Infect. Immun. 63:1173–1175

Allan RJ, Rowe A, Kwiatkowski D, 1993. *Plasmodium falciparum* varies in its ability to induce tumor necrosis factor. Infect Immun. 61:4772–4776

Allison AC, Hendrickse RG, Edington GM, Houba V, Petris SD, Adeniyi A, 1969. Immune complexes in the nephrotic syndrome of African children. Lancet 1:1232–1237

Alves W, Schinazi LA, Aniceto F, 1969. *Plasmodium ovale* infections in the Philippines. Bull. World Health Org. 39:494–495

Archibald HM, 1956. The influence of malarial infection of the placenta on the incidence of prematurity. Bull. World Health Org. 15:842–845

Baird JK, Masbar P, Masbar S, 1990. *Plasmodium ovale* in Indonesia. Southeast Asian J. Trop. Med. Public Health 21:541–544

Bazin C, Lamy C, Piette M, Gorenflot A, Duhamel C, Valla A, 1976. Un nouveau cas de babesiose humeine. Nouv. Presse Med. 5:799–800

Beaver PC, Jung RC, Cupp EW, 1984. *Clinical Parasitology*. Philadelphia: Lea & Febiger

Benach JL, Coleman JL, Habicht GS, MacDonald AAGE, Giron JA, 1985. Serological evidence for simultaneous occurrences of Lyme disease and babesiosis. J. Infect. Dis. 152:473–477

Benach JL, Habicht GS, 1981. Clinical characteristics of human babesiosis. J. Infect. Dis. 144:481

Benach JL, Habicht GS, Hamburger MI, 1982. Immunoresponsiveness in acute babesiosis in humans. J. Infect. Dis. 146:369–380

Benezra D, Brown AE, Polsky B, Gold JW, Armstrong D, 1987. Babesiosis and infection with human immunodeficiency virus (HIV). Ann. Intern. Med. 107:944

Berendt AR, Ferguson DJP, Newbold CI, 1990. Sequestration in *Plasmodium falciparum* malaria: sticky cells and sticky problems. Parasitol. Today 6:247–254

Berendt AR, Turner GDH, Newbold CI, 1994. Cerebral malaria: the sequestration hypothesis. Parasitol. Today 10:412–414

Bhamarapravati N, Boonpucknavig S, Boonpucknavig V, Yaemboonruang C, 1973. Glomerular changes in acute *Plasmodium falciparum* infection: an immunopathologic study. Arch. Pathol. 96:289–293

Boonpucknavig V, Sitprija V, 1979. Renal disease in acute *Plasmodium falciparum* infection in man. Kidney Int. 16:44–52

Bouoma MJ, Dye C, 1997. Cycles of malaria associated with El Niño in Venezuela: brief report. JAMA 278:1772–1774

Bouvier P, Breslow N, Doumbo O, Robert CF, Picquet M, Mauris A, Dolo A, Dembele HK, Delley V, Rougemont A, 1997a. Seasonality, malaria, and impact of prophylaxis in a West African village II. Effect on birthweight. Am. J. Trop. Med. Hyg. 56:384–389

Bouvier P, Doumbo O, Breslow N, Robert CF, Picquet M, Mauris A, Piquet M, Kouriba B, Dembele HK, Delley V, Rougemont A, 1997b. Seasonality, malaria, and impact of prophylaxis in a West African village I. Effect on anemia in pregnancy. Am. J. Trop. Med. Hyg. 56:378–383

Brasseur P, Gorenflot A, 1992. Human babesiosis in Europe. Mem. Inst. Oswaldo Cruz 87 Suppl 3:131–132

Brasseur P, Gorenflot A, 1996. Human babesial infections in Europe. Rocz. Akad. Med Bialymst. 41:117–122

Bredt AB, Weinstein WM, Cohen S, 1981. Treatment of babesiosis in asplenic patients. JAMA 245:1938–1939

Brito RD, Meira JA, Bassoi ON, 1962. Contribuicao ao estudo da malaria. II. Patologia do figado na malaria aguda. Rev. Inst. Med. Trop. Sao Paulo 4:105–111

Bruckner DA, Garcia LS, Shimizu RY, Goldstein EJC, Murray PM, Lazar GS, 1985. Babesiosis: problems in diagnosis using autoanalyzers. Am. J. Clin. Pathol. 83:520–521

Butcher GA, 1992. HIV and malaria: a lesson in immunology. Parasitol. Today 8:307–311

Cahill KM, Benach JL, Reich LM, Bilmes E, Zins JH, Siegel FP, Hochweis S, 1981. Red cell exchange: treatment of babesiosis in a splenectomized patient. Transfusion 21:193–198

Carme B, Bouquety JC, Plassart H, 1993. Mortality and sequelae due to cerebral malaria in African children in Brazze Ville, Congo. Am. J. Trop. Med. Hyg. 48:216–221

Carsley J, MacLean JD, 1997. Malaria in Canada. Can. Med. Assoc. J. 156:57–58

CDC, 1986a. *Plasmodium vivax* malaria—San Diego County, California, 1986. Morb. Mort. Weekly Rep. 35:679–681

CDC, 1986b. Outbreak of malaria imported from Kenya. Morb. Mort. Weekly Rep. 35:567–573

CDC, 1997. Probable locally acquired mosquito-transmitted *Plasmodium vivax* infection—Georgia, 1996. Morb. Mort. Weekly Rep. 46:264–267

Chisholm ES, Ruebush II, Sulzer AJ, 1978. *Babesia microti* infection in man: evaluation of an indirect imunofluorescent antibody test. Am. J. Trop. Med. Hyg. 27:14–19

Chisholm ES, Sulzer AJ, Ruebush TKI, 1986. Indirect imunofluorescence test for human *Babesia microti* infection: antigenic specificity. Am. J. Trop. Med. Hyg. 35:921–925

Clark IA, Cowden WB, Rockett KA, 1994. The pathogenesis of human cerebral malaria. Parasitol. Today 10:417–418

Clark IA, Rockett KA, 1994. The cytokine theory of human cerebral malaria. Parasitol. Today 10:410–412

Clark IA, Rockett KA, Cowden WB, 1991. Proposed link between cytokines, nitric oxide and human cerebral malaria. Parasitol. Today 7:205–207

Collins WE, Jeffery GM, 1996. Primaquine resistance in *Plasmodium vivax*. Am. J. Trop. Med. Hyg. 55:243–249

Cooke BM, Coppel RL, 1995. Cytoadhesion and *falciparum* malaria: going with the flow. Parasitol. Today 11:282–287

Corliss JO, 1994. An interim utilitarian ("user-friendly") hierarchical classification and characterization of the protists. Acta Protozool. 33:1–51

Cot M, Abel L, Roisin A, Barro D, Yada A, Carnevale P, Feingold J, 1993. Risk factors of malaria infection during pregnancy in Burkina Faso: suggestion of a genetic influence. Am. J. Trop. Med. Hyg. 48:358–364

Crawley J, Smith S, Kirkham F, Muthinji P, Waruiru C, Marsh K, 1996. Seizures and status epilepticus in childhood cerebral malaria. Q. J. Med. 89:591–597

Dammin GJ, Spielman A, Benach JL, Piesman J, 1981. The rising incidence of clinical *Babesia microti* infection. Hum. Pathol. 12:398–400

Day NP, Pham TD, Phan TL, Dinh XS, Pham PL, Ly VC, Tran TH, Nguyen TH, Bethell DB, Nguyan HP, White NJ, 1996. Clearance kinetics of parasites and pigment-containing leukocytes in severe malaria. Blood 88:4694–4700

Deaton JG, 1970. Fatal pulmonary edema as a complication of acute falciparum malaria. Am. J. Trop. Med. Hyg. 19:196–201

Dover AS, Schultz MG, 1971. Transfusion-induced malaria. Transfusion 11:353–357

Etrican JH, Williams H, Cook IA, Lancaster WM, Clarck JC, Joiner LP, Lewis D, 1979. Babesiosis in man. A case from Scotland. Br. Med. J. 2:474

Falagas ME, Klempner MS, 1996. Babesiosis in patients with AIDS: a chronic infection presenting as fever of unknown origin. Clin. Infect. Dis. 22:809–812

Fernandez Villar B, White DJ, Benach JL, 1991. Human babesiosis. Prog. Clin. Parasitol. 2:129–143

Field JW, Sandosham AA, Fong YL, 1963. *The Microscopical Diagnosis of Human Malaria*. I. *A Morphological Study of the Erythrocytic Parasites in Thick Blood Films*. Kuala Lumpur: Economy Printers Ltd.

Field JW, Shute PG, 1956. *The Microscopic Diagnosis of Human Malaria*. II—*A Morphological Study of the Erythrocytic Parasites*. Kuala Lumpur: Government Press

Filstein MR, Benach JL, White DJ, Brody BA, Goldman WD, Bakal CW, Schwartz RS, 1980. Serosurvey for human babesiosis in New York. J. Infect. Dis. 141:518–521

Fitzpatrick JEP, Kennedy CC, McGeown MG, Oreopoulos DG, Robertson GH, Soyannwo MA, 1969. Further details of third recorded case of redwater (babesiosis) in man. Br. Med. J. 4:770–772

Foster SO, 1996. Malaria in the pregnant African woman: epidemiology, practice, research and policy. Am. J. Trop. Med. Hyg. 55:1

Fujioka H, Aikawa M, 1996. The molecular basis of pathogenesis of cerebral malaria. Microbiol. Pathogen. 20:63–72

Gerber MA, Shapiro ED, Krause PJ, Cable RG, Badon SJ, Ryan RW, 1994. The risk of acquiring Lyme disease or babesiosis from a blood transfusion. J. Infect. Dis. 170:231–234

Gigioli G, 1962a. Malaria and renal disease, with special reference to British Guiana I. Introduction. Ann. Trop. Med. Parasitol. 56:101–109

Gigioli G, 1962b. Malaria and renal disease, with special reference to British Guiana II. The effect of malaria eradication on the incidence of renal disease in British Guiana. Ann. Trop. Med. Parasitol. 56:225–241

Gilles HM, Hendrickse RG, 1960. Possible aetiological role of *Plasmodium malariae* in "nephrotic syndrome" in Nigerian children. Lancet 1:806–807

Gilles HM, Hendrickse RG, 1963. Nephrosis in Nigerian children: role of *Plasmodium malariae*, and effect of antimalarial treatment. Br. Med. J. 2:27–31

Gilles HM, Warrell DA, 1993. *Bruce-Chwatt's Essential Malariology*. London: Edward Arnold

Gombert ME, Goldstein EJC, Benach JL, Tenenbaum MJ, Grunwaldt E, Kaplan MH, Eveland LK, 1982. Human babesiosis: clinical and therapeutic considerations. JAMA 248:3005–3007

Gordon S, Cordon RA, Mazdzer EJ, Valigorsky JM, Blagg NA, Barnes SJ, 1984. Adult respiratory distress syndrome in babesiosis. Chest 86:633–634

Grabowski EF, Giardina PJ, Goldberg D, Masur H, Read SE, Hirsch RL, Benach JL, 1982. Babesiosis transmitted by a transfusion of frozen-thawed blood. Ann. Intern. Med. 96:466–467

Grau GE, Kossodo SD, 1994. Cerebral malaria: mediators, mechanical obstruction or more? Parasitol. Today 10:408–409

Greenberg AE, Nsa W, Ryder RW, Medi M, Nzeza M, Kitadi N, Baangi M, Malanda N, Davachi F, Hassig SE, 1991. *Plasmodium falciparum* malaria and perinatally acquired human immunodeficiency virus type 1 infection in Kinshasa, Zaire. N. Engl. J. Med. 325:105–109

Grunwaldt E, 1977. Babesiosis on Shelter Island. N.Y. State J. Med. 77:1320–1321

Grundwalt E, Barbour AG, Benach JL, 1983. Correspondence. Simultaneous occurrence of babesiosis and Lyme disease. N. Engl. J. Med. 308:1166

Gupta P, Hurley RW, Helseth PH, Goodman JL, Hammerschmidt DE, 1995. Pancytopenia due to hemophagocytic syndrome as the presenting manifestation of babesiosis. Am J Hematol. 50:60–62

Gutierrez Y, Aikawa M, Fremount HN, Sterling CR, 1976. Experimental infection of *Aotus* monkeys with *Plasmodium falciparum*. Light and electron microscopic changes. Ann. Trop. Med. Parasitol. 70:25–44

Harambasic H, Krsnjavi B, Urbanke A, 1976. The second case of human babesiosis (piroplasmosis) in Yugoslavia. Acta Parasitol. Iugoslav. 7:37–41

Healy G, 1989. The impact of cultural and environmental changes on the epidemiology and control of human babesiosis. Trans. R. Soc. Trop. Med. Hyg. 83 Suppl: 35–38

Healy GR, Ruebush TK II, 1980. Morphology of *Babesia microti* in human blood smears. Am. J. Clin. Pathol. 73: 107–109

Healy GR, Walzer PD, Sulzer AJ, 1976. A case of asymptomatic babesiosis in Georgia. Am. J. Trop. Med. Hyg. 25:376–378

Hedberg K, Shaffer N, Davachi F, Hightower A, Lyamba B, Paluku MP, Nguyen-Dinh P, Breman JG, 1993. *Plasmodium falciparum*–associated anemia in children at a large urban hospital in Zaire. Am. J. Trop. Med. Hyg. 48:365–371

Hendrickse RG, Adeniyi A, 1979. Quartan malarial nephrotic syndrome in children. Kidney Int. 16:64–74

Herwaldt B, Persing DH, Precigout EA, Goff WL, Mathiesen DA, Taylor PW, Eberhard ML, Gorenflot AF, 1996. A fatal case of babesiosis in Missouri: identification of another piroplasm that infects humans. Ann. Intern. Med. 124:643–650

Hoare CA, 1981. On the status of *Entopolypoides* (Piroplasmida). In: Anonymous, *Parasitology Topics. Presentation Volume to P. C. C. Garnham FRS*. Society of Protozoologists Special Publication No 1, pp. 112–116

Hollingdale MR, 1985. Malaria and the liver. Hepatology 5:327–335

Holzer BR, Gluck Z, Zambelli D, Fey M, 1985. Transmission of malaria by renal transplantation. Transplantation 39:315–316

Houba V, Allison AC, Adeniyi A, Houba JE, 1971. Immunoglobulin classes and complement in biopsies of Nigerian children with the nephrotic syndrome. Clin. Exp. Immunol. 8:761–774

Imbert P, Sartelet I, Rogier C, Ka S, Baujat G, Candito D, 1997. Severe malaria among children in a low seasonal transmission area, Dakar, Senegal: influence of age on clinical presentation. Trans. R. Soc. Trop. Med. Hyg. 91:22–24

Jacoby GA, Hunt JV, Kosinski KS, Demirjian ZN, Huggins C, Etkind P, Marcus LC, Spielman A, 1980. Treatment of transfusion-transmitted babesiosis by exchange transfusion. N. Engl. J. Med. 303:1098–1100

Jelinek T, Proll S, Hess F, Kabagambe G, von Sonnenburg F, Loscher T, Kilian AH, 1996. Geographic differences in the sensitivity of a polymerase chain reaction for the detection of *Plasmodium falciparum* infection. Am. J. Trop. Med. Hyg. 55:647–651

Jervis HR, Sprinz H, Johnson AJ, 1972. Experimental infection with *Plasmodium falciparum* in *Aotus* monkeys. II. Observations on host pathology. Am. J. Trop. Med. Hyg. 21:272–281

Karunaweera ND, Grau GE, Gamage P, Carter R, Mendis KN, 1992. Dynamics of fever and serum levels of tumor necrosis factor are closely associated during clinical paroxysms in *Plasmodium vivax* malaria. Proc. Natl. Acad. Sci. USA 89:3200–3203

Kibukamusoke JW, Hutt MSR, 1967. Histological features of the nephrotic syndrome associated with quartan malaria. J. Clin. Pathol. 20:117–123

Krause PJ, Telford SR, Pollack RJ, Ryan R, Brassard P, Zemel L, Spielman A, 1992. Babesiosis: an underdiagnosed disease of children. Pediatrics 89:1045–1048

Krause PJ, Telford SR, Ryan R, Conrad PA, Wilson M, Thomford JW, Spielman A, 1994. Diagnosis of babesiosis: evaluation of a serologic test for the detection of *Babesia microti* antibody. J. Infect. Dis. 169:923–926

Krause PJ, Telford SR, Spielman A, Sikand V, Ryan R, Christianson D, Burke G, Brassard P, Pollack R, Peck J, Persing DH, 1996. Concurrent Lyme disease and babesiosis. Evidence for increased severity and duration of illness. JAMA 275:1657–1660

Krogstad DJ, 1996. Malaria as a reemerging disease. Epidemiol. Rev. 18:77–89

Kwiatkowski D, 1995. Malarial toxins and the regulation of parasite density. Parasitol. Today 11:206–212

Leeflang P, Oomen JMV, Zwart D, Meuwissen JHET, 1976. The prevalence of *Babesia* antibodies in Nigerians. Int. J. Parasitol. 6:159–161

Lefrere F, Besson C, Datry A, Chaibi P, Leblond V, Binet JL,

Sutton L, 1996. Transmission of *Plasmodium falciparum* by allogeneic bone marrow transplantation. Bone Marrow Transplant. 18:473–474

Leopardi O, Naughten W, Salvia L, Colecchia M, Matteelli A, Zucchi A, Shein A, Muchi JA, Carosi G, Ghione M, 1996. Malaric placentas. A quantitative study and clinicopathological correlations. Pathol. Res. Pract. 192:892–898

Lobel HO, Campbell CC, Schwartz IK, Roberts JM, 1985. Recent trends in the importation of malaria caused by *Plasmodium falciparum* into the United States from Africa. J. Infect. Dis. 152:613–617

Looareesuwan S, Ho M, Wattanagoon Y, White NJ, Warrell DA, Bunnag D, Harinasuta T, Wyler DJ, 1987. Dynamic alteration in splenic function during acute *falciparum* malaria. N. Engl. J. Med. 317:675–679

Maitland K, Williams TN, Bennett S, Newbold CI, Peto TE, Viji J, Timothy R, Clegg JB, Weatherall DJ, Bowden DK, 1996. The interaction between *Plasmodium falciparum* and *P. vivax* in children on Espiritu Santo island, Vanuatu. Trans. R. Soc. Trop. Med. Hyg. 90:614–620

Maldonado YA, Nahlen BL, Roberto RR, Ginsberg M, Orellana E, Mizrahi M, McBarron K, Lobel HO, Campbell CC, 1990. Transmission of *Plasmodium vivax* malaria in San Diego County, California, 1986. Am. J. Trop. Med. Hyg. 42:3–9

Marcus LC, Steere AC, Duray PH, Anderson AE, Mahoney EB, 1985. Fatal pancarditis in a patient with coexistent Lyme disease and babesiosis. Ann. Intern. Med. 103:374–376

Marsaudon E, Camenen J, Testou D, Bourree P, Samson P, Luneau F, 1995. Une babesiose humaine a *Babesia canis*, responsable d'une anurie de 40 jours. Ann. Med. Interne 146:451–452

Marsden PD, Connor DH, Voller A, Kelly A, Schofield FD, Hutt MSR, 1967. Splenomegaly in New Guinea. Bull. World Health Org. 36:901–911

Marsden PD, Hutt MSR, Wilks NE, Voller A, Blackman V, Shah KK, Connor DH, Hamilton PJS, Banwell JG, Lunn HF, 1965. An investigation of tropical splenomegaly at Mulago hospital, Kampala, Uganda. Br. Med. J. 1:89–92

Marsh K, English M, Crawley J, Peshu N, 1996. The pathogenesis of severe malaria in African children. Ann. Trop. Med. Parasitol. 90:395–402

Mathewson HO, Anderson AE, Hazard GW, 1984. Self-limited babesiosis in a splenectomized child. Pediatr. Infect. Dis. 3:148–149

Matteelli A, Donato F, Shein A, Muchi JA, Abass AK, Mariani M, Leopardi O, Maxwell CA, Carosi G, 1996. Malarial infection and birthweight in urban Zanzibar, Tanzania. Ann. Trop. Med. Parasitol. 90:125–134

Mattia AR, Waldron MA, Sierra LS, 1993. Use of the quantitative buffy coat system for detection of parasitemia in patients with babesiosis. J. Clin. Microbiol. 31:2816–2818

McDermott JM, Wirima JJ, Steketee RW, Breman JG, Heymann DL, 1997. The effect of placental malaria infection on perinatal mortality in rural Malawi. Am. J. Trop. Med. Hyg. 55:61–65

Mendis KN, Carter R, 1995. Clinical disease and pathogenesis in malaria. Parasitol. Today 11:PTI 2–PTI 15

Miller LH, 1972. The ultrastructure of red cells infected by *Plasmodium falciparum* in man. Trans. R. Soc. Trop. Med. Hyg. 66:459–462

Miller LH, 1984. Malaria. In: Warren KS, Mahmoud AAF (eds), *Tropical and Geographical Medicine*. New York: McGraw-Hill Book Company, pp. 223–230

Miller LH, Mason SJ, Dvorak JA, Shiroishi T, McGinniss M, 1977a. Erythrocytic receptors for malarial merozoites and the Duffy blood group system. Human blood groups. In Miller LH, Pino JA, McKelvey JJ Jr (eds), *Proceedings of the 5th International Convocation of Immunology*. pp. 394–400

Miller LH, McAuliffe FM, Mason SJ, 1977b. Erythrocyte receptors for malaria merozoites. Am. J. Trop. Med. Hyg. 26:204–208

Muller O, Moser R, 1990. The clinical and parasitological presentation of *Plasmodium falciparum* malaria in Uganda is unaffected by HIV-1 infection. Trans. R. Soc. Trop. Med. Hyg. 84:336–338

Muntendam AH, Jaffar S, Bleichrodt N, van Hansbrock M, 1996. Absence of neuropsychological sequelae following cerebral malaria in Gambian children. Trans. R. Soc. Trop. Med. Hyg. 90:391–394

Newton CR, Marsh K, Peshu N, Kirkham FJ, 1996. Perturbations of cerebral hemodynamics in Kenyans with cerebral malaria. Pediatr. Neurol. 15:41–49

Nyirjesy P, Kavasya T, Axelrod P, Fischer PR, 1993. Malaria during pregnancy: neonatal morbidity and mortality and the efficacy of chloroquine chemoprophylaxis. Clin. Infect. Dis. 16:127–132

Ockenhouse CF, Tegoshi T, Maeno Y, Benjamin C, Ho M, Kan KE, Thway Y, Win K, Aikawa M, Lobb RR, 1992. Human vascular endothelial cell adhesion receptors for *Plasmodium falciparum*–infected erythrocytes: roles for endothelial leukocyte adhesion molecule 1 and vascular cell adhesion molecule 1. J. Exp. Med. 176:1183–1189

Ong KR, Stavropoulos C, Inada Y, 1990. Correspondence. Babesiosis, asplenia, and AIDS. Lancet 336:112

Ortiz JM, Eagle RC Jr, 1982. Ocular findings in human babesiosis (Nantucket fever). Am. J. Ophthalmol. 93:307–311

Osorno BM, Vega C, Ristic M, Robles C, Ibarra S, 1976. Isolation of *Babesia* spp. from asymptomatic human beings. Vet. Parasitol. 2:111–120

Oteo JA, Estrada A, 1992. Babesiosis humana. Estudio de vectores. Enferm. Infecc. Microbiol. Clin. 10:466–469

Persing DH, Herwaldt BL, Glaser C, Lane RS, Thomford JW, Mathiesen D, Krause PJ, Phillip DF, Conrad PA, 1995. Infection with a *Babesia*-like organism in northern California. N. Engl. Med. 332:298–303

Piesman J, Mather TN, Dammin GJ, Telford SR, Lastavica CC, Spielman A, 1987. Seasonal variation of transmission risk of Lyme disease and human babesiosis. Am. J. Epidemiol. 126:1187–1189

Pitney WR, 1968. The tropical spenomegaly syndrome. Trans. R. Soc. Trop. Med. Hyg. 62:717–728

Popovsky MA, Lindberg LE, Syrek AL, Page PL, 1988. Prevalence of *Babesia* antibody in a selected blood donor population. Transfusion 28:59–61

Pruthi RK, Marshall WF, Wiltsie JC, Persing DH, 1995. Human babesiosis. Mayo Clin. Proc. 70:853–862

Punyagupta S, Srichaikul T, Nitlyanant P, 1974. Acute pulmonary insufficiency in *falciparum* malaria: summary of 12 cases with evidence of disseminated intravascular coagulation. Am. J. Trop. Med. Hyg. 23:551–559

Quick RE, Herwaldt BL, Thomford JW, Garnett ME, Eberhard ML, Wilson M, Spach DH, Dickerson JW, Telford SR, Steingart KR, et al, 1993. Babesiosis in Washington State: a new species of *Babesia*? Ann. Intern. Med. 119:284–290

Ranque P, 1986. A simple method for post-mortem confirmation of the diagnosis of cerebral malaria: transethmoidal puncture of the brain. Trans. R. Soc. Trop. Med. Hyg. 80:663

Raucher HS, Jaffin H, Glass JL, 1984. Babesiosis in pregnancy. Obstet. Gynecol. 63:7S–9S

Reiter I, Weiland G, 1989. Recently developed methods for the detection of babesial infections. Trans. R. Soc. Trop. Med. Hyg. 83 Suppl:21–23

Roberts DD, Sherwood JA, Spitalnik SL, 1985. Thrombospondin binds *falciparum* malaria parasitized erythrocytes and may mediate cytoadherence. Nature 318:64–66

Rosner F, Zarrabi MH, Benach JL, Habicht GS, 1984. Babesiosis in splenectomized adults: review of 22 reported cases. Am. J. Med. 76:696–701

Ruebush TK II, Juranek DD, Chisholm ES, 1977a. Human babesiosis on Nantucket Island. Evidence for self-limited and subclinical infections. N. Engl. J. Med. 297:825–827

Ruebush TK II, Cassaday PB, Marsh HJ, Lisker SA, Voorhees DB, Mahoney EB, Healy GR, 1977b. Human babesiosis on Nantucket Island. Ann. Intern. Med. 86:6–9

Ruebush TK II, Juranek DD, Spielman A, Piesman J, Healy GR, 1981a. Epidemiology of human babesiosis on Nantucket Island. Am. J. Trop. Med. Hyg. 30:937–941

Ruebush TK II, Piesman J, Collins WE, Spielman A, Warren M, 1981b. Tick transmission of *Babesia microti* to *Rhesus* monkeys (*Macaca mulatta*). Am. J. Trop. Med. Hyg. 22:555–559

Sanders M, 1998. *Ixodes dammini*: a junior synonym for *Ixodes scapularis*. Emerg. Infect. Dis. 4:132

Scholtens RG, Braff EH, Healy GR, Gleason N, 1968. A case of babesiosis in man in the United States. Am. J. Trop. Med. Hyg. 17:810–813

Shih CM, Liu LP, Chung WC, Ong SJ, Wang CC, 1997. Human babesiosis in Taiwan: asymptomatic infection with a *Babesia microti*-like organism in a Taiwanese woman. J. Clin. Microbiol. 35:450–454

Shulman CE, Graham WJ, Jilo H, Lowe BS, New L, Obiero J, Snow RW, Marsh K, 1996. Malaria is an important cause of anaemia in primigravidae: evidence from a district hospital in coastal Kenya. Trans. R. Soc. Trop. Med. Hyg. 90:535–539

Skrabalo Z, Deanovic Z, 1957. Piroplasmosis in man. Report on a case. Doc. Med. Geogr. Trop. 9:11–16

Slovut DP, Benedetti E, Matas AJ, 1996. Babesiosis and hemophagocytic syndrome in an asplenic renal transplant recipient. Transplantation 62:537–539

Soothill JF, Hendrickse RG, 1967. Some immunological studies of the nephrotic syndrome of Nigerian children. Lancet 2:629–636

Spielman A, 1976. Human babesiosis on Nantucket Island: transmission by nymphal *Ixodes* ticks. Am. J. Trop. Med. Hyg. 25:784–787

Spielman A, Etkind P, Piesman J, Ruebush TK II, Juranek DD, Jacobs MS, 1981. Reservoir hosts of human babesiosis on Nantucket Island. Am. J. Trop. Med. Hyg. 30:560–565

Steketee RW, Eckman MR, Burgess EC, Kuritsky JN, Dickerson J, Schell WL, Godsey MS Jr, Davis JP, 1985. Babesiosis in Wisconsin: a new focus of disease transmission. JAMA 253:2675–2678

Sturchler D, 1989. Correspondence. How much malaria is there worldwide? Parasitol. Today 5:39–40

Taylor F, 1996. Transfusion-associated malaria. Emerg. Infect. Dis. 2:152

Telford SR, 1998. The name *Ixodes dammini* epidemiologically justified. Emerg. Infect. Dis. 4:132–133

Thomford JW, Conrad PA, Telford SR, Mathiesen D, Bowman BH, Spielman A, Eberhard ML, Herwaldt BL, Quick RE, Persing DH, 1994. Cultivation and phylogenetic characterization of a newly recognized human pathogenic protozoan. J. Infect. Dis. 169:1050–1056

Tran TH, Day NP, Ly VC, Nguyen TH, Pham PL, Nguyen HP, Bethell DB, Dihn XS, White NJ, 1996. Blackwater fever in southern Vietnam: a prospective descriptive study of 50 cases. Clin. Infect. Dis. 23:1274–1281

Turkmen A, Sever MS, Ecder T, Yildiz A, Aydin AE, Erkoc R, Eraksoy H, Eldegez U, Ark E, 1996. Posttransplant malaria. Transplantation 62:1521–1523

Walter PR, Garin Y, Blot P, 1982. Placental pathologic changes in malaria: a histologic and ultrastructural study. Am. J. Pathol. 109:330–342

WHO, 1987. The biology of malaria parasites. Tech. Rep. Series No. 743. Geneva: World Health Organization

Wilson LB, Chowning WM, 1904. Studies in *Pyroplasmosis hominis* ("spotted fever" or "tick fever" of the Rocky Mountains). J. Infect. Dis. 1:31–57

Wittner M, Rowin KS, Tanowitz HB, Hobbs JF, Saltzman S, Wenz B, Hirsch R, Chisholm E, Healy GR, 1982. Successful chemotherapy of transfusion babesiosis. Ann. Intern. Med. 96:601–604

Wolf RE, Gleason NN, Schoenbaum C, Western KA, Klein CA, Healy GR, 1978. Intraerythrocytic parasitosis in humans with *Entopolypoides* species (family Babesiidae): association with hepatic dysfunction and serum factors inhibiting lymphocyte response to phytohemagglutin. Ann. Intern. Med. 88:769–773

Woods GL, Gutierrez Y, 1993. *Diagnostic Pathology of Infectious Diseases*. Philadelphia: Lea & Febiger

Wozniak EJ, Lowenstine LJ, Hemmer R, Robinson T, Conrad PA, 1996. Comparative pathogenesis of human WA1 and *Babesia microti* isolates in a Syrian hamster model. Lab Animal Sci. 46:507–515

Zucker JR, 1996. Changing patterns of autochthonous malaria transmission in the United States: a review of recent outbreaks. Emerg. Infect. Dis. 2:37–43

11

THE CILIATES

Balantidium coli belongs to the phylum Ciliophora of the kingdom Protista, which comprises all protozoa with cilia and mitochondria with tubular, often curved cristae, which in anaerobic species may be replaced by hydrogenosomes (Corliss, 1994). These protozoa have one or more diploid micronuclei and one or more polyploid macronuclei. Conjugation or another related process used in sexual reproduction is also present in this group. Most species of the Ciliophora are free-living, and a few are parasitic; all species of the genus *Balantidium* are parasitic. The taxonomy of this genus is difficult to determine, and the genus is not well defined. One species, *B. coli*, has been recognized in the large intestine of many animals, including rats (Awakian, 1937), in primates suffering from diarrhea (Cockburn, 1948), and in humans (Beaver et al. 1984).

Balantidium coli—Balantidiasis

Life Cycle. The life cycle of *Balantidium* involves a trophozoite stage in the lumen of the large intestine and a cyst formed in the colon. Evacuated trophozoites die soon afterward (Arean, Koppisch, 1956), but the cysts

are resistant to environmental conditions. It appears that ingestion of cysts with contaminated water or food produces the infection.

Morphology. *Balantidium coli* is the largest protist found in humans, measuring 50 to 200 μm in length $\times$ 40 to 70 μm in width. However, the size of *Balantidium* reported in several textbooks by different authors varies considerably (Sargeaunt, 1971). Conjugation of two individuals (exchange of genetic material) seems to be the form of reproduction, occurring between a small and a large trophozoite (Sargeaunt, 1971). The trophozoites are oval, with a slightly pointed anterior end and a broadly rounded posterior end. On the anterior end, just to the side of the longitudinal axis, the trophozoites have a cytostome (mouth), seen as a funnel-shaped structure lined inside with cilia. The entire body is covered by shorter cilia than those seen in the cytostome; in fresh isotonic solution preparations of stool samples, the cilia are seen moving actively with a wave-like motion. The cytoplasm of the trophozoites has numerous granules and food vacuoles in addition to one or two larger contractile vacuoles at the posterior end. The contractile vacuoles fill with fluid and are emptied periodically through a small opening in the cell membrane (Zaman, 1970a). A conspicuous beam-shaped macronucleus and a smaller structure, the micronucleus, are located at the center of the body. The cyst is spherical, with a thick wall, and averages 45 to 75 μm in diameter. Inside the cyst, the parasite resembles a small trophozoite with a macronucleus, a micronucleus, and cilia (Fig. 11–1 A–C).

In electron micrographs the parasite has a body wall consisting of an irregular pellicle (the outermost layer), forming ridges and furrows, below which lies the plasma membrane. Beneath the plasma membrane is a system of microtubules, and slightly below microtubules is a band made of fibrils. The pellicle, the plasma membrane, and the band of microtubules comprise the ectoplasm of the organism, which is filled with loose ribosomes, a granular endoplasmic reticulum, and membrane-bound vacuoles. The cilia arise from basal bodies, or kinetosomes, located in the cytoplasm; the cilium has an arrangement of nine double filaments and two single filaments at the center. The endoplasm contains the macronucleus, which has a double-layered membrane with pores, and the nucleoplasm contains the chromatin coils. The nucleolus is dense and compact. The micronucleus has a matrix filled with fine, moderately dense granules (Kan, 1971; Zaman, 1970b).

Geographic Distribution and Epidemiology. *Balantidium coli* has an extensive distribution throughout the tropics and subtropics, where it is highly prevalent in hogs and other animals. Human infections are relatively unusual; both single cases and clusters of small number of cases are recorded sporadically, more often in warmer climates. It was estimated that up to 1960, fewer than 700 cases of balantidiasis in humans had been recorded (Biagi, 1970). An epidemic on the island of Truk, with about 110 infected individuals, occurred after a devastating typhoon (Walzer et al. 1973). The relationship between infections in hogs and infections in humans is not well understood. In some communities without hogs there are human infections (Forsyth, 1954; McCarey, 1952), and in some communities with large numbers of infected hogs, human infections are rare (Awakian, 1937; Radford, 1973). Only in about one-fourth of human infections has an association with hogs been established (Young, 1950). These observations have prompted some investigators to believe that the balantidia in pigs and in humans are two different species. Immobilization tests using specific antisera have shown that isolates from pigs and humans are different (Zaman, 1964). Attempts to transmit the infection from human to human using both trophozoites and cysts have failed (Young, 1950). The prevalence of balantidiasis in the general population in endemic areas is not known; probably less than 0.1 of 1.0% of individuals are infected (Arean, Koppisch, 1956). Surveys of some villages of New Guinea have shown that 28% of the inhabitants are infected, while in neighboring villages the parasite is unknown (Couvee, Rijpstra, 1961; Ewers, 1972). In the United States, *Balan-*

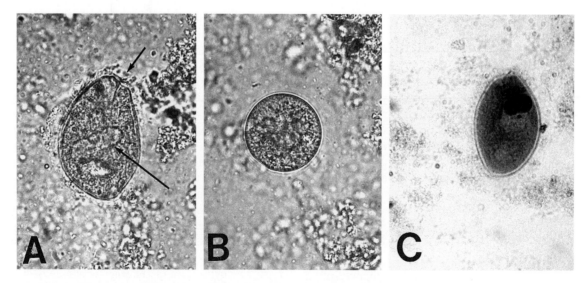

Fig. 11–1. *Balantidium coli*, diagnostic stages. *A* and *B.* Wet mounts, unstained. *A*, Trophozoite with cytostome in the anterior end (short arrow) and macronucleus to- ward the center (long arrow). A large vacuole is seen below the macronucleus. *B*, Cyst. *C*, Trophozoite stained with iron hematoxylin stain, all ×450.

tidium was recorded sporadically until the 1950s, when a review of the literature collected 61 cases in the country (Arean, Koppisch, 1956), mainly from the southern states; one-fourth of the cases occurred in Louisiana (Swartzwelder, 1950). The decrease in the number of cases of balantidiasis in the United States probably parallels the decrease in other intestinal parasites due to improved sanitation and socioeconomic conditions.

Pathogenesis and Immunity. Little data are available on the pathogenesis of and the immunity to *Balantidium* infections in animals or humans. It appears that the parasite has a low infectivity rate, judging by the rarity of human cases. Infected baboons in captivity lose the infection in about 2 months (Myers, Kuntz, 1968), but similar studies in hogs or humans are not available. Hogs infected under natural conditions do not have serum antibodies against *Balantidium* detected by the immunofluorescence antibody test (Dzbenski, 1966), and their infections are invariably asymptomatic.

Clinical Findings. Asymptomatic infections with *Balantidium* are common (Baskerville et al. 1970; van der Hoeven, Rijpstra, 1957), but in persons with symptoms, the disease may range from mild to fulminant (Dorfman et al. 1984b). Patients acute dysentery (Kennedy, Stewart, 1957) are indistinguishable from those with other forms of colitis, including amebic colitis. In milder infections, the individual has chronic intermittent symptoms such as episodes of diarrhea, epigastric distress, abdominal pain, and several bowel movements per day, with mucus and rarely with blood, alternating with episodes of constipation. Intermittent fever and vomiting in infants have been described (Woody, Woody, 1960). The dysenteric form usually has a sudden onset, with up to 20 bowel movements per day with blood and mucus, as well as abdominal pain and loss of weight (Castro et al. 1983; Lara, Bernal, 1974). Fulminant cases have been observed in debilitated, emaciated, and immune-deficient persons (Iglezias, 1980), with death occurring 3 to 5 days later. In some cases, the clinical course and the gross and microscopic findings of fulminant balantidiasis parallel those of fulminant amebiasis, with per

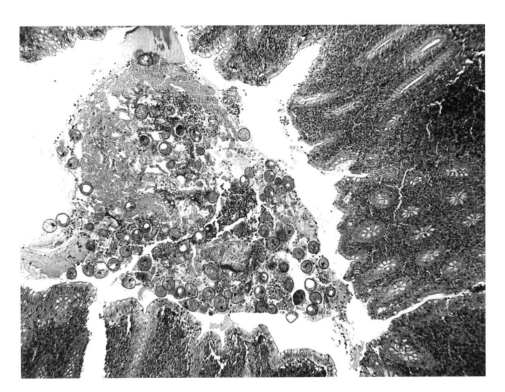

Fig. 11–2. *Balantidium coli*, section of appendix showing a colony of trophozoites in the lumen, section stained with hematoxylin and eosin stain. No mucosal alterations are seen, ×100. (Courtesy of V.M. Arean, M.D., Department of Pathology, Saint Anthony's Hospital, St. Petersburg, Florida.)

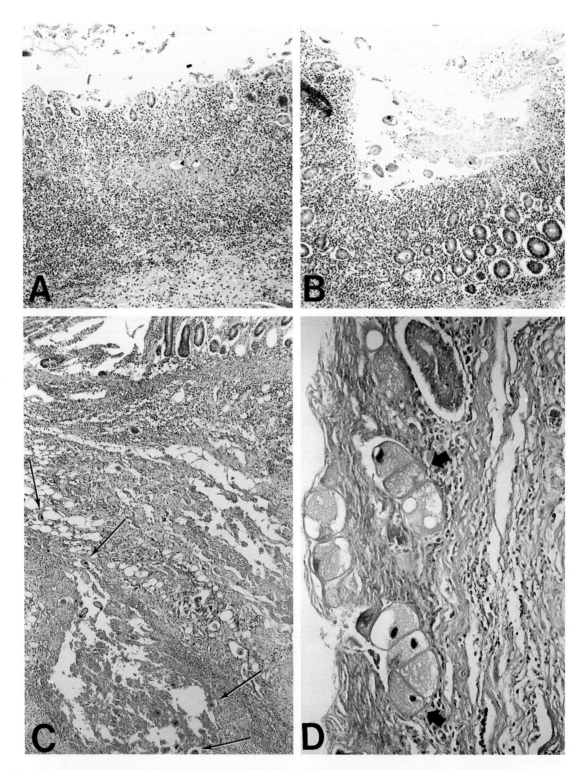

Fig. 11–3. *Balantidium coli* in large intestine, sections stained with hematoxylin and eosin stain. *A* and *B*, Low-power views showing the superficial ulceration; in *B* it extends halfway down into the mucosal layer, ×70. *C*, Deeper area of necrosis involving the submucosa showing parasites (arrows), ×55. *D*, Necrotic parasites (postmortem changes) (arrow) in a patient with superficial ulceration and postmortem autolysis of the mucosa, ×180.

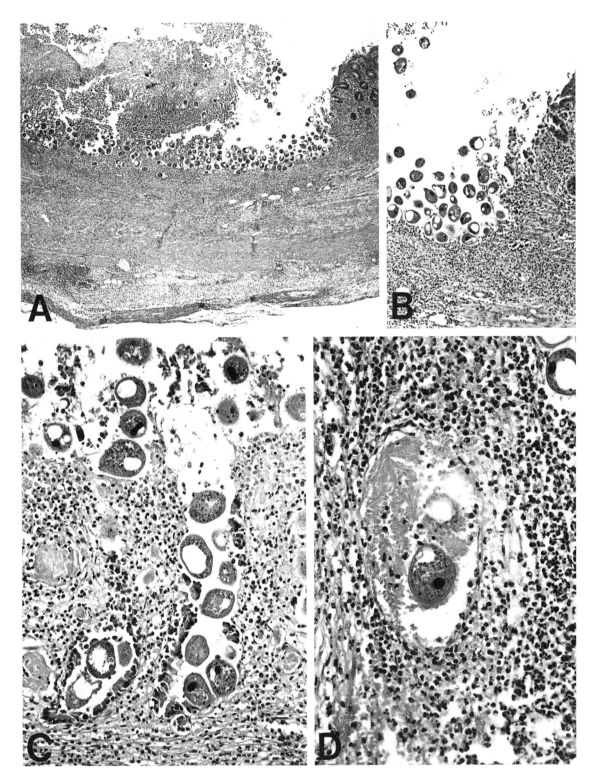

Fig. 11–4. *Balantidium coli* in human appendix, sections stained with hematoxylin and eosin stain. *A*, Low-power view of a typical ulcer with numerous organisms, ×28. *B*, Detail of the ulcer's edge, ×70. *C*, Ulcer showing parasites deep within the crypts, ×180. *D*, Small vessel with a trophozoite in the lumen. Note the marked polymorphonuclear cell and the less pronounced mononuclear cell infiltrate, ×450. (Preparation courtesy of V.M. Arean, M.D., Department of Pathology, Saint Anthony's Hospital, St. Petersburg, Florida.)

267

foration of the bowel and peritonitis. Acute appendicitis, more often in children than in adults, is a known manifestation of balantidiasis (Dorfman et al. 1984a, 1984b; Gonzalez Sanchez, 1978).

Peritonitis due to intestinal perforation and peritonitis in cases of *Balantidium* infection have been described. Outside the gastrointestinal tract, infections have been reported rarely in the vagina, producing vaginitis (Isaza-Mejia, 1955); in two women with intestinal balantidiasis, asymptomatic vaginal infections occurred (Norman, Jessop, 1973). Two other reports of cervicovaginal balantidiasis are mistaken identifications of the parasite. In one, the structures depicted in the photograph are too large (Rutschow, 1976); in the other, too small (Rivasi, Giannotti, 1983), and both are outside the known size range of *Balantidium*. There are also cases of urinary tract infection (Maliwa, Von Haus, 1920), liver abscess (Auz, 1984), and infection of the liver capsule alone (Cespedes et al. 1967). A few cases of pulmonary invasion have been recorded. In one case, the patient had disseminated peritoneal, pleural, and pulmonary disease (Cespedes et al. 1967). In two other cases of lung involvement, the parasites were not illustrated (Daoudal, 1986; Dorfman et al. 1984b), and in another, the objects depicted did not resemble *Balantidium* (Ladas et al. 1989). In the last three cases, the identification of the parasite in the lungs remains doubtful.

Pathology. In acute balantidiasis the entire colon is affected, often with greater involvement of the rectosigmoid (Arean, Koppisch, 1956). Grossly, the ulcers resemble those of amebiasis, varying from small and crater-like to large areas of ulceration with ragged edges filled with necrotic material. The healthy-appearing

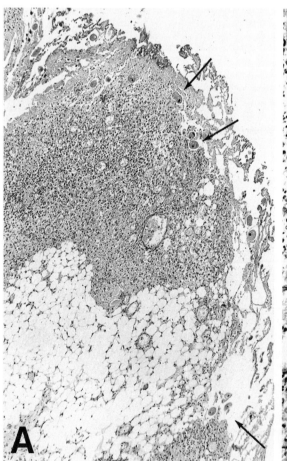
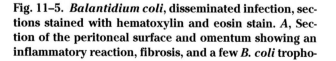
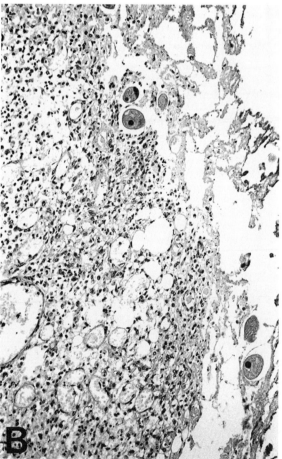

Fig. 11–5. *Balantidium coli*, disseminated infection, sections stained with hematoxylin and eosin stain. *A*, Section of the peritoneal surface and omentum showing an inflammatory reaction, fibrosis, and a few *B. coli* trophozoites (arrows), ×55. *B*, Higher magnification showing greater detail, ×140. (Preparation courtesy of J. Ro, M.D., Department of Pathology, M.D. Anderson Cancer Center, Houston, Texas.)

mucosa has no undermining below, as in *Entamoeba histolytica* infections. The ulcers may extend to deeper layers of the colon, sometimes with perforation, but they usually do not extend laterally in the submucosa.

Microscopically, sections of the colon have *Balantidium* in the lumen (Fig. 11–2), on the mucosa, and deep in the crypts, often producing no damage in asymptomatic patients. Individuals with symptoms invariably have tissue invasion by the parasites. At first, focal destruction of the upper layers of the mucosa occurs (Fig. 11–3 *A*), progressing to ulceration of the whole mucosa and later of the submucosa (Fig. 11–3 *B*). The ulcer produced by *Balantidium* has a wide opening, appearing as a shallow indentation, usually filled with necrotic debris, with trophozoites located at the edge and bottom of the ulcer in varying numbers, some deep in the crypts (Figs. 11–3 *B* and 11–4 *A*). Infiltration by mononuclear cells (lymphocytes and plasma cells) and a few polymorphonuclear cells accompanies the lesion (Fig. 11–3 *C–D*). Concurrent bacterial infections may manifest as an abundant polymorphonuclear cell infiltrate. Involvement of small blood vessels in the wall of the intestine (Fig. 11–4 *D*) is shown by the formation of thrombi containing parasites. In most cases, the ulcer extends down to the muscular layers (Fig. 11–4 *A–C*), but in severe infections the parasites occur throughout the entire thickness of the wall, including the surface of the serosa. In cases of perforation, either gross or microscopic (Fig. 11–5 *A–B*), the parasites are found in the peritoneal surface, the omentum, and the mesenteric adipose tissue; extension to other organs may occur (Japp et al. 1972). Patients with peritonitis also have prominent inflammatory changes due to the concomitant bacterial infection. In at least one immune-deficient individual, the parasites were found in the esophagus, stomach, small intestine, and colon (Iglezias, 1980). In other cases, they were located in the lymph nodes.

Diagnosis. Balantidiasis is difficult to diagnose on clinical grounds because the symptoms are nonspecific. Recovery and identification of trophozoites and cysts in the stools by the clinical laboratory is necessary for specific diagnosis. *Balantidium* is one of the most misidentified human parasites because laboratory personnel are not familiar with its diagnostic characteristics (Fig. 11–1 *A–C*). Moreover, there are many freeliving ciliated organisms that superficially resemble *Balantidium*. They are sometimes found in water and reagents and may contaminate clinical samples, leading to misdiagnosis.

In tissues, only the trophozoites are present, with the same morphologic characteristics described above. The size of the parasite allows numerous histologic sections of a single organism in different planes; therefore, there is marked variability in the size, shape, and internal structures of the parasite in each section. In hematoxylin and eosin–stained sections, the nuclei stain black and the cytoplasm stains red; the cilia are apparent. The contractile vacuole of the trophozoite is usually found in the posterior half of the body; it is seen as a large, empty space. In cases of peritonitis, *Balantidium* has been recovered and diagnosed cytologically in specimens stained with Papanicolaou stain (Lahiri et al. 1977). No serologic tests are available for the diagnosis of balantidiasis.

References

Arean VM, Koppisch E, 1956. Balantidiasis. A review and report of cases. Am. J. Clin. Pathol. 32:1089–1115

Auz JL, 1984. Abcesso hepatico balantidiano. Rev. Med. Panama 9:51–55

Awakian A, 1937. Studies on the intestinal protozoa of rats. II. Rats as carriers of *Balantidium*. Trans. R. Soc. Trop. Med. Hyg. 31:93–98

Baskerville L, Ahmed Y, Ramchand S, 1970. *Balantidium* colitis: report of a case. Dig. Dis. 15:727–731

Beaver PC, Jung RC, Cupp EW, 1984. *Clinical Parasitology*. Philadelphia: Lea & Febiger

Biagi FF, 1970. Unusual isolates from clinical material—*Balantidium coli*. Ann. N.Y. Acad. Sci. 174:1023–1026

Castro J, Vazquez-Iglesias JL, Arnal-Monreal F, 1983. Dysentery caused by *Balantidium coli*—report of two cases. Endoscopy 15:272–274

Cespedes R, Rodriguez O, Valverde O, Fernandez J, Gonzalez UF, Jara PJW, 1967. Balantidiosis: Estudio de un caso anatomoclinico masivo con lesiones y presencia del parasito en el intestino delgado y pleura. Acta Med. Costar. 10:135–151

Cockburn TA, 1948. *Balantidium* infection associated with diarrhoea in primates. Trans. R. Soc. Trop. Med. Hyg. 42:291–293

Corliss JO, 1994. An interim utilitarian ("user-friendly") hierarchical classification and characterization of the protists. Acta Protozool. 33:1–51

Couvee LMJ, Rijpstra AC, 1961. The prevalence of *Balantidium coli* in the central highlands of Western New Guinea. Trop. Geogr. Med. 13:284–286

Daoudal P, 1986. Balantidiose pulmonaire. Un cas en Franche-Comte. Presse Med. 15:257

Dorfman S, Gil De Salazar F, Bravo LG, 1984a. Balantidiasis apendicular. Aportacion de dos casos. Rev. Esp. Enferm. Apar. Dig. 65:167–170

Dorfman S, Rangel O, Bravo LG, 1984b. Balantidiasis: report of a fatal case with appendicular and pulmonary involvement. Trans. R. Soc. Trop. Med. Hyg. 78: 833–834

Dzbenski TH, 1966. Immuno-fluorescent studies on *Balantidium coli*. Trans. R. Soc. Trop. Med. Hyg. 60: 387–389

Ewers WH, 1972. Parasites of man in Papua-New Guinea. Southeast Asian J. Trop. Med. Public Health 2:79–86

Forsyth DM, 1954. Correspondence. Balantidiasis. Lancet 1:628–629

Gonzalez Sanchez O, 1978. Apendicitis aguda por *Balantidium coli*. Rev. Cubana Med. Trop. 30:9–13

Iglezias SD, 1980. Exacerbacao de balantidiase e estrongiloidiase em paciente corn penfigo foliaceo sul Americano na vigencia de corticoidoterapia. Rev. Hosp. Clin. Fac. Med. Sao Paulo 35:88–90

Isaza-Mejia G, 1955. Balantidiasis vaginal. Antioquia Med. 5:488–491

Japp HH, Moraes WC, Rabello Filho M, Miziara HL, 1972. Balantidiose. Apresentacao de um caso com perfuracao intestinal. Rev. Assoc. Med. Brasil 18:129–132

Kan SP, 1971. Electron microscopic study of *Balantidium* from man. Southeast Asian J. Trop. Med. Public Health 2:1–8

Kennedy CC, Stewart RC, 1957. Balantidial dysentery: a human case in northern Ireland. Trans. R. Soc. Trop. Med. Hyg. 51:549–558

Ladas SD, Savva S, Frydas A, Kaloviduris A, Hatzioannou J, Raptis S, 1989. Invasive balantidiasis presented as chronic colitis and lung involvement. Dig. Dis. Sci. 34:1621–1623

Lahiri VL, Elhence BR, Agarwal BM, 1977. *Balantidium* peritonitis diagnosed on cytologic material. Acta Cytol. 21:123–124

Lara AR, Bernal RM, 1974. Sindrome disenterico por *Balantidium coli* en ninos. Bol. Med. Hosp. Infant. Mexico 31:779–784

Maliwa E, Von Haus V, 1920. Uber Balantidien-infektion der Harnwege. Z. Urol. 14:495–501

McCarey AG, 1952. Balantidiasis in South Persia. Br. Med. J. 1:629–631

Myers BJ, Kuntz RE, 1968. Intestinal protozoa of the baboon *Papio doguera* Pucheran, 1856. J. Protozool. 15:363–365

Norman JG, Jessop P, 1973. *Balantidium coli* in a cervico-vaginal smear. Med. J. Aust. 1:694–696

Radford AJ, 1973. Balantidiasis in Papua New Guinea. Med. J. Aust. 1:238–241

Rivasi F, Giannotti T, 1983. *Balantidium coli* in cervico-vaginal cytology. A case report. Pathologica 75:439–442

Rutschow H, 1976. *Balantidium-coli* infektion des welblichen Genitale. Geburtshilfe. Frauenheilkd. 36:348–351

Sargeaunt PG, 1971. The size range of *Balantidium coli*. Trans. R. Soc. Trop. Med. Hyg. 65:428

Swartzwelder JC, 1950. Balantidiasis. Am. J. Dig. Dis. 17: 173–179

van der Hoeven JA, Rijpstra AC, 1957. Intestinal parasites in the central mountain district of Netherlands New-Guinea. Trop. Geogr. Med. 13:225–228

Walzer PD, Judson FN, Murphy KB, Healy GR, English DK, Schultz MG, 1973. Balantidiasis outbreak in Truk. Am. J. Trop. Med. Hyg. 22:33–41

Woody NC, Woody HB, 1960. Balantidiasis in infancy: review of the literature and report of a case. J. Pediatr. 56:485–489

Young MD, 1950. Attempts to transmit human *Balantidium coli*. Am. J. Trop. Med. Hyg. 30:71–72

Zaman V, 1964. Studies on the immobilization reaction in the genus *Balantidium*. Trans. R. Soc. Trop. Med. Hyg. 58:255–259

Zaman V, 1970a. Activity of contractile vacuole in the parasitic ciliate, *Balantidium coli*. Experientia 26:806–807

Zaman V, 1970b. Ultrastructure of *Balantidium*. Southeast Asian J. Trop. Med. Public Health 1:225–230

Part II

The Nematodes

The helminths are metazoan organisms (bodies with many cells) commonly referred to as *worms*. For practical purposes, all worms of medical importance belong to one of two groups: the nematodes or *roundworms* and the Platyhelminths or *flatworms*. The flatworms belong to two groups, the Trematoda or flukes (see the introduction to Part III) and the Cestoda or tapeworms (see the introduction to Part IV). In the following paragraphs, the morphology and biology of nematodes of human medical importance are discussed. This information is not intended to apply to all known groups of nematodes. It is provided as an aid to the recognition of those species encountered in humans.

The nematodes include the largest number of helminth species and are by far the most commonly found parasites of humans. Morphologically, they are characterized by an elongated body, round on cross section, and by a general body cavity, the *pseudocoelom* (see below). The main biologic characteristics of the nematodes are two sexes and the existence of both free-living and parasitic species of plants and animals. The life cycle of nematodes varies from a simple adult-egg-adult pattern to more complicated ones requiring an obligatory intermediate host or hosts in which a larval stage develops. Humans are definitive hosts for an array of nematodes, but for some of them, humans behave as intermediate hosts. Humans are not intermediate hosts of parasites because predation of humans seldom occurs; thus, the intermediate stages in humans generally do not pass to their definitive hosts. For example, humans infected with *Echinococcus granulosus* (hydatid cysts) behave as intermediate hosts, but seldom is the cyst ingested by dogs or cats, the definitive hosts of the parasites (see Chapter 27). In these cases, we refer to humans as *final hosts*. For some larval stages of certain species of nematodes, humans can also behave as *paratenics* (see below, under classification Ascaridida). Nematodes in general produce infections that vary from asymptomatic to oligosymptomatic to life-threatening. Some nematode infections are often restricted to certain geographic areas of the world; others are widely distributed in the tropical and semitropical areas as well.

Adult

The morphology of adult nematodes is quite variable and probably depends on their adaptation to a parasitic or free-living existence or to the organ in which they reside. Nematode species of medical importance have sizes that vary from barely visible with the naked eye (*Halicephalobus = Micronema*) to 1.2 m in length (*Dracunculus*). The general shape of nematodes is cylindrical, and sometimes the body is notably more slender in its anterior half—for example in *Trichinella*, some capillarids, and *Trichuris*. In general, the body of female nematodes is straight, while that of males is curved ventrally on the posterior end. In some groups, the posterior end of the males has a *copulatory bursa*, seen as a circular or oval expansion of the body, supported by chitinous rays. The main structures of the body of nematodes, used in their identification in tissue sections, are reviewed below.

Cuticle

The cuticle of nematodes is an important structure for their recognition in tissue sections. The cuticle is complex. It is always composed of several layers when viewed under the electron microscope, but it is often seen as a single layer under the light microscopy. Some genera have defined cuticular layers, the number varying from one genus to another and from the larva to the adult stage. Under the cuticle is a zone, the *hypodermis*, visible in some groups with the light microscope (see below).

The layers of the cuticle and the hypodermis are seen only when the worm is viewed on cross sections or longitudinal sections. The general thickness of the cuticle varies from less than 1 μm, as in *Wuchereria* (Fig. II–1 *A*), *Brugia*, and other filariids, to 500 μm or more in *Ascaris* (Fig. II–1 *B*). The cuticles of *Ascaris*, *Dirofilaria*, *Loa*, *Onchocerca*, and others have distinct layers (Fig. II–1 *B–E*). The layers of the cuticle of *Dirofilaria* and *Loa* (Fig. II–1 *C–D*), two closely related genera, are conspicuous, especially on the lateral aspects of the worm, because usually the cuticle is thicker on this aspect of the body. Two layers of the cuticle of *Dirofilaria* consist of oblique fibers running perpendicular to each other, a feature seen in tangential sections (see Fig. 20–22 *D*).

The external surface of the cuticle of most nematodes found in humans is generally smooth on cross sections and longitudinal sections (Fig. II–1 *A*, *B*, and *E*). Some groups have *ridges* seen as regularly spaced, rounded knobs or spikes on either cross sections or longitudinal sections. Most species of *Dirofilaria* (Fig. II–1 *C*) have distinct *longitudinal ridges*. *Loa* has *bosses*—small, irregularly scattered, round protuberances (Fig. II–1 *E*). *Onchocerca* has *transverse ridges* seen on oblique and longitudinal sections (Fig. II–1 *D*), and *Enterobius* and some larval stages of ascariids have lateral alae (Fig. II–1 *F*). These characteristics are important for diagnosis in tissue sections. The internal surface of the cuticle is generally smooth in most species, but *Dirofilaria* has a thickening on the lateral aspects, the *internal ridge* or *internal thickening* (Fig. II–1 *C*).

Another structure found in the cuticle of nematodes is the *bacillary band*, a characteristic of the Trichinelloidea (*Trichuris*, *Trichinella*, some capillariids, and others) (Fig. II–2 *A–B*). The bacillary band is composed of cuticular pores, each with a glandular cell located in the hypodermis (Fig. II–2 *B*). Bacillary bands may occur as a single band along the entire body of the worm, such as in *Trichuris* (Fig. II–2 *A*), or as several bands, such as in some capillariids.

Subcuticle or Hypodermis

The hypodermis, located below the cuticle, is composed of a syncytium of cytoplasmic extensions of cells arranged in four groups of variable size projecting into the body cavity of the worm. These four projections are located on the dorsal, ven-

───────────────────────────────▶

Fig. II–1. The cuticle and lateral cords of some nematodes of importance in human medicine, sections stained with hematoxylin and eosin stain. A, *Wuchereria bancrofti* in cross section. Note the cuticle, which is less than 1 μm thick (short arrow); the contractile portion of the muscle cells (long arrow); the wide and low lateral cords (between arrowheads); and the uterus with microfilariae, ×705. B, *Ascaris lumbricoides* in cross section. Note the cuticle, which is approximately 50 μm thick; the hypodermis (short arrows), and the cytoplasm of the hypodermis cells forming the lateral cord (long arrow), ×70. C, *Dirofilaria ursi* in cross section. The cuticle is layered, with longitudinal ridges (small arrows), and with an internal thickening or ridge in the interior aspect (long arrow). The lateral cord (c) is clearly divided into ventral (v) and dorsal (d) aspects, ×350. D, *Onchocerca volvulus* in longitudinal section. The transverse ridges of the cuticle (short arrows) are evidence of longitudinal sections. The cuticle is layered, and the inner layer has the striae (long arrows) in a pattern of two striae for each ridge, ×705. E, *Loa loa* in cross section. Note the cuticle with bosses (short arrow) and its layered nature. The lateral cords are clearly divided into ventral and dorsal portions, and each portion has a small nucleus. The muscle cells are clearly seen, ×350. F, *Enterobius vermicularis* in cross section. Note the prominent lateral alae (short arrow). The lateral cord is low (long arrow) and has two excretory canals, seen as two open spaces (ec1 and ec2), ×550.

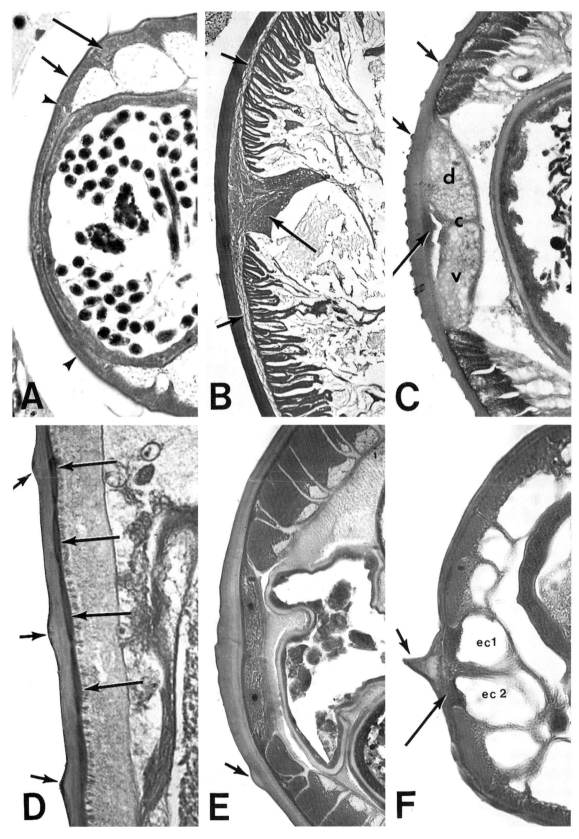

Fig. II–1.

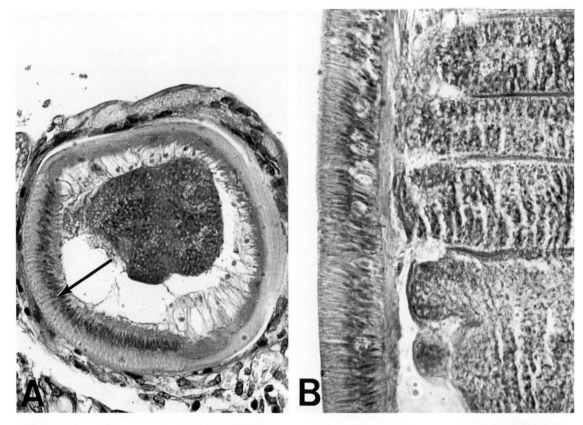

Fig. II–2. *Trichuris trichiura*, cross section and longitudinal section at the level of the esophagus, hematoxylin and eosin stain. *A*, Cross section showing the bacillary band, comprising one-third of the circumference of the worm (arrow). Note that the bacillary band is composed of many cells with nuclei, which are arranged in a palisade. Each cell is located around a minute pore, which is barely visible on light microscopy. The glandular esophagus (stichosome) is located at the center of the worm, ×450. *B*, Longitudinal section illustrating similar structures. Note that the esophagus is composed of stichocytes, which are lobulated and appear segmented on some longitudinal sections, ×705.

tral, and lateral aspects of the worm, forming *dorsal*, *ventral*, and *lateral cords*, respectively. These cords are characteristic of nematodes and divide the somatic muscles into four fields or quadrants (see Figs. 11–3 *A–B* and 19–18 *A*).

The lateral cords are important for diagnosis of nematodes in sections. Thus, one should become acquainted with their morphology, their size, and the number of nuclei present in each cross section. The lateral cords form the canals of the excretory system of the worm when present, but they are not generally seen with light microscopy. The excretory system of *Enterobius* is large, with two wide-open tubes on each lateral cord (Fig. II–3 *A*). Excretory tubes are absent in the Trichinelloidea, and in other groups a single tube is found. The lateral cords in general are prominent, while the dorsal and ventral cords are relatively inconspicuous (Fig. II–3 *A–B*). The lateral cords are usually located as high as the muscles, sometimes higher; others have a Y shape, as in *Anisakis* (see Fig. 16–19 *D*). In filarial worms the lateral cords may be low and wide, for example in *Wuchereria* (Fig. II–1 *A*); they are narrow and high in *Dirofilaria* (Fig. II–1 *C*). Often the lateral cords have two distinct fields, ventral and dorsal (Fig. II–1 *C* and *E*).

Muscles

Nematodes have only longitudinal muscle fibers that run from one end of the worm to the other; no transverse muscles are present. As stated above, the muscle mass of nematodes is divided into four quadrants by the cells of the hypodermis (Fig. II–3 A–B). Each muscle cell is composed of two distinct portions: the contractile portion, located at the base of the cell body, lying against the hypodermis, and the cytoplasmic portion above, facing the body cavity and often appearing as an empty space (Fig. II–3 A). The number of muscle cells in a nematode is of diagnostic value; this number is usually expressed as the number per quadrant.

Depending on the number of muscle cells, nematodes are *meromyarian* if there are two to five cells per quadrant, as in *Oesophagostomum* and *Enterobius* (Fig. II–2 A), or *polymyarian* if there are numerous cells per quadrant, as in *Ascaris* (Fig. II–3 B). In addition, muscle cells are platymyarian if their contractile fibrils are at the base, against the hypodermis, or *coelomyarian* if the fibrils extend along the sides of the cell membrane toward the body cavity.

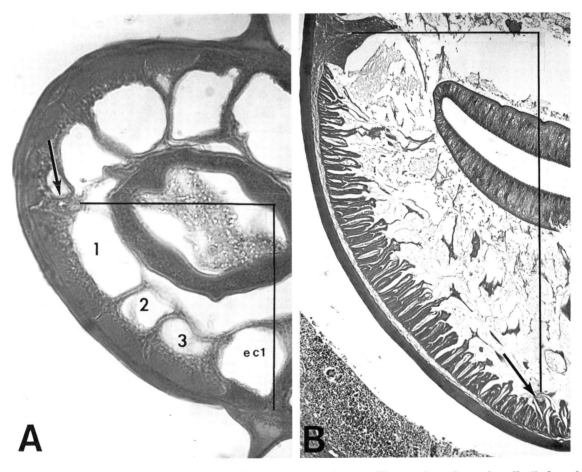

A

B

Fig. II–3. *Enterobius vermicularis and Ascaris lumbricoides* on cross section illustrating some of the nematode muscle nomenclature, hematoxylin and eosin stain. A, *Enterobius vermicularis*, showing one quadrant of the musculature (between the right angle lines). The lateral cord at the bottom shows one of the excretory channels (ec1); the dorsal cord (arrow) is smaller, often in- conspicuous. The number of muscle cells (1, 2, and 3) is small (meromyarian), ×705. B, *Ascaris lumbricoides*, also showing one quadrant of muscle cells. The lateral cord is on the left and the ventral cord (inconspicuous) is at the bottom (arrow). The muscle cells are numerous in one quadrant (polymyarian), ×55.

Body Cavity

The body cavity of nematodes is limited by the muscle cells and is referred to as the *pseudocoelom* or *pseudocele* because it lacks a mesothelial lining. The body cavity contains the digestive and reproductive systems of the worm. The spaces between these systems are filled with fluid, the amount of which is controlled by the excretory system of the worm (Fig. II–3).

Digestive System. In general, the digestive system of nematodes is composed of the *buccal cavity*, that portion between the beginning of the esophagus and the *oral opening* on the anterior tip of the worm. The *buccal capsule* is an enlarged buccal cavity with sclerotized walls. The oral opening is sometimes surrounded by three lips and at other times by small protrusions, the oral papillae. The *esophagus* (see Fig. 15–3 *A–B* and *color plate* VII *A*) is most commonly a cylindrical muscular structure; at other times, it is composed of three distinct parts: the *corpus*, the *isthmus*, and the *pseudobulb*. The pseudobulb is a rounded, muscular dilation before the intestinal–esophageal junction; on cross section, the esophagus has a Y-shaped lumen (see Figs. 15–13 *D* and 15–18 *D*). In some groups the esophagus is divided into two parts, the anterior muscular and the posterior glandular, sometimes referred to as the *ventriculus*. The esophagus in *Trichuris*, *Trichinella*, the capillariids, and other related forms is known as the *stichosome*. It is composed entirely of glandular cells, the *stichocytes*, that form the capillary esophageal lumen (Fig. II–2 *A–B*; see also Fig. 21–2 *D–E*). The *intestine* or *midgut* is variable in structure. It is composed of cells with a brush border (*microvilli*) that is often apparent on sections of the worm (see Figs. 1–5 *D* and 15–10 *D*). In the anterior portion of the intestine, near the intestinal–esophageal junction, some species have a cecum that extends anteriorly. The number of cells forming the intestine (as seen on cross sections) and their arrangement—either as a syncytium, as in *Angiostrongylus* (see Fig. 13–14 *C*), or as cells with well-defined cell borders (see Fig. 18–6 *D*)—is of diagnostic importance. In some groups the intestine is large; in others it is an inconspicuous tube. One characteristic of the intestine is that it is firmly anchored to the body at the mouth and the anus. In addition, when a nematode is cut in two, each portion of the intestine remains in position; the anterior half is attached to the oral opening, the posterior half to the anus. Thus, the intestine is always present in cross sections. The *rectum* in females is the last portion of the intestine. The rectum opens at the posterior end of the worm through the *anal pore*, located at some distance from the posterior tip. In males the rectum is transformed into a cavity, the *cloaca*, where the male genital system and the intestine join; the anal pore is often surrounded by papillae, the *anal papillae*. The oral and anal papillae are important morphologic characteristics for classification of nematodes in toto but seldom in tissue sections.

Reproductive System

The anatomic and histologic structures of the reproductive system of nematodes are complicated; on cross section they often appear as a series of tubular structures. In general, the male reproductive system is composed of a single tube, which usually begins in the anterior half of the body as the *testis*. The testis is followed by the *vas deferens*, the *seminal vesicle*, and finally the *ejaculatory duct* at the posterior end of the worm in the cloaca.

The female reproductive system is more complicated. In most nematodes it is composed of two tubes, each beginning with the *ovary* and continuing with the *oviduct*, the *seminal receptacle*, the *uterus*, the *vagina*, and the *genital pore*, a small opening on the ventral side of the body. Usually one set of reproductive organs is located in the anterior half of the body and the other in the posterior half. The two sets join in the midbody, or thereabout, to form the vagina, which terminates in the vulva. In some groups, for example *Trichinella*, *Trichuris*, and the capillariids, the female genital system is composed of only one tube. Both the male and female genital systems are folded on themselves one or more times; thus, in cross sections they appear as several structures.

The genital system is anchored to the body of the worm only at the vulva in the female and at the cloaca in the male. Therefore, when a nematode is cut in two, the part of the genital system not anchored to the body may often fall, leaving a pseudocoelom with only the intestinal tube (see Fig. 19–10 A–D). This usually happens at the surgical desk when the specimen is sectioned for processing and embedding. Often parts of the genital tract are found adjacent to the worm in the tissues, raising questions that confuse the diagnostician unfamiliar with the worm.

Although the different components of the genital system of nematodes are histologically characteristic and are recognizable on microscopic examination, their description is outside the scope of this discussion. For identification purposes, the most important structure of the genital system is the uterus because it may contain mature eggs (see Figs. 15–13 D and 17–7 B), larvae (see Fig. 22–6 F), or microfilariae (see Figs. 18–10 B and 19–16 C–D). Any of these findings is helpful in identifying the organism in question. Often the female uterus is empty or contains only immature cells, indicating that the worm under study is nonfertilized, either because of the absence of males or because it is prepuberal (see Fig. 19–12 B).

Larva

Most nematodes parasitic in humans produce eggs that are evacuated with the feces (intestinal nematodes), the sputum (*Mamommonogamus laryngeus*), or the urine (*Dioctophyme renale*) to continue their development in the environment. Others produce larvae (*Strongyloides stercoralis*), which usually require further development outside of the body before entering a new host. Finally, some tissue nematodes such as the filarial worms produce *microfilariae*, embryos beyond the egg stage but not fully developed larvae. The development of larvae and microfilariae continues through several stages, each stage emerging from the previous one by *molting* (shedding their cuticle) until they become adults. Eggs evacuated with feces often require development under appropriate conditions, resulting in a first-, second-, and third-stage larva inside the egg (*Ascaris*, *Trichuris*, and *Toxocara*). Some eggs may hatch and produce free-living larvae, which develop in soil to the third stage (*Ancylostoma* and *Necator*). Larvae evacuated with the feces also develop to the third stage as free-living organisms in soil (*Strongyloides*). The microfilariae require arthropods as obligatory intermediate hosts in which they develop to the third stage (*Wuchereria*, *Brugia*, and *Loa*). Other nematodes that shed larvae in water need aquatic arthropods for development of infective larvae (*Dracunculus medinensis*).

The *third-stage* larva of nematodes is the infective stage. This stage has to be ingested with soil (*Ascaris* and *Toxocara*) or with the intermediate host (*Dracunculus*) or must enter through the skin (*Necator*, *Ancylostoma*, and *Strongyloides*) to reach its location in the new host and develop to an adult. In some nematodes, such as *Enterobius* and *Trichuris*, the infective eggs (with a third-stage larva) hatch after ingestion and develop directly into adults in the intestine. In others, such as, *Ascaris*, the infective eggs reach the intestine, hatch, and produce larvae that have an obligatory developmental phase in the lungs before migrating to the intestine to become adults. Larvae entering through the skin, such as those of *Necator*, *Ancylostoma*, and *Strongyloides*, migrate through the blood vessels to the lungs and via the trachea to the intestine. The infective larvae of filarial worms are deposited on the skin by their vectors, enter through the skin, and migrate through the tissues before reaching the site where they develop to adults. Development to adulthood occurs after the third-stage larva molts to the fourth and then to the fifth or adult stage.

The larval stages of nematodes vary in size from microscopic (*Ascaris*, *Toxocara*, *Strongyloides*, and *Ancylostoma*) (see Fig. 17–4 C) to 2 to 3 cm in length (*Anisakis*, *Pseudoterranova*, and others) (see Fig. 16–17). Since some nematode larvae occur in humans and produce morbidity (*Toxocara* and *Anisakis*) and mortality (*Baylisascaris*), it is important to recognize their basic morphology in cross sections for diagnostic purposes.

The larvae of nematodes have the same general internal organization as the adults, except that the male or female genital system has not developed (see Fig. 12–11). Often rudimentary structures or groups of cells (the *genital primordium*) are the only representatives of sex organs (see Fig. 12–11). In addition, in smaller larval forms the body cavity is not apparent, a feature that confuses the neophyte. The important features of the larval stages are the *cuticle*, often less than 1 μm thick, and the *lateral alae*, either single (*Toxocara*, *Baylisascaris*, and *Ascaris*; see Figs. 16–5 C, 16–10, 15–12 D–E and 15–20 C–D) or double (*Strongyloides*, *Pelodera*, *Ancylostoma*, and *Necator*) (see Figs. 11–7 B, 11–15 D, and 13–9). The *muscles* are usually rudimentary and sometimes are not easily differentiated from the cuticle (see Fig. 17–4 C). The *lateral cords* are also rudimentary, with small nuclei (see Fig. 16–22). The *excretory columns*, located on the lateral cords, are often prominent, with or without a discernible lumen. The *intestine* may have a lumen with ingested material or may be closed. The larvae of *Toxocara*, *Strongyloides*, *Ancylostoma*, and *Necator* are usually less than 24 μm in diameter. The larvae of *Ascaris* and *Baylisascaris* are generally between 50 and 65 μm in diameter. The larvae of *Anisakis*, *Pseudoterranova*, and others are 0.2 to 0.8 mm in diameter (see Fig. 16–19 D).

LIFE CYCLES

The life cycles of nematodes can be direct, with no intermediate hosts, such as in *Enterobius*. Some nematodes have a life cycle that requires a phase of development in soil. In these instances, soil is akin to an intermediate host because its conditions are specific for the development of the parasite, hence the term *soil transmitted helminths*.

Some nematodes have obligatory intermediate hosts. *Angiostrongylus* requires slugs and snails. The filarial worms depend on blood-sucking arthropods to move from one host to another. *Aonchoteca* (= *Capillaria*) *philippinensis* needs freshwater fish, and *Anisakis* and *Pseudoterranova* require marine fish and crustaceans. *Dracunculus* uses freshwater crustaceans, while *Gnathostoma* requires a crustacean as a first intermediate host and a fish as a second intermediate host.

Classification

The zoologic classification of nematodes is outside the scope of this discussion. Thus, only some of the basic arrangements of the medically important nematodes are provided to understand their relationships. The important nematodes belong to six orders: Rhabditida, Strongylida, Oxyurida, Ascaridida, Spirurida, and Enoplida. The main characteristics will be outline here, and each group is studied in the following chapters.

1. *Rhabditida:* Rhabditida comprises the free-living nematodes, some of which have a phase adapted to a parasitic existence, for example *Strongyloides.* The species of *Strongyloides* have larval stages in soil; these larvae infect their hosts through the skin. Other free-living nematodes produce sporadic infections in humans and animals, for example *Halicephalobus* (= *Micronema*) and *Pelodera.*

2. *Strongylida:* The species of Strongylida are commonly known as *hookworms.* They are characterized by having larvae as their infective stages. There are two types of larvae. One type is free-living and enters the new host through the skin, such as in *Ancylostoma* and *Necator,* or through the mouth, such as in *Trichostrongylus* and *Ancylostoma.* The other type of larvae requires intermediate hosts that, when ingested, produce the infection (*Angiostrongylus*). Those forms, which gain access to the host through the skin, are classically associated with cutaneous larva migrans. Some members of the Strongylida may undergo paratenesis (see below, Ascaridida).

3. *Oxyurida:* Oxyurida has two parasitic forms generally recognized in humans: *Enterobius vermicularis,* the common pinworm, and *Syphacia,* the pinworm of the mouse, which sometimes produces human infections.

4. *Ascaridida:* Ascaridida has many species of medical importance, the adults of which generally inhabit the gastrointestinal tract of most vertebrates. The infective stages of some genera of Ascaridida develop in soil (*Ascaris* and *Toxocara*). In others, there is an obligatory intermediate host (*Anisakis* and *Pseudoterranova*). In both instances, ingestion of the infective stage is necessary to produce a new infection. Most genera of Ascaridida must migrate through the tissues before reaching the adult stage in the intestine.

   Certain members of the Ascaridida can remain as infective forms in the tissues of abnormal hosts. This association is known as *paratenesis* and the abnormal host as a *paratenic* host. Larval stages in paratenic hosts remain alive and unchanged for long periods, probably for the life of the paratenic host. These ascariids (*Toxocara*) are responsible for the production of visceral larva migrans in humans.

5. *Spirurida:* Spirurida is probably the largest group of parasitic nematodes of humans. Many genera require an arthropod intermediate host in their life cycles. Members of Spirurida occur in the wall of the gastrointestinal tract (*Gnathostoma*), the squamous epithelium of the mouth and esophagus (*Gongylonema*), the subcutaneous tissue (*Dracunculus, Onchocerca, Loa,* and *Dirofilaria*), the lymphatics (*Wuchereria* and *Brugia*), the brain (*Meningonema*), and other tissues and organs. *Gnathostoma* in abnormal hosts remains in the infective stage (paratenesis) and produces both cutaneous and visceral larva migrans. By far the most important group of Spirurida are the filarial worms, with many parasitic forms in humans and animals. In humans they produce morbidity and mortality, which in certain geographic areas constitute problems of public health importance.

6. *Enoplida:* Enoplida has two superfamilies with species important for humans: Trichinelloidea and Dioctophymatoidea. Trichinelloidea has parasitic forms in the intestine (*Trichuris, Trichinella,* and *Aonchoteca* [= *Capillaria*] *philippinensis*), the respiratory passages (*Eucoleus aerophilus* [= *Capillaria aerophila*]), the viscera (*Calodium hepaticum* [= *Capillaria hepatica*]), the skin (*Anatrichosoma*), and other sites. In general, Trichinelloidea produces infections by ingestion of infective eggs with soil (*Trichuris* and some species of capillariids) or infective larvae in intermediate hosts (*Trichinella* and *Aonchoteca philippinensis*). Dioctophymatoidea has many species parasitic in animals; sporadic *Dioctophyme renale* and *Eustrongylides* infections in humans have been reported.

═══ Part II ═══
Geographic Distribution

The parasitic nematodes of humans have a worldwide distribution. The soil-transmitted nematodes occur more frequently in areas where hygienic habits are poor and the conditions for development of infective stages in soil are most suitable (tropical and temperate zones). Those nematodes requiring blood-sucking arthropods, such as the filarial worms, have a mostly tropical distribution. Zoonotic infections produced by many species of filariids are infrequent in the tropical and the temperate zones. The prevalence of nematode infections is linked to the food habits of the population in certain geographic areas. *Anisakis* and *Pseudoterranova* infections are due to consumption of raw marine fish in Japan and other places, and *Aonchoteca philippiensis* infections to consumption of raw freshwater fish in the Philippines.

12

RHABDITIDA

Rhabditida comprises all of the free-living forms, one of the largest groups of nematodes. Some genera have a parasitic phase, while others are only facultative parasites. One important member of Rhabditida is *Strongyloides*, with at least seven species known in humans, producing intestinal and dermal infections. One species, *S. stercoralis* in the intestine, may become opportunistic in certain immune-suppressed hosts to produce infections that are lethal if not treated. *Halicephalobus* (= *Micronema*) *deletrix* produces sporadic, isolated cases of facultative parasitism in humans, establishing colonies in the tissues of parasitic females that produce eggs and larvae. Finally, *Pelodera strongyloides* has a larval stage that parasitizes the skin of humans and animals.

Strongyloides

The genus *Strongyloides* has many species infecting animals and one species well known as a parasite of humans: *S. stercoralis*, which is endemic in tropical and subtropical areas. Other species are *S. fuelleborni*, a parasite of Old World primates (chimpanzees and African baboons), which produces intestinal infections in some populations in parts of Africa, and its subspecies, *S. fuelleborni kellyi* (Viney et al. 1991) in Papua, New Guinea. *Strongyloides myopotami* from nutria and *S. procyonis* from raccoons are responsible for cases of cutaneous larva migrans in the southeastern United States (Little, 1965). Finally, *S. websteri* of horses, *S. ramsoni* of pigs, and *S. papillosus* of sheep (Roeckel, Lyons, 1977) also produce cutaneous larva migrans (see Chapter 14). Experimental infections of humans with *S. ramsoni* (Matuzenko, 1971) and *S. myopotami* (Little, 1965) produce transient patent infections, as demonstrated by the recovery of larvae in the stools (Freedman, 1991). Most species of *Strongyloides* have relatively low host specificity, and other animal species probably produce zoonotic infections in humans (Beaver et al. 1984), perhaps explaining different clinical syndromes. These infections are difficult to study because in general the different stages of the life cycle of *Strongyloides* are morphologically alike, so distinction of the zoonotic species on these grounds is difficult.

Strongyloides Stercoralis—Strongyloidiasis

Strongyloides stercoralis was discovered over 120 years ago in the stools of French troops suffering from diarrhea in Cochin-China (modern Vietnam), and the disease it produces was known for many years as *Cochin-China diarrhea*. The elucidation of the complete life cycle, as described below, required 50 years after the discovery of the worm. Dogs served as experimental models for the infection, and much of our knowledge of the biology of *S. stercoralis* is derived from studies in these animals. In certain forms of immune suppression *Strongyloides* becomes opportunistic, producing a disease that is fatal if not treated; this makes the worm of paramount importance in human medicine.

Morphology and Life Cycle. The parasitic females of *S. stercoralis* are up to 2.7 mm in length by 30 to 40 μm in maximum diameter. No males occur in the intestine or other tissues, and the females multiply by parthenogenesis. The females of *Strongyloides* are buried deep in the crypts of the duodenum and upper jejunum; sometimes they are found in the terminal portion of the stomach. In the mucosa, they lay eggs that develop rapidly into larvae, which gain access to the lumen and, carried with the intestinal contents, are evacuated with the feces. Once in the environment, the larvae continue to mature in appropriate soil to become infective larvae capable of penetrating the skin, gaining access to the bloodstream, and traveling to the lungs. Once in the pulmonary capillaries, the larvae break into the alveoli, migrate to the epiglottis, and are swallowed, to reach the duodenum and mature to adult females (Fig. 12–1 a; Beaver et al. 1984).

The larvae evacuated in the feces are known as *rhabditoid* larvae. They measure 380 μm in length by 20 μm in width and have a well-defined, muscular esophagus with a prominent esophageal bulb (see Fig. 11–10 A–C). Rhabditoid larvae feed in soil before evolving into infective *filariform* larvae, characterized by a slender esophagus (without a bulb) that occupies at least the anterior half of the body. They also have a notched posterior end and are about 630 μm in length by 16 μm in width (Fig. 12–10 D–F; Beaver et al. 1984).

Two aspects of the life cycle of *S. stercoralis* are important. First, the rhabditoid larvae passed in the feces may develop in soil to males and females, known as the *free-living generation* of the parasite. This development

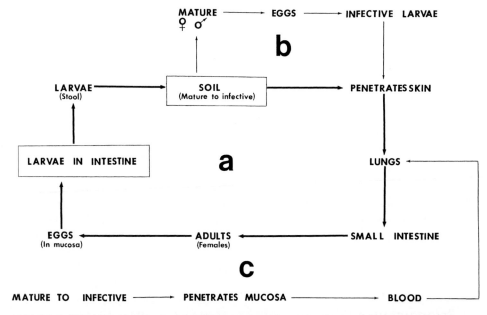

Fig. 12–1. Life cycle of *Strongyloides stercoralis*. The main cycle is as depicted in (a). The route followed by the parasite in (b) occurs in soil under certain conditions, in humid tropical countries, and results in the free-living generation of the parasite. The route in (c) is more important in human medicine; it depicts the autoinfection, in which larvae in the intestine become infective, enter the colonic mucosa, and via the general circulation gain access to the lungs and travel back to the intestine. These larvae complete the life cycle within the same host.

occurs in the feces and in soil with abundant moisture, principally in tropical climates; it is the main form of the parasite's development, and it is probably repeated under optimal conditions (Fig. 12–1 *B*). Second, the rhabditoid larvae may develop to infective stages *within the intestine*. In this case, they enter the intestinal mucosa, gain access to the general circulation, and travel to the lungs to complete their life cycle. This type of development is known as *autoinfection*. It is sometimes referred to as *internal autoinfection* to differentiate it from infections due to larvae that mature in the anus and produce *external autoinfection* (Fig. 12–1 *C*). The reason for autoinfection is not known, but is suggested that a prolonged intestinal transit time may be responsible because it gives the larvae time to develop in the intestine. Another explanation for autoinfection, especially in patients receiving steroid therapy, is that the larvae are stimulated by a metabolite produced by degradation of the steroid. This metabolite is antigenically similar to ecdysone or 20-hydroxyecdysone, the hormone that promotes molting (Genta, 1992). Neither explanation is supported experimentally or accounts for autoinfection in all cases. It is more likely that autoinfection is a normal biologic characteristic of the parasite, and that it occurs at low levels in all infections and is responsible for the longevity of *Strongyloides* infections (Gill, Bell, 1979; Gill et al. 1977). Thus, new females arrive in the duodenum in numbers just large enough to replace senescent ones, keeping the infection alive for many years. It is believed that in certain types of immune impairment, autoinfection results in *hyperinfection* or massive strongyloidiasis (opportunistic disease). In this case, more larvae complete the life cycle and, over a period of time, numerous parasites come to reside in the intestine. These parasites produce significant morbidity, which is fatal if untreated. Since in this situation host immunity is important in maintaining autoinfection at a manageable level, the immune response appears to modulate autoinfection. However, the view that immune impairment of the host is responsible for autoinfection has been challenged (Genta, 1992).

Biology. Since *S. stercoralis* is classified in the Rhabditida, it is by definition a free-living nematode with a parasitic phase. The parasitic phase starts when filariform larvae enter through the skin or mucosa of the mouth. In the skin, some larvae enter through the hair follicles and others through the bare epithelial cells about 15 minutes after contact, producing irritation, redness, and petechiae, depending on the number of larvae present. The larvae migrate from the entry site through the blood vessels, and some may reach the muscles (Ashford et al. 1978) or other organs, where they remain for several days. But eventually they reach the lungs, the obligatory route for passage into the intestine. This obligatory pulmonary passage has been proven several times, even in experiments in which infective larvae were introduced into the intestine in several places (Galliard, 1950). These experiments, and the classic experiments of Fuelleborn (1929) on the migration of *Strongyloides* larvae, are often ignored in modern reports dealing with the life cycle of the parasite. Yet, the classic view has been challenged based on experimental infections of dogs using radiolabeled larvae. It is now proposed that infective larvae entering the skin (or the intestine in autoinfection) migrate randomly to many other organs and reach the intestine without necessarily going through the lungs (Schad et al. 1989). This contrarian view is not supported by any of the many studies of patients dying of autoinfection, who usually have no parasites outside the intestinal tract or the respiratory tree (Haque et al. 1994). This view is even more remarkable when we consider that most of these studies used autopsy material and that larvae continue migrating after death, dispersing to many sites in the body. Only on a few occasions have biopsy specimens from patients infected with *Strongyloides* revealed larvae in the skin and in autopsy material from liver, brain, or other organs (see below).

A biologic feature of *S. stercoralis* rarely mentioned in the clinical literature is its capacity to mature to adulthood in the bronchial epithelium, where it produces eggs and larvae. Invasion of the bronchial mucosa by *Strongyloides* has been demonstrated histologically in animal models (Faust, 1935) and has been mentioned, without histologic confirmation, as occurring in humans (Craven et al. 1971; De Paola, 1962). It has also been reported to occur in the bronchial epithelium of autopsied patients, but there is no photographic documentation of this situation (Haque et al. 1994). The best proof available is the finding of eggs and rhabditoid larvae in the sputum of patients suffering from chronic bronchitis or asthmatic symptoms (Nwokolo, Imohiosen, 1973; Shiroma, 1964) and in a patient with a pulmonary abscess (Seabury et al. 1971) (Fig. 12–2 A–C).

The longevity of the parasitic females of *S. stercoralis* is not known. The longevity of the infection, at least in British (Gill, Bell, 1979, 1987; Gill et al. 1977), Australian (Grove, 1980), Canadian (Proctor et al. 1985), and American (Pelletier, 1984) World War II prisoners of the Japanese, has been found to be several decades. Transmission of *Strongyloides* and other nematodes by maternal milk has been documented in animals (Lyons et al. 1970); in humans one species,

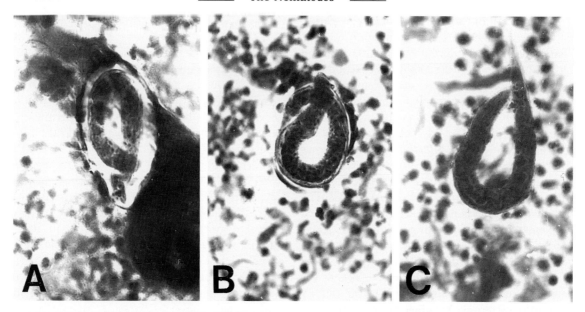

Fig. 12–2. *Strongyloides stercoralis*, eggs and larvae in sputum of individual with bronchial colonization by adult parasites, preparation stained with Papanicolaou stain. *A* and *B*, Eggs with developed larva. *C*, Recently hatched larva, all ×400. (Courtesy of P.C. Beaver, Ph.D., School of Tropical Medicine and Public Health, Tulane University, New Orleans, Louisiana.)

probably *S. fuelleborni*, has been found in the milk of lactating women (Brown, Girardeau, 1977). Circulating larvae explain the transmission of the parasite from a cadaver organ donor to two renal transplant recipients (Hoy et al. 1981). In addition, in a nonendemic area, eggs, larvae, and in one case adult worms were recovered from patients' stool samples, suggesting infections with animal species of *Strongyloides* (zoonotic) (Boram et al. 1981).

In spite of all the advances in elucidating the biology of *Strongyloides*, many questions remain. For example, what is the fate of the male worms during the parasitic cycle? How does *Strongyloides* produce disease in humans? What is the exact mode of transmission (in spite of the accepted notion that it is solely through the skin)? What stimulates the transformation from rhabditiform to filariform larvae in the intestine of some individuals? What determines the proportion of larvae maturing to infective stages and reaching the lungs under normal conditions and in autoinfection? And, above all, do one or several species of *Strongyloides* infect humans, some of which may be zoonotic? Answers to any of these questions would provide information relevant to human strongyloidiasis. Recent studies of strains isolated from humans and animals with the polymerase chain reaction hold promise for the identification of the species (Ramachandran et al. 1997).

Epidemiology. The prevalence of strongyloidiasis is not known; estimates vary from 3 to 30 million (Genta, 1989) to no less than 100 million (Jorgensen et al. 1996) infected individuals worldwide (Genta, 1989), usually in rural communities. The disease is more prevalent in developing countries of the tropical zone, but its geographic distribution also includes parts of the temperate zone. In general, the epidemiology of strongyloidiasis parallels that of hookworm infection. However, in some areas where *Strongyloides* is present, hookworms are few or absent, and vice versa. Several surveys of strongyloidiasis have been carried in many places, showing prevalence rates that vary from less than 1% to 80%, with the highest rates found in tropical countries; it is likely than in most places the prevalence is less than 20% (Faust, Giraldo, 1960). In institutions for the mentally retarded there are clusters of strongyloidiasis cases (Braun et al. 1988; Huminer et al. 1992; Proctor et al. 1987).

In the United States, several surveys of schoolchildren have revealed prevalences of 4.0% in Harlan County, Kentucky (Fulmer, Huempfner, 1965), 0.9% in Williamson County, Tennessee (Quinn, 1971), and 0.3% in Clay County, Kentucky (Walzer et al. 1982). Among patients of Charity Hospital in New Orleans, the prevalence was 0.4% (Hubbard et al. 1974). At King's County Hospital in New York City the prevalence was 1.0% (Eveland et al. 1975), and at the University of Kentucky Medical Center it was 2.5% (Walzer et al. 1982). The patients at the Veterans Medical Center at Mountain Hope, Tennessee, had a rate of 3.0% (Reddy et al. 1983), and those at the Johnson City Veterans Hospital in eastern Tennessee had a rate of 4.0% (Berk et al. 1987). It is evident that foci of active *Strongyloides* transmission exist in the area where the four corners of Kentucky, Tennessee, Virginia, and North Carolina meet (Berk et al. 1987), as well as in other regions of the southern United States. Humans are the most important natural host of *S. stercoralis*, although infections occur naturally in dogs (Georgi, Sprinkle, 1974). Higher percentages of infection than expected in the male gay population have been reported (Phillips et al. 1981). Transmission from an infected gay man to two of his partners in Los Angeles suggests that sexual transmission must occur (Sorvillo et al. 1983).

Strongyloidiasis is reported from time to time as a locally acquired infection in many countries. Examples include Switzerland (Berthoud, Berthoud, 1975); Romania, where foci of endemicity revealed up to 7% positivity in the populations tested (Dancesco, 1968); France (Doury, 1993); Spain and Italy (Junod, 1987b); northern Italy (Scaglia et al. 1984); and England (Sprott et al. 1987), countries that are not generally consider endemic. The bulk of the cases seen in Europe occur in immigrants from tropical countries and in travelers to endemic areas.

Pathogenesis. *Strongyloides* is a pathogen with low to medium virulence in the immune-competent population, especially judging by the number of asymptomatic infections in endemic areas. In some hosts, the great majority of whom receive steroids, the infection becomes opportunistic. It is also opportunistic in persons suffering from adult T-cell leukemia produced by the human T-lymphocyte leukemia virus (HTLV-1), in whom the infection is difficult to treat (see below). The mechanism by which *Strongyloides* produces disease in humans and experimental animals is not known. In hyperinfection, large numbers of larvae in the lungs cause alveolar hemorrhage due to damage of the alveolar wall when larvae pass from the capillaries into the respiratory tree. At the beginning of the infection, hypereosinophilia is common due to migration of larvae through the tissues, a feature also common with hyperinfection for the same reason. Symptoms of allergy and high levels of immunoglobulin E (IgE) commonly occur in infected patients with manifestations of asthma, wheezing, bouts of coughing, and skin allergies. Sometimes these symptoms last for long periods (decades) as the sole manifestation of the infection.

Immunity. The immunity to *Strongyloides* infections in humans has not been well studied. Most knowledge has been gained from animal models, mainly rats infected with *S. ratti*. The persistence of the infection in humans for many years (see above) indicates that the immune system of the host is not effective on three fronts: (*1*) inability to eliminate adult worms from the gut; (*2*) inability to prevent reinfection by larvae maturing in the intestine; and (*3*) inability to destroy the larvae once they reenter the intestinal mucosa (Neva, 1986). In the rat, infections produced by large numbers of larvae resulted in spontaneous expulsion of the adult worms from the gut about 3 weeks after infection. This effect was associated with an increase in the mast cell population of the gut. The mastositosis and the self-cure can be reversed with steroid therapy (Olson, Schiller, 1978a, 1978b). Other experimental data show a relationship between larval antigens and the development of humoral and cellular responses to the infection that result in expulsion of the worms from the intestine (Genta et al. 1983a). Since rats do not develop hyperinfection, they are not a good model for studying other aspects of the immune response (Neva, 1986).

Other animals used to study strongyloidiasis are the dog and the monkey (*Erythrocebus patas*). In the monkey, low-level autoinfection occurs during the infection. If steroids are administered, monkeys develop hyperinfection similar to that of humans. In the monkey, immunity to reinfection is demonstrated when the animals are cured of their primary infection and are reexposed later to infective larvae (Neva, 1986). Monkeys were used to study the role of mast cells in the intestine. The results were similar to those in rats, in which infection and challenge to the infection are always associated with an increase in the mast cell population of the intestine. The mast cells release histamine in response to the parasite's antigens, but they lost the capacity to respond when the animals receive steroids, resulting in hyperinfection. Prolonged steroid therapy of infected monkeys eventually results in death. One monkey that developed hyperinfection spontaneously had a mast cell population that did not respond to the parasite's antigens (Barrett et al. 1988). These observations have been applied to humans in the form of a test for diagnosis: mast cells from the patient degranulate when antigens extracted from larvae are added (Deluol et al. 1984). The test is highly specific because tests of patients infected with other intestinal nematodes are always negative.

Information on immunity to strongyloidiasis in humans is limited, and the assumption that hyperinfection is based on an alteration of the host's cellular immunity has not been fully explored. The belief that altered cellular immunity does *not* play a role in hyperinfection is confirmed indirectly by the rarity of opportunistic strongyloidiasis in patients with acquired immune deficiency syndrome (AIDS). Moreover, in patients with uncomplicated strongyloidiasis, there is little or no cellular response in vitro to larval antigens, suggesting that factors other than cellular immunity are responsible for protection against the disease (Genta et al. 1983b).

Regarding the humoral response, it is known that individuals with strongyloidiasis have specific antibodies to larval antigens. The total amount of such antibodies is higher in patients with uncomplicated strongyloidiasis than in those with hyperinfection (Genta et al. 1983c). The same is true of IgG4 and IgG2; the IgG4 fraction reacted with antigens of the parasite more than any of the other immunoglobulins (Genta, Lillibridge, 1989). In addition, IgE and IgA are elevated in infected individuals (Genta, Weil, 1982; Grove et al. 1986; McRury et al. 1986). However, the presence or absence of antibodies does not correlate with the presence or absence of hyperinfection (Genta, Lillibridge, 1989).

Clinical Findings. The symptoms and signs of strongyloidiasis vary, depending on the immune status of the host. The presence of rhabditoid larvae in the feces of asymptomatic individuals living in endemic areas is a common finding. A 2-year longitudinal follow-up of a rural population in Colombia with a prevalence of approximately 30% did not show a single case of overt symptoms during the observation period (Little, Gutierrez, 1968).

Immune-Competent Hosts. The prepatent period of *Strongyloides* varies from 3 days (Sandground, 1926) to 27 days (Tanaka, 1966) after exposure to larvae in human experimental infections. Local reaction to the larvae in some individuals is immediate, lasting for 21 days as a skin eruption. The passage of larvae through the lungs manifests 6 to 9 days after infection with coughing and tracheal irritation. The intestinal symptoms, consisting of epigastric pain, bouts of diarrhea, and constipation, begin 18 days after exposure (Tanaka, 1966). In clinical observations of patients with *S. stercoralis*, some individuals present with epigastric pain simulating peptic ulcer (Brasitus et al. 1980), or with epigastric pain and diarrhea, often accompanied by nausea and vomiting, and on occasion with massive upper gastrointestinal bleeding (Bhatt et al. 1990; Brasitus et al. 1980). Other patients have chronic mild diarrhea with duodenitis that is sometimes

visible on radiographs of the duodenum (Brasitus et al. 1980), and bloody stools 1 month after exposure to larvae may persist for several weeks (Tanaka, 1966). Other abnormalities seen on radiographs are nodular defects, thickening or effacement of the mucosal folds, and narrowing of the lumen with rigidity of the viscus (Arantes Pereira et al. 1960; Berkmen, Rabinowitz, 1972). If the symptoms persist, weight loss and signs of malabsorption may develop (Alcorn, Kotcher, 1961), but no malabsorption is produced by the parasite per se; instead, malabsorption is due to a concomitant protein malnutrition (Garcia et al. 1977). The epigastric pain of strongyloidiasis in the adult has been described as a sharply localized burning sensation or a deep, dull, aching pain sometimes radiating to other parts of the abdomen and becoming more intense after a meal (Jones, 1950). The combination of diarrhea and symptoms of gastric ulcer in the adult suggests strongyloidiasis (Coulaud et al. 1980; Tham, 1979). In one patient the infection in the lower stomach was associated with a bleeding ulcer (Dees et al. 1990). Some patients present with a gastric outlet obstruction (Adetiloye, 1992) or duodenal obstruction simulating a malignancy (Schanaider, Madi, 1996). Others present with stenosis of the distal common bile duct, enlargement of the head of the pancreas, and jaundice (Pijls et al. 1986) or with stenosis of the sphincter and jaundice (Delarocque et al. 1994). Subacute intestinal obstruction (Al-Bahrani ZR et al. 1995) and ileus (Bannon et al. 1995) are the presenting symptoms in other patients. In the intestinal mucosa in various patients, endoscopic findings include inflammation, edema, bleeding, ulcerations, and small, raised nodular lesions (Choudhry et al. 1995). A study of 56 patients in the United States showed similar clinical findings in adults. It was estimated that between 2% and 3% of these patients had hyperinfection.

The peripheral eosinophilia varies throughout the course of the infection. It may be high at the beginning, during larval migration, but may drop to normal when the parasites are established in the intestine in asymptomatic individuals. In symptomatic patients from nonendemic areas, peripheral eosinophilia is on average 16%, with the highest rate being 77%. In symptomatic patients living in endemic areas it is less than 10%, with the highest rate being 50% (Junod, 1987a). Allergic skin manifestations are common in some patients, sometimes lasting for decades if strongyloidiasis is not diagnosed and treated. The combination of diarrhea or gastrointestinal symptoms and skin eruptions is a clue to the infection (Leighton, MacSween, 1990). Other cutaneous lesions are petechiae and purpura (see below). Cutaneous larva migrans due to maturation of larvae on the perianal folds and their entry into the skin produces *larva currens* (see Chapter 14). The skin symptoms and signs may be the first manifestation of the infection (Amer et al. 1984; Brumpt, Sang, 1973) and sometimes the only manifestation (Pelletier, Gabre Kidan, 1985). In other cases, cough, wheezing, or chronic asthma, often lasting for many years, may be the only symptoms of the disease. The asthma seen in some cases often manifests soon after the patient is placed on steroid therapy for other conditions (Dunlap et al. 1984). However, sometimes it occurs together with other signs and symptoms of hyperinfection (Strazzella, Safirstein, 1989). In these cases, rhabditoid larvae usually are present in the stools or in duodenal aspirates (Fig. 12–12).

Immune-Compromised Hosts. The forms of immune impairment that predispose to hyperinfection are varied. Malignancies, especially certain lymphomas (Pagliuca et al. 1988) and leukemias, prolonged steroid therapy, and radiation therapy and chemotherapy for malignancies are common causes. Other causes are immune-suppressive therapy in organ transplant patients (Morgan et al. 1986), malnutrition, chronic infections, and probably senescence. In areas endemic for strongyloidiasis, the disease is strongly prevalent in patients with hematologic malignancies (Nucci et al. 1995). In many immune-compromised patients, the symptoms of strongyloidiasis are often masked by preexisting medical problems; thus, the clinical diagnosis is often not made. The main biologic features of the infection in these hosts are the large number of parasites in the gastrointestinal tract and the large number of larvae migrating through the lungs. The symptoms are related to the intestine, the lungs, and other organs. Epigastric pain, profuse diarrhea, weight loss, nausea, and vomiting, sometimes alternating with periods of constipation, are common. Pulmonary symptoms are productive cough, respiratory failure in advanced cases (Venizelos et al. 1980), or asthma alone (Dunlap et al. 1984) and areas of pneumonic consolidation on chest radiographs (Berger et al. 1980). In one case, pulmonary abscesses were attributed to *Strongyloides* without convincing evidence (Ford et al. 1981); it is unlikely that the parasite produced such lesions. Continuous migration of infective larvae through the lungs results in respiratory failure (Mejia et al. 1992), and if the patient is not treated, the disease is fatal. However, larval migration through the lungs never produces restrictive pulmonary disease, as some investigators claim (Lin et al. 1995). Peripheral eosinophilia in hyperinfection is often absent (Berger et al. 1980; Purtilo et al. 1974), especially in patients with prolonged cortico-steroid therapy or bone marrow suppression; sometimes the eosinophilia is masked by the high white blood cell count in leukemic patients. Intercurrent bacterial, fungal, and other infections are often found at autopsy.

In recent years, a number of patients with advanced hyperinfection have rapidly developed (in less than 12 hours) a rash, usually periumbilical, extending to other parts of the abdomen, the chest, and sometimes the legs. The rash has been described as petechial hemorrhages (Yim et al. 1984), nonpalpable purpuric eruption (Kalb, Grossman, 1984), petechial rash (von Kuster, Genta, 1984), periumbilical purpura (Ronan et al. 1984), resembling multiple purpuric thumbprints (Bank et al. 1984), ecchymotic eruption or progressive petechial purpuric eruption (Purvis et al. 1984), reticular nonblanching, nonpalpable petechial-to-purpuric rash (Simpson et al. 1984), and diffuse erythematous, nonpruritic petechial eruption (Gordon et al. 1994). In most of these patients, skin biopsy specimens revealed numerous *Strongyloides* larvae within the interstitium, sometimes in the capillaries (Fig. 12–3 *A–B*). In some patients, the larvae elicited a granuloma formation (Gordon et al. 1994); in others, there was a perivascular lymphocytic infiltrate and numerous eosinophils with dilation, congestion, and microscopic hemorrhages of the capillary bed. The larvae presumably arrived at the skin via the circulation, but the reason for the peculiar distribution in the periumbilical area remains obscure.

Strongyloidiasis in AIDS Patients. At the beginning of the AIDS epidemic, disseminated strongyloidiasis was thought to be an important coinfection, but in 1987 it was removed from the list of AIDS-defining illnesses by the Centers for Disease Control and Prevention. About two dozen reports of patients with AIDS and strongyloidiasis have been published. This is a minuscule number if one considers the high prevalence of human immune deficiency virus (HIV) and *Strongyloides* infections in the general populations of some African and Latin American countries (Moura et al. 1989), which would suggest a large number of cases of opportunistic strongyloidiasis. Moreover, studies of patients with AIDS enteropathy in Africa have revealed cases of asymptomatic strongyloidiasis (Conlon et al. 1990). Since AIDS does not promote opportunistic strongyloidiasis (Colebunders et al. 1988; Lucas, 1990), it is obvious that the depletion of $CD4^+$ T lymphocytes plays no role in the disease. Disseminated strongyloidiasis in patients with AIDS must occur in a subset of individuals with other conditions (Gompels et al. 1991), such as steroid therapy for lymphoma (Dutcher

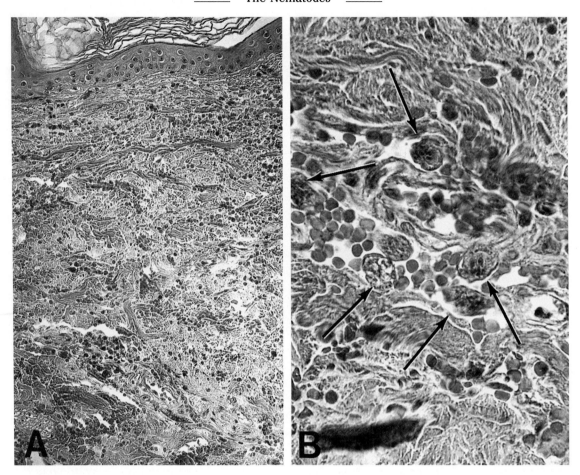

Fig. 12–3. *Strongyloides stercoralis* **larvae in periumbilical purpura. Sections stained with hematoxylin and eosin.** *A,* **Low-power view showing the hemorrhagic** area, ×180. *B,* **higher magnification illustrating the larvae (cross sections) within the extravasated blood (arrows), ×700.**

et al. 1990), marked weight loss (Harcourt Webster et al. 1991), and other intercurrent infections (Jain et al. 1994; Maayan et al. 1987).

Strongyloidiasis in HTLV-1 Infections. The human T-lymphocyte virus type 1 is a retrovirus that causes adult T-cell leukemia, especially in the southwestern islands of Japan, Taiwan, the Caribbean region, and some parts of Africa. In the mid-1980s, a study of carriers of *S. stercoralis* in Japan revealed that these individuals were two to three times more likely to have antibodies for HTLV-1 (Nakada et al. 1984b). A large recent survey in Okinawa, Japan, produced similar findings (Hayashi et al. 1997). There are also reports of individual cases (Newton et al. 1984; Patey et al. 1984; Phelps et al. 1984) and clusters of cases (Dixon et al. 1984; Plumelle et al. 1984) of *Strongyloides* hyperinfection in patients with adult T-cell leukemia in which the parasite behaved more aggressively, was dif-

ficult to treat, and recurred over several years. In another study, patients with HTLV-1 infection and *Strongyloides* were found to excrete more larvae in their stools (Robinson et al. 1984).

In spite of these data, other investigators were unable to confirm these findings with studies done in the same area (Arakaki et al. 1984a, 1984b) and in Jamaica (Neva et al. 1984). It appears, then, that these two infections coexist in some patients and that in some of them, *Strongyloides* is more aggressive. Whether the HTLV-1 infection predisposes to hyperinfection by *Strongyloides* or whether both infections are cofactors that lead to the development of the T-cell leukemia has not been determined (Nakada et al. 1984a; Patey et al. 1984). Immunologic studies in one patient carrier of HTLV-1 with *Strongyloides* hyperinfection followed for several years revealed a decrease in *Strongyloides*-specific IgG until it became undetectable despite the presence of the parasite. Treatment cleared the infec-

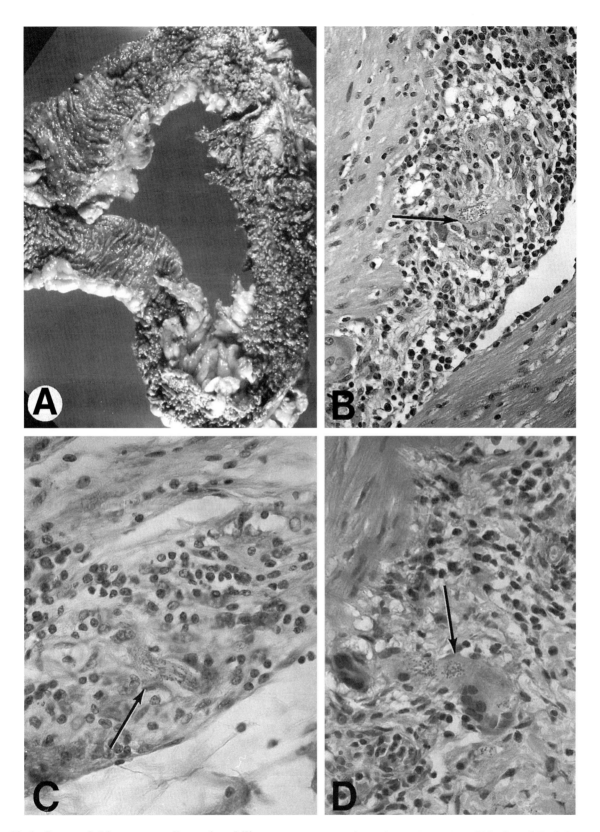

Fig. 12–4. *Strongyloides stercoralis*, eosinophilic granulomatous enterocolitis. *A*, Gross lesions in resected colon of a patient diagnosed as having ulcerative colitis. *B–D*, Histologic preparations stained with hematoxylin and eosin stain. *B*, Granuloma within the peritoneal lining consisting of histiocytes engulfing and destroying a larva (arrow), ×280. *C* and *D*, Other granulomas with larvae being destroyed within giant cells (arrows), ×450. (Reported by: Gutierrez, Y., Bhatia, P., Garbadawala, S.T., et al. 1996. *Strongyloides stercoralis* eosinophilic granulomatous enterocolitis. Am. J. Surg. Pathol. 20:603–612.)

tion, but the worms reappeared as soon as it was stopped; IgE was also undetected, and immediate skin hypersensitivity to specific *Strongyloides* antigens was negative (Newton et al. 1984). The relation between decreased IgE and *Strongyloides* exacerbation in patients with HTLV-1 was also suggested by other workers (Robinson et al. 1984) and confirmed by still others (Newton et al. 1992). Studies of patients with adult T-cell leukemia, with or without *Strongyloides* and high eosinophilia, showed that the *Strongyloides* group survived longer, that hypereosinophilia without *Strongyloides* infection has no influence on the evolution of the leukemia, and that patients with *Strongyloides* without eosinophilia do even better (Plumelle et al. 1984, 1997).

Eosinophilic Granulomatous Enterocolitis. A type of colitis was observed in a series of elderly patients, most of who were receiving steroid therapy. In addition, some of these patients were suffering from a disease clinically characterized as ulcerative colitis in some or as Crohn's disease in others. Some patients underwent resection of the colon, or segments of colon, or of small intestine (Fig. 12–4 *A*). Some patients died at the beginning of their intestinal illness from other unrelated causes; others died of their disease; and some, diagnosed on the basis of pathology specimens as suffering from strongyloidiasis, were treated and recovered. Study of the surgical specimens and biopsy specimens revealed that all patients were suffering from *Strongyloides* eosinophilic granulomatous enterocolitis, which manifested clinically as one of the diseases mentioned above. In all specimens from these patients, *Strongyloides* larvae were found in the intestinal wall, producing a granulomatous inflammation (*color plate* VI *G–H*). The larvae in the granulomas were in different stages of disintegration (Fig. 12–4 *B–D*) and were found within an intense infiltration of the wall by eosinophils. The granulomas varied from poorly to well formed, with giant cells, and were located in all layers of the viscus, some on the peritoneal surface and the adjacent fatty tissue

(Fig. 12–4 *C–D*). The histologic picture was consistent with strong hypersensitivity to the parasite, with massive tissue eosinophilia and granulomatous inflammation of the invading larvae (*color plate* VI *I–J*). The eosinophils were degranulating in large numbers, which led to the conclusion that the ulcerative lesions in the intestinal wall were probably due to tissue lysis by the major basic protein released by the eosinophils (Gutierrez et al. 1996).

Hepatitis. In cases of hyperinfection studied at autopsy, the presence of larvae in the liver has been mentioned sporadically (Hartz, 1946, 1954). In at least one report, the finding in four children was reported as visceral larva migrans rather than hyperinfection (Buitrago, Gast-Galvis, 1965a, 1965b). A few reports provided a more detailed description of this finding as a granulomatous hepatitis seen in children and adults suffering from hyperinfection (Lopez et al. 1984; Poltera, 1974; Poltera, Katsimbura, 1974). The larvae are found in branches of the portal vein and in the portal spaces, sometimes without eliciting an inflammatory response. In other cases, the larvae are found among infiltrating cells and some times in granulomas. The larvae in blood vessels or lymphatics appear to be viable; those within inflammatory cells and especially within granulomas are disintegrating, particularly if eosinophils are present (Fig. 12–9 *A–B*).

Pathology

Immune-Competent Hosts. The gross and microscopic changes in strongyloidiasis in immunologically intact hosts range from minimal to marked, depending on the severity of the disease (Coutinho et al. 1996). In patients with mild symptoms, the duodenal mucosa is grossly normal or slightly edematous. Microscopically, only the presence of parasites calls attention to the infection (Fig. 12–5 *A–B*). The female parasites are located deep in the crypts (Fig. 12–5 *A* and *C*), surrounded by groups of eggs in different stages of matu-

---

Fig. 12–5. *Strongyloides stercoralis* in a duodenal biopsy specimen of an adult with symptoms of peptic ulcer, sections stained with hematoxylin and eosin stain. *A,* Low magnification showing the location of the female parasite deep in the crypts (short arrow) and developing larvae (long arrow), ×140. *B,* Another area of the mucosa with several developing larvae within the eggs, ×140. *C* and *D,* Higher magnification illustrating four cross sections of a female within the crypt (*C*). Note the delicate cuticle and weak muscle layer (short arrows). The internal organs seen in cross section are the intestine (long arrow), the uterus and ovary. (Note that in *Strongyloides* one set of ovary and uterus extends anteriorly from the vulva and the other set extends posteriorly.) On cross section the uterus is a single tube; the ovary is convoluted and appears as single or double (open arrow, bottom). Developing larvae within the eggs are shown in *D.* Note the lack of an inflammatory infiltrate, ×450. (Courtesy of R. Lash, M.D., Department of Pathology, The Cleveland Clinic Foundation, Cleveland, Ohio.)

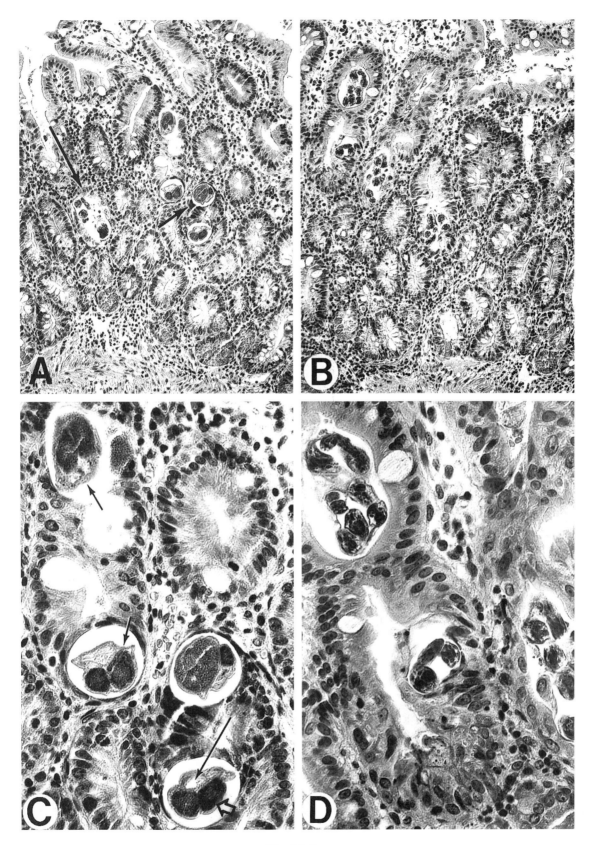

Fig. 12–5.

ration and by larvae in the interstitium (Fig. 12–5 A–D; Stemmermann, 1967). The mucosal architecture is normal, with little or no cellular infiltration (Fig. 12–5 C–D). The infiltration consists of mononuclear cells and rare polymorphonuclear leukocytes, some of which are eosinophils. In patients with severe clinical disease the mucosa is flattened, with loss of villi and marked infiltration by lymphocytes. The most striking changes are those observed with cytochemical staining of the intestinal mucosa, changes that increase progressively from minimal to severe disease. The infiltrating plasma cells stain with IgA stain. They are found in the epithelium, the lamina propria, and the crypts of the secretory unit of Brunner's gland. A secretory component is seen in the plasma cells but not in the epithelial cells. In contrast, human lymphocyte antigen-DR (HLA-DR) positivity of the epithelial cell lining decreases progressively with the severity of the disease, following a pattern opposite to that of the secretory component (Coutinho et al. 1996).

Immune-Compromised Hosts. Hyperinfection or massive strongyloidiasis involves histologic changes in several organ systems. These changes have been studied in experimental animals (Faust, Kagy, 1933; Harper et al. 1984) and in humans (Hartz, 1954; Purtilo et al. 1974).

Gastrointestinal tract. The gross appearance of the small intestine is sometimes unremarkable; in other cases, signs of duodenitis are seen, with edema of the mucosal folds.. The main microscopic finding is a large number of parasites in the pyloric region of the stomach (Imasato et al. 1968; Tham, 1979; Wurtz et al. 1994), duodenum, and upper jejunum (Fig. 12–6 A–C). Necrosis, ulceration, or hemorrhage is usually not associated with the parasites. The inflammatory infiltrate varies with the host's bone marrow status and often consists of mononuclear and polymorphonuclear cells. In autopsy specimens, larvae are often observed in the lymphatics of the submucosa, the muscularis, and other sites due to postmortem migration (Fig. 12–6 D). The colon has ulcerations varying from 2 to 20 mm in diameter, hyperemic erosions of the cecum, and deep ulcerations (Hartz, 1954; Purtilo et al. 1974). The cecum may be slightly thickened because of edema, usually with ulcerations and numerous filariform larvae in all layers (Fig. 12–7 A–D; Hartz, 1954; Purtilo et al. 1974).

Lungs. The gross changes of the lungs are a combined weight of over 1000 g, uniform consolidation of all lobes, hemorrhagic cut surfaces, and bronchi filled with inspissated mucus. The microscopic changes are hemorrhage and a variable inflammatory reaction, depending on the underlying disease and other intercur-

rent infections (Fig. 12–8 A–B). The main feature is the presence of *Strongyloides* larvae in the tissues, the alveolar spaces, and the bronchi. Often the parasites are found within mucous plugs in the respiratory tree (Fig. 12–8 C–D).

Brain. The number of reported cases of brain involvement by *Strongyloides* is less than 10 (Morgello et al. 1993). In most of these cases the diagnosis was circumstantial, based on clinical grounds, with no support from tissues to confirm the clinical impression (Meltzer et al. 1979; Schindzielorz et al. 1991; Vishwanath et al. 1982). Some patients presented with other infections of the central nervous system; others showed larvae in the spinal fluid, and the disease was considered strongyloidiasis of the brain (Belani et al. 1987). In one patient studied clinically, a cerebral vasculitis-like syndrome was attributed to *Strongyloides*, also based on circumstantial evidence (Wachter et al. 1984). Two documented cases occurred in patients with AIDS (Morgello et al. 1993).

In those cases in which the brain was available for study, the gross changes were unremarkable, in one instance consisting of petechial hemorrhages, edema, and focal necrosis (Neefe et al. 1973). Microscopically, larvae may be seen in brain tissue with no surrounding inflammation (Fig. 12–9 C–D); less often, they are found in microscopic areas of necrosis, apparently produced by blockage of blood vessels. Other larvae are seen degenerating in an inflammatory reaction consisting of mononuclear and polymorphonuclear cells resembling granulomas (Neefe et al. 1973) or in granulomas (Morgello et al. 1993). In one case, a brain abscess was attributed to *Strongyloides* infection based on the presence of larvae. However, since *Candida*, a well-known invader of blood vessels resulting in infarcts and abscesses, also present, it is likely that *Strongyloides* was an innocent bystander, not the cause of the abscess (Masdeu et al. 1982).

Other Organs. *Strongyloides* larvae have been found in every other organ system and tissue, usually as viable organisms, with no surrounding inflammatory reaction, a finding best explained by postmortem migration of the parasites. Only on one occasion were they found in the heart, lungs, lymph nodes, esophagus, stomach, small and large intestines, pancreas, skeletal muscles, and thoracic and abdominal vascular adventitia within granulomas in all stages of formation (Morgello et al. 1993).

Diagnosis. *Strongyloides* is diagnosed in the clinical laboratory by finding rhabditoid larvae in fecal specimens (Fig. 12–10 A–C). The larvae must be distin-

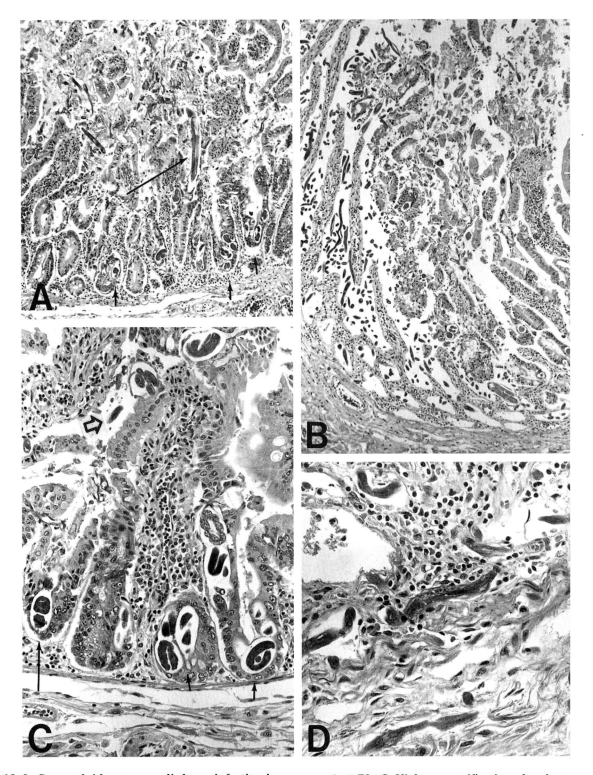

Fig. 12–6. *Strongyloides stercoralis* hyperinfection in a patient with lymphocytic leukemia, sections stained with hematoxylin and eosin stain. *A* and *B*, Low-power magnification showing a large number of parasites, mostly larval stages; one female is seen in *A* (long arrow), as are several developing eggs deep in the crypts (small arrows), ×70. *C*, Higher magnification showing recently laid eggs (long arrows), developing larvae (small arrows), and larvae on their way to the lumen (open arrow), ×180. *D*, Larvae deep in the lamina propria and submucosa representing postmortem migration. The infiltrating cells correspond to leukemic cells, ×280.

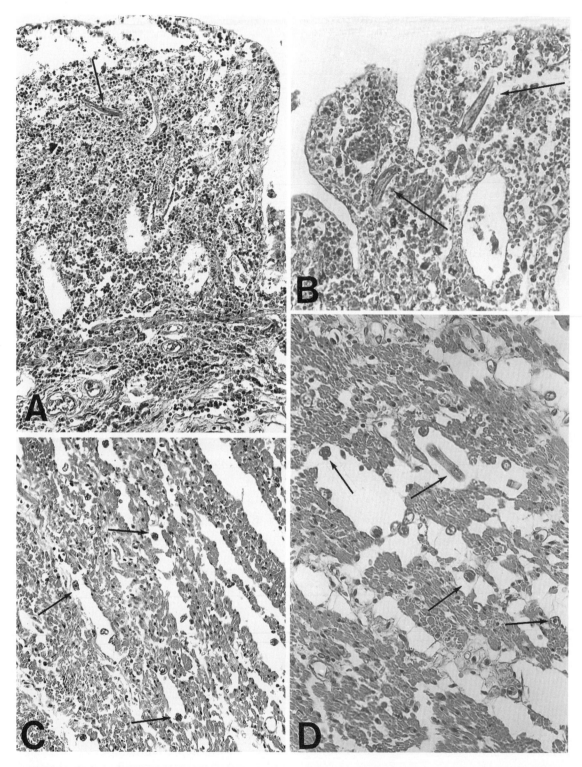

Fig. 12–7. *Strongyloides stercoralis* in the colonic wall, hyperinfection in the same patient in Figure 12–6, sections stained with hematoxylin and eosin stain. *A* and *C*, Low-power magnification showing superficial ulceration of the mucosa with a larva (*A*) and muscle layer with numerous filariform larvae (*C*) (arrows) on their way to the lung, ×180. *B* and *D*, Higher magnification showing the parasites (arrows), ×480.

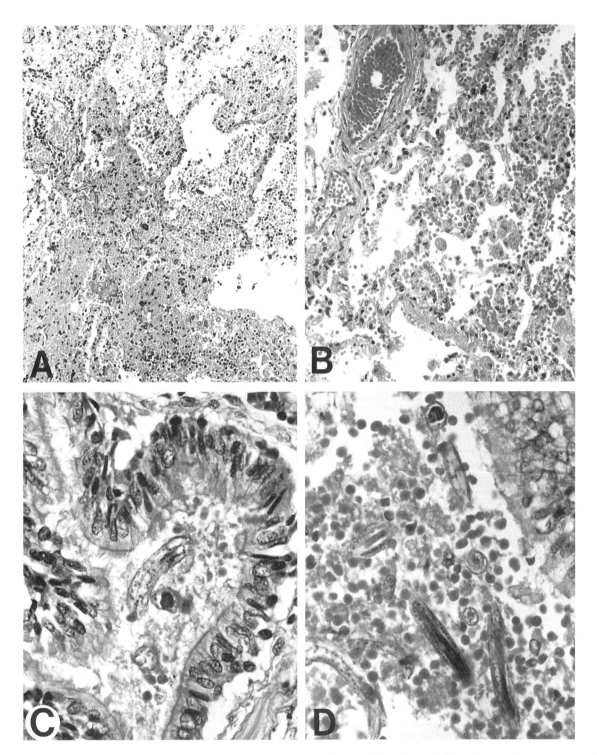

Fig. 12–8. *Strongyloides stercoralis* in lung, hyperinfection in the same patient in Figure 12–6, sections stained with hematoxylin and eosin stain. *A*, Low magnification showing hemorrhage of lung, ×140. *B*, Detail showing intact septa, macrophages, and alveolar hemorrhage. The few infiltrating cells correspond to leukemic cells, ×220. *C* and *D*, Higher magnification of smaller bronchi with cross and oblique section of *S. stercoralis* larvae, ×550.

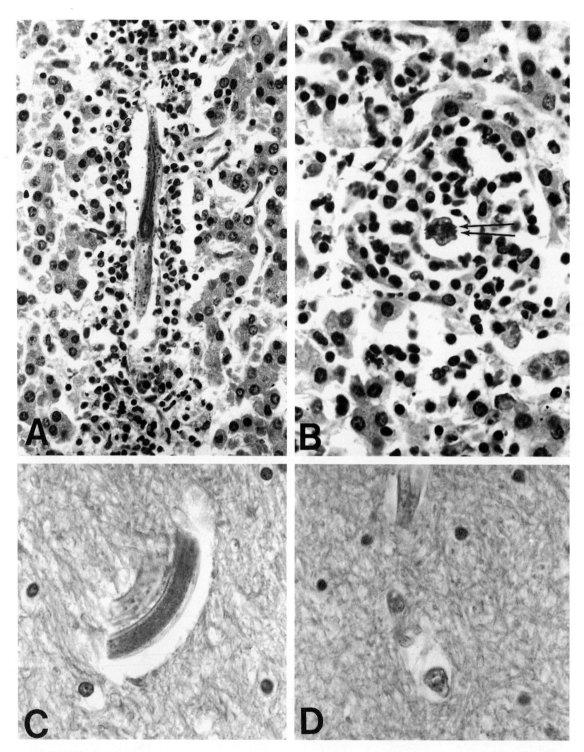

Fig. 12–9. *Strongyloides stercoralis* in various organs, sections stained with hematoxylin and eosin stain. *A* and *B*. Larvae in liver within a poorly formed granuloma. *A*, Longitudinal section showing the esophagus and the intestine, ×450. *B*, Cross section showing two minute lateral alae on each side (arrows). Note the infiltrate, composed mostly of mononuclear cells, ×705. (Preparation courtesy of B. Buitrago, M.D., Instituto Nacional de Salud, Bogota, Colombia. Reported by: Buitrago, B., and Gast-Galvis, A. 1965. Sindrome larva migrans visceral (granulomatosis larvaria) en Colombia. Rev. Soc. Colomb. Pediatr. Pueric. 6:89–95.) *C* and *D, S. stercoralis* in brain, sections stained with hematoxylin and eosin stain. Oblique and cross sections of larvae within brain tissue of patient with hyperinfection, ×705. (Preparation courtesy of H.J. Manz, M.D., Department of Pathology, Georgetown University Medical Center, Washington, D.C. Reported by: Neefe, L.I., Pinilla, O., Garagusi, V.F., et al. 1973. Disseminated strongyloidiasis with cerebral involvement. A complication of corticosteroid therapy. Am. J. Med. 55:832–838.)

guished from rhabditoid larvae of hookworms that sometimes develop in stool samples at room temperature (Fig. 12–11). Duodenal aspirates are rarely needed when stool samples are negative. In duodenal aspirates, all stages of the parasite are found: females, eggs, and larvae in different stages of development (Fig. 12–12).

Stool Samples. The direct fecal smear, either unstained or stained with iodine, and similar preparations of concentrated stools are good basic tools. Concentration by the Baermann technique and the Harada Mori fecal culture (Beaver et al. 1984) also produce good results when larvae are not recovered with standard methods. Direct fecal smears revealed 73% of 122 cases of strongyloidiasis (Milder et al. 1981) and 60% of 1350 cases in another study (Sato et al. 1995). The Baermann concentration has been found to be 3.6 times more efficient than the direct smear (de Kaminsky, 1993).

Agar Plate Culture. The newest method for detection of larvae in feces is the *bacterial colony displacement* or *agar plate culture* technique. The basis for this technique was the observation that sputum plated in agar plates for bacteriologic studies show a peculiar displacement of the colonies, visible with the naked eye, produced by larvae of *Strongyloides* (Panosian et al. 1986). This observation led to the use of this method for detection of larvae in feces (Koga et al. 1990, 1991). The advantage of this method is that 2 g of stool is easily examined. One disadvantage is that other nematodes (hookworm, *Trichostrongylus*, *Oesophagostomum*, *Ternidens*, free-living nematodes, and others) that occur as eggs in the stools will have time to incubate and

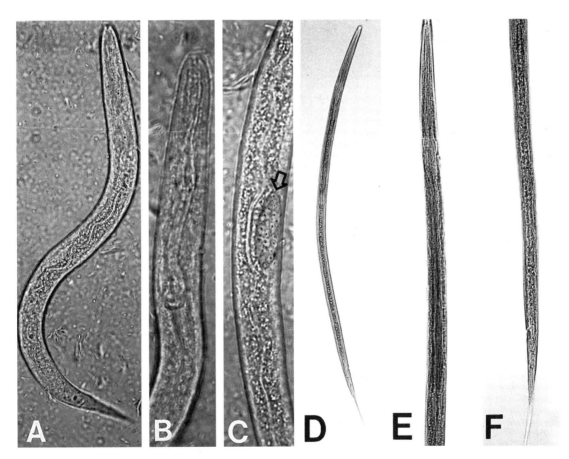

Fig. 12–10. *Strongyloides stercoralis*, **rhabditoid and filariform larvae.** *A–C.* **Rhabditoid larvae in stools.** *A,* **Larva showing relative esophageal and intestinal length,** ×450. *B,* **Anterior portion illustrating the rhabditoid esophagus. Note the length of the buccal cavity, which** is shorter than the diameter of the worm at this level, ×705. *C,* **The genital primordium (arrow),** ×705. *D–F,* **Filariform larva.** *D,* **Larva illustrating the general shape and body proportions,** ×180. *E,* **Anterior portion showing filariform esophagus,** ×350. *F,* **Posterior end,** ×350.

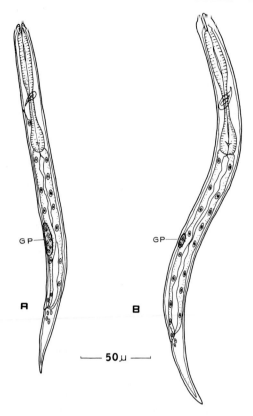

Fig. 12–11. *Strongyloides stercoralis*, line drawing of first-stage larvae (*A*) and hookworm larva (*B*) in human stools. Note the size of both the buccal cavity and the genital primordium (GP), which are necessary for their diagnosis. (In: Smith, J.W., and Gutierrez, Y. 1984. Medical parasitology. In: Henry, J.B. (ed.), *Clinical Diagnosis and Management by Laboratory Methods*, 18th ed. Philadelphia: W.B. Saunders, p. 1193. Reproduced with permission.)

hatch, producing larvae that must be differentiated from *Strongyloides*. Nevertheless, the agar plate culture method is superior to all others (de Kaminsky, 1993; Koga et al. 1990; Sato et al. 1995; Sukhavat et al. 1994).

The diagnosis of hyperinfection in the clinical laboratory is based on the *recovery of filariform larvae* from stools and their examination under the microscope immediately after collection (Fig. 12–10 D–F); (Eveland et al. 1975). Immediate examination is more important for stool samples because rhabditoid larvae may transform into filariform larvae in feces at room temperature within a few hours (Fig. 12–11). The presence of *Strongyloides* larvae in other fluids and eggs (see above) in the sputum is also diagnostic of hyperinfection.

Other Fluids. Duodenal aspirate is the fluid most commonly used for diagnosis of strongyloidiasis, especially when the stools of immune-competent hosts are negative. In patients with hyperinfection, duodenal aspirates usually yield a large number of organisms (Fig. 12–12 *A*). The second most commonly used fluid for diagnosis of hyperinfection is sputum, where larvae are easily seen in wet preparations or in smears stained with Papanicolaou stain (Chaudhuri et al. 1980; Humpherys, Hieger, 1979; Wang et al. 1980; *color plate* VI *E–F*). In all cases where *Strongyloides* larvae are found in sputum, especially in individuals with complaints of chronic asthma, care should be taken to determine if the bronchial epithelium has been colonized (see above; Fig. 12–2 A–C; Nwokolo, Imohiosen, 1973). Less commonly used are bronchial brushings (Harris et al. 1980) and bronchoalveolar lavage fluid (Kramer et al. 1990; Mejia et al. 1992; Schainberg, Scheinberg, 1989). Lar-

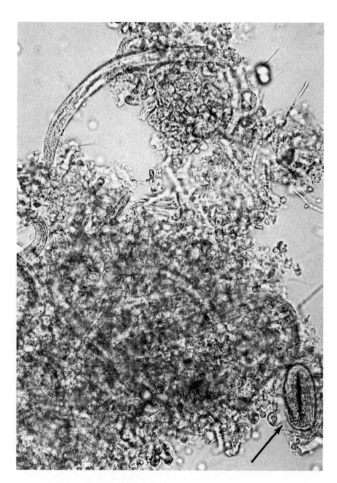

Fig. 12–12. *Strongyloides stercoralis*, duodenal aspirate in a case of hyperinfection, unstained. Note the larval stages among the debris. One stage with a larva inside is seen (arrow), ×310.

vae detected in routine cervicovaginal smears or collected for other reasons (Avram et al. 1984; Murty et al. 1994 are always an accidental finding and are most likely due to migration from the perineum into the vagina. Larvae in pleural, peritoneal (Avagnina et al. 1980), and spinal fluid also are always an incidental finding. Larvae found in the urine of a patient were due to a vesicocolic fistula (Downs, Frye, 1970), and larvae found in a gastric aspirate were probably due to parasitization of the lower stomach (Yassin, Garret, 1980).

Tissue Sections. *Strongyloides* is sometimes found in small intestinal biopsy specimens taken for reasons other than the diagnosis of strongyloidiasis. Although the presence of the parasite often explains the clinical symptoms, usually only a few organisms are found (Fig. 12–5 A–D). In cross sections and oblique sections the females are up to 35 μm in diameter. Structures recognized in the females include the intestine, the gonads, and sometimes immature eggs in the uterus (Fig. 12–5 C). Recently laid eggs are oval or rounded masses of eosinophilic granular material within a thin, barely visible egg shell; they measure 52 × 33 μm. Slightly older eggs are in the early stages of cleavage; the oldest ones have developmental embryos and larvae (Fig. 12–6 C). Hatched rhabditoid larvae are located in the mucosa near the lumen and measure up to 14 μm in diameter (Fig. 12–6 D).

Serology. Serologic tests for the diagnosis of strongyloidiasis are available, but in the past they showed little specificity. Recently, an enzyme-linked immunosorbent assay test using *S. stercoralis* antigen has been found positive in 97% and negative in 95% of samples from individuals with proven infection (Genta, 1988; Lindo et al. 1994). Other serologic tests, all greatly improved, are also available, but their use in the routine clinical laboratory is far from standard.

Strongyloides fuelleborni fuelleborni and *S. f. kellyi*

Strongyloides f. fuelleborni and *S. f. kellyi* (*S. fuelleborni* and *S. kellyi* for short; Fig. 12–13) are parasites of the small intestine of certain primates in Africa and of humans in Asia. Infections with *S. fuelleborni* in humans have been reported from many countries of central, eastern and southern Africa (Pampiglione, Ricciardi, 1971). The prevalence of the infection in some

forest communities is up to 50%, while in the savanna it is sporadic (Pampiglione, Ricciardi, 1972b). Infections with *S. kellyi* in Papua, New Guinea, have been reported with a prevalence of 18% (Kelly et al. 1976; Kelly, Voge, 1973).

The symptoms produced by *S. fuelleborni* are known from one experimental infection in a human subject exposed to 300 larvae (Pampiglione, Ricciardi, 1972a), a large inoculum that would seldom occur in nature all at once. The larvae entering the skin produced intense burning and itching within 15 minutes that lasted for 4 hours, and reappeared at times over the next 24 hours. Pinpoint redness and streaking occurred at the site of inoculation. Pulmonary symptoms consisting of a nonproductive cough occurring in in-

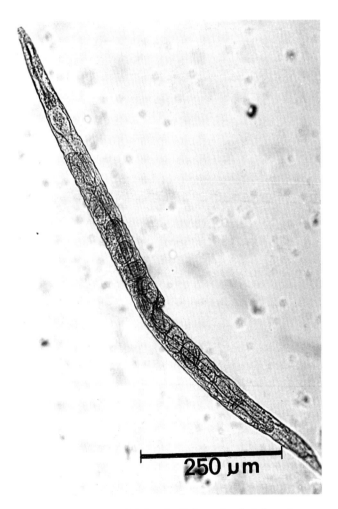

Fig. 12–13. *Strongyloides fuelleborni*, **adult female, unstained. Note the postvulvar constriction of the body. (In: Hira, P.R., and Patel, B.G. 1977.** *Strongyloides fuelleborni* **infections in man in Zambia. Am. J. Trop. Med. Hyg. 26:640–643. Reproduced with permission.)**

tense bouts of short duration developed during the fifth day of exposure and lasted for about 2 hours. The cough was followed by a burning sensation of the palate with red streaking of the pharyngeal region and a burning sensation at the sternal margin, especially after swallowing food. Chest x-radiograms were negative. Intestinal symptoms began the 20th day after exposure, with cramp-like pain in the epigastrium that lasted for several weeks; on the 28th day, eggs appeared in the stools. Allergic symptoms were also evident, and peripheral eosinophilia began increasing on the 26th day, reaching 48% on the 56th day after infection and then decreasing spontaneously, becoming almost normal 12 months later. Therapy was given on the 61st day after infection, resulting in a complete cure (Pampiglione, Ricciardi, 1972a). Clinical studies of naturally acquired infections are difficult to conduct because the study populations usually have several intestinal parasites.

In Papua, New Guinea, it is believed that *S. kellyi* is responsible for a syndrome known as *swollen belly sickness* in children. The disease, which is fatal in infants 2 to 6 months of age, usually presents with abdominal distention, respiratory distress, generalized edema, and gastrointestinal symptoms (Barnish, Barker, 1987; Vince et al. 1979). Other less common symptoms are vomiting, constipation, diarrhea, and signs of hepatomegaly, splenomegaly and fever on hospital admission (Vince et al. 1979). Autopsies in fatal cases have revealed nonspecific changes; the gross appearance of the bowel was normal, and no evidence of dissemination of the infection was found (Vince et al. 1979).

Lesions produced by *S. fuelleborni* in humans have not been described. The diagnosis is based on the presence of eggs in the stools (Fig. 12–14 A–B) measuring 48 to 54 × 32 to 35 μm, usually in an early stage of cleavage. The eggs of *S. fuelleborni* and *S. kellyi* are slightly smaller than hookworm eggs, and the specific identification of the parasite is based on the developmental stages (larvae) in fecal specimens at room temperature or in cultures (Hira, Patel, 1977, 1980; Kelly et al. 1976).

Other Free-living Nematodes

As stated above, under special circumstances, other free-living nematodes invade the tissues and organs of humans and animals. *Halicephalobus* (= *Micronema*) invades the internal organs; *Diploscapter coronata* in-

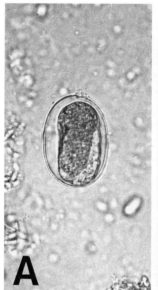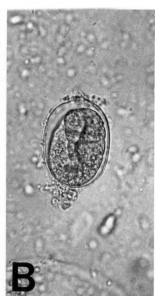

Fig. 12–14. *Strongyloides fuelleborni. A* and *B*, Eggs in stools of an individual from Papua, New Guinea, unstained, ×495. (Courtesy of M.D. Little, Ph.D., School of Tropical Medicine and Public Health, Tulane University, New Orleans, Louisiana.)

vades the urinary bladder (Witenberg, 1951) and stomach of achlorhydric patients (Chandler, 1938), producing no symptoms; and *Pelodera strongyloides* invades the skin. Since *Halicephalobus* and *Pelodera* are found in tissues, they will be discussed in some detail.

Micronema (= *Halicephalobus*) Species

Besides *Strongyloides, Halicephalobus* is the most important free-living nematode because it produces fatal infections. *Halicephalobus* is a genus of small, free-living nematodes inhabiting humus and other decaying organic material, and occasionally the tissues of animals and humans (Fig. 12–15 A–B). There are three reported human infections with *Halicephalobus*, classified twice as *Micronema* (= *Halicephalobus*) *deletrix* and once simply as a *Micronema* (= *Halicephalobus*) species. The original description of *H. deletrix* (Anderson, Bemrick, 1965) is based on females, eggs, and larvae recovered from bilateral growths in the nares of a horse; the females measured 250 μm in length by 17 μm in width and the eggs 9 to 11 × 32 to 46 μm. Since the worms found in all human patients appear to be larger than those in animals, their classification as *H. deletrix* seems presumptive at present; classification simply as a *Halicephalobus* species seems a more correct diagnosis. Infections in animals result in gingivitis (Cho et al. 1985), mastitis (Greiner et al. 1991), or disseminated disease (Alstad et al. 1979; Spalding et al. 1990), all of which are well known in veterinary practice.

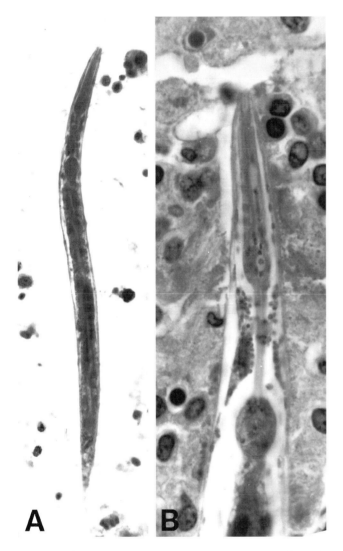

Fig. 12–15. *Halicephalobus* **species, adult parasites.** *A,* **Adult female recovered from the sediment of centrifuged formalin in which the brain was fixed, ×460.** *B,* **Longitudinal section of an adult in brain. Note that the esophagus follows the buccal cavity and is composed of a corpus, isthmus, and bulb from anterior to posterior, ×1,040. (In: Hoogstraten, J., and Young, W.G. 1975. Meningoencephalomyelitis due to the saprophagous nematode,** *Micronema deletrix.* **Can. J. Neurol. Sci. 2:121–126. Reproduced with permission.)**

Clinical Findings. The three known human cases of *Halicephalobus* infection have involved the brain, and all were fatal. The first patient, a 5-year-old boy from Canada who suffered an accident in a manure spreader, had a meningoencephalomyelitis with abundant nematodes in the brain (Hoogstraten, Young, 1975). The second, 47-year-old man in Texas, entered the hospital with leg pain and mental confusion; the symptoms progressed, and he died 19 days later (Shadduck et al. 1979). The third, a 54-year-old man from Washington, D.C., had a long history of chronic medical problems and alcoholism. He was admitted to the hospital acutely ill, with low weight and decubitus ulcers, and died 11 days later (Gardiner et al. 1981).

Pathology. The changes in the central nervous system in all three patients with *Micronema* infection are similar. The brain was soft, fragmenting, and swollen, with flattened gyri and a dusky brown color, with characteristics of a "respirator brain." Coronal sections showed similar changes throughout, as well as focal hemorrhages and hyperemia.

On microscopic examination, extensive inflammatory infiltration of the meninges (Fig. 12–16 *A–B*), the perivascular spaces, and other areas of brain tissue was found (Fig. 12–17 *B–C*). These areas of inflammation occurred around foci of necrosis, with infiltration by mononuclear and polymorphonuclear neutrophils (Fig. 12–17 *B–C*) and macrophages in other older areas. Cross sections and oblique sections of numerous adult females were seen in most areas of necrosis (Fig. 12–17 *A* and *D*), together with eggs and larvae in different stages of development (Fig. 12–16 *B*). In some cases, the parasites were found in areas with a marked chronic inflammatory reaction and fibrosis; in others, granulomas with multinucleated foreign giant cells were observed. Outside the central nervous system parasites were found only in the heart, but in animals they have been reported in kidneys (Alstad et al. 1979), maxillae (Johnson, Johnson, 1966), kidneys and brain (Rubin, Woodard, 1974), and other tissues.

Diagnosis. The diagnosis of *Halicephalobus* in all known cases has been made in tissue sections. In some instances, the worms were recovered from the sediment of formalin fixing the organs and tissues. The histologic characteristic of *Halicephalobus* infection is the presence of small adult females, together with eggs and developmental larval stages (Fig. 12–16 *B–D*). The females are up to 450 μm in length by 24 μm in diameter (Gardiner et al. 1981), with a characteristic rhab-

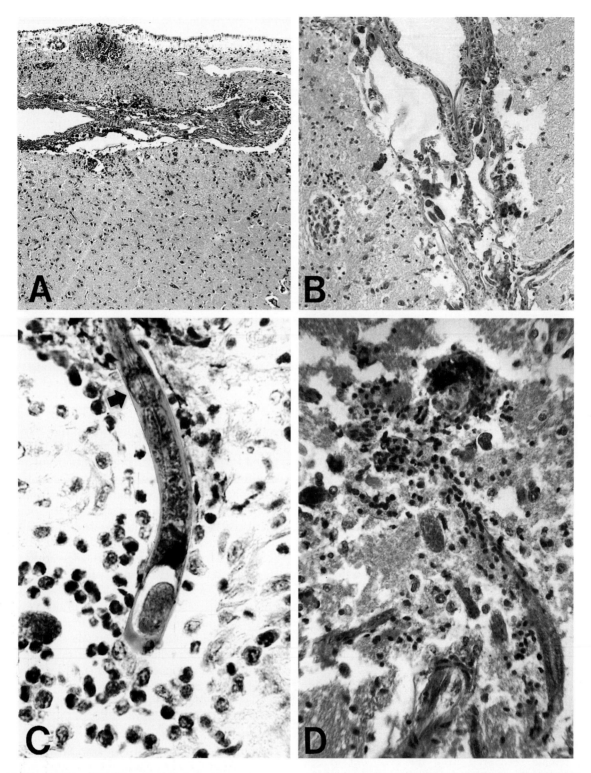

Fig. 12–16. *Halicephalobus* species in a horse, hematoxylin and eosin stain. *A*, Low-power view showing inflammation of the meninges, ×55. *B*, Eggs and developing larvae in meninges, ×280. *C*, Longitudinal section of a female showing the esophageal bulb (arrow), the intestine, and a single developed egg in the uterus (open arrow) ×705. *D*, Eggs and developing larvae, ×350.

(Courtesy of A.D. Alstad, D.V.M., Ph.D., North Dakota Veterinary Diagnostic Laboratory, North Dakota State University, Fargo, North Dakota. Reported by: Alstad, A.D., Berg, I.E., and Samuel, C. 1979. Disseminated *Micronema deletrix* infection in the horse. J. Am. Vet. Med. Assoc. 174:264–266.)

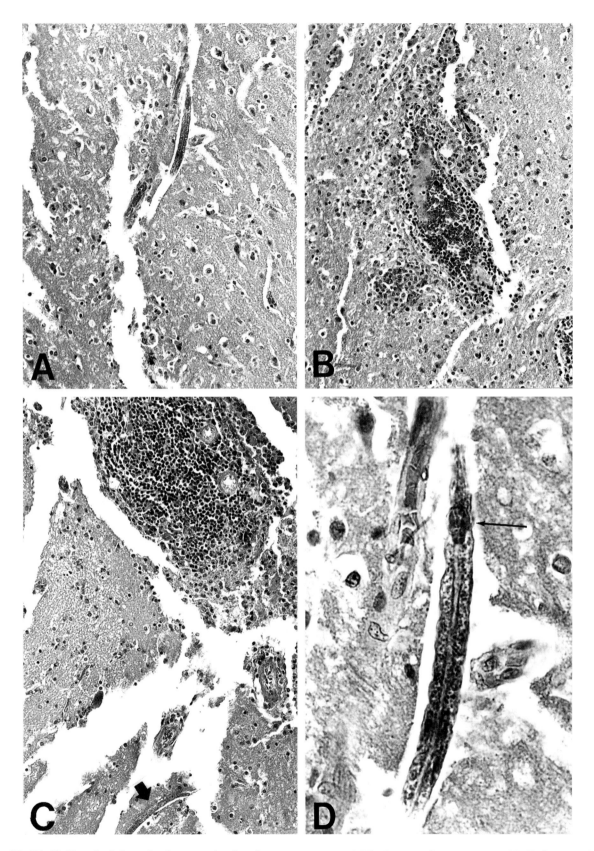

Fig. 12–17. *Halicephalobus* in human brain, hematoxylin and eosin stain. *A* and *B*, Low-power view of brain showing a larva (*A*) and necrosis with an inflammatory reaction around a small vessel (*B*), ×180. *C*, Another area with a mononuclear cell infiltrate (top) and a larva (arrow, bottom), ×705. *D*, Longitudinal section of a larva showing the lower part of the esophagus (arrow), ×705. (Preparation courtesy of D.H. Connor, M.D., Division of Geographic Pathology, Armed Forces Institute of Pathology, Washington, D.C. Reported by: Hoogstraten, J., and Young, W.G. 1975. Meningoencephalomyelitis due to the saprophagous nematode, *Micronema deletrix*. Can. J. Neurol. Sci. 2:121–126.)

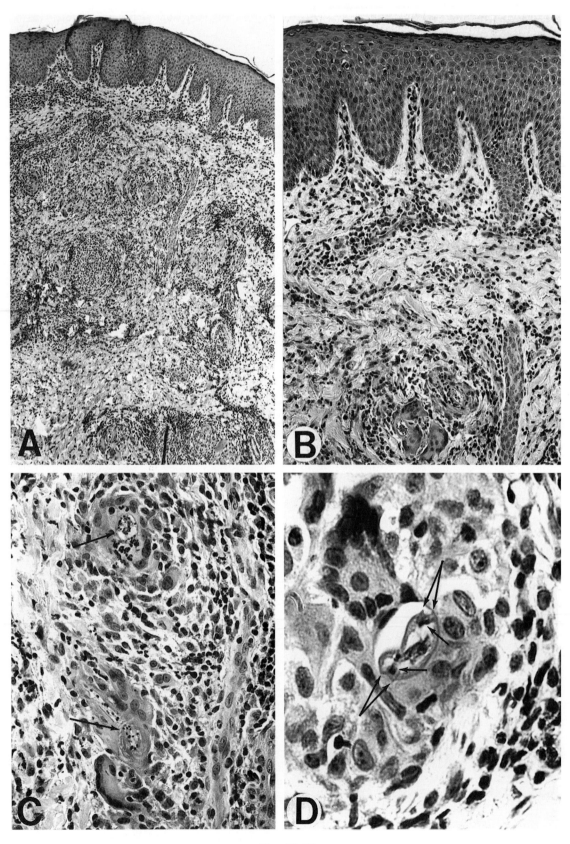

Fig. 12–18.

ditiform esophagus consisting of three areas: the corpus, isthmus, and bulb (Figs. 12–15 A–B and 14–16 C). The uterus has only one fully developed egg (Fig. 12–16 C). The eggs in tissues measure 35 by 17 μm; they have one or more cells or larvae in different stages of development (Fig. 12–16 B).

Pelodera strongyloides

Pelodera species are small, free-living nematodes, the larval stages of which produce dermatitis in humans and animals. *Pelodera* has been found in dogs, cattle, sheep, and horses, causing significant dermatitis. There are two well-documented reports of this infection in humans (Ginsburg et al. 1984; Pasyk, 1978). Both patients were children, one 11 years of age and the other 6 months old. The older child had a dermatitis of 1 month's duration, as well as pruritic lesions on the trunk and lower limbs; the infant had hyperpigmented papular nodules on the lower abdomen and thighs. A third report of a 20-year-old landscape worker in Houston, Texas, did not include a description of the parasite or the characteristics of the parasite that allowed its identification as *Pelodera* (Jones et al. 1991).

Histologically, the lesions in the 6-month-old infant were limited to the epidermis, with larvae in necrotic hair follicles accompanied by an infiltration of mononuclear cells and eosinophils. In some areas, the infiltrate extended deep into the hair follicles and around the small vessels in the upper subcutaneous tissues. The histologic lesions of the 11-year-old child were superficial pustules with polymorphonuclear cells, necrotic debris, and keratinocytes extending throughout the dermis into the subcutaneous tissues (Fig. 12–18 A) as a granulomatous inflammation (Fig. 12–18 B–C). Some granulomas contained dead larvae (Fig. 12–18 B–C) and others living larvae identified as *Pelodera* (Fig. 12–18 D).

The diagnosis is based on the morphologic characteristics of the larvae, which measure 25 μm in diameter at the base of the esophagus. Cross sections of the midbody reveal two lateral alae, one on either side of the body, up to 1 μm high and 2 μm apart (see Fig. 12–18 D). The body wall is 2 to 3 μm thick, and the lateral cords are noted by the presence of one or two dense nuclei (see Fig. 12–18 D; Ginsburg et al. 1984).

References

Adetiloye VA, 1992. A case of fatal gastrointestinal strongyloidiasis in an otherwise healthy Nigerian, masquerading as gastric outlet obstruction. Trop. Geogr. Med. 44:60–62

Al-Bahrani ZR, al Saleen T, al Gailiani M, 1995. Sub-acute intestinal obstruction by *Strongyloides stercolaris*. J. Infect. 30:47–50

Alcorn MO Jr, Kotcher E, 1961. Secondary malabsorption syndrome produced by chronic strongyloidiasis. South. Med. J. 54:193–197

Alstad AD, Berg IE, Samuel C, 1979. Disseminated *Micronema deletrix* infection in the horse. JAVMA 174: 264–266

Amer M, Attia M, Ramadan AS, Matout K, 1984. Larva currens and systemic disease. Int. J. Dermatol. 23: 402–403

Anderson RV, Bemrick WJ, 1965. *Micronema deletrix* n. sp., a saprophagous nematode inhabiting a nasal tumor of a horse. Proc. Helminthol. Soc. Wash. 32:74–75

Arakaki T, Asato R, Ikeshiro T, Sakiyama K, Iwanaga M, 1984a. Is the prevalence of HTLV-1 infection higher in *Strongyloides* carriers than in non-carriers? Trop. Med. Parasitol. 43:199–200

Arakaki T, Kohakura M, Asato R, Ikeshiro T, Nakamura S, Iwanaga M, 1984b. Epidemiological aspects of *Strongyloides stercoralis* infection in Okinawa, Japan. J. Trop. Med. Hyg. 95:210–213

Arantes Pereira O, Oliveira AD, Barretto Netto M, 1960. Es-

◄────

Fig. 12–18. *Pelodera strongyloides* **in human skin, hematoxylin and eosin stain.** *A,* **Low-power view of skin showing the florid granulomatous inflammation, ×55.** *B,* **Higher magnification showing well-preserved epidermis and two granulomas (bottom) composed of multinucleated foreign body giant cells, histiocytes, and epithelioid cells. The inflammatory reaction is composed of mononuclear cells, ×140.** *C,* **Higher magnification showing two granulomas containing small pyknotic nuclei corresponding to disintegrating larvae (arrows), ×280.** *D,* **A granuloma with a well-preserved larva cut on cross section. Note the double alae (arrows in V), widely separated, and the lateral columns with dark-staining nuclei (arrows), ×705. (Slide courtesy of P.C. Beaver, Ph.D., School of Public Health and Tropical Medicine, Tulane University, New Orleans, Louisiana. Reported by: Ginsburg, B., Beaver, P.C., Wilson, E.R., et al. 1984. Dermatitis due to larvae of a soil nematode,** *Pelodera strongyloides.* **Pediatr. Dermatol. 2:33–37.)**

trongiloidose intestinal: correlacao anatomo-radiologica de um caso fatal. Rev. Brasileira Radiol. 3:127–142

Ashford RW, Vince JD, Gratten MJ, Miles WE, 1978. *Strongyloides* infection associated with acute infantile disease in Papua New Guinea. Trans. R. Soc. Trop. Med. Hyg. 72:554

Avagnina MA, Elsner B, Iotti RM, Re R, 1980. *Strongyloides stercoralis* in Papanicolaou-stained smears of ascitic fluid. Acta Cytol. 24:36–39

Avram E, Yakovlevitz M, Schachter A, 1984. Cytologic detection of *Enterobius vermicularis* and *Strongyloides stercoralis* in routine cervicovaginal smears and urocytograms. Acta Cytol. 28:468–470

Bank DE, Grossman ME, Kohn SR, Rabinowitz AD, 1984. The thumbprint sign: rapid diagnosis of disseminated strongyloidiasis. J. Am. Acad. Dermatol. 23:324–326

Bannon JP, Fater M, Solit R, 1995. Intestinal ileus secondary to *Strongyloides stercoralis* infection: case report and review of the literature. Am. Surg. 61:377–380

Barnish G, Barker J, 1987. An intervention study using thiabendazole suspension against *Strongyloides fuelleborni*-like infections in Papua New Guinea. Trans. R. Soc. Trop. Med. Hyg. 81:60–63

Barrett KE, Neva FA, Gam AA, Cicmanec J, London WT, Phillips JM, Metcalfe DD, 1988. The immune response to nematode parasites: modulation of mast cell numbers and function during *Strongyloides stercoralis* infections in nonhuman primates. Am. J. Trop. Med. Hyg. 38:574–581

Beaver PC, Jung RC, Cupp EW, 1984. *Clinical Parasitology*. Philadelphia: Lea & Febiger

Belani A, Leptrone D, Shands JWJ, 1987. *Strongyloides* meningitis. South. Med. J. 80:916–918

Berger R, Kraman S, Paciotti M, 1980. Pulmonary strongyloidiasis complicating therapy with corticosteroids. Report of a case with secondary bacterial infections. Am. J. Trop. Med. Hyg. 29:31–34

Berk SL, Verghese A, Alvarez S, Hall K, Smith B, 1987. Clinical and epidemiologic features of strongyloidiasis. A prospective study in rural Tennessee. Arch. Intern. Med. 147:1257–1261

Berkmen YM, Rabinowitz J, 1972. Gastrointestinal manifestations of strongyloidiasis. Am. J. Roentgenol. Radiol. Ther. Nuclear Med. 115:306–311

Berthoud F, Berthoud S, 1975. A propos de18 cas d'anguillulose diagnostique a Geneve. Schweiz. Med. Wochenschr. 105:1110–1115

Bhatt BD, Cappell MS, Smilow PC, Das KM, 1990. Recurrent massive upper gastrointestinal hemorrhage due to *Strongyloides stercoralis* infection. Am. J. Gastroenterol. 85:1034–1036

Boram LH, Keller KF, Justus DE, Collins JP, 1981. Strongyloidiasis in immunosuppressed patients. Am. J. Clin. Pathol. 76:778–781

Brasitus TA, Gold RP, Kay RH, Magun AM, Lee WM, 1980. Intestinal strongyloidiasis: a case report and review of the literature. Am. J. Gastroenterol. 73:65–69

Braun TI, Fekete T, Lynch A, 1988. Strongyloidiasis in an institution for mentally retarded adults. Arch. Intern. Med. 148:634–636

Brown RC, Girardeau HF, 1977. Transmammary passage of *Strongyloides* sp. larvae in the human host. Am. J. Trop. Med. Hyg. 26:215–219

Brumpt LC, Sang HT, 1973. Larva currens seul signe pathognomonique de la strongyloidose. Ann. Parasitol. Hum. Comp. 48:319–328

Buitrago B, Gast-Galvis A, 1965a. Presentacion de cuatro casos del sindrome larva migrans visceral. Antioquia Med. 15:342–343

Buitrago B, Gast-Galvis A, 1965b. Sindrome larva migrans visceral (granulomatosis larvaria) en Colombia. Rev. Soc. Col. Pediatr. Pueric. 6:89–95

Chandler AC, 1938. *Diploscapter coronata* as a facultative parasite of man, with a general review of vertebrate parasitism by rhabditoid worms. Semin. Respir. Infect. 30:44–55

Chaudhuri B, Nanos S, Soco JN, McGrew EA, 1980. Disseminated *Strongyloides stercoralis* infestation detected by sputum cytology. Acta Cytol. 24:360–362

Cho DY, Hubbard RM, McCoy DJ, Stewart TB, 1985. *Micronema* granuloma in the gingiva of a horse. JAVMA 187:505–507

Choudhry U, Choudhry R, Romeo DP, Cammerer RC, Gopalswamy N, 1995. Strongyloidiasis: new endoscopic findings. Gastrointest. Endosc. 42:170–173

Colebunders R, Lusakumuni K, Nelson AM, Gigase P, Lebughe I, van Marck E, Kapita B, Francis H, Salaun JJ, Quinn TC, Piot P, 1988. Persistent diarrhoea in Zairian AIDS patients: an endoscopic and histological study. Gut 29:1687–1691

Conlon CP, Pinching AJ, Perera CU, Moody A, Luo NP, Lucas SB, 1990. HIV-related enteropathy in Zambia: a clinical, microbiological, and histological study. Am. J. Trop. Med. Hyg. 42:83–88

Coulaud JP, Mercher YL, Tessier S, Mechali D, 1980. Analyse epidemiologique, clinique et therapeutique de 427 cas d'anguilluloses observes a Paris. Bull. Soc. Pathol. Exot. 73:100–108

Coutinho HB, Robalinho TI, Coutinho VB, Almeida JR, Filho JT, King G, Jenkins D, Mahida Y, Sewell HF, Wakelin D, 1996. Immunocytochemistry of mucosal changes in patients infected with the intestinal nematode *Strongyloides stercoralis*. J. Clin. Pathol. 49:717–720

Craven JL, Cantrell EO, Lewis MO, 1971. *Strongyloides stercoralis* infection presenting as necrotizing jejunitis. Trans. R. Soc. Trop. Med. Hyg. 65:532–533

Dancesco P, 1968. Recherches sur un foyer endemizue de strongyloidose de la zone temperee. Bull. Soc. Pathol. Exot. 61:651–661

de Kaminsky RG, 1993. Evaluation of three methods for laboratory diagnosis of *Strongyloides stercoralis* infection. J. Parasitol. 79:277–280

De Paola D, 1962. Pathology of strongyloidiasis. Bol. Centro. Estudos. Hos. Servidores. Estado. 14:3–98

Dees A, Batenburg PL, Umar HM, Menon RS, Verweij J, 1990. *Strongyloides stercoralis* associated with a bleeding gastric ulcer. Gut 31:1414–1415

Delarocque AE, Hadengue A, Degott C, Vilgrain V, Erlinger S, Benhamou JP, 1994. Biliary obstruction resulting from *Strongyloides stercoralis* infection. Report of a case. Gut 35:705–706

Deluol AM, Colin Y, Penalba C, Cenac J, Leynadier F, Dry J, Coulaud JP, 1984. Le test de degranulation des basophiles humains (TDBH) applique au diagnostic de l'anguillulose. Resultats preliminaires. Bull. Soc. Pathol. Exot. 77:360–362

Dixon AC, Yanagihara ET, Kwock DW, Nakamura JM, 1984. Strongyloidiasis associated with human T-cell lymphotropic virus type I infection in a nonendemic area. West. J. Med. 151:410–413

Doury P, 1993. Anguillulose autochthone en France. Bull. Soc. Pathol. Exot. 86:116

Downs RA, Frye IL, 1970. Vesicocolic fistula: *Strongyloides stercoralis* in the urine (a case report). J. Ark. Med. Soc. 67:193–195

Dunlap NE, Shin MS, Polt SS, Ho KJ, 1984. Strongyloidiasis manifested as asthma. South. Med. J. 77:77–78

Dutcher JP, Marcus SL, Tanowitz HB, Wittner M, Fuks JZ, Wiernik PH, 1990. Disseminated strongyloidiasis with central nervous system involvement diagnosed antemortem in a patient with acquired immunodeficiency syndrome and Burkitts' lymphoma. Cancer 66:2417–2420

Eveland LK, Kenney M, Yermakov V, 1975. Laboratory diagnosis of autoinfection in strongyloidiasis. Am. J. Clin. Pathol. 63:421–425

Faust EC, 1935. Experimental studies on human and primate species of *Strongyloides*: IV. The pathology of *Strongyloides* infection. Arch. Pathol. 19:769–806

Faust EC, Giraldo LE, 1960. Parasitological surveys in Cali, Departamento del Valle, Colombia. VI. Strongyloidiasis in Barrio Siloe, Cali, Colombia. Trans. R. Soc. Trop. Med. Hyg. 54:556–563

Faust EC, Kagy ES, 1933. Experimental studies on human and primate species of *Strongyloides*. I. The variability and instability of types. Am. J. Trop. Med. 13:47–65

Ford J, Reiss-Levy E, Clark E, Dyson AJ, Schonell M, 1981. Pulmonary strongyloidiasis and lung abscess. Chest 79:239–240

Freedman DO, 1991. Experimental infection of human subject with *Strongyloides* species. Rev. Infect. Dis. 13:1221–1226

Fuelleborn F, 1929. On the larval migration of some parasitic nemtatodes in the body of the host and its biological significance. J. Helminthol. 7:15–26

Fulmer HS, Huempfner HR, 1965. Intestinal helminths in Eastern Kentucky: a survey in three rural counties. Am. J. Trop. Med. Hyg. 14:269–275

Galliard H, 1950. Recherces sur l'infestation experimentale a *Strongyloides stercoralis* au Tonkin. 1re Note. Ann. Parasitol. Hum. Comp. 25:441–473

Garcia FT, Sessions JT, Strum WB, Schweistris E, Tripathy K, Bolanos O, Lotero H, Duque E, Ramelli D, Mayoral LG, 1977. Intestinal function and morphology in strongyloidiasis. Am. J. Trop. Med. Hyg. 26:859–865

Gardiner CH, Koh DS, Cardella TA, 1981. *Micronema* in man: third fatal infection. Am. J. Trop. Med. Hyg. 30:586–589

Genta RM, 1988. Predictive value of an enzyme-linked immunosorbent assay (ELISA) for the serodiagnosis of strongyloidiasis. Am. J. Clin. Pathol. 89:391–394

Genta RM, 1989. Global prevalence of strongyloidiasis: critical review with epidemiologic insights into the prevention of disseminated disease. Rev. Infect. Dis. 11:755–767

Genta RM, 1992. Dysregulation of strongyloidiasis: a new hypothesis. Clin. Microbiol. Rev. 5:345–355

Genta RM, Lillibridge JP, 1989. Prominence of IgG4 antibodies in the human responses to *Strongyloides stercoralis* infection. J. Infect. Dis. 160:692–699

Genta RM, Ottesen EA, Gam AA, Neva FA, 1983a. Immunologic responses to experimental strongyloidiasis in rats. Z. Parasitenk. 69:667–675

Genta RM, Ottesen EA, Neva FA, Walzer PD, Tanowitz HB, Wittner M, 1983b. Cellular responses in human strongyloidiasis. Am. J. Trop. Med. Hyg. 32:990–994

Genta RM, Ottesen EA, Poindexter R, Gam AA, Neva FA, Tanowitz HB, Wittner M, 1983c. Specific allergic sensitization to *Strongyloides* antigens in human strongyloidiasis. Lab. Invest. 48:633–638

Genta RM, Weil GJ, 1982. Antibodies to *Strongyloides stercoralis* larval surface antigens in chronic strongyloidiasis. Lab. Invest. 47:87–90

Georgi JR, Sprinkle CL, 1974. A case of human strongyloidosis apparently contracted from asymptomatic colony dogs. Am. J. Trop. Med. Hyg. 23:899–901

Gill GV, Bell DR, 1979. *Strongyloides stercoralis* infection in former Far East prisoners of war. Br. Med. J. 2:572–574

Gill GV, Bell DR, 1987. *Strongyloides stercoralis* infection in Burma Star veterans. Br. Med. J. Clin. Res. Ed. 294:1003–1004

Gill GV, Bell DR, Reid HA, 1977. Strongyloidiasis in ex–Far East prisoners of war. Br. Med. J. 1:1007

Ginsburg B, Beaver PC, Wilson ER, Whitley RJ, 1984. Dermatitis due to larvae of a soil nematode, *Pelodera strongyloides*. Pediatr. Dermatol. 2:33–37

Gompels MM, Todd J, Peters BS, Main J, Pinching AJ, 1991. Disseminated strongyloidiasis in AIDS: uncommon but important. AIDS 5:329–332

Gordon SM, Gal AA, Solomon AR, Bryan JA, 1994. Disseminated strongyloidiasis with cutaneous manifestations in an immunocompromised host. J. Am. Acad. Dermatol. 31:255–259

Greiner EC, Mays MBC, Smart GC Jr. Weisbrode SE, 1991. Verminous mastitis in a mare caused by a free-living nematode. J. Parasitol. 77:320–322

Grove DI, 1980. Strongyloidiasis in Allied ex-prisoners of war in south-east Asia. Br. Med. J. 280:598–601

Grove DI, Northern C, Heenan PJ, 1986. *Strongyloides stercoralis* infections in the muscles of mice: a model for investigating the systemic phase of strongyloidiasis. Pathology 18:72–76

Gutierrez Y, Bhatia P, Garbadawala ST, Dobson JR, Wallace TM, Carey TE, 1996. *Strongyloides stercoralis* eosinophilic granulomatous enterocolitis. Am. J. Surg. Pathol. 20:603–612

Haque AK, Schnadig V, Rubin SA, Smith JH, 1994. Pathogenesis of human strongyloidiasis: autopsy and quantitative parasitological analysis. Mod. Pathol. 7:276–288

Harcourt Webster JN, Scaravilli F, Darwish AH, 1991. *Strongyloides stercoralis* hyperinfection in an HIV positive patient. J. Clin. Pathol. 44:346–348

Harper JS III, Genta RM, Gam A, London WT, Neva FA, 1984. Experimental disseminated strongyloidiasis in *Erythrocebus patas*. I. Pathology. Am. J. Trop. Med. Hyg. 33:431–443

Harris RA Jr, Musher DM, Fainstein V, Young EJ, Clarridge J, 1980. Disseminated strongyloidiasis. Diagnosis made by sputum examination. JAMA 244:65–66

Hartz PH, 1946. Human strongyloidiasis with internal autoinfection. Arch. Pathol. 41:601–611

Hartz PH, 1954. Strongyloidiasis with internal autoinfection in children. Doc. Med. Geogr. Trop. 6:61–68

Hayashi J, Kishihara Y, Yoshimura E, Furusyo N, Yamaji K, Kawakami Y, Murakami H, Kashiwagi S, 1997. Correlation between human T cell lymphotropic virus type-1 and *Strongyloides stercoralis* infections and serum immunoglobulin E responses in residents of Okinawa, Japan. Am. J. Trop. Med. Hyg. 56:71–75

Hira PR, Patel BG, 1977. *Strongyloides fulleborni* infections in man in Zambia. Am. J. Trop. Med. Hyg. 26:640–643

Hira PR, Patel BG, 1980. Human strongyloidiasis due to the primate species *Strongyloides fulleborni*. Trop. Geogr. Med. 32:23–29

Hoogstraten J, Young WG, 1975. Meningo-encephalomyelitis due to the saprophagous nematode, *Micronema deletrix*. Can. J. Neurol. Sci. 2:121–126

Hoy WE, Roberts NJ Jr, Bryson MF, Bowles C, Lee JC, Rivero AJ, Ritterson AL, 1981. Transmission of strongyloidiasis by kidney transplant? Disseminated strongyloidiasis in both recipients of kidney allografts from a single cadaver donor. JAMA 246:1937–1939

Hubbard DW, Morgan PM, Yaeger RG, Unglaub WG, Hood MW, Willis RA, 1974. Intestinal parasite survey of kindergarten children in New Orleans. Pediatr. Res. 8:652–658

Huminer D, Symon K, Groskopf I, Pietrushka D, Kremer I, Schantz PM, Pitlik SD, 1992. Seroepidemiologic study of toxocariasis and strongyloidiasis in institutionalized mentally retarded adults. Am. J. Trop. Med. Hyg. 46:278–281

Humpherys K, Hieger LR, 1979. *Strongyloides stercoralis* in routine Papanicolaou-stained sputum smears. Acta Cytol. 23:471–476

Imasato K, Ninomiya F, Noro S, Yonekura A, Shindo N, 1968. Two cases of *Strongyloidosis stercoralis*: larvae recognized in the mucosa propria of stomach. J. Kurume Med. Assoc. 31:78–82

Jain AK, Agarwal SK, El-Sadr W, 1994. *Streptococcus bovis* bacteremia and meningitis associated with *Strongyloides stercoralis* colitis in a patient infected with human immunodeficiency virus. Clin. Infect. Dis. 18:253–254

Johnson KH, Johnson DW, 1966. Granulomas associated with *Micronema deletrix* in the maxillae of a horse. JAVMA 149:155–159

Jones CA, 1950. Clinical studies in human strongyloidiasis. I. Semeiology. Gastroenterology 16:743–756

Jones CC, Rosen T, Greenberg C, 1991. Cutaneous larva migrans due to *Pelodera strongyloides*. Cutis 48:123–126

Jorgensen T, Montresor A, Savioli L, 1996. Correspondence. Effectively controlling strongyloidiasis. Parasitol. Today 12:164

Junod C, 1987a. Etude retrospective de 1,934 cas de strongyloidose diagnostique a Paris (1970–1986). II. Diagnostic. Eosinophilie. Traitement. Bull. Soc. Pathol. Exot. 80:370–382

Junod C, 1987b. Etude retrospective de 1,934 cas de strongyloidose diagnostiques a Paris (1970–1986). I. Origin geographic. Epidemiologie. Bull. Soc. Pathol. Exot. 80:357–369

Kalb RE, Grossman ME, 1984. Periumbilical purpura in disseminated strongyloidiasis. JAMA 256:1170–1171

Kelly A, Little MD, Voge M, 1976. *Strongyloides fulleborni*–like infections in man in Papua New Guinea. Am. J. Trop. Med. Hyg. 25:694–699

Kelly A, Voge M, 1973. Report of a nematode found in humans at Kiunga, Western District. Papua New Guinea Agr. J. 16:59

Koga K, Kasuya S, Khamboonruang C, Sukhavat K, Ieda M, Takatsuka N, Kita K, Ohtomo H, 1991. A modified agar plate method for detection of *Strongyloides stercoralis*. Am. J. Trop. Med. Hyg. 45:518–521

Koga K, Kasuya S, Khamboonruang C, Sukavat K, Nakamura Y, Tani S, Ieda M, Tomita K, Tomita S, Hattan N, et al, 1990. An evaluation of the agar plate method for the detection of *Strongyloides stercoralis* in northern Thailand. J. Trop. Med. Hyg. 93:183–188

Kramer MR, Gregg PA, Goldstein M, Llamas R, Krieger BP, 1990. Disseminated strongyloidiasis in AIDS and non-AIDS immunocompromised hosts: diagnosis by sputum and bronchoalveolar lavage. South. Med. J. 83:1226–1229

Leighton PM, MacSween HM, 1990. *Strongyloides stercoralis*. The cause of an urticarial-like eruption of 65 years' duration. Arch. Intern. Med. 150:1747–1748

Lin AL, Kessimian N, Benditt JO, 1995. Restrictive pulmonary disease due to interlobular septal fibrosis associated with disseminated infection by *Strongyloides stercoralis*. Am. J. Res. Crit. Care Med. 151:205–209

Lindo JF, Conway DJ, Atkins NS, Bianco AE, Robinson RD, Bundy DA, 1994. Prospective evaluation of enzyme-linked immunosorbent assay and immunoblot methods for the diagnosis of endemic *Strongyloides stercoralis* infection. Am. J. Trop. Med. Hyg. 51:175–179

Little MD, 1965. Dermatitis in a human volunteer infected with *Strongyloides* of nutria and raccoon. Am. J. Trop. Med. Hyg. 14:1007–1009

Little MD, Gutierrez Y, 1968. Soil relations in the epidemiology of strongyloidiasis. In: *Proceedings of the Eighth International Congress on Tropical Medicine and Malaria*. 8:221–222.

Lopez JE, Marcano Torres M, Pena JR, Quintini A, Malpica CC, Lopez Salazar Y, 1984. Hepatitis granulomatosa producida por el *Strongyloides stercoralis*. Presentacion de un caso con confirmacion histopatologica. GEN 38:133–143

Lucas SB, 1990. Missing infections in AIDS. Trans. R. Soc. Trop. Med. Hyg. 84(Suppl):1:34–38

Lyons ET, Drudge JH, Tolliver SC, 1970. *Strongyloides* larvae in milk of sheep and cattle. Mod. Vet. Pract. 51:65–68

Maayan S, Wormser GP, Widerhorn J, Sy ER, Kim YH, Ernst JA, 1987. *Strongyloides stercoralis* hyperinfection in a patient with the acquired immune deficiency syndrome. Am. J. Med. 83:945–948

Masdeu JC, Tantulavanich S, Gorelick PP, Maliwan N, Heredia S, Martinez Lage JM, Rubino FA, Ross E, Mamdani M, 1982. Brain abscess caused by *Strongyloides stercoralis*. Arch. Neurol. 39:62–63

Matuzenko VA, 1971. On human invasion with the agent of swine strongyloidoisis [in Russian; English summary]. Med. Parazitol. 40:427–431

McRury J, De Messias IT, Walzer PD, Huitger T, Genta RM, 1986. Specific IgE responses in human strongyloidiasis. Clin. Exp. Immunol. 65:631–638

Mejia JH, Denis M, Leleu G, Roux P, Mayaud C, Akoun G, 1992. Insuffisance respiratoire aigue liee a un anguillulose d'hyperinfestation. Diagnostique par LBA et evolution favorable. Rev. Pneumol. Clin. 48:75–78

Meltzer RS, Singer C, Armstrong D, Mayer K, Knapper WH, 1979. Antemortem diagnosis of central nervous system strongyloidiasis. Am. J. Med. Sci. 277:91–98

Milder JE, Walzer PD, Kilgore G, Rutherford I, Klein M, 1981. Clinical features of *Strongyloides stercoralis* infection in an endemic area of the United States. Gastroenterology 80:1481–1488

Morgan JS, Schaffner W, Stone WJ, 1986. Opportunistic strongyloidiasis in renal transplant recipients. Transplantation 42:518–524

Morgello S, Soifer FM, Lin CS, Wolfe DE, 1993. Central nervous system *Strongyloides stercoralis* in acquired immunodeficiency syndrome: a report of two cases and review of the literature. Acta Neuropathol. 86:285–288

Moura H, Fernandes O, Viola JP, Silva SP, Passos RH, Lima DB, 1989. Enteric parasites and HIV infection: occurrence in AIDS patients in Rio de Janeiro, Brazil. Mem. Inst. Oswaldo Cruz 84:527–533

Murty DA, Luthra UK, Sehgal K, Sodhani P, 1994. Cytologic detection of *Strongyloides stercoralis* in a routine cervicovaginal smear. A case report. Acta Cytol. 38:223–225

Nakada K, Kohakura M, Komoda H, Hinuma Y, 1984a. Correspondence. High incidence of HTLA antibody in carriers of *Strongyloides stercoralis*. Lancet 1:633

Nakada K, Yamaguchi K, Furugen S, Nakasone T, Nakasone K, Oshiro Y, Kohakura M, Hinuma Y, Seiki M, Yoshida M, Matutes E, Catovsky D, Ishii T, Kakatsuki K, 1984b. Monoclonal integration of HTLV-I proviral DNA in patients with strongyloidiasis. Int. J. Cancer 40:145–148

Neefe LI, Pinilla O, Garagusi VF, Bauer H, 1973. Disseminated strongyloidiasis with cerebral involvement: a complication of corticosteroid therapy. Am. J. Med. 55:832–838

Neva FA, 1986. Biology and immunology of human strongyloidiasis. J. Infect. Dis. 153:397–406

Neva FA, Murphy EL, Gam A, Hanchard B, Figueroa JP, Blattner WA, 1984. Correspondence. Antibodies to *Strongyloides stercoralis* in healthy Jamaican carriers of HTLV-1. N. Engl. J. Med. 320:252–253

Newton RC, Limpuangthip P, Greenberg S, Gam A, Neva FA, 1984. *Strongyloides stercoralis* hyperinfection in a carrier of HTLV-I virus with evidence of selective immunosuppression. Am. J. Med. 92:202–208

Newton RC, Limpuangthip P, Greenberg S, Gam A, Neva FA, 1992. *Strongyloides stercoralis* hyperinfection in a carrier of HTLV-I virus with evidence of selective immunosuppression. Am. J. Med. 92:202–208

Nucci M, Portugal R, Pulcheri W, Spector N, Ferreira SB, de Castro M, Noe R, de Oliveira OH, 1995. Strongyloidiasis in patients with hematologic malignancies. Clin. Infect. Dis. 21:675–677

Nwokolo C, Imohiosen EAE, 1973. Strongyloidiasis of respiratory tract presenting as "asthma." Br. Med. J. 2:153–154

Olson CE, Schiller EL, 1978a. *Strongyloides ratti* infections in rats I. Immunopathology. Am. J. Trop. Med. Hyg. 27:521–526

Olson CE, Schiller EL, 1978b. *Strongyloides ratti* infections in rats II. Effects of cortisone treatment. Am. J. Trop. Med. Hyg. 27:527–531

Pagliuca A, Layton DM, Allen S, Mufti GJ, 1988. Hyperinfection with *Strongyloides* after treatment for adult T cell leukaemia-lymphoma in an African immigrant. Br. Med. J. 297:1456–1457

Pampiglione S, Ricciardi ML, 1971. The presence of *Strongyloides fuelleborni* von Linstow, 1905, in man in Central and East Africa. Parassitologia 13:257–269

Pampiglione S, Ricciardi ML, 1972a. Experimental infestation with human strain *Strongyloides fulleborni* in man. Lancet 1:663–665

Pampiglione S, Ricciardi ML, 1972b. Geographic distribution of *Strongyloides fulleborni* in humans in tropical Africa. Parassitologia 14:329–338

Panosian KJ, Marone P, Edberg SC, 1986. Elucidation of *Strongyloides stercoralis* by bacterial-colony displacement. J. Clin. Microbiol. 24:86–88

Pasyk K, 1978. Dermatitis rhabditidosa in an 11-year-old girl. A new cutaneous parasitic disease of man. Br. J. Dermatol. 98:107–112

Patey O, Gessain A, Breuil J, Courillon Mallet A, Daniel MT, Miclea JM, Roucayrol AM, Sigaux F, Lafaix C, 1984. Seven years of recurrent severe strongyloidiasis in an HTLV-I-infected man who developed adult T-cell leukaemia. AIDS 6:575–579

Pelletier LL Jr, 1984. Chronic strongyloidiasis in World War II Far East ex-prisoners of war. Am. J. Trop. Med. Hyg. 33:55–61

Pelletier LL Jr, Gabre Kidan T, 1985. Chronic strongyloidiasis in Vietnam veterans. Am. J. Med. 78:139–140

Phelps KR, Ginsberg SS, Cunningham AW, Tschachler E, Dosik H, 1984. Case report: adult T-cell leukemia/lymphoma associated with recurrent *Strongyloides* hyperinfection. Am. Med. Sci. 302:224–228

Phillips SC, Mildvan D, William DC, Gelb AM, White MC, 1981. Sexual transmission of enteric protozoa and helminths in a venereal-disease-clinic population. N. Engl. J. Med. 305:603–606

Pijls NH, Yap SH, Rosenbusch G, Prenen H, 1986. Pancreatic mass due to *Strongyloides stercoralis* infection: an unusual manifestation. Pancreas 1:90–93

Plumelle Y, Gonin C, Edouard A, Bucher BJ, Thomas L, Brebion A, Panelatti G, 1984. Effect of *Strongyloides stercoralis* infectin and eosinophilia on age at onset and prognosis of adult T-cell leukemia. Am. J. Clin. Pathol. 107:81–87

Plumelle Y, Gonin C, Edouard A, Bucher BJ, Thomas L, Brebion A, Panelatti G, 1997. Effect of *Strongyloides stercoralis* infection and eosinophilia on age at onset and prognosis of adult T-cell leukemia. Am J Clin. Pathol 107:81–87

Plumelle Y, Pascaline N, Nguyen D, Panelatti G, Jouannelle A, Jouault H, Imbert M, 1984. Adult T-cell leukemia-lymphoma: a clinico-pathologic study of twenty-six patients from Martinique. Hematol. Pathol. 7:251–262

Poltera AA, 1974. Fatal strongyloidiasis in Uganda. Ann. Trop. Med. Parasitol. 68:81–90

Poltera AA, Katsimbura N, 1974. Granulomatous hepatitis due to *Strongyloides stercoralis*. J. Pathol. 113:241–246

Proctor EM, Isaac Renton JL, Robertson WB, Black WA, 1985. Strongyloidiasis in Canadian Far East war veterans. Can. Med. Assoc. J. 133:876–878

Proctor EM, Muth HA, Proudfoot DL, Allen AB, Fisk R, Isaac Renton J, Black WA, 1987. Endemic institutional strongyloidiasis in British Columbia. Can. Med. Assoc. J. 136:1173–1176

Purtilo DT, Meyers WM, Connor DH, 1974. Fatal strongyloidiasis in immunosuppressed patients. Am. J. Med. 56:488–493

Purvis RS, Beightler EL, Diven DG, Sanchez RL, Tyring SK, 1984. *Strongyloides hyperinfection* presenting with petechiae and purpura. Int. J. Dermatol. 31:169–171

Quinn RW, 1971. The epidemiology of intestinal parasites of importance in the United States. South. Med. Bull. 59:20–30

Ramachandran S, Gam AA, Neva FA, 1997. Molecular differences between several species of *Strongyloides* and comparison of selected isolates of *S. stercoralis* using a polymerase chain reaction-linked restriction fragment length polymorphism approach. Am. J. Trop. Med. Hyg. 56:61–65

Reddy KR, Laurain AR, Thomas E, 1983. Strongyloidiasis: when to suspect the wily nematode. Postgrad. Med. 74:273–282

Robinson RD, Lindo JF, Neva FA, Gam AA, Vogel P, Terry SI, Cooper ES, 1984. Immunoepidemiologic studies of *Strongyloides stercoralis* and human T lymphotropic virus type I infections in Jamaica. J. Infect. Dis. 169:692–696

Roeckel IE, Lyons ET, 1977. Cutaneous larva migrans, an occupational disease. Ann. Clin. Lab. Sci. 7:405–410

Ronan SG, Reddy RL, Manaligod JR, Alexander J, Fu T, 1984. Disseminated strongyloidiasis presenting as purpura. J. Am. Acad. Dermatol. 21:1123–1125

Rubin HL, Woodard JC, 1974. Equine infection with *Micronema deletrix*. JAVMA 165:256–258

Sandground JH, 1926. Biological studies on the life-cycle in the genus *Strongyloides* Grassi, 1879. Am. J. Hyg. 6:337–383

Sato Y, Kobayashi J, Toma H, Shiroma Y, 1995. Efficacy of stool examination for detection of *Strongyloides* infection. Am. J. Trop. Med. Hyg. 53:248–250

Scaglia M, Brustia R, Bernuzzi AM, Strosselli M, Malfitano A, Capelli D, 1984. Autochthonous strongyloidiasis in Italy: an epidemiological and clinical review of 150 cases. Bull. Soc. Pathol. Exot. 77:328–332

Schad GA, Aikens LM, Smith G, 1989. *Strongyloides stercoralis*: is there a canonical migratory route through the host? J. Parasitol. 75:740–749

Schainberg L, Scheinberg MA, 1989. Recovery of *Strongyloides stercoralis* by bronchoalveolar lavage in a patient with acquired immunodeficiency syndrome. Am. J. Med. 87:486

Schanaider A, Madi K, 1996. Intestinal strongyloidiasis mimicking a tumour. Eur. J. Surg. 162:429–430

Schindzielorz A, Edberg SC, Bia FJ, 1991. *Strongyloides stercoralis* hyperinfection and central nervous system involvement in a patient with relapsing polychondritis. South. Med. J. 84:1055–1057

Seabury JH, Abadie S, Savoy F Jr, 1971. Pulmonary strongyloidiasis with lung abscess: ineffectiveness of thiabendazole therapy. Am. J. Trop. Med. Hyg. 20:209–211

Shadduck JA, Ubelaker J, Telford VQ, 1979. *Micronema deletrix* meningoencephalitis in an adult man. Am. J. Clin. Pathol. 72:640–643

Shiroma Y, 1964. Studies on human strongyloidiasis in Okinawa, Ryukyu. Kagoshima Med. J. 34:243–246

Simpson WG, Gerhardstein DC, Thompson JR, 1984. Disseminated *Strongyloides stercoralis* infection. South. Med. J. 86:821–825

Sorvillo F, Mori K, Sewake W, Fishman L, 1983. Correspondence. Sexual transmission of *Strongyloides stercoralis* among homosexual men. Br. J Vener. Dis. 59:342

Spalding MG, Greiner EC, Green SL, 1990. *Halicephalobus (Micronema) deletrix* infection in two half-sibling foals. JAVMA. 196:1127–1129

Sprott V, Selby CD, Ispahani P, Toghill PJ, 1987. Indigenous strongyloidiasis in Nottingham. Br. Med. J. 294:741–742

Stemmermann GN, 1967. Strongyloidiasis in migrants. Pathological and clinical considerations. Gastroenterology 53:59–70

Strazzella WD, Safirstein BH, 1989. Asthma due to parasitic infestation. N.J. Med 86:947–949

Sukhavat K, Morakote N, Chaiwong P, Piangjai S, 1994. Comparative efficacy of four methods for the detection of *Strongyloides stercoralis* in human stool specimens. Ann. Trop. Med. Parasitol. 88:95–96

Tanaka H, 1966. Genus *Strongyloides*. In: Morishita KKYMH (ed), *Progress of Medical Parasitology in Japan*, Vol 3. Tokyo: Meguro Parasitological Museum, pp. 591–638

Tham KT, 1979. *Strongyloides* gastritis—report of a case. J. Trop. Med. Hyg. 82:21–22

Venizelos PC, Lopata M, Bardawil WA, Sharp JT, 1980. Respiratory failure due to *Strongyloides stercoralis* in a patient with a renal transplant. Chest 78:104–106

Vince JD, Ashford RW, Gratten MJ, Bana Koiri J, 1979. *Strongyloides* species infestation in young infants of Papua, New Guinea: association with generalized oedema. Papua New Guinea Med. J. 22:120–127

Viney ME, Ashford RW, Barnish G, 1991. A taxonomic study of *Strongyloides* Grassi, 1879 (Nematoda) with special reference to *Strongyloides fuelleborni* von Linstow, 1905 in man in Papua New Guinea and the description of a new subspecies. Systematic Parasitol. 18:95–109

Vishwanath S, Baker RA, Mansheim BJ, 1982. *Strongyloides* infection and meningitis in an immunocompromised host. Am. J. Trop. Med. Hyg. 31:857–858

von Kuster LC, Genta RM, 1984. Cutaneous manifestations of strongyloidiasis. Arch. Dermatol. 124:1826–1830

Wachter RM, Burke AM, MacGregor RR, 1984. *Strongyloides stercoralis* hyperinfection masquerading as cerebral vasculitis. Arch. Neurol. 41:1213–1216

Walzer PD, Milder JE, Banwell JG, Kilgore G, Klein M, Parker R, 1982. Epidemiologic features of *Strongyloides stercoralis* infection in an endemic area of the United States. Am. J. Trop. Med. Hyg. 31:313–319

Wang T, Reyes CV, Kathuria S, Strinden C, 1980. Diagnosis of *Strongyloides stercoralis* in sputum cytology. Acta Cytol. 24:40–43

Witenberg G, 1951. Some unusual observations on helminthiasis in Israel. Harefuah 41:178–180

Wurtz R, Mirot M, Fronda G, Peters C, Kocka F, 1994. Short report: gastric infection by *Strongyloides stercoralis*. Am. J. Trop. Med. Hyg. 51:339–340

Yassin SM, Garret M, 1980. Parasites in cytodiagnosis: a case report of *Strongyloides stercoralis* in Papanicolaou smears of gastric aspirate, with a review of the literature. Acta Cytol. 24:539–544

Yim Y, Kikkawa Y, Tanowitz H, Wittner M, 1984. Fatal strongyloidiasis in Hodgkin's disease after immunosuppressive therapy. J. Trop. Med. Hyg. 73:245–249

13

STRONGYLIDA—HOOKWORMS, *OESOPHAGOSTOMUM, TRICHOSTRONGYLUS, ANGIOSTRONGYLUS,* AND OTHERS

The order Strongylida has four superfamilies that contain all the families and genera of a group of nematodes characterized by a bursa on the posterior end of the male; thus they are known as the *bursate* nematodes. The bursa in some groups is visible with the naked eye, giving the worm the appearance of a broken stick with several splinters extending out of the broken end. These "splinters" are the rays that support the bursa, a bell-shaped, symmetrical structure produced by the cuticle of the worm, which contains the anus and the copulatory portion of the genital system. The bursa's function during copulation is to keep the male attached to the female. The Strongylida is one of the largest groups of nematodes occurring naturally in most vertebrates, and humans have at least two species of their own. In addition, humans have about three dozen other species that have been reported at various times as zoonotic infections. For didactic purposes, members of the Strongylida that are important in human medicine are classified as follows (Beaver et al. 1984):

Superfamily: Ancylostomatoidea
 Family: Ancylostomatidae
  Genus: *Ancylostoma* (*A. duodenale, A. ceylanicum, A. braziliense,* and *A. caninum*)
 Family: Buonostomidae
  Genus: *Necator* (*N. americanus*)

Superfamily: Strongyloidea
 Family: Chabertiidae
  Genus: *Ternidens* (*T. deminutus*)
 Family: Oesophagostomidae
  Genus: *Oesophagostomum* (*Oe. stephanostomum, Oe. aculeatum, Oe. bifurcum* [= *brumpti*], *Oe. oesophagostomum,* and *Oe. venulosum*)
 Family: Syngamidae
  Genus: *Mammomonogamus* (*M. laryngeus*)

Superfamily: Trichostrongyloidea
 Family: Trichostrongylidae

Genus: *Trichostrongylus* (*T. orientalis*, *T. colubriformis*, *T. vitrinus*, *T. probolurus*, *T. axei*, *T. brevis*, *T. skrjabini*, and *T. instabilis*)

Superfamily: Metastrongyloidea

Family: Metastrongylidae

Genus: *Angiostrongylus* (*A. cantonensis* and *A. costaricensis*)

Each of these genera is discussed in this chapter because their members produce important diseases in humans. Some, like *Ancylostoma duodenale* and *Necator americanus*, the two parasites of humans, are responsible for large numbers of cases in tropical and subtropical areas. The others are nonhuman parasites and occur less often as zoonotic infections usually restricted to specific areas, where they produce important morbidity and in some instances mortality. Most of the bursate nematodes found in humans produce infections of the gastrointestinal tract; one species, *Mammomonogamus laryngeus*, is found in the upper respiratory tract; and species of *Angiostrongylus* occur in the circulatory system and the tissues. Most strongylids infecting humans have life cycles in soil, from which infective larvae reach the skin of their hosts; others, like the angiostrongylids, require intermediate hosts.

Hookworms—Ancylostomiasis and Necatoriasis

As stated above, the important hookworms of humans are *A. duodenale* and *N. americanus*, which together with *A. ceylanicum* from animals are parasites of the small intestine. In addition to these species, many other species of animal hookworms parasitize humans, producing zoonotic infections that manifest mostly as cutaneous larva migrans (see Chapter 14). One biologic characteristic of some species of hookworms is the capacity of their larval stages to remain "arrested" in the skeletal muscles and other tissues of the definitive host. The larvae in the tissues can produce infections in the fetus or can mature to adults at a later time under suitable conditions. The same thing happens when larvae enter abnormal hosts. In this case, the larvae mature to adults only when the abnormal host is ingested by the natural definitive host of the parasite. Whether human infections occur by ingestion of animal meat needs demonstration; this route of infection is possible. This phenomenon, known as *paratenism*, is the biologic basis for the production of visceral larva migrans (see Chapter 17). The main morphologic characteristic of the members of the superfamily Ancylostomatoidea is a wide globular buccal capsule bearing teeth in *Ancylostoma* and cutting plates in *Necator* (Beaver et al. 1984). These genera belong to two different families (see above) because their morphologic characteristics and their life cycles are different.

Necator is parasitic in herbivores and *Ancylostoma* in carnivores. *Necator* is less virulent than *Ancylostoma*, probably because humans acquired *Necator* earlier in their evolution, before they became scavengers of dead animals and later hunters. This pattern of evolution makes humans suitable for the acquisition of *Ancylostoma* when they became carnivores.

Hookworms have produced human disease since time immemorial in communities in where human excreta was not disposed of properly or was used as fertilizer. The infection was common in coal miners of Europe and the United States, who suffered severe morbidity. Only after the discovery of the worms and the elucidation of their life cycles were effective control measures slowly adopted. In recent decades, the importance of hookworms as agents of human disease has declined in most parts of the world because the conditions for their endemicity have decreased. This has happened not only because of control campaigns but also because of steady improvement in socioeconomic conditions in many parts of the world. Nevertheless, areas of high endemicity, limited mostly to the poor rural areas of the tropics, still exist.

Morphology. The adults of the species regularly found in humans vary from 0.7 to 1.3 cm in length, the largest being *A. duodenale*. Grossly, the female worms have a cylindrical, whitish, slightly curved body, while the males are straight and bear the bursa at the posterior end. On gross examination, the worms are identified easily as hookworms. However, determination of the species is difficult and requires knowledge, a microscope, well-fixed and well-prepared specimens, and especially the males to determine the minute difference in the shape of the bursa's rays. Because hookworms are rarely identified in tissue sections, their microanatomy is outside this discussion. A recently developed polymerase chain reaction distinguishes the two human hookworms and *A. caninum* and can detect mixed infections (Hawdon, 1996).

The other stage of hookworms important in human disease is the eggs evacuated in the stools. The eggs are delicate, with a thin, transparent shell containing a mass of dark granular cells. The cells divide rapidly, and in stool samples left at room temperature, tadpole embryos develop in few hours. The eggs measure about 60 to 76 × 35 to 40 μm (Fig. 13–4 A–B), and in the species that infect humans, they are identical. Therefore, the usual diagnosis of hookworm eggs, when they are found in stools is correct.

Life Cycle and Biology. The adult females in the upper part of the small intestine lay nonembryonated eggs that are evacuated with the intestinal contents (Fig. 13–4 A–B). In soil with optimal moisture and temperature conditions, larvae develop in the eggs and hatch in about 2 days as rhabditiform larvae. They feed in soil and evolve as free-living larvae, molting twice and becoming infective filariform larvae in about 7 to 10 days. Infective larvae enter the skin of susceptible hosts, travel through the circulation, and arrive in the lungs, where they rapidly break the capillary vessels to enter the alveolar spaces. They then migrate to the upper respiratory airways, the epiglottis, the esophagus, stomach, and finally the small intestine, where they mature to adults (Fig. 13–1). Passage through the lungs occurs 3 to 5 days after penetration of the skin by the larvae. The adults live in the intestine for periods ranging from 1 to 17 years, the last figure confirmed in a light *Necator* infection (Beaver, 1988). From egg to egg, the hookworm cycle takes approximately 6 weeks. A fundamental difference between the life cycles of *Ancylostoma* and *Necator* is that if the larvae of *Ancylostoma* are ingested and reach the small intestine, they develop to adults directly in the intestine, omitting the pulmonary migration. *Necator* has obligatory migration through the lungs.

In an experimental infection with *A. duodenale* in a human volunteer, a slight increase in the eosinophil count (to about 600/mm) occurred during an 8-month period; eggs were not present in the stools. At the eighth

month of infection the eosinophil count rose rapidly (to over 5000/mm), and eggs appeared in the stools. The number of eggs per gram of feces reached over 2500 during the 75th week after the infection (Nawalinski, Schad, 1974). This experiment, and others, demonstrate that larvae of *A. duodenale* have an arrested phase in the tissues, an adaptation of the worm to areas where rainy and dry seasons alternate (Schad, 1991; Schad et al. 1973). In these cases, the worms acquired toward the end of the rainy season are arrested and migrate to the intestine months later, coinciding with the next rainy season favorable for development of the eggs in the environment (Schad, 1991; Schad et al. 1973). An arrested phase in the tissues also explains the transmammary passage of the infection to infants.

Geographic Distribution and Epidemiology. The geographic distribution of hookworms is mostly tropical and subtropical. *Necator americanus* predominates in the African and American continents (Fig. 13–2); *Ancylostoma duodenale* predominates in southern Europe, northern Africa, and parts of the Middle East (Fig. 13–3); and *Necator* and *A. duodenale* overlap in the Asian and Southeast Asian countries. *Ancylostoma ceylanicum* occurs sporadically, usually producing infections with a low worm burden in China, Southeast Asia, and Surinam (WHO, 1981). The prevalence of hookworm infection depends on the suitability of the soil for development of the larvae, contamination of the environment with human excreta, and the amount of contact between soil and the skin or mouth. Humans are the sole hosts for *A. duodenale* and *N. americanus*, and in endemic areas humans develop a relationship with these hookworms that results in infections with low worm burdens that are well tolerated; heavy symptomatic infections are unusual. In the latter circumstances, the parasite in heavily infected individuals must be identified in the laboratory on the basis of the egg count in the stools. Surveys of populations in endemic areas without egg counts have little meaning; assessment of the impact of the infection in any given population requires the separation of individuals with light, medium, and heavy infections.

Hookworms are soil-transmitted helminths that in most tropical areas infect their hosts continuously throughout the year; in areas with rainy and dry seasons, they produce infections mainly during the rainy season. Epidemiologically, they are closely associated with other soil-transmitted helminths, especially *Ascaris lumbricoides* and *Trichuris trichiura*, which are commonly found infecting the same hosts. In endemic areas the prevalence of hookworm increases with age,

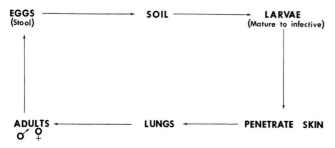

Fig. 13–1. Hookworms, schematic life cycle. Note that species of *Ancylostoma* can be acquired either by ingestion of larvae, without requiring pulmonary migration (see text), or through the skin.

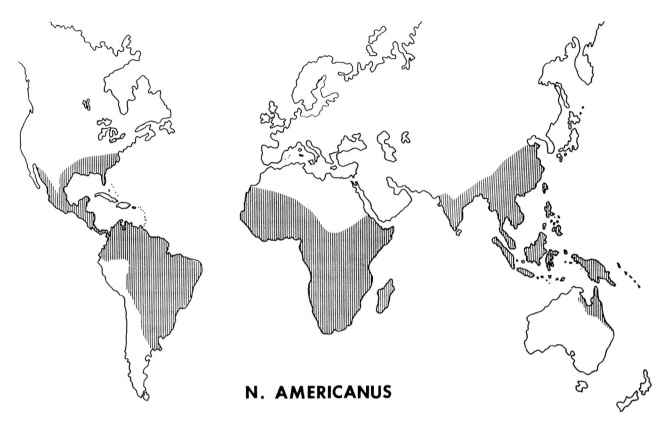

Fig. 13–2. Approximate geographic distribution of *Necator americanus*.

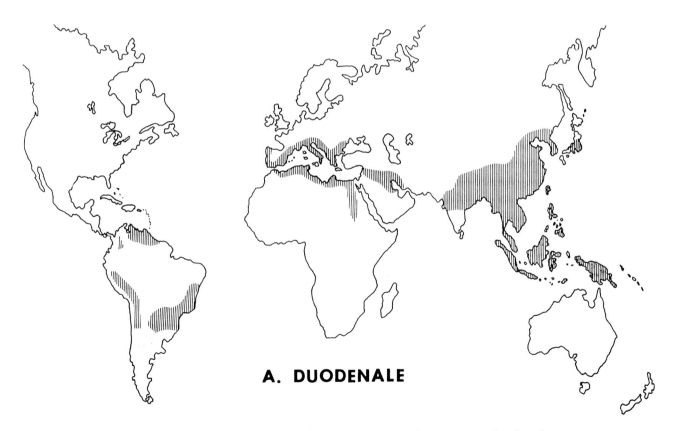

Fig. 13–3. Approximate geographic distribution of *Ancylostoma duodenale*.

as does the worm burden. Heavy infections are prob ably acquired under natural conditions by some indi viduals, a few worms at a time. A study of a popula tion with *Necator* infections showed that in a treated group that reacquired the infection, the infection rose to its original level in about 2 years; the average num ber of worms gained per person per year was eight or nine (Quinnell et al. 1993). Infection by ingestion of infective *A. duodenale* larvae with contaminated food occurs often, but as stated earlier, *Necator* must enter the skin to complete its life cycle. Infants in endemic areas acquire *A. duodenale* infections through their mother's milk (Nwosu, 1978) but not *Necator* infec tions. The failure of *A. duodenale* to become widely es tablished in the southeastern United States is believed to be due to its greater dependence on the oral route for transmission (WHO, 1964). The rate of prevalences in endemic areas can be up to 90%; in Europe as re cently as 1956, the rate in coal miners in Portugal was 75%, but the importance of the infection throughout Europe is now minimal. The prevalence of *Necator* in a community of Zimbabwe was 80% in the adult pop ulation. The average number of worms per person was about 8, and the maximum number in one patient was 70 (Bradley et al. 1992). These are very low, well-tol erated infections. In Bali, Indonesia, as expected, the prevalence of hookworm infection was higher in wet than in dry environments, and three-fourths of the in fections were light to very light (Bakta et al. 1993). In the United States, a survey of school children revealed prevalences in different counties varying between 0% and 12%; of a total of 172 children infected, 48 had moderate to heavy infections (Martin, 1972a). Similar survey in adults living in 27 counties revealed that 16% of whites and 8% of blacks were infected; the preva lence in men was twice that in women (Martin, 1972b). In McCreary County, Kentucky, the rate of infection in school children was 15% (Gloor et al. 1970). More recently, there was an outbreak of hookworm infection in military personnel during operations in Grenada (Kelley et al. 1989). In general, in most areas of the world, especially in cities, prevalence rates and worm burdens have steadily declined due to improved hy giene.

Pathogenesis. The ancylostomids in the small intes tine become attached to the mucosa when the worm "sucks" a tuft of mucosal enterocytes into the spa cious buccal cavity. The tuft of cells is digested and their products are ingested by the worm, a process that is repeated every 10 minutes (*color plate* VII A; Carroll et al. 1984; Kalkofen, 1970). The process of attaching to the mucosa for feeding produces lacera tions and rupture of capillaries that bleed. This bleed ing is aggravated by an anticoagulant (ancylostom atin) produced by the worm, as shown in *A. caninum* (Eiff, 1966). This anticoagulant is a 8.7 kDa peptide that appears to inhibit factor Xa (Cappello et al. 1995). The site of the worm's attachment continues to bleed for some time after the worm moves to an other place. Blood lost as food for the worm proper is insignificant (Kalkofen, 1970), but since attach ment to the mucosa changes constantly throughout the life of the worm, the many lacerations produced result in significant bleeding. The degree of laceration depends on the age of the infection and the degree of crowding of the worms; crowding, in turn, depends both on the number of worms and on their distribu tion in the intestine (Krupp, 1961). Attachment to the mucosa is more active in the early stages of the in fection when maturation to adulthood and synchro nous copulation are occurring (Beaver et al. 1964). The effects of mucosal bleeding depend on the nutri tional status of the host (Tripathy et al. 1971). This bleeding eventually results in a hypochromic micro cytic anemia referred to as *hookworm disease*.

The amount of intestinal bleeding also depends on the species and on the number of worms in the intes tine at any given time. The number of worms in the intestine can be estimated roughly from the total num ber of eggs eliminated in the feces every 24 hours di vided by the number of eggs laid by a single female. No good estimates are available for the number of eggs laid by *A. duodenale*, but about 25,000 to 30,000 per female is the figure most quoted. In light infec tions with *Necator*, the females lay about 20,000 to 50,000 eggs per day, depending on the age of the worm. This is a more reliable figure and corresponds roughly to 500 eggs per gram of stool per worm in young worms, declining to 200 eggs per gram per senescent female (Beaver, 1955). The amount of bleed ing in a given patient is estimated on the basis of the number of eggs per gram of feces in 24 hours (Layrisse, Roche, 1964).

Clinical Findings. Hookworm infections occur equally in men and women if exposure is equal, but because men work outside the house, the clinical infection is seen mostly in young adult men, less often in children. The clinical manifestations of ancylostomiasis are sometimes first noted at the site of larval penetration through the skin, a form of cutaneous larva migrans known as *ground itch* (see Chapter 14). The second set of symp toms (Loeffler's syndrome) occurs in about 70% of in dividuals due to the migration of larvae through the lungs (see Chapter 16).

The clinical symptoms of the intestinal phase vary with the number of worms in the intestine, the species, the duration of the infection, and the nutritional status of the host, and usually consist of fatigue, nausea, vomiting, and abdominal pain (Rogers, Dammin, 1946). Diarrhea without mucus or blood can also be a symptom; abdominal pain occurs in 86% of patients, weight loss in 80%, and vomiting in 58%. Sporadic cases in adults have presented with significant blood loss through the gastrointestinal tract (De La Riva et al. 1981; Hollander et al. 1973; McDowell, 1981; Naik et al. 1976; Walker, Bellmaine, 1975). However, this condition is mostly seen in neonates and is sometimes fatal (5% mortality in a large series in China) (Alvarez-Pagan, Torrez De Vega, 1963; Yu et al. 1995). The infections in China were produced exclusively by *A. duodenale*. High peripheral eosinophilia is usually present during the migratory phase of the worms and lasts for 3 to 4 months, after which it begins decreasing until the eosinophil level becomes normal. Thus, during the chronic phase of hookworm infection, there usually is no significant eosinophilia, and if reinfection occurs, the eosinophilia does not reach the peak of the first infection (Lavier, Brumpt, 1944). Chronic hookworm infection, without gastrointestinal symptoms, is characterized by profound microcytic hypochromic anemia due to chronic blood loss (Borrero et al. 1961; see above), the aforementioned hookworm disease.

Wakana Disease. A constellation of pulmonary and intestinal symptoms, seen in Japanese patients during late summer and early autumn soon after ingesting green vegetables, is known by the Japanese name *Wakana-Byo* (*Waka* = green; *Na* = vegetable; and *Byo* = disease) (Harada, 1962). These symptoms are due to infective larvae of *A. duodenale* ingested with the vegetables and consist of three clinical stages. (*1*) The digestive stage, soon after consumption of the vegetables, includes abdominal pain, salivation, nausea, and vomiting. (*2*) The oropharyngeal stage consists of dryness, itching, and pain in the throat, dryness of the mouth, and hoarseness. (*3*) The most important stage consists of pulmonary symptoms of persistent asthmatic productive cough, dyspnea, fever, hypereosinophilia, and pulmonary infiltration, lasting for several days (Harada, 1962). The digestive symptoms are due to larvae reaching the intestine and developing directly into adults. The oropharyngeal symptoms are due to larvae entering the buccal and pharyngeal mucosae and migrating to the lungs to complete the cycle. The

pulmonary symptoms are due to passage of the larvae through the respiratory tree to the intestine. Examination of the sputum reveals the larvae. On follow-up, these patients invariably develop ancylostomiasis (Harada, 1962; Matsusaki, 1966).

Ancylostoma caninum. Asymptomatic human infections with adult *A. caninum* worms have been recorded, usually after the worms were expelled by treatment, recovered, and properly classified (Lie, Bras, 1950; Manalang, 1925; Mao, 1945; Pereira-Barreto, Amaral, 1944). In these infections, only two or three worms were recovered from the stools in the laboratory; in one case, the worms were brought to the physician (in these instances, there is always the question of whether the worm was truly in the patient's stool). The rarity of these reports is striking (about five patients in the most of this century) because parasitologists commonly examine recovered worms to determine their species. There is also a report of three worms of *A. duodenale* in the rectum recovered during sigmoidoscopy from a patient with symptoms consistent with a heavy hookworm infection and typical eggs in the stools (Yong et al. 1992).

Ancylostoma caninum Enterocolitis. In recent years, a number of patients living in Brisbane, Australia, have been reported, either individually or as series, with an eosinophilic enterocolitis attributed to *A. caninum* (Croese, 1988; Croese et al. 1990, 1994a, 1994b; Prociv, Croese, 1990; Walker et al. 1995). Two such infections were reported in the United States. No worms were recovered, leaving only the patients' history, speculation, and positive serology as the basis for the diagnosis (Khoshoo et al. 1994, 1995). The age of the Australian patients varied from 9 to 86 years (mean about 43 years of age), with a male:female ratio of 2:1 (Walker et al. 1995). The clinical presentation consisted of abdominal pain, small bowel obstruction, diarrhea, rectal bleeding, and high peripheral eosinophilia. Endoscopic findings were mucosal edema with inflammation, ulceration, mucosal nodules, and bowel stricture. In addition, surgical exploration revealed, lymphadenopathy and ascitis in some cases, and some patients required bowel resection; all of these clinical findings were non-specific. The resected specimens were portions of ileum, large intestine, and appendix. Their histologic appearance varied with the area studied; the greatest changes were seen in the stenotic area of bowel. These changes consisted of dilated lymphatics, congestion, and heavy infiltration by eosinophils; the serosal surface showed fibrin deposition, inflammation, and reactive mesothelial cells. The draining lymph nodes showed numerous eosinophils in the sinuses, medullary cords, and paracortical areas. In a few instances, an area of attachment of a worm showed superficial lacerations, villous atrophy, and crypt cell hyperplasia (Walker et al. 1995). In even fewer cases, a worm recovered from some patients was identified as *A. caninum*. Serologic studies of patients diagnosed clinically with the condition showed that they had specific antibodies against *A. caninum* larvae, while diverse control groups were negative (Croese et al. 1994b; Loukas et al. 1992, 1994). Further studies of this condition, including a more precise description of the recovered worms stating the basis for their identification, as well as the relationship of the worm to the lesion, are necessary. Moreover, the occurrence of the infection in a single geographic area needs a rational explanation that likely rests on the worm, the habits of the exposed population, or both.

Pathology. The gross pathologic changes of the small intestine in hookworm infections consist of focal hemorrhages in the duodenum, jejunum, and ileum; the parasites are seen attached to the mucosa throughout these organs. *Necator americanus* is usually found in the duodenum and jejunum, and *A. duodenale* inhabits the jejunum and proximal ileum (Rep, 1975). The attachment site shows the portion of mucosa in the buccal cavity. The lamina propria below the attachment site shows intense infiltration by neutrophils, eosinophils, and plasma cells (Carroll et al. 1984).

Few studies of the microscopic lesions in the human intestine are available. One study of intestinal biopsy specimens from 22 heavily infected individuals (more than 5000 hookworm eggs per gram of feces) showed few nonspecific changes in 18, mainly slightly dilated crypts, decreased mucus production, and minimal epithelial cell turnover (Layrisse et al. 1964). The biopsy specimen from 1 one of these 18 subjects contained one adult hookworm, with no inflammatory reaction of the surrounding tissues. Biopsy specimens from the other four subjects showed marked mucosal atrophy in one, flattening and fusion of villi in another, and infiltration by polymorphonuclear cells in two. Another study of patients with necatoriasis showed similar results, and the report stated that there was no relationship between the severity of the clinical symptoms and the changes in the mucosa. However, no egg counts were made to determine the severity of the infection (Cantor et al. 1966). Thus, it appears that on the basis of these studies, the histologic changes in the small intestine in hookworm infections are minimal and inespecific.

Mucosal and submucosal nodules or abscesses measuring up to 1.0 cm in diameter and containing an adult

hookworm (*A. duodenale* or *A. ceylanicum*) have been described (Biagi et al. 1957; Elmes, McAdam, 1954).

Diagnosis. In the clinical laboratory, hookworm infection is diagnosed by recovery and identification of the eggs in the stools. All hookworm eggs need careful measurement and should fall within the range of 60 to 76 × 35 to 40 μm (Fig. 13–4 *A–B*). Care is needed to distinguish these eggs from those of related species such as *Ternidens deminutus* (see below) and *Trichostrongylus* (see below). Hookworms are rarely diagnosed in histologic sections. In stool samples left at room temperature for more than 24 hours, hookworm eggs develop into larvae that begin to hatch in 48 hours. The larvae measure 250 to 300 μm in length, with a long, narrow buccal chamber and a small genital primordium (see Fig. 12–11). These larvae should be distinguished from those of *Strongyloides stercoralis* (see Chapter 12) and from those of free-living nematodes sometimes occurring in stool samples contaminated with soil.

The standard direct fecal smears and concentration techniques used in the clinical laboratory are still the methods used for diagnosis. Egg counts made in the laboratory and reported to the clinician are necessary for assessment of the intensity of the infection. The Kato thick smear, which examines about 65 mg of feces and allows quantification of the eggs, is an easy and convenient method (Beaver et al. 1984; Martin, Beaver, 1968).

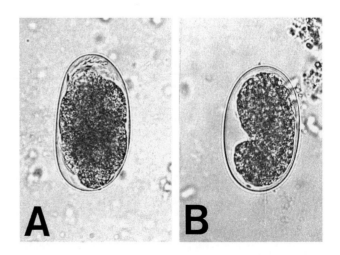

Fig. 13–4. Hookworm eggs in human stools, unstained. *A*, Recently passed egg, ×495. *B*, Several hours later showing the beginning of larva formation (tadpole stage), ×55.

Oesophagostomum—Oesophagostomiasis

The genus *Oesophagostomum* has many species parasitic in primates in Africa, Asia, and South America; swine and sheep are also hosts of the parasite. The genus *Oesophagostomum* is related to the hookworms, and the worms grossly resemble them in form and size. Close study reveals the differences in the buccal cavity, which is cylindrical and has a crown of bristles, the corona radiata. The anterior end of the worm has a semiglobose appearance due to transversal constriction of the cuticle just behind the anterior end.

Life Cycle and Biology. The adult parasites are about two to three times larger than hookworms; they live attached to the mucosa of the large intestine, where they produce eggs that are evacuated with feces. In appropriate soil, the eggs embryonate and produce larvae that live in and become infective in soil. The larvae require ingestion by the appropriate hosts to produce the infection. In the colon the developing worms bury themselves in the wall, forming an abscess where they mature into adults; after maturation, the adult worms leave the abscess, attach to the colonic mucosa, and start laying eggs. The eggs in soil develop to infective larvae, and humans acquire the infection by ingesting these infective larvae from soil or with food or water. The number of eggs produced by each female during a 24-hour period is estimated at 16 to 68 per gram of feces.

Geographic Distribution and Epidemiology. Human infections are known in Uganda (Anthony, McAdam, 1972; Elmes, McAdam, 1954; Welchman, 1966), Togo and Ghana (Haaf, Van Soest, 1964; Krepel et al. 1992; Polderman et al. 1991), Rhodesia (Gordon et al. 1969), Sudan (Jacques, Lynch, 1964), Kenya (Kaminsky, Ndinya-Achola, 1977), Nigeria (Leiper, 1911), the Ivory Coast (Chabaud, Lariviere, 1958), Indonesia (Kwo, 1972; Tan, Lie, 1953), and Brazil (Railliet, Henry, 1909; Thomas, 1910). In Nova Scotia, Canada, *Oe. venulosum* eggs and adults were recovered after treatment from the feces of nine siblings living on a farm (Embil et al. 1982). Recent studies in Togo and Ghana have shown that the prevalence of *Oe. bifurcum* varies among different communities, with the highest prevalence being 59%. The infection usually occurs in association with hookworm; it is uncommon in children less than 5 years of age, and women are more likely to be infected than men (Krepel et al. 1992; Polderman et al. 1991). In areas of high endemicity, the prevalence of the infection increased rapidly from 3 to 10 years of age, at which point it levels off (Krepel et al. 1992). The transmission pattern closely follows that of the hookworm and occurs mainly during the rainy season (Krepel et al. 1995).

Clinical Findings. The only known clinical symptoms of oesophagostomiasis are those produced by the immature worms while developing in the intestinal wall, serosa, or peritoneal cavity. All these cases are acute, with a gradual onset, continuous pain, and tenderness, often with guarding in the right lower quadrant, resulting in the need for surgical intervention. Some patients have vomiting and slight fever. On clinical examination, a mass is palpable in the abdomen. Laboratory tests are normal except for a slight eosinophilia (Anthony, McAdam, 1972). One patient presented with marked rectal bleeding (Leoutsakos et al. 1977). The condition is one of continuous deterioration necessitating exploratory surgery. Resection of an inflammatory tumor within the wall of the terminal ileum, ileocecal region, colon, mesentery, or abdominal wall is usually necessary. The clinical symptoms produced by worms after they leave the abscesses in the wall and attach to the mucosa not known. The difficulties are due to the common coexistence in patients of hookworms and *Oesophagostomum*.

Pathology. Most descriptions of the gross and microscopic changes of oesophagostomiasis are based on surgically resected specimens. The lesion is characterized as an inflammatory mass of the gut (*color plate* VII *B*). In some patients, multiple masses are present (Barrowclough, Crome, 1979; Leoutsakos et al. 1977); in others, the entire colon is affected (Jacques, Lynch, 1964). In the resected portion of intestine with the mass, measuring about 4 to 6 cm in diameter, the surface of the mucosa is usually normal. However, the wall is markedly thickened and usually shows one or more abscesses, 1 to 2 cm in diameter, filled with necrotic debris and sometimes with the parasite. The abscesses are located in the wall, in the submucosa, or on the peritoneal surface. In some cases there is a track leading from the abscess down into the muscular layer. The surrounding lymph nodes are enlarged; the peritoneum shows focal peritonitis; and on occasion an *Oesophagostomum* worm has been found crawling on the peritoneal surface during surgery (Fig. 13–5 *A*). In one patient the parasite was recovered from a subcutaneous nodule on his back; the nodule had lasted for 9 months without producing symptoms but had recently become larger, prompting the patient to consult his physician (Ross et al. 1989).

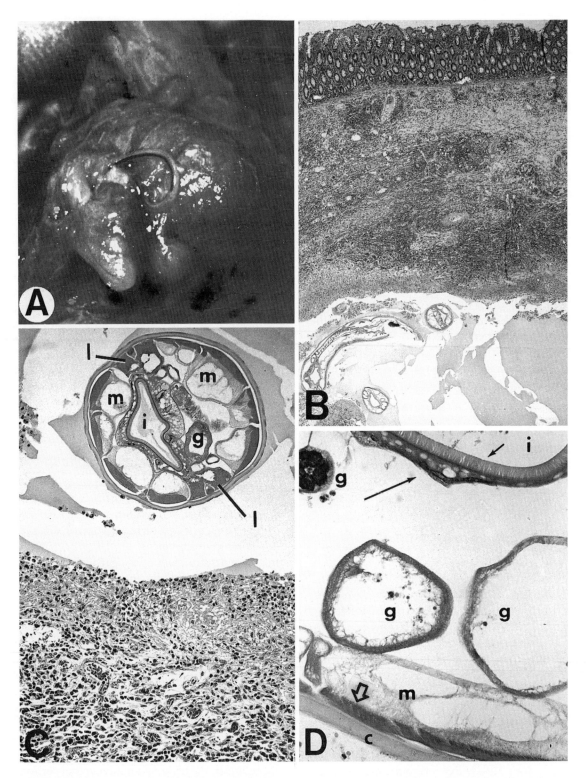

Fig. 13–5. *Oesophagostomum* lesions in humans. *A*, Appendix of a patient undergoing surgical resection showing acute inflammation and an *Oesophagostomum* worm on the serosal surface. *B–D*. Sections stained with hematoxylin and eosin stain. *B*, Low-power view of a colon with an abscess within the wall, with the worm at its center, ×12. *C*, Higher magnification showing the worm with some of its internal organs: i, intestine; g, gonads; m, muscle cells; l, lateral cords, ×70. *D*, Higher magnification showing some detail of the worm: i, intestine with fused cells (long arrows) and a well-developed brush border (short arrow); g, gonads; m, muscle cell with low contractile elements (open arrow); c, cuticle, ×280. (*A* courtesy of P.P. Anthony, M.D., Area Department of Pathology, Exeter, England.)

The gross lesions produced by *Oesophagostomum* are of three types: (*1*) a mass consisting of a central abscess containing the living worm (Fig. 13–5 *B–D* and *color plate* VII *B*); (*2*) a mass with an abscess and tracts but with no parasite (Fig. 13–6 *A–B*); or (*3*) an inflammatory mass on the serosal surface, omentum, or abdominal wall, adherent to surrounding structures, with no parasite (Fig. 13–6 *C–D*; Anthony, McAdam, 1972).

Microscopically, the lesion has central necrosis and organization toward the periphery, with granulation tissue, macrophages, and chronic inflammation (Fig. 13–6 *C–D*). Tissue eosinophils are present in small to moderate numbers, and Charcot-Leyden crystals are often abundant. In some cases, cross sections of the parasite are seen (Fig. 13–5 *B–D*); lesions involving the omentum have fat necrosis (Fig. 13–6 *C–D*).

Diagnosis. The clinical diagnosis of *Oesophagostomum* infection is difficult because the eggs of the hookworm and *Oesophagostomum* cannot be separated (Krepel, Polderman, 1992). Moreover, as stated previously, the two infections often coexist. Coprocultures of stool samples and study of the infective larvae are necessary for proper identification of either genus, but the species are impossible to separate on the basis of the characteristics of the larvae (Krepel et al. 1995). The guidelines provided by Little should be followed for proper identification (WHO, 1981), and worm burdens can be estimated on the basis of the number of larvae recovered in the cultures (Krepel et al. 1995). The serologic diagnosis based on enzyme-linked immunosorbent assay tests for immunoglobulin G4 (IgG4) is specific in 95% of cases (Polderman et al. 1993).

On histologic sections, the only possible identification of the parasite is to the level of the genus *Oesophagostomum*. In areas where cases are detected regularly, the specific diagnosis in surgical specimens lacking the worms is often presumptive. Exact species identification requires recovery of male worms and their study in toto. It is suggested that human infection by *Oesophagostomum* in South America is produced by *Oe. stephanostomum*; in Asia by *Oe. aculeatum*; and in Africa by *Oe. bifurcum* (= *Oe. brumpti*) and *Oe. oesophagostomum* (Beaver et al. 1984; Chabaud, Lariviere, 1958).

The worms found in cross sections are somewhat immature and are smaller than those found in the intestine. In sections they are up to 0.7 mm in diameter, depending on the degree of development. The cuticle is smooth, measuring 14 μm in average thickness; the hypodermis is thin and not easily apparent, except at the lateral cords, which show the lateral excretory ducts to be somewhat dilated (Fig. 13–5 *C–D*). There are usually two muscle cells per quadrant (Fig. 13–5 *C*), with a contractile portion that is uniformly low; and the rest of the cytoplasmic substance appears as empty spaces (Fig. 13–5 *C–D*). The most characteristic feature of the group is the intestine, formed by a syncytium of cells with a few nuclei per histologic section and a well-developed brush border (Fig. 13–5 *D*). The gonads are small tubular structures (Fig. 13–5 *C–D*), and the esophagus is muscular.

Mammomonogamus laryngeus—Gapeworm Infection

Members of the family Syngamidae are parasites of the respiratory tracts of animals, including birds, cats, and cattle, and are known as *gapeworms*. The genus *Mammomonogamus* occurs naturally in the upper airways of cats, cattle, and water buffaloes in some tropical areas. One species, *M. laryngeus*, produces sporadic infections in humans. The genus *Syngamus*, a parasite of birds, was once considered the species occurring in humans, hence the name *syngamosis* found in some texts.

Morphology and Life Cycle. The gross morphology of the parasites is striking because the male is about one-half the length of the female. Males and females attach to the tracheal mucosa by their thick-walled buccal capsule that opens directly anteriorly. In addition, the male is permanently attached in copula at the middle of the female's body by its posterior bursa, giving the two worms a Y shape (Fig. 13–7 *A*). The freshly recovered worms are red before fixation. The life cycle of *M. laryngeus* is not known, but species of the related genus *Syngamus* have earthworms as intermediate hosts for their development.

Epidemiology and Geographic Distribution. Human infections are uncommon; fewer than 100 cases have been reported. At least one-half of the cases occurred in Martinique alone (Nosanchuk et al. 1995), and only one each has occurred in the Philippines (St. John et al. 1929) and in Thailand (Pipitgool et al. 1992). Many of the infections have been diagnosed in France (Dufat et al. 1971; Junod et al. 1970; Sang et al. 1970), England (Baden et al. 1974), Canada (Leers et al. 1985), Australia (Birrell et al. 1978), and the United States (Gardiner, Schantz, 1983; Nosanchuk et al. 1995; Timmons et al. 1983; Weinstein, Molavi, 1971), either in tourists

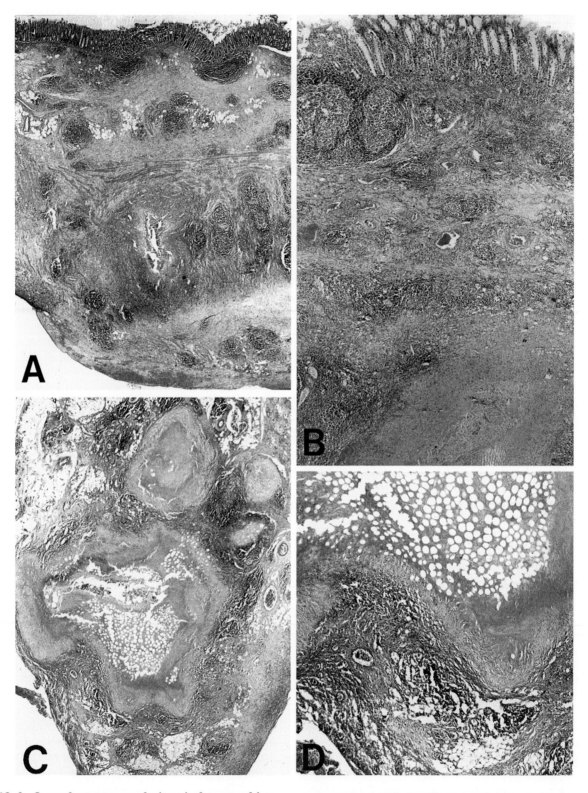

Fig. 13–6. *Oesophagostomum* lesions in humans, histologic sections stained with hematoxylin and eosin stain. *A* and *B*, Intestinal lesions with no parasite, attributed to *Oesophagostomum* in an area where cases are seen frequently. *A* ×12; *B* ×28; *C* and *D*, Omental lesions with no worm. *C* ×12; *D* ×70. (Preparations courtesy of P.P. Anthony, M.D., Area Department of Pathology, Exeter, England.)

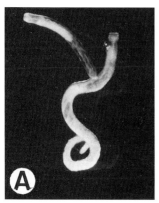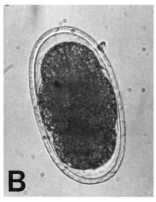

Fig. 13–7. *Mammomonogamus laryngeus*. A, Adult male and female worms *in copula*, removed at bronchoscopy from the mucosa of a bronchus of Australian woman who visited Guyana, ×6. (In: Birrel, D.J., Moorhouse, D.E., Gardner, M.A.H., and May, C.S. 1978. Chronic cough and hemoptysis due to a nematode, "*Syngamus laryngeus*." Aust. N.Z. J. Med. 8:168–170. Reproduced with permission.) B, Egg, ×465. (In: Beaver, P.C., Jung, R.C., and Cupp, E.W. 1984. *Clinical Parasitology*, 9th edition. Philadelphia, Lea & Febiger, p. 289. Reproduced with permission.)

to the Caribbean or in immigrants from that region. Countries where the infection has been reported include Martinique (Magdeleine et al. 1974; Mornex et al. 1980), Brazil (de Lara et al. 1993; Londero, Lauda, 1967; Santos et al. 1986; Severo et al. 1988), Puerto Rico (Font, 1943; Hoffman, 1932), Dominica West Indies (Grell et al. 1978), Santa Lucia (Leiper, 1913; Wells, 1951), Trinidad (Hoffman, 1932), Guayana (Leiper, 1925), and Guadaloupe (Cunnac et al. 1988).

Clinical Findings. The clinical diagnosis of gapeworm infection is very difficult; it must be considered in any patient who returns from an endemic area and presents with a dry cough, at times paroxysmal, often at night, and sometimes with scant sputum. A few individuals complain of hemoptysis and weight loss (Birrell et al. 1978), pleuritic pain (Weinstein, Molavi, 1971), and nausea (Machado De Mendonca et al. 1962). Physical examination is unremarkable; peripheral eosinophilia is up to 23% (Junod et al. 1970). If sputum is recovered, a differential count reveals up to 70% of eosinophils.

Bronchoscopic examination of the upper respiratory tract shows a red, slightly edematous mucosa and usually one pair of firmly attached parasites forming the characteristic Y shape. In one case, the worms were

found within a cyst (Gardiner, Schantz, 1983). Removal of the parasites usually results in complete remission of the symptoms in 24 hours or less.

Diagnosis. The diagnosis is made by identification of the recovered adult parasites. Examination of the patient's stool or sputum may reveal the characteristic eggs, which resemble hookworm eggs, except for the thicker shell of *Mammomonogamus* eggs (Fig. 13–7 *B*).

Trichostrongylus—Trichostrongyliasis

The genus *Trichostrongylus* has many species that infect animals, herbivorous animals, worldwide; they are economically important because of the infections they produce in cattle, sheep, goats, and other animals. Infections in humans received some attention in past decades, but the interest in trichostrongyliasis has waned in recent times, perhaps because of the decreasing number of cases or because the infection continues to be misdiagnosed as hookworm infection.

Morphology and Life Cycle. *Trichostrongylus* species are small nematodes that inhabit the small intestine, where they live embedded in the mucosa. The worms are slender and delicate, lack a buccal capsule, and have a distinct notch in the anterior portion of the body. The females lay eggs that have morphologic characteristics of the genus; no separation of the species is possible. The eggs are 90 to 95 μm in their greatest dimension (Fig. 13–8 *A–B*). They are larger than the eggs of hookworms, are tapered slightly more at each end, and have a thicker shell. The eggs are evacuated with the feces. Under proper soil and environmental conditions they embryonate, hatch, and produce infective larvae in about 60 hours. These larvae are more resistant to desiccation than those of hookworms. When ingested by the appropriate host, they develop into adult worms directly in the intestine in about 3 to 4 weeks without migrating through the lungs.

Geographic Distribution and Epidemiology. Infections in humans occur in large numbers in certain areas, but they have been described sporadically worldwide, especially when the infection is looked for. The species responsible for human infections are *T. colu-*

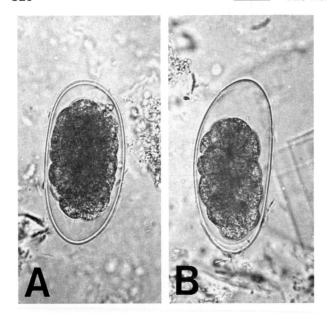

Fig. 13–8. *A* and *B*, *Trichostrongylus* eggs in human stools, unstained, ×495.

briformis, T. orientalis, T. vitrinus, T. probolurus, T. axei, T. brevis, T. skrjabini, and *T. instabilis.* These species are often highly prevalent in parts of the Middle East (Egypt, Iran, Iraq, and Armenia), India, Australia, North Africa, Siberia, Japan, Java, China, and Taiwan. Some *Trichostrongylus* species have a wide geographic range of distribution; others are more restricted to certain places; and still others have a wide overlap in their distribution. In some localities in Japan the prevalence rate is up to 40% (Otsuru, 1962), and in Iraq it is up to 25% (Watson, 1953). In many other places the infection has been recorded as *Trichostrongylus,* for example in the United States, Chile, Israel, Fiji, Hawaii, the Democratic Republic of Congo, Zimbabwe, Peru, and Thailand.

Clinical Findings. The clinical symptoms of trichostrongyliasis in two cases reported from California of a husband and wife who became ill were abdominal pain, diarrhea, weakness, and profound eosinophilia. The husband had 52% eosinophils of 17,900 white blood cells and the wife 71% eosinophils of 35,750 white blood cells. *Trichostrongylus* eggs were found in the stools of both patients, who tended a garden and used sheep manure as fertilizer. The patients were treated, but small numbers of eggs were present 1 month later (Wallace et al. 1956). Slight blood loss through the intestine has been found in patients with *Trichostrongylus* who passed 100 to 400 eggs per gram of feces (Arakawa, 1961).

Pathology and Diagnosis. There are no histologic studies of the small intestine in *Trichostrongylus* infections in humans. In laboratory animals infected with 500 larvae, only minor lesions were observed histologically, but infections with 50,000 larvae produced marked lesions, as expected. The diagnosis is made in the clinical laboratory by recovery of eggs with the typical morphology described above (Fig. 13–8 *A–B*).

Angiostrongylus

The family Metastrongylidae has genera and species that inhabit the pulmonary airways, pulmonary parenchyma, and blood vessels of their hosts. The classification of the different genera of this family is controversial, and there is no consensus among different writers. The Metastrongylidae have a heteroxenous (two-host) life cycle, requiring gastropods (snails and slugs) as their intermediate hosts. The genus *Angiostrongylus* has several species, most of which are found in the circulatory systems of their definitive hosts. Some of these species have low host specificity, infecting several species of animals. Two species are known to occur in humans: *A. cantonensis,* producing eosinophilic meningitis and other central nervous system syndromes, and *A. costaricensis,* producing abdominal angiostrongyloidiasis. An undetermined species of *Angiostrongylus* produced a fatal infection in a man in Italy, in whom the worms matured to adults in the pulmonary arteries and produced apparently viable larvae (Fig. 13–9 *A–D*; Pirisi et al. 1995).

Angiostrongylus cantonensis— Eosinophilic Meningitis

Angiostrongylus cantonensis is a parasite of the pulmonary arteries of many species of rats, mainly *Rattus norvegicus, R. rattus,* species of *Bandicota,* and other rodents, especially in eastern Africa, the Pacific Islands, Southeast Asia, and Australia. Two related species, *A. mackerrasae* (Bhaibulaya, 1968) and *A. malaysiensis* (Bhaibulaya, Cross, 1971; Cross, Bhaibulaya, 1974), occur in the same hosts and have a geographic distribution in Southeast Asia similar to that of *A. cantonensis* (Bhaibulaya, 1979; Carney, Stafford, 1979). No human infections with either one of these species have been recorded, but they are expected; the study of worms recovered from infected individuals is necessary

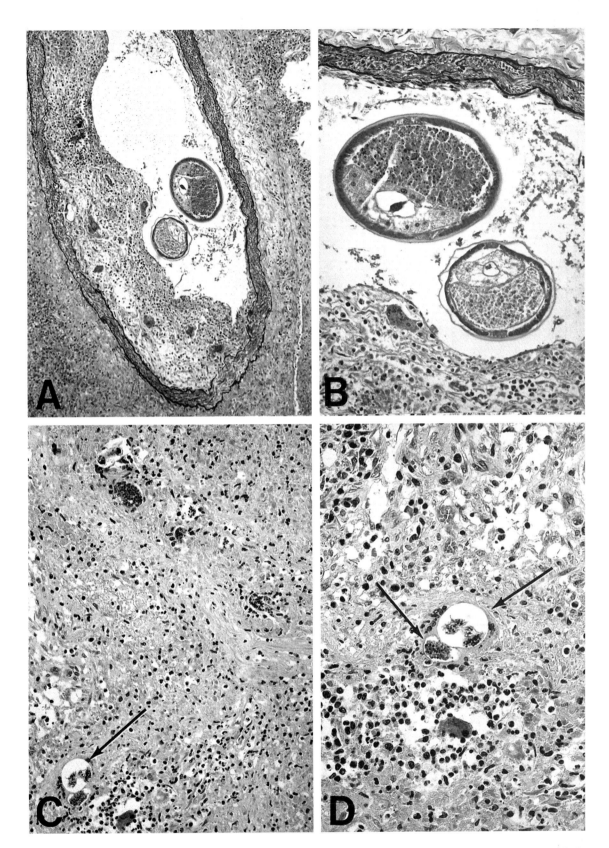

Fig. 13–9. *Angiostrongylus* species in pulmonary arteries of a man from Italy. Preparations stained with hematoxylin and eosin stain. *A*, Low-power view of worms in a pulmonary artery. Note the arteritis with mural thrombus, ×70. *B*, Higher magnification illustrating cross sections of a male, ×180. *C* and *D*, Areas of lung consolidation, with fibrosis and developing eggs (arrows), ×180. (Reported by Pirisi, M., Gutierrez, Y., Minini, C., et al. 1994. Fatal human pulmonary infection caused by an *Angiostrongylus*-like nematode. Clin. Infect. Dis. 20:59–65.)

for speciation, a difficult task because most infections are not fatal. An infection with a species of *Parastrongylus*, a genus related to *Angiostrongylus*, was reported in West Africa (Ivory Coast) in a 10-year-old boy who ingested an *A. fulica* snail. The child had meningitis with marked eosinophilia and recovered in about 3 weeks. The diagnosis was based on a 10 mm worm recovered during the spinal tap (Nozais et al. 1980).

The first documented cases of *A. cantonensis* infection were reported by Rosen et al. (1962) in two Filipino men who died in a mental hospital in Hawaii. The histologic study of their brain tissue showed an eosinophilic meningoencephalitis, and young adult worms were recovered from the preserved brains, identified, and illustrated. These patients came to the attention of Rosen while he was investigating an outbreak of eosinophilic meningitis in Tahiti (Rosen et al. 1961). A previous case in Taiwan in 1944, recorded in Japanese in a local journal, was lost until the report was translated into English 20 years later (Beaver, Rosen, 1964). Since the time of Rosen's findings, the clinical disease, the epidemiology, the geographic extent of the infection, and the modes of transmission have been extensively studied.

Morphology and Life Cycle. *Angiostrongylus cantonensis* organisms are 17 to 25 mm in length and 0.26 to 0.36 mm in width, the males being smaller than the females. The worms are delicate and slightly tapered at the ends, and the males have a rudimentary bursa. Fresh specimens show the intestine as a dark, wavy tube extending from the anterior to the posterior end.

The adult worms of *A. cantonensis* (Fig. 13–10) live in the pulmonary arteries, where they lay eggs. The eggs become trapped in the capillary bed of the lung, where they develop larvae that hatch and migrate via the respiratory tree to the epiglottis, esophagus, and intestine to be evacuated with feces. The larvae are ingested by several species of slugs or land snails (the giant African land snail, *Achatina fulica*, is one of the most common intermediate hosts). In the gastropod, the larvae develop to the infective stage in about 2 weeks. On ingestion by the rodent or by humans, the larvae migrate to the central nervous system, where they mature. The invasion of brain tissue lasts for approximately 10 days, after which the larvae migrate to the meninges (subarachnoid space), where they grow for about 3 weeks. When the worms are 12 to 13 mm in length, they migrate once more through the venous system, reaching the heart and finally the branches of the pulmonary arteries, to become adults and begin oviposition (Alicata, Jindrak, 1970; MacKerras, Sandars, 1954, 1955).

Humans are abnormal hosts for *A. cantonensis*, and the parasite does not develop to adulthood. The worms migrate from the brain toward the branches of the pulmonary arteries, but they die during migration. Rarely, the worms locate in the pulmonary arteries (Sonakul, 1978; Yii et al. 1968a).

Geographic Distribution and Epidemiology. The geographic distribution of *A. cantonensis* has steadily expanded during the last 200 years. It began on the east coast of Africa, moved east, and presently includes most of Southeast Asia, India, and the Pacific basin, including Hawaii. This migration coincided with the expansion of one of the main intermediate hosts of the parasite, *Achatina fulica*, known as the *giant land snail* (Mead, 1961). Although infections due to ingestion of

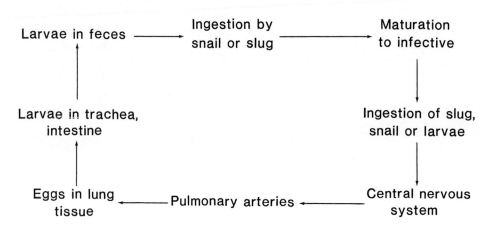

Fig. 13–10. *Angiostrongylus cantonensis*, schematic life cycle.

A. fulica by humans are documented, *A. fulica* is more important in nature for maintaining the life cycle between the rodents. Species of *Pila* and related snails are more important in transmission of the disease to humans, at least in Thailand and other Southeast Asian countries, because humans customarily eat these snails (Bhaibulaya, 1979; Hongladarom, Indarakoses, 1966; Punyagupta et al. 1970). Infected rodents have been found in Louisiana, in the United States (Campbell, Little, 1988), where a human case was reported recently (New et al. 1995); in Cuba (Aguiar et al. 1981), with several cases reported in humans (Pascual et al. 1981); in Egypt (Yousif, Ibrahim, 1978); and in Puerto Rico (Andersen et al. 1986).

The prevalence of *A. cantonensis* in humans is not known; human infections occur sporadically or regularly in some places in endemic areas (Franco et al. 1960) and less often in epidemic outbreaks (Rosen et al. 1961). In contrast, there have been many surveys of the prevalence of the parasite among the local rodent population and the gastropods' intermediate hosts, most of them showing a high prevalence of the infection among the natural hosts.

Human infections are acquired by the ingestion of raw, infected snails and slugs, sometimes for medicinal purposes. Other animals such as freshwater prawns, shrimp, crabs, terrestrial planarians, and frogs harbor the infective larvae, some acting as paratenic hosts of the parasite. Ingestion of the snails, the natural hosts, usually results in heavy infections that may be fatal. Most infections in humans occur by ingestion of vegetables or water contaminated with larvae shed in the mucus of the snail. In northern Thailand, an apparently important source of infection is well water contaminated with drowned *A. fulica* (Crook et al. 1968). The larvae survive free in water for 12 days (Crook et al. 1968) to 21 days (Richards, Merrit, 1967); experimental inoculation of rats with larvae that survived for 60 hours in water produced infections (Crook et al. 1971). More important is the fact that larvae survive in chlorinated water and are only partially susceptible to iodine treatment (Crook et al. 1971).

Clinical Findings. The incubation period of *A. cantonensis* infection in humans varies from 12 to 28 days. Some patients have a history of eating raw or improperly cooked snails or slugs. However, most do not; they probably acquire the infection by accidental ingestion of larvae in vegetables or water, or by ingestion of infected paratenic hosts harboring the larvae. In Thailand, men are infected more often than women; the

male:female ratio is 2:1 (Punyagupta et al. 1970). *Angiostrongylus* produces several clinical syndromes in humans.

Eosinophilic Meningoencephalitis. Prodromal symptoms of eosinophilic meningoencephalitis include vomiting, vague abdominal discomfort, shortness of breath, a feeling of heaviness, and occasionally low fever. The main symptoms include headache, nuchal rigidity, photophobia, vision impairment, and facial paresthesias and paralysis. In some patients, facial paralysis may be the only presenting symptom (Cross, 1978; Jindrak, 1975). Most patients have other neurologic abnormalities such as vertigo, loss of balance, and meningismus. The symptoms usually last for a few days to 1 month, running a benign course and leaving no sequelae. The mortality, of about 1%, is probably related to the large number of larvae ingested (Punyagupta et al. 1970b); geographic variations in the severity of the disease have been found. Recurrence of symptoms in some patients is frequent and is probably due to reinfection

The cerebrospinal fluid pressure is mildly elevated; the fluid is clear, hazy, or sometimes cloudy, with increased white blood cells, sometimes up to 3400 per cubic millimeter. In 80% of cases the white blood cell count in the spinal fluid ranges between 150 and 1500, with eosinophilia greater than 20% in 95% of cases (Kuberski, Wallace, 1979). The levels of cerebrospinal fluid proteins are slightly increased; and bacterial and viral cultures are negative. The parasites are sometimes recovered from the cerebrospinal fluid (Bunnag et al. 1969; Chiu et al. 1981; Kuberski et al. 1979; Nitidandhaprabhas et al. 1975) when a syringe with a 20- to 23-gauge needle is used to aspirate the fluid, mainly from children (Cross, 1978; Yii, 1976). Blood eosinophilia greater than 3% is present in over 90% of cases, and white blood cell counts range from 7000 to 24,500 per cubic millimeter. In some patients the infection presents with high fever, high cerebrospinal fluid pressure with low sugar, and marked elevation of protein and white blood cells resembling bacterial meningitis (Chotmongkol, Tiamkao, 1992).

Eosinophilic Myeloencephalitis. A few cases of *Angiostrongylus* myeloencephalitis have been reported, mostly from Thailand. These cases, associated with eating raw or pickled snails, are generally fatal. The symptoms and the eosinophilia are more pronounced than those in meningoencephalitis (Punyagupta, 1965).

Eosinophilic Radiculomyeloencephalitis. This syndrome is characterized by exquisite pain and paresthesias of the lower extremities and by sensory symptoms in the arms, trunk, or other locations (Punyagupta et al. 1968). In an outbreak in which 16 persons with a history of eating raw land snails (*Achatina fulica*) were infected, the pain did not extend above the T7 sensory level. Some patients had constipation; others had urinary incontinence or retention. There were no ocular symptoms or vomiting (Kliks et al. 1982).

Ocular Angiostrongyloidiasis. Ocular symptoms are found in up to 16% of cases, bilaterally in more than one-half, with diplopia and abnormal visual fields being the main complaints. Examination of the eye may reveal an abnormal fundus in 12% of the patients and a blurred disc or papilledema in others. The worms may also be found in the eye; sometimes they are clearly seen in the anterior chamber or the iris with the naked eye (Fig. 13–11). Worms clearly visible in the anterior chamber are usually in advanced stages of development, measure over 1 cm in length, and are recovered relatively easily by the ophthalmologist (Chiu et al. 1981; Le-Van-Hoa et al. 1974; Prommindaroj et al. 1962; Sunardi et al. 1977; Widagdo et al. 1977; Fig. 13–11). Worms located in the retina or in the posterior pole of the eye are smaller. They are either infective larvae that migrate to the eye soon after infection (Nelson et al. 1988) or slightly more developed worms (Kanchanaranya et al. 1972; Kanchanaranya, Punyagupta,

1971) that usually are found soon after the symptoms start (Nelson et al. 1988).

Pathology. Pathologic examination of the central nervous system has been done in a few cases of *A. cantonensis* infection. Grossly, the brain has a mild to moderate meningeal exudate, hyperemia, and focal areas of hemorrhage. Worms, measuring up to 12 mm in length, are found in the subarachnoid spaces; in heavy infections, up to 600 worms have been recovered at autopsy (Cross, 1978; Yii et al. 1968b). The worms recovered from humans are generally longer than those of the same age found in rats (Punyagupta, Bunnag, 1970). Coronal sections reveal small petechial hemorrhages through the white and gray matter. In addition, necrosis with hemorrhages up to 4 mm in diameter are found in some areas of the brain and the spinal cord. These lesions, which correspond to small tracks made by the migrating parasites can be followed on close examination of thin slices.

The main histologic finding is marked infiltration of the meninges by eosinophils, plasma cells, and lymphocytes (Fig. 13–12 *A*; Nye et al. 1970). Cross, oblique, and longitudinal sections of the parasites may be seen in the subarachnoid spaces (see Fig. 12–13

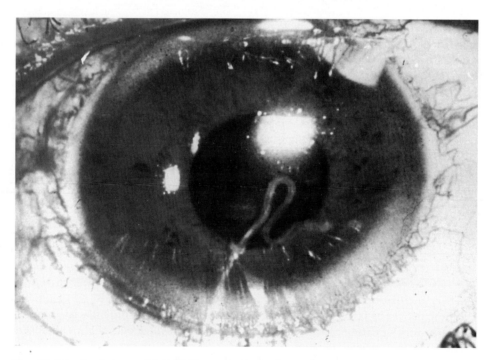

Fig. 13–11. *Angiostrongylus* in the eye. Note the parasite floating in the anterior chamber of the eye of a 34-year-old man in Bangkok, Thailand. (In: Beaver, P.C., Jung, R.C., and Cupp, E.W. 1984. *Clinical Parasitology*, 9th edition. Philadelphia, Lea & Febiger, p. 293. Reproduced with permission.)

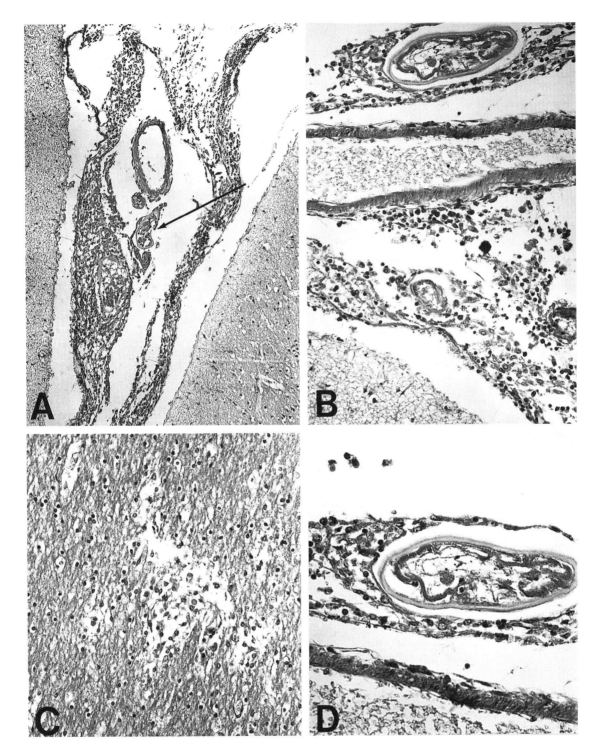

Fig. 13–12. *Angiostrongylus cantonensis* in human brain, sections stained with hematoxylin and eosin stain. *A*, Low-power view of meninges showing an inflammatory infiltrate. An oblique section of an *A. cantonensis* larva is seen (arrow), ×70. *B*, Higher magnification showing the infiltrate and the worm (top), ×180. *C*, Small tunnel-like lesion in brain tissue. Note the scant infiltrate, ×180. *D*, Higher magnification of an oblique section of the worm, ×280.

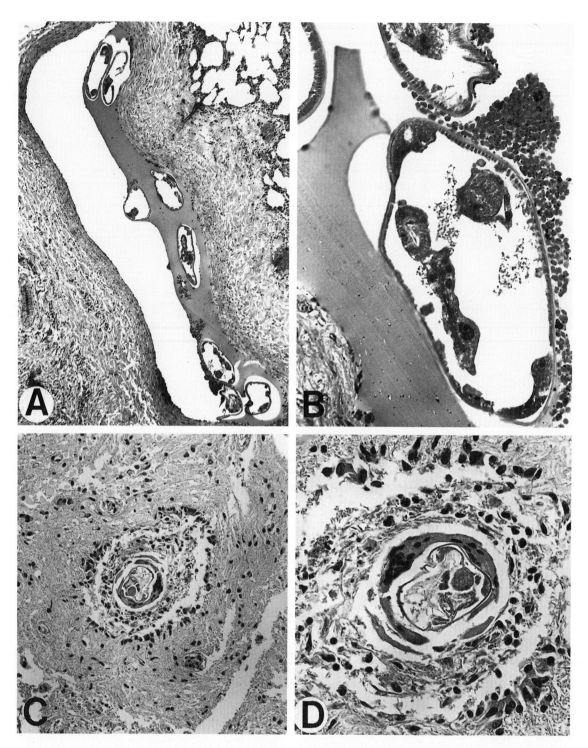

Fig. 13–13. *Angiostrongylus cantonensis* in human tissues, sections stained with hematoxylin and eosin stain. *A* and *B*. Pulmonary artery. *A*, Low-power view of a branch of a pulmonary artery showing eight cross and oblique sections of juvenile *A. cantonensis* in a 5-year-old girl who died of a heavy infection, ×27. *B*, Higher magnification showing one slightly oblique section of one worm, ×360. *C* and *D*. Spinal cord. *C*, Low-power view showing the ependymal canal with the worm within a granuloma, ×140. *D*, Higher magnification showing the worm almost surrounded by a multinucleated foreign body giant cell. Note the disruption of the ependymal cells at the periphery, ×360. (Preparations courtesy of J.H. Cross, Ph.D., Navy Medical Research Unit, Taipei, Taiwan. Reported by: Yii, C.Y., Chen, C.Y., Fresh, J.W., et al. 1968. Human angiostrongyliasis involving the lungs. Chin. J. Microbiol. 1:148–150.)

B–D), the ventricles, and the ependymal canal (Fig. 13–13 *C–D*). Small areas of necrosis (Fig. 13–12 *C*) with a scant polymorphonuclear and mononuclear cell infiltrate produced by migrating larvae within the brain are common. Individuals dying with heavy infections have many recent tracks of necrosis and hemorrhage, in some instances with worms; polymorphonuclear cells, mostly eosinophils; and abundant Charcot-Leyden crystals. Parasites may also be present in the meningeal spaces, sometimes in large numbers, and the meninges have marked polymorphonuclear cell infiltration (Sonakul, 1978). Adult worms have been found occasionally in the pulmonary arteries in massive fatal infections with adult females containing immature larvae in their uteri (Fig. 13–13 *A–B*; Cross, 1978; Yii et al. 1968b). In another case, the eggs and larvae were found in the capillary bed, but adult worms were not mentioned (Phan Trinh et al. 1967).

Diagnosis. In endemic areas the diagnosis of *A. cantonensis* is made on clinical grounds in persons with characteristic central nervous system symptoms and cerebrospinal fluid eosinophilia. A history of eating raw snails or having been in contact with the snails or other animal sources of the infection strongly suggests the infection (Cross, 1978). Other helminths producing cerebrospinal fluid eosinophilia and central nervous system symptoms must be excluded. *Gnathostoma* (see Chapter 18), *Baylisascaris* (see Chapter 16), and *Toxocara*, especially in children, which produce myeloencephalitis should be carefully ruled out, especially where they are endemic. Larval stages and adult worms can be recovered from the cerebrospinal fluid (Bunnag et al. 1969; Kuberski et al. 1979; Nitidandhaprabhas et al. 1975) and in rare instances from the eye, providing a specific diagnosis (Prommindaroj et al. 1962; Yii, 1976).

The diagnosis is not made in tissues, except for autopsy material; in a few autopsies of individuals dying with overwhelming infections, parasites were recovered in toto, or were found in tissue sections of the central nervous system. Rarely are the worms found in the lungs (Fig. 13–13 *A–B*). In cross sections, *A. cantonensis* is indistinguishable from related species; thus, only a generic diagnosis is possible.

In sections, the parasite is usually well preserved (Fig. 13–14 *A–D*). Larvae and young adults are often located within the subarachnoid spaces 10 to 12 days after infection (Fig. 13–14 *B–D*). At this time, only empty tracks left by the worms are found in the brain

tissue (Fig. 13–12 *C*). In cross sections the worms measure up to 124 μm in diameter; the cuticle is thin and delicate, with fine longitudinal striations (Fig. 13–14 *C*). The muscles (Fig. 13–14 *D*) are uniformly lower than the lateral cords, which appear rounded and prominent, with about two to four nuclei per histologic section (Fig. 13–14 *C–D*). The intestine is a syncytium of cells without cell junctions, with two to five nuclei per histologic section (Fig. 13–14 *C–D*). In young adults the gonads are immature; the uteri consist of a pair of tubes with 5 to 12 densely stained cells (Fig. 13–14 *D*), and the male has a single genital tube (Otsuru, 1978).

Serologic testing is available in certain laboratories, especially in endemic areas. An enzyme-linked immunosorbent assay test has been developed and used, with satisfactory results (Cross, Chi, 1982; Yen et al. 1989). Specific immunoglobulins are detected in both the sera and spinal fluid of patients (Tungkanak et al. 1972).

Angiostrongylus costaricensis— Abdominal Angiostrongyloidiasis

Angiostrongylus costaricensis (Morera, Cespedes, 1971) is a parasite of the cotton rat (*Sigmodon hispidus*) and the black rat (*Rattus rattus*); it occurs in the branches of the mesenteric arteries. A related species, *A. siamensis*, described in several species of rats in Southeast Asia, produces infections in these animals similar to those of *A. costaricensis*.

Morphology and Life Cycle. The male of *A. costaricensis* is 22 mm long by 140 μm wide, and the female is 42 mm long by 350 μm wide. The worms are slender and filariform, with slightly tapered ends and an inconspicuous bursa in the males. As stated previously, the life cycle of *A. costaricensis* requires two hosts (Fig. 13–15). Eggs deposited in the mesenteric arteries are carried with the blood flow to the capillaries in the intestinal wall and develop to larvae. After hatching, the larvae migrate through the tissues to reach the intestinal lumen and be evacuated in the feces. The larvae in soil are ingested by slugs (*Vaginulus plebeius* and other species), the intermediate hosts, and become infective. Ingestion of the slug frees the larvae in the intestine. The larvae then migrate through the tissues and enter the mesenteric vessels to become adults (Morera, 1973).

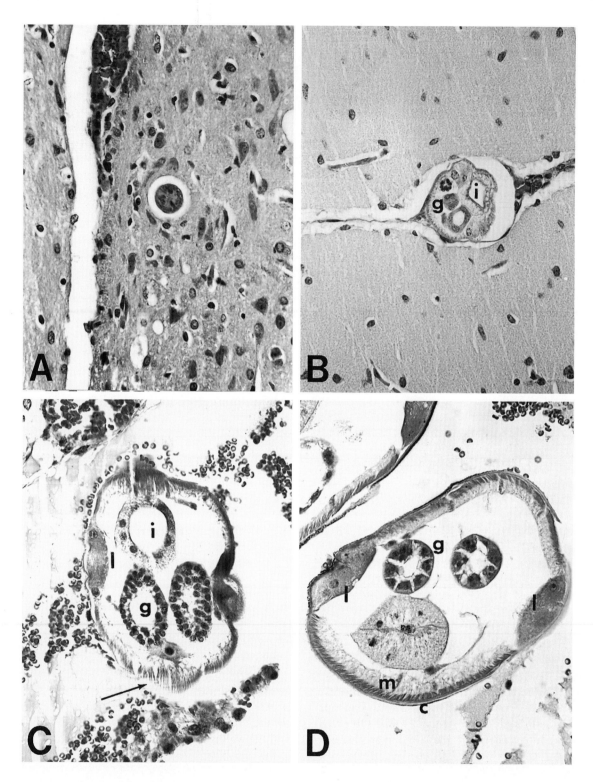

Fig. 13–14. *Angiostrongylus*, diagnostic characteristics. Parasites in cross sections of rat brain, infected experimentally and sacrificed at different time intervals, sections stained with hematoxylin and eosin stain. All ×360 to demonstrate the worm's growth. *A*, Young larva at 7 days after infection in brain tissue; note the lack of an in-

flammatory reaction. *B*, Eleven days after infection. Note the worm already located in a brain sulcus. The intestine, the immature gonads, the thin cuticle and muscle layer, and the lateral cords are well defined. *C*, Sixteen days after infection. Note the larger size of the worm showing the minute longitudinal striations of the cuticle (arrow).

(continued)

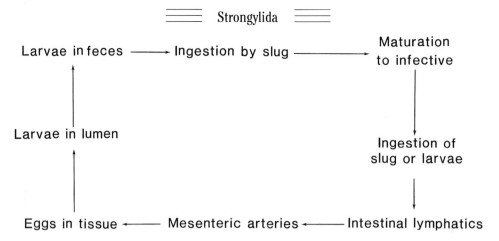

Fig. 13–15. *Angiostrongylus costaricensis*, schematic representation of the life cycle.

Geographic Distribution and Epidemiology. Humans are accidental hosts that probably acquire the infection by ingestion of fruits and vegetables contaminated with infective larvae shed by the slugs in their mucus. Human infections have been reported from Costa Rica (Cespedes et al. 1967), Honduras (Sierra, Morera, 1972; Zuniga et al. 1983), Nicaragua (Vasquez et al. 1993), Brazil (Iabuki, Montenegro, 1979; Rojas Ayala, 1987; Rojas Ayala et al. 1982), Venezuela (Salfelder et al. 1970; Zambrano et al. 1975), Colombia (Malek, 1981), Ecuador (Lazo et al. 1995; Morera et al. 1983), and Mexico (Zavala-Velazquez et al. 1974). One case from the Democratic Republic of Congo (formerly Zaire), Africa, diagnosed in histologic sections was questionably identified, on the basis of the length of the larvae alone, as *A. costaricensis* (Baird et al. 1987). In the United States, the parasite occurs in naturally infected cotton rats in Texas (Ubelaker, Hall, 1979).

Clinical Findings. Most human infections with *A. costaricensis* occur in children. A review of 116 patients diagnosed in Costa Rica between 1966 and 1976 found abdominal pain in the right iliac fossa in 84%, anorexia in 61%, vomiting in 45%, diarrhea in 34%, constipation in 14%, and abdominal rigidity in 4%. On palpation of the abdomen there was pain, and in at least one-half of the cases, a tumor-like mass was felt in the right lower quadrant. There was usually a temperature of 38°C to 38.5°C of up to 4 weeks' duration without chills; rectal examination was painful in half of the patients. The general clinical picture was that of moderate appendicitis (Iabuki, Montenegro, 1979); significant laboratory findings included peripheral eosinophilia ranging from 11% to 61% in 75% of cases and leukocyte counts of 10,000 to 30,000 per cubic millimeter in 43%, more than 30,000 per cubic millimeter in 15%, and more than 50,000 per cubic millimeter in 5%. Radiologic films showed changes in the terminal ileum, appendix, cecum, or ascending colon such as spasticity, filling defects, and reduced lumen of the terminal ileum. A majority of the patients required appendectomy; others underwent ileocecal resection, hemicolectomy, or colostomy (Loria-Cortes, Lobo-Sanahuja, 1980).

Pathology. In humans, *A. costaricensis* occurs in the branches of the mesenteric artery irrigating the terminal ileum, appendix, and cecum, where the majority of the lesions occur. The small intestine shows thickening and edema of the wall. The serosal surface has white, small granulomas resembling small grains of salt; the predominant gross finding is inflammation of the intestine. The mucosal surface usually has ulcerations, and the wall is three to four times its normal thickness;

The intestine has six nuclei in this section; intestinal cell boundaries are not discernible. The two tubes representing the immature ovaries have numerous nuclei. The lateral cords are prominent; the one on the left is well defined and has two nuclei. Muscle cells not well defined on this section. The cuticle is thin and delicate. *D*, Twenty-one days after infection. The uteri are represented by two tubes with 10 to 12 dark-staining nuclei. The lateral cords are large and oval, with visible nuclei (usually two to four). The muscle cells are polymyarian, and the cuticle is delicate. Abbreviations: c, cuticle; g, gonads; i, intestine; l, lateral cord; m, muscle cell.

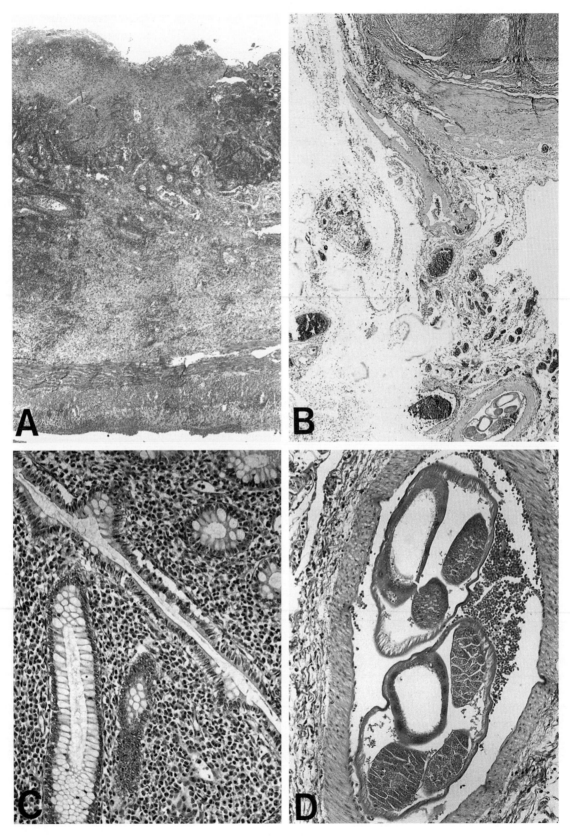

Fig. 13–16.

regional lymph nodes are enlarged. Advanced cases have necrosis of the intestinal wall, fistula formation, and peritonitis, probably due to thrombosis of larger vessels producing infarction of the bowel (Cespedes et al. 1967; Loria-Cortes, Lobo-Sanahuja, 1980).

The striking histologic features of *A. costaricensis* infection in humans are the exuberant tissue eosinophilia, edema of all layers of the intestinal wall (Fig. 13–16 *A* and *C*), and granulomas around the eggs. The granulomas formed by histiocytes have a few mononuclear cells and abundant eosinophils, and the eggs in the granulomas may have developing larvae. Some granulomas are empty because the larvae migrate to the lumen; however, larvae do not generally occur in the stools of infected humans. The vessels containing the adult parasites (Fig. 13–16 *B* and *D*) may be infiltrated by eosinophils; sometimes they are thrombosed and may contain a dead *Angiostrongylus* worm. The lymph nodes draining the affected area are hyperplastic, with many eosinophils in the sinusoids. In chronic cases, fibrosis of the intestinal wall contributes to its thickening. Recorded aberrant locations of adult *A. costaricensis* include the spermatic artery (Ruiz, Morera, 1983), liver (Morera et al. 1982), omentum and testis (Loria-Cortes, Lobo-Sanahuja, 1980), lymph nodes, and a hernial sac.

Diagnosis. The clinical diagnosis of intestinal angiostrongyloidiasis is difficult. Stool samples rarely show the larvae, as is always the case in the rodent natural hosts. Histologically, the granulomatous inflammation produced by eggs measuring 60 to 45 μm, in different stages of development, free larvae 13 μm in diameter, and marked tissue eosinophilia are diagnostic. The adult parasites are sometimes dead and necrotic. In sections, *A. costaricensis* (Fig. 13–16 *D*) measures up to 240 μm in the maximum diameter. The cuticle is smooth and delicate. The muscle layer is low and weak, and the lateral cords are inconspicuous (Fig. 13–16 *D*). The intestine is well developed and occupies one-third to one-half of the worm's body cavity; it consists of a syncytium with several nuclei in each histo-

logic section (Fig. 13–16 *D*). The gonads consist of several tubular structures containing developing eggs in the female.

References

Aguiar PH, Morera P, Pascual J, 1981. First record of *Angiostrongylus cantonensis* in Cuba. Am. J. Trop. Med. Hyg. 30:963–965

Alicata JE, Jindrak K, 1970. *Angiostrongylosis in the Pacific and Southeast Asia*. Springfield, Illinois: Charles C Thomas

Alvarez-Pagan M, Torrez De Vega CA, 1963. Fatal intestinal hemorrhage due to hookworm in infants. Bol. Soc. Med. Puerto Rico 55:456–462

Andersen EM, Gubler DJ, Sorensen K, Beddard J, Ash LR, 1986. First report of *Angiostrongylus cantonensis* in Puerto Rico. Am. J. Trop. Med. Hyg. 35:319–322

Anthony PP, McAdam IWJ, 1972. Helminthic pseudotumours of the bowel: thirty-four cases of helminthoma. Gut 13:8–16

Arakawa H, 1961. A study on fecal blood loss associated with *Ancylostoma duodenale*, *Necator americanus* and *Trichostrongylus orientalis* infections. Niigata Igakkai Zasshi 75:1068–1092

Baird JK, Neafie RC, Lanote L, Connor DH, 1987. Abdominal angiostrongylosis in an African man: case study. Am. J. Trop. Med. Hyg. 37:353–356

Bakta IM, Widjana IDP, Sutisna P, 1993. Some epidemiological aspects of hookworm infection among the rural population of Bali, Indonesia. Southeast Asian J. Trop. Med. Public Health 24:87–93

Barrowclough H, Crome L, 1979. Oesophagostomiasis in man. Trop. Geogr. Med. 31:133–138

Basden RDE, Jackson JW, Jones EI, 1974. Gapeworm infestation in man. Br. J. Dis. Chest 68:207–209

Beaver PC, 1955. Observations on *Necator* infections resulting from exposure to three larvae. Tomo extraordinario, Marzo 1955. Rev. Iberica. Parasitol. 1–9

Beaver PC, 1988. Light, long-lasting *Necator* infection in a volunteer. Am. J. Trop. Med. Hyg. 39:369–372

Beaver PC, Jung RC, Cupp EW, 1984. *Clinical Parasitology*. Philadelphia: Lea & Febiger

Fig. 13–16. *Angiostrongylus costaricensis* in humans, sections stained with hematoxylin and eosin stain. *A,* Low-power view of a section of ileum from a patient with *A. costaricensis* infection. Note the inflammatory infiltrate in all layers of the viscus. At the bottom there is an indication of peritonitis, ×28. *B–D,* Appendix. *B,* Mesoappendix showing a portion of an enlarged, hyperplastic lymph node (top) and an artery with two sections of an adult worm (bottom), ×28. *C,* Higher magnification of appendiceal mucosa showing the florid eosinophil infiltrate, ×180. *D,* Small artery with two sections of a female *A. costaricensis*. Compare and contrast the morphology with that of *A. cantonensis* (Fig. 13–13); note the inconspicuous lateral cords; the gonads are well developed (adult worm); the muscles, cuticle, and intestine are similar, ×70. (Preparations courtesy of J.K. Frenkel, M.D., Department of Pathology, University of Kansas Medical Center, Kansas City, Kansas.)

Beaver PC, Rosen L, 1964. Memorandum on the first report of *Angiostrongylus* in man, by Nomura and Lin, 1945. Am. J. Trop. Med. Hyg. 13:589–590

Beaver PC, Yoshida Y, Ash LR, 1964. Mating of *Ancyloatoma caninum* in relation to blood loss in the host. J. Parasitol. 50:286–295

Bhaibulaya M, 1968. A new species of *Angiostrongylus* in an Australian rat, *Rattus fuscipes*. Semin. Respir. Infect. 58:789–799

Bhaibulaya, M. 1979. Geographical distribution of *Angiostrongylus* and angyostrongyliais in Thailand, Indo-China and Australia. In: Cross JH (ed), *Studies on Angiostrongyliasis in Eastern Asia and Australia*. NAMRU-2 Special Pub. No. 44. Taipei, Taiwan: NAMRU-2, pp. 49–52

Bhaibulaya M, Cross JH, 1971. *Angiostrongylus malaysiensis* (Nematoda: Metastrongylidae), a new species of rat lung-worm from Malaysia. Southeast Asian J. Trop. Med. Public Health 2:527–533

Biagi FF, Villa TS, Alvarez G, 1957. Nodulos en la submucosa intestinal producidos por *Ancylostoma duodenale* (Dubini, 1843). Rev. Biol. Trop. 5:35–43

Birrell DJ, Moorhouse DE, Gardner MAH, May CS, 1978. Chronic cough and haemoptysis due to a nematode, "*Syngamus laryngeus*." Aust. NZ. J. Med. 8:168–170

Borrero J, Restrepo A, Botero D, Latorre G, 1961. Clinical and laboratory studies on hookworm disease in Colombia. Am. J. Trop. Med. Hyg. 10:735–741

Bradley M, Chandiwana SK, Bundy DAP, Medley GF, 1992. The epidemiology and population biology of *Necator americanus* infection in a rural community in Zimbabwe. Trans. R. Soc. Trop. Med. Hyg. 86:73–76

Bunnag T, Benjapong W, Noeypatimanond S, Punyagupta S, 1969. The recovery of *Angiostrongylus cantonensis* in the cerebrospinal fluid of a case of eosinophilic meningitis. J. Med. Assoc. Thailand 52:665–672

Campbell BG, Little MD, 1988. The finding of *Angiostrongylus cantonensis* in rats in New Orleans. Am. J. Trop. Med. Hyg. 38:568–573

Cantor DS, Biempica L, Toccalino H, O'Donnel JC, 1966. Estudios de intestino delgado en pacientes afectados de necatoriasis y parasitos multiple. Bol. Chil. Parasitol. 21:70–76

Cappello M, Vlasuk GP, Bergum PW, Huang S, Hotez PJ, 1995. *Ancylostoma caninum* anticoagulant peptide: a hookworm-derived inhibitor of human coagulation factor Xa. Proc. Natl. Acad. Sci. USA 92:6152–6156

Carney WP, Stafford EE, 1979. Angiostrongyliasis in Indonesia. A review. In: Cross JH (ed), *Studies on Angiostrongyliasis in Eastern Asia and Australia*. NAMRU-2 Special Pub. No. 44. Taipei, Taiwan: NAMRU-2, pp. 14–25

Carroll SM, Robertson TA, Papadimitriou JM, Grove DI, 1984. Transmission electron microscopical studies of the site of attachement of *Ancylostoma ceylanicum* to the small bowel mucosa of the dog. J. Helminthol. 58:313–320

Cespedes R, Salas J, Makbel S, Troper L, Mullner F, Morera P, 1967. Granulomas entericos y linfaticos con intensa eosinophilia tisular producidos por un estrongildeo (strongylata). I. Patologia. Acta Med. Costar. 10:235–255

Chabaud AG, Lariviere M, 1958. Sur les oesophagostomes parasites de l'homme. Bull. Soc. Pathol. Exot. 51:384–393

Chiu JK, Huang WH, Cheng KH, Chang IH, Teng WH, Kao TH, 1981. Three cases of worm proven human angiostrongyliasis in Taiwan. Chin. J. Microbiol. Immunol. 14:247–250

Chotmongkol V, Tiamkao S, 1992. Unusual manifestation of eosinophilic meningitis. Southeast Asian J. Trop. Med. Public Health 23:539–540

Correa de Lara, T de A, Aparecida Barbosa M, Rodrigues de Oliveira M, Godoy ID, Queluz TT, 1993. Human syngamosis: two cases of chronic cough caused by *Mammomonogamus laryngeus*. Chest 103:264–265

Croese J, Loukas A, Opdebeeck J, Fairley S, Prociv P, 1994a. Human enteric infection with canine hookworms. Ann. Intern. Med. 120:369–374

Croese J, Loukas A, Opdebeeck J, Prociv P, 1994b. Occult enteric infection by *Ancylostoma caninum*: a previously unrecognized zoonosis. Goastroenterology 106:3–12

Croese J, Prociv P, Maguire EJ, Crawford AP, 1990. Eosinophilic enteritis presenting as surgical emergencies: a report of six cases. Med. J. Aust. 153:415–417

Croese J, 1988. Eosinophilic enteritis—a recent North Queensland experience. Aust. NZ. J. Med. 18:848–853

Crook JR, Fulton SE, Supanwong K, 1968. Ecological studies on the intermediate and definitive hosts of *Angiostrongylus cantonensis* (Chen, 1935) in Thailand. Ann. Trop. Med. Parasitol. 62:27–44

Crook JR, Fulton SE, Supanwong K, 1971. The infectivity of third stage *Angiostrongylus cantonensis* larvae shed from drowned *Achatina fulica* snails and the effect of chemical agents on infectivity. Trans. R. Soc. Trop. Med. Hyg. 65:602–605

Cross JH, 1978. Clinical manifestations and laboratory diagnosis of eosinophilic meningitis syndrome associated with angiostrongyliasis. Southeast Asian J. Trop. Med. Public Health 9:161–170

Cross JH, Bhaibulaya M, 1974. Validity of *Angiostrongylus malaysiensis* Bhaibulaya and Cross, 1971. Southeast Asian J. Trop. Med. Public Health 5:374–378

Cross JH, Chi JCH, 1982. ELISA for the detection of *Angiostrongylus cantonensis* antibodies in patients with eosinophilic meningitis. Southeast Asian J. Trop. Med. Public Health 13:73–76

Cunnac M, Magnaval JF, Cayarci D, Leophonte P, 1988. A propos de 3 cas de syngamose humaine en Guadeloupe. Revue de Pneumologie Clinique 44:140–142

De La Riva H, Gomez Escamilla D, Frati AC, 1981. Acute massive intestinal bleeding caused by hookworm. JAMA 246:69

Dufat R, Sang HT, Herrenschmidt JL, Vergez P, Andre J, 1971. A propos d'un nouveau cas de syngamose bronchique humaine en provenance de la Martinique. J. Fr. Med. Chir. Thorac. 25:547–554

Eiff JA, 1966. Nature of an anticoagulant from the cephalic

glands of *Ancylostoma caninum*. J. Parasitol. 52:833–843

Elmes BGT, McAdam IWJ, 1954. Helminthic abscess, a surgical complication of oesophagostomes and hookworms. Ann. Trop. Med. Parasitol. 48:1–7

Embil JA, Salisbury S, Meerovitch E. 1982. Familial infection with *Oesophagostomum venulosum*. In: Mueller M, Gutteridge W, Koehler P (eds), *Proceedings of the 5th International Congress Parasitology*. Toronto and Amsterdam: Elsevier Biochemical Press, p. 289

Font JH, 1943. *Syngamus laryngeus* in man. Report on three additional cases from Puerto Rico. Bol. Asoc. Med. Puerto Rico 35:331–333

Franco R, Bories S, Couzin B, 1960. A propos de 142 cas de meningite a eosinophiles observes a Tahiti et en Nouvelle-Caledonie. Med. Trop. 20:41–55

Gardiner CH, Schantz PM, 1983. *Mammomonogamus* infection in a human. Report of a case. Am. J. Trop. Med. Hyg. 32:995–997

Gloor RF, Breyley ER, Martinez IG, 1970. Hookworm infection in a rural Kentucky county. Am. J. Trop. Med. Hyg. 19:1007–1009

Gordon JA, Ross CM, Affleck H, 1969. Abdominal emergency due to an oesophagostome. Ann. Trop. Med. Parasitol. 63:161–164

Grell GAC, Watty EI, Muller RL, 1978. Syngamus in a West Indian. Br. Med. J. 2:1464

Haaf E, Van Soest AH, 1964. Oesophagostomiasis in man in North Ghana. Trop. Geogr. Med. 16:49–53

Harada Y, 1962. Wakana disease and hookworm allergy. Yonago Acta Med. 6:109–118

Hawdon JM, 1996. Differentiation between the human hookworms *Ancylostoma duodenale* and *Necator americanus* using PCR-RFLP. J. Parasitol. 82:642–647

Hoffman WA, 1932. Gapeworm infestation of man. Bol. Asoc. Med. Puerto Rico 24:703–704

Hollander M, Tabingo R, Stankewick WR, 1973. Successful treatment of massive intestinal hemorrhage due to hookworm infection in a neonate. J. Pediatr. 82:332–334

Hongladarom T, Indarakoses A, 1966. Eosinophilic meningoencephalitis caused by *Pila* snail ingestion in Bangkok. J. Med. Assoc. Thailand 49:1–9

Iabuki K, Montenegro MR, 1979. Apendicite por *Angiostrongylus costaricensis*. A presentacao de um caso. Rev. Inst. Med. Trop. Sao Paulo 21:33–36

Jacques JE, Lynch JB, 1964. Massive oesophagostomiasis of the colon. Gut 5:80–82

Jindrak K, 1975. Angiostrongyliasis cantonensis (eosinophilic meningitis, Alicata's disease). In: Hornabrook R (ed), *Topics on Tropical Neurology*, Vol. 12. Philadelphia: F.A. Davis Co., pp. 133–164

Junod C, Philbert M, Sang HT, 1970. Une observation de syngamose humaine a localisation bronchique. Premier cas traite et gueri par le thiabendazole. Bull. Soc. Pathol. Exot. 63:483–488

Kalkofen UP, 1970. Attachment and feeding behavior of *Ancylostoma caninum*. Z. Parasitenk. 33:339–354

Kaminsky RG, Ndinya-Achola JO, 1977. *Oesophagostomum* sp. from Kenya. Identification through tissue sections. E. Afr. Med. J. 54:296–297

Kanchanaranya C, Prechanond A, Punyagupta S, 1972. Removal of living worm in retinal *Angiostrongylus cantonensis*. Am. J. Ophthalmol. 74:456–458

Kanchanaranya C, Punyagupta S, 1971. Case of ocular angiostrongyliasis associated with eosinophilic meningitis. Am. J. Ophthalmol. 71:931–934

Kelley PW, Takafuji ET, Wiener H, Milhous W, Miller R, Thompson NJ, Schantz P, Miller RN, 1989. An outbreak of hookworm infection associated with military operations in Grenada. Milit. Med. 154:55–59

Khoshoo V, Craver R, Schantz P, Loukas A, Prociv P, 1995. Correspondence. Abdominal pain, pan-gut eosinophilia, and dog hookworm infection. J. Pediatr. Gastroenterol. Nutr. 21:481

Khoshoo V, Schantz P, Craver R, Stern GM, Loukas A, Prociv P, 1994. Dog hookworm: a cause of eosinophilic enterocolitis in humans. J. Pediatr. Gastroenterol. Nutr. 19:448–452

Kliks MM, Kroenke K, Hardman JM, 1982. Eosinophilic radiculomyeloencephalitis: an angiostrongyliasis outbreak in American Samoa related to ingestion of *Achatina fulica* snails. Am. J. Trop. Med. Hyg. 31:1114–1122

Krepel HP, Baeta S, Kootstra CJ, Polderman AM, 1995. Reinfection patterns of *Oesophagostumum bifurcum* and hookworm after anthelmintic treatment. Trop. Geogr. Med. 47:160–163

Krepel HP, Baeta S, Polderman AM, 1992. Human *Oesophagostomum* infection in northern Togo and Ghana: epidemiological aspects. Ann. Trop. Med. Parasitol. 86:289–300

Krepel HP, Polderman AM, 1992. Egg production of *Oesophagostomum bifurcum*, a locally common parasite of humans in Togo. Am. J. Trop. Med. Hyg. 46:469–472

Krepel HP, Velde EA vd, Baeta S, Polderman AM, 1995. Quantitative interpretation of coprocultures in a population infected with *Oesophagostomum bifurcum*. Trop. Geogr. Med. 47:157–159

Krupp IM, 1961. Effects of crowding and of superinfection on habitat selection and egg production in *Ancylostoma caninum*. J. Parasitol. 47:957–961

Kuberski T, Bart RD, Briley JM, Rosen L, 1979. Recovery of *Angiostrongylus cantonensis* from cerebrospinal fluid of a child with eosinophilic meningitis. J. Clin. Microbiol. 9:629–631

Kuberski T, Wallace GD, 1979. Clinical manifestations of eosinophilic meningitis due to *Angiostrongylus cantonensis*. Neurology 29:1566–1570

Kwo EH, 1972. Parasitic infection in man in North Sumatra, Indonesia. Yonsei Rep. Trop. Med. 3:23–25

Lavier G, Brumpt LC, 1944. L'evolution de l'eosinophilie au cours de l'ankylostomose. Sang 16:97–102

Layrisse M, Blummenfeld N, Carbonell L, Desenne J, Roche N, 1964. Intestinal absorption tests and biopsy of the jejunum in subjects with heavy hookworm infection. Am. J. Trop. Med. Hyg. 13:297–305

Layrisse M, Roche M, 1964. The relationship between anemia and hookworm infection. Results of surveys of rural Venezuelan population. Am. J. Hyg. 79:279–301

Lazo RF, Cedeno C, Llaguno M, 1995. Angiostrongylosis abdominal: Dos nuevos casos en Ecuador. *Proceedings of the XII Congreso Latinoamericano de Parasitologia.* Santiago, Chile: p. 305.

Le-Van-Hoa, Ho-Van-Tri, Huynh-Ngoc-Phuong, 1974. L'angiostrongylose oculaire chez l'homme au sud Viet-Nam. Bull. Soc. Pathol. Exot. 66:743–746

Leers WD, Sarin MK, Arthurs K, 1985. Syngamosis, an unusual cause of asthma: the first reported case in Canada. Can. Med. Assoc. J. 132:269–270

Leiper RT, 1911. The occurrence of *Oesophagostomum apiostomum* as an intestinal parasite of man in Nigeria. J. Trop. Med. Hyg. 14:116–118

Leiper RT, 1913. Gapes in man, an occasional helminthic infection. A notice of its discovery by Dr. A. King in St. Lucia. Lancet 1:170

Leiper RT, 1925. *Syngamus kingi*, a second case in man. Trans. R. Soc. Trop. Med. Hyg. 19:279

Leoutsakos B, Agnadi N, Kolisiatis S, 1977. Rectal bleeding due to *Oesophagostomum brumpti*: report of a case. Dis. Colon Rectum 20:632–634

Lie KJ, Bras G, 1950. *Ancylostoma caninum* in Indonesia. Doc. Neerl. Indones. Morb. Trop. 2:288

Londero AT, Lauda P, 1967. Infeccao humana por *Syngamus laryngeus*. Hospital 72:1267–1269

Loria-Cortes R, Lobo-Sanahuja JF, 1980. Clinical abdominal angiostrongylosis. A study of 116 children with intestinal eosinophilic granuloma caused by *Angiostrongylus costaricensis*. Am. J. Trop. Med. Hyg. 29:538–544

Loukas A, Croese J, Prociv P, 1992. Detection of antibodies to secretions of *Ancylostoma caninum* in human eosinophilic enteritis. Trans. R. Soc. Trop. Med. Hyg. 86:650–653

Loukas A, Opdebeeck J, Croese J, Prociv P, 1994. Immunologic incrimination of *Ancylostoma caninum* as a human enteric pathogen. Am. J. Trop. Med. Hyg. 50:69–77

Machado De Mendonca J, Davidson S, Loures JDC, 1962. Mais um caso brasileiro de singamose humana. Atas Soc. Biol. Rio. Jan. 6:18–20

MacKerras MJ, Sandars DF, 1954. Life history of the rat lung-worm and its migration through the brain of its host. Nature 173:956–957

MacKerras MJ, Sandars DF, 1955. The life history of the rat lung-worm *Angiostrongylus cantonensis* (Chen) (Nematoda: Metastrongylidae). Aust. J. Zool. 3:1–21

Magdeleine J, Magnaval JF, Brossard B, Michel M, Turiaf J, 1974. La syngamose humaine a la Martinique. Med. Afr. Noire 21:651–655

Malek EA, 1981. Presence of *Angiostrongylus costaricensis* Morera and Cespedes 1971 in Colombia. Am. J. Trop. Med. Hyg. 30:81–83

Manalang C, 1925. Studies on ankylostomiasis in the Philippines. In: *Proceedings of the 6th Congress Far East Association Tropical Medicine Abstracts Scientific Papers,* Tokyo, October 12–16, pp. 351–357.

Mao CP, 1945. Occurrence of dog hookworm (*Ancylostoma caninum*) in man. Chinese Med. J. 63:130–132

Martin LK, 1972a. Hookworm in Georgia. I. Survey of intestinal helminth infections and anemia in rural school children. Am. J. Trop. Med. Hyg. 21:919–929

Martin LK, 1972b. Hookworm in Georgia. II. Survey of intestinal helminth infections in members of rural households of southeastern Georgia. Am. J. Trop. Med. Hyg. 21:930–943

Martin LK, Beaver PC, 1968. Evaluation of Kato thick-smear technique for quantitative diagnosis of helminth infections. Am. J. Trop. Med. Hyg. 17:382–391

Matsusaki G, 1966. Hookworm disease and prevention. In: Morishita K, Komiya Y, Matsufbayashi H (eds), *Progress of Medical Parasitology in Japan*, vol. 3. Tokyo: Meguro Parasitological Museum, pp. 187–282

McDowell DE, 1981. Intestinal bleeding caused by hookworm. JAMA 246:2806

Mead AR, 1961. *The Giant African Snail: A Problem of Economic Malacology.* Chicago: University of Chicago Press

Morera P, 1973. Life history and redescription of *Angiostrongylus costaricensis* Morera and Cespedes, 1971. Am. J. Trop. Med. Hyg. 22:613–621

Morera P, Cespedes R, 1971. *Angiostrongylus costaricensis* n. sp. (Nematoda: Metastrongyloidea), a new lungworm occurring in man in Costa Rica. Rev. Biol. Trop. 18: 173–185

Morera P, Lazo R, Urquizo J, Llaguno M, 1983. First record of *Angiostrongylus costaricensis* Morera and Cespedes, 1971 in Ecuador. Am. J. Trop. Med. Hyg. 32:1460–1461

Morera P, Perez F, Mora F, Castro L, 1982. Visceral larval migrans-like syndrome caused by *Angiostrongylus costaricensis*. Am. J. Trop. Med. Hyg. 31:67–70

Mornex JF, Magdeleine J, De Thore J, 1980. La syngamose humaine (*Mammomonogamus nasicola*) cause de toux chronique en Martinique. 37 observations recentes. Nouv. Presse Med. 9:3628

Naik SR, Mitra SK, Mehta S, 1976. Massive intestinal haemorrhage due to infection with *Ancylostoma duodenale*. J. Trop. Med. Hyg. 79:2–5

Nawalinski TA, Schad GA, 1974. Arrested development in *Ancylostoma duodenale*: course of a self-induced infection in man. Am. J. Trop. Med. Hyg. 23:895–898

Nelson RG, Warren RC, Scotti FA, Call TG, Kim BS, 1988. Ocular angiostrongyliasis in Japan: a case report. Am. J. Trop. Med. Hyg. 38:130–132

New D, Little MD, Cross J, 1995. Correspondence. *Angiostrongylus cantonensis* infection from eating raw snails. N. Engl. Med, 332:1105–1106

Nitidandhaprabhas P, Harnsomburana K, Thepsitthar P, 1975. *Angiostrongylus cantonensis* in the cerebrospinal fluid of an adult male patient with eosinophilic meningitis in Thailand. Am. J. Trop. Med. Hyg. 24:711–712

Nosanchuk JS, Wade SE, Landolf M, 1995. Case report of and description of parasite *Mammomonogamus laryngeus* (human syngamosis) infection. J. Clin. Microbiol. 33:998–1000

Nozais JP, Moreau J, Morlier G, Kouame J, Doucet J, 1980. Premier cas de meningite a eosinophiles en Cote-d'Ivoire avec presence d'un *Parastrongylus* sp. dans le liquide cephalo-rachidien. Bull. Soc. Pathol. Exot. 73:179–182

Nwosu ABC, 1978. Human neonatal infections with hookworms in an cndcmic area—a possible transmammary route. *In: Proceedings of the 4th International Congress of Parasitology.* Warsaw, Poland. Section C, p. 10.

Nye SW, Tangchai P, Sundarakiti S, Punyagupta S, 1970. Lesions of the brain in eosinophilic meningitis. Arch. Pathol. 89:9–19

Otsuru M, 1962. Studies on *Trichostrongylus* (Nematoda: Trichostrongylidae) of man and animals. Kiseichugaku Zasshi 11:244–248

Otsuru M, 1978. *Angiostrongylus cantonensis* and angiostrongyliasis in Japan, with those of neighbouring Taiwan. In: Morishita K, Komiya Y, Matsubayashi H (eds), *Progress of Medical Parasitology in Japan*, Vol. 6. Tokyo: Meguro Parasitological Museum, pp. 225–274.

Pascual JE, Bouli RP, Aguiar H, 1981. Eosinophilic meningoencephalitis in Cuba, caused by *Angiostrongylus cantonensis.* Am. J. Trop. Med. Hyg. 30:960–962

Pereira-Barreto M, Amaral ADF, 1944. Sobre dois casos de parasitismo do homem pelo *Ancylostoma caninum.* (Ercolani, 1859) Hall, 1913. Rev. Clin. Sao Paulo 16:235–240

Phan Trinh, Hoang-Thuc-Thuy, Nguyen-Huu-Binh, 1967. Un cas de meningoencephalite a eosinophiles, de bronchopneumonie et de myocardite interstitielle du a *Angiostrongylus cantonensis*, Chen 1935. Bull. Soc. Pathol. Exot. 67:298–304

Pipitgool V, Chaisiri K, Visetsupakarn P, Srigan V, Maleewong W, 1992. Case report: *Mammonogamus (syngamus) laryngeus* infection: a first case report in Thailand. Southeast Asian J. Trop. Med. Public Health 23:336–337

Pirisi M, Gutierrez Y, Minini C, Dolcet F, Beltrami CA, Pizzolito S, Pitzus E, Bartoli E, 1995. Fatal human pulmonary infection caused by an *Angiostrongylus*-like nematode. Clin. Infect. Dis. 20:59–65

Polderman AM, Krepel HP, Baeta S, Blotkamp J, Gigase P, 1991. Oesophagostomiasis, a common infection of man in northern Togo and Ghana. Am. J. Trop. Med. Hyg. 44:336–344

Polderman AM, Krepel HP, Verweij JJ, Baeta S, Rotmans JP, 1993. Serological diagnosis of *Oesophagostomum* infections: serological diagnosis of *Oesophagostomum* infections. Trans. R. Soc. Trop. Med. Hyg. 87:433–435

Prociv P, Croese J, 1990. Human eosinophilic enteritis caused by dog hookworm *Ancylostoma caninum.* Lancet 335:1299–1302

Prommindaroj K, Leelawongs N, Pradatsundarasar A, 1962. Human angiostrongyliasis of the eye in Bangkok. Am. J. Trop. Med. Hyg. 11:759–761

Punyagupta S, 1965. Eosinophilic meningoencephalitis in Thailand: summary of nine cases and observations on *Angiostrongylus cantonensis* as a causative agent and *Pila ampullacea* as a new intermediate host. Am. J. Trop. Med. Hyg. 14:370–374

Punyagupta S, Bunnag T, 1970. Growth rate of *Angiostrongylus cantonensis* in man and rat. J. Parasitol. 56(Sect 2):274–275

Punyagupta S, Bunnag T, Juttijudata P, Rosen L, 1970. Eosinophilic meningitis in Thailand. Epidemiologic studies of 484 typical cases and the etiologic role of *Angiostrongylus cantonensis*. Am. J. Trop. Med. Hyg. 19:950–958

Punyagupta S, Limtrakul C, Vichipanthu P, Karuchanchetanee C, Nye SW, 1968. Radiculomyeloencephalitis associated with eosinophilic pleocytosis. Report of nine cases. Am. J. Trop. Med. Hyg. 17:551–560

Quinnell RJ, Slater AFG, Tighe P, Walsh EA, Keymer AE, Pritchard DI, 1993. Reinfection with hookworm after chemotherapy in Papua New Guinea. Semin. Respir. Infect. 106:379–385

Railliet A, Henry A, 1909. Description of Thomas' oesophagostome. Trans. R. Soc. Trop. Med. Hyg. 3:49–52

Rep BH, 1975. The topographic distribution of *Necator americanus* and *Ancylostoma duodenale* in the human intestine. Trop. Geogr. Med. 27:169–176

Richards CS, Merrit JW, 1967. Studies on *Angiostrongylus cantonensis* in molluscan intermediate hosts. J. Parasitol. 53:382–388

Rogers AM, Dammin GJ, 1946. Hookworm infection in American troops in Assam and Burma. Am. J. Med. Sci. 211:531–538

Rojas Ayala MA, 1987. Angiostrongiloidiase abdominal. Seis casos observados no parana e em Santa Catarina, Brasil. Mem. Inst. Oswaldo Cruz 82:29–36

Rojas Ayala MA, Guerra IF, Schir RA, Motizuki A, 1982. Angiostrongiloidose abdominal. Mem. Inst. Oswaldo Cruz 77:189–193

Rosen L, Chappell R, Laqueur GL, Wallace GD, Weinstein PP, 1962. Eosinophilic meningoencephalitis caused by a metastrongylid lung-worm of rats. JAMA 179:620–624

Rosen L, Laigret J, Bories S, 1961. Observations on an outbreak of eosinophilic meningitis on Tahiti, French Polynesia. Am. J. Hyg. 74:26–42

Ross RA, Gibson DI, Harris EA, 1989. Cutaneous oesophagostomiasis in man. J. Helminthol. 63:261–265

Ruiz PJ, Morera P, 1983. Spermatic artery obstruction caused by *Angiostrongylus costaricensis* Morera and Cespedes. Am. J. Trop. Med. Hyg. 32:1458–1459

Salfelder K, Deliscano TR, Ortiz AD, Barreto LF, Calderon RG, 1970. Ileitis regional eosinofilica de origen parasitario. GEN 25:131–140

Sang HT, Junod C, Philbert M, 1970. Notes parasitologiques sur *Syngamus laryngeus* Railliet, 1899 et la syngamose humaine. A propos d'un cas de syngamose bronchique chez l'homme. Bull. Soc. Pathol. Exot. 63:488–497

Santos VA, Villela MSH, Serra RG, 1986. Ocorrencia de um novo caso de Singamose humana em Sao Paulo, Brasil. Rev. Inst. Med. Trop. Sao Paulo 28:358–363

Schad GA, 1991. Hooked on hookworm: 25 years of attachement. J. Parasitol. 77:179–186

Schad GA, Chowdhury AB, Dean CG, Kochar VK, Nawalinski TA, Thomas J, Tonascia JA, 1973. Arrested development in human hookworm infections: an adaptation to a seasonally unfavorable external environment. Science 180:502–504

Severo LC, Conci LMA, Camargo JJP, Andre-Alves MR, Palombini BC, 1988. Syngamosis: two new Brazilian cases and evidence of a possible pulmonary cycle. Trans. R. Soc. Trop. Med. Hyg. 82:467–468

Sierra E, Morera P, 1972. Angiostrongilosis abdominal. Primer caso humano encontrado en Honduras (Hospital Evangelico de Siguatepeque). Acta Med. Costar. 15:95–99

Sonakul D, 1978. Pathological findings in four cases of human angiostrongyliasis. Southeast Asian J. Trop. Med. Public Health 9:220–227

St John JH, Simmons JS, Gardner LL, 1929. Infestation of the lung by a nematode of the genus *Cyathostoma*. JAMA 92:1816–1818

Sunardi W, Lokollo DM, Margono SS, 1977. Ocular angiostrongyliasis in Semarang, Central Java. Am. J. Trop. Med. Hyg. 26:72–74

Tan KS, Lie KJ, 1953. Redescription of *Oesophagostomum apiostomum* (Willach, 189 Railliet and Henry, 1905) from man and monkeys in Indonesia. Doc. Med. Geogr. Trop. 5:123–127

Thomas HW, 1910. The pathological report of a case of oesophagostomiasis in man. Ann. Trop. Med. Parasitol. 4:57–88

Timmons RF, Bowers RE, Price DL, 1983. Infection of the respiratory tracts with *Mammomanogamus* (*Syngamus*) *laryngeus*: a new case in Largo, Florida, and a summary of previously reported cases. Am. Rev. Respir. Dis. 128:566–569

Tripathy K, Tuffi Garcia F, Lotero H, 1971. Effect of nutritional repletion on human hookworm infection. Am. J. Trop. Med. Hyg. 20:219–223

Tungkanak R, Sirisinha S, Punyagupta S, 1972. Serum and cerebrospinal fluid in eosinophilic meningoencephalitis: immunoglobulins and antibody to *Angiostrongylus cantonensis*. Am. J. Trop. Med. Hyg. 21:415–420

Ubelaker JE, Hall NM, 1979. First report of *Angiostrongylus costaricensis* Morera and Cespedes, 1971 in the United States. J. Parasitol. 65:307–317

Vasquez JJ, Boils PL, Sola JJ, Carbonell F, de Juan Burgueno M, Giner V, Berenguer-Lapuerta J, 1993. Angiostrongyliasis in a European patient: a rare cause of gangrenous ischemic enterocolitis. Gastroenterology 105:1544–1549

Walker AC, Bellmaine SP, 1975. Severe alimentary bleeding associated with hookworm infestation in aboriginal infants. Med. J. Aust. 1:751–752

Walker NI, Croese J, Clouston AD, Loukas A, Prociv P, 1995. Eosinophilic enteritis in northeastern Australia. Pathology, association with *Ancylostoma caninum*, and implications. Am. J. Surg. Pathol. 19:328–337

Wallace L, Henkin R, Mathies AW, 1956. *Trichostrongylus* infestation with profound eosinophilia. Ann. Intern. Med. 45:146–150

Watson JM, 1953. Human trichostrongylosis and its relationship to ancylostomiasis in southern Iraq, with comments on world incidence. Semin. Respir. Infect. 43:102–109

Weinstein LP, Molavi A, 1971. *Syngamus laryngeus* infection (syngamosis) with chronic cough. Ann. Intern. Med. 74:577–580

Welchman JM, 1966. Helminthic abscess of the bowel. Br. J. Radiol. 39:372–376

Wells AV, 1951. Identity of hookworm in the throat. Br. Med. J. 1:952

WHO, 1964. Soil-transmitted helminths. Technical Report Series No. 277. Geneva: WHO, 1–70

WHO, 1981. Intestinal protozoan and helminthic infections. Technical Report Series No. 666. Geneva: WHO, 1–150

Widagdo, Sunardi, Lokollo DM, Margono SS, 1977. Ocular angiostrongyliasis in Semarang, Central Java. Am. J. Trop. Med. Hyg. 26:72–74

Yen C, Chen ER, Kojima S, Kobayashi M, 1989. Preparation of monoclonal antibody against *Angiostrongylus cantonensis* antigen. Southeast Asian J. Trop. Med. Public Health 20:19–124

Yii CY, 1976. Clinical observations on eosinophilic meningitis and meningoencephalitis caused by *Angiostrongylus cantonensis* on Taiwan. Am. J. Trop. Med. Hyg. 25:233–249

Yii CY, Chen CY, Fresh JW, Chen T, Cross JH, 1968a. Human angiostrongyliasis involving the lungs. Chinese J. Microbiol. 1:148–150

Yii CY, Chen CY, Hsieh HC, Shih CC, Fresh JW, Chen T, 1968b. Report of fatal case of eosinophilic meningoencephalitis caused by *Angiostrongylus cantonensis*. J. Formosan Med. Assoc. 67:4–4

Yong TS, Shin HJ, Im KI, Kim WH, 1992. An imported human case of hookworm infection with worms in the rectum. Korean J. Parasit. 30:59–62

Yousif F, Ibrahim A, 1978. The first record of *Angiostrongylus cantonensis* from Egypt. Z Parasitenkd. 56:73–80

Yu SH, Jiang ZX, Xu LQ, 1995. Infantile hookworm disease in China. A review. Acta Trop. 59:265–270

Zambrano Z, Diaz I, Salfelder K, 1975. Ileocolitis seudotumoral eosinofilica de origen parasitario. GEN 29:87–96

Zavala-Velazquez J, Ramirez-Baquedano W, Reyes-Perez A, Bates-Flores M, 1974. *Angiostrongylus costaricensis*. Primeros casos Mexicanos. Rev. Invest. Clin. 26:389–394

Zuniga SR, Cardona Lopez V, Alvarado QD, 1983. Angiostrongilosis abdominal. Rev. Med. Hondur. 51:184–192

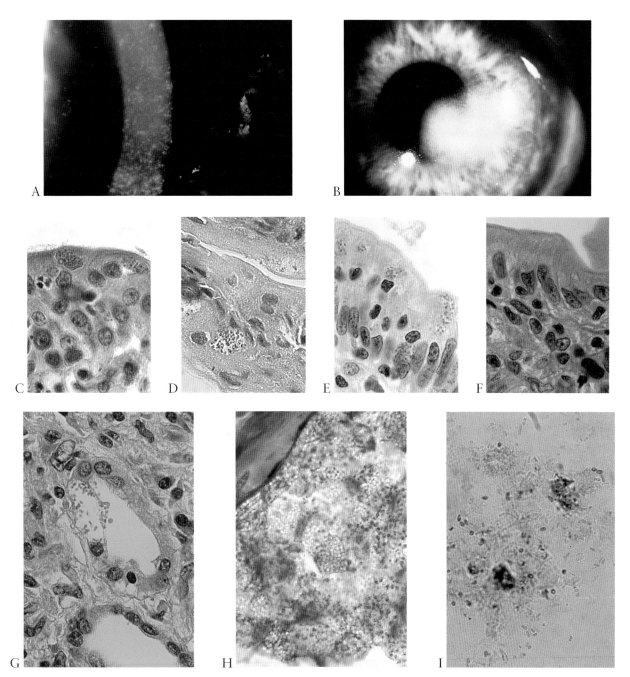

Color Plate 1. *A, Encephalitozoon,* keratitis. Note the punctate lesions which are seen more clearly when illuminated with the slit lamp. (Courtesy of C. Y. Lowder, M.D., Division of Ophthalmology, The Cleveland Clinic Educational Foundation, Cleveland, Ohio.) *B, Vittafforma corneae* keratitis. The lesion produced by this species is more extensive and causes perforation of the cornea. (Courtesy of R. Font, M.D., Cullen Eye Institute, Baylor College of Medicine, Houston, Texas. Reported by: Davis, R. M., Font, R. L., Keisler, M. S., et al. Corneal microsporidiosis. A case report including ultrastructural observations. Ophthalomology 97:953–957.) *C–D, Encephalitozoon,* infection of the cornea and extension to the nasal cavity in a patient with acquired immune deficiency syndrome (AIDS), sections stained with hematoxylin and eosin stain. *C,* Biopsy specimen of cornea. Note the parasites within a vacuole in the epithelial cell, ×640. *D,* Within the nasal epithelium, where the parasite produced large inflammatory polyps. Also, note the presence of two infected epithelial cells, ×640. *E–F,* Intestinal microsporidia, sections stained with hematoxylin and eosin stain. *E, Encephalitozoon intestinalis;* note the location of the parasite in vacuoles within epithelial cells and the nuclear deformation in the center of the cell, ×640. *F, Enterocytozoon bieneusi.* Note the parasites within the cytoplasm of the enterocytes, the lack of vacuole formation, and the cupping of the apex of the nuclei of infected cells. Also, compare the size of these spores (1μm) with the size of the spores of *E. intestinalis* (2μm) in *E,* ×640. *G, Encephalitozoon cuniculi* in kidney tubular epithelial cells of a patient with disseminated infection, section stained with hematoxylin and eosin stain, ×640. *H, Pleistophora* in skeletal muscle, section stained with periodic acid–Schiff stain, ×640. *I, Enterocytozoon bienusi* in fecal smear stained with trichrome stain. Note that the parasites are located within an epithelial cell, which is still recognizable by its nucleus, ×1,120.

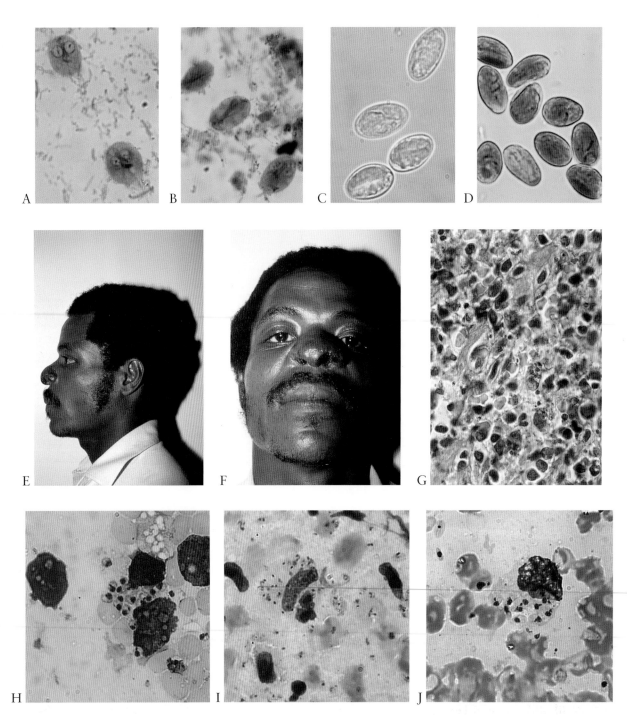

Color Plate II. *A–B, Giardia lamblia* in fecal smears, stained with iron-hematoxylin stain. *A,* Trophozoite in the anteroposterior view. *B,* Cysts, ×1,120. *C–D, Giardia lamblia* cysts in a smear of a fecal sample concentrate. *C,* Unstained. *D,* Iodine stained, ×1,120. *E–F,* American mucocutaneous leishmaniasis. Typical metastasis to the nose by *L. braziliensis.* Note the configuration of the nose in profile ("tapir nose"). (Courtesy of A. D'Alessandro, M.D., CIDEIM, Cali, Colombia, and Tulane University School of Public Health and Tropical Medicine, New Orleans, Louisiana.) *G,* Cutaneous leish-maniae. Section stained with immunoperoxidase stain and counterstained with hematoxylin and eosin stain, ×640. *H–J,* Leishmania amastigotes in diagnostic smears, preparations stained with Giemsa stain, all ×1,120. *H,* Imprint of spleen in visceral leishmaniasis. Note the macrophages with numerous amastigotes. *I,* Imprint of a cutaneous lesion from a patient with diffuse cutaneous leishmaniasis. Note the large number of parasites, many of which appear artifactually outside the cells. *J,* Smear from the border of a skin ulcer. (Preparations courtesy of N. Saravia, Ph.D, CIDEIM, Cali, Colombia, and Tulane University School of Public Health and Tropical Medicine, New Orleans, Louisiana.)

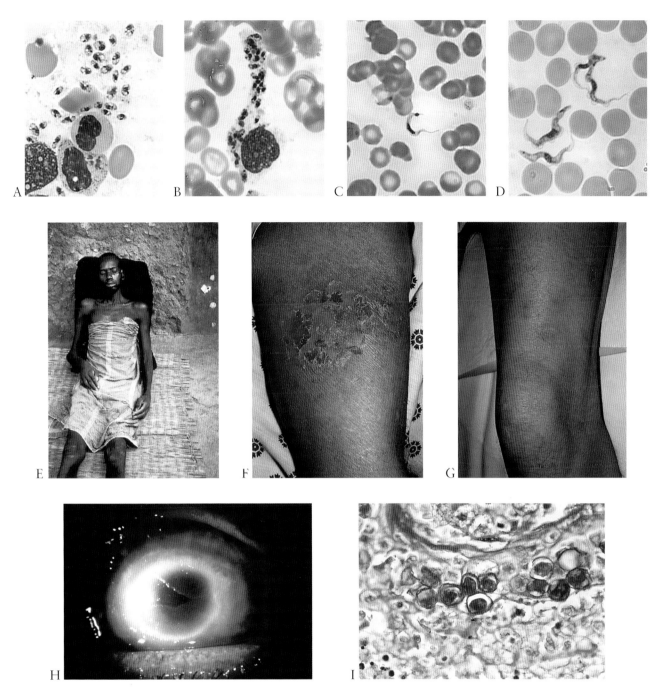

Color Plate III. *A–B*, Visceral leishmaniasis in a bone marrow smear stained with Giemsa stain, ×1,120. Note the broken histiocytes with scattered amastigotes next to them and the typical morphologic characteristics of the amastigotes, mainly the kinetoplast. *C, Trypanosoma cruzi* in blood smear of an experimentally infected mouse, stained with Giemsa stain. Note the C shape of the parasite and its large kinetoplast, ×1,120. *D, Trypanosoma brucei* in blood smear of an experimentally infected animal, stained with Giemsa stain. Note the small kinetoplast and the fact that one parasite is undergoing division, ×1,120. *E, Trypanosoma b. gambiense* infection. Severely ill African male with central nervous system involvement. (Courtesy of W. Peters, M.D., Department of Medical Protozoology, London School of Hygiene and Tropical Medicine, London.) *F–G*, African trypanosomiasis, inoculation chancre. Note the indurated area (*F*) with superfiicial desquamation of the upper epidermis and the rash over the rest of the leg. (Courtesy of R. Cochran, M.D., Houston, Texas. From: Cochran, R., and Rosen, T. 1983. African trypanosomiasis in the United States. Arch. Dermatol. 119:670–674. Reproduced with permission.) *H, Acanthamoeba polyphaga* keratitis. Corneal ulceration and marked keratitis with conjunctivitis. (Courtesy of H. Levine, M.D., Department of Pathology, Cleveland Clinic Educational Foundation, Cleveland, Ohio.) *I*, Acanthamebid around a blood vessel in the brain, demonstrating the characteristic morphology of the cysts in tissues, ×400.

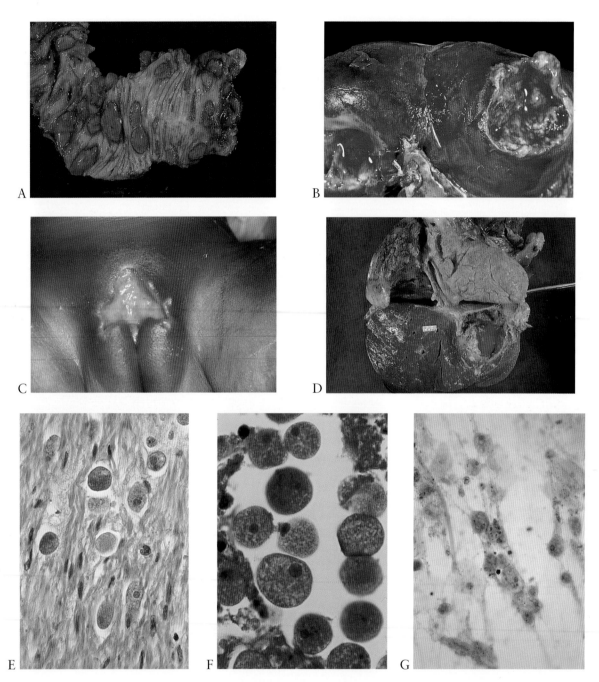

Color Plate IV. *A–D, Entamoeba histolytica,* gross lesion in several organs. *A,* Colon showing extensive ulceration in a patient who underwent emergency colectomy. *B,* Hepatic liver abscess in a 2-year-old infant born and raised in the United States. *C,* Vulva of an infant with a large ulcer. Note the sharp edges and clean base with granulation tissue. (Photograph in *C* courtesy Of A. D'Alessandro, M.D., School of Public Health and Tropical Medicine, Tulane University, New Orleans, Louisiana. Patient at Universidad de Valle, Cali, Colombia.) *D,* Heart showing a rupture of the left lobe of the liver and abscess into the pericardium with purulent pericarditis. Note the connection between the abscess and the pericardial cavity (shown by the probe). (Courtesy of N. Gispert, M.D., Mexico City, Mexico.) *E–F, Entamoeba histolytica* in colon (*E*) and cervix (*F*), demonstrating the morphology of the parasites, sections stained with hemotoxylin and eosin stain. Note the following: the location of the parasite within an empty space, the smooth cell membrane, the finely vacuolated cytoplasm, the nucleus measuring up to 4 μm (absent in some specimens because of the plane of sectioning), and the size (up to 25 μm due to shrinkage during fixation and processing). Note that with hematoxylin and eosin stain, the nucleus of *E. histolytica* stains acidophilically and the cytoplasm slightly basophilically. The reverse is true for histiocytes. *G, Entamoeba histolytica* in a vaginal smear, stained with Papanicolaou stain, from a patient with amebiasis of the cervix. Note the parasites, with the typical nucleus and phagocytized red blood cells (arrows), which stain discretely with Papanicolaou stain, ×250.

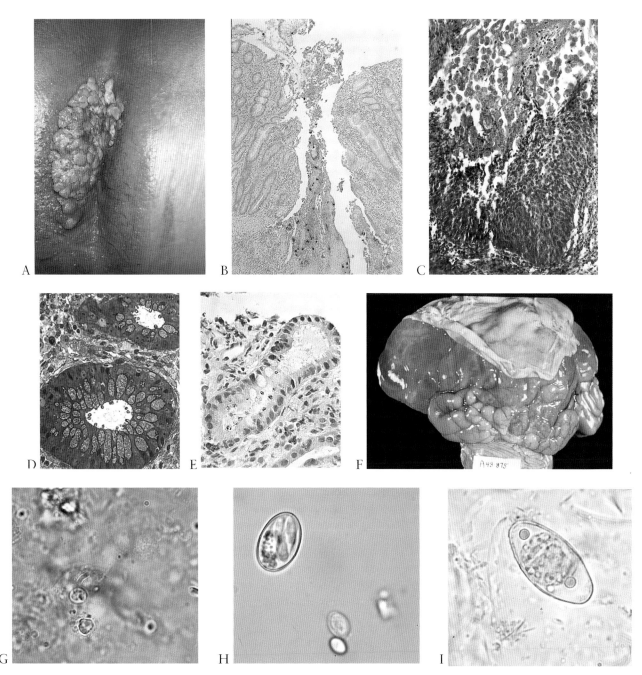

Color Plate V. *A, Entamoeba histolytica.* Pseudocondylomatous lesion of the anus. Note the lack of ulceration, an uncommon finding in these cases. (Courtesy of A. D'Alessandro, M.D., School of Public Health and Tropical Medicine, Tulane University, New Orleans, Louisiana. Patient at Universidad de Valle, Cali, Colombia.) *B, Entamoeba histolytica,* section of colonic ulcer stained with immunoperoxidase stain, ×32. *C, Entamoeba histolytica* in an anal ulcerated growth in a male homosexual, diagnosed as amebic based on fresh mounts from scrapings of the surface. The biopsy specimen shows the coexistence of a squamous cell carcinoma (bottom) and the amebic infection (top), section stained with hematoxylin and eosin stain, ×125. *D–E, Cryptosporidium parvum* in intestine. *D,* In biopsy specimen of colon, embeddded in plastic and stained with hematoxylin and eosin stain, ×260. *E,* In biopsy specimen of small intestine, stained with immunoperoxidase stain, ×260. *F, Toxoplasma gondii,* congenital infection. Gross appearance of the external surface of the brain. Note the effacement of the gyra at the frontotemporal lobes. (Courtesy of U. Roessmann, M.D., Institute of Pathology, Case Western Reserve University, Cleveland, Ohio). *G–I,* Oocysts and sporocyst of intestinal apicomplexan parasites. *G,* Oocyst of *Cryptosporidium,* fresh mount, unstained, ×1,120. *H,* Sporocyst of *Sarcosystis bovicanis,* fresh mount, unstained. This sporocyst, recovered from the feces of a dog, is morphologically similar to sporocysts of *S. hominis* and *S. suihominis* in feces of humans, ×1,120. (Sample courtesy of R. Fayer, Ph.D., Animal Parasitology Institute, United States Department of Agriculture, Beltsville, Maryland.) *I,* Oocyst of *Isospora belli,* fresh mount, stained with iodine stain, ×1,120. (Sample courtesy of R. G. Yaeger, Ph.D., Tulane University, School of Public Health and Tropical Medicine, New Orleans, Louisiana.)

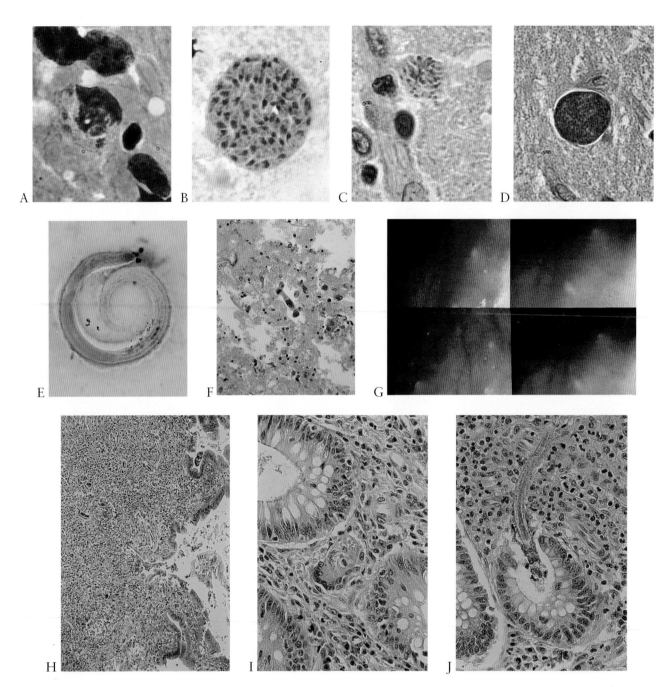

Color Plate VI. *A–D, Toxoplasma gondii*. Diagnostic stages. *A–B*. Tissue imprints stained with Giemsa stain. *A*, Trophozoites (tachyzoites) in imprint of brain from a mouse infected experimentally. *B*, Cyst in imprint of brain from case in Figures 10–11 *B* and 10–14. Note the morphologic characteristics of well-preserved individual trophozoites, which are easy to demonstrate because in smears they have little shrinkage due to fixation. *C–D*, Toxoplasma in histologic sections of brain. *C*, Trophozoites in a pseudocyst, thin paraffin-embedded section stained with hematoxylin and eosin stain. Note that in this section the individual tachyzoites are well delineated. *D*, Cyst in section stained with periodic acid–Schiff stain. Note that the cyst is positive because the bradyzoites (and tachyzoites) have periodic acid–Schiff positive granules. Compare the size and the morphologic elements in the tissue and the imprint stages, all ×1,120. *E–F, Strongyloides stercoralis* in sputum of patients with hyperinfection. *E*, Larva stained with Papanicolaou stain, ×320. (Preparation courtesy of J. Buchino, M.D., Department of Pathology, Children's Hospital, Louisville, Kentucky.) *F*, Cell block in another patient showing sections of larvae, hematoxylin and eosin stain, ×160. *G–J, Strongyloides stercoralis* and eosinophilic granulomatous enterocolitis. *G*, Gross lesions, early in the disease, showing the granulomas underneath the mucosal cell layer. Note that ulceration has not yet occurred. *H–J*, Histologic appearance of colon in sections stained with hematoxylin and eosin stain. *H*, Low magnification showing one ulcer with a marked inflammatory reaction, ×62. *I*, A giant cell in the submucosa with an engulfed, disintegrating larva, ×260. *J*, A longitudinal section of a larva entering the mucosa. Note the numerous eosinophils covering the parasite, most of which are undergoing degranulation, ×260. (Reported by Gutierrez, Y., Bhatia, P., Garbadawala, S. T., et al. 1996. *Strongyloides stercoralis* eosinophilic granulomatous enterocolitis. Am. J. Surg. Pathol. 20:603–612.)

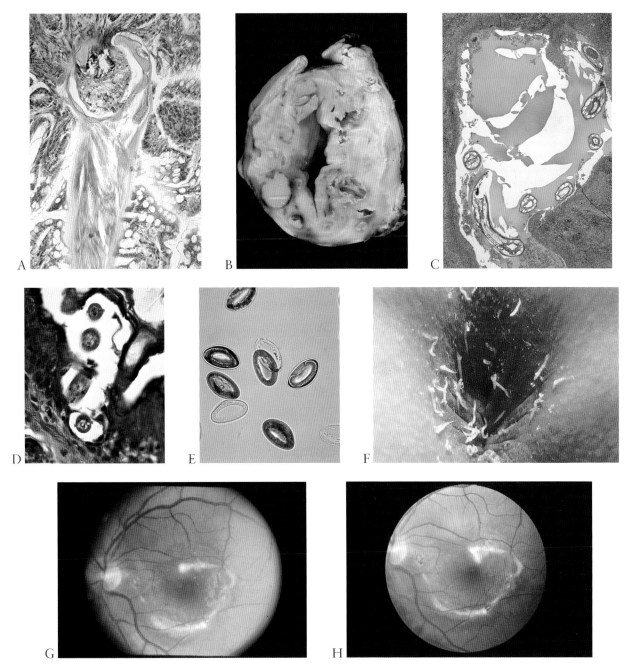

Color Plate VII. *A,* Hookworm, adult attached to intestinal mucosa, section stained with hematoxylin and eosin stain. Note the portion of intestinal mucosa within the buccal cavity of the worm, ×160. (Courtesy of P. C. Beaver, Ph.D., School of Public Health and Tropical Medicine, Tulane University, New Orleans, Louisiana.) *B–D, Oesophagostomum* in humans. *B,* Transverse section of colon shows the enormous thickening of the wall and the abscesses produced by the worms. *C,* Histologic section, stained with hematoxylin and eosin stain, illustrates worms within the abscess, ×16. *D, Ancylostoma braziliense,* experimental infection in mouse, section stained with hematoxylin and eosin stain. Note the location of the larva within the epidermal layer, ×320. (Preparation courtesy of D. E. Norris, Ph.D., Department of Biology, University of South Mississippi, Hattiesburg, Mississippi. Reported by: Norris, D. E. 1971. The migratory behavior of the infective-stage larvae of *Ancylostoma braziliense* and *Ancylostoma tubae-forme* in rodent paratenic hosts. J. Parasitol. 57:988–1009.) *E, Enterobius vermicularis* eggs in Scotch Tape preparation, unstained, ×200. *F, Enterobius vermicularis.* Adult worms in the anus of a 5-year-old child who was crying and restless and complained of abdominal pain. Note the female parasites in the perianal skin, some of which appear spent after having deposited their eggs. Masses of eggs are seen as small white clumps. (In: 1993. Images in clinical medicine, N. Engl. J. Med. 328: 927. Reproduced with permission.) *H–I, Toxocara* ocular lesion. Retinal tract in a 16-year-old boy followed for 4 years. The ocular lesion had periods of quiescence due to encapsulation of the larva and periods of activity due to its reemergence and continued migration in the retina. *H,* The lesion on December 20. *I,* Two months later. (Courtesy of E. M. Sorr, M.D., Department of Ophthalmology, St. Francis General Hospital, Pittsburgh, Pennsylvania. In: Sorr, E. M., 1984. Meandering ocular toxocariasis. Retina 4:90–96. Reproduced with permission.)

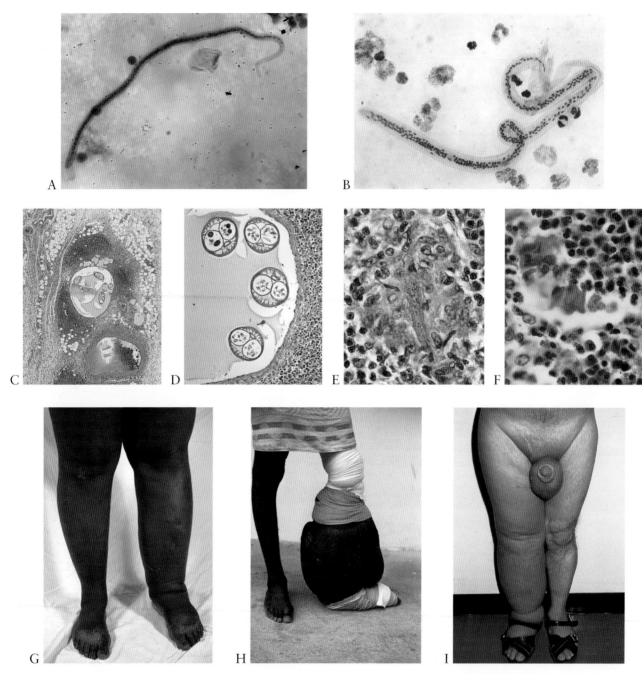

Color Plate VIII. *A–B,* Lymphatic filariae and microfilariae. *A, Brugia malayi,* stained with periodic acid–Schiff hematoxylin stain, ×320. *B, Wuchereria bancrofti,* stained with hematoxylin stain, ×500. *C–D, Brugia malayi,* lesions in experimental animals, sections stained with hematoxylin and eosin stain. *C,* Low magnification showing a dilated lymphatic vessel with cross sections of the worm. Note the inflammatory reaction around the vessel, ×16. *D,* Higher magnification demonstrating the worm within the lymphatic vessel and the inflammatory reaction, ×100. (Preparations courtesy of A. Ewert, Ph.D., Department of Microbiology, University of Texas Medical Branch, Galveston, Texas.) *E–F,* Meyers-Kouwenaar syndrome. Sections of lymph node, stained with hematoxylin and eosin stain. *E,* Microfilaria being destroyed within a granuloma; note the inflammatory eosinophils, ×400. *F,* The M-K body consists of an amorphous mass of eosinophilic material, ×500. *G–I, Wuchereria bancrofti* infection producing different degrees of elephantiasis in individuals from Haiti (*G* and *H*) and in a Turkish man with elephantiasis of the leg and scrotum (*I*). (*D* Courtesy of C. Karaffa-Myles, M.D., Department of Medicine, The Cleveland Clinic Educational Foundation, Cleveland, Ohio.)

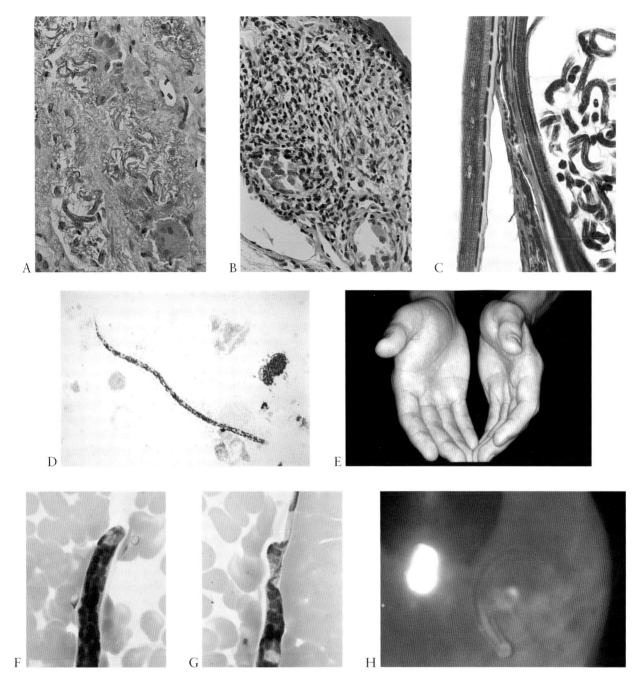

Color Plate IX. *A–B, Onchocerca volvulus,* corneal lesions, sections stained with hematoxylin and eosin stain. Note the microfilariae in the cornea, showing some imflammation and giant cells (*A*) and a strong inflammatory reaction in the cornea of another patient (*B*), ×260. *C, Onchocerca volvulus* in tissues cut longitudinally, section stained with trichrome stain, demonstrating the striae, ×400. *D, Onchocerca volvulus* microfilaria stained with Giemsa stain, ×200. *E, Loa loa* infection in a man with swelling of the left hand (Calabar swelling). (Courtesy of R. Silverman, Department of Dermatology, School of Medicine, Case Western Reserve University, and University Hospitals of Cleveland, Cleveland, Ohio.) *F–G,* Microfilaria of *Loa loa* stained with Giemsa stain, demonstrating the anterior (*F*) and posterior (*G*) ends. Note that the sheath does not stain with Giemsa stain but is revealed by the displacement of the red blood cells, ×630. *H, Gnathostoma* in the eye of a patient in Ecuador. (Courtesy of R. Lazo S., M.D., Centro de Investigacion de Enfermedades Parasitarias y por Hongoes, Quito, Ecuador.)

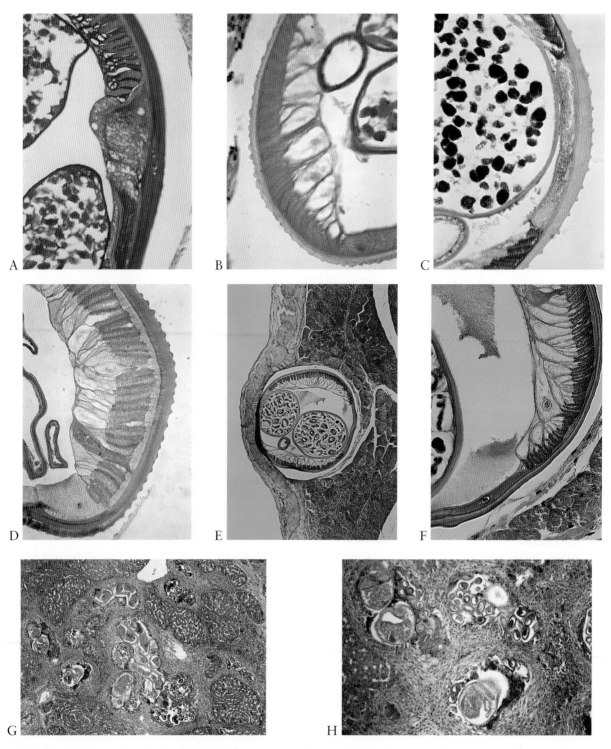

Color Plate X. *A–F,* Subcutaneous zoonotic filariae of humans, detail of the cuticle. *A, Dirofilaria immitis* from an infected dog. The section shows the lack of visible longitudinal ridges. Note the layers of the cuticle, seen better at the level of the lateral chords, and the internal thickening of the cuticle, ×200. *B, Dirofilaria tenuis* from a human infection of subcutaneous tissues. Note the longitudunal ridges and their crowded character (no separation between them), ×260. *C, Dirofilaria ursi,* from a naturally infected porcupine. Observe the cuticular ridges and their wide separation from one another, ×250. *D, Dirofilaria repens* from a human patient, demonstrating the longitudinal ridges. Note that the ridges are separated from one another but are more robust. Contrast these ridges with the sharp ridges of *D. ursi,* ×200. *E–F, Dirofilaria striata* from a naturally infected animal. Note the location of the parasite under the muscle fascia and the smooth character of the cuticle *(E).*The lateral ridge of the cuticle is demonstrated in *(F),* right lower portion, ×260. The section in *C* is stained with trichrome stain; all other sections are stained with hematoxylin and eosin stain. *G–H, Capillaria hepatica* in a rat liver, sections stained with hematoxylin and eosin stain. *G,* Low-magnification photograph showing numerous sections of adult worms and eggs. Note the marked fibrosis around the worms, ×31. *H,* Higher magnification illustrating the marked fibrosis with disruption of the hepatic architecture, ×80.

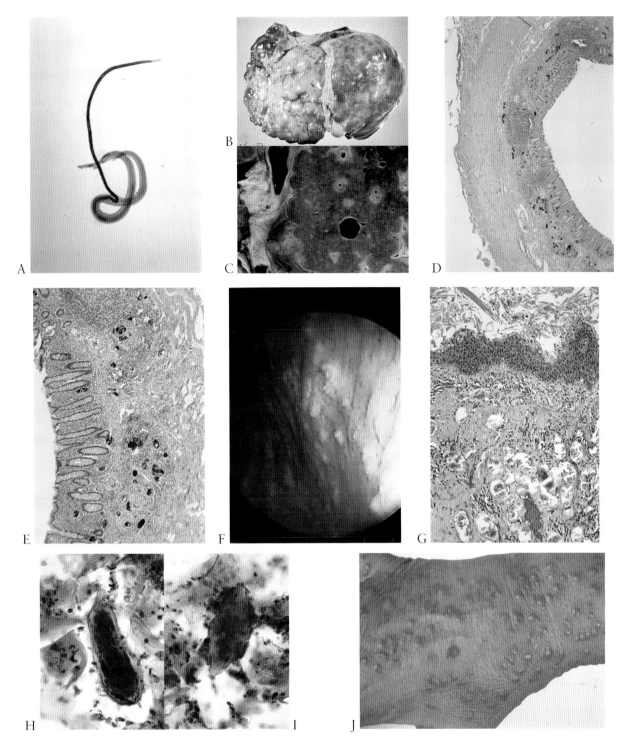

Color Plate XI. *A, Schistosoma mansoni* adults, stained with acetic-alum carmine stain. Note the male and female worms; the female is longer and more slender, and in this case has only the anterior portion of the body in the male's gynecophorous canal, ×72. *B–C, Schistosoma mansoni,* gross appearance of the liver. *B,* The liver shows marked fibrosis. *C,* Close-up view of the cut surface shows fibrosis around the portal system (pipesteam fibrosis) and a slightly nodular appearance. (Courtesy of R. Falzoni, M.D., Department of Pathology, Hospital das Clinicas da Faculdade de Medicina da Universidade de São Paulo, Brazil.) *D–I, Schistosoma haematobium* in humans. *D–E,* In human appendix, section stained with hematoxylin and eosin stain. *D,* Low-power view showing calcified eggs, ×12. *E,* Higher magnification of mucosa with calcified eggs. Note the absence of granulomas and the moderate inflammatory infiltrate, consisting mostly of mono-nuclear cells and a few polymorphs, ×30. *F–G,* In urinary bladder. *F,* Granulomatous appearance of the urinary bladder epithelium. (Courtesy of N. Cornish, M.D., Department of Clinical Pathology, Cleveland Clinic Educational Foundation, Cleveland, Ohio.) *G,* Histologic appearance of the lesions, note the large number of eggs and the inflammatory infiltrate, ×80. *H–I,* In a vaginal smear stained with Papanicolaou stain. *H,* Miracidium artifactually broken out of its shell at the time the smear was prepared. Note the cilia and the metazoan characteristics (multiple nuclei) of the larva. *I,* Egg showing a small terminal spine (bottom end). Note the numerous cells still attached to the eggshell, ×260. *J,* Schistosomal dermatitis produced by a zoonotic infection with any of several bird schistosomes capable of causing the lesion. (Courtesy of J. Pilz, M.D., Facharzt fur Dermatologie, Allergologie und Umweltmedizin, Munich, Germany.)

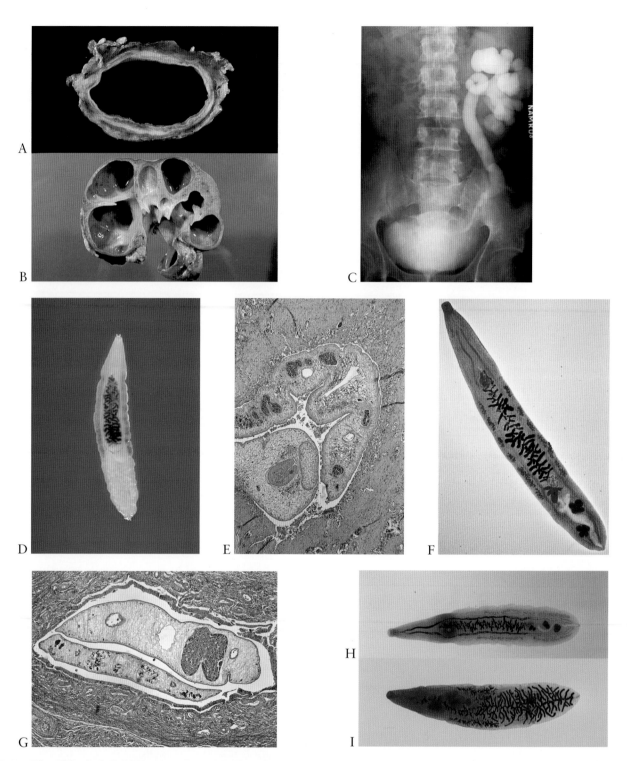

Color Plate XII. *A–C, Schistosoma haematobium* infection producing obstructive uropathy. *A,* Urinary bladder showing thickening and calcification of the wall. *B,* The kidney shows significant dilation of the pelvis and the caliceal system. *C,* A pyelogram demonstrates obstruction of the lower left ureter. (Courtesy of J. H. Smith, M.D., Department of Path-ology and Laboratory Medicine, College of Medicine, Texas A & M University, College Station, Texas.) *D–E, Clonorchis sinensis. D,* Adult worm, unstained, ×2. *E,* Liver section from an infected human, stained with hematoxylin and eosin stain, demonstrating the worms in the bile duct and the marked fibrosis of the duct, ×30. *F–G, Opistorchis viverrini.* Adult worm stained with acetic-alum carmine, ×12 (*F*) and worm in the bile duct (*G*). The worm in this section is difficult to identify, but it is probably an *Opistorchis.* Section stained with hematoxylin and eosin stain, ×40. *H, Amphimerus pseudophelineus.* Adult worm stained with hematoxylin stain, x6.4. *I, Dicrocoelium dendriticum.* Adult worm stained with acetic-alum carmine stain, ×6.4.

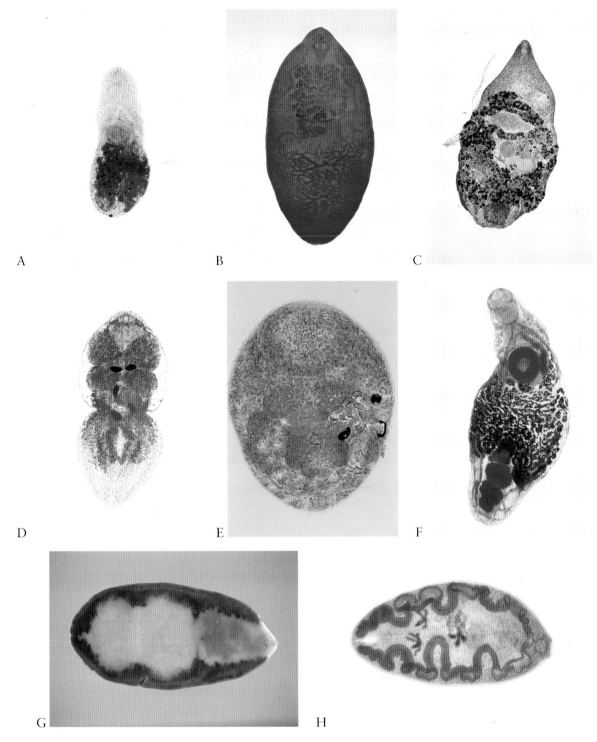

Color Plate XIII. *A, Heterophyes heterophyes.* Adult worm stained with acetic-alum carmine stain, ×40. (Preparation courtesy of E. A. Malek, Ph.D., School of Public Health and Tropical Medicine, Tulane University, New Orleans, Louisiana.) *B, Fasciolopsis buski.* Adult worm stained with acetic-alum carmine stain, ×2. *C, Metagonimus yokogawai.* Adult worm stained with acetic-alum carmine stain, ×40. *D, Neodiplostomum (= Fibricola) seoulensis.* Adult worm stained with acetic-alum carmine stain, ×40. (Preparation for *C* and *D* courtesy of S. Huh, M.D., Department of Parasitology, College of Medicine, Hallym University, Chunchon, Korea.) *E, Gymnophalloides seoi.* Adult worm stained with acetic-alum carmine stain, ×260. (Preparation courtesy of S. H. Lee, Department of Parasitiology, College of Medicine, Seoul National University, Seoul, Korea.) *F, Philophthalmus* species. Adult worm recovered from the eye of a man in Ohio, stained with acetic-alum carmine stain, ×12.5. (Reported by: Gutierrez, Y., Grossniklaus, H. E., and Annable, W. L. 1987. Human conjunctivitis caused by the bird parasite *Philophthalmus.* Am. J. Ophthalmol. 104:417–419.) *G, Fasciolopsis buski.* Adult worm, unstained, ×2. *H, Paragonimus westermani.* Adult worm stained with acetic-alum carmine stain, ×16. (Preparation courtesy of S. Huh, M.D., Department of Parasitology, College of Medicine, Hallym University, Chunchon, Korea.)

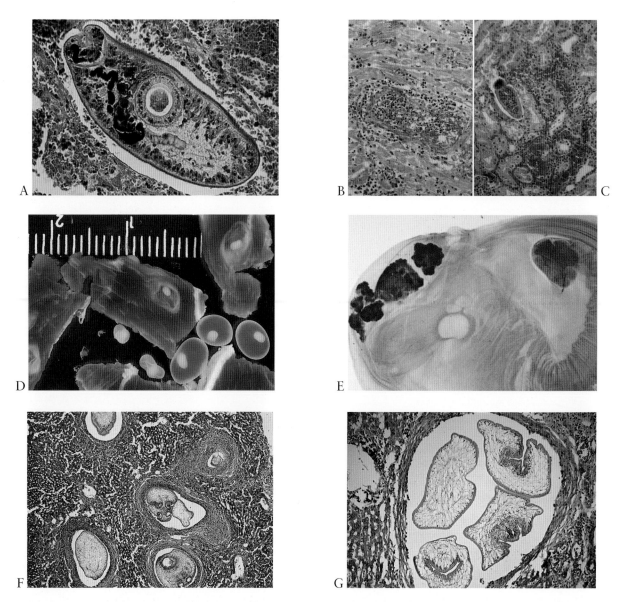

Color Plate XIV. *A–C, Alaria americana* in a man with systemic infection, sections stained with hematoxylin and eosin stain. *A,* Metacercaria in the lung, cut longitudinally. Note the oral sucker at the anterior aspect (upper right) and the ventral sucker at the midportion of the body, ×950. *B,* Microscopic lesions in the heart representing tracks left by the metacercariae during their migration, ×160. *C,* Similar lesions and the parasite in the kidney, ×160. (Reported by: Fernandez, B. J., Cooper, J. D., Cullen, J. B., et al. 1976. Systemic infection with *Alaria americana* (Trematoda). Can. Med. Assoc. J. 115:1111–1114. Courtesy of B. J. Fernandez, M.D., Department of Pathology, Mount Sinai Hospital, Toronto, Canada.) *D–E, Taenia saginata* cysticerci in muscle and dissected out. Note the translucent nature of the cysts, which allows visualization of the scolex inside. *E,* Whole mount of a cysticercus of *T. solium* stained with acetic-alum carmine stain. Visualized here are the scolex and the neck of the parasite, ×8. *F–G, Tetrathyridium* larva of *Mesocestoides* in the liver of an experimentally infected animal. This strain of the parasite was multiplying asexually, *F* ×32, *G* ×64.

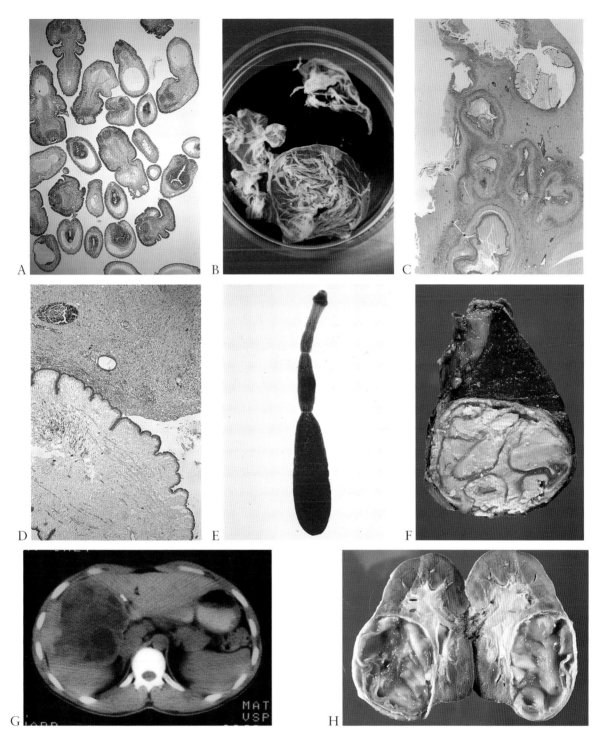

Color Plate XV. *A, Cysticercus longicollis* of *Taenia crassiceps,* section stained with hematoxylin and eosin stain. Note the cysticerci with scolices, some of which are budding, ×12.5. *B, Cysticercus racemosus* from a human case. Note the absence of a scolex and the outgrowths of the cyst. (Courtesy of P. Torres, Dr.Sc., Instituto de Parasitilogia, Universidad Austral de Chile, Valdivia, Chile. Reported by: Ortega, E., and Torres, P. 1991. Un caso de infeccion humana por cysticerco racemoso de localizacion parenquimatosa en Valdivia, Chile. Rev. Inst. Med. Trop. S. Paulo. 33:227–331. Reproduced with permission.) *C–D, Sparganum* in the brain, section stained with hematoxylin and eosin stain. *C,* Low magnification illustrating the damage produced by the larva. Note that the parasite is viable in some places and completely disintegrated in others. This is a feature of tapeworms parasites, whose bodies may contain both dead and living portions, ×5. *D,* Higher magnification illustrating the larva with its characteristic longitudinal muscles, ×32. *E–H,Echinococcus granusus. E,* Adult showing the scolex, followed by the neck and three proglottids: one immature, one mature, and one gravid, ×20. *F,* Computed tomogram of a cyst in the liver. *G,* Dead, degenerating cyst in the spleen. (Courtesy of J. Torrado, M.D.). *H,* Viable cyst in the kidney. Note the white acellular membrane and the daughter cysts. (Courtesy of Ariel Gutierrez-Hoyos, M.D.) (Both authors at Servicio de Patologia, Hospital Aranzazu, San Sabastian, Universidad del Pais Vasco, Spain.)

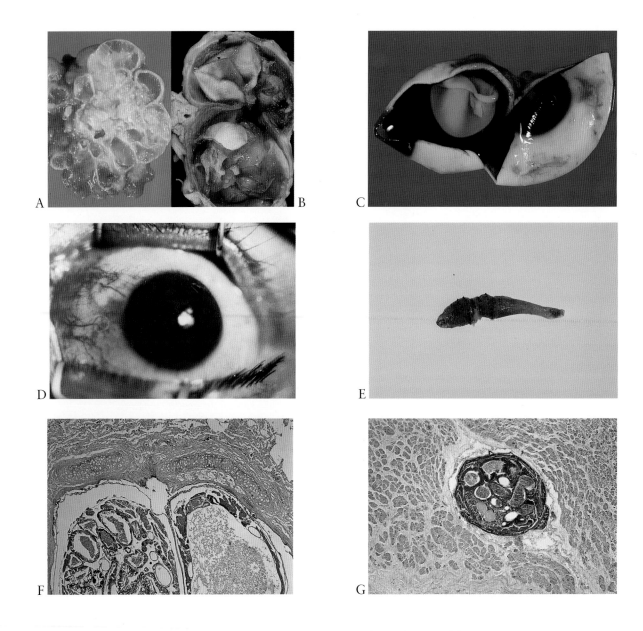

Color Plate XVI. *A–D, Echinococcus* cysts, gross appearance. *A, Echinococcus vogeli* in liver; note its polycystic nature. (Courtesy of A. D'Alessandro, M.D., CIDEIM, Cali, Colombia, and Tulane University School of Public Health and Tropical Medicine, New Orleans, Louisiana.) *B,* Viable *Echinococcus granulosus* in pancreas. *C, Echinococcus granulosus* in the eye. (Courtesy of Ariel Gutierrez-Hoyos, M.D., Servicio de Patologia, Hospital Aranzazu, San Sabastian, Universidad del Pais Vasco, Spain.) *D, Linguatula serrata* in the eye of an Ecuadorian patient. The parasite is barely visible at the upper left of the dilated pupil. (Courtesy of R. Lazo S., M.D., Centro de Investigacion de Enfermedades Parasitarias y por Hongos, Quito, Ecuador.) *E, Dermatobia hominis,* second-stage larva, recovered from a furuncle of a patient who had recently traveled to Central America. Note the rows of spines around the body. *F–G,* Maggots in dead people. *F,* Maggot in the bronchus and *G* in the heart of an individual found 3 days after his death, sections stained with hematoxylin and eosin stain. Note the autolysis and the lack of inflammation. (Courtesy of R. C. Challener, M.D., Cuyahoga County Coroner's Office, Cleveland, Ohio.)

14

CUTANEOUS LARVA MIGRANS

The parasitic species associated with infections under natural, accidental laboratory, or experimental conditions, with cutaneous larva migrans and their definitive hosts are the following:

Hookworms

Genus: *Ancylostoma* (hookworm)

Species: *A. braziliense* (cats and dogs), *A. caninum* (dogs), *A. duodenale* (humans), and *A. ceylanicum* (dogs, cats, and humans)

Genus: *Necator* (hookworm)

Species: *N. americanus* (humans)

Genus: *Uncinaria* (hookworm)

Species: *U. stenocephala* (dogs)

Genus: *Bunostomum* (hookworm)

Species: *B. phlebotomum* (cattle)

Strongyloides

Genus: *Strongyloides*

Species: *S. stercoralis* (human), *S. myopotami* (nutria), *S. procyonis* (raccoons), *S. ramsoni* (pigs), *S.*

websteri (horses), and *S. papillosus* (sheep and goats)

Spiruriids

Genus: *Gnathostoma* (stomach worm)

Species: *G. spinigerurn* (cats)

Insects

Genus: *Gasterophilus* (insect)

Species: *G. intestinalis*, *G. nasalis*, and *G. hemorrhoidalis* (horse botflies)

Genus: *Hypoderma* (insect)

Species: *H. bovis* and *H. lineatus* (cattle warble flies)

Biology. The port of entry to the definitive host by infective larvae of hookworms (see Chapter 13) and of *Strongyloides* (see Chapter 12) is the skin; species of *Ancylostoma* may also use the oral route (see Chapter 13). In both cases the larvae migrate to the intestine and develop into adults. In nature, the larvae of these parasitic species may accidentally or purposely invade hosts other than their normal definitive hosts, remaining dormant in the tissues (see Chapter 13). For example, the larvae of *A. caninum* in abnormal hosts migrate from the skin and distribute throughout the skeletal muscle cells (Lee et al. 1973, 1975; Nichols, 1956), and the larvae of *A. tubaeforme* of cats invade the salivary glands and nasopharyngeal epithelium (Norris, 1973). In these tissues, the larvae remain in a state of paratenism. (The larvae remain in the muscles and when, through carnivorism, the paratenic host is ingested by the appropriate final host for the parasite, they complete their life cycle.)

Species of *Strongyloides* infecting hosts other than their normal definitive hosts may complete their development and produce intestinal infections because they generally have low host specificity. Species of *Gnathostoma* and other related spiruriids in abnormal hosts also become paratenic (see Chapter 18). Moreover, species of *Gasterophilus* and *Hypoderma* enter the skin of their normal hosts, migrating in the tissues and reaching the intestinal tract to continue their life cycle (see Chapter 28). All these species (hookworms, *Strongyloides Gnathostoma*, *Gasterophilus*, and *Hypoderma*) in humans, abnormal hosts, produce lesions while traveling through the skin referred to as *cutaneous larva migrans* (Beaver, 1956). The first known description of the disease used the name *creeping eruption* (Lee, 1874), but later the term *cutaneous larva migrans* was introduced (Crocker, 1893). The pioneer work of Kirby-Smith and colleagues (Kirby-Smith et al. 1926) and that of White and Dove (White, Dove, 1928, 1929) demonstrated that the infective larvae of animal hookworms are the main producer of the disease.

The development of cutaneous larva migrans requires persistence of the larvae in the skin for periods longer than those normally required to enter the general circulation to continue their life cycles. Hookworm and *Strongyloides* larvae in the skin may persist when they are located in abnormal hosts or in normal hosts that have become sensitized to the parasite's antigens. The larval stages of *Gnathostoma* (see Chapter 18) migrate in the tissues, including the skin, in their paratenic hosts.

The majority of cases of cutaneous larva migrans are therefore zoonotic. Most of these cases are due to *A. braziliense* and *A. caninum*, both of which have a worldwide distribution. In Europe, cutaneous larva migrans is also produced by *Uncinaria stenocephala*, and in southern Louisiana and Texas, some cases are due to animal *Strongyloides* (Burks, Jung, 1960; Little, 1965). In areas endemic for *A. duodenale*, *A. ceylan-*

icum, *N. americanus*, and *S. stercoralis*, cutaneous larva migrans is also due to these organisms.

The mechanism responsible for the production of cutaneous larva migrans in humans by *A. duodenale*, *N. americanus*, and *S. stercoralis* is not well known. Allergic sensitization to the parasite and its antigens, produced by repeated exposure to the larvae, has some supportive evidence. Repeated experimental exposure of the skin to infective larvae of *N. americanus* produced an increased skin reaction with successive exposures (Beaver, 1944). Similarly, the development of a skin rash in a volunteer exposed to *Strongyloides* of animals necessitated several exposures before the lesions developed (Little, 1965). Whether animal hookworms and other species of animal *Strongyloides* require sensitization of the host before producing lesions is not known. The mere fact that they are not native human species, and thus that humans are unsuitable hosts, may explain some wandering through the skin.

Geographic Distribution and Epidemiology. Cutaneous larva migrans occurs throughout the tropical and subtropical areas of the world, especially where moist, sandy coastal soil is present. In the United States most infections occur in the southeastern states, especially Florida (Donaldson et al. 1950), but they are also found sporadically elsewhere. The incidence of the infection is unknown, mainly because many cases do not come to the attention of physicians; in 1950 over 7000 cases were reported in Florida (Wilson, 1952). In recent years, cases of cutaneous larva migrans acquired by American tourists (Caumes et al. 1995; CDC, 1981; Jelinek et al. 1994) and European tourists to the Caribbean or to African countries (Barriere, 1974; Rubio et al. 1992) have been reported with more frequency (Barriere, 1974). Large outbreaks usually occur in groups of individuals such as soldiers during field exercises (Hume, 1930) or in groups of travelers (Huber, 1972).

Clinical Findings. Larva migrans is clinically a dermatitis anywhere in the skin; it is more common in skin areas likely to be in contact with soil, such as the extremities (Fig. 14–1 A–B). In experimental infections with 50 larvae, the symptoms begin a few minutes after exposure with a prickling sensation; 10 minutes later, small wheals up to the size of a pinhead develop. A few hours later reddish papules replace the initial wheals; the papules then coalesce to form a confluent erythemato-papular eruption. At 24 hours minute vesicles appear, becoming an erythemato-papular-vesicular

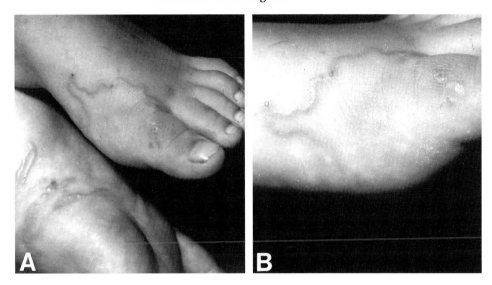

Fig. 14–1. Cutaneous larva migrans, lesions in a 3-year-old child. *A,* **Serpiginous tracks in both feet. Note the difference in the lesions between the right foot (top) and the left (bottom).** *B,* **Right foot showing a single track corresponding to one larva migrating in the epidermis; the lesion began in the toe, and this portion of the lesion is the oldest part of the track; the newer portion is less well-defined.**

dermatitis that itches intensively. At the fifth day postinfection, definitive serpiginous, linear, tortuous advancing tracts appear, consisting of fine, wavy, raised linear tracks containing small, erythematous papules with excoriations (Africa, 1932). The lesion, or lesions, advances steadily through the skin at a rate that depends on the species of the parasite producing the infection. The appearance of the tracks changes with their age: the most recent portions consist of narrow, erythematous formations that fade toward their ends. Portions of the lesion 24 to 48 hours old consist of a well-defined track that is slightly raised, easily palpated, and 1 to 2 mm wide, punctuated with small, pearly-looking vesicles filled with fluid. These vesicles may become secondarily infected. The 48 to 72 hour lesion is dry, consisting of a collapsed track with a crust that desquamates. If the lesion is scratched, the vesiculo-pustular dermatitis reappears; completely healed tracts may show depigmentation of the skin (Africa, 1932). The tracks may be numerous in heavy infections, but a few tracks or even only one track may be present; each track corresponds to a larva migrating through the skin. Superimposed bacterial infections due to continuous scratching of the lesion are common, these infections change the appearance of the dermatitis. Peripheral eosinophilia of between 6% and 19% was found in a series of patients studied in a tropical area; the total leukocyte counts were less than 10,000 per cubic millimeter (Homez, 1954). Massive eosinophilia

is uncommon; it occurs in heavily infected individuals (Homez, 1967)

Depending on the species responsible for the lesion and the clinical appearance, cutaneous larva migrans can be grouped into several types. Classification promotes understanding of the disease and management of the patient. Sometimes the type of lesion suggests the identity of the larva.

Type I. Animal Hookworms. Ancylostoma braziliense, *A. caninum,* and probably other animal hookworms produce cutaneous larva migrans characterized by well-defined tracks that extend several centimeters from their point of origin. The lesions may disappear for days and then reappear at other places. The infection can be chronic, lasting for many months in spite of treatment. Most important, these larvae migrate at a rate of 3.5 to 5 cm per 24 hours (Figs. 14–1 *A–B*).

Type II. Human Hookworms. Ancylostoma duodenale and *N. americanus* produce these lesions. They are characterized by marked blister formation, short tracks around the site of entry of larvae, and intense itching. Biologically, they are characterized by eventual migration to the lungs and intestine, where the parasites mature to adults. This type of larva migrans is known commonly as *ground itch.* The patient invariably shows hookworm eggs in feces approximately 5 weeks later (Fig. 14–2; see Chapter 13 Beaver, 1944; Yoshida et

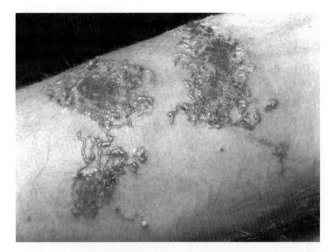

Fig. 14–2. *Necator americanus*, **experimental infection with 200 larvae applied to the skin at three locations. Photographs were taken 63 hours later. Note the numerous blisters and the small tracks produced by this human hookworm. (Courtesy of P.C. Beaver, Ph.D., School of Public Health and Tropical Medicine, Tulane University, New Orleans, Louisiana. In: Beaver, P.C. 1964. Cutaneous larva migrans. Indust. Med. Surg. 33:319–321. Reproduced with permission.)**

patent infection, as has been shown with *S. ramsoni* (Matuzenko, 1971) and *S. myopotami* (Little, 1965). Infections with *S. myopotami* and *S. procyonis* are known only in the Gulf Coast states of the United States from clinical cases (Burks, Jung, 1960) and experimental infections (Little, 1965). The lesion is an erythematous, macular, nonscaly, circinate eruption resembling erythema multiforme. Examination with indirect light shows the characteristic burrows of migrating larvae (Burks, Jung, 1960). It is believed that the lesions are acquired while standing immersed in water. The initial distribution of the lesions is below the line of submersion; later the lesions may extend to other areas of the body (Figs. 14–4 *A–B*; Little, 1965).

al. 1971). In endemic areas of hookworm the condition is seen often, with the largest number of cases occurring in infants less than 2 years old (Bada, 1971).

Type III. Strongyloides stercoralis. Human *Strongyloides* produces a type of cutaneous larva migrans known as *larva currens* because it advances at a rate of up to 5 cm per hour (Arthur, Shelley, 1958; Brumpt, Sang, 1973). Often the lesion begins in the perineal area and then advances to the lower extremities, the back, or the front of the abdomen, sometimes reaching the chest. The tract is wide, poorly defined (Fig. 14–3), and sometimes fairly long; often the patient complains of other allergic cutaneous manifestations (Amer et al. 1984). The patient usually has a patent *Strongyloides* infection that is diagnosed by the cutaneous presentation. *Strongyloides* larvae within the perineal region become infective, penetrate the skin, and produce the lesions (see Chapter 12).

Type IV. Animal Strongyloides. Cutaneous larva migrans produced by *Strongyloides* of animals is variable. The few reports of larva migrans due to accidental laboratory infections with *S. ramsoni*, *S. papillosus*, and *S. websteri* (Maligin, 1958; Roeckel, Lyons, 1977) indicate that the lesions are similar to those seen in *S. stercoralis*. Also important is the fact that some of these species may be able to reach the intestine and produce

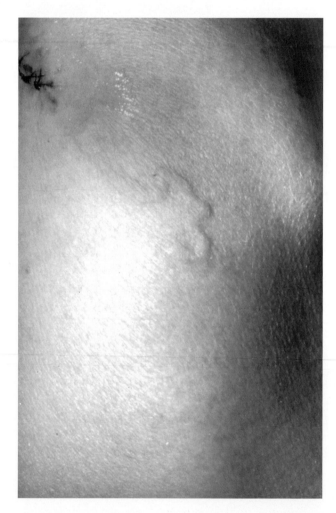

Fig. 14–3. *Strongyloides stercoralis*, **larva currens in a Southeast Asian man who presented with rash and was biopsied (surgical sutures at top). One hour later he had developed a 7 cm track produced by a migrating larva. (Courtesy of B.R. Davis, M.D., Department of Dermatology, Cleveland Metropolitan Hospital, Cleveland, Ohio.)**

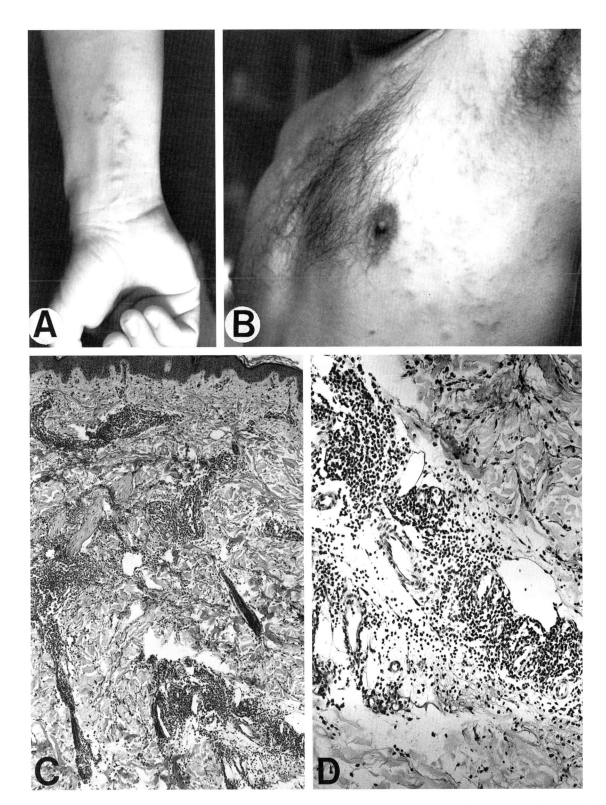

Fig. 14–4. *Strongyloides procyonis* and *S. myopotami*, lesions produced experimentally. *A*, Gross lesion of the arm. Note the tracks produced by the larvae. *B*, Chest lesions. *C* and *D*. Histologic appearance, sections stained with hematoxylin and eosin stain. *C*, Low-power view of skin showing large foci of inflammatory cells in the dermis, ×55. *D*, Higher magnification of an infiltrate showing its distribution around the small blood vessels, ×140. (Gross photographs and preparation courtesy of M.D. Little, Ph.D., School of Public Health and Tropical Medicine, Tulane University, New Orleans, Louisiana. Reported by: Little, M.D. 1965. Dermatitis in a human volunteer infected with *Strongyloides* of nutria and raccoon. Am. J. Trop. Med. Hyg. 14:1007–1009. Reproduced with permission.)

Type V. Gnathostoma. Cutaneous larva migrans produced by species of *Gnathostoma* and other non-speciated spiruriids (see Chapter 18) is usually seen in Japan and Thailand and less often in other countries of Southeast Asia (Bhaibulaya, Charoenlarp, 1983; Daengsvang, 1980; Miyazaki, 1960). Parasitic invasion occurs not only from below the skin (by ingested larvae that migrate from the intestine to the skin), but also probably from direct penetration of the parasite through the skin while handling animal flesh (Daengsvang et al. 1970). The rate of migration of the larvae is variable and may depend on their location in the skin. In the epidermis, larvae travel at a rate of up to 4.5 cm in 24 hours (Tamura, 1921), while in the dermis they travel at a rate of about 3.0 cm per hour.

The lesions produced by *Gnathostoma* in the skin are usually wide tracks similar to those of *A. braziliense,* disappearing and reappearing at a distant location and often lasting for several months. Sometimes after the larvae disappear from the skin, an inflammatory nodule forms somewhere in the subcutaneous tissues (see Chapter 18). The parasites have been found migrating both in the epidermis (Tamura, 1921) and in the dermis (Nagao, 1955; Pinkus et al. 1981);

because of their size, *Gnathostoma* larvae can be visualized easily with the naked eye and recovered in toto if a small incision is made (Bhaibulaya, Charoenlarp, 1983).

Type VI. Insect Larvae. Some species of *Gasterophilus* and *Hypoderma* have been found migrating through the skin and producing linear lesions originally described by the term *creeping eruption.* These lesions are now referred to as *myiasis,* a group of infections produced by the larvae of flies, and sometimes as *myiasis linearis* (see Chapter 28). The characteristic lesion produced by *Gasterophilus* and *Hypoderma* consists of a single continuous track without blister formation moving at a rate of 3 cm (Rudell, 1913) to 7.5 cm (Schalek, 1923) per 24 hours. In all cases, the larva is found at the end of the track. It is easily seen by rubbing the skin with mineral oil (Austman, 1926) or by blanching the skin with slight pressure from a small magnifying glass. The larva is usually located in the epidermis, (Selisky, 1926), sometimes in the upper dermis (Darier, 1920; Heath et al. 1968; Montgomery, 1930), and can always be extracted intact by exscoriating the superficial epidermis.

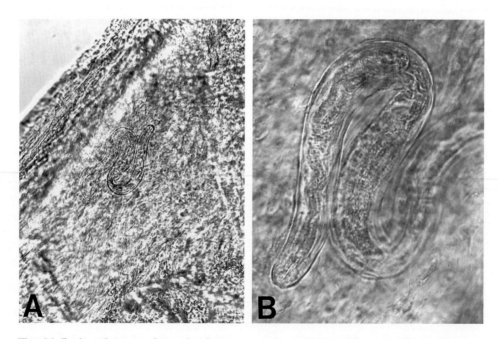

Fig. 14–5. *Ancylostoma* **larva in the cornea of a patient with corneal opacities requiring a transplant.** *A* **and** *B,* **Different magnifications of the larva mounted in toto. (Photographs courtesy of P.C. Beaver, Ph.D., School of Public Health and Tropical Medicine, Tulane University, New Orleans, Louisiana. Reported by: Nadbath, R.P., and Lawlor, P.P. 1965. Nematode (Ancylostoma) in the cornea. A case report. Am. J. Ophthalmol. 59:486–490. Reproduced with permission.)**

Other Manifestations of Cutaneous Larva Migrans. There are other aspects of cutaneous larva migrans that should be considered. As stated above, the human hookworms, *S. stercoralis*, and other animal *Strongyloides* species eventually gain access to the lungs. They may produce Loeffler's syndrome (see Chapter 16) and complete their life cycles. The animal hookworms may also reach the lungs in humans and produce Loeffler's syndrome, but they do not mature to adults in the intestine (Butland, Coulson, 1985; Horton, 1949; Wright, Gold, 1946). In some individuals with cutaneous larva migrans and pulmonary infiltrates (Kalmon, 1954) or pulmonary symptoms, the larvae can be recovered from sputum (Muhleisen, 1953).

Another aspect of cutaneous larva migrans is the migration of the larvae through the cornea, producing inflammation that results in opacities (Figs. 14–5 A–B; Beaver, 1969; Nadbath, Lawlor, 1965). Finally, there is an eosinophilic myositis following cutaneous larva migrans, probably caused by *A. caninum.* After the typical skin lesions disappear, the parasites invade the deep muscles of the thigh, producing a myositis (Fig. 14–6) with generalized symptoms (Little et al. 1983). In one case, fever, cough, chest pain, and pulmonary infiltrates that persisted for several weeks developed, and the peripheral eosinophilia reached 31% of 38,000 white blood cells. Following these symptoms, swelling over the right thigh, effusion over the right knee, and right inguinal lymphadenopathy developed. After approximately 3 months of continuous and incapacitating disease, a muscle biopsy was performed. One year later, the affected thigh was still tender and enlarged in spite of several treatments (Fig. 14–6). The behavior of the larvae in this case is similar to the behavior expected in a paratenic host (Lee et al. 1973): encapsulation in the muscle mass. Technically, the lesion is another form of visceral larva migrans (see Chapter 17).

Pathology. The best-known pathologic changes in cutaneous larva migrans are those produced by hookworm larvae in experimental and natural infections and by *Strongyloides* in experimental ones. All hookworm larvae appear to migrate through the epidermis in the stratum of Malpighi (between the granular cell layer and the stratum basale), where they burrow a tunnel (see Fig. 15–7 A). Larval stages are seldom seen in tissue sections because the clinical lesion develops long after the larva has passed through; it is located away from the visible end of the track in an area of normal-looking skin. Biopsy specimens of the lesions usually show only the empty tunnel (Fig. 14–7 B), with a polymorphonuclear cell infiltrate consisting mainly of eosinophils and a few mononuclear cells in the dermis (Fig. 14–7 B). If the larva is found, it is located in a burrow (Fig. 14–7 C) or in a hair follicle without inflammation.

Strongyloides is located in the upper dermis just below the epidermis. The larva has not been found in biopsy specimens of skin in clinical cases, and in experimental infections there is only an inflammatory reaction noted in the dermis, similar to that seen in hookworms (Figs. 14–4 C–D). In cases of *Strongyloides* infection, larvae were present in skin biopsy specimens taken from periumbilical purpuric rashes in different patients. These patients had disseminated infection, and the parasite reached the dermis through the circulation,

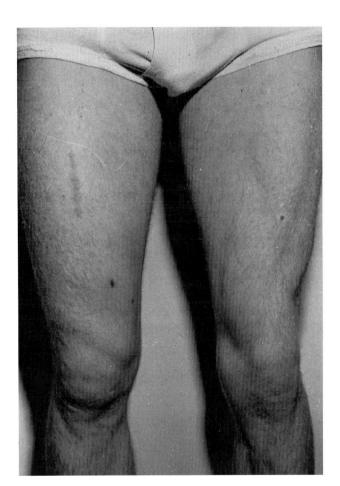

Fig. 14–6. Myositis caused by *A. caninum* larvae. Man with swelling of the right thigh. (Courtesy of M.D. Little, Ph.D., School of Public Health and Tropical Medicine, Tulane University, New Orleans, Louisiana. Reported by: Little, M.D., Halsey, N.A., Cline, B.L., et al. 1983. *Ancylostoma* larva in a muscle fiber of a man following cutaneous larva migrans. Am. Trop. Med. Hyg. 32:1285–1288. Reproduced with permission.)

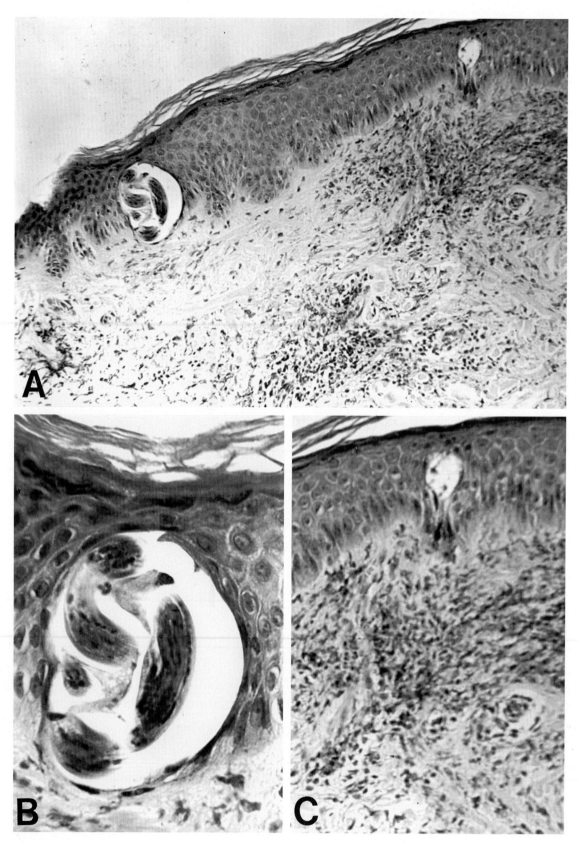

Fig. 14–7. Histologic appearance of cutaneous larva migrans produced by hookworm larvae, hematoxylin and eosin stain. *A*, Low-power view of a section from a skin biopsy specimen showing the location of the hookworm larva (*Ancylostoma*) within the epidermis. On the right is the empty track through which the larva migrated and the inflammatory reaction in the dermis. Note the lack of inflammation around the larva, ×200. *B*, Higher magnification of the larva, ×320. *C*, Empty track and inflammatory reaction, ×150. (Photograph courtesy of H. Blank, M.D., Department of Dermatology, Miami School of Medicine, Miami, Florida.)

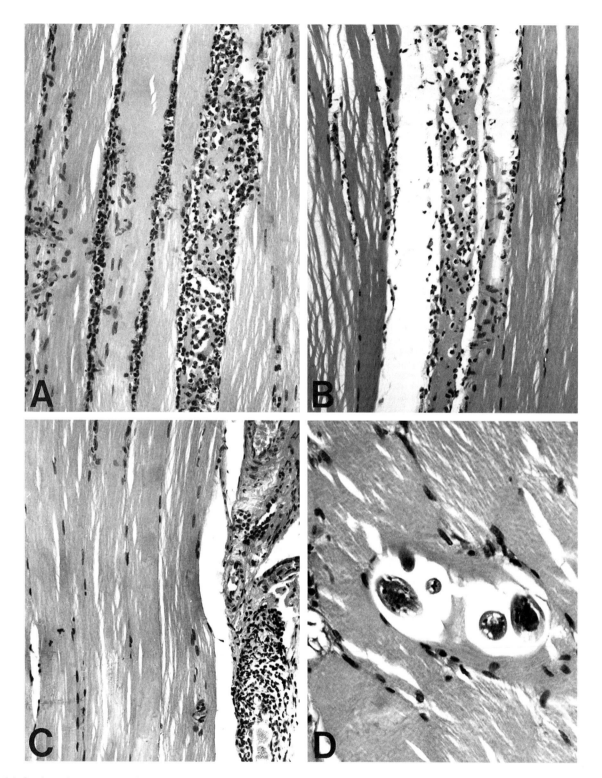

Fig. 14–8. *Ancylostoma caninum*, myositis following cutaneous larva migrans, hematoxylin and eosin stain. *A* and *B*, Low-power view of affected muscle fibers. Note the complete destruction and the inflammatory reaction, consisting mostly of eosinophils, ×180. *C*, Another area showing the perivascular infiltrate in the interfascicular connective tissue; at the bottom there is a vasculitis, ×180. *D*, Detail of a larva inside a muscle fiber. Note the lack of inflammatory reaction. (Preparation courtesy of M.D. Little, Ph.D., School of Public Health and Tropical Medicine, Tulane University, New Orleans, Louisiana. From the same patient shown in Fig. 14–6.)

not through active skin penetration (see Chapter 12; Kalb, Grossman, 1984). The larvae of *Gnathostoma* (see Chapter 18 and Fig. 18–4), *Gasterophilus*, and *Hypoderma* (see Chapter 28) can be found in the epidermis and dermis.

The eosinophilic myositis produced by *Ancylostoma* larvae (probably *A. caninum*) consists of inflammatory changes around and within dead muscle fibers. The characteristic histologic picture consists of single fiber degeneration, with large numbers of eosinophils and an inflammatory infiltrate of the interstitium of adjacent muscles and around blood vessels (Figs. 14–8 *A–C*), often involving the vessel wall itself (vasculitis) (Fig. 14–8 *C*). The larvae are located inside the muscle fiber and do not produce an inflammatory reaction (Fig. 14–8 *D*).

Diagnosis. The diagnosis of cutaneous larva migrans is usually made clinical grounds, based on the patient's history and the clinical appearance of the skin lesions. Rarely, histologic sections show pathologic changes in the skin produced by the larva; even more rarely, the larva is found (Figs. 14–7 *A–B* and *color plate* VII *D*). If there is a larva in the epidermis, it may correspond to hookworm, *Gasterophilus*, *Hypoderma*, *Gnathostoma*, or another spiruriid nematode. Hookworm larvae in cross section measure up to 24 Fm wide and have small, double lateral alae (*color plate* VII *D*), but it is impossible to identify the different species of hookworm larvae in cross sections (Nichols, 1956). *Gasterophilus*, *Hypoderma* (see Chapter 28), and *Gnathostoma* (see Chapter 18) are larger and have distinct morphologic features. *Strongyloides* larvae in cases of larva currens are located below the epidermis; their maximum diameter at midgut is between 14 and 16 Fm (Nichols, 1956).

References

Africa CM, 1932. Studies on experimental creeping eruption in the Philippines. Philipp. J. Sci. 48:89–101

Amer M, Attia M, Ramadan AS, Matout K, 1984. Larva currens and systemic disease. Int. J. Dermatol. 23:402–403

Arthur RP, Shelley WB, 1958. Larva currens. A distinctive variant of cutaneous larva migrans due to *Strongyloides stercoralis*. Arch. Dermatol. 78:186–190

Austman KJ, 1926. Creeping eruption: report of first case from Manitoba. JAMA 87:1196–1200

Bada JL, 1971. Larva "migrans" cutanea. (Estudio de cien casos). Med. Trop. 47:124–133

Barriere H, 1974. Creeping disease, myase cutanee. Une nouvelle pathologie de vacances. Semin. Hop. Paris 50:827–829

Beaver PC, 1944. Immunity to *Necator americanus* infection. J. Parasitol. 31(Sect 2):18

Beaver PC, 1956. Parasitological review. Larva migrans. Exp. Parasitol. 5:587–621

Beaver PC, 1969. The nature of visceral larva migrans. J. Parasitol. 55:3–12

Bhaibulaya M, Charoenlarp P, 1983. Creeping eruption caused by *Gnathostoma spinigerum*. Southeast Asian J. Trop. Med. Public Health 14:266–268

Brumpt LC, Sang HT, 1973. Larva currens seul signe pathognomonique de la strongyloidose. Ann. Parasitol. Hum. Comp. 48:319–328

Burks JW, Jung RC, 1960. A new type of water dermatitis in Louisiana. South. Med. J. 53:716–719

Butland RJA, Coulson IH, 1985. Pulmonary eosinophilia associated with cutaneous larva migrans. Thorax 40:76–77

Caumes E, Carriere J, Guermonprez G, Bricaire F, Danis M, Gentilini M, 1995. Dermatoses associated with travel to tropical countries: a prospective study of the diagnosis and management of 269 patients presenting to a tropical disease unit. Clin. Infect. Dis. 20:542–548

CDC, 1981. Cutaneous larva migrans in American tourists—Martinique and Mexico. Morb. Mort. Weekly Rep. 30:308, 313

Crocker HR, 1893. Larva migrans. In: *Diseases of the Skin*, 2nd ed. Philadelphia: 926–927

Daengsvang S, 1980. *A Monograph on the Genus* Gnathostoma *and Gnathostomiasis in Thailand*. Tokyo: Southeast Asian Medical Information Center

Daengsvang S, Sermswatsri B, Youngyi P, Guname D, 1970. Penetration of the skin by *Gnathostoma spinigerum* larvae. Ann. Trop. Med. Parasitol. 64:399–402

Darier J, 1920. Cas de creeping disease (larva migrans) contracte a Paris. Ann. Dermatol. Syphilogr. 1:113–120

Donaldson AW, Steele JH, Scatterday JE, 1950. Creeping eruption in the southeastern United States. *Proceedings of the 87th Annual Meeting of the American Veterinary Association*, Section of Public Health, pp. 83–89

Heath ACG, Elliott DC, Dreadon RG, 1968. *Gasterophilus intestinalis*, the horse bot-fly as a cause of cutaneous myasis in man. N.Z. Med. J. 68:31–32

Homez J, 1954. La dermatitis verminosa serpiginosa (creeping disease) en Maracaibo. Estudio sobre doscientos casos. Rev. Soc. Med. Quir. Zulia 28:41–61

Homez J, 1967. Dermatitis larvaria verminosa migrans (creeping eruption). Med. Cutan. 2:263–276

Horton SH, 1949. Creeping eruption. Report of a case with Loeffler's syndrome. U.S. Naval Med. Bull. 49:703–706

Huber HP, 1972. Epidemieartiges Auftreten von creeping diesase. Dermatologica 145:88–91

Hume EE, 1930. Wet sand creeping eruption at the largest American army station. Trans. R. Soc. Trop. Med. Hyg. 24:313–326

Jelinek T, Maiwald H, Nothdurft HD, Loscher T, 1994. Cutaneous larva migrans in travelers: synopsis of histories, symptoms, and treatment of 98 patients. Clin. Infect. Dis. 19:1062–1066

Kalb RE, Grossman ME, 1984. Periumbilical purpura in disseminated strongyloidiasis. JAMA 256:1170–1171

Kalmon EH, 1954. Creeping eruption associated with transient pulmonary infiltrations. Radiology 62:222–226

Kirby-Smith JL, Dove WE, White GF, 1926. Creeping eruption. Arch. Dermatol. Syphilogr. 13:137–175

Lee KT, Little MD, Beaver PC, 1973. Intra-cellular (muscle-fiber) habitat of *Ancylostoma caninum* larvae in the vertebrate host. Yonsei Rep. Trop. Med. 4:155

Lee KT, Little MD, Beaver PC, 1975. Intracellular (muscle-fiber) habitat of *Ancylostoma caninum* in some mammalian hosts. J. Parasitol. 61:589–598

Lee RJ, 1874. Case of creeping eruption. Trans. Clin. Soc. 8:44–45

Little MD, 1965. Dermatitis in a human volunteer infected with *Strongyloides* of nutria and raccoon. Am. J. Trop. Med. Hyg. 14:1007–1009

Little MD, Halsey NA, Cline BL, Katz SP, 1983. *Ancylostoma* larva in a muscle fiber of man following cutaneous larva migrans. Am. J. Trop. Med. Hyg. 32:1285–1288

Maligin SA, 1958. A case of cutaneous form of strongyloidiasis caused by larvae of *S. ransomi, S. websteri* and *S. papilosus*. Med. Parasitol. 4:446–447

Matuzenko VA, 1971. On human invasion with the agent of swine strongyloidoisis [in Russian. English summary]. Med. Parazitol. 40:427–431

Miyazaki I, 1960. On the genus *Gnathostoma* and human gnathostomiasis with special reference to Japan. Exp. Parasitol. 9:338–370

Montgomery H, 1930. Larva migrans (creeping eruptions). Arch. Dermatol. Syphilogr. 22:813–821

Muhleisen JP, 1953. Demonstration of pulmonary migration of the causative organism of creeping eruption. Ann. Intern. Med. 38:595–600

Nadbath RP, Lawlor PP, 1965. Nematode (*Ancylostoma*) in the cornea. A case report. Am. J. Ophthalmol. 59:486–490

Nagao M, 1955. A case of creeping disease caused in man by a larval *Gnathostoma spinigerum*. Fukuoka Acta Med. 46:207–214

Nichols RL, 1956. Etiology of visceral migrans. II. Comparative larval morphology of *Ascaris lumbricoides, Necator americanus, Strongyloides stercoralis,* and *Ancylostoma caninum*. J. Parasitol. 42:363–399

Norris DE, 1973. Migratory behavior of infective stage larvae of *Ancylostoma* species in rodent paratenic hosts. *Proc. 9th Int. Cong. Trop. Med. Mal.* 1:175–176

Pinkus H, Fan J, Degiusti D, 1981. Creeping eruption due to *Gnathostoma spinigerum* in a Taiwanese patient. Int. J. Dermatol. 20:46–49

Roeckel IE, Lyons ET, 1977. Cutaneous larva migrans, an occupational disease. Ann. Clin. Lab. Sci. 7:405–410

Rubio S, Ruiz L, Gascon J, Corachan M, 1992. Lava migrans cutanea en viajeros. Med. Clin. Barcelona 98:224–226

Rudell GL, 1913. Creeping eruption. Two cases with recovery of the larvae. JAMA 61:247

Schalek A, 1923. First report of case of creeping disease. Neb. Med. J. 8:38–39

Selisky AB, 1926. Zur histologie der creeping disease. Arch. Dermatol. Syphilogr. 152:123–125

Tamura H, 1921. On creeping disease. Br. J. Dermatol. Syphilogr. 33:81–151

White GF, Dove WE, 1928. The causation of creeping eruption. JAMA 90:1701–1704

White GF, Dove WE, 1929. A dermatitis caused by larvae of *Ancylostoma caninum*. Arch. Dermatol. Syphilogr. 20:191–200

Wilson JF, 1952. The treatment of larva migrans with stibanose. A preliminary report. South. Med. J. 45:127–130

Wright DO, Gold EM, 1946. Loeffler's syndrome associated with creeping eruption (cutaneous helminthiasis). Report of twenty-six cases. Arch. Intern. Med. 78:303–312

Yoshida Y, Okamoto K, Chiu JK, 1971. Experimental infection of man with *Ancylostoma ceylanicum* Looss, 1911. Chinese J. Microbiol. 4:157–167

15

OXYURIDA—*ENTEROBIUS VERMICULARIS*– ENTEROBIASIS OR OXYURIASIS

The family Oxyuridae, has the order Oxyurida, which contains two genera with parasitic species in humans: *Enterobius* and *Syphacia*. The most important species is *E. vermicularis*, referred to commonly as *pinworm* because of the characteristic needle-like posterior end of the female. Another species, *E. gregorii*, was characterized on the basis of minute morphologic differences of the spicule (part of the copulatory organ of the male) (Hugot, 1983; Hugot, Tourte Schaefer, 1985). However, careful study has shown that the differences in the spicules are due to differences in the worm's age (Hasegawa et al. 1998). *Enterobius* occurs in every place where it has been searched for, always in coinfections (sympatrically) with *E. vermicularis* (Ashford et al. 1988; Chittenden, Ashford, 1987; Hasegawa, Kinjo, 1996). The genus *Syphacia* is parasitic in mice; in only one case, worms and eggs of *S. obvelata* were recovered from a child in the Philippines (Riley, 1919).

Morphology and Life Cycle. On gross examination *E. vermicularis* appear as delicate, small white nematodes. The male is 2 to 5 mm long by 0.2 mm wide, with the posterior end curved ventrally; the female is larger, 8 to 13 mm long by 0.5 mm wide, with a sharply pointed posterior end. Both sexes have a cephalic bladder-like cuticular inflation. Under the microscope, well-fixed, cleared specimens show a muscular esophagus with a large terminal bulb; gravid females usually have uteri greatly expanded by a large number of eggs. The eggs are translucent, often with a developing embryo or a fully developed larva; they have a thick shell that is flattened on one side, and they measure 50 to 60 μm × 20 to 30 μm (Beaver et al. 1984).

Enterobius vermicularis inhabits the colon, especially the cecal portion, but whether it lives within the intestinal contents or within the mucus close to the wall, as *Syphacia* does in the mouse, is unknown. Members of the Oxyurida have only one host in their life cycles (Fig. 15–1). After the worms copulate, the gravid *Enterobius* females migrate from the cecum to the anus and out to the perianal skin, where they lay eggs that develop to infective stages in the moist perianal skin folds (*color plate* VII *E–F*). After infective eggs are ingested by a susceptible host, the larvae develop to adults in the intestine, probably within the mucosal crypts of the ileum, cecum, and appendix. These are immature worms, which after maturation leave the mucosa and locate in the lumen (Duran-Jorda, 1957). In the lumen,

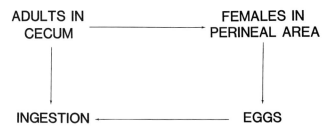

Fig. 15–1. *Enterobius vermicularis*, **schematic representation of the life cycle.**

the normal habitat of the parasites, they ingest colonic contents (Mya, 1955). The entire cycle is reportedly complete within 4 to 6 weeks, with 30 days being the best estimate (Cho et al. 1981).

Geographic Distribution and Epidemiology. *Enterobius vermicularis* has a worldwide distribution. It is acquired by contamination and thus is common among persons living in close contact. It occurs with equal frequency in both sexes. Enterobiasis has been shown repeatedly to be an infection that tends to occur in all persons within a household. Deworming of a population with a single dose of medication resulted 10 months later in a higher prevalence rate and higher worm burdens (Haswell Elkins et al. 1987). It has been repeatedly suggested that the prevalence of enterobiasis is lower in the tropics (WHO, 1981), but this conclusion appears to be due to poor survey methodologies (Haswell Elkins et al. 1987). In several studies, the prevalence of enterobiasis has been shown to decrease with increasing age (Cram, Reardon, 1939; Hayashi et al. 1959; Rahman, 1991), suggesting that it is an infection mostly of children. However, in surveys made in India, the prevalence of the infection was similar in all age groups (Haswell Elkins et al. 1987). *Enterobius* occurs in 24% of Eskimos and Aleutians, as shown by a study of appendices removed surgically (Ashburn, 1941). In a shantytown in Lima, Peru, the prevalence in school children was 42% (Gilman et al. 1991), comparable to the 40% rate found in a similar group in Indonesia (Norhayati et al. 1994). The prevalence of enterobiasis is significantly lower in blacks than in whites; the reason for this difference is unknown (Cherubin, Shookhoff, 1963; Cram, 1943). In an orthopedic ward of a children's hospital in Liverpool, England, the prevalence of *E. vermicularis* was 55% (Ashford et al. 1988). The parasite is transmitted from person to person through contaminated hands, clothes, and fomites. In a study of children from two elementary schools in southern California, the prevalence of *Enterobius* was 12% and 22%, but these rates represented a significant

decline from those found in a study performed two decades earlier. Extrapolation of these data to the country at large indicates that there are at least 4.5 million children with enterobiasis in the United States (Wagner, Eby, 1983).

Clinical Findings. The main symptom of enterobiasis is pruritus, mostly in the evening, probably due to the migration of female pinworms during oviposition. The disease causes continuous scratching of the perineal area, which can result in superimposed bacterial infections. Peripheral eosinophilia is absent because the worms normally do not migrate through the tissues. Women may develop vulvovaginitis (Kacker, 1973). Other symptoms of enterobiasis are due to the migration of female worms from the perineal area into the vagina and other organs. This is discussed below under Ectopic Locations and Clinicopathologic Correlation.

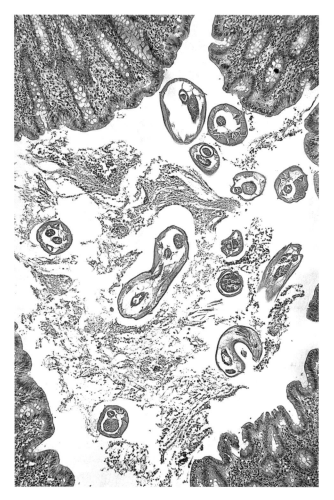

Fig. 15–2. *Enterobius vermicularis* **in the lumen of the appendix. Section stained with hematoxylin and eosin stain, ×60.**

Pathology. There are usually no histologic changes in the large intestine associated with *Enterobius*. The parasites are often found in the lumen of the appendix (Figs. 15–2 and 15–3 *A–F*; Sinniah et al. 1991); in rare cases, they are buried in the mucosa (Fig. 15–4 *A–D*). The second most common location is in the abdominal cavity, especially the pelvic peritoneum (see below). On occasion, worms are found within the mucosa of the small intestine (see Fig. 14–3 *A*), the colon, and the appendix, generally with no inflammatory reaction; in a few instances, they are found within an acute abscess (Fig. 15–4 *D*; see below).

A report of an emaciated, chronically ill 46-year-old man, with dysentery and massive enterobiasis of the ileum and colon, with numerous ulcerations, led the author to conclude that the ulcers were unrelated to the parasite (Bijlmer, 1946). This interpretation should be revised because of similar cases reported recently (Beattie et al. 1995; Liu et al. 1995a; Liu et al. 1995b; Surmont & Liu 1995) and an unpublished case of a patient observed by this writer. The patient was a mentally impaired young man admitted to the hospital with a clinical diagnosis of enterocolitis. Examination of his stool revealed numerous immature and mature male and female *Enterobius* organisms, abundant eosinophils, and Charcot-Leyden crystals.

Ectopic Locations and Clinicopathologic Correlation.

As stated above, female worms lay their eggs in the perianal and perineal skin, where they move. This movement puts the worms in the path of various structures and organs, which predisposes them to locate ectopically. In women the worms may enter the vagina, and through the cervical os to the uterine cavity, fallopian tubes, ovaries, and peritoneal cavity. The worms release eggs during their migration and die anywhere in their path. The released eggs may be found in clinical samples taken at the time, such as in vaginal and cervical smears. Eggs released in the peritoneal cavity elicit a granulomatous reaction. The dead worm may also produce an inflammatory reaction and, depending upon the location of the necrosis, may cause abscess formation and finally organization, leaving a residual, collagenized granuloma measuring up to 2 cm in diameter. In addition to migrating through the genital tract of women, the worms may enter other structures and organs, where the pathophysiology of the tissue reaction is harder to explain. These ectopic locations of *Enterobius* are discussed in the following paragraphs.

Perianal and Perineal Skin. In the perianal (Mattia, 1992) and perineal (Shiraki et al. 1974; Sinniah et

al. 1991) skin, as well as on the surface of the rectum (Chandrasoma, Mendis, 1977), the parasites produce inflammatory nodules, abscesses, and cellulitis. Surgical resection of these lesions reveals the dead worm, or the uterus full of eggs, or a mass of eggs, depending on how much time has elapsed since the worm gained access to the area. It should be kept in mind that *Enterobius* cannot damage the skin; thus, the worms must enter a normal or, probably more likely, an inflamed and dilated gland. This is indicated by one case in which a perianal mass with cellulitis showed the worm within areas of squamous epithelium on histologic sections (Mattia, 1992). However, the presence of epithelia near the worm has been neither seen nor commented on in other similar cases (Chandrasoma, Mendis, 1977; Mortensen, Thomson, 1984; Sinniah et al. 1991). In a series of 259 pathologic specimens with lesions produced by *Enterobius*, the prevalence of perineal lesions was over 1% (Sinniah et al. 1991).

Urinary Bladder and Urethra. The most important ectopic location of *Enterobius* is the urinary bladder, especially in young girls. That the worms enter the urethra and urinary bladder of females was confirmed by the case of a small girl with acute urinary symptoms. The exit of an adult *Enterobius* from the urethra was witnessed by a physician, the father of the girl (Broadbent, 1975). Moreover, *Enterobius* eggs have been recovered in the urine of young girls (Adungo et al. 1986). Presumably, worms entering the urinary bladder carry intestinal bacteria. This was shown in one study revealing a higher incidence of urinary tract infections (60%) caused by *Escherichia coli* in young girls with a coexisting *Enterobius* infection. This association was statistically significant when compared to only 5% in an age-matched control group (Simon, 1974). This original conclusion that worms entering the urinary bladder carry intestinal bacteria was firmly established by a study of girls in whom nocturia, enuresis nocturna, and bacteriuria were significantly higher in those with enterobiasis. The authors of this study suggest screening for pinworm in all girls with urinary symptoms (Gokalp et al. 1991). Recurrent urinary tract infections have also been found more commonly in girls with enterobiasis (Kropp et al. 1978). Sudden nocturnal and diurnal enuresis and frequent urination have been suggested to be associated with enterobiasis (Sachdev, Howards, 1975).

Prostate. The presence of prostatic lesions (Symmers, 1957) produced by *Enterobius*, with symptoms of prostatitis and with eggs in urine (Raymond et al. 1979), was difficult to explain in the past but not anymore.

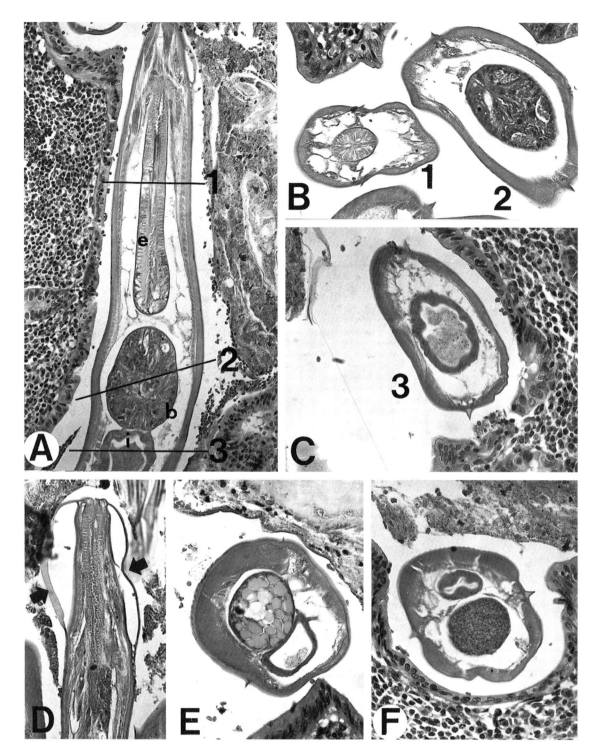

Fig. 15–3. *Enterobius vermicularis* in human appendix, sections stained with hematoxylin and eosin stain. *A*, Longitudinal section, slightly off center, showing the muscular esophagus (e), the bulb (b), and the most anterior portion of the intestine (i). The lines numbered 1, 2, and 3 correspond to the levels of the cross sections 1, 2, and 3, shown in *B* and *C*, ×180. *B*, Cross sections at the level of the esophagus (1) and the bulb (2). Note the lateral alae, ×280. *C*, Cross section at the level of the intestine (3), ×280. *D*, Longitudinal section of the cephalic end showing the mouth opening, with no buccal capsule, and the cephalic inflations (bladder-like expansions of the cuticle) (arrows), ×280. *E*, Cross section of a female at the midbody showing the uterus with immature eggs and the intestine, ×280. *F*, Cross section of a male with the seminal vesicle filled with spermatozoa, ×280.

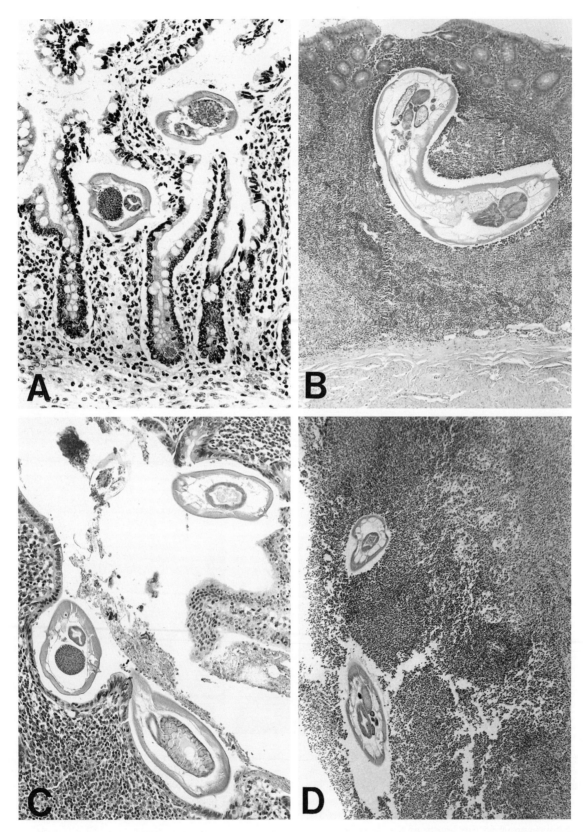

Fig. 15–4. *Enterobius* in intestinal mucosa, sections stained with hematoxylin and eosin stain. *A*, Young adult deep in the crypt of the ileal mucosa, probably developing before reaching the cecum as a fully grown adult; note the lack of an inflammatory response, ×180. *B*, Oblique section of a worm buried in the mucosa of the appendix. Note the normal appendiceal architecture, without inflammation, ×55. *C*, Within the lumen of the appendix, ×140. *D*, Worm within an abscess in an appendix with suppuration; however, the worm is not the cause of the inflammation. The parasites are located within an abundant polymorphonuclear cell infiltrate, ×55.

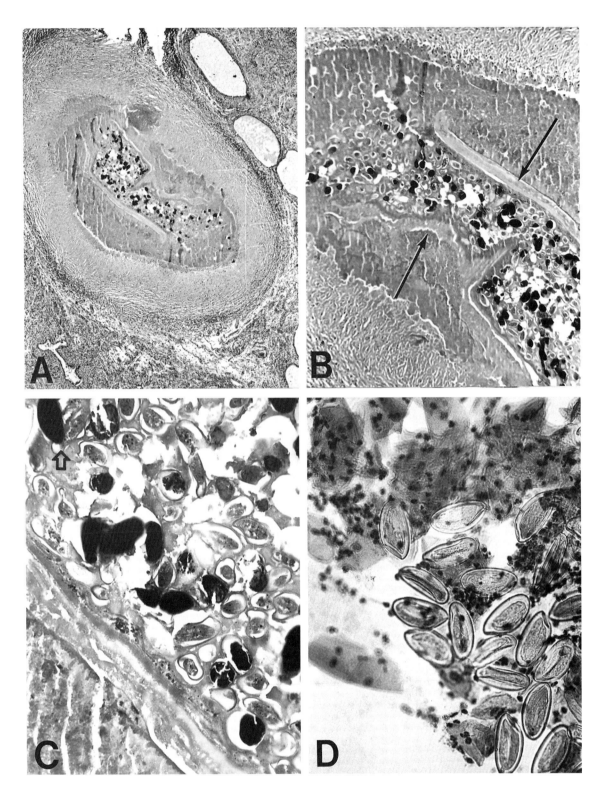

Fig. 15–5. *Enterobius*, ectopic location. *A–C.* Sections stained with hematoxylin and eosin stain. *A,* Ovarian granuloma deep in the parenchyma, ×28. *B,* Higher magnification showing the center of the granuloma with numerous calcified eggs. Remnants of the uterine wall of the worm are still present (arrows), ×63. *C,* Detail showing the eggs, composed of a thick shell and a cell mass. Darkly stained eggs are calcified; some have a shape suggesting *Enterobius* eggs, ×250. *D,* Papanicolaou stain of a vaginal smear with numerous *E. vermicularis* eggs, ×80. (Papanicolaou stain courtesy of A. Aaoki, M.D., Department of Pathology, Sheppard Air Force Base, Wichita Falls, Texas.)

An adult *Enterobius* was found in the anterior urethra of a homosexual man (Al Allaf, Hayatee, 1977) and in the urethra of a another homosexual man who presented with irritation 4 hours after anal intercourse (Ogunji, 1983). This finding provides a rational explanation.

Vulva. Studies of large series of women with pruritus vulvae have shown that enterobiasis is a notable extravaginal cause of the symptom (Pumpianski, Sheskin, 1965). Individual cases of vulvovaginitis where the worms were found in the vagina have been reported (Chung et al. 1997; Deshpande, 1992; Kacker, 1973). Lesions similar to those in the perianal and perineal skin are also known to occur in the vulva (Sun et al. 1991), probably caused by the worm entering one of the vestibular glands.

Vagina. Both adults and eggs of *Enterobius* have been found repeatedly in Papanicolaou smears (Fig. 15–5 *D*) from women with vaginitis (Garud et al. 1980; Langlinais, 1969; Moscolo et al. 1979; Mossop, 1978), with acute vulvovaginitis (Kacker, 1973), and with cervicitis that in some cases resembled a carcinoma (Symmers, 1950). An inflammatory lesion in the wall of the vagina, similar to those described above, suggested that the worm was located in a Bartholin gland (Snow et al. 1978).

Uterus. *Enterobius* has been found to produce an abscess in the wall of the uterus, resulting in gynecologic symptoms (Fatherree et al. 1951). It has also been found as an asymptomatic nodule in the cervix (Campbell et al. 1981). In endometrial curettings from a woman suffering from metrorrhagia, a dead *Enterobius* was found (Sogbanmu, 1976). Finally, the extraordinary finding of a 2 cm macerated human embryo with an *Enterobius* located in its peritoneal and abdominal cavities, has been reported (Mendoza et al. 1987).

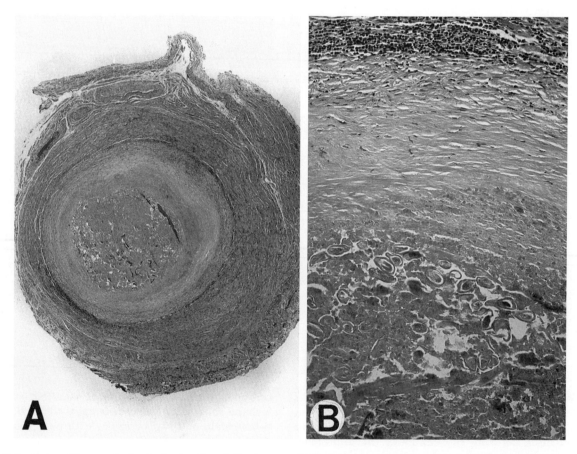

Fig. 15–6. *Enterobius vermicularis* in the fallopian tube, sections stained with hematoxylin and eosin stain. *A*, Low-power view of a tube obstructed by a granuloma elicited by an ectopic worm, ×22. *B*, Higher magnification showing the fibrous wall of the granuloma and the eggs of the parasite, which are still identifiable, ×140.

Fallopian Tubes. Acute unilateral (Saffos, Rhatigan, 1977) or bilateral (Kogan et al. 1983) salpingitis has often been associated with *Enterobius*, frequently in combination with pelvic inflammatory disease (see below). The salpingitis may produce a walled-off abscess sometimes associated with the ovary (Khan et al. 1981; Shroff, Deodhar, 1984) or with an abundant exudate in the lumen (Schnell et al. 1992). Both types of cases are diagnosed because the abscess or the exudate contains eggs of the parasite. Chronic salpingitis can also be unilateral (Tsung, Loh, 1979) or bilateral; it is usually produced by the dead worm in the lumen, resulting in a granuloma that obstructs the tube (Fig. 15–6 A–B; Tsung, Loh, 1979). In some of these cases, it is not clear whether the worm was directly responsible for the lesion or whether it arrived at an already diseased fallopian tube. One should exercise caution in interpreting these findings.

Ovary. Granulomas on the surface of the ovary or in the ovarian parenchyma (Fig. 15–5 A–C) are incidental findings in autopsy or surgical specimens. Those found within the parenchyma are thought to result from the worm entering a recently ruptured Graafian follicle and eventually becoming organized (Beckman, Holland, 1981). In some cases, the lesion is bilateral (Dalrymple et al. 1986; Hernandez Rodriguez, Vinuela Herrero, 1977); in others, it produces adhesions between the ovary and the pelvic cavity (McMahon et al. 1984).

Pelvic Cavity. Because of the significant morbidity produced, invasion of the pelvic cavity by wandering *Enterobius* has some importance. The lesions can be produced either by individual eggs or by the dead worm. The individual eggs laid in a relatively large area of the pelvic peritoneum result in a granulomatous inflammation with clinical manifestations of pelvic inflammatory disease (Pearson et al. 1981). Observers of the gross lesions at surgery refer to their appearance as multiple 1 to 2 mm pearly, white nodules (Brooks et al. 1962), or as 3 to 10 mm white nodules (Dalrymple et al. 1986) sometimes simulating carcinomatosis (Dalrymple et al. 1986; FitzGerald et al. 1974) or pinhead nodules (Ruiter et al. 1962). The distribution of the lesions is variable (reviewed by Sjovall, Akerman, 1968), involving any combination of the pelvic organs and structures or the entire pelvic peritoneum down to the pouch of Douglas (Dalrymple et al. 1986). In some cases, there are adhesions of the adnexa (Brooks et al. 1962) or of other organs; in one patient, the uterus was fixed on retroversion (FitzGerald et al. 1974). Microscopic study of these lesion reveals the granulomas at different stages of evolution; the earlier ones with abundant eosinophils, are referred to as *eosinophilic granulomas* (Fig. 15–7 C–D; Dalrymple et al. 1986). One patient with extensive pelvic involvement had a ruptured appendix 18 months earlier, indicating that the worms had seeded the peritoneal cavity at the time of the rupture (Dalrymple et al. 1986). In another case of perforated appendix, the worms were found in histologic sections outside the appendix (Chandrasoma, Mendis, 1977). This summary is biased toward the symptomatic cases because those are the ones reported. The proportion of asymptomatic versus symptomatic cases is unknown because series of cases are difficult to collect. A literature review of 18 cases showed that one-third had important symptoms (Symmers, 1950).

Larger granulomas, up to 1 cm in diameter, are usually incidental findings. They are produced by the dead worm, and they contain numerous eggs. They are found anywhere in the pelvic cavity and are usually single, though sometimes multiple. They may be found together with the granulomatous inflammation produced by the eggs. The granulomas are attached to any of the organs, especially the uterus (Mayayo et al. 1986), the falciform ligament (Wille-Jorgensen et al. 1982), the serosal surface of the fallopian tubules (Saffos, Rhatigan, 1977; Symmers, 1950), and the area near the appendix (Chandrasoma, Mendis, 1977).

Peritoneum and Omentum. *Enterobius* in the peritoneum, other than in the pelvic cavity peritoneum, is almost always an incidental finding during abdominal surgery or at autopsy. Grossly, the lesions are smooth, hard nodules, whitish in color, loosely or firmly attached to any organ covered by the peritoneum (Biagi, Delgado y Garnica, 1964; Sjovall, Akerman, 1968). On section, the nodule may have a necrotic center or may consist of a collagenized tissue mass (Fig. 15–7 A). Microscopically, these nodules are usually burned out granulomas with remnants of a worm in its terminal stages of degeneration; sometimes only one to several pockets with eggs representing the remains of the female uteri are found (Fig. 15–7 B). An 11-year-old girl with symptoms of acute appendicitis had an inflammatory omental granuloma produced by the worm (Nutting et al. 1980). Granulomas have also been found in an inguinal hernia (Tornieporth et al. 1992).

Intestinal Wall. Nodules and abscesses produced by *Enterobius* associated with the intestinal wall have been reported on several occasions. The nodules are more often found on the peritoneal surface (see above), but

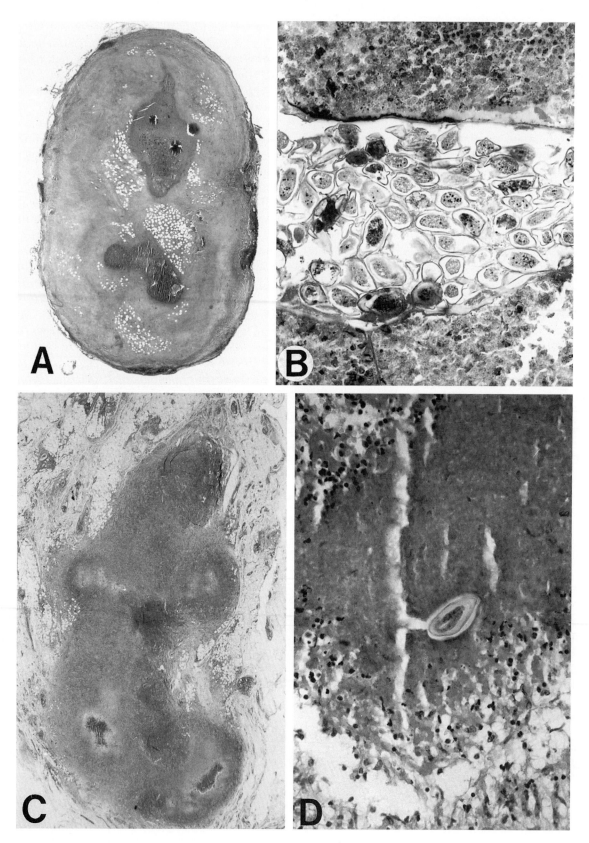

Fig. 15–7.

sometimes they are located in inflammatory lesions within the wall itself (Fig. 15–4 C–D). Once more, the pathogenesis of inflammatory lesions must be interpreted with caution. It was stated above that immature *Enterobius* tend to enter the intestinal crypts, probably as part of their life cycle (Duran-Jorda, 1957; Fig. 15–4 A–B). It is conceivable, but not proven, that in rare instances inflammation may result from bacterial infection, the worm, or both. It is also likely that the worms enter an already diseased area of the intestinal wall, such as an inflamed diverticulum (McDonald, Hourihane, 1972). In some cases, the lesion is a perforated ileum (Chandrasoma, Mendis, 1977; Patterson et al. 1993); in others, the anal wall (Chandrasoma, Mendis, 1977; Vafai, Mohit, 1983), the wall of the ascending colon (Chandrasoma, Mendis, 1977; Shiraki et al. 1974), or the sigmoid (Shiraki et al. 1974) is affected. In one case, the worms were collected from the opening of a persistent onphalomesenteric duct (Mulchandani, 1966).

Other Sites. *Enterobius* has been found in other anatomic sites where its presence is more difficult to explain, such as the liver (Daly, Baker, 1984; Little et al. 1973; Mondou, Gnepp, 1989; Slais, 1962) and lung (Beaver et al. 1973; Brandt, 1949).

Diagnosis. The diagnosis of *Enterobius* is usually clinical, based on a history of perineal itching. In the clinical laboratory, the diagnosis is confirmed by finding the eggs (*color plate* VII G) or the adults in perianal samples taken with the Scotch Tape anal swab. No recommendations exist concerning the number of anal swabs needed for the diagnosis of 100% of infections. In one study, six swabs were enough (Sadun, Melvin, 1956); in another, the prevalence of enterobiasis increased steadily in a cohort of children, from 17% with the first swab to 44% with the eighth swab (Fan, Chan, 1990). In a survey in Peru, two swabs detected 75% of the cases in children examined with five swabs (Gilman et al. 1991). From these data, it can be concluded that if the clinical symptoms indicate, repeated swabs should be taken to confirm the clinical diagnosis.

Adult *E. vermicularis* are occasionally found in tissue sections from appendices removed surgically or at autopsy. The estimated percentage of this finding varies from less than 1% (Collins, 1965) to 3% (Ashburn, 1941). However, if the appendiceal contents are examined together with the tissue section, the prevalence rises to about 8% (Ashburn, 1941). In many of these cases the appendix is normal, but in others a histologic picture of appendicitis may be found (Boulos, Cowie, 1973; Bouree, Dubourdieu, 1984); in either case, worms may be embedded in the wall of the appendix. The relationship between the worms and appendicitis has been explored many times; the consensus is that the worms do not produce the inflammatory reaction and are only innocent bystanders (Budd, Armstrong, 1987). The identification of *Enterobius* in tissue sections is based on its characteristic microanatomy (Fig. 15–2 A–F). The diameter of the worm is variable, depending on the level of the section, the sex of the worm, and its stage of maturation. The females measure up to 350 μm in diameter at midbody and the males up to 150 μm. The cuticle of the worms is 6 to 7 μm thick and has transverse striations 3 μm apart. The characteristic lateral alae, sharply pointed, not easily deformed, and appearing as transparent structures (Fig. 15–2 B–F), are 26 μm high by 20 to 28 μm at the base in the female and much less in the male. The lateral cords are low, with one or two nuclei; the muscle layer has at least four cells per quadrant. The esophagus has three regions: the corpus, the isthmus, and the bulb (Fig. 15–2 A–B). It is followed by the intestine, which consists of cells without well-defined cell borders, with one to four nuclei per histologic section. The brush border is low and inconspicuous. The gonads are represented by tubular structures (Fig. 15–2 E–F); in gravid females, the uterus contains numerous eggs.

In aberrant locations a degenerating female is usually found, often consisting of only remnants of uteri with eggs or eggs alone. The diagnosis is based on the eggs' measurements (50 to 60 × 20 to 30 μm) and their typical morphology, with one side slightly flattened, as seen in some sections (Figs. 15–5 C and 15–7 B and D). The eggs have been found in smears of aspirated

Fig. 15–7. *Enterobius vermicularis* in other ectopic locations, sections stained with hematoxylin and eosin stain. *A,* Peritoneal granuloma produced by an *Enterobius* adult worm. Note the central necrotic areas and some remnants of adipose tissue. Most of the granuloma is composed of mature collagen, with no inflammatory reaction except at the periphery, where a slight lymphocytic infiltrate is seen with higher magnification, ×8. *B,* Detail of a similar granuloma from another individual showing the worm's uterus filled with eggs, ×280. *C,* Multiple small granulomas produced by eggs freed from a dead *Enterobius* female in the peritoneal cavity, ×8. *D,* Detail of one granuloma, ×280. (Preparation of *C* and *D* courtesy of A. Gutierrez-Hoyos, M.D., Servicio de Patologia, Hospital Aranzazu, San Sebastian, Universidad del Pais Vasco, Spain.)

material from an ovarian granuloma (Donofrio et al. 1994).

In wet preparations of cervical and vaginal smears, the eggs of *Enterobius* have their normal translucent appearance (San Cristobal, de Mundi, 1976); in preparations stained with Papanicolaou stain, the eggs have a bright golden yellow tint (Fig. 15–5 D). In some cases, empty egg shells are found. This is an artifact that results from preparation of the smear; larvae outside the empty shells may be seen, especially if the smears are stained with acridine orange for examination under fluorescent light (San Cristobal, de Mundi, 1976).

References

Adungo NI, Ondijo SO, Pamba HO, 1986. Observation of *Enterobius vermicularis* ova in urine: 3 case reports. E. Afr. Med. J. 63:676–678

Al Allaf GA, Hayatee ZG, 1977. Recto-urethral migration of *Enterobius vermicularis*. Trans. R. Soc. Trop. Med. Hyg. 71:351

Ashburn LL, 1941. Appendiceal oxyuriasis: its incidence and relationship to appendicitis. Am. J. Pathol. 17:841–856

Ashford RW, Hart CA, Williams RG, 1988. *Enterobius vermicularis* infection in a children's ward. J. Hosp. Infect. 12:221–224

Beattie RM, Walker SJ, Domizio P, 1995. Ileal and colonic ulceration due to enterobiasis. J. Pediatr. Gastroenterol. Nutr. 21:232–234

Beaver PC, Jung RC, Cupp EW, 1984. *Clinical Parasitology*. Philadelphia: Lea & Febiger

Beaver PC, Kriz JJ, Lau TJ, 1973. Pulmonary nodule caused by *Enterobius vermicularis*. Am. J. Trop. Med. Hyg. 22:711–713

Beckman EN, Holland JB, 1981. Ovarian enterobiasis—a proposed pathogenesis. Am. J. Trop. Med. Hyg. 30:74–76

Biagi FF, Delgado y Garnica R, 1964. Problemas quirurgicos por *Enterobius vermicularis*. Rev. Fac. Med. Mexico 6:251–260

Bijlmer J, 1946. An exceptional case of oxyuriasis of the intestinal wall. J. Parasitol. 32:359–366

Boulos PB, Cowie AGA, 1973. Pinworm infestation of the appendix. Br. J. Surg. 60:975–976

Bouree P, Dubourdieu M, 1984. Les appendicites parasitaires. A propos de 4 observations d'appendicite aigue. Bull. Soc. Pathol. Exot. 77:81–89

Brandt M, 1949. Parasitare Lungenfibrose durch *Oxyuris (Enterobius) vermicularis*. Tuberkulosearzt 3:685–688

Broadbent V, 1975. Children's worms. Br. Med. J. 2:89

Brooks TJ Jr, Goetz CC, Plauche WC, 1962. Pelvic granuloma due to *Enterobius vermicularis*. JAMA 179:492–494

Budd JS, Armstrong C, 1987. Role of *Enterobius vermicularis* in the aetiology of appendicitis. Br. J. Surg. 74:748–749

Campbell JS, Mandavia S, Threlfall W, McCarthy P, Loveys CNR, 1981. Pinworm granuloma of cervix uteri—incidental observation following IUD use and cone biopsy. J. Trop. Med. Hyg. 84:215–217

Chandrasoma PT, Mendis KN, 1977. *Enterobius vermicularis* in ectopic sites. Am. J. Trop. Med. Hyg. 26:644–649

Cherubin CE, Shookhoff HB, 1963. The prevalence of enterobiasis, with regard to population group, among 500 children in New York City. Am. J. Trop. Med. Hyg. 12:69–72

Chittenden AM, Ashford RW, 1987. *Enterobius gregorii* Hugot 1983; first report in the U.K. Ann. Trop. Med. Parasitol. 81:195–198

Cho SY, Hong ST, Kang SY, 1981. Morphological observation of *Enterobius vermicularis* expelled by various anthelmintics. Korean J. Parasitol. 19:18–26

Chung DI, Kong HH, Yu HS, Kim J, Cho CR, 1997. Live female *Enterobius vermicularis* in the posterior fornix of the vagina of a Korean woman. Korean J. Parasitol. 35:67–69

Collins DC, 1965. A study of 50,000 specimens of the human vermiform appendix. Surg. Gynecol. Obstet. 101:437–445

Cram EB, 1943. Studies on oxyuriasis XXVIII. Summary and conclusions. Am. J. Dis. Child. 65:46–59

Cram EB, Reardon L, 1939. Studies on oxyuriasis XII. Epidemiological findings in Washington, D.C. Am. J. Hyg. 29:17–24

Dalrymple JC, Hunter JC, Ferrier A, Payne W, 1986. Disseminated intraperitoneal *Oxyuris* granulomas. Aust. N.Z. Obstet. Gynaecol. 26:90–91

Daly JJ, Baker GF, 1984. Pinworm granuloma of the liver. Am. J. Trop. Med. Hyg. 33:62–64

Deshpande AD, 1992. Correspondence. *Enterobius vermicularis* live adult worms in the high vagina. Postgrad. Med J. 68:690–691

Donofrio V, Insabato L, Mossetti G, Boscaino A, de Rosa G, 1994. Correspondence. *Enterobius vermicularis* granuloma of the ovary: report of a case with diagnosis by intraoperative cytology. Diagn. Cytopathol. 11:205–206

Duran-Jorda F, 1957. Appendicitis and enterobiasis in children. Arch. Dis. Child. 32:208–215

Fan PC, Chan CH, 1990. Consecutive examinations by scotch-tape perianal swabs in diagnosis of enterobiasis. Kaohsiung J. Med. Sci. 6:647–652

Fatherree JP, Carrera GM, Beaver PC, 1951. *Enterobius vermicularis* in the human uterus. Mississippi Doctor 29:159–161

FitzGerald TB, Mainwaring AR, Ahmed A, 1974. Pelvic peritoneal oxyuriasis simulating metastatic carcinoma: a case report. Br. J. Obstet. Gynaecol. 81:248–250

Garud MA, Saraiya U, Paraskar M, Khokhawalla J, 1980. Vaginal parasitosis. Acta Cytol. 24:34–35

Gilman RH, Marquis GS, Miranda E, 1991. Prevalence and symptoms of *Enterobius vermicularis* infections in a Peruvian shanty town. Trans. R. Soc. Trop. Med. Hyg. 85:761–764

Gokalp A, Gultekin EY, Kirisci MF, Ozdamar S, 1991. Relation between *Enterobius vermicularis* infestation and dysuria, nocturia, enuresis nocturna and bacteriuria in primary school girls. Indian Pediatr. 28:948–950

Hasegawa H, Kinjo T, 1996. Human pinworms collected from a chimpanzee, *Pan troglodytes*, in a zoo of Okinawa, Japan. J. Helminthol. Soc. Wash. 63:272–275

Hasegawa H, Takao Y, Nakao M, Fukuma T, Tsuruta O, Ide K, 1998. Is *Enterobius gregorii* Hugot, 1983 (Nematoda: Oxyuridae) a distinct species? J. Parasitol. 84: 131–134

Haswell Elkins MR, Elkins DB, Manjula K, Michael E, Anderson RM, 1987. The distribution and abundance of *Enterobius vermicularis* in a South Indian fishing community. Semin. Respir. Infect. 95:339–354

Hayashi S, Sato K, Takada A, Shirasaka R, Fukui M, Sasa M, Sukigara H, Hiraka K, 1959. Studies on the epidemiology of pinworm (*Enterobius vermicularis*) in Japan. Jpn. J. Exp. Med. 29:213–250

Hernandez Rodriguez JL, Vinuela Herrero A, 1977. Hallazgo de huevos de oxiuros en ambos ovarios. Acta Obstet. Ginecol. Hisp. Lusit. 25:41–50

Hugot JP, 1983. *Enterobius gregorii* (Oxyuridae, Nematoda), un nouveau parasite humain. Ann. Parasitol. Hum. Comp. 58:403–404

Hugot JP, Tourte Schaefer C, 1985. Etude morphologique des deux Oxyures parasites de l'homme: *Enterobius vermicularis et E. gregorii*. Ann. Parasitol. Hum. Comp. 60:57–64

Kacker PP, 1973. Vulvo-vaginitis in an adult with threadworms in the vagina. Br. J. Vener. Dis. 49:314–315

Khan JS, Steele RJC, Stewart D, 1981. *Enterobius vermicularis* infestation of the female genital tract causing generalised peritonitis. Br. J. Obstet. Gynaecol. 88:681–683

Kogan J, Alter M, Price H, 1983. Bilateral *Enterobius vermicularis* salpingo-oophoritis complicated with *Bacteroides fragilis* septicemia. Postgrad. Med. 73: 305–310

Kropp KA, Cichocki GA, Bansal NK, 1978. *Enterobius vermicularis* (pinworms), introital bacteriology and recurrent urinary tract infection in children. J. Urol. 120:480–482

Langlinais PC, 1969. *Enterobius vermicularis* in a vaginal smear. Acta Cytol. 13:40–41

Little MD, Cuello CJ, D'Alessandro A, 1973. Granuloma of the liver due to *Enterobius vermicularis*. Report of a case. Am. J. Trop. Med. Hyg. 22:567–569

Liu LX, Chi J, Upton MP, Ash LR, 1995a. Eosinophilic colitis associated with larvae of the pinworm *Enterobius vermicularis*. Lancet 346:410–412

Liu LX, Chi JY, Upton MP, Ash LR, 1995b. Molecular identification of *Enterobius vermicularis* larvae as a cause of human eosinophilic ileocolitis. Joint meeting of the American Society of Parasitology and American Association of Veterinary Parasitology, Pittsburgh, Pennsylvania, p. 107

Mattia AR, 1992. Perianal mass and recurrent cellulitis due to *Enterobius vermicularis*. Am. J. Trop. Med. Hyg. 47:811–815

Mayayo E, Mestres M, Sarmiento J, Camblor G, 1986. Pelvic oxyuriasis: case report. Acta Obstet. Gynecol. Scand. 65:805–806

McDonald GS, Hourihane DO, 1972. Ectopic *Enterobius vermicularis*. Gut 13:621–626

McMahon JN, Connolly CE, Long SV, Meehan FP, 1984. *Enterobius* granulomas of the uterus, ovary and pelvic peritoneum. Two case reports. Br. J. Obstet. Gynaecol. 91:289–290

Mendoza E, Jorda M, Rafel E, Simon A, Andrada E, 1987. Invasion of human embryo by *Enterobius vermicularis*. Arch. Pathol. Lab. Med. 111:761–762

Mondou EN, Gnepp DR, 1989. Hepatic granuloma resulting from *Enterobius vermicularis*. Am. J. Clin. Pathol. 91:97–100

Mortensen NJ, Thomson JP, 1984. Perianal abscess due to *Enterobius vermicularis*: report of a case. Dis. Colon Rectum 27:677–678

Moscolo G, Pizzinato U, Novelli GG, 1979. Correspondence. Colpocytologic observation of eggs of *Enterobius vermicularis*. Acta Cytol. 23:425–426

Mossop RT, 1978. Threadworm vaginitis. Cent. Afr. J. Med. 24:10–11

Mulchandani HJ, 1966. Roundworm infestation of Meckel's diverticulum. J. Indian Med. Assoc. 46:262

Mya, M. 1955. Life cycle studies on the mouse pinworm *Syphacia obvelata* and *Aspicularis tetraptera*. M.S. thesis, Tulane University

Norhayati M, Hayati MI, Oothuman P, Azizi O, Fatmah MS, Ismail G, Minudin YM, 1994. *Enterobius vermicularis* infection among children aged 1–8 years in a rural area in Malaysia. Southeast Asian J. Trop. Med. Public Health 25:494–497

Nutting SA, Murphy F, Inglis FG, 1980. Abdominal pain due to *Enterobius vermicularis*. Can. J. Surg. 23:286–287

Ogunji FO, 1983. Postcoital pinworm infection. J. Hyg. Epidemiol. Microbiol. Immunol. 27:103–105

Patterson LA, Abedi ST, Kottmeier PK, Thelmo W, 1993. Perforation of the ileum secondary to *Enterobius vermicularis*: report of a rare case. Mod. Pathol. 6:781–783

Pearson RD, Irons RP Sr, Irons RP, Jr, 1981, Chronic pelvic peritonitis due to the pinworm *Enterobius vermicularis*. JAMA 245:1340–1341

Pumpianski R, Sheskin J, 1965. Pruritus vulvae: a five-year survey. Dermatologica 131:446–451

Rahman WA, 1991. Prevalence of *Enterobius vermicularis* in man in Malaysia. Trans. R. Soc. Trop. Med. Hyg. 85:249

Raymond G, Toubol J, Pastorini P, Kermarec Y, Varini JP, LeFichoux Y, Dellamonica P, 1979. Prostatite a eosinophiles avec presence d'oeufs d'oxyure dans les urines. J. Urol. Nephrol. Paris 85:228–230

Riley WA, 1919. A mouse oxyurid, *Syphacia obvelata*, as a parasite of man. J. Parasitol. 6:89–93

Ruiter HD, Rijpstra AC, Swellengrebel NH, 1962. Ectopic *Enterobius vermicularis*. Variations in its pattern. Trop. Geogr. Med. 14:375–380

Sachdev YV, Howards SS, 1975. *Enterobius vermicularis* infestation and secondary enuresis. J. Urol. 113:143–144

Sadun EH, Melvin DM, 1956. The probability of detecting infections with *Enterobius vermicularis* by successive examinations. J. Pediatr. 48:438–441

Saffos RO, Rhatigan RM, 1977. Unilateral salpingitis due to *Enterobius vermicularis*. Am. J. Clin. Pathol. 67:296–299

San Cristobal A, de Mundi A, 1976. Correspondence. *Enterobius vermicularis* larvae in vaginal smears. Acta Cytol. 20:190–192

Schnell VL, Yandell R, Van Zandt S, Dinh TV, 1992. *Enterobius vermicularis* salpingitis: a distant episode from precipitating appendicitis. Obstet. Gynecol. 80:553–555

Shiraki T, Otsuru M, Kenmotsu M, Kihara T, Hisayasu N, Motoyama N, 1974. Invasion of *Enterobius vermicularis* into the human tissues—a report of 4 cases of eosinophilic granulomas caused by adult *Enterobius* in the intestines and their adjacent tissues. Jpn. J. Parasitol. 23:125–137

Shroff CP, Deodhar LP, 1984. Oxyuric salpingitis (a case report). J. Postgrad. Med. 30:51–52

Simon RD, 1974. Pinworm infestation and urinary tract infection in young girls. Am. J. Dis. Child. 128:21–22

Sinniah B, Leopairut J, Neafie RC, Connor DH, Voge M, 1991. Enterobiasis: a histopathological study of 259 patients. Ann. Trop. Med. Parasitol. 85:625–635

Sjovall A, Akerman M, 1968. Peritoneal granulomas in women due to the presence of enterobius S. oxyuris vermicularis. Acta Obstet. Gynecol. Scand. 47:361–372

Slais J, 1962. Zur Pathogenese der Oxyurengranulome. Zentralbl. Allg. Pathol. 103:214–222

Snow P, Cartwright G, Rumbaugh R, 1978. Correspondence. *Enterobius* in an unusual location. JAMA 240:2046

Sogbanmu MO, 1976. Pelvic inflammatory disease associated with *Enterobius vermicularis* in the endometrium. E. Afr. Med. J. 53:702–706

Sun T, Schwartz NS, Sewell C, Lieberman P, Gross S, 1991. *Enterobius* egg granuloma of the vulva and peritoneum: review of the literature. Am. J. Trop. Med. Hyg. 45:249–253

Surmont I, Liu LX, 1995. Correspondence. Enteritis, eosinophilia, and *Enterobius vermicularis*. Lancet 346:1167

Symmers WSC, 1950. Pathology of oxyuriasis. With special reference to granulomas due to the presence of *Oxyuris vermicularis* (*Enterobius vermicularis*) and its ova in the tissues. Arch. Pathol. 50:475–516

Symmers WSC, 1957. Two cases of eosinophilic prostatitis due to metazoan infestation (with *Oxyuris vermicularis*, and with a larva of *Linguatula serrata*). J. Pathol. Bacteriol. 73:549–555

Tornieporth NG, Disko R, Brandis A, Barutzki D, 1992. Ectopic enterobiasis: a case report and review. J. Infect. 24:87–90

Tsung SH, Loh WP, 1979. Invasion of the fallopian tube by *Enterobius vermicularis*. Ann. Clin. Lab. Sci. 9: 393–395

Vafai M, Mohit P, 1983. Granuloma of the anal canal due to *Enterobius vermicularis*. Dis. Colon Rectum 26:349–350

Wagner ED, Eby WC, 1983. Pinworm prevalence in California elementary school chidlren, and diagnositc methods. Am. J. Trop. Med. Hyg. 32:998–1001

WHO, 1981. Intestinal protozoan and helminthic infections. Technical Report Series No 666 1–150. Geneva: WHO

Wille-Jorgensen P, Hesselfeldt P, Ravn V, 1982. *Enterobius vermicularis* in the falciform ligament. Dan. Med. Bull. 29:83–84

16

ASCARIDIDA

The order Ascaridida comprises a large number of relatively large nematodes that parasitize many groups of animals; those that are important to humans belong in the superfamily Ascaridoidea. Two families of the Ascaridoidea, Ascarididae and Anisakidae, have all the species important in human medicine, and most of them inhabit the gastrointestinal tract as adult worms. The life cycles of these parasites are either direct or indirect. Parasites with direct cycles have eggs that require development in soil to become infective and must be ingested by the final host to complete their cycles. Parasites with indirect cycles also pass eggs that require maturation in soil, but they are ingested by intermediate hosts, where the larvae usually encapsulate in the tissues, to infect the predator final host when they are ingested. In some species of the Ascaridoidea with direct life cycles, the infective eggs may be ingested by unnatural hosts. In these cases, the eggs produce larvae in the intestine that migrate through the tissues and encapsulate in the muscles in a state of paratenesis, and the unnatural host becomes a paratenic host. This is a feature of the life cycle of species of *Toxocara*, a feature that is important in medicine because it is the biologic basis for the production of visceral larva migrans (see Chapter 17).

Some members of the Ascaridoidea are parasites as adult worms in the intestine of humans, such as *Ascaris*, or in the tissues, such as *Lagochilascaris*. However, most species of the Ascaridoidea found in humans are parasites as larval stages: *Toxocara*, *Anisakis*, *Pseudoterranova*, and *Baylisascaris*.

Ascaris lumbricoides—Ascariasis

Ascaris lumbricoides is the largest nematode of the gastrointestinal tract of humans. It normally inhabits the lumen of the duodenum and upper jejunum. A related species that occurs in pigs, *A. suum*, is morphologically almost identical to *A. lumbricoides*; experimentally, it has produced infections in humans (Takata, 1951). However, in humans, *A. suum* usually does not progress beyond the pulmonary phase (Phills et al. 1972). Ascariasis is an important disease especially in children, who may suffer significant morbidity when heavily infected and sometimes mortality due to intestinal obstruction or extraintestinal locations of the worm.

Morphology. The adult female of *Ascaris* is up to 35 cm in length, and the male is up to 31 cm; their maximum diameter is about 0.6 and 0.4 cm, respectively. Both females and males are cylindrical, with tapering ends, but the male is tightly curved ventrally at the posterior end. The female has a slight, wide, annular depression anterior to the midpart of the body referred to as the *genital girdle*; this is the area where the vulva is located. Worms that are alive when recovered from the intestine or the stools move actively; dead worms have a flaccid appearance, and when fixed in formalin, they become stiff and wiry-looking.

Life Cycle. The females lay their eggs in the duodenum, to be evacuated with the feces. If the eggs reach appropriate soil, they develop to the infective stage in approximately 3 to 4 weeks. Ingestion of soil contaminated with infective eggs places the eggs in the stomach and small intestine, where they hatch, freeing larvae that penetrate the viscus wall to enter the circulatory and lymphatic systems and migrate to the liver and lungs. In the pulmonary capillary bed, the worms have an obligatory phase of growth and development that lasts for 10 to 14 days. The young larvae grow to about 2 mm in length and undergo physiologic adaptations that allow them to survive in the intestine. When the larvae are ready, they break the alveolar septae, enter the alveolus, and moves through the tracheobronchial tree to reach the epiglottis, esophagus, and duodenum, where they grow to adults in 8 to 12 weeks (Fig. 16–1; Beaver et al. 1984).

Geographic Distribution and Epidemiology. Ascariasis is a common infection in the tropics and subtropics. Transmission occurs throughout the year in some places. In others it is interrupted by cold, dry seasons or by dry, rainy seasons. The epidemiology of *Ascaris* in most places closely parallels that of *Tricuris trichiura*

(Asaolu et al. 1992). Ascariasis is a soil-transmitted helminthiasis; children are the group most heavily infected and have the highest prevalence rates, which vary with the socioeconomic status (Holland, Asaolu, 1990). It is estimated that children living in two institutions in Jamaica were ingesting 9 to 20 infective eggs of *Ascaris* per year (Wong et al. 1991). Estimates of the number of persons infected with *Ascaris* worldwide vary, but about one-fourth of the population is a widely quoted figure. The prevalence in Nigeria, the most populous country in Africa, ranges from 10% to 96%, depending on the group studied (Holland, Asaolu, 1990). In the United States the prevalence of *Ascaris* has decreased considerably, but areas of low endemicity are still found in the southeastern states, and sporadic cases are seen in other parts of the country. A study of worms evacuated by persons in the United States indicates that, on the basis of their rDNA, they are mostly pig *Ascaris* (Anderson, 1995).

Clinical Findings. The first symptoms produced by *Ascaris* in humans are respiratory, due to the passage of larvae through the lungs; the disease manifests as a benign pneumonitis known as *Loeffler's syndrome* (see below). The intestinal symptoms of ascariasis vary, depending on the number of worms. The heaviest infections are found mainly in small children because of their proclivity to ingest soil. The main symptoms in children are abdominal pain, loss of appetite, and failure to thrive. In children, ingestion of only 50 worms may produce significant symptoms, especially if their diet is also deficient in calories and proteins (Beaver, 1975). In heavy infections the abdomen protrudes. Nutritional impairment usually accompanies the infection due to altered carbohydrate absorption and increased fecal nitrogen and fat, which correlate with the number of worms in the intestine (Tripathy et al. 1971; Tripathy et al. 1972). The long-term effect of impaired nutrition is growth and developmental retardation (Crompton,

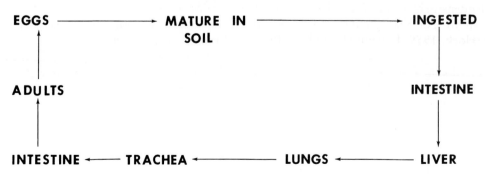

Fig. 16–1. *Ascaris lumbricoides*, schematic representation of the life cycle.

1992; Stephenson, 1980; Stephenson et al. 1980). Lactose maldigestion is found in infected children compared with controls, which disappears after deworming (Carrera et al. 1984). Allergic manifestations in ascariasis are common. They begin at the time of the pulmonary infection and continue during the intestinal phase, usually manifesting as asthma and skin hives that are alleviated by specific treatment (Chacko, 1970). In older children and adults, the infection is usually clinically silent because of the smaller worm burden; often the presence of eggs or adult worms in the feces is the only sign of infection. In computed tomograms of the abdomen in a patient with intestinal complications after surgery, the worms appeared as cylindrical filling defects (Beitia et al. 1997; Hommeyer et al. 1995).

Ectopic Lesions. *Ascaris* has a propensity to migrate from its usual duodenal location to other organs, producing diverse symptoms and signs that are sometimes life-threatening. Migration of worms from the intestine occurs as a result of temperature changes in the host (fever, low postmortem temperature), drugs such as general anesthesia tics, and the need for copulation in the female worms (Beaver, 1964). A good example of postmortem migration is that of worms in the paranasal sinuses (Naravane et al. 1997).

Stomach. *Ascaris* may enter the stomach and produce emesis that often carries the worm into the vomitus (Atias et al. 1959) or may produce trauma of the mucosa that results in bleeding (Wilairatana et al. 1994). The worms have been known to enter a nasogastric tube and obstruct it (Golz et al. 1982; Ortega, 1992).

Esophagus and upper airways. Migration of *Ascaris* through the esophagus to the epiglottis and upper airways produces respiratory difficulties in some cases (Moyes, Rogers, 1971). In others, it produces cardiopulmonary arrest (Mimpriss, 1972; Mittal et al. 1976; Moyes, Rogers, 1971). One patient coughed up the worm during an episode of acute stridor and cyanosis in the intensive care unit (Faraj, 1993). Worms are also known to exit through the nares and the lacrimal duct (Hock, 1959; Kanapumbi, Lubeji, 1996; Kaplan et al. 1956). On rare occasions they enter the eustachian tube, producing perforation of the tympanic membrane (Shah, Desai, 1969) and otitis media and exiting through the ear (Fagan, Prescott, 1993).

Intestine. Migration to the lower intestine is probably the most frequent and most important complication of ascariasis. In this case, a tangled mass of adult worms (Fig. 16–2 *A*) usually moves from the duodenum to lodge in the ileocecal valve (Jenkins, Beach, 1954; Ochola-Abila, Barrack, 1982). This complication occurs more often in children (Villamizar et al. 1996) under 5 years of age but also in adults (Akgun, 1996). It is estimated that in an area of the southeastern United States where prevalence rates of infection varied from 8% to 28%, intestinal obstruction due to *Ascaris* occurred in 1 of every 1000 children infected, (Bernstein, 1977). In Calabar, Nigeria, *Ascaris* was responsible for 25% of intestinal obstructions seen during a 10-year period (Archibong et al. 1994). The symptoms of ascariasis are vomiting, abdominal pain and distention, and constipation, with partial or total intestinal obstruction demonstrated on plain abdominal radiographs (Fig. 16–2 *B*; Appleby et al. 1982; Blumenthal, Schultz, 1975). Abdominal ultrasonograms reveal the worms as tubular structures (Coskun et al. 1996).

Pancreatic duct. *Ascaris* enters the pancreatic duct directly from the duodenum to produce marked pancreatitis (Chen, Li, 1994; Khuroo et al. 1993; Schuster et al. 1977). In a series of 42 patients, most were young women with severe, acute upper abdominal pain, tenderness, and raised serum amylase levels; the diagnosis was often made on the basis of ultrasonographic demonstration of the worms (Chen, Li, 1994; Larrubia et al. 1996). Necrotizing pancreatitis does not often result from worms in the pancreas; therefore, conservative management is recommended (Chen, Li, 1994).

Biliary ducts and gallbladder. The common bile duct, the gallbladder, and the intrahepatic biliary tree can be affected, with the majority of cases seen in childhood (Louw, 1974). However, persons of any age can be affected. During clinical management of these patients, the worms have been retrieved during endoscopy (Saul et al. 1984). In any of these locations the worms produce symptoms of acute pancreatitis, acute cholecystitis, or acute cholangitis (Fig. 16–2 *C*; Fontes et al. 1984; Khuroo, Zargar, 1985; Khuroo et al. 1990). Ultrasonograms in these patients clearly reveal the worms and confirm the diagnosis (de-Andrade et al. 1992; de la Cruz Alvarez et al. 1996; Filice et al. 1995). Chronic disease may also result if the obstruction is intermittent or partial.

Liver. The worms may reach the liver parenchyma, forming abscesses that sometimes perforate into the pleural cavity, the lungs (Chao et al. 1965), and the pericardium (Joshi et al. 1961). In endemic areas, ascariasis should be considered in any patient with biliary symptoms, especially if the patient is a child. After abdominal surgery, *Ascaris* may migrate to the peritoneal cavity or the skin wound through the sutures (Hakami et al. 1976) and, after biliary surgery, to the gallbladder or a T-tube, producing important morbidity and mortality (Fig. 16–2 *D*).

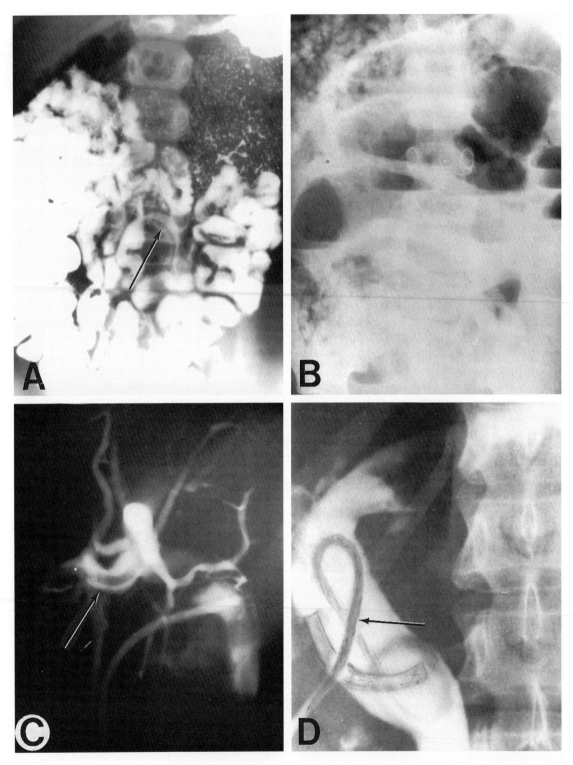

Fig. 16–2. *Ascaris lumbricoides*, roentgenograms showing aberrant locations. *A*, Adult *Ascaris* in jejunum (arrow). *B*, Intestinal obstruction produced by *A. lumbricoides* in the ileocecal valve. (Courtesy of A. D'Alessandro, M.D., School of Public Health and Tropical Medicine, Tulane University, New Orleans, Louisiana. In: Beaver, P.C., Jung, R.C., and Cupp, E.W. 1984. *Clinical Parasitology*, 9th ed. Philadelphia: Lea & Febiger. Reproduced with permission.) *C*, Operative cholangiogram showing an adult *Ascaris* in the common bile duct (arrow). *D*, *Ascaris* adult worm in a greatly dilated common bile duct with a T-tube placed after gallbladder surgery. The worm (arrow) has entered the T-tube, producing obstruction and requiring repeat surgery.

Abdominal cavity. Adult *Ascaris* migrates to the peritoneal cavity through intestinal ulcerations and sutures after recent intestinal surgery. The clinical presentation in most cases consists of a tumor mass anywhere in the abdomen (Adebamowo et al. 1993). In other patients, it may appear as a granulomatous peritonitis (see below; Mello et al. 1992).

Other sites. In clinical practice, worms have been seen in many locations, always unexpectedly. In one case, the worms passed through a fistula between the intestine and the ureter to gain access to the kidney, moving from the kidney through a sinus tract into ulcerated skin above the left gluteal region (Bustamante-Sarabia et al. 1977). In other cases, worms exited out through an open onphalomesenteric duct (Perera, 1993) and from a fistula of an ulcerated inguinal hernia (Correa-Henao, 1957). In one patient, the worm passed through a fistula between the intestine and the urinary bladder and was evacuated with the urine (Pamba, Musangi, 1978). The most baffling case is one in which the worms were located in the placenta, and were passed spontaneously and recovered from the vagina by the physician. Moreover, the baby, born by cesarean section, had worms in the intestine, passing a 30 cm *Ascaris* male on the second day of life and a 28 cm *Ascaris* female on the sixth day (Chu et al. 1972). How the worms reached the placenta and the intestine of the baby is unknown. The only thing left is to speculate that the mother acquired the infection while pregnant, and that the larvae migrated to the lungs of the fetus and completed the life cycle in its intestine. The adult worms were passed by the fetus in utero through the anus, the mouth, or both, and from the amniotic sac were passed into the vagina. At birth, the baby still had the two worms that were expelled later.

Pathology. The gross appearance of the small intestine in ascariasis is usually unremarkable, except for the presence of the parasites (Fig. 16–3). The microscopic changes in the intestine have rarely been studied. A normal mucosa (Maxwell et al. 1968) or nonspecific elongation of the crypts, a decreased villus-crypt ratio, and a mononuclear cell infiltrate of the lamina propria that reverted to normal after deworming have been found. These changes persisted after the patients were placed on a special hospital diet, indicating that the worms, and not the patients' nutritional status, were responsible for the histologic changes (Tripathy et al. 1972).

Ectopic Ascaris. The pathologic changes of ectopic ascariasis vary, depending on the time that has elapsed between the arrival of the parasite at a given location

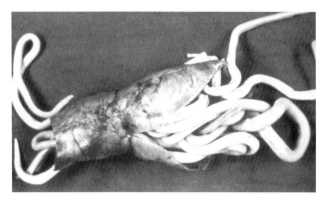

Fig. 16–3. *Ascaris lumbricoides*, segment of duodenum with several adult worms. (Photograph courtesy of M.I.S. Duarte, M.D., Department of Pathology, Medical Center, São Paulo State University, São Paulo, Brazil).

and its retrieval. Patients with worms in the biliary tree or the peritoneal cavity usually have other concomitant medical problems, so interpretation of the morbidity produced by the worm, or by associated bacterial infections, is difficult. The main sites where *Ascaris* have been found in humans will now be discussed.

Appendix. Adult *Ascaris* in the appendix (Fig. 16–4 A–B) or in a Meckel's diverticulum (Fig. 16–5 A–B) produces obstruction and symptoms of appendicitis, sometimes with perforation and peritonitis (Fig. 16–5 C–D; Smedresman, 1977).

Peritoneal cavity. Adult *Ascaris* worms may enter the peritoneal cavity through perforations or recent surgical sutures, often producing fatal peritonitis due to bacterial contamination. Perforation of the small intestine by the worms themselves appears to be rare but apparently has occurred (Ihekwaba, 1979). If the wandering worm is a female, it may lay eggs that produce a granulomatous inflammation (Fig. 16–6 A–B) of the serosal surface (Cooray, Panaboicke, 1960). The worm eventually dies and produces a large abscess that manifests as a mass somewhere in the abdominal cavity (Chandrasoma et al. 1978). The mass often simulates a tumor (Adebamowo et al. 1993; Bambirra et al. 1985; Formiga Ramos et al. 1980). In acute cases, the surgeon may find the perforation and one to several worms in the peritoneal cavity (Odaibo, Awogun, 1988), sometimes alive (Atias et al. 1959). The granulomas produced by eggs in the peritoneal cavity appear grossly as numerous white nodules less than 0.5 mm in diameter resembling miliary tuberculosis (Chandrasoma et al. 1978; Winslow et al. 1958). Microscopically, each granuloma contains one egg at the center; its appearance depends on the time of evolution of the lesion. In experimental conditions, the eggs in tissues of different

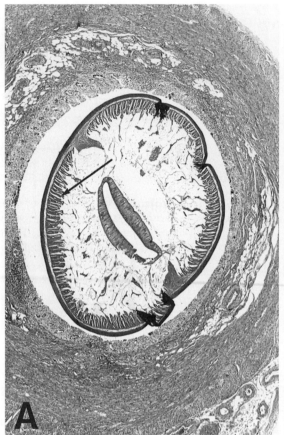

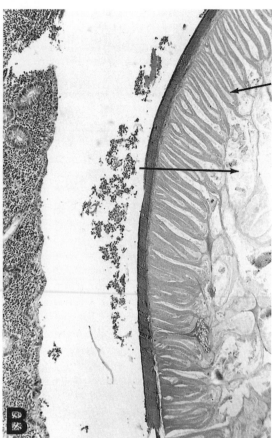

Fig. 16–4. *Ascaris lumbricoides* in the appendix, sections stained with hematoxylin and eosin stain. *A*, Low-power view of the appendix with a cross section of the adult worm; at this level, only intestine and muscle cells (arrow) are shown, ×22. *B*, Detail of the worm showing the cuticle and part of the muscle cells with the contractile portion (short arrow) and cytoplasm (long arrow), ×70.

animals elicited a cellular response with eosinophils and neutrophils within 2 hours, and a microabscess was formed by the sixth hour. At 4 days the histologic picture was that of a granulomatous reaction, with well-formed granulomas containing epithelioid and multinucleated foreign body giant cells (Arean et al. 1962). The eggs of *Ascaris* in the peritoneum have been mistaken for *Coccidioides immitis* (Lacaz et al. 1982).

Biliary tree. The biliary tree is probably the most common location for ectopic ascariasis. In a series of 437 pathologic specimens with *Ascaris* submitted for

examination to the Armed Forces Institute of Pathology, 38 produced fatal complications and 21 occurred in the biliary tree (Piggott et al. 1970). Through the sphincter of Oddi the worms enter the pancreatic duct, the common bile duct, and the biliary tree, producing obstruction of the duct, dilation, and an inflammatory reaction. In the pancreatic duct, they cause pancreatitis (Bernstein, 1977; Capallo, Gongaware, 1984). Some of these cases have been diagnosed by visualizing the worms on plain radiographs or on endoscopic retrocholecystopancreatograms (Bernstein, 1977). The

Fig. 16–5. *Ascaris lumbricoides* in Meckel's diverticulum. *A*, Gross appearance of the viscus after removal showing hyperemia and serositis. *B*, Viscus opened longitudinally, showing one adult parasite. The thread-like structures protruding from the sectioned ends of the worms (arrows) correspond to the gonads. *C* and *D*. Microscopic view of section stained with hematoxylin and eosin stain. *C*, Low-power view showing necrosis of the wall and marked infiltration by polymorphonuclear cells down to the serosal surface, ×70. *D*, Higher magnification showing necrosis of the mucosa, ×180. (Gross photographs and preparations courtesy of M.E. Bush, M.D., Department of Pathology, Norwalk Hospital, Norwalk, Connecticut.)

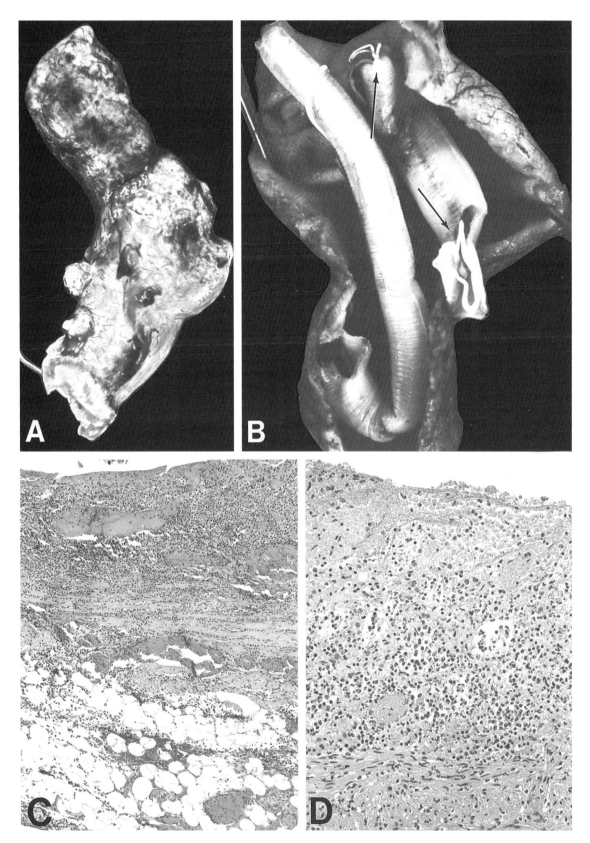

Fig. 16–5.

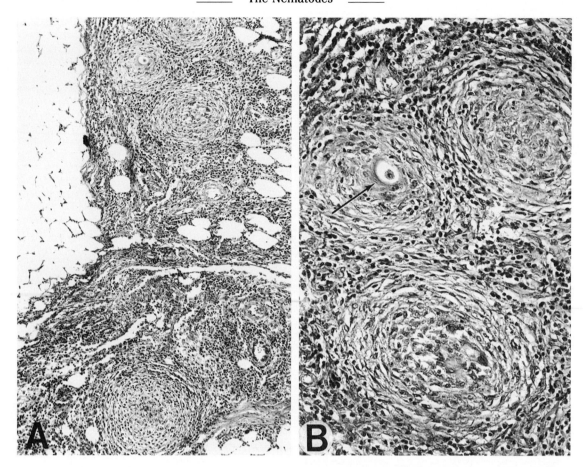

Fig. 16–6. *Ascaris lumbricoides* eggs laid by a wandering female worm in the peritoneal cavity, producing peritonitis, section stained with hematoxylin and eosin stain. *A*, Low-power view showing several granulomas, ×70. *B*, Higher magnification. One granuloma shows the typical *Ascaris* egg in tissues (arrow), without the outer mammillated layer of the shell, ×180. (Preparation from H. Estrada, M.D., Department of Pathology, School of Medicine, Universidad de Caldas, Manizales, Colombia.)

symptoms vary in accordance with the location of the worm and the time that has elapsed since its arrival, but in general they are those of either acute or chronic cholecystitis. Dead worms in the common bile duct and the gallbladder (Fig. 16–7 *A–B*) are a nidus for deposition of bile salts, leading to the formation of stones (Choi et al. 1993; Kalejaiye et al. 1977). In endemic areas, *Ascaris* is a cause of lithiasis of the common bile duct, the gallbladder, and the intrahepatic ducts. In comparison with nonendemic areas, the disease is usually seen in younger patients (Cobo et al. 1964). Sections of calculi produced by *Ascaris* show the mineralized parasite (Fig. 16–7 *C–D*). From the common bile duct, the migrating worm may enter the intrahepatic bile ducts (Fig. 16–9 *A–B*) and the hepatic parenchyma to produce one or more abscesses (Figs. 16–8 *A–E* and 16–10; Correa-Henao, 1957; Rossi, Bisson, 1983; Santillan Doherty et al. 1986). In debilitated patients and in small children (Fig. 16–9 *C–D*) this complication is often fatal. An abscess may perforate into the pleural cavity (Chao et al. 1965), lungs, and pericardium (Joshi et al. 1961). If the patient survives, the dead worm in the liver results in the formation of a granuloma, which often calcifies, leaving only eggs remaining (Fig. 16–10 *B–D*; Correa-Henao, 1957).

Postmortem migration. After death, the worms leave the intestine and wander into any of the organs described above (Fig. 16–11 *A–D*). Thus, ectopic *Ascaris* found at autopsy must be evaluated within this context and requires microscopic study for histologic evidence of inflammatory changes indicative of premortem migration.

Diagnosis. The diagnosis of ascariasis is often made on clinical grounds, especially in children living in en-

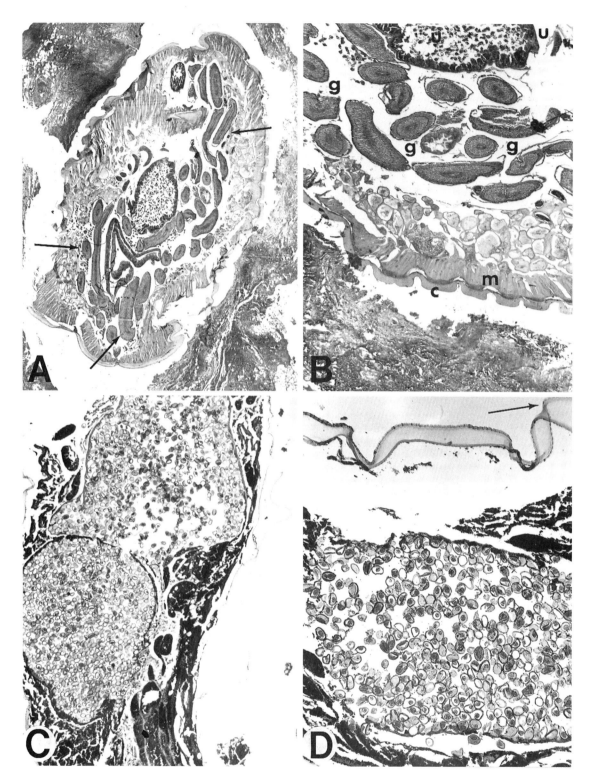

Fig. 16–7. *Ascaris lumbricoides* in the gallbladder, sections stained with hematoxylin and eosin stain. *A*, Low-power view of a section of a gallbladder neck showing significant inflammation and a cross section of a recently dead *Ascaris* from a 25-year-old woman who had symptoms of acute epigastric pain, fever, and vomiting of 10 days' duration. The round, elongated structures (arrows) correspond to cross sections and oblique sections of the gonads of the parasite, ×8. *B*, Higher magnification illustrating the cuticle (c), muscle cells (m), the gonads (g), and a section of the uterus (u) with immature eggs (top), ×22. (Preparation from N.A. Sustento, M.D., Department of Pathology, College of Medicine, University of the Philippines.) *C* and *D*, Oblique sections of a mineralized *Ascaris* found in a gallbladder removed because of chronic cholecystitis. Note the section of the uterus containing numerous eggs. A longitudinal section of the cuticle shows the typical cross striations. *C* ×28; *D* ×55. (Preparation courtesy of H. Estrada, M.D., Department of Pathology, School of Medicine, Universidad de Caldas, Manizales, Colombia.)

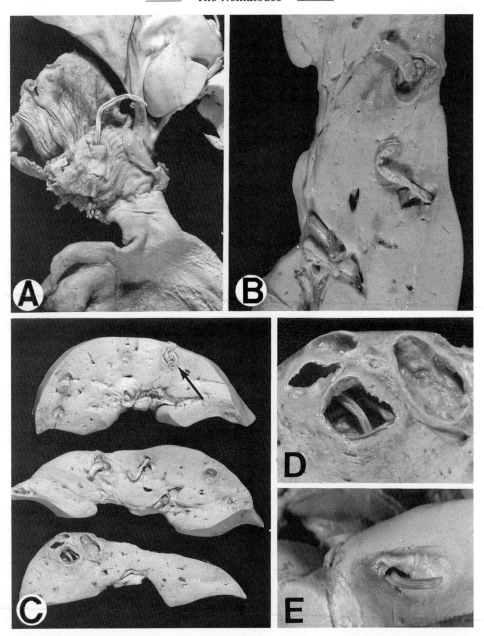

Fig. 16–8. *Ascaris lumbricoides*, lesions in liver produced by ectopic adult worms in a 21-month-old boy brought to the emergency room with fever, abdominal pain, stupor, and progressive lost of weight. *A,* Adult worm in the papilla of Vater. *B* and *C,* Sections of liver showing the multiple abscesses (*C*) and detail of some of them (*B*). *D* and *E,* Higher magnification of some of the abscesses. (In: Rossi, M.A., and Bisson, F.W. 1983. Fatal case of multiple liver abscesses caused by adult *Ascaris lumbricoides*. Am. J. Trop. Med. Hyg. 32: 523–525. Reproduced with permission.)

demic areas. More often *Ascaris* is diagnosed in the laboratory by finding the characteristic eggs, which measure up to 75 × 60 μm, in stool samples (Fig. 16–12 *A–B*). Ideally, counts or estimates of eggs per gram of feces should be made to assess the level of the infec-

tion. Often adult worms are received in the laboratory for diagnosis. All these "worms" require careful examination because patients sometimes bring earthworms or roundworms from animals and sometimes even objects that to the untrained eye resemble worms,

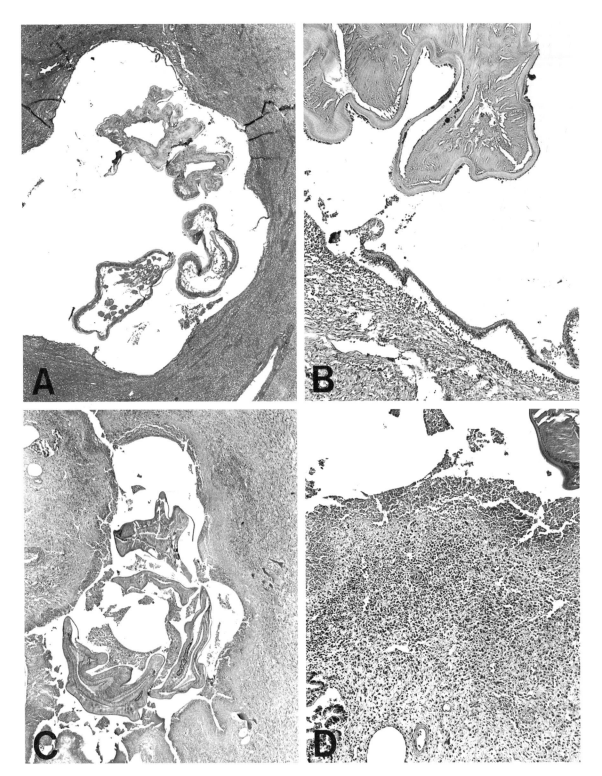

Fig. 16–9. *Ascaris lumbricoides*, recent migration to the liver, sections stained with hematoxylin and eosin stain. *A*, Largely dilated intrahepatic bile duct with four oblique sections of a necrotic, immature *Ascaris*, ×12. *B*, Higher magnification showing a portion of the parasite (top), part of the bile epithelium (bottom), and the acute inflammatory reaction, ×70. (Preparation from N.A. Sustento, M.D., Department of Pathology, College of Medicine, University of the Philippines.) *C*, Slightly older lesion from another autopsy showing early organization around the dead worm, ×22. *D*, Necrosis (top) and granulation tissue with an inflammatory infiltrate (bottom) are seen, ×70.

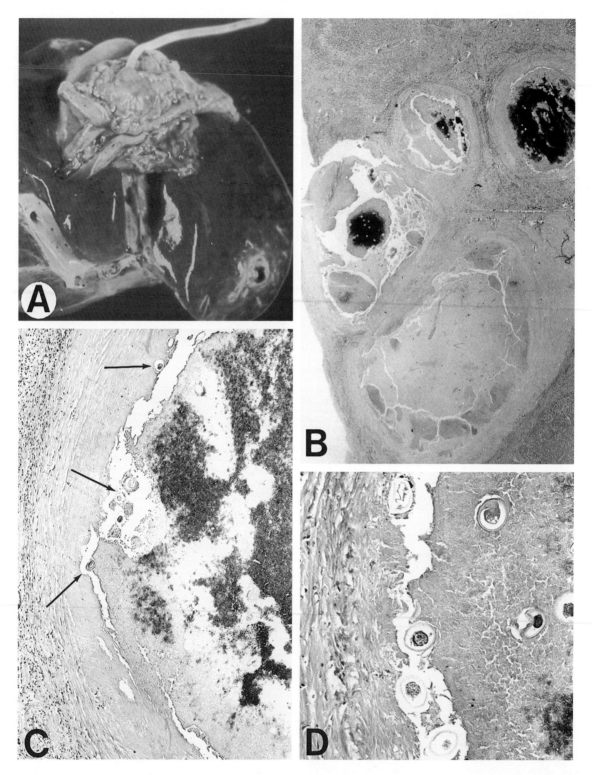

Fig. 16–10. *Ascaris lumbricoides* in liver. *A*, Gross picture of a liver abscess with the worm. (Courtesy of M.I.S. Duarte, M.D., Department of Pathology, Medical Center, São Paulo State University, São Paulo, Brazil.) *B–D*. Granulomas, sections stained with hematoxylin and eosin stain. *B*, Low-power view of liver granulomas showing fibrosis and calcification, ×12. *C*, Medium-power view of one granuloma showing the fibrous wall and a portion of the central calcified region. Some eggs (arrows) are seen at this magnification, ×70. *D*, Higher magnification showing the eggs, ×180.

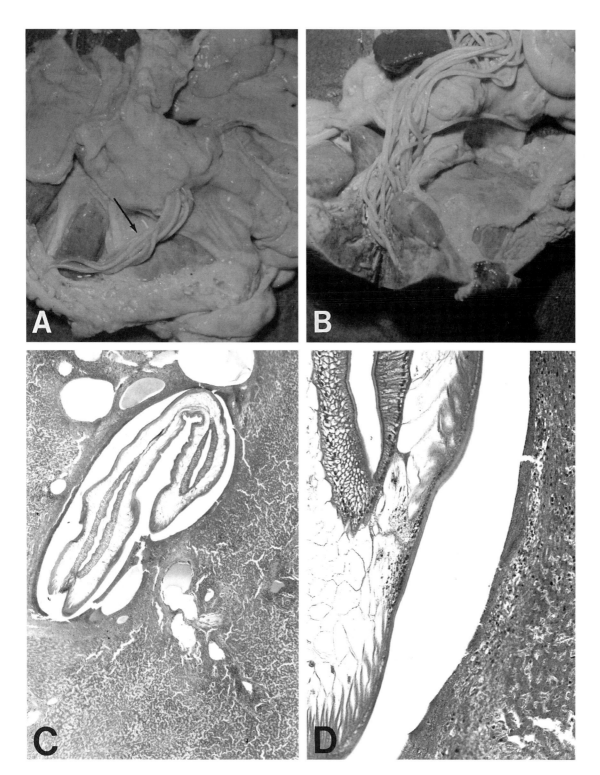

Fig. 16–11. *Ascaris lumbricoides*, postmortem migration. *A*, Gross picture of an open bile duct with several adult *Ascaris* worms (arrow). *B*, Another view showing the parasites reaching into the liver. (Courtesy of H. Estrada, M.D., Department of Pathology, School of Medicine, Universidad de Caldas, Manizales, Colombia.) *C* and *D*. Sections stained with hematoxylin and eosin stain. *C*, Low-power view of a liver section from another autopsy showing an immature *Ascaris*. Note the surrounding tissue lysis (postmortem) and the lack of inflammation. The empty spaces correspond to overgrowth of gas-producing bacteria, ×8. *D*, Higher magnification showing the lack of tissue response, ×140.

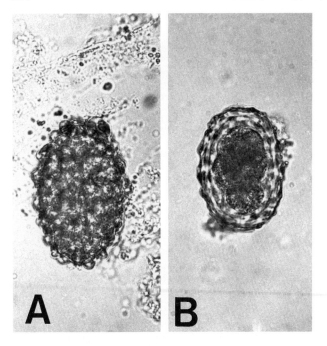

Fig. 16–12. *Ascaris lumbricoides* eggs in stools, unstained, ×495. *A*, Unfertilized. *B*, Fertilized.

claiming that they were passed by the patient. The reliability of the history of the parasite in question should always be considered, and any retrieval of a worm without a credible witness should be suspected until the worm is conclusively identified.

In tissue sections, adult worms are most commonly found in the appendix, the common bile duct, and the liver, but they may also occur in other organs. The size of the worm in cross sections varies from 0.5 to 6 mm, depending on its maturity and sex. In sections, the worms have a multilayered outer cuticle ranging from 8 μm in thickness in small specimens to 50 μm in larger ones (Figs. 16–4 *A–B* and 16–7 *A–B*). The cuticle has transverse striations up to 15 μm apart that are especially evident on oblique and longitudinal cuts (Fig. 16–7 *D*). The subcuticle or hypodermis is as thick as the cuticle and is composed of small fibers. The muscles are well developed, with cells possessing a sarcoplasm larger than the contractile portion extending into the body cavity (Fig. 16–4 *A–B*). The lateral cords are prominent, with a rudimentary excretory tube (Fig. 16–4 *A*), and the intestine, usually oval, is composed of a single layer of numerous columnar cells with short microvilli (Fig. 16–11 *D*). The gonads are seen as numerous sections of small, rounded tubules with tall cells containing nuclei located toward the bases (Fig. 16–7 *A–B*). The uteri are two tubes filled with eggs in dif-

ferent stages of development, depending on the level of the section.

The identification of *Ascaris* eggs in tissue sections, usually within granulomas (Fig. 16–6 *A–B*), is based on their size, which must be comparable to the size of eggs in stools. The eggs in the peritoneal cavity contain developing larvae (embryonates), but these larvae probably do not survive for long (Africa, Garcia, 1936). The eggs usually lack the outer mammillated layer; if present, this layer is often swollen, greatly widened, and distorted. The innermost lipoid vitelline membrane appears as a smooth double wall containing a mass of cytoplasm; often the eggs are calcified.

Loeffler's Syndrome—Nematode Pneumonitis

The condition known as *Loeffler's syndrome* was described in 1932 as "pulmonary transitory shadows or infiltrations" quickly appearing and diminishing, seen bilaterally on chest radiograms. This condition was discovered during fluoroscopic surveys of tuberculosis patients in Zurich; no definitive cause was given, but some investigators suggested that *Ascaris* might be responsible for the symptoms (Loeffler, 1956). Similar symptoms had been reported in Japan by Koino (Koino, 1922), who studied experimental infections of *Ascaris* in humans and referred to the pulmonary symptoms as *Ascaris pneumonia*. After the clinical description, Loeffler carried out experimental work in laboratory animals and concluded that *Ascaris* was indeed the cause of the syndrome named after him. In his work, Loeffler suggested an allergic component, and he referred to the worms as the *antigen*. The monumental work of Vogel and Minning in 1942 in human experimental infections established that an allergic component was at work because as few as six *Ascaris* larvae migrating through the lungs produced significant symptoms (Vogel, Minning, 1942).

Loeffler's syndrome is a self-limited, benign clinicopathologic entity that lasts for about 10 days. It is characterized by mild to moderate bronchitis, peripheral eosinophilia, and fleeting pulmonary infiltrates seen on two or more chest radiograms taken 2 to 3 days apart (Loeffler, 1956). The peripheral eosinophilia is generally between 4000 and 8000 per cubic millimeter, rarely exceeding 40% of the total white blood cell count. The most important causes of Loeffler's syndrome are larvae of parasitic nematodes migrating through the lungs. These include *A. lumbricoides* and

A. *suum* of pigs; the hookworms of humans (*Ancylostoma duodenale*, *A. ceylanicum*, and *Necator americanus*); the hookworms of animals (*A. caninum* and *A. braziliense*); and *Strongyloides stercoralis* and *S. fuelleborni*. Pollen of certain plants may also produce Loeffler's syndrome-like symptoms. However, it appears that the most important cause of Loeffler's syndrome is *Ascaris* because, of all the helminths traveling through the respiratory system, *Ascaris* is the only one that requires a developmental phase in the lungs, which lasts for up to 2 weeks. Loeffler's syndrome in humans has been produced in experimental infections with *A. lumbricoides* (Koino, 1922; Patz, 1959; Vogel, Minning, 1942) and *A. suum* (Takata, 1951); in natural infections (Gelpi, Mustafa, 1968; Spillmann, 1975) sometimes producing outbreaks (Barlow et al. 1961); and in accidental infections with *A. suum* (Phills et al. 1972).

The infective larvae of *Ancylostoma*, *Necator*, and *Strongyloides* reaching the lungs must also migrate from the circulatory system to the alveoli, tracheobronchial tree, and intestine, but they lack a phase of development in the lungs. However, these parasites often produce Loeffler's syndrome, generally less intense than that produced by *Ascaris* (see Chapters 12 and 13). This has been shown in experimental infections with human hookworms (Kendrick, 1934) and *Strongyloides* (Faust, 1935; Pampiglione, Ricciardi, 1972), as well as in hundreds of iatrogenic infections produced with human hookworms for the treatment of polycythemia vera (Brumpt, 1952; Lavier, Brumpt, 1944) and in natural infections with zoonotic hookworms that produce cutaneous larva migrans (Little et al. 1983; Muhleisen, 1953; Wright, Gold, 1945). Although the number of larvae migrating through the lungs at any given time plays a role in the intensity of the symptoms, sensitization to the parasite is more important. As stated, a few larvae of *Ascaris* are capable of producing a full-blown case of Loeffler's syndrome (Vogel, Minning, 1942).

Clinical Findings. Loeffler's syndrome produced by *Ascaris* lasts for about 10 days and manifests with productive or nonproductive cough, dyspnea, cyanosis, and, in some cases, internal discomfort. If the cough is productive, the mucus may be blood-tinged. Marked tracheitis, with sloughing of fragments of respiratory epithelium in the mucus, has been recorded, and some individuals have abundant sputum 5 to 8 days after the onset of the symptoms; pleuritis and generalized urticaria have also been observed. The physical examination is unremarkable, though some individuals with heavy infections (45 larvae) have fever. White blood cell counts of 20,000 to 25,000 per cubic millimeter and up to 70% eosinophilia were recorded in Saudi Arabia (Gelpi, Mustafa, 1967, 1968). The x-ray films are the best guides to assess the severity of the illness.

Loeffler's syndrome caused by human hookworms manifests with irritation of the trachea, larynx, and pharynx, producing the sensation of suffering from a cold. On the fourth day of infection the patient complaint of mild retrosternal and thoracic pain, accompanied by dry cough, hoarseness, and, in some cases, aphonia. The cough and pain are usually nocturnal, producing insomnia. Physical examination reveals a hyperemic larynx, and chest roentgenograms taken daily show infiltrates after the third day (Brumpt, 1952; Kendrick, 1934; Lavier, Brumpt, 1944; Rogers, Dammin, 1946). In Wakana disease (see Chapter 13), acute gastrointestinal symptoms precede the pulmonary manifestations. This happens because, in these cases, the larvae of *Ancylostoma* are ingested and locate directly in the intestine, and some enter the mucosa of the mouth and esophagus and migrate through the lungs (Harada, 1962). The zoonotic hookworms responsible for cutaneous larva migrans appear to produce more intense and more prolonged pulmonary symptoms (Muhleisen, 1953; Wright, Gold, 1945), with pulmonary infiltrates seen even in mild infections (see Chapter 14).

Loeffler's syndrome produced by the larvae of *Strongyloides* is rather mild. In an experimental infection, 500 infective larvae of *S. stercoralis* produced only minimal subjective and objective evidence of pulmonary involvement (Faust, 1935). About 320 larvae of *S. fuelleborni* produced only an unproductive cough starting on the fifth day, and chest radiograms were negative (Pampiglione, Ricciardi, 1972). Hyperinfection with *S. stercoralis* usually manifests with pulmonary symptoms, but the worms move through the lungs continuously for a long period of time (see Chapter 12).

It should be stressed that the main characteristics of the syndrome are the pulmonary infiltrations and their fleeting character, the peripheral eosinophilia, the mildness of the disease, and its short duration. The radiologic picture plus eosinophilia alone does not constitute Loeffler's syndrome. It is unfortunate to see the term *Loeffler's syndrome* often misused for infiltrates of longer duration. In reality, the diagnosis cannot be made on the basis of anatomic specimens, or by a clinician on the basis of the clinical symptoms, or by a radiologist with only one chest radiogram.

Pathology. There are two studies of histologic changes in individuals dying of *Ascaris* pneumonia (Beaver, Danaraj, 1958; Piggott et al. 1970), the first in a 30-year-old man with symptoms of tropical eosinophilia (see Chapter 19) and the second in a 12-month-old infant. In both cases, the gross appearance of the lungs consisted of patchy consolidation with a thick, tenacious, yellowish exudate filling the bronchi in the man and diffuse consolidation with small gray densities in the infant.

At autopsy, both patients were found to have had an eosinophilic pneumonia with abundant polymorphonuclear cells (Fig. 16–13 C). Eosinophils were present in the alveoli, in the bronchi, and in the well-preserved septae. A fibrinous exudate, Charcot-Leyden crystals, and hemorrhages were seen in the alveolar spaces (Fig. 16–13 A–B), and *Ascaris* larvae were found in the interstitium, the alveoli, and the lumen of the bronchi (Fig. 16–13 C–E). The picture is that of both alveolar and interstitial disease.

Diagnosis. Loeffler's syndrome is diagnosed by the radiologist using two or more chest radiograms taken 2 or 3 days apart and the clinical history of the patient. Recovery of nematode larvae in the sputum or gastric washings of the patient (Gelpi, Mustafa, 1967; Proffit, Walton, 1962) confirms the diagnosis in the laboratory. Examination of sputum reveals numerous eosinophils and Charcot-Leyden crystals on direct examination. *Ascaris* larvae are rarely found in histologic sections of the lungs. They are identified on the basis of their diameter, approximately 60 μm; the thin cuticle (the cuticle plus muscle fibers are less than 4 μm thick); and the lateral alae, 7 to 10 μm high (Fig. 16–13 C–E). The muscle layer has three or four cells per quadrant (Fig. 16–13 E). The lateral cords are well developed, with approximately three nuclei in each section (Fig. 16–13 D–E). The intestinal tract is composed of seven or eight cells per histologic section and has an open lumen without food particles (Fig. 16–13 E; Beaver, Danaraj, 1958).

Lagochilascaris minor— Lagochilascariasis

The genus *Lagochilascaris* belongs to the Ascarididae and has five known species in wild carnivores in Africa and on the American continent. One species, *L. minor*, has been reported in humans; it also occurs in dogs and cats (Campos et al. 1992). The main morphologic characteristics of the genus are some features of the lips surrounding the oral opening; they have a harelip appearance and are separated from the body by a deep groove or collar (Sprent, 1971).

Morphology and Life Cycle. The adult females measure 20 to 60 × 0.20 to 0.80 mm and the males 5 to 17 × 0.19 to 0.60 mm (Sprent, 1971). The life cycle of *L. minor* has only recently been studied. The adult worms live in tunnels and abscesses of tumor masses in the anterior part of the body of cats, mainly in the tissues around the esophagus, trachea, rhinopharynx, and cervical lymph nodes. Some of the abscesses open to the skin (sinus tracks) of the neck and drain pus. The eggs produced by the females pass in the pus draining from the sinuses and embryonate in soil. Experimentally, mice have been used as intermediate hosts, in which ingested embryonated eggs hatch and produce larvae that encapsulate in the tissues. When the cat ingests the infected mouse, an infection with adult worms is produced. Cats do not become directly infected by ingesting infective eggs (Campos et al. 1992). How humans become infected is not known, but it now appears that it occurs by swallowing infective eggs from soil, as was suggested previously (Smith et al. 1983).

Clinical Symptoms and Pathology. The majority of known cases of lagochilascariasis have occurred in Brazil (Campos et al. 1992; Correa et al. 1978; Moraes et al. 1983, 1985). The rest are from Mexico (Mar-

---

Fig. 16–13. ***Ascaris lumbricoides*** **pneumonia, sections stained with hematoxylin and eosin stain. A,** Low-power view of a medium-sized bronchus filled with mucus containing many eosinophils, ×70. **B,** Higher magnification of the same bronchus showing the mucus, abundant polymorphonuclear eosinophils, and four oblique sections and cross sections of *Ascaris* larvae (arrows), ×180. **C,** Higher magnification of pulmonary parenchyma showing two cross sections of a larva in the air spaces. Note the inflammatory exudate, ×280. **D** and **E,** Detail of a larva in cross sections. Note the lateral alae (short arrows), the open intestine, with a substance in the lumen (long arrow), the large lateral cords with up to three nuclei (open arrow), and the muscle layer, ×705. (Preparation AFIP No. 1282192. Reported by: Piggot, J., Hansbarger, E.A., Jr., and Neafie, R.C. 1970. Human ascariasis. Am. J. Clin. Pathol. 53:223–234.)

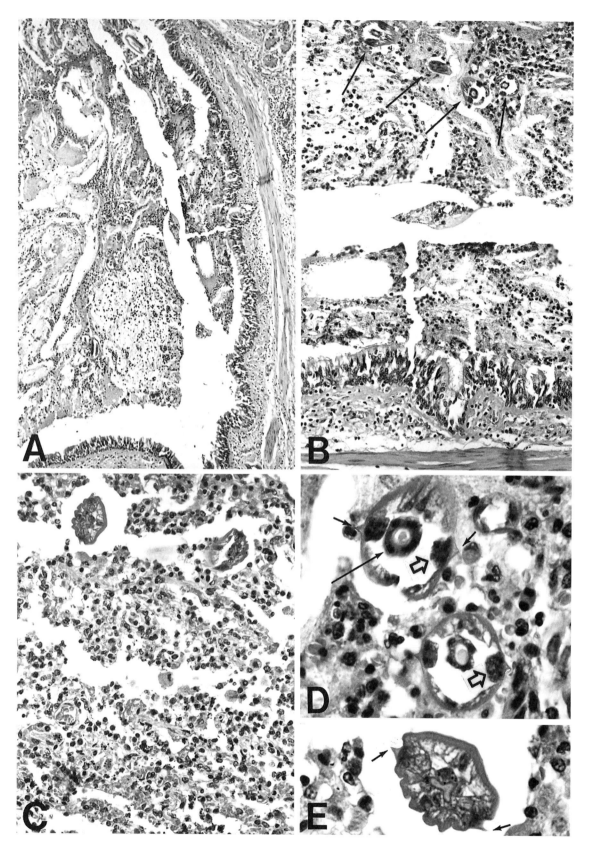

Fig. 16–13.

tinez, 1980), Colombia (Botero, Little, 1984), Venezuela (Orihuela et al. 1987; Volcan et al. 1982), Bolivia (Olle Goig et al. 1996), Costa Rica (Brenes-Madrigal, Brenes, 1961), Trinidad (Leiper, 1909; Pawan, 1926, 1927), Tobago (Draper, 1963; Draper, Buckley, 1963), and Surinam (Oostburg, Varma, 1968). The known cases of *Lagochilascaris* infections in humans are fewer than 50. Clinically, the disease presents as tissue swelling due to chronic inflammation, sometimes resembling a tumor. The compromised organs are the nasal sinuses, rhino- and oropharynx, middle ear (mastoid), cervical region, dental alveolus, lungs, central nervous system, and the sacral region. Some patients have sinus tracks that open to the skin or the oropharynx at the time of presentation; others develop the sinuses later. The condition progresses slowly over a period of several months; fever and pain are absent. A man in Brazil developed an encephalopathy and died; parasites were recovered as mature and immature adults from multiple abscesses in his lungs and brain (Fig. 16–14 *A–D*; Rosemberg et al. 1986). The histologic picture is that of necrosis (Fig. 16–14 *A*), acute and chronic inflammation, abscesses, and sinus tracks containing larvae and adults (Fig. 16–14 *B–D*) and eggs.

Diagnosis. Physicians familiar with the infection can make the diagnosis of lagochilascariasis on clinical grounds by examining pus discharged through the sinuses. The pus reveals eggs with a characteristic number of pits at the circumference of the eggshell, which allow identification of the species. *Lagochilascaris minor* eggs have 15 to 16 pits at the circumference, which are seen clearly on scanning electron micrographs (Bowman et al. 1983; Sprent, 1971).

In sections of tissues from the sinuses and the inflammatory mass, eggs, larval stages, and adults are usually recognized. The eggs show the pits in some sections (Fig. 16–14 *D*). The larvae of *L. minor* in humans are in different stages of development and measure up to approximately 200 μm in diameter at midbody (Fig. 16–14 *B*). The cuticle is 2 to 3 μm thick, with translucent lateral alae, sometimes flexed dorsally and measuring 13 μm in height, and striae about 1 μm in height that are evident in some longitudinal sections (Fig. 16–14 *B*). The muscle cells are numerous and relatively small, with a contractile portion about one-third the height of the cell, which is about 32 μm. The lateral cords of the hypodermis are usually as tall as the muscle cells. They are divided into two distinct portions (Fig. 16–14 *B*), each with three to five small nuclei, usually toward the base. The esophagus is not circular in transverse section for the first 30 μm, but instead has a cloverleaf shape; the remainder is circular. The esophagus is muscular, with a triangular lumen (Fig. 16–14 *D*). The intestine is often one-half or more the diameter of the worm. It is composed of many tall columnar cells with small nuclei at the base (Fig. 16–14 *B* and *D*). The microvilli are tall, especially in the posterior intestine (Bowman, 1987).

The adults have a similar morphology in cross section, but are larger, up to 0.5 mm in diameter, with a cuticle 7 to 8 μm thick and distinct lateral alae up to 35 μm in height. The most conspicuous characteristic of adult worms is the genital organs; in the females, the uterus has numerous eggs (Fig. 16–14 *D*).

Anisakis and *Pseudoterranova*— Anisakiasis and Pseudoterranoviais

Anisakis and *Pseudoterranova* are genera of the family Anisakidae within the superfamily Ascaridoidea. These ascariids parasitize the stomach of marine mammals, their natural definitive hosts. The larval stages of some species in these two genera are medically important because they occur in humans. The names of the genera and the species of *Anisakis* and *Pseudoterranova* have been changed several times as knowledge of

---

Fig. 16–14. *Lagochilascaris minor*, infection in the cerebellum. *A*, Gross appearance of the cerebellum showing areas of necrosis (open arrows) and hemorrhage (black). *B–D*. Histologic appearance, sections stained with hematoxylin and eosin stain. *B*, Cross section of an adult worm illustrating the intestine (i), sex organs (s), cuticle (c), lateral alae (la), and muscle cells (m), ×140. *C*, Low-power view of the cerebellum with necrosis, hemorrhage, and five cross sections of adult worms, ×22. *D*, Higher magnification showing two cross sections of a female worm. The section at the bottom is through the esophagus (e). The section on top is through the midbody. Note the intestine (i), sections of the sex organs (s), and the uterus (u) with eggs showing the characteristic pitted shell, ×140. (Preparations courtesy of S. Rosemberg, M.D., Faculdade de Medicina da Universidade de São Paulo, São Paulo, Brazil. Reported by: Rosemberg, S., Lopes, M.B.S., Mazuda, Z., et al. 1986. Fatal encephalopathy due to *Lagochilascaris minor* infection. Am. J. Trop. Med. Hyg. 35:575–578.)

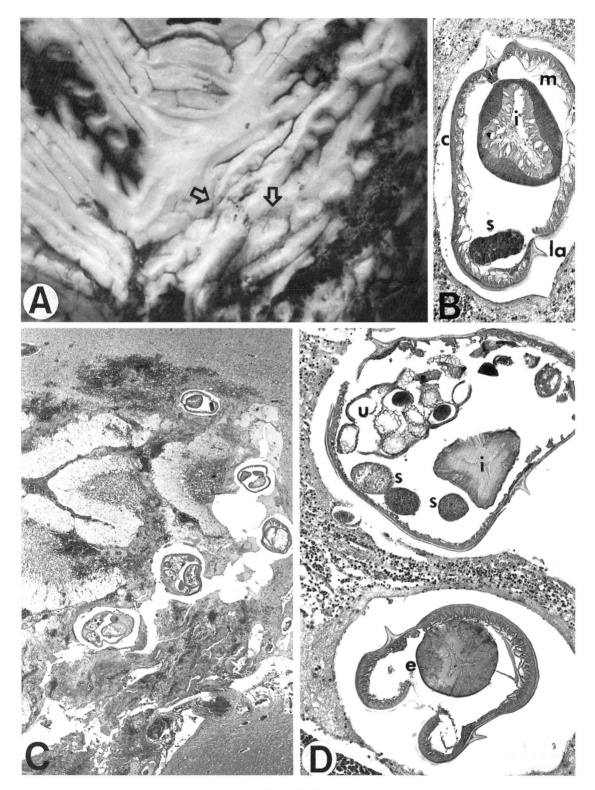

Fig. 16–14.

their biology and their taxonomic relationships has increased, creating confusion among nonexperts. Today it is believed that *Anisakis* has two species important in humans: *A. simplex* and *A. physeteris*, the larval stages of which were known in humans as *type I* and *type II*, respectively (Ishikura et al. 1992). *Anisakis* are parasites of Cetacea (whales, porpoises, dolphins, and others) and of Pinnipedia (seals, sea lions, walruses, and others). The genus *Pseudoterranova* (referred to at different times in the past as *Ascaris, Porracecum, Terranova,* and *Phocanema*) has one species, *P. decipiens,* which occurs exclusively in the Pinnipedia (Correa et al. 1980); formerly, its larval stages in humans were referred to as *Terranova type A.* The first cases of anisakiasis were reported from the Netherlands, and the larvae (*Anisakis*) recovered from the patients were identified as *Eustoma rotundatum* (Van Thiel et al. 1960). All of these names have been used in the medical literature for the worms that cause the infection and are mentioned here only for clarification. The larval stages of *Anisakis* are usually found in mackerel and herring, and those of *P. decipiens* are found in cod and pollock, hence the names *herring worm disease* and *codworm disease,* plus other similar ones.

Morphology. Anisakiid worms (a name used here for simplicity and to denote both *Anisakis* and *Pseudoterranova*) are large nematodes that grossly resemble *Ascaris.* The particulars of the adult stages are of no importance for this discussion, but the larval stages found in humans have practical interest because they are often brought to the physician by the patient or are found in anatomic specimens by the pathologist. In general, anisakiid larvae are up to 3 cm in length by less than 1 mm in diameter. The cephalic end has the three lips characteristic of the Ascaridoidea, as well as a small tooth, the *boring tooth.* The esophagus is divided into two portions, the anterior muscular part and the posterior glandular part known as the *proventriculus.* Some species have a cecum that arises at the junction of the esophagus and the intestine, running frontward along the esophagus. At the posterior end, some species have a pointed structure, the *mucron.* Most larvae recovered from human infections lasting for less than 3 days are third-stage larvae. Larvae from longer-lasting infections have molted to the fourth stage and sometimes to the fifth stage. There are morphologic differences in these various stages, but they are outside the scope of this discussion. The most practical approach is to determine the genus, which is identified on the basis of the characteristics of the esophagus and the intestine. The larvae of

Pseudoterranova have a short cecum, while those of *Anisakis* do not.

Life Cycle and Biology. The life cycles of the different anisakiids of medical importance have small variations. In general, the adults live in the host's stomach, with their cephalic end buried in the mucosa, sometimes forming large tumor-like masses containing many worms. Eggs are evacuated with the feces into seawater, where they embryonate and hatch, releasing free-living larvae. These larvae are swallowed by any of the many species of small marine invertebrates, such as amphypods, decapods, caridean prawns, euphausiids, and others. The euphausiids are considered important intermediate hosts for *Anisakis*, while copepods and larger macroinvertebrates are important for *Pseudoterranova.* In the intermediate hosts the infective larvae develop; however, many species of fish and squid serve as transport hosts for the parasite. (Transport hosts are those that acquire infective larvae, which may increase in size and encapsulate in the tissues but do not grow to the next stage.) Small fish, the transport hosts, are ingested by larger fish, where the larvae reencapsulate in the tissues or the viscera. This mechanism ensures their movement and their concentration (increased numbers) as they progress through the food chain. The definitive hosts become infected by ingesting the intermediate hosts or any of the many transport hosts. Transport hosts (fish) are the main source of human infections (Fig. 16–15).

Geographic Distribution and Epidemiology. Human infections with anisakiids occur when raw squid or marine fish bearing the infective larvae are ingested. Infections are especially common in Japan, where dishes of raw fish such as sushi, sashimi, oka, and poison crewe are common in the daily diet (Oshima, 1972, 1987). In the Netherlands, anisakiasis became common in the 1950s, but preventive measures brought a de-

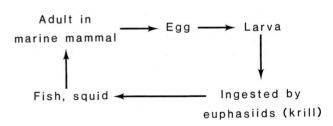

Fig. 16–15. *Anisakis,* **schematic representation of life cycle.**

cline and disappearance of the infection by the 1970s (Van Thiel, 1976). Sporadic cases of anisakiasis have been reported in many other countries, including the United States. In the United States, several cases of upper airway disease, with few or no symptoms, have been reported (Chitwood, 1970, 1975; Juels et al. 1975; Kates et al. 1973; Kliks, 1983; Little, Most, 1973). In most of these cases, the patient felt the worm in the buccal cavity and retrieved it or coughed it up. In most cases, the parasites were identified as *Pseudoterranova*. The cases reported with worms in the intestinal tract were probably due to *Anisakis* (Appelby et al. 1982; Deardorff et al. 1986; Hsiu et al. 1986; Pinkus et al. 1975; Sakanari et al. 1988; Valdiserri, 1981). Ingestion of anisakiid larvae without apparent morbidity must be common because, in Eskimos, the worms have been recovered from the stools during surveys of intestinal parasites (Hitchcock, 1950; Rausch et al. 1967). A report of pulmonary anisakiasis diagnosed on the basis of serology alone is dubious (Kobayashi et al. 1985). In addition, a case mistakenly diagnosed as *A. costarricensis* in California (Hulbert et al. 1992) is actually a case of *Anisakis* (Ash, 1993).

Clinical Findings. Anisakiasis and pseudoterranoviasis cannot be distinguished clinically; thus, the generic term *anisakiasis* is used to refer to both infections. Only when the larva has been recovered and identified is the distinction made. In general, the disease is either intestinal or extraintestinal. In the intestinal tract, the worms are found anywhere from the mouth to the colon; the stomach is the most important location (remember, this is the natural habitat of the worm), followed by the intestine, the esophagus, and the oral cavity. Extraintestinal anisakiasis occurs most commonly in the pharynx, followed by the abdominal cavity; on rare occasions, the worm has been found in most other organs of the peritoneal cavity.

Because the great majority of cases occur in the gastrointestinal tract, intestinal anisakiasis is the most important form of the disease. Invasions outside the intestine are extremely rare. In an extensive review of cases in Japan, 117 extraintestinal cases were reported; they included 24 in the esophagus, 3 in the oral cavity, and 1 each in the tongue and uvula. This leaves only 88 cases that are truly extraintestinal (Ishikura et al. 1992). The clinical manifestations of anisakiasis are summarized in the following paragraphs. Those who wish to study the disease in depth should consult the exhaustive works of Ishikura and Namiki on gastric anisakiasis (Ishikura, Namiki, 1989) and those of

Ishikura and Kokichi on intestinal anisakiasis (Ishikura, Kikuchi, 1990).

The clinical presentation of anisakiasis varies, depending on the duration of the infection, the location of the worm in the intestine, the species, and probably hosts factors such as sensitization to the parasite. The acute symptoms of anisakiasis start 4 to 12 hours after eating a meal of raw fish and may last for months (Muraoka et al. 1996; Yokogawa, Yoshimura, 1965). The patient often presents with acute, severe abdominal and epigastric pain, nausea, vomiting, and abdominal distention. On clinical examination, a movable soft mass or induration is felt. The abdominal distention is found to be due to gas in the intestine and fluid in the peritoneal cavity. Intermittent bouts of diarrhea with blood and constipation due to intestinal obstruction may occur; mild fever may also be present. Laboratory tests reveal leukocytosis with eosinophilia, but in general they are not helpful. The most important tests are radiograms and ultrasonograms (Fig. 16–19 *A*), which may reveal edema and ulceration of the affected bowel and sometimes shadows of the larva when a contrast medium is used. Tomograms may reveal a tumor-like mass on the wall (Fig. 16–16 *A*). In the stomach, the tumor may not be seen in follow-up radiograms; this is the so-called vanishing tumor of the stomach in the Japanese literature. Endoscopic studies may reveal erosion, ulceration, and hemorrhagic lesions, and sometimes the worm, which can be retrieved, curing the patient (Fig. 16–17 *A–B*; Akasaka et al. 1977). High-resolution ultrasound and contrast radiographs of the intestine can often secure the diagnosis, avoiding surgery (Shirahama et al. 1992).

A worm in the small intestine produces lesions resembling those of regional ileitis (Hayasaka et al. 1971; Ishikura et al. 1967). The symptoms vary with the location of the parasite, usually consisting of sudden, violent abdominal pain, nausea, vomiting, and signs of peritoneal irritation. On palpation, a poorly defined area of induration is felt. The leukocyte count is up to 15,000 per cubic millimeter, with a high percentage of polymorphonuclear cells. Exploratory laparotomy reveals 200 to 500 ml of straw-colored fluid in the peritoneal cavity and a segment of inflamed intestine.

The symptoms produced by the worm in the oropharynx consist of sudden episodes of coughing, and some patients cough up the worm. Other patients feel the worm in the mouth or throat and retrieve it with the fingers. Most cases of anisakiid larvae reported in the United States have occurred in the upper respiratory tract and the mouth (Chitwood, 1970, 1975; Juels et al. 1975; Kates et al. 1973; Kliks, 1983; Little, Most, 1973). However, cases in the upper respiratory

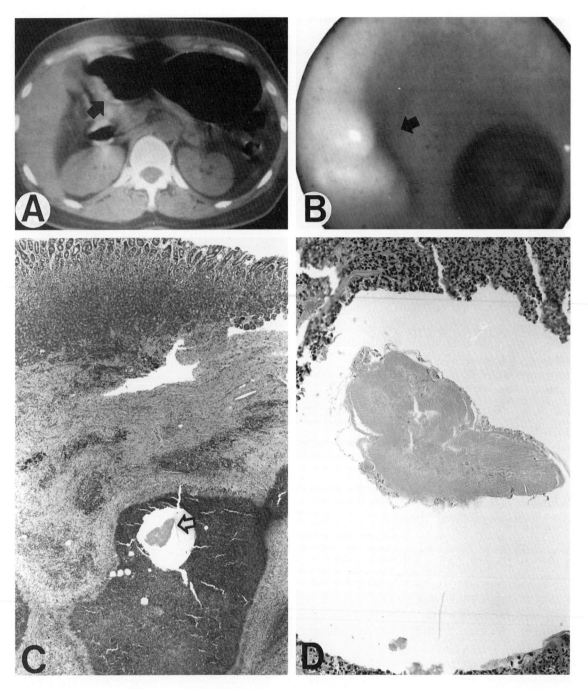

Fig. 16–16. *Anisakis* in stomach. *A*, Computed tomographic scan showing thickening of the stomach wall (arrow). *B*, Gastroscopic picture showing presumed tumor within the gastric wall (arrow). *C* and *D*. Sections stained with hematoxylin and eosin stain. *C*, Low-power view of the stomach wall with an abscess in the submucosa showing a necrotic anisakiid larva (arrow), ×28. *D*, Higher magnification of the worm showing lack of histologic detail. Under the microscope, the worm was still identifiable by the muscle layer and a faint lateral cord, ×220. (Gross photographs and preparations courtesy of J.G. Hsieu, M.D., Department of Pathology, De Paul Hospital, Norfolk, Virginia. Reported by: Hsiu, J.G., Gamsey, A.J., Ives, C.E., et al. 1986. Gastric anisakiasis: Report of a case with clinical, endoscopic, and histological findings. Am. J. Gastroenterol. 81:1185–1187. *A* and *B* reproduced with permission.)

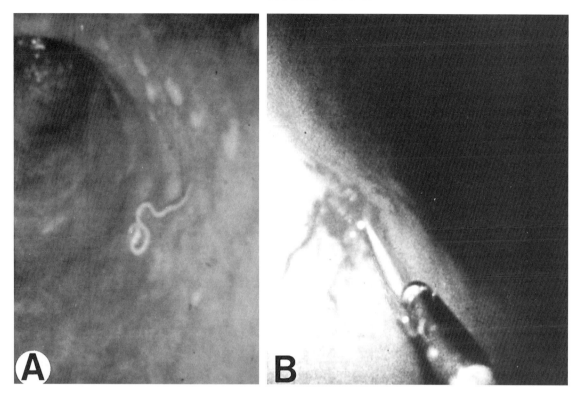

Fig. 16–17. *Anisakis* in the stomach. *A*, Larva in the stomach as seen with the gastroscope. The anterior end is buried in the mucosa. *B*, Extraction of the larva dur-ing endoscopy. (Courtesy of T. Oshima, M.D., Department of Parasitology, School of Medicine, University of Shinshu, Matsumoto, Japan.)

tract have also been reported in other countries, mostly in Japan (Ishikura et al. 1992; Tanaka et al. 1968). One recent case reported as *Anisakis* in the tonsils, identified in tissue sections, is an artifact, not a worm (Bhargava et al. 1996).

Pathology. Anisakiid larvae may be found in surgical specimens lodged anywhere in the gastrointestinal tract. Rarely is more than one larva present; a case reported with 56 larvae of *A. simplex* in the stomach is extraordinary (Kagei, Isogaki, 1992). The surgeon may retrieve the worm from the peritoneal cavity and submit it with the surgical specimen. Geographic differences in the distribution of the larvae in the intestine have been observed. In Japan, the stomach is affected in about 65% of the cases (Yokogawa, Yoshimura, 1967); in the Netherlands, in about 7% (Van Thiel, Van Houten, 1967). In the intestine, the worms occur mainly in the last 100 cm of the small bowel; a few have been found in the cecum and the ileum (Ishikura, Kikuchi, 1990).

Grossly, the segment of stomach or intestine removed surgically due to anisakiasis has a markedly thickened wall; the serosal surface is edematous and hyperemic, with focal areas of hemorrhage and signs of peritonitis. Lymph nodes, if present, are enlarged, and in a few cases contain the worm. An area of intestinal perforation is often seen as a small focus of necrosis, and sometimes the parasite is seen protruding into the peritoneal cavity. When the resected intestinal segment is opened, the mucosa is found to be hyperemic and edematous. It usually contains the parasite buried in the mucosa, with its posterior end free in the lumen. Grossly, the appearance of the resected bowel sometimes resembles Crohn's disease.

Four types of microscopic lesions have been described in intestinal anisakiasis, depending upon the stage of evolution: (*1*) a phlegmon characterized by a well-preserved larva located among abundant inflammation and erosion of the mucosa, hemorrhage, and diffuse infiltration by eosinophils and mononuclear cells (Figs. 16–18 *A–D* and 16–19 *B–D*; (*2*) an abscess containing a dead, degenerating parasite at the center, with granulation tissue at the periphery and abundant infiltration by eosinophils (Fig. 16–16 *C–D*; (*3*) abscess with a necrotic center and a thick capsule of granulation tissue, with good numbers of eosinophils still pres-

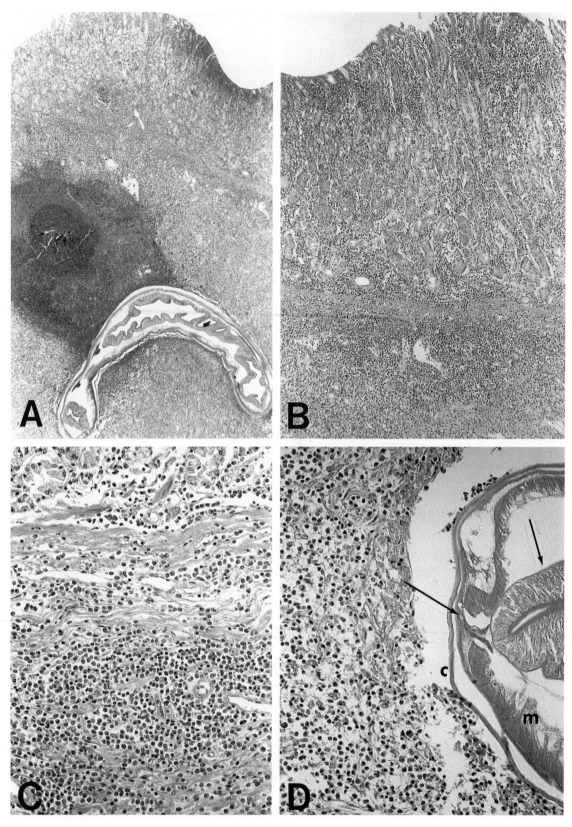

Fig. 16–18. *Anisakis* in the stomach, sections stained with hematoxylin and eosin stain. *A*, Low-power view of the gastric wall with an abscess and a larva deep in the submucosa, ×22. *B*, Detail of the mucosa showing the inflammatory reaction, mainly eosinophils, ×55. *C*, Higher magnification, ×180. *D*, Detail of the worm showing the cuticle (c), the lateral cords in the form of a Y (long arrow), the intestine (short arrow), and the muscle cells (m). (Preparation courtesy of T. Oshima, M.D., Department of Parasitology, School of Medicine, University of Shinshu, Matsumoto, Japan.)

ent throughout the thickness of the intestinal wall; at the center may be remains of a parasite, which is hard or impossible to identify; (4) a granuloma, which is a healed lesion consisting of granulation tissue and a few infiltrating cells, some of which are eosinophils (Kojima, 1966).

Diagnosis. The larva recovered from humans belongs either to *Anisakis* or to *Pseudoterranova*. As stated above, if the infection is of short duration (2–3 days), the larva is a third-stage (infective) larva. In longer-lasting infections, the larva has time to molt to the fourth or even the fifth stage (Ishikura et al. 1995; Kliks, 1983, 1986). Distinguishing the larvae of *Anisakis* from those of *Pseudoterranova* is based on the characteristics of the esophagus and the intestine (Oshima, 1972; Sohn, Seol, 1994), and their examination requires special preparation of the worm. A larva received in the laboratory can be placed in 3 or 4 ml of a mixture of 70% alcohol and 5% glycerol in a small vial left open to allow the alcohol to evaporate; this occurs in a couple of days. When the larva is in the glycerol (which does not evaporate), it can be examined under the microscope to determine its internal structures. The main feature of *Pseudoterranova* is the presence of an intestinal cecum, which is absent in *Anisakis*. Several other morphologic differences exist between these two larvae, but they are less obvious to the nonspecialist.

In tissue sections all anisakiids have characteristic structures. These structures allow the general diagnosis of anisakiid larva or less precise *Anisakis* species, which suffices for general clinical purposes. A generic diagnosis may be made in some cases, depending on the plane of section and the region of the worm sectioned, but this requires examination by personnel familiar with the morphology of the larvae. The anisakiids in tissue sections are generally 250 to 800 μm in diameter. The cuticle is moderately thick, with transverse striations 7 to 9 μm wide (Figs. 16–18 D, and 16–19 D) that are better appreciated in oblique and longitudinal sections. The lateral cords are probably the most distinctive structure in this group, appearing as a Y continuing with the hypodermis (subcuticle) at the base, with the two arms of the Y free in the cavity (Figs. 16–18 D and 16–19 D). The muscle cells are numerous. The excretory cell (renette cell) is present only in sections of the anterior portion of the worm (Fig. 16–19 D). The intestinal tract of the parasite is composed of the esophagus, with its two distinct muscular and glandular sections (see above); the intestine consists of a single layer of tall columnar epithelial cells, with no substantial intestinal lumen (Oshima, 1972; Shiraki,

1974). The cecum of *Pseudoterranova* may be seen if the worm is sectioned at that level, which is helpful in identifying this genus.

Baylisascaris—Baylisascariasis

The genus *Baylisascaris* of the family Ascarididae has fewer than a dozen species that occur in small to large wild carnivorous mammals; they are found in every geographic area where they have been investigated. *Baylisascaris* are large ascariids that superficially resemble the human *Ascaris*, but they possess distinct morphologic features that enable their specific identification, a subject outside this discussion.

Life Cycle and Biology. The life cycle of most species of *Baylisascaris* is not known; one species studied is *B. melis*, from the badger in the Old World, which was shown to require an intermediate host (Mozgovoi, Shakhmatova, 1979). Another species, *B. procyonis*, also requires an intermediate host. In general, the life cycle of *Baylisascaris* is as follows: adult worms in the small intestine pass eggs, which are evacuated in the feces to embryonate in soil and become infective for small animals. Upon ingestion by these animals, the eggs hatch and the larvae migrate in the tissues, grow, and encapsulate before they become infective for their final hosts. Through predation, the larvae reach the intestine of their definitive hosts, where they grow to adults. The species found in the raccoon, *B. procyonis*, and in the skunk, *B. columnaris*, produce massive damage during their migration through the tissues of their intermediate hosts. One system especially affected is the central nervous system, often resulting in the death of the intermediate host. The number of larvae migrating through the tissues and the size of the infected animal are important in producing morbidity in the animal; a single larva of *B. procyonis* or *B. columnaris* is capable of killing a mouse in 7 to 12 days.

There are at least four species of *Baylisascaris* in North America: *B. procyonis* in raccoons, *B. columnaris* in skunks, *B. transfuga* in bears, and *B. laevis* in martens. Infections with *Baylisascaris* larvae have been found in many animals, sometimes producing outbreaks of veterinary and economic importance (Dade et al. 1977; Jacobson et al. 1976; Kazacos et al. 1983). There are three recorded human infections with *Baylisascaris* larvae in the tissues; two were fatal. In these patients, the larvae were found and identified on

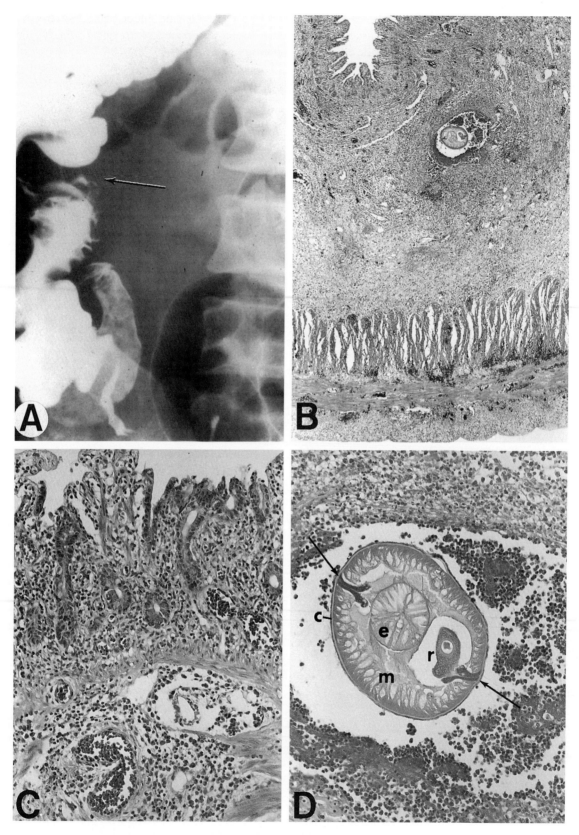

Fig. 16–19.

the basis of circumstantial evidence as *B. procyonis*, without taking into account that other species of *Baylisascaris* or of related ascarids cannot be ruled out conclusively (Fox et al. 1985; Huff et al. 1984). In these two human infections the parasites behaved as they would have in their natural intermediate hosts. Thus, in humans, the host–parasite relationship is not one of paratenesis; therefore, *Baylisascaris* does not produce, sensu strictu, visceral larva migrans (see Chapter 17). The third case was diagnosed only on the basis of serology. The patient was treated and recovered (Cunningham et al. 1994).

The occurrence of *Baylisascaris* larvae in the eye of subhuman primates under experimental conditions has been described (Kazacos et al., 1984a, 1984b). Nematode larvae larger than those of *Toxocara* (see Chapters 17 and 21) have been found in the retina of humans, sometimes producing diffuse unilateral subacute neuroretinitis syndrome (Gass, Braunstein, 1983), but the nematode responsible for this lesion has not been conclusively identified. Therefore, although *Baylisascaris* appears to be the species involved in some cases (Kazacos et al. 1984a, 1984b, 1985), this conclusion is not justified at present.

Clinical Findings. The clinical picture of the two fatal cases of baylisascariasis has many similarities. One patient was a 10-month-old infant, the other an 18-month-old child with Down's syndrome. Both infants had an acute upper respiratory illness followed by symptoms in the central nervous system. One infant was lethargic, irritable, and obtunded, with loss of most spontaneous movements. On physical examination he was semicomatose, with extensor posturing, hyperactive deep tendon reflexes, and positive bilateral Babinski signs. The other infant was also lethargic at the time of hospital admission, with a supple neck, mild hepatomegaly, a vertical nystagmus, and right arm hypertonicity. The laboratory findings in both children were similar. The white blood cell counts were 10,000 and 17,000 per cubic millimeter, with 37% and 27% eosinophilia, respectively. The cerebrospinal fluid con-

tained 5 and 92 white blood cells, respectively, and no pathogenic organisms were found. Serologic tests for different parasitic infections were negative. One infant died 6 days after arriving at the hospital, the other at home 14 months after the onset of illness.

The third child, a 13-month-old boy, was brought to the hospital because he refused to walk, and had right-sided torticollis and right-sided gaze preference, together with symptoms of an upper respiratory tract infection. The larvae were not detected, but specific antibodies to larval antigens were found in the spinal fluid; again, specific identification of the parasite was based on circumstantial evidence. The patient was treated and left the hospital with severe neurologic sequelae (Cunningham et al. 1994). A fourth case was reported as *Baylisascaris* based on the study of a presumably necrotic larva that was too degenerated for identification. The presumed larva had produced an eosinophilic pseudotumor in the heart, which protruded into the left ventricle and resulted in the sudden death of a 10-year-old boy in Massachusetts (Boschetti, Kasznica, 1995). This case should not be included in the casuistic of baylisascariasis.

Pathology. Grossly, the main changes produced by baylisascariasis occur in the brain. The infant dying in the hospital of the acute infection had congestion of the meninges, swelling and softening of the brain, and cerebellar herniation. On coronal sections the brain tissue was found to be necrotic, especially in the inner third of the periventricular white matter (Fig. 16–20 A), which clearly showed numerous track-like lesions. The infant dying 14 months later with chronic baylisascariasis infection had a small brain weighing 810 g (normal = 1065 g) with thick gray meninges, especially at the base of the brain and the spinal cord. Coronal sections revealed severe atrophy of both cerebral hemispheres, the corpus callosum, basal ganglia, thalami, massa intermedia, cerebellum, brain stem, and spinal cord. The white matter was reduced in mass, pale, and hard, and the cortex showed small cavitations. Outside the central nervous system, other organs in both pa-

Fig. 16–19. *Anisakis* in the intestine. *A*, X-ray film showing a filling defect (arrow) due to inflammation of the colonic wall. *B–D*. Histology, sections stained with hematoxylin and eosin stain. *B*, Low-power view of the intestinal wall, resected from another patient, showing inflammation, edema, and a cross section of an anisakiid larva in the submucosa, ×12. *C*, Higher magnification showing an inflammatory exudate, ×180. *D*, Detail of the worm cut at the level of the esophagus. Note the cuticle (c), the muscle cells (m), the esophagus (e), and the excretory rennete cell (r); lateral cords are conspicuous (arrows), with the characteristic Y-shaped morphology. (Preparation courtesy of T. Oshima, M.D., Department of Parasitology, School of Medicine, University of Shinshu, Matsumoto, Japan.)

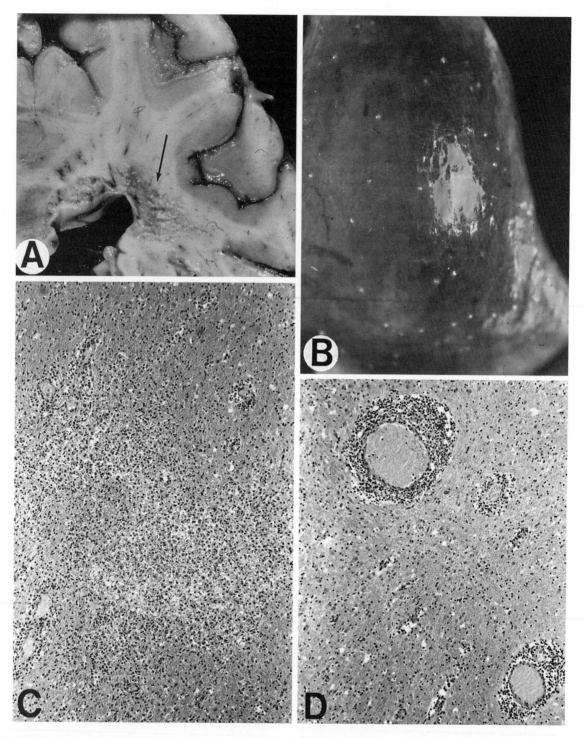

Fig. 16–20. *Baylisascaris* infection in a man. *A*, Coronal section of brain with acute infection showing necrosis around the ventricle (arrow). *B*, Pleural surface showing the small granulomas. *C* and *D*. Microscopic brain appearance, sections stained with hematoxylin and eosin stain. *C*, Low-power view showing necrosis and an inflammatory infiltrate, ×70. *D*, Higher magnification illustrating the perivascular infiltrate, ×70. (Photographs and preparations courtesy of N.S. Gould, M.D., Department of Pathology, Michael Reese Hospital and Medical Center, Chicago, Illinois. Reported by: Fox, A.S., Kazacos, K.R., Gould, N.S., et al. 1985. Fatal eosinophilic meningoencephalitis and visceral larva migrans caused by the raccoon ascariid *Baylisascaris procyonis*. N. Engl. J. Med. 312:1619–1623. *B* reprinted with permission.)

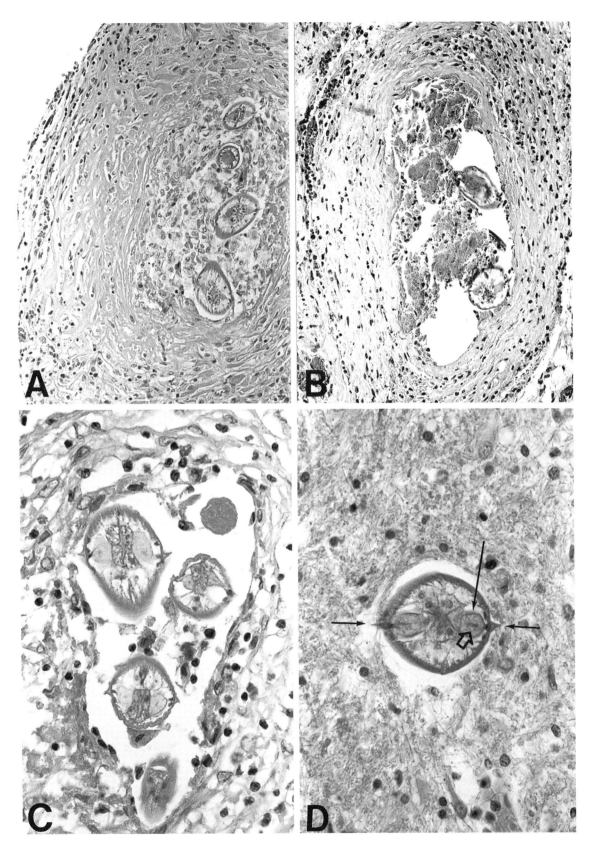

Fig. 16–21. *Baylisascaris* in human tissues, sections stained with hematoxylin and eosin stain, same infant as in Figure 15–19. *A* and *B*, Low-power view showing an encapsulated, coiled larva in the pleura (*A*) and the omentum (*B*), ×180. *C* and *D*, Larvae in the heart and brain showing the morphologic characteristics. Note that the larva in the brain is not encapsulated (*D*). The well-developed lateral alae (short arrows) are evident; the lateral cords have two to three nuclei (long arrow); the excretory columns have a dot-like lumen (open arrow); the intestine at the center is composed of four to six cells with well-defined cell borders, ×450.

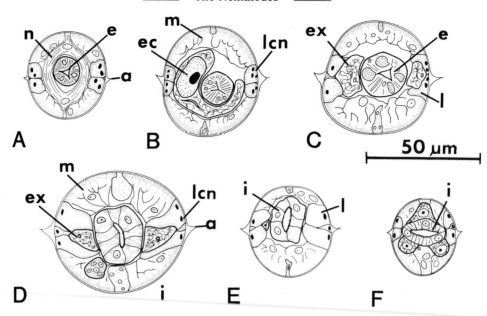

Fig. 16–22. *Baylisascaris procyonis*, histologic anatomy of the larva in cross sections. From experimentally infected mice at 14 days postinfection. *A*, Transverse section at the level of the nerve ring. *B*, At the level of the excretory commissure showing the excretory cell nucleus. *C*, At the base of the esophagus. *D*, At the midbody showing the genital primordium. *E* and *F*, At the posterior end. Abbreviations: a, alae; e, esophagus; ec, excretory cell nucleus; ex, excretory columns; i, intestine; l, lateral cords; lcn, lateral cord nuclei; m, muscle cells; n, nerve ring. (Courtesy of D. Bowman, Ph.D., Department of Microbiology, Immunology, and Parasitology, New York State College of Veterinary Medicine, Cornell University, Ithaca, New York. In: Bowman, D. 1987. Diagnostic morphology of four larval ascaridoid nematodes that may cause visceral larva migrans: *Toxascaris leonina*, *Baylisascaris procyonis*, *Lagochilascaris sprenti*, and *Hexametra leidyi*. J. Parasitol. 73:1198–1215. Reproduced with permission.)

tients showed granulomas 1.0 to 1.5 mm in diameter, which were most evident on the serosal surfaces (Fig. 16–20 *B*).

Microscopically, the brain of the infant with acute disease had marked necrosis of the white matter, the meninges, and especially the Virchow-Robin spaces (Fig. 16–20 *C–D*). Numerous macrophages, eosinophils, and lymphocytes with occasional plasma cells were present. Larvae were not encapsulated in the brain, and were present in both necrotic and healthy tissue (Fig. 16–21 *D*), but other organs contained numerous encapsulated larvae (Fig. 16–21 *A–C*).

The brain of the child with chronic infection had many granulomas, mostly around the periventricular white matter and the cerebral and cerebellar cortices. Whether these granulomas contained larvae was not reported. Encapsulated larvae were found in many other tissues and organs.

Diagnosis. The diagnosis of baylisascariasis is made by identifying encapsulated or nonencapsulated parasites in tissue sections. Encapsulated larvae are located in granulomas composed of fibrous tissue. In the granuloma the larva is at the center, coiled, and usually cut at three to five body levels. Sections through the midbody of *Baylisascaris* vary from 50 to 65 m in diameter (Fig. 16–21 *C–D*). The cuticle is about 1 μm thick, with transverse striae 1 μm in height and prominent pointed lateral alae (Fig. 16–21 *D*). The lateral cords are also prominent, with a minute excretory canal and two or three small, hyperchromic nuclei per section. The muscles, four to six per quadrant, are well developed. The intestine has four to six cells per section and is open; well-developed larvae contain food particles in the lumen (Fig. 16–22; Bowman, 1987). This description applies generally to *B. procyonis*, *B. columnaris*, and *B. transfuga*, which show no differences on cross sections (personal observations); larval stages of other species of *Baylisascaris* have not been studied on cross sections. In related ascariids, only the larval stages of *Lagochilascaris sprenti* and *Hexametra leydyi* have been studied.

References

Adebamowo CA, Akang EE, Ladipo JK, Ajao OG, 1993. Ascarid granuloma presenting as pseudotumour. Trop. Geogr. Med. 45:86–88

Africa CM, Garcia EY, 1936. Embryonated eggs of *Ascaris lumbricoides* in the mesenteric tissue of man, with special reference to the possibility of autoinfestation. J. Philipp. Isl. Med. Assoc. 16:461–467

Akasaka Y, Matsuno K, Yoshida Y, Arizono N, Ikai T, Ogino K, Takeuchi S, Yamada M, 1977. Endoscopical treatment of gastric anisakiasis with special reference to ecdysis of *Anisakis* type I larva in the human stomach. J. Kyoto Pref. Univ. Med. 86:257–260

Akgun Y, 1996. Intestinal obstruction caused by *Ascaris lumbricoides*. Dis. Colon Rectum 39:1159–1163

Anderson TJ, 1995. *Ascaris* infections in humans from North America: molecular evidence for cross-infection. Semin. Respir. Infect. 110:215–219

Appelby D, Kapoor W, Karpf M, Williams S, 1982. Anisakiasis nematode infestation producing small-bowel obstruction. Arch. Surg. 117:836

Archibong AE, Ndoma ER, Asindi AA, 1994. Intestinal obstruction in southeastern Nigerian children. E. Afr. Med. J. 71:286–289

Arean VM, Castells J, Herron C, Crandall C, 1962. Further studies on the pathogenesis of the ascaridic granuloma. Am. J. Trop. Med. Hyg. 11:731–738

Asaolu SO, Holland CV, Jegede JO, Fraser NR, Stoddard RC, Crompton DWT, 1992. The prevalence and intensity of soil-transmitted helminthiases in rural communities in Southern Nigeria. Ann. Trop. Med. Parasitol. 86:279–287

Ash LR, 1993. Human anisakiasis misdiagnosed as abdominal angiostrongyliasis. Clin. Infect. Dis. 16:332–333

Atias A, Hermosilla M, Alessandrini H, 1959. Ascaridiasis peritoneal. Descripcion de tres casos. Bol. Chil. Parasitol. 14:13–15

Bambirra EA, Margarida A, Nogueira MF, Andrade IED, 1985. Tumoral form of ascariasis: report of a case. J. Trop. Med. Hyg. 88:273–276

Barlow JB, Pocock WA, Tabatznik BA, 1961. An epidemic of 'acute eosinophilic pneumonia' following 'beer drinking' and probably due to infestation with *Ascaris lumbricoides*. S. Afr. Med. J. 35:390–394

Beaver PC, 1964. *Ascaris* strangled in a shoe-eyelet. Am. J. Trop. Med. Hyg. 13:295–296

Beaver PC, 1975. Biology of soil-transmitted helminths: The massive infection. Health Lab. Sci. 12:116–125

Beaver PC, Danaraj TJ, 1958. Pulmonary ascariasis resembling eosinophilic lung. Autopsy report with description of larvae in the bronchioles. Am. J. Trop. Med. Hyg. 7:100–111

Beaver PC, Jung RC, Cupp EW, 1984. *Clinical Parasitology*. Philadelphia: Lea & Febiger

Beitia AO, Haller JO, Kantor A, 1997. CT findings in pediatric gastrointestinal ascariasis. Comput. Med. Imaging Graph. 21:47–49

Bernstein RB, 1977. Biliary ascariasis diagnosed by ERCP with chronic dilatation of the biliary system. Am. J. Dig. Dis. 22:391–394

Bhargava D, Raman R, El Azzouni MZ, Bhargava K, Bhusnurmath B, 1996. Anisakiasis of the tonsils. J. Laryngol. Otol. 110:387–388

Blumenthal DS, Schultz MG, 1975. Incidence of intestinal obstruction in children infected with *Ascaris lumbricoides*. Am. J. Trop. Med. Hyg. 24:801–805

Boschetti A, Kasznica J, 1995. Visceral larva migrans induced eosinophilic cardiac pseudotumor: a cause of sudden death in a child. J. Forensic Sci. 40:1097–1099

Botero D, Little MD, 1984. Two cases of human *Lagochilascaris* infection in Colombia. Am. J. Trop. Med. Hyg. 33:381–386

Bowman DD, 1987. Diagnostic morphology of four larval ascaridoid nematodes that may cause visceral larva migrans: *Toxascaris leonina*, *Baylisascaris procyonis*, *Lagochilascaris sprenti*, and *Hexametra leidyi*. J. Parasitol. 73:1198–1215

Bowman DD, Smith JL, Little MD, 1983. *Lagochilascaris sprenti* sp. n. (Nematoda: Ascarididae) from the opossum, *Didelphis virginiana* (Marsupialia: Didelphidae). J. Parasitol. 69:754–760

Brenes-Madrigal RR, Brenes AF, 1961. Lagochilascariasis humana en Costa Rica. Programa General y Resumen de Trabajos del Congreso Latinoamericana y Nacional de Microbiologia, Costa Rica, Dec. 10–17, p. 35

Brumpt LC, 1952. Deductions cliniques tirees de cinquante cas d'ankylostomose provoquez. Ann. Parasitol. Hum. Comp. 27:237–249

Bustamante-Sarabia J, Martuscello-Q A, Tay J, 1977. Ectopic ascariasis: report of a case with adult worms in the kidney. Am. J. Trop. Med. Hyg. 26:568–569

Campos DM, Freire Filha LG, Vieira MA, Paco JM, Maia MA, 1992. Experimental life cycle of *Lagochilascaris minor* Leiper, 1909. Rev. Inst. Med. Trop. Sao Paulo 34:277–287

Capallo DV, Gongaware RD, 1984. Biliary ascariasis. South. Med. J. 77:1201–1202

Carrera E, Nesheim MC, Crompton DWT, 1984. Lactose maldigestion in *Ascaris*-infected preschool children. Am. J. Clin. Nutr. 39:255–264

Chacko DD, 1970. Correspondence. Intestinal parasites and asthma. N. Engl. J. Med. 283:101

Chandrasoma PT, De Silva S, Yoganathan M, 1978. Roundworm granuloma of the anterior abdominal wall. Postgrad. Med. J. 54:103–107

Chao TC, Ewert A, Zaman V, 1965. *Ascaris lumbricoides*

eggs in liver and lungs of 2 year old boy at necropsy; confirmation by experimental inoculations of animals. Med. J. Malaya 20:340–341

Chen D, Li X, 1994. Forty-two patients with acute *Ascaris* pancreatitis in China. J. Gastroenterol. 29:676–678

Chitwood MB, 1970. Nematodes of medical significance found in market fish. Am. J. Trop. Med. Hyg. 19:599–602

Chitwood MB, 1975. *Phocanema*-type larval nematode coughed up by a boy in California. Am. J. Trop. Med. Hyg. 24:710–711

Choi MH, Park IA, Hong IK, Chai JY, Lee SH, 1993. A case of biliary ascariasis accompanied by cholelithiasis. Korean J. Parasitol. 31:71–74

Chu WG, Chen PM, Huang CC, Hsu CT, 1972. Neonatal ascariasis. J. Pediatr. 81:785

Cobo A, Hail RC, Torres E, Cuello CJ, 1964. Intrahepatic calculi. Arch. Surg. 89:936–941

Cooray GH, Panaboicke RO, 1960. Granulomatous peritonitis caused by *Ascaris* ova. Trans. R. Soc. Trop. Med. Hyg. 54:358–361

Correa-Henao A, 1957. Lesiones por *Ascaris lumbricoides* erraticos. Antioquia Med. 7:144–157

Correa LL, Yamanaka MT, Correa M, Silfa M, Silva R, 1980. Ocorrencia de ovos grandes de *Trichuris trichiura* em fezes humanas. Rev. Inst. Adolfo Lutz Sao Paulo 40:59–64

Correa MOA, Hyakutake S, Brandi AJ, Monteiro CG, 1978. Novo caso de parasitismo humano por *Lagochilascaris minor* Leiper, 1909. Rev. Inst. Adolfo Lutz Sao Paulo 38:59–65

Coskun A, Ozcan N, Durak AC, Tolu I, Gulec M, Turan C, 1996. Intestinal ascariasis as a cause of bowel obstruction in two patients: sonographic diagnosis. J. Clin. Ultrasound 24:326–328

Crompton DWT, 1992. Ascariasis and childhood malnutrition. Trans. R. Soc. Trop. Med. Hyg. 86:577–579

Cunningham CK, Kazacos KR, McMillan JA, Lucas JA, McAuley JB, Wozniak EJ, Weiner LB, 1994. Diagnosis and management of *Baylisascaris procyonis* infection in an infant with nonfatal meningoencephalitis. Clin. Infect. Dis. 18:868–872

Dade AW, Williams JF, Trapp AL, Ball WH, 1977. Cerebral nematodiasis in captive nutria. JAVMA 171:885–886

de Andrade DR, Jr, Karam JA, Warth M do, de Merca AF, Jukemura J, Machado MC, Rocha AD, 1992. Massive infestation by *Ascaris lumbricoides* of the biliary tract: report of a successfully treated case. Rev. Inst. Med. Trop. Sao Paulo 34:71–75

de la Cruz Alvarez JR, Pineda Marino J, Sanchez Miguez J, Vilaplana JC, Dominguez Rodriguez F, Hermo Brion JA, Otero I, 1996. Ascariasis biliopancreatica: una entida infrecuente en nuestro medio. Gastroenterol. Hepatol. 19:210–212

Deardorff TL, Fukumura T, Raybourne RB, 1986. Invasive anisakiasis. A case report from Hawaii. Gastroenterology 90:1047–1050

Draper JW, 1963. Infection with *Lagochilascaris minor*. Br. Med. J. 1:931–932

Draper JW, Buckley JJC, 1963. *Lagochilascaris minor* (Leiper) from a patient in Tobago. Trans. R. Soc. Trop. Med. Hyg. 57:7

Fagan JJ, Prescott CA, 1993. Ascariasis and acute otitis media. Int. J. Pediatr. Otorhinolaryngol. 26:67–69

Faraj JH, 1993. Correspondence. Upper airway obstruction by *Ascaris* worm. Can. J Anaesth. 40:471

Faust EC, 1935. Experimental studies on human and primate species of *Strongyloides*: IV. The pathology of *Strongyloides* infection. Arch. Pathol. 19:769–806

Filice C, Marchi L, Meloni C, Patruno SF, Capellini R, Bruno R, 1995. Ultrasound in the diagnosis of gallbladder ascariasis. Abdom. Imaging 20:320–322

Fontes B, Utiyama EM, Morimoto RY, Pires PWA, Birolini D, de Oliveira MR, 1984. Ascariasis of the gallbladder: report of two cases and review of the literature. Int. Surg. 69:335–338

Formiga Ramos CC, de Olviera Ramos AM, de Carvalho ARL, 1980. Pseudotumorous form of ascariasis. Am. J. Trop. Med. Hyg. 29:795–798

Fox AS, Kazacos KR, Gould NS, Heydemann PT, Thomas C, Boyer KM, 1985. Fatal eosinophilic meningoencephalitis and visceral larva migrans caused by the raccoon ascarid *Baylisacaris procyonis*. N. Engl. J. Med. 312:1619–1623

Gass JDM, Braunstein RA, 1983. Further observations concerning the diffuse unilateral subacute neuroretinitis syndrome. Arch. Ophthalmol. 101:1689–1697

Gelpi AP, Mustafa A, 1967. Seasonal pneumonitis with eosinophilia. A study of larval ascariasis in Saudi Arabs. Am. J. Trop. Med. Hyg. 16:646–657

Gelpi AP, Mustafa A, 1968. *Ascaris* pneumonia. Am. J. Med. 44:377–389

Golz A, Merzbach D, Eliachar I, Joachims HE, 1982. Nasogastric tube obstruction by *Ascaris lumbricoides*. Ann. Trop. Med. Parasitol. 76:581–582

Hakami M, Kharrad M, Mosavy SH, 1976. Escape of ascarides through herniorrhaphy wounds. Am. J. Proctol. 27:47–48

Harada Y, 1962. Wakana disease and hookworm allergy. Yonago Acta Med. 6:109–118

Hayasaka H, Ishikura H, Takayama T, 1971. Acute regional ileitis due to *Anisakis* larvae. Int. Surg. 55:8–14

Hitchcock DJ, 1950. Parasitological study on the Eskimos in the Bethel area of Alaska. J. Parasitol. 36:232–234

Hock CC, 1959. *Ascaris* in the right lacrimal duct of a child. Proc. Alum. Assoc. Malaya 12:109–110

Holland CV, Asaolu SO, 1990. Ascariasis in Nigeria. Parasitol. Today 6:143–147

Hommeyer SC, Hamill GS, Johnson JA, 1995. CT diagnosis of intestinal ascariasis. Abdom. Imaging 20:315–316

Hsiu JG, Gamsey AJ, Ives CE, D'Amato NA, Hiller AN, 1986. Gastric anisakiasis: report of a case with clinical, endoscopic, and histological findings. Am. J. Gastroenterol. 81:1185–1187

Huff DS, Neafie RC, Binder MJ, De Leon GA, Brown LW, Kazacos KR, 1984. The first fatal *Baylisascaris* infection in man: an infant with eosinophilic meningo-encephalitis. Pediatr. Pathol. 2:345–352

Hulbert TV, Larsen RA, Chandrasoma PT, 1992. Abdominal angiostrongyliasis mimicking acute appendicitis and Meckel's diverticulum: report of a case in the United States and review. Clin. Infect. Dis. 14:836–840

Ihekwaba FN, 1979. *Ascaris lumbricoides* and perforation of the ileum: a critical review. Br. J. Surg. 66:132–134

Ishikura H, Hayasaka H, Kikuchi Y, 1967. Acute regional ileitis at Iwanai in Hokkaido with special reference to intestinal anisakiasis. Sapporo Med. J. 32:183–196

Ishikura H, Kikuchi K, 1990. *Intestinal Anisakiasis in Japan.* Tokyo: Springer-Verlag.

Ishikura H, Kikuchi K, Akao N, Doutei M, Yagi K, Takahashi S, Sato N, 1995. Parasitologic significance of the alteration of the causative Anisakidae worm and of the *Pseudoterranova decipiens* female immature adult worm, casting off the cuticles, and excreted from human in Kanazawa City. Hokkaido. [in Japanese English summary]. Igaku. Zasshi. 70:667–685

Ishikura H, Kikuchi K, Nagasawa K, Ooiwa T, Takamiya H, Sato N, Sugane K, 1992. Anisakidae and anisakidosis. Prog. Clin. Parasitol. 3:43–102

Ishikura H, Namiki M, 1989. *Gastric Anisakiasis in Japan. Epidemiology, Diagnosis, Treatment.* Tokyo: Springer-Verlag

Jacobson HA, Scanlon PF, Nettles VF, Davidson WR, 1976. Epizootiology of an outbreak of cerebrospinal nematodiasis in cottontail rabbits and woodchucks. J. Wildlife Dis. 12:357–360

Jenkins MQ, Beach MW, 1954. Intestinal obstruction due to ascariasis: report of thirty-one cases. Pediatrics 13:419–425

Joshi BN, Nair B, Gadgil RK, 1961. Roundworm induced abscess liver with secondary pericarditis. J.J.J. Group Hosp. Grant Med. Coll. 6:63–64

Juels CW, Butler W, Bier JW, Jackson GJ, 1975. Temporary human infection with *Phocanema* sp. larva. Am. J. Trop. Med. Hyg. 24:942–944

Kagei N, Isogaki H, 1992. A case of abdominal syndrome caused by the presence of a large number of *Anisakis* larvae. Int. J. Parasitol. 22:251–253

Kalejaiye EO, Solanke TF, Adekunle OO, Ogunbiyi O, 1977. Biliary lithiasis associated with ascariasis in a Nigerian woman. Arch. Surg. 112:645–647

Kanapumbi N, Lubeji K, 1996. Un ascaris dans les voies lacrymales. A propos d'un cas zairois. Sante 6:258–259

Kaplan CS, Freedman L, Elsdon-Dew R, 1956. A worm in the eye: a familiar parasite in an unusual situation. S. Afr. Med. J. 30:791–792

Kates S, Wright KA, Wright R, 1973. A case of human infection with the cod nematode *Phocanema* sp. Am. J. Trop. Med. Hyg. 22:606–608

Kazacos KR, Raymond LA, Kazacos EA, Vestre WR, 1985. The raccoon ascarid. A probable cause of human ocular larva migrans. Ophthalmology 92:1735–1744

Kazacos KR, Reed WM, Kazacos EA, Thacker HL, 1983. Fatal cerebrospinal disease caused by *Baylisascaris procyonis* in domestic rabbits. JAVMA 183:967–971

Kazacos KR, Vestre WA, Kazacos EA, 1984a. Raccoon ascarid larvae (*Baylisascaris procyonis*) as a cause of ocular larva migrans. Invest. Ophthalmol. Vis. Sci. 25:1177–1183

Kazacos KR, Vestre WA, Kazacos EA, Raymond LA, 1984b. Diffuse unilateral subacute neuroretinitis syndrome: probable cause. Arch. Ophthalmol. 102:967

Kendrick JF, 1934. The length of life and the rate of loss of the hookworms, *Ancylostoma duodenale* and *Necator americanus*. Am. J. Trop. Med. 363:379

Khuroo MS, Zargar SA, 1985. Biliary ascariasis: a common cause of biliary and pancreatic disease in an endemic area. Gastroenterology 88:418–423

Khuroo MS, Zargar SA, Mahajan R, 1990. Hepatobiliary and pancreatic ascariasis in India. Lancet 335:1503–1506

Khuroo MS, Zargar SA, Yattoo GN, Javid G, Dar MY, Boda MI, Khan BA, 1993. Worm extraction and biliary drainage in hepatobiliary and pancreatic ascariasis. Gastrointest. Endosc. 39:680–685

Kliks MM, 1983. Anisakiasis in the western United States: four new case reports from California. Am. J. Trop. Med. Hyg. 32:526–532

Kliks MM, 1986. Human anisakiasis: an update. JAMA 225:2605

Kobayashi A, Tsuji M, Wilbur DL, 1985. Probable pulmonary anisakiasis accompanying pleural effusion. Am. J. Trop. Med. Hyg. 34:310–313

Koino S, 1922. Experimental infection with *Ascaris* in human body with special reference to the clinical symptoms of *Ascaris* pneumonia. A preliminary report. Tokyo. Iji Shiushi 2299:197–1978. (Summary in Trop. Dis. Bull. 21:570, 1923.)

Kojima K, 1966. Histopathological findings of the *Anisakis*-like larva infection. Jpn. J. Parasitol. 15(Suppl):284–285

Lacaz C de S, Pettinati AH, Paula AB de, Souza DI, Zandin R, 1982. Granuloma solitario, por *Ascaris lumbricoides*, de localizacao intraperitoneal, simulando coccidioidomicose. Rev. Inst. Med. Trop. Sao Paulo 24:378–384

Larrubia JR, Ladero JM, Mendoza JL, Morillas JD, Diaz RM, 1996. The role of sonography in the early diagnosis of biliopancreatic *Ascaris* infestation. J. Clin. Gastroenterol. 22:48–50

Lavier G, Brumpt LC, 1944. L'evolution de l'eosinophilie au cours de l'ankylostomose. Sang 16:97–102

Leiper RT, 1909. A new nematode worm from Trinidad, *Lagochilascaris minor* sp. n. Oroc. Zool. Soc. London 4:35–36

Little MD, Halsey NA, Cline BL, Katz SP, 1983. *Ancylostoma* larva in a muscle fiber of man following cutaneous larva migrans. Am. J. Trop. Med. Hyg. 32:1285–1288

Little MD, Most H, 1973. Anisakid larva from the throat of a woman in New York. Am. J. Trop. Med. Hyg. 22:609–612

Loeffler W, 1956. Transient lung infiltrations with blood eosinophilia. Int. Arch. Allergy 8:54–59

Louw JH, 1974. Biliary ascariasis in childhood. S. Afr. J. Surg. 12:219–225

Martinez M, 1980. Parasitos animales de la region buconasofaringea. Rev. Assoc. Dental Mex. 37:340–369

Maxwell JD, Murray D, Ferguson A, Calder E, 1968. *Ascaris lumbricoides* infestation associated with jejunal mucosal abnormalities. Scot. Med. J. 13:280–281

Mello CM, Briggs MD, Venancio ES, Brandao AB, Queiroz FC, 1992. Granulomatous peritonitis by *Ascaris*. J. Pediatr. Surg. 27:1229–1230

Mimpriss TJ, 1972. Correspondence. Respiratory obstruction due to a round worm. Br. J. Anesth. 44:413

Mittal VK, Dhaliwal R, Yadav RVS, Sahariar S, 1976. Fatal respiratory obstruction due to round worm. Med. J. Aust. 2:210–212

Moraes MAP, Arnaud MVC, De Lima PE, 1983. Novos casos de infeccao humana por *Lagochilascaris minor* Leiper, 1909, encontrados no Estado do Para, Brasil. Rev. Inst. Med. Trop. Sao Paulo 25:139–146

Moraes MAP, Arnaud MVC, MacEdo RC de, Anglada AE, 1985. Infeccao pulmonar fatal por *Lagochilascaris* sp., provavelmente *Lagochilascaris minor* Leiper, 1909. Rev. Inst. Med. Trop. Sao Paulo 27:46–52

Moyes DG, Rogers MA, 1971. Respiratory obstruction due to a round worm. Case report. Br. J. Anesth. 43:1099

Mozgovoi AA, Shakhmatova VI, 1979. The life-cycle of the ascarid from badgers, *Baylisascaris melis* (Gedoelst, 1920) Sprent, 1968. Trudy Biol. Inst. Sibirskogo Otdeleniya Akad. Nauk. 38:104–113

Muhleisen JP, 1953. Demonstration of pulmonary migration of the causative organism of creeping eruption. Ann. Intern. Med. 38:595–600

Muraoka A, Suehiro I, Fujii M, Nagata K, Kusunoki H, Kumon Y, Shirasaka D, Hosooka T, Murakami K, 1996. Acute gastric anisakiasis: 28 cases during the last 10 years. Dig. Dis. Sci. 41:2362–2365

Naravane A, Lindo JF, Williams LA, Gardener MT, Fletcher CK, 1997. *Ascaris lumbricoides* in the paranasal sinuses of a Jamaican adult. Trans. R. Soc. Trop. Med. Hyg. 91:37

Ochola-Abila P, Barrack SM, 1982. Round worm intestinal obstruction in children at Kenyatta National Hospital, Nairobi. E. Afr. Med. J. 59:113–118

Odaibo SK, Awogun IA, 1988. Small intestinal perforation by *Ascaris lumbricoides*. Trans. R. Soc. Trop. Med. Hyg. 82:154

Olle Goig JE, Recacoechea M, Feeley T, 1996. First case of *Lagochilascaris minor* infection in Bolivia. Trop. Med. Int. Health 1:851–853

Oostburg BFJ, Varma AAO, 1968. *Lagochilascaris minor* infection in Surinam. Report of a case. Am. J. Trop. Med. Hyg. 17:548–550

Orihuela R, Botto C, Delgado O, Ortiz A, Suarez JA, Arguello C, 1987. *Lagochilascaris* humana en Venezuela: descripcion de un caso fatal: relatos de casos. Rev. Soc. Bras. Med. Trop. 20:217–221

Ortega R, 1992. Correspondence. An unusual cause of nasogastric tube obstruction. Anesth. Analg. 75:147–148

Oshima T, 1972. *Anisakis* and anisakiasis in Japan and adjacent area. In: Morishita K, Komiya Y, Matasubayashi H (eds), *Progress of Medical Parasitology in Japan*, Vol. 4. Tokyo: Meguro Parasitological Museum, pp. 301–393

Oshima T, 1987. Anisakiasis—is the sushi bar guilty? Parasitol. Today 3:44–48

Pamba HO, Musangi EM, 1978. Urogenital ascariasis. Case report. E. Afr. Med. J. 55:596–597

Pampiglione S, Ricciardi ML, 1972. Experimental infestation with human strain *Strongyloides fulleborni* in man. Lancet 1:663–665

Patz IM, 1959. Acute eosinophilic pneumonia possibly due to infection with *Ascaris lumbricoides*. Cent. Afr. J. Med. 5:399–404

Pawan JL, 1926. A case of infection with *Lagocheilascaris minor* (Leiper). Ann. Trop. Med. Parasitol. 20:201–202

Pawan JL, 1927. Another case of infection with *Lagocheilascaris minor* (Leiper). Ann. Trop. Med. Parasitol. 21:45–46

Perera J, 1993. Patent vitello-intestinal duct: an unusual presentation. Ceylon Med. J. 38:140–142

Phills JA, Harrold AJ, Whiteman GV, Perelmutter L, 1972. Pulmonary infiltrates, asthma and eosinophilia due to *Ascaris suum* infestation in man. N. Engl. J. Med. 286:965–970

Piggott J, Hansbarger EA Jr, Neafie RC, 1970. Human ascariasis. Am. J. Clin. Pathol. 53:223–234

Pinkus GS, Coolidge C, Little MD, 1975. Intestinal anisakiasis. First case report from North America. Am. J. Med. 59:114–120

Proffit RD, Walton MB, 1962. *Ascaris* pneumonia in a two year old girl. Diagnosis by gastric aspirate. N. Engl. J. Med. 266:931–934

Rausch RL, Scott EM, Rausch VR, 1967. Helminths in Eskimos in western Alaska, with particular reference to *Diphyllobothrium* infection and anaemia. Trans. R. Soc. Trop. Med. Hyg. 61:351–357

Rogers AM, Dammin GJ, 1946. Hookworm infection in American troops in Assam and Burma. Am. J. Med. Sci. 211:531–538

Rosemberg S, Lopez MBS, Mazuda Z, Campos R, Vieira Bressan MCR, 1986. Fatal encephalopathy due to *Lagochilascaris minor* infection. Am. J. Trop. Med. Hyg. 35:575–578

Rossi MA, Bisson FW, 1983. Fatal case of multiple liver abscesses caused by adult *Ascaris lumbricoides*. Am. J. Trop. Med. Hyg. 32:523–525

Sakanari JA, Loinaz HM, Deardorff TL, Raybourne RB, McKerrow JH, Frierson JG, 1988. Intestinal anisakiasis. A case diagnosed by morphologic and immunologic methods. Am. J. Clin. Pathol. 90:107–113

Santillan Doherty P, Juarez de la Cruz F, Guraieb Barragan E, Gallo Reynoso S, Rosa Laris C de I, 1986. Parasitosis de vias biliares: *Ascaris lumbricoides*. Rev. Invest. Clin. 38:297–302

Saul C, Pias VM, Jannke HA, Braga NHM, 1984. Endoscopic removal of *Ascaris lumbricoides* from the common bile duce. Am. J. Gastroenterol. 79:725–727

Schuster DI, Belin RP, Parker JC, Burke JA, Jona JZ, 1977. Ascariasis—its complications, unusual presentations and surgical approaches. South. Med. J. 70:176–178

Shah KN, Desai MP, 1969. *Ascaris lumbricoides* from the right ear. Indian Pediatr. 6:92–93

Shirahama M, Koga T, Ishibashi H, Uchida S, Ohta Y, Shimoda Y, 1992. Intestinal anisakiasis: US in diagnosis. Radiology 185:789–793

Shiraki T, 1974. Larval nematodes of family Anisakidae (Nematoda) in the Northern Sea of Japan—as a causative agent of eosinophilic phlegmone or granuloma in the human gastrointestinal tract. Acta Med. Biol. 22:57–98

Smedresman P, 1977. *Ascaris lumbricoides* as an unusual cause of appendicitis in an 8-year-old girl. Clin. Pediatr. 16:197

Smith JL, Bowman DD, Little MD, 1983. Life cycle and development of *Lagochilascaris sprenti* (Nematoda: Ascarididae) from opossums (Marsupialia: Didelphidae) in Louisiana. J. Parasitol. 69:736–745

Sohn WM, Seol SY, 1994. A human case of gastric anisakiasis by *Pseudoterranova decipiens* larva. Korean J. Parasitol. 32:53–56

Spillmann RK, 1975. Pulmonary ascariasis in tropical communities. Am. J. Trop. Med. Hyg. 24:791–800

Sprent JFA, 1971. Speciation and development in the genus *Lagochilascaris*. Semin. Respir. Infect. 62:71–112

Stephenson LS, 1980. The contribution of *Ascaris lumbricoides* to malnutrition in children. Semin. Respir. Infect. 81:221–233

Stephenson LS, Crompton DWT, Latham MC, Schulpen TWJ, Nesheim MC, Jansen AAJ, 1980. Relationships between *Ascaris* infections and growth of malnourished preschool children in Kenya. Am. J. Clin. Nutr. 33:1165–1172

Takata I, 1951. Experimental infection of man with *Ascaris* of man and the pig. Kitasato Arch. Exp. Med. 23:49–59

Tanaka H, Takata S, Nishimura T, Watanabe S, 1968. A case report of *Anisakis* larva penetration in the pharynxmucosa. Jpn. J. Parasitol. 17(Suppl):641

Tripathy K, Duque E, Bolanos O, Lotero H, Mayoral LG, 1972. Malabsorption syndrome in ascariasis. Am. J. Clin. Nutr. 25:1276–1281

Tripathy K, Gonzalez F, Lotero H, Bolanos O, 1971. Effects of *Ascaris* infection on human nutrition. Am. J. Trop. Med. Hyg. 20:212–218

Valdiserri RO, 1981. Intestinal anisakiasis. Report of a case and recovery of larvae from market fish. Am. J. Clin. Pathol. 76:329–334

Van Thiel PH, 1976. The present state of anisakiasis and its causative worms. Trop. Geogr. Med. 28:75–85

Van Thiel PH, Kuipers FC, Roskam RTh, 1960. A nematode parasitic to herring, causing acute abdominal syndromes in man. Trop. Geogr. Med. 12:97–113

Van Thiel PH, Van Houten H, 1967. The localization of the herringworm *Anisakis marina* in and outside the human gastrointestinal wall (with a description of the characteristics of its larval and juvenile stages). Trop. Geogr. Med. 19:56–62

Villamizar E, Mendez M, Bonilla E, Varon H, de Onatra S, 1996. *Ascaris lumbricoides* infestation as a cause of intestinal obstruction in children: experience with 87 cases. J. Pediatr. Surg. 31:201–204

Vogel H, Minning W, 1942. Beitrage zur klinik der lungenascariasis und Frage der fluchtigen eosinophilen Lungeninfiltrate. Beitr. Klin. Tuberkulose 98:624–654

Volcan GS, Ochoa FR, Medrano CE, Devalera Y, 1982. *Lagochilascaris minor* infection in Venezuela. Report of a case. Am. J. Trop. Med. Hyg. 31:1111–1113

Wilairatana P, Wilairatana S, Charoenlarp P, 1994. Gastric ascariasis associated with upper gastrointestinal hemorrhage. Southeast Asian J. Trop. Med. Public Health 25:401

Winslow DJ, Hankins JR, Steuer GZ, 1958. Granulomatous peritonitis due to *Ascaris* ova: report of a case simulating tuberculous peritonitis. Med. Ann. District Columbia 27:298–302

Wong MS, Bundy DA, Golden MH, 1991. The rate of ingestion of *Ascaris lumbricoides* and *Trichuris trichiura* eggs in soil and its relationship to infection in two children's homes in Jamaica. Trans. R. Soc. Trop. Med. Hyg. 85:89–91

Wright DO, Gold EM, 1945. Loeffler's syndrome associated with creeping eruption (cutaneous helminthiasis). JAMA 128:1082–1083

Yokogawa M, Yoshimura H, 1965. *Anisakis*-like larvae causing eosinophilic granulomata in the stomach of man. Am. J. Trop. Med. Hyg. 14:770–773

Yokogawa M, Yoshimura H, 1967. Clinicopathologic studies on larval anisakiasis in Japan. Am. J. Trop. Med. Hyg. 16:723–728

17

VISCERAL LARVA MIGRANS

Certain genera of the Ascaridoidea, Strongylina, and Spirudidea—for example, *Toxocara*, *Ancylostoma*, and *Gnathostoma*, respectively—have species with the ability to maintain a host–parasite relationship known as *paratenesis* (Beaver, 1969). Paratenesis occurs when the infective stages of the parasite (infective eggs of *Toxocara* or infective larvae of *Ancylostoma*) accidentally enter hosts other than their natural definitive hosts. In these nonnatural hosts, the larvae migrate through the tissues without undergoing development and eventually encapsulate, remaining indefinitely as infective larvae in the tissues. (Note that the differences between paratenic and intermediate hosts are that intermediate hosts are obligatory hosts in which the larvae change and grow into the infective stage for the definitive host. By contrast, paratenic hosts are not obligatory, and no transformation of the larvae occurs.) Migration of these larvae through the tissues produces an inflammatory reaction that results in the syndrome known as *visceral larva migrans*. However, the inflammation is always insufficient to destroy the larvae, which eventually encapsulate in the tissues (usually the muscles), remaining unchanged for the life of the paratenic host. By predation and cannibalism, a larva may pass through a series of paratenic hosts, but ingestion of the paratenic host by the natural definitive host of the larva in question results in completion of the larval life cycle. Humans behave as paratenic hosts for *Toxocara*, *Ancylostoma*, *Gnathostoma*, and other genera, and develop visceral larva migrans.

Under the concept of paratenesis outlined above, the species of nematodes producing visceral larva migrans in humans include *Toxocara canis* and *T. cati*. Some animal hookworms persist in tissues, such as *Ancylostoma braziliense* and *A. caninum* (see Chapter 13), the sparganum stage of species of *Spirometra* (see introduction to Part IV), and the mesocercaria stage of *Alaria* (see introduction to Part III). However, since the original name of the disease referred to children infected with *Toxocara*, the clinical meaning of visceral larva migrans in human medicine should be reserved for infections with *Toxocara*, such as those due to *T. canis* and *T. cati*.

Nonproducers of visceral larva migrans, sensu strictu, are certain parasites causing diseases that clinically resemble visceral larva migrans but in which the host–parasite relationship is not one of paratenesis. These parasites include *Capillaria hepatica*, which invades the viscera of humans but attains maturity as it does in its natural hosts (see Chapter 22); *Anisakis*, which develops somewhat but perishes sometime after its acquisition (see Chapter 16); and *Baylisascaris*, which develops to the infective stage in humans, behaving as it does in its natural intermediate hosts (see Chapter 16). Finally, there are other parasites that develop somewhat to advanced larval or juvenile adult stages without acquiring full maturity. In this chapter, the discussion of visceral larva migrans in humans is limited to the invasion and migration of *Toxocara* in the tissues; the other species are presented in other chapters. *Toxocara pteropodis* from bats was thought to produce visceral larva migrans in Palm Island, Australia (Moorhouse, 1982), but this theory was later disproved (Prociv et al. 1986). It should be emphasized that the biologic definition of visceral larva migrans used in this book does not preclude a wider definition by clinicians during their *workup of patients* with high peripheral eosinophilia and other clinical manifestations consistent with larva migrans. Once the true nature of the infection is established, the term *visceral larva migrans* should not be applied to infections other than those produced by species of *Toxocara*.

Toxocara canis and *T. cati* toxocariasis and Visceral Larva Migrans

The so-called roundworms of dogs and cats are well known by the general public because they occur commonly in these animals and because of the morbidity and mortality they produce. These roundworms have been assigned to the genus *Toxocara* of the family Ascarididae (see Chapter 16) on the basis of their morphologic characteristics. The infection they produce in dogs and cats, referred to as *toxocariasis*, involves the adult stages of the parasite. In humans *Toxocara* generally does not mature into adult worms in the intestine, remaining as larval stages in the tissues, and the infection produced is known as *visceral larva migrans*. Technically, the term *toxocariasis* should not apply to the human infection.

Geographic Distribution and Epidemiology. *Toxocara canis* of dogs and *T. cati* of cats are widely distributed throughout most regions of the world, parasitizing both domestic and wild canids and felids. Since both animals and humans acquire the infection by ingesting infective eggs in soil, *Toxocara* is another soil-transmitted helminth. The epidemiology of *Toxocara*

infections in humans resembles that of *Ascaris* and *Trichuris* in the sense that the infection is primarily found in infants and small children. Visceral larval migrans occurs in both tropical and subtropical countries, often in places where *Ascaris* is less prevalent or nonexistent. In the United States, the prevalence of *Toxocara* infection among children has been estimated to be approximately 5%. The main risk factors for infection in urban children are geophagia and having a litter of puppies at home (Marmor et al. 1987).

The prevalence of toxocariasis in animals has been widely studied, with surveys carried out in many places worldwide. The rates of prevalence are highly variable, depending not only on the true prevalence of the parasite, but also on the methodology used in the studies, the group of animals studied, the age of the animals, and other factors. A comprehensive review of the literature (Barriga, 1988) reveals a prevalence in the developed countries of between 4% and 50%; it is much higher in tropical developing countries, where rates of 80% have been recorded. The percentage of soil con-tamination (positive stools found on the ground) has also been studied and, as expected, it parallels the prevalence in animals (Barriga, 1988). Soil contamination studies based on positive stools have little relevance to the epidemiology of visceral larva migrans in humans because they do not reflect the amount of fecal contamination of the soil.

Seroepidemiologic studies in humans to determine the prevalence of specific antibodies to *Toxocara* have been carried out in many places. The results of these studies are also variable, depending mostly on the group of individuals tested, but in general, the prevalence of these antibodies is less than 5% in most places (range, 1% to 16%) (Barriga, 1988; Hermann et al. 1985). One feature of the epidemiology of visceral larva migrans observed in an area with extremely high seroprevalence is that the prevalence decreased with age. The seropositivity in two villages of Santa Lucia, the West Indies, peaked at 40% and 50% at about 10 years of age and steadily declined to 10% and 20%, respectively, at 45 years of age (Bundy et al. 1987). The same pattern was observed in Brazil, where the overall prevalence was less than 4% (Chieffi et al. 1990), and in Spain, where, in addition, higher seroprevalence was found among children living in cities than in those from rural areas (Conde Garcia et al. 1989). Contamination of soil with *Toxocara* eggs is also more common in urban than in rural communities (Mizgajska, 1997), probably because there are more dogs per square mile and less space for them to defecate.

Life Cycle and Biology. The biologic relationship between these nematodes and their natural hosts is rather complex, with several types of transmission (Fig. 17–1) that are outside the scope of this discussion. The natural definitive hosts acquire the infection by ingesting soil contaminated with the infective eggs. In *T. canis* the eggs hatch in the intestine, freeing the larvae, which migrate through the intestinal wall, liver, lungs, respiratory tree, esophagus, and intestine in a manner similar to that of *Ascaris* in humans. Once in the intestine, they develop into adults and produce eggs that are evacuated with the feces, to mature to infective stages in the environment (see Fig. 16–1 *A* and *C*).

In humans and in paratenic animal hosts, the ingested *T. canis* eggs hatch in the intestine. The larvae enter the intestinal wall, migrate to the liver and somehow "recognize" that their host is not their natural definitive host. They then arrest their development and migrate through the viscera until they eventually encapsulate in the muscles, retaining their infectivity for their final hosts. If a paratenic host is ingested by another abnormal host, the larvae repeat the process of tissue migration and encapsulation (Fig. 17–1 *B*). If the

paratenic host is ingested by the natural final host, the life cycle of the parasite is completed after it follows the normal migratory pathway, resulting in adult worms in the intestine.

Immunity. Little information about the immunology of visceral larva migrans in humans is available. Specific antibodies to *Toxocara* larvae are known to be elicited by the infection, and their titers are known to decrease slowly in patients followed for 5 years after their clinical disease (Fenoy et al. 1992). Similarly, antibody levels decrease slowly over time, as shown in seroepidemiologic studies (Bundy et al. 1987; Chieffi et al. 1990). Whether these antibodies are protective is not known. The bulk of the literature, dating back to 1958, deals with animal models and studies in classical immune reactions.

Clinical Findings. Visceral larva migrans is a disease of children, typically 1 to 4 years old (peak age, 2 years), who are brought to the physician because of pica, cough, wheezing, slight to moderate fever, and sometimes convulsions. The child becomes irritable, does not eat or sleep well, and fails to thrive. Noted on physical examination are moderate hepatomegaly and pulmonary rales or wheezes; chest radiograms often show infiltrates (Fig. 17–2 *A–B*). The disease occurs more often in boys than in girls and sometimes simultaneously in siblings or playmates of the child (Pena-Pereiro et al. 1978). (Before the infection was recognized, these cases were known as *benign eosinophilic leukemia, familial eosinophilia*, and so on.) The oldest known case of visceral larva migrans, diagnosed on sound clinical grounds, is that of a 7$^{1}/_{2}$-year-old hyperkinetic, mentally retarded, psychotic boy with a history of pica. Proven cases of visceral larva migrans in adults have never been reported, that is, the presence of the larva in tissues has never been demonstrated satisfactorily, and such cases are not expected to occur. This statement is made with full knowledge of the numerous cases in the literature of visceral larva migrans in adults, based on findings of peripheral eosinophilia and a positive serologic test for *Toxocara*. Probably a mentally retarded adult, with continuous access to contaminated soil, will someday become infected with *Toxocara* and develop symptoms of visceral larva migrans.

The most frequent laboratory finding is peripheral eosinophilia, which should be over 30% before the clinical diagnosis of visceral larval migrans is made (Snyder, 1961). Half of the patients have eosinophilia of over 50%, and in some cases it reaches 90% (Snyder,

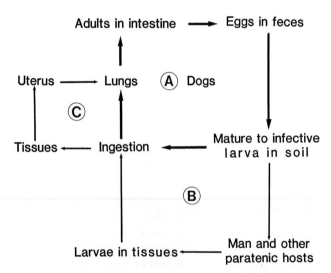

Fig. 17–1. *Toxocara* life cycle. (A) the usual cycle, using soil for maturation of eggs to the infective stage. Ingestion of infective eggs produces an intestinal infection with adult worms in the dog after pulmonary migration. (B) transmission of *Toxocara* through paratenic hosts. In mammals other than dogs, the ingested eggs contain larvae that remain in the tissues without further development. Ingestion of these hosts by dogs results in an infection with adult *Toxocara* in the intestine. In humans, the parasite acquired in this manner produces visceral larva migrans. (C) Another form of transmission from the bitch to its offspring.

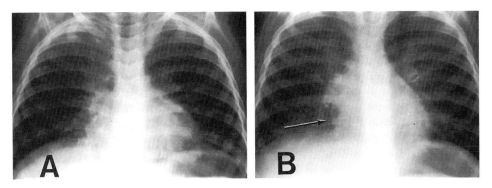

Fig. 17–2. *Toxocara.* **Pulmonary infiltrates in visceral larval migrans.** *A,* **Moderate hilar infiltrate.** *B,* **Two weeks later, the infiltrate has resolved almost completely. Note the now visible right heart border (arrow).**

1961). The white blood cell count is 20,000 to 60,000 per cubic millimeter in 55% of cases, and a few patients may have counts of up to 150,000 per cubic millimeter (Fig. 17–3 *C–D*; Huntley et al. 1965). Anemia is present in most children. Serum gammaglobulin levels are elevated, especially IgG, and anti-A and anti-B isohemagglutinin titers are increased. The enzyme-linked immunosorbent assay is positive, but this test is not necessary for the clinical diagnosis, which can be based on the above findings alone.

The disease is self-limited. In patients who were observed before the parasitic nature of the disease was known and who did not received treatment for such disease, the eosinophilia steadily decreased and became normal 6 to 8 months later. Similar observations have been made in asymptomatic children (who had only high peripheral eosinophilia and positive serology) who were followed for up to 1 year. On the enzyme-linked immunosorbent assay, the titers also fell steadily, paralleling the fall of the eosinophil level (Bass et al. 1987). The main organs involved in visceral larva migrans will now be discussed.

Heart. Involvement of the heart is variable and is usually not apparent clinically, although patients with myocarditis and congestive heart failure requiring hospitalization have been described (Vargo et al. 1977). Electrocardiographic abnormalities and cardiomegaly are common (Friedman, Hervada, 1960). Less frequent findings are gallop rhythm, low-voltage QRS, and T waves accompanying a dilated and poorly contracting ventricle (Vargo et al. 1977).

Lungs. Probably one-third to one-half of the children with visceral larva migrans have pulmonary symptoms (Beaver, 1962; Snyder, 1961) varying from mild to life-threatening; in at least one patient, severe granuloma-

tous involvement of the lungs was fatal (Brill et al. 1953). The usual clinical symptom is a chronic cough lasting for 3 weeks or more, sometimes paroxysmal and associated with recurrent wheezing; in one series, a few children required hospitalization because of their respiratory distress (Huntley et al. 1965). The chest x-ray films may show bilateral peribronchial infiltrations or patchy infiltration of the perihilar areas (Fig. 17–2 *A–B*; Beshear, Hendley, 1973).

Brain. Often the symptom of central nervous system visceral larva migrans is convulsions (Huntley et al. 1965); on several occasions, this disease produced a fatal encephalopathy (Beautyman et al. 1966; Fortenberry et al. 1991; Mikhael et al. 1974; Schochet, 1967). A case of hemiplegia was probably, in retrospect, an infection with *Baylisascaris* (Anderson et al. 1975), and a case of encephalopathy attributed to *Toxocara* was *Calodium* (= *Capillaria*) *hepaticum* infection (Sumner, Tinsley, 1967; see Chapter 22).

Eye. Ocular visceral larva migrans occurs at any age, but the group more often affected is older children, with an average age of 7.5 years at presentation. The disease is more predominant in boys. The main complaints are unilateral strabismus and failing vision. A few children may have a previous history of visceral larva migrans, but rarely do the ocular symptoms parallel the visceral disease; peripheral eosinophil levels are rarely elevated. The three main presentations of ocular *Toxocara* visceral larva migrans are chronic endophthalmitis with retinal detachment (Fig. 17–8 *B*), posterior pole granuloma (Fig. 17–8 *A*), and peripheral granuloma. Less common manifestations are vitreous abscess, pars planitis, optic neuritis, keratitis (especially caused by hookworm larvae; see Chapter 14), uveitis, and hypopyon (Brown, 1970; Molk, 1983). In some

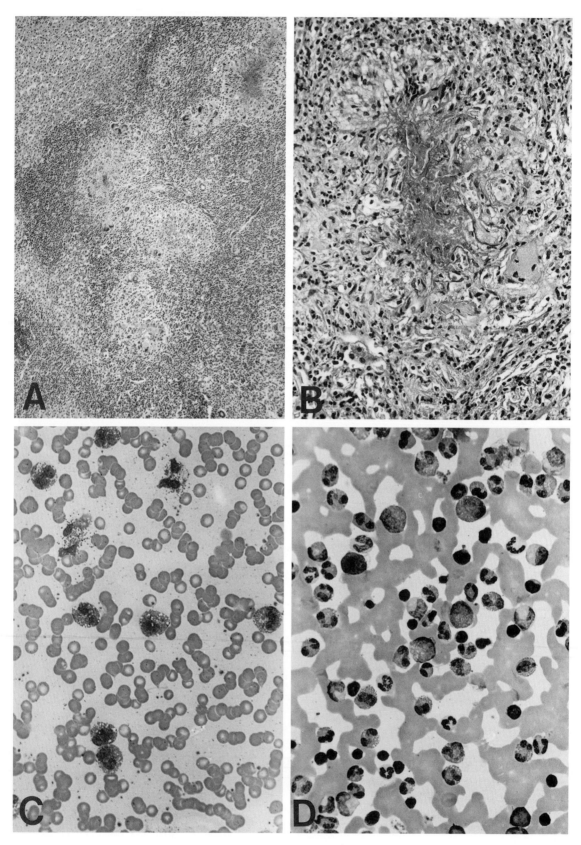

Fig. 17–3. *Toxocara*. Pathologic abnormalities usually associated with visceral larva migrans. *A* and *B*. Liver biopsy specimen, sections stained with hematoxylin and eosin stain. *A*, Low-power view showing numerous granulomas in different stages of evolution, ×55. *B*, Higher magnification showing one granuloma. The presence of granulomas without a larva is the most common finding, ×220. *C* and *D*, Peripheral blood smear and bone marrow stained with Wright stain. Note the marked eosinophilia, ×450.

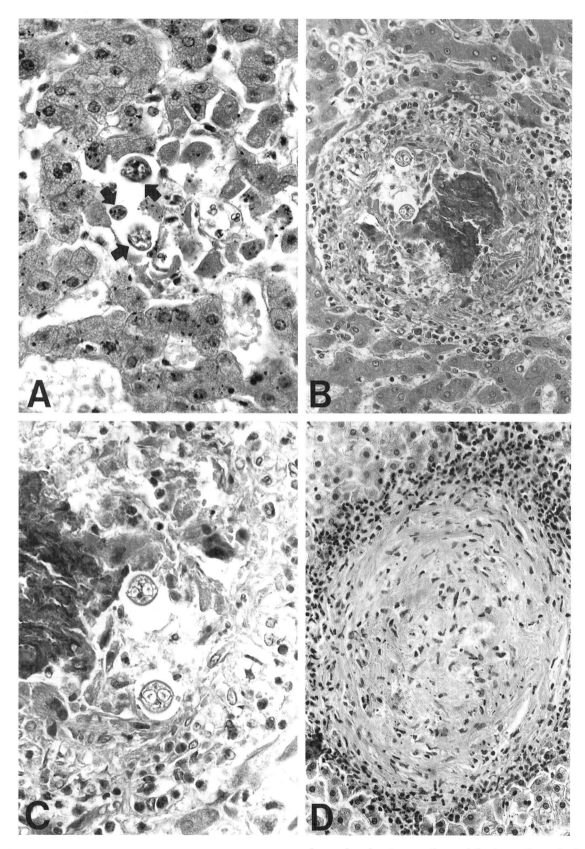

Fig. 17–4. *Toxocara* in liver, sections stained with hematoxylin and eosin stain. *A*, Section of a larva in the liver, with no inflammatory reaction, indicating that the parasite is moving through the tissues. There are three sections of the larva (arrows), ×440. *B*, Well-formed granuloma showing two sections of the larva through the midbody, ×220. *C*, Higher magnification showing the morphology of the parasite on cross section (compare this with line drawing No. 8 of Figure 17–9), ×450. *D*, Mature, mostly collagenized granuloma without a larva, ×220.

cases a nematode larva, sometimes motile, has been observed in the retina (Parsons, 1952; Rubin et al. 1968), the vitreus, the iris (Baldone et al. 1964), or the cornea (Baldone et al. 1964) during the eye examination, resulting in a clinical diagnosis of *Toxocara* without a solid basis. The tracks of the migrating larva have also been observed in the retina, progressing slowly over several months, with periods of activity and quiescence (*color plate* VII *G–H*; Sorr, 1984).

Before the recognition of nematode endophthalmitis in 1950 (Wilder, 1950), lesions produced by *Toxocara* in the eye, especially those seen as a mass, were invariably diagnosed as retinoblastomas, and the eye was enucleated. The pathologist's finding of inflammatory tissue or a granuloma usually resulted in a diagnosis of pseudoglioma (Kogan, Boniuk, 1962). Enucleation of eyes due to *Toxocara* has greatly decreased, but even today, the clinical diagnosis of retinoblastoma is incorrect in over 55% of the cases, 26% of which are due to *Toxocara* infection (Shields, 1984).

Pathology. The main changes observed in visceral larva migrans are seen in the liver, where the largest concentration of larvae occurs during the active infection, but almost any other organ system may be affected. Grossly, the liver is slightly increased in size and appears mottled, with white plaques randomly distributed over the surface and, on section, throughout the entire parenchyma. These plaques are 0.5 to 3.0 mm in diameter, and on close inspection they have irregular borders. The consistency of the liver is usually soft. The gross appearance of other organs is unremarkable, although sometimes the heart appears soft, with evidence of myocarditis, and patients with central nervous system involvement may have small areas of necrosis in the brain. In a child with visceral larva migrans who died of serum hepatitis, the number of larvae was estimated by digestion of the tissues in artificial gastric juice. There were 60 larvae per gram of liver tissue, 5 larvae per gram of skeletal muscle, and 3 to 5 larvae per gram of brain (Dent et al. 1956).

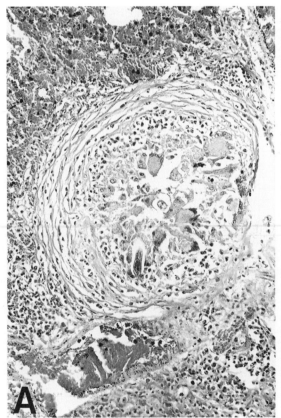
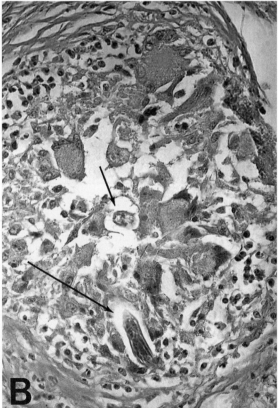

Fig. 17–5. *Toxocara* in the lung, sections stained with hematoxylin and eosin stain. *A*, Low-power view of a granuloma, ×140. *B*, Higher magnification with one oblique section (short arrow) and one longitudinal section (long arrow) of a larva, ×280.

The basic microscopic lesion in most organs is a granulomatous inflammation (Fig. 17–3 *A–B*). In the liver, these granulomas correspond to the white plaques observed grossly. Serial section reconstruction shows that they are tortuous, irregular track lesions filled with necrotic material produced by the migration of a larva (Beaver et al. 1952).

The earliest lesion seen in the liver is minimal disruption of the parenchyma accompanied by a few inflammatory cells and a larva (Fig. 17–5 *A*). This lesion progresses to more advanced cellular necrosis with infiltration by polymorphonuclear cells, mainly eosinophils, histiocytes, and lymphocytes (Fig. 17–4 *B–C*). The granuloma becomes well formed, with multinucleated foreign body giant cells, epithelioid cells, and mononuclear and polymorphonuclear cell infiltrates (Figs. 17–3 *B* and 17–4 *B–C*). In these granulomas the larva is usually viable and appears to be in command of the lesion (Fig. 16–5 *B–C*). The larva may leave the granuloma and relocate in an-

other part of the liver or later in a different tissue, where it apparently becomes encapsulated and dormant, possibly remaining so for the life of the host. Granulomas without the parasite (Fig. 17–4 *D*) resolve, with complete healing; no residual *Toxocara* lesions in the liver or other organs have been observed.

In other organs, the histologic appearance of *Toxocara* infection is similar to that described in the liver. In the lungs, granulomas with and without larvae are found (Fig. 17–5 *A–B*), sometimes in abundance, producing a histologic picture of allergic granulomatosis, with numerous eosinophils throughout the parenchyma (Brill et al. 1953). In the brain the parasites do not encapsulate readily. Usually only tracks are found. The tracks are seen as small areas of tissue necrosis and a few infiltrating cells, both polymorphonuclear eosinophils and lymphocytes. These lesions have been studied in children dying of encephalopathy, in whom the larvae were identified only after numerous sections were examined (Beautyman

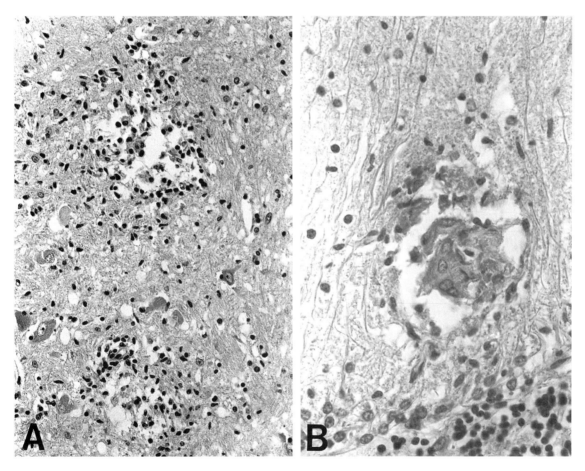

Fig. 17–6. *Toxocara* **lesions in the brain of an experimentally infected baboon, sections stained with hematoxylin and eosin stain.** *A* **and** *B*, **Different magnification** of tracks made by the migrating larva, ×220 and ×450, respectively.

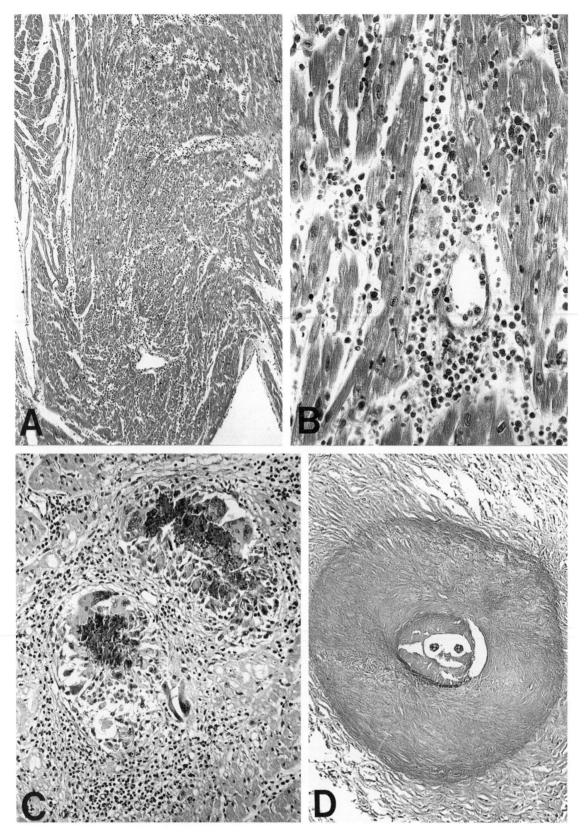

Fig. 17–7. *Toxocara* in the heart, sections stained with hematoxylin and eosin stain. *A*, Low-power view showing a focus of myocarditis, ×55. *B*, Higher magnification illustrating the infiltrate, composed of mononuclear cells and eosinophils, ×280. *C*, Two granulomas without larvae, ×180. (Preparation courtesy of M.J. Finegold, M.D., Department of Pathology, Baylor College of Medicine, Texas Children's Hospital, Houston, Texas. Reported by: Vargo, T.A., Singer, D.B., Gillette, P.C., et al. 1977. Correspondence. Myocarditis due to visceral larva migrans. J. Pediatr. 90:322–323.) *D*, Encapsulated larva in pericardium, ×125. (Courtesy of P.C. Beaver, School of Public Health and Tropical Medicine, Tulane University, New Orleans, Louisiana. In: Correa, P., Gonzales-Mugaburu, L., and D'Alessandro, A. 1966. Primer caso Colombiano de toxocarosis. Antioquia Med. 16:487–497. Reproduced with permission.)

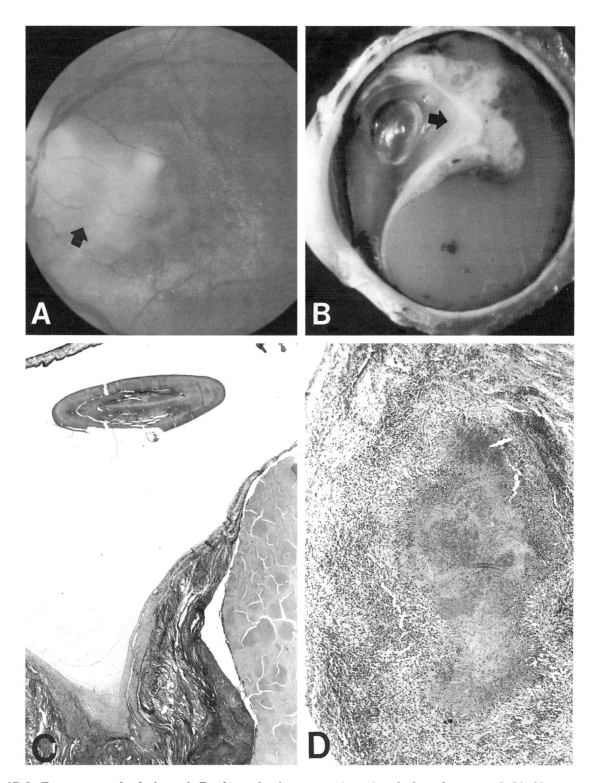

Fig. 17–8. *Toxocara*, ocular lesions. *A*, Fundoscopic picture of ocular toxocariasis. Note the large granuloma represented by the white area (arrow). *B*, Section through the midportion of an enucleated eye from a patient with *Toxocara* infection. The clinical diagnosis was malignancy. Note the fibrous tissue mass, seen as a white and light gray area (arrow) and a large hematoma behind it, represented by the dark gray area. *C* and *D*. Sections stained with hematoxylin and eosin stain. *C*, Low-power view showing the lens (top), granulation tissue (bottom), and part of the hematoma (right), ×9. *D*, Higher magnification of the granuloma. No larva is seen in this section, ×55.

411

et al. 1966; Mikhael et al. 1974), as well as in experimental animals (Fig. 17–6 A–B). In all cases in which tracks or granulomas without larvae are found in the tissues, the specific diagnosis of toxocariasis is not warranted unless the larva has been found in other tissues.

In the heart the parasite rarely encapsulates, but in one case encapsulation occurred in the pericardium (Fig. 16–7 D) (Correa et al. 1966). However, granulomas without parasites and myocarditis in children with visceral larva migrans and cardiac symptoms have been described. The myocarditis is usually focal (Fig. 17–7 A–B), with marked edema and infiltration by mononuclear cells and eosinophils. In some areas, granulomas, sometimes well formed and containing multinucleated foreign body giant cells, are observed. In one report, granulomas found in biopsy specimens of the heart taken during cardiac surgery in small children were at-

tributed to *Toxocara* even though the larvae were not found (Dao, Virmani, 1986). The cause of the granulomas in these cases should remain open.

In the eye, one larva is usually present, producing an inflammatory reaction (Fig. 17–8 B–D) that, depending on its location and intensity, results in the different clinical pictures described above. The larva usually enters the eye via the retinal circulation, producing the more common chronic endophthalmitis with retinal detachment or granuloma in the posterior pole. Uveitis is seen in 10% of patients with ocular *Toxocara* infection (Perkins, 1966), and in one case, the larva produced optic neuritis (Bird et al. 1970). The larva has not been recovered in toto and identified due to its small size. In one case, pars plana vitrectomy was done to relieve the inflammation. The material that was collected showed the larva in the Millipore filter used to

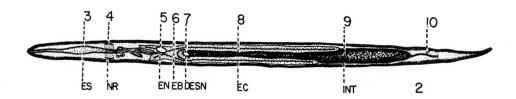

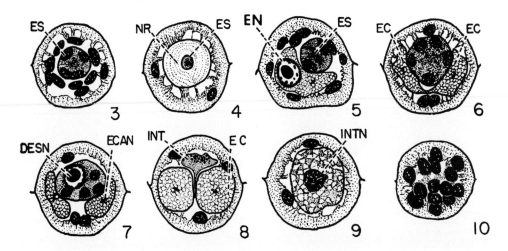

Fig. 17–9. *Toxocara canis* microanatomy in cross sections, as found in paratenic hosts. The diagram shows anatomy at different levels; all drawings were made with a camera lucida. Abbreviations: es, esophagus; nr, nerve ring; en, excretory nucleus; eb, esophageal bulb; ec, excretory columns; desn, nucleus of dorsal esophageal gland; int, intestine; intn, nucleus of intestinal cell. (In: Nichols, R.L. 1956. The etiology of visceral larva migrans. I. Diagnostic morphology of infective second-stage *Toxocara* larvae. J. Parasitol. 42:349–362. Reproduced with permission.)

concentrate the removed inflamed vitreus (Maguire et al. 1990).

Diagnosis. The diagnosis of visceral larva migrans is usually based on the patient's clinical presentation; several serologic tests have been used and improved, becoming more reliable. The enzyme-linked immunosorbent assay is presently the best test, but positive serology does not confirm the diagnosis of toxocariasis. Needle biopsy of the liver is not recommended because the probability of recovering a larva is low, and open liver biopsy for the sole purpose of confirming the diagnosis generally is not justified. Elevated isoagglutinin titers (anti-A and anti-B), especially anti-A, suggest *Toxocara* infection.

If tissues are available and parasites are present, they are identified on the basis of features evident in cross sections through the midgut (Fig. 17–4 C); oblique and longitudinal sections rarely permit specific identification of the larva. In tissue sections, the diameter of *T. canis* varies from 18 to 20 μm and that of *T. cati* from 14 to 16 μm. The length of both larvae is 290 to 350 μm. The larvae have small lateral alae that appear in most cross sections of the body, except at the most anterior and posterior parts. The cuticle is better seen on transverse sections at the level of the lateral alae; the muscles appear as an irregular layer below the cuticle. The excretory columns are evident and appear as two large, rounded structures (Fig. 17–9; Nichols, 1956b). It is possible to distinguish morphologically between *T. canis* and other larvae potentially found in humans (Nichols, 1956a).

References

Anderson DC, Greenwood R, Fishman M, Kagan IG, 1975. Acute infantile hemiplegia with cerebrospinal fluid eosinophilic pleocytosis: an unusual case of visceral larva migrans. J. Pediatr. 86:247–249

Baldone JA, Clark WB, Jung RC, 1964. Nematode ophthalmitis: report of two cases. Am. J. Ophthalmol. 57:763–766

Barriga OO, 1988. A critical look at the importance, prevalence and control of toxocariasis and the possibilities of immunological control. Vet. Parasitol. 29:195–234

Bass JL, Mehta KA, Glickman LT, Blocker R, Eppes BM, 1987. Asymptomatic toxocariasis in children. Clin. Pediatr. 26:441–446

Beautyman W, Beaver PC, Buckley JJC, Woolf AL, 1966. Review of a case previously reported as showing an ascarid larva in the brain. J. Pathol. Bacteriol. 91:271–273

Beaver PC, 1962. Toxocarosis (visceral larva migrans) in relation to tropical eosinophilia. Bull. Soc. Pathol. Exot. 55:555–576

Beaver PC, 1969. The nature of visceral larva migrans. J. Parasitol. 55:3–12

Beaver PC, Snyder CH, Carrera GM, Dent JH, Lafferty JW, 1952. Chronic eosinophilia due to visceral larva migrans. Report of three cases. Pediatrics 9:7–19

Beshear JR, Hendley JO, 1973. Severe pulmonary involvement in visceral larva migrans. Am. J. Dis. Child. 125:599–600

Bird AC, Smith JL, Curtin VT, 1970. Nematode optic neuritis. Am. J. Ophthalmol. 69:72–77

Brill R, Churg J, Beaver PC, 1953. Allergic granulomatosis associated with visceral larva migrans. Case report with autopsy findings of *Toxocara* infection in a child. Am. J. Clin. Pathol. 23:1208–1215

Brown DH, 1970. Ocular *Toxocara canis*. Part II. Clinical review. J. Pediatr. Ophthalmol. 7:182–191

Bundy DAP, Thompson DE, Robertson BD, Cooper ES, 1987. Age-relationships of *Toxocara canis* seropositivity and geohelminth infection prevalence in two communities in St. Lucia, West Indies. Trop. Med. Parasitol. 38:309–312

Chieffi PP, Ueda M, Camargo ED, de Souza AM, Guedes ML, Gerbi LJ, Spir M, Moreira AS, 1990. Visceral larva migrans: a seroepidemiological survey in five municipalities of Sao Paulo state, Brazil. Rev. Inst. Med. Trop. Sao Paulo 32:204–210

Conde Garcia L, Muro Alvarez A, Simon Martin F, 1989. Epidemiological studies on toxocariasis and visceral larva migrans in a zone of western Spain. Ann. Trop. Med. Parasitol. 83:615–620

Correa P, Gonzalez-Mugaburu L, D'Alessandro A, 1966. Primer caso Colombiano de toxocarosis. Breve actualizacion del sindrome de larva migratoria visceral. Antioquia Med. 16:489–497

Dao AH, Virmani R, 1986. Visceral larva migrans involving the myocardium: report of two cases and review of the literature. Pediatr. Pathol. 6:449–456

Dent JH, Nichols RL, Beaver PC, Carrera GM, Staggers RJ, 1956. Visceral larva migrans with a case report. Am. J. Pathol. 32:777–803

Fenoy S, Cuellar C, Aguila C, Guillen JL, 1992. Persistence of immune response in human toxocariasis as measured by ELISA. Int. J. Parasitol. 22:1037–1038

Fortenberry JD, Kenney RD, Younger J, 1991. Visceral larva migrans producing static encephalopathy in an infant. Pediatr. Infect. Dis. J. 10:403–406

Friedman S, Hervada AR, 1960. Severe myocarditis with recovery in a child with visceral larva migrans. J. Pediatr. 56:91–96

Hermann N, Glickman NT, Schantz PM, Weston MG, Domanski LM, 1985. Seroprevalence of zoonotic toxocariasis in the United States: 1971–1973. Am. J. Epidemiol. 122:890–896

Huntley CC, Costas MC, Lyerly AD, 1965. Visceral larva migrans syndrome: clinical characteristics and immunologic studies in 51 patients. Pediatrics 36:523–536

Kogan L, Boniuk M, 1962. Causes for enucleation in childhood with special reference to pseudogliomas and unsuspected retinoblastomas. Int. Ophthalmol. Clin. 2: 507–524

Maguire AM, Green WR, Michels RG, Erozan YS, 1990. Recovery of intraocular *Toxocara canis* by pars plana vitrectomy. Ophthalmology 97:675–680

Marmor M, Glickman L, Shofer F, Faich LA, Rosemberg C, Cornblatt B, Friedman S, 1987. *Toxocara canis* infection of children: epidemiologic and neuropsychologic findings. Am. J. Public Health 77:554–559

Mikhael NZ, Montpetit VJA, Orizaga M, Rowsell HC, Richard MT, 1974. *Toxocara canis* infestation with encephalitis. Can. J. Neurol. Sci. 1:114–120

Mizgajska H, 1997. The role of some environmental factors in the contamination of soil with *Toxocara* spp. and other geohelminth eggs. Parasitol. Int. 46:67–72

Molk R, 1983. Ocular toxocariasis: a review of the literature. Ann. Ophthalmol. 15:216–231

Moorhouse DE, 1982. Toxocariasis. A possible cause of the Palm Island mystery. Med. J. Aust. 1:172–173

Nichols RL, 1956a. Etiology of visceral migrans. II. Comparative larval morphology of *Ascaris lumbricoides, Necator americanus, Strongyloides stercoralis,* and *Ancylostoma caninum*. J. Parasitol. 42:363–399

Nichols RL, 1956b. The etiology of visceral larva migrans. I. Diagnostic morphology of infective second-stage *Toxocara* larvae. J. Parasitol. 42:349–362

Parsons HE, 1952. Nematode chorioretinitis. Report of a case, with photographs of a viable worm. Arch. Ophthalmol. 47:799–800

Pena-Pereiro A, Ramos-Garcia A, Sanchez-Miranda JM, 1978. Larva migrans visceral. Rev. Cubana Med. Trop. 30:59–67

Perkins ES, 1966. Pattern of uveitis in children. Br. J. Ophthalmol. 50:169–185

Prociv P, Moorhouse DE, Wah MJ, 1986. Toxocariasis—an unlikely cause of Palm Island disease. Med. J. Aust. 145:14–15

Rubin ML, Kaufman HE, Tierney JP, Lucas HC, 1968. An intraretinal nematode. (A case report). Trans. Am. Acad. Ophthalmol. Otolaryngol. 72:855–866

Schochet SS, 1967. Human *Toxocara canis* encephalopathy in a case of visceral larva migrans. Neurology 17:227–229

Shields JA, 1984. Ocular toxocariasis. A review. Surv. Ophthalmol. 28:361–381

Snyder CH, 1961. Visceral larva migrans. Ten years' experience. Pediatrics 28:85–91

Sorr EM, 1984. Meandering ocular toxocariasis. Retina 4:9096

Sumner D, Tinsley EGF, 1967. Encephalopathy due to visceral larva migrans. J. Neurol. Neurosurg. Psychiatry 30:580–584

Vargo TA, Singer DB, Gillette PC, Fernbach DJ, 1977. Correspondence. Myocarditis due to visceral larva migrans. J. Pediatr. 90:322–323

Wilder HC, 1950. Nematode endophthalmitis. Trans. Am. Acad. Ophthalmol. Otolaryngol. 55:99–109

18

SPIRURIDA—*DRACUNCULUS, GNATHOSTOMA,* AND OTHERS

The order Spirurida comprises one of the largest groups of nematodes. These worms are characterized biologically by requiring one or more intermediate hosts in their life cycles and morphologically by having a cephalic end with bilateral, symmetric structures and an esophagus divided into two portions, the anterior muscular and the posterior glandular. The members of the order Spirurida occur in the gastrointestinal tract and other tissues; those important in human medicine belong to the following superfamilies (Beaver et al. 1984):

Order: Spirurida
  Superfamily: Dracunculoidea
    Genera: *Dracunculus* and *Phylometra*
  Superfamily: Gnathostomatoidea
    Genera: *Gnathostoma* and *Physaloptera*
  Superfamily: Rictularioidea
    Genus: *Rictularia*
  Superfamily: Thelazoidea
    Genus: *Thelazia*
  Superfamily: Spiruroidea
    Genera: *Gongylonema* and *Spirocerca*

  Superfamily: Acuarioidea
    Genus: *Cheilospirura*
  Superfamily: Filarioidea (see Chapters 19–21)

In this chapter, some species of the first five superfamilies are discussed; those of the superfamily Filarioidea will be discussed in Chapters 19–21 because of the large number of species and their importance in human medicine.

Dracunculus medinensis— Dracunculiasis or Guinea Worm Infection

The superfamily Dracunculoidea includes genera and species that usually inhabit the tissues of animals and humans. Two of its genera have species that occur in humans: *Dracunculus medinensis*, which is by far the most important, and a species of *Phylometra*, found once in an open lesion of the hand (Deaedorff et al. 1986).

Morphology and Life Cycle. *Dracunculus medinensis* has a marked sexual dimorphism. The females are very long, 70 to 120 cm long by 0.7 to 1.7 mm wide. The males are very small and have not been completely studied; they are reported to be 4 cm or less in length.

The life cycle of *Dracunculus* is similar to that of other spiruriids (Fig. 18–1). The adult female lives in the subcutaneous tissues, usually those of the lower extremities. When gravid, the female produces an ulceration of the skin through which larvae are freed to enter fresh water; the larvae are ingested by small crustaceans, mostly of the genus *Cyclops*, where they develop and become infective. Human infections are acquired by drinking water with *Cyclops* containing infective larvae. Once in the intestine, the larvae become free and migrate through the intestinal wall to reach the connective tissues of the retroperitoneum. In the retroperitoneum, the larvae become young worms that migrate to the subcutaneous tissues and complete their development in about 1 year (Beaver et al. 1984).

Geographic Distribution and Epidemiology. Dracunculiasis is an infection that has been energetically targeted for eradication, and both its geographic distribution and its prevalence are changing rapidly (Hopkins et al. 1997; Peries, Cairncross, 1997). The infection occurred mainly in the tropics and subtropics. Africa is the main area of endemicity, in a region extending from the west to the east coast, limited on the north by the Sahara and on the south by the equatorial line. In this region there were areas of high endemicity interspersed with areas of low endemicity and still other areas with only sporadic cases (Hopkins et al. 1997). In 1987 the number of cases in Africa was estimated to be about 3.32 million (Watts, 1987). In addition, the Middle East, Saudi Arabia, Iran, Afghanistan, Pakistan, and the southern countries of the former Soviet Union had foci of endemicity. India

also had extensive areas of endemicity, and cases had been reported from Indonesia, probably imported from India. Sporadic cases of guinea worm in humans have also been reported from China, South Korea, and Japan (Kobayashi et al. 1986). Imported cases have rarely been found in the United States (CDC, 1998). However, the endemic areas of dracunculiasis are decreasing rapidly due to the control programs undertaken by many countries under the auspices of the World Health Organization. The target date for total eradication was 1995, but war in some countries and lack of funds in others delayed the program (Hopkins et al. 1993; Hopkins, Ruiz-Tiben, 1990; Muller, 1992). The infection is linked to poor drinking water supplies, providing the opportunity to interrupt the cycle in humans relatively easily. In some places transmission of the infection is seasonal, peaking during periods of below-average rainfall, when *Cyclops* reaches its highest concentration in ponds and wells (Belcher et al. 1975). *Dracunculus insignis* is commonly found in raccoons, minks, and other wild animals from Louisiana to Canada, and *D. lutrae* is found in otters in Canada. *Dracunculus insignis* is morphologically indistinguishable from *D. medinensis*, but whether it is a different species has not been completely established (Beverley Burton, Crichton, 1976).

Clinical Findings. The symptoms of dracunculiasis vary with the acute or chronic phase of the infection. Migration of the larvae to the retroperitoneum and later to the subcutaneous tissues produces no symptoms. The first symptoms appear about 1 year after the ingestion of infective larvae, when the worms are located in the subcutaneous tissues, and coincide with the need of the gravid female to discharge the larvae into water.

The final location of the parasite in 85% of cases is the lower extremities (Fig. 18–2 *A–B*), often the ankle or between the metatarsal bones, but almost any other place in the body is suitable for the worm (Roussel, 1987). When the gravid female needs to discharge the larvae, it moves the anterior portion of its body from below the subcutaneous tissues toward the skin and produces a local inflammatory reaction. Local signs in the area are induration and redness, preceded by slight fever and urticaria and followed by the formation of a small blister that produces intense irritation and a burning sensation. The patient has an extreme urge to immerse the affected area in water, rapidly breaking the blister. The skin break results in an ulcer through which a few centimeters of the anterior body of the female protrude (Fairley, 1924). Soon afterward, a loop of the uterus breaks through the body wall of the worm to discharge hundreds of larvae into the water. Swelling, inflamma-

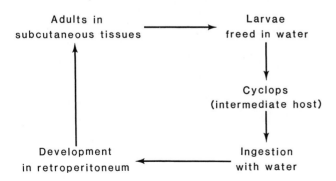

Fig. 18–1. *Dracunculus medinensis*, schematic representation of the life cycle.

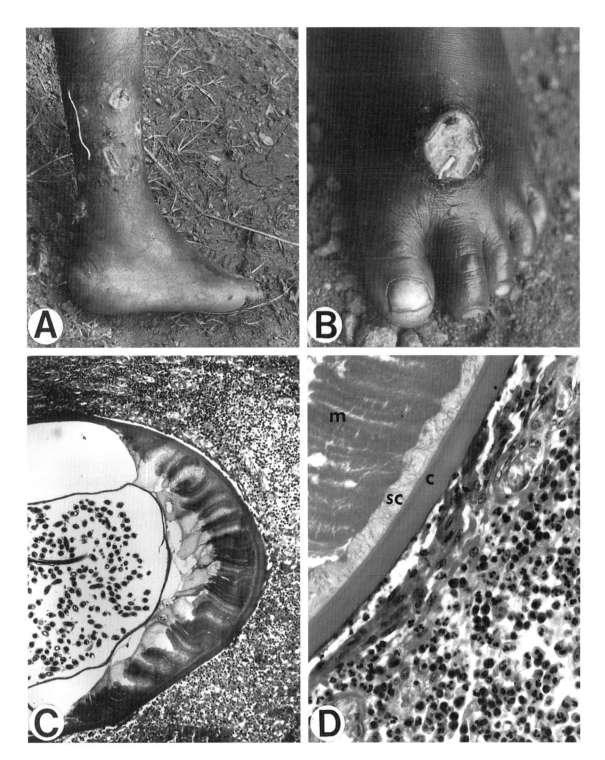

Fig. 18–2. *Dracunculus medinensis*. *A* and *B*, Lesions in feet of two individuals from Nigeria. Note the anterior portion of the female protruding in the skin ulcers of both patients. *C*, Cross section of a *Dracunculus* female from a human host. Note the surrounding inflammatory reaction. The somatic muscles of *Dracunculus* are clearly divided between ventral and dorsal fields, separated by thin, wide lateral cords. One such muscle field and one of the two uteri filled with larvae are seen here, ×100. *D*, Detail of a worm cuticle (c) showing the smooth cuticle and subcuticle (sc). The contractile portion of the muscles (m) is seen, ×400. (Courtesy of R. Muller, Ph.D., Commonwealth Institute of Parasitology, St. Albans, Herts, England.)

tion, and, later, secondary bacterial infections are responsible for subsequent symptoms and the incapacitation produced by the disease (Adeyeba, 1985). Although usually one worm develops in a patient, there are cases of multiple infections. In Nigeria the disease produces up to 100 days of work loss per year in infected individuals (Kale, 1977) and up to 25% absenteeism in infected school children (Ilegbodu et al. 1986).

If the worm is injured or dies in the subcutaneous tissue, it may provoke an anaphylactic reaction. However, more often it produces a strong inflammatory reaction (Fairley, 1924), with formation of an abscess; eventually the worm may calcify (Zaman et al. 1985). Sometimes the inflammation involves the joints, producing arthritis, synovitis, and contraction of muscles and tendons, with resultant ankylosing of the joints.

Migration of the parasite from the retroperitoneum to the subcutaneous tissues results in aberrant locations of the worm, with production of unusual clinical syndromes. Some of these syndromes are constrictive pericarditis (Kinare et al. 1962), extradural compression or abscesses (Adeloye, 1983; Reddy, Valli, 1967), and abscesses in the spinal canal (Donaldson, Angelo, 1961; Mathur et al. 1981; Odaibo et al. 1986), the periorbital tissues (Verma, 1966, 1968), the testis (Pendse et al. 1982, 1987), and other sites (Kobayashi et al. 1986).

The chronic manifestations of the infection are usually sequelae produced by the dead, calcified worms in the tissues and may appear up to 20 years later (McLaughlin et al. 1984). The most common complaints are rheumatic, usually of the lower extremities or the spinal column. Calcified worms around joints or other body structures are common findings in radiographs (el Garf, 1985; McLaughlin et al. 1984).

Pathology and Diagnosis. The main histopathologic manifestation of *Dracunculus* infection is the formation of a soft tissue abscess anywhere the worm dies and disintegrates. The diagnosis is sometimes based on worms recovered while draining the abscess; it is rarely based on examination of tissue sections (Fig. 18–2 C–D). Living parasites located in the subcutaneous tissues probably elicit little inflammation, except at the anterior portion of the worm, where blister formation and breakage of the skin occur. Calcified worms may be surrounded by fibrous connective tissue and chronic inflammation.

Gnathostoma—Gnathostomiasis

The superfamily Gnathostomatoidea has two genera of importance for human medicine: *Gnathostoma* and

Physaloptera. These genera are parasitic in animals, and both are accidental parasites in humans. *Gnathostoma* and *Physaloptera* inhabit the gastrointestinal tract of their definitive hosts, where they usually live buried in the intestinal wall. The adults of *Gnathostoma* are located in the stomach, producing a tumor-like thickening. *Physaloptera* adults may occur at various levels of the gastrointestinal tract, with their anterior end buried in the mucosa. There are a few reports of human infections with *Physaloptera caucasica* in several parts of the world (Apt et al. 1965; Carney et al. 1977; Witemberg, 1951). Most of these infections occur in Africa, where adult worms have been recovered from the intestines of patients with infarction of the bowel (Nicolaides et al. 1977). The adults of *Physaloptera* are easily mistaken for immature *Ascaris*, which makes it possible that *Physaloptera* infection is underreported worldwide.

The genus *Gnathostoma* has fewer than ten species, four of which are recorded in humans. *Gnathostoma spinigerum*, is commonly found in wild and domestic cats and dogs in India, China, Japan, and Southeast Asia (Radomyos, Daengsvang, 1987). *Gnathostoma hispidum* inhabits the gastric mucosa of wild and domestic pigs in Europe, Asia, and Australia (Taniguchi, Ando, 1992). *Gnathostoma doloresi* is found in wild boars in southern Japan (Nawa et al. 1989; Ogata et al. 1988; Seguchi et al. 1995), and *G. nipponicum* is found in weasels in Japan (Ando et al. 1988, 1990; Sato et al. 1992). Other species of *Gnathostoma* are known on the American continent, such as *G. procyonis* in raccoons, *G. didelphis* (= *G. turgida*) in opossums, and a recently described species, *G. binucleatum*. The last species occurs in ocelots in Mexico. The presence of *G. spinigerum* on the American continent has been questioned; no credible evidence of its presence on this continent appears to be available (Ash, 1962). Worms recovered and identified from the humans infections occurring in Central and South America have been identified as *G. spinigerum* (Ollague et al. 1988). However, no definitive conclusion can be drawn about the species infecting humans on the American continent (Ogata et al. 1998). The species producing human infections in Latin America must be one of the known indigenous species on this continent or one not yet described.

In addition to these known species of *Gnathostoma* in humans, a series of infections with other spiruriid larvae has been described recently in Japan. These larvae have morphologic characteristics that permit their classification within the order Spirurida, but they are clearly not *Gnathostoma* because their bodies are devoid of spines (Ando et al. 1992; Kagei, 1991; Kagei et al. 1992; Okazaki et al. 1993; Taniguchi, Katsuhiko,

1994). The identification of these larvae is being pursued. Ando and coworkers (Ando et al. 1992) have suggested that they are at least morphologically similar to larvae from marine fish described as larva "X." These larvae have a strong capacity to invade tissues (Hasegawa, 1978).

Morphology. The type species of the genus *Gnathostoma* is *G. spinigerum.* Adult male worms range from 11 to 25 mm in length and adult females from 25 to 54 mm, varying with the size of their host. In smaller hosts the parasites are stout, while in larger ones they are longer and more slender. The worms may be reddish, sometimes whitish, and always curved ventrally. Their main morphologic characteristics are the subglobose cephalic end, separated from the body by a constriction, and the spines covering the anterior half of the body. The surface of the subglobose cephalic end

is covered with several rows of sharp, curved hooks and the anterior half of the body with flat, leaf-like spines that are broader at the base, with one, two, or three serrations at the end. The number of serrations varies with the area of the body, being three behind the cephalic end and one in the middle of the worm; the posterior half of the parasite is devoid of spines. The number of rows of hooks and the character of the spines are valuable in identifying the species. The internal anatomy of the worm is similar to that of other nematodes. One exception is the presence of four glands or cervical sacs in the anterior two-thirds of the esophagus, which on cross section are seen as empty spaces.

Most of the worms in humans are usually recovered from the skin, the subcutaneous tissues, and the eye, and most specimens are advanced third-stage larvae or very young adult worms (Radomyos, Daengsvang, 1987). The general morphology of the larva is similar to that of the adult (Fig. 18–3 *A–C*), with its subglobose cephalic

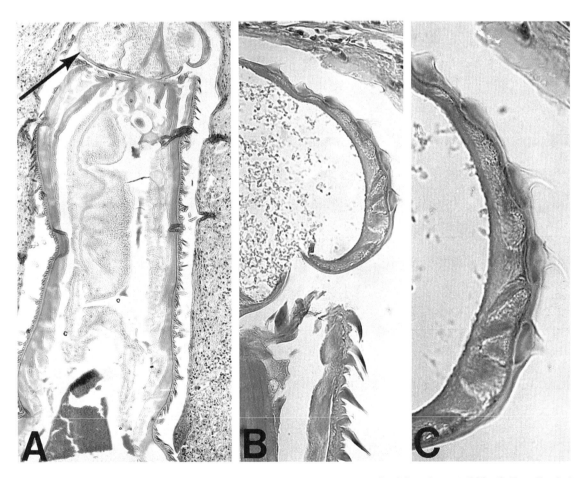

Fig. 18–3. *Gnathostoma,* **adult worm in the stomach wall of an animal, preparation stained with hematoxylin stain.** *A,* **Anterior portion buried in the wall. Note the globose anterior end (arrow), ×52.** *B,* **Higher magnification showing the anterior end and the cuticle of the worm covered with spines, ×280.** *C,* **Detail of the globose portion showing the spines, ×570. (Preparation courtesy of M.D. Little, Ph.D., School of Public Health and Tropical Medicine, Tulane University, New Orleans, Louisiana.)**

end containing rows of hooks and its body containing spines in its anterior half. The esophagus and the four sacs around it are seen, and no developed sexual organs are present. These larvae are identified on the basis of several characteristics: (1) the shape of the body, (2) the number of rows of hooks at the cephalic end (Fig. 18–3 C), (3) the number of hooks in each row, (4) the character of the spines covering the body, and (5) the extent to which the body is covered by the spines (Daengsvang, 1981). Identification of these larvae is a difficult task that is outside the scope of this discussion. If the pathologist receives such a larva or recovers it from a surgical specimen, the larva should not be sectioned but should be referred to an expert on this group of parasites. The morphology in tissue sections is discussed below (see Diagnosis).

Life Cycle. The life cycle of *Gnathostoma* has been studied extensively. It may involve one intermediate host and one final host or two intermediate hosts and one final host; in addition, many paratenic hosts aid its transmission through predation (Fig. 18–4; Daengsvang, 1980). The worms pass eggs in the feces of the definitive host. In water they mature and produce first-stage larvae that are ingested by small arthropods of the genus *Cyclops*. In the body cavity of the arthropod, the larvae mature first to the early third stage and then to the late third stage. If freshwater fish or other animals swallow the infected *Cyclops*, the larvae are freed in the intestine and migrate through the tissues to encapsulate in the muscles and remain infective for their final hosts. Cats and dogs ingest larvae encapsulated in the animal muscles.

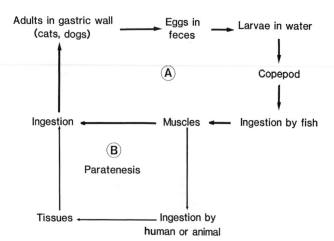

Fig. 18–4. *Gnathostoma*, schematic representation of the life cycle. (A) the usual pathway followed by the worm. (B) Many animals help with transmission by paratenesis.

The larvae are freed once more in the stomach and the intestine, migrate to the liver and the abdominal cavity, and finally move to the wall of the stomach, where they grow to adults (Fig. 18–3 A). The inflammatory tissue reaction produces marked thickening of the stomach wall resembling a tumor. A small opening in the mucosa overlying the tumor allows the eggs of the worm to pass to the stomach and be evacuated with the feces. Ingestion of encapsulated larvae in fish by humans and other unnatural hosts produces infection and migration of the larvae through the tissues. Ingestion of water with *Cyclops* harboring advanced third-stage larvae also produces the infection in humans. In abnormal hosts, including humans, the larvae generally do not develop. Thus, they are paratenic hosts, and gnathostomiasis is a type of visceral larva migrans sensu latu (see Chapter 17).

Geographic Distribution and Epidemiology. Human infections with *Gnathostoma* have been described in India, Japan, the Philippines, Thailand (where most human infections have been recorded), Mexico (Martinez-Cruz et al. 1989; Pelaez, Perez-Reyes, 1970), Guatemala (Mazariegos-Bonilla, 1987), and Ecuador (Ollague, 1985). In the United States (Horohoe et al. 1984; Kagen et al. 1984; Pinkus et al. 1981; Stowens, Simon, 1981) and other countries (Chabasse et al. 1988), *Gnathostoma* has been reported sporadically among Southeast Asian immigrants. In these cases, the disease may manifest in immigrants years after their arrival at the nonendemic area. The disease is also acquired by eating raw or uncooked fish, frogs, and snakes; in Southeast Asia, several species of *Ophicephalus*, freshwater fish, are responsible for most human infections (Miyazaki, 1960).

After *Gnathostoma* larvae are ingested by humans, they reach the intestine, probably migrate to the liver, and travel from there to almost any place in the body. The aimless migration through the tissues produces damage and symptoms that are variable and difficult to diagnose clinically; if the larva reaches the brain, it may cause death. The *Gnathostoma* worms recovered from humans are 2.5 to 12.5 mm long by 0.4 to 1.2 mm wide (Radomyos, Daengsvang, 1987). Depending on the location and the extent of migration of the parasite, different clinical syndromes are produced.

Clinical Findings. The initial clinical symptoms of gnathostomiasis usually begin soon after ingestion of the larva and are due to migration of the larva through the intestinal wall and liver. Some individuals complain of epigastric pain, nausea, and vomiting that sometimes lasts for 2 to 3 weeks. After the initial symptoms occur, manifestations in any other organ system appear either soon afterward or months or even years later. In one case, it was certain that $3^1/_2$ years had elapsed between ingestion of the larva and ocular manifestations of the infection in one patient (Tudor, Blair, 1971). It is also likely that the infection was once acquired in-utero (Daengsvang, 1981). The main organs affected will now be discussed.

Subcutaneous Tissues. The most common location of the parasite is the subcutaneous tissue, where it produces indurations due to edema and inflammation. This syndrome is known by several local names, such as *Yangtze River's edema* and *Shangai's rheumatism* in China, *tuao chid* in Japan, and *paniculitis nodular migratoria eosinofilica* in Latin America. A pruritic, erythematous skin reaction often accompanies the induration. The swelling lasts for 1 to 2 weeks, then dis-

appears and reappears later, either nearby or in other locations. As time passes, the lesions and the symptoms become less frequent and less intense until they finally vanish. The swelling is due to mechanical damage, and the allergic reaction is caused by the worm and its products (Daengsvang, 1980; Miyazaki, 1960, 1966).

Skin. A form of creeping eruption, or cutaneous larva migrans (see Chapter 14), is sometimes produced by the larva of *Gnathostoma* migrating through the skin (Fig. 18–5 *A–B*). The larva reaches the skin from the muscles and the subcutaneous tissues, but it probably gains access by direct penetration when fish and animals are handled during food preparation (Daengsvang et al. 1970). A wide serpiginous track forms in the skin, at the end of which the larva is sometimes seen with the naked eye. The larva is recovered after a small incision of the epidermis (Bhaibulaya, Charoenlarp, 1983).

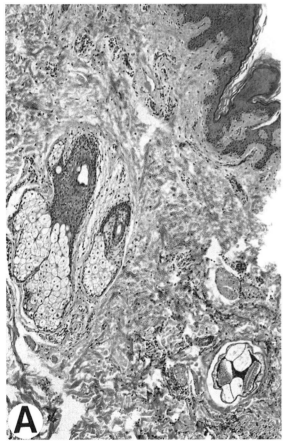
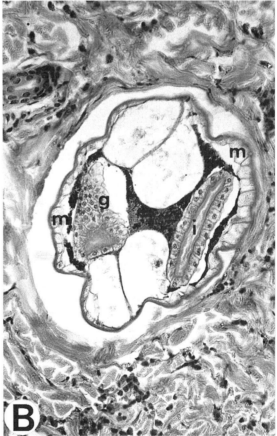

Fig. 18–5. *Gnathostoma* in skin, sections stained with hematoxylin and eosin stain. *A,* Low-power view of skin section with a larva of *Gnathostoma* in the dermis. Note the scant inflammatory reaction, ×85. *B,* Higher magnification of the larva. Note the developing muscles (m), the intestine (i), and the gonad of the worm (g), ×280. (Preparation courtesy of P.C. Beaver, Ph.D., School of Public Health and Tropical Medicine, Tulane University, New Orleans, Louisiana.)

Central Nervous System. Gnathostoma in the central nervous system produces radiculomyelitis, radiculomyeloencephalitis, and subarachnoid hemorrhages (Boongird et al. 1977), usually with radicular pain, headache, or both. Radicular pain is thought to result from migration of the larvae through the spinal root nerves on their way to the spinal canal and brain; the pain usually lasts for 1 to 5 days (Boongird et al. 1977; Punyagupta et al. 1968, 1990). This pain is often accompanied by paralysis of one or more extremities; paraplegia is not uncommon, followed by triplegia and quadriplegia. The degree of paralysis varies from minimal to extreme weakening. Patients with *Gnathostoma* encephalitis have cranial nerve symptoms, often following paralysis of the extremities. Cranial nerve palsies, nystagmus, and meningeal irritation may be the only findings, but in most cases the symptoms have a clear migratory pattern, which is considered characteristic of gnathostomiasis (Boongird et al. 1977). The clinical distinction between central nervous system gnathostomiasis and eosinophilic meningoencephalitis produced by *Angiostrongylus* (see Chapter 13) is that in *Gnathostoma* there is acute nerve root pain, signs of spinal cord compromise, and hemorrhagic or xantochromic spinal fluid (Punyagupta et al. 1990). In some cases, further symptoms reappear after 2 weeks due to migration and relocation of the larva. The laboratory data usually are not helpful. The cerebrospinal fluid pressure is often increased; the fluid is hemorrhagic or xanthochromic. Eosinophilia is present in all cases, and the total white blood cell count is less than 500 per cubic millimeter. Peripheral eosinophilia may be present. In children, *Gnathostoma* is an important cause of spontaneous subarachnoid hemorrhage (Visudhiphan et al. 1980).

Eye. The eye is the only organ where *Gnathostoma* is visualized, producing an inflammatory reaction; often the larva is recovered intact (*color plate* IX *H*; Biswas et al. 1994). For this reason, literature reports of eye infections with *Gnathostoma* are numerous. Another reason is that the eye is a site of the body (together with the breast and the genitals) that produces great concern in patients, inducing them to consult a physician for the slightest ailment. The manifestations of ocular gnathostomiasis vary, depending on the location of the worm and its route to the eye. In one patient, the ocular manifestations were accompanied by a Bell's palsy. In another patient with loss of vision and the sensation of a worm-like particle in the eye, the worm was seen in the retina attached to a blood vessel (Bathrick et al. 1981). The worms are often seen in the anterior chamber of the eye attached to the iris, producing uveitis (Chen, 1949; Seal et al. 1969; Sen,

Ghose, 1945), anterior uveitis (Choudhury, 1970; Kittiponghansa et al. 1987), or hemorrhage (Gyi, 1960). The worms are also seen in the cornea with perforation (Tansuphasiri, 1974) and glaucoma (Kittiponghansa et al. 1987).

Lungs. Pulmonary gnathostomiasis is usually diagnosed clinically, based on a history of subcutaneous swellings, eosinophilia, and an unexplained unilateral pleural effusion (Nagler et al. 1983; Thuraisingam et al. 1969). Some patients with cough, chest pain, and lesions visible on chest x-ray films recovered after expectoration of the worm (Vibulseth, Leelarasamee, 1980); in others, spontaneous pneumothorax was the main finding (Kangsadal, Bovornkitti, 1960).

Gastrointestinal Tract. A common gastrointestinal symptom is acute abdomen due to obstruction. X-ray films may show thickening of the wall with narrowing of the lumen (Fig. 18–6 *A*; Kurathong et al. 1979; Laohapand et al. 1981; Sirikulchayanonta, Chongchitnant, 1979). The laboratory tests in these cases show pronounced leukocytosis and eosinophilia. In one case the worm was located in the ascending colonic wall, producing intestinal obstruction (Seguchi et al. 1995).

Other Organs. Other organs invaded by larvae of *Gnathostoma* are the female genital tract (Hadidjaja et al. 1979), the urinary system (Migasena et al. 1964; Nitidandhaprabhas et al. 1975b), the male genitalia (Piyaratn, Samranwetaya, 1971), the trachea, with expectoration of the worm (Nitidandhaprabhas et al. 1975a), the ear (Prasansuk, Hinchcliffe, 1975), the tongue (Srisawai et al. 1988), and the breast (Tesjaroen et al. 1990).

Pathology. The pathologic manifestations of *Gnathostoma* consist of inflammation, edema, and tissue destruction in the path of the larva. Much of the tissue reaction is believed to be allergic, but the size of the larva is also an important factor. The greatest amount of tissue destruction is produced in the brain, where the larva may migrate extensively.

Subcutaneous Tissues. The main microscopic change in the subcutaneous tissues is an intense inflammatory reaction seen as edema and infiltration by polymorphonuclear cells, eosinophils, and histiocytes, sometimes extending deep into adipose tissue and muscles. The lesion usually resolves without sequelae if the larva relocates, but it may become an abscess, organize, and remain as a hard nodule with a necrotic center surrounded by fibrous tissue (Bovornkitti, Tandhanand, 1959; Kangsadal, Bovornkitti, 1960).

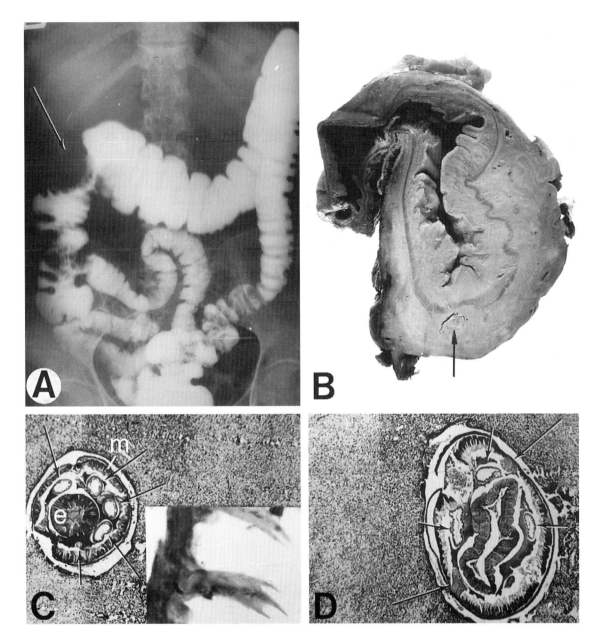

Fig. 18–6. *Gnathostoma* in the colonic wall of an individual from Thailand with clinical symptoms and signs of a malignancy. *A*, Barium enema showing a filling defect in the hepatic flexure (arrow). *B*, Gross specimen, sectioned through the center of the mass, showing necrosis with the worm barely visible (arrow), cut across. Note the thickening of the submucosa, muscle, and peritoneal layers. *C* and *D*. Microscopic features of the lesion, sections stained with hematoxylin and eosin stain. *C*, Cross section of the worm through the muscular esophagus (e), the four cervical sacs (long arrows), a section of the developing genital tract (short arrow), and the muscle layer (m), ×35.

Inset: cuticular spines with three teeth found at a level of the worm that corresponds to about the midesophagus, ×450. *D*. Transverse section of the worm at the midbody level showing the intestine and the tubes (short arrows) from which the reproductive tract will evolve. Note the cuticle, muscle layer, and lateral cords (long arrows), ×35. (Courtesy of T. Laohapand, M.D., Department of Pathology. Faculty of Medicine, Siriraj Hospital, Mahidol University, Bangkok, Thailand. Reported by: Laohapand, T., Sonakul, D., Lolekha, S., et al. 1981. Gnathostomiasis of the colon simulating malignancy. A case report. J. Med. Assoc. Thai. 64:192–195. Reproduced with permission.)

Central Nervous System. The external appearance of the brain may be hemorrhagic, with flattened gyri due to edema, and often with signs of herniation. Worms have been seen moving freely on the meningeal surface of the brain, spinal cord, and other places (Bunnag et al. 1970; Punyagupta et al. 1968). In coronal sections of brain and in sections of spinal cord, hemorrhagic track-like lesions measuring approximately 1 mm in diameter have been observed. Some tracks appeared to be filled with clotted blood. In cases of myelitis, the worm tracks have been followed from below, in the spinal cord, up to the midbrain. Sometimes the tracks in the cord are only 1 cm or less in length, disappearing into the surface of the cord and then reentering at a higher level. Larger areas of hemorrhage may be present in the brain due to disruption of blood vessels; sometimes these hemorrhages are large enough to fill the ventricles (Chitanondh, Rosen, 1967; Punyagupta, Juttijudata, 1967). Gross areas of white and gray matter necrosis without hemorrhage occur in some cases. The microscopic changes consist of areas of necrosis and hemorrhage corresponding to the tracks seen grossly, with loss of tissue, small numbers of macrophages filled with phagocytized, degenerated myelin, and adjacent neurons with eosinophilic degeneration; tracks cut longitudinally are found to have identical changes. Older lesions are filled with red blood cells and chronic inflammatory infiltrates consisting mainly of histiocytes, lymphocytes, plasma cells, and a variable number of eosinophils. The larger hemorrhagic areas in white and gray matter may have different degrees of organization. Larvae are rarely seen in histologic sections of brain tissue.

Gastrointestinal Tract. A segment of gastrointestinal tract is often removed when the viscus wall is invaded by *Gnathostoma.* Grossly, the intestine has an inflammatory thickening of the wall with reduction of the lumen, usually without mucosal ulceration (Fig. 18–6 *B*). The parasite is often found in the inflammatory mass, from which it can be recovered in toto. Histologic examination reveals an abscess with eosinophils, poly-

morphonuclear cells, lymphocytes, and sometimes the parasite in the center of the abscess (Figs. 18–6 *C–D* 18–7 *A–D*). Edema is present in the surrounding tissues. Organizing older lesions have multinucleated foreign body giant cells and fibrosis.

Diagnosis. In endemic areas, the clinical diagnosis of gnathostomiasis is often based on the patient's history of eating raw fish, the clinical symptoms, the skin manifestations, and the presence of subcutaneous migratory swellings. The clinical diagnosis is usually not based on recovery of the worm. In rare cases in which the worm is recovered, a definitive diagnosis is based on study of the worm in toto that hopefully results in its exact classification (Daengsvang, 1980; Miyazaki, 1960, 1966). A study of *Gnathostoma* worms retrieved from a large number of patients, showed advanced third-stage larvae, as well as immature and mature males and females (Radomyos, Daengsvang, 1987), indicating that *Gnathostoma* appears to develop beyond the third stage in humans.

Gnathostoma larvae recovered from humans are recognized on the basis of the external morphologic characteristics outlined above, which are best seen under a stereoscope. As stated, they measure up to 12.5 mm long by up to 1.2 mm wide; they are white-reddish when first isolated from tissues and often have a dark intestinal tract. The internal structures of the larva consist of a large esophagus occupying the anterior third of the body, with a slender, muscular anterior portion and a thicker, glandular posterior portion. Extending posteriorly alongside the muscular esophagus are four cervical sacs or glands.

The identification of *Gnathostoma* in tissue sections is sometimes necessary when surgical specimens are submitted for histologic diagnosis. The worm may be found, usually alive, producing some inflammation. *Gnathostoma* can be recognized on cross sections based on the following characteristics. The larva is up to 350 μm in diameter. Sections through the anterior esophagus show the four cervical sacs as rounded structures close to the

---

Fig. 18–7. ***Gnathostoma*** **in the large intestine, sections stained with hematoxylin and eosin stain.** ***A*,** **Low-power view of the colonic wall, with a significant inflammatory reaction and a cross section of the worm located in the internal muscle layer, ×11.** ***B*,** **Higher magnification of the lesion without the worm, ×22.** ***C*,** **The parasite showing the thick cuticle (c), the muscle layer (m) with approximately 15 cells per quadrant, and the large intestine (i) with cells with well-defined borders, ×70.** ***D*,** **Detail of** ***Gnathostoma*** **in cross section. Note the muscle cells with a contractile portion at least one-third the** height of the cell (short arrows). The muscle fibers (contractile portion) have a U shape. The developing genital tract (long arrows) are small tubular structures. The intestinal cells are of different heights, with coarsely granular cytoplasm and a clear brush border, ×140. (Preparation courtesy of P.C. Beaver, Ph.D., School of Public Health and Tropical Medicine, Tulane University, New Orleans, Louisiana. Reported by: Fontan, R., Beauchamp, F., and Beaver, P.C. 1975. Sur quelques helminthiases humaines nouvelles au Laos. I. Nematodes. Bull. Soc. Pathol. Exot. 68:557–566.)

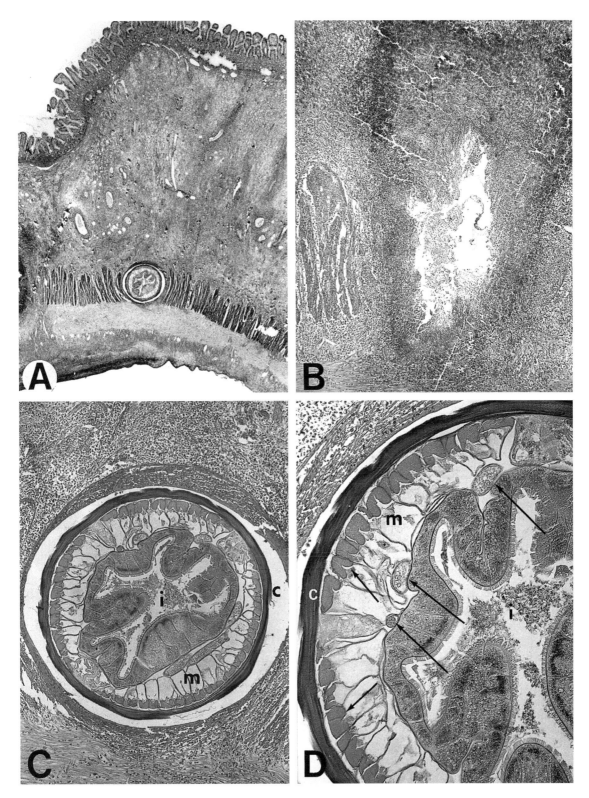

Fig. 18–7.

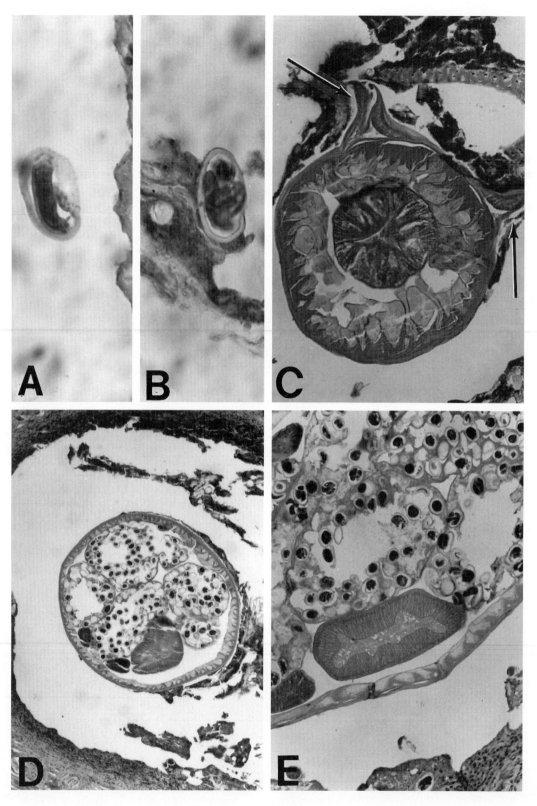

Fig. 18–8. *Rictularia* in the appendix, sections stained with hematoxylin and eosin stain. *A* and *B*, Sections of eggs showing the thick shell and a fully developed larva, ×400. *C*, Cross section of the worm through the anterior end showing the esophagus of the parasite. Note the subventral combs of the parasite (arrows), ×40. *D*, Section through the middle of the worm showing the uterus filled with eggs, ×20. *E*, Higher magnification illustrating the intestine of the worm, the uterus, and the developing eggs, ×100. (In Kenney, M., Eveland, L.K., Yermakov, M., et al. 1975. A case of *Rictularia* infection of a man in New York. Am. J. Trop. Med. Hyg. 24:596–599. Reproduced with permission.)

esophagus (Fig. 18–6 C). The cuticle is thick, with spines in the anterior portion, and the subcuticle (hypodermis) is relatively thin (Fig. 18–7 C–D). The lateral cords are prominent (Fig. 18–7 D). The muscle cells total 10 to 15 per quadrant, have well-defined cell borders, and have a large cytoplasmic portion and low muscle fibers (Fig. 18–7 C–D). The intestine is well developed and has coarsely granular cells with a well-defined brush border. The intestinal cells are either columnar or spherical. There are 10 to 30 cells per histologic section and a variable number of nuclei (Figs. 18–6 D and 18–7 C–D). The developing genital tract is seen as tube-like structures between the intestine and the muscle cells (Figs. 18–6 C–D and 18–7 C–D).

Japanese authors have made great progress in distinguishing the species of *Gnathostoma* in cross sections, especially those species occurring in their country and in Southeast Asia. The number of intestinal cells, their shape, and the number of their nuclei appear to be helpful differentiating characteristics. Both *G. spinigerum* and *G. nipponicum* have columnar intestinal cells; 21 to 29 in *G. spinigerum* and half as many in *G. nipponicum.* Both *G. hispidum* and *G. doloresi* have roughly the same number of spherical intestinal cells: usually with one nucleus per cell in *G. hispidum* and two in *G. doloresi* (Akahane, Mako, 1986; Taniguchi, Ando, 1992). The microscopic anatomy in cross sections of other species of *Gnathostoma* has not yet been studied.

A species of the genus *Rictularia,* in the superfamily Rictularioidea, was found in the appendix of a 90-year-old-man during a routine autopsy in New York City. This genus, which parasitizes rodents and bats, is characterized by two subventral rows of spines (Fig. 18–8 A–E; Kenney et al. 1975).

Thelazia—Thelaziasis

The genus *Thelazia* comprises several species of spruriid nematodes adapted to live in the conjunctival sac of mammals such as dogs and rabbits, in species of birds, and accidentally in humans. *Thelazia callipaeda* has been recovered from humans in China (Hsiang, 1955), Japan (Mimori et al. 1991), Korea (Hong et al. 1995; Im et al. 1974), Russia (Kozlov, 1962; Miroshnichenko et al. 1988), Indonesia (Kosin et al. 1989), and Thailand (Bhaibulaya et al. 1970; Yospaiboon et al. 1989), and *T. californiensis* has been recovered in the United States (Chiapella et al. 1976; Doezie et al. 1996; Kirschner et al. 1990; Knierim, Jack, 1975). A species of *Thelazia* that was impossible to identify was

described in a man in Assam (Mahanta et al. 1996). Other species found in Kentucky, the United States, are *T. lacrimalis* in horses (Lyons, Drudge, 1975) and *T. gulosa* and *T. skrjabini* in cattle.

The life cycle of *Thelazia* species affecting humans and the circumstances in which humans acquire the infection are unknown. The adult worms deposit their eggs in the conjunctiva. The intermediate hosts are probably flies, in which the eggs develop to infective larvae (Kozlov, 1962). *Thelazia* infections in humans produce excessive lacrimation, and migration of the worms in the conjunctiva may produce scarifications of the cornea. Removal of the parasites from the lacrimal sac and the surface of the eye is the treatment of choice; specific diagnosis is made by identification of the worms.

Gongylonema—Gongylonematosis

The superfamily Spiruroidea has two genera, *Gongylonema* and *Spirocerca,* each with one species described in humans: *G. pulchrum* and *S. lupi. Gongylonema* is a parasite of pigs, monkeys, sheep, cattle, and bears. In humans the infection has been reported fewer than three dozen times, mostly from Austria (Rysavy et al. 1969), Bulgaria (Sliwensky, 1941), Germany (Jelinek, Loscher, 1994; Weber, MacHe, 1973), Hungary (Amaszta et al. 1972), Italy (Ghetti, 1925; Rossi-Espagnet, Salera, 1955), Russia (Bulcheva, Augustina, 1962; Engelshtein, Kigel, 1965; Gefter, Nemirovskaia, 1965), Spain (Illescas-Gomez et al. 1988), Morocco (Gaud, 1952; Pages, Gaud, 1951), China (Ch'En et al. 1958; Feng et al. 1955), New Zealand (Johnston, 1936), Sri Lanka (Crusz, Sivalingam, 1950), and the United States (Dismuke, Routh, 1963; Ransom, 1923; Stiles, Baker, 1928). *Spirocerca* occurs naturally in wild and domestic dogs. Only once has the infection been reported in humans, in an infant in Italy who acquired it in utero and developed gastrointestinal symptoms soon after birth. Mature worms were found in the wall of the ileum (Biocca, 1959).

Gongylonema lives in tunnels within the squamous epithelium of the esophagus and the oral cavity of the definitive hosts (Fig. 18–9 A–B). The male is up to 6.3 cm long and the female is up to 14.5 cm long by 0.3 and 0.5 mm wide, respectively. Eggs laid within the tunnels in the squamous epithelium are eventually sloughed off into the lumen of the esophagus and are evacuated, fully embryonated, with the feces. An intermediate host, usually a dung beetle or a cockroach, is required. Ingestion of infected intermediate hosts pro-

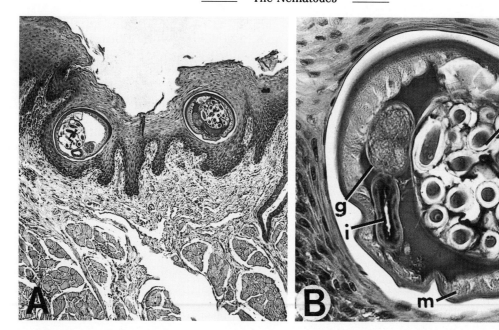

Fig. 18–9. *Gongylonema* in the tongue of a monkey, sections stained with hematoxylin and eosin stain. *A*, Low-power view of the tongue with two cross sections of *Gongylonema* in the squamous epithelium. Note the lack of inflammatory reaction, ×70. *B*, Higher magnification of one section of a female worm showing the uterus filled with eggs (u), the gonads (g), the intestine (i), and the muscle layer (m). Note the tunnel in the squamous epithelium and the lack of inflammation, ×350. (Preparation courtesy of P.C. Beaver, Ph.D., School of Public Health and Tropical Medicine, Tulane University, New Orleans, Louisiana.)

duces the infection in the natural definitive hosts or in humans.

Clinical Findings, Pathology, and Diagnosis. Some individuals suffering from gongylonematosis have the sensation of a worm moving through the mucosa of the buccal cavity (Gaud, 1952; Johnston, 1936; Thomas, 1952; Young, Hayne, 1953). Examination shows a rounded, linear induration making several loops back and forth in the mucosa, and scarification of the surface reveals the worm (Dismuke, Routh, 1963; Feng et al. 1955; Ward, 1916). Some patients develop pharyngitis and small abscess-like lesions containing the parasites (Stiles, 1921a, 1921b; Waite, Gorrie, 1935); others cough up the worm. Histologic abnormalities have not been described in patients with *Gongylonema* infections. In one case, a biopsy specimen taken from a mucosal erosion 1.0 cm in diameter revealed *Gongylonema* eggs in the squamous epithelium (Feng et al. 1955). The diagnosis is made clinically, based on the typical location of the worm within the squamous epithelium; by recovery and study of the adult worms; or, rarely, in tissue sections containing the parasite. In one case, eggs were visualized in sputum samples (Feng et

al. 1955); however, stool examination usually does not show eggs because they occur in small numbers.

Finally, a species of *Cheilospirura*, a genus of the superfamily Acuarioidea, was reported once from the eye of a man in the Philippines (Africa, Garcia, 1936).

References

Adeloye A, 1983. Correspondence. Extradural compression by Guinea worm. Surg. Neurol. 19:482–483

Adeyeba OA, 1985. Secondary infections in dracunculiasis: bacteria and morbidity. Int. J. Zoonoses 12:147–149

Africa CM, Garcia EY, 1936. A new nematode parasite (*Cheilospirura* sp.) of the eye of man in the Philippines. J. Philipp. Isl. Med. Assoc. 16:603–607

Akahane H, Mako T, 1986. Studies on the life cycle of *Gnathostoma hispidum* Fedtschenko, 1872 (2). The experimental infection of a pig with the early third-stage larvae from loaches. Jpn. J. Parasitol. 35:161–164

Amaszta M, Hollo F, Miskolczy L, Strobl I, 1972. First incidence of human gongylonematosis in Hungary. Parasitol. Hung. 5:239–246

Ando K, Sato Y, Miura K, Chinzei Y, Ogawa S, 1992. Further observation on the larva of the suborder Spirurina suspected as the causative agent of creeping eruption. Jpn. J. Parasitol. 41:384–389

Ando K, Tanaka H, Taniguchi Y, Shimizu M, Kondo K, 1988. Two human cases of gnathostomiasis and discovery of a second intermediate host of *Gnathostoma nipponicum* in Japan. J. Parasitol. 74:623–627

Ando K, Tokura H, Chinzei Y, 1990. Morphological features in cross section of early and advanced third-stage larvae of *Gnathostoma nipponicum.* Jpn. J. Parasitol. 39:482–487

Apt W, Sapunar J, Doren J, Rojo M, 1965. *Physaloptera caucasica.* Primeros casos humanos en Chile. Bol. Chil. Parasitol. 20:111–113

Ash LR, 1962. Migration and development of *Gnathostoma procyonis* Chandler, 1947 in mammalian hosts. J. Parasitol. 48:306–313

Bathrick ME, Mango CA, Mueller JF, 1981. Intraocular gnathostomiasis. Am. Acad. Ophthalmol. 88:1293–1295

Beaver PC, Jung RC, Cupp EW, 1984. *Clinical Parasitology.* Philadelphia: Lea & Febiger

Belcher DW, Wurapa FK, Ward WB, Lourie IM, 1975. Guinea worm in southern Ghana: its epidemiology and impact on agricultural productivity. Am. J. Trop. Med. Hyg. 24:243–249

Beverley Burton M, Crichton VF, 1976. Attempted experimental cross infections with mammalian guinea-worms, *Dracunculus* spp. (Nematoda: Dracunculoidea). Am. J. Trop. Med. Hyg. 25:704–708

Bhaibulaya M, Charoenlarp P, 1983. Creeping eruption caused by *Gnathostoma spinigerum.* Southeast Asian J. Trop. Med. Public Health 14:266–268

Bhaibulaya M, Prasertsilpa S, Vajrasthira S, 1970. *Thelazia callipaeda* Railliet and Henry, 1910 in man and dog in Thailand. Am. J. Trop. Med. Hyg. 19:476–479

Biocca E, 1959. Infestazione umana prenatale da *Spirocerca lupi* (Rud., 1809). Parassitologia 1:137–142

Biswas J, Gopal L, Sharma T, Badrinath SS, 1994. Intraocular *Gnathostoma spinigerum.* Clinicopathologic study of two cases with review of literature. Retina 14:438–444

Boongird P, Phanpradit P, Siridej N, Chirachariyavej T, Chuahirun S, Vejjajiva A, 1977. Neurological manifestations of gnathostomiasis. J. Neurol. Sci. 31:279–291

Bovornkitti S, Tandhanand S, 1959. A case of spontaneous pneumothorax complicating gnathostomiasis. Dis. Chest 35:328–331

Bulcheva NA, Augustina TI, 1962. A case of *Gongylonema* infection in man. Med. Parasitol. 31:611–612

Bunnag T, Comer DS, Punyagupta S, 1970. Eosinophilic myeloencephalitis caused by *Gnathostoma spinigerum.* Neuropathology of nine cases. J. Neurol. Sci. 10:419–434

Carney WP, Van Peenen PFD, See R, Hagelstein E, Lima B, 1977. Parasites of man in remote areas of Central and South Sulawesi, Indonesia. Southeast Asian J. Trop. Med. Public Health 8:380–389

CDC, 1998. Imported dracunculiasis—United States, 1995 and 1997. Morb. Mort. Weekly Rep. 47:209–211

Ch'En KH, Wang SP, Yu MH, Liu TS, 1958. *Gongylonema* infestation. A case report with morphologic study. Chin. Med. J. 77:254–256

Chabasse D, Cauchy AC, De Gentile L, Bouchara JP, 1988. Gnathostomose humaine revele par un syndrome de larva migrans cutanee. A propos d'une observation. Bull. Soc. Pathol. Exot. 81:326–331

Chen HT, 1949. A human ocular infection by *Gnathostoma* in China. J. Parasitol. 35:431–433

Chiapella KJ, Weinman C, Roberto R, 1976. Thelaziasis—California. Morb. Mort. Weekly Rep. 25:367

Chitanondh H, Rosen L, 1967. Fatal eosinophilic encephalomyelitis caused by the nematode *Gnathostoma spinigerum.* Am. J. Trop. Med. Hyg. 16:638–645

Choudhury AR, 1970. Ocular gnathostomiasis. Am. J. Ophthalmol. 70:276–278

Crusz H, Sivalingam V, 1950. A note on the occurrence of *Gongylonema pulchrum* Molin, 1857, in man in Ceylon. J. Parasitol. 36:25–26

Daengsvang S, 1980. *A Monograph on the Genus* Gnathostoma *and Gnathostomiasis in Thailand.* Tokyo: Southeast Asian Med Information Center

Daengsvang S, 1981. Gnathostomiasis in Southeast Asia. Southeast Asian J. Trop. Med. Public Health 12:319–332

Daengsvang S, Sermswatsri B, Youngyi P, Guname D, 1970. Penetration of the skin by *Gnathostoma spinigerum* larvae. Ann. Trop. Med. Parasitol. 64:399–402

Deaedorff TL, Overstreet RM, Okihiro M, Tam R, 1986. Piscine adult nematode invading an open lesion in a human hand. Am. J. Trop. Med. Hyg. 35:827–830

Dismuke JC Jr, Routh CF, 1963. Human infection with *Gongylonema* in Georgia. Am. J. Trop. Med. Hyg. 12:73–74

Doezie AM, Lucius RW, Aldeen W, Hale DV, Smith DR, Mamalis N, 1996. *Thelazia californiensis* conjunctival infestation. Ophthalmic Surg. Lasers 27:716–719

Donaldson JR, Angelo TA, 1961. Quadriplegia due to Guinea-worm abscess. J. Bone Joint. Surg. 197:198

el Garf A, 1985. Parasitic rheumatism: rheumatic manifestations associated with calcified Guinea worm. J. Rheumatol. 12:976–979

Engelshtein AS, Kigel RM, 1965. A case of *Gongylonema pulchrum* in man. Med. Parasitol. 34:163–164

Fairley NH, 1924. Studies in dracontiasis. Part IV. The clinical picture—an analysis of 140 cases. Indian J. Med. Res. 12:351–367

Feng LC, Tung MS, Su SC, 1955. Two Chinese cases of *Gongylonema* infection. A morphological study of the parasite and clinical study of the cases. Chinese Med. J. 73:149–162

Gaud J, 1952. Gongylonemose humaine au Maroc. Bull. Inst. Hyg. Maroc. 12:83–86

Gefter VA, Nemirovskaia OI, 1965. Human gongylonematosis. Med. Parasitol. 34:158–163

Ghetti G, 1925. A proposito del *Gongylonema neoplasticum* ricerche nello stomaco umano. Pathologica 17:520–523

Gyi K, 1960. Intra-ocular gnathostomiasis. Br. J. Ophthalmol. 44:42–45

Hadidjaja P, Margono SS, Moeloek FA, 1979. *Gnathostoma spinigerum* from the cervix of a woman in Jakarta. Am. J. Trop. Med. Hyg. 28:161–162

Hasegawa H, 1978. Larval nematodes of the superfamily Spiruroidea—a description, identification and examination of their pathogenicity. Acta Med. Biol. 26: 79–116

Hong ST, Park YK, Lee SK, Yoo JH, Kim AS, Chung YH, Hong SJ, 1995. Two human cases of *Thelazia callipaeda* infection in Korea. Korean J. Parasitol. 33:139–144

Hopkins DR, Ruiz-Tiben E, 1990. Dracunculiasis eradication: target 1995. Am. J. Trop. Med. Hyg. 43:296–300

Hopkins DR, Ruiz-Tiben E, Kaiser RL, Agle AN, Withers JPC, 1993. Dracunculiasis eradication: beginning of the end. Am. J. Trop. Med. Hyg. 49:281–289

Hopkins DR, Ruiz-Tiben E, Ruebush TK, 1997. Dracunculiasis eradication: almost a reality. Am. J. Trop. Med. Hyg. 57:252–259

Horohoe JJ, Ritterson AL, Chessin LN, 1984. Urinary gnathostomiasis. JAMA 251:255–256

Hsiang HF, 1955. *Thelazia callipaeda* in human eye: report of one case. Chinese J. Ophthalmol. 5:58–59

Ilegbodu VA, Kale OO, Wise RA, Christensen BL, Steele JH Jr, Chambers LA, 1986. Impact of guinea worm disease on children in Nigeria. Am. J. Trop. Med. Hyg. 35:962–964

Illescas-Gomez MP, Rodriguez Osorio M, Gomez Garcia V, Gomez Morales MA, 1988. Human *Gongylonema* infection in spain. Am. J. Trop. Med. Hyg. 38:363–365

Im KI, Kim SJ, Min DY, Kim SD, Lew IIM, 1974. A human infection with *Thelazia* sp. in Korea. Yonsei Rep. Trop. Med. 5:136–139

Jelinek T, Loscher T, 1994. Human infection with *Gongylonema pulchrum*: a case report. Trop. Med. Parasitol. 45:329–330

Johnston TH, 1936. A note on the occurrence of the nematode *Gongylonema pulchrum* in man in New Zealand. N.Z. Med. J. 35:172–176

Kagei N, 1991. Morphological identification of parasites in biopsied specimens from creeping disease lesions. Jpn. J. Parasitol. 40:437–445

Kagei N, Kumazawa H, Miyoshi K, Kosugi I, Ishih A, 1992. A case of ileus caused by a spiruroid nematode. Int. J. Parasitol. 22:839–841

Kagen CN, Vance JC, Simpson M, 1984. Gnathostomiasis. Infestation in an Asian immigrant. Arch. Dermatol. 120:508–510

Kale OO, 1977. The clinico-epidemiological profile of Guinea worm in the Ibadan district of Nigeria. Am. J. Trop. Med. Hyg. 26:208–214

Kangsadal P, Bovornkitti S, 1960. A case of gnathostomiasis with spontaneous hydropneumothorax. J. Trop. Med. Hyg. 63:67–70

Kenney M, Eveland LK, Yermakov V, Kassouny DY, 1975. A case of *Rictularia* infection of man in New York. Am. J. Trop. Med. Hyg. 24:596–599

Kinare SG, Parulkar GB, Sen PK, 1962. Constrictive pericarditis resulting from dracunculosis. Br. Med. J. 1:845

Kirschner BI, Dunn JP, Ostler HB, 1990. Correspondence. Conjunctivitis caused by *Thelazia californiensis*. Am. J. Ophthalmol. 110:573–574

Kittiponghansa S, Prabriputaloong A, Pariyanonda S, Ritch R, 1987. Intracameral gnathostomiasis: a cause of anterior uveitis and secondary glaucoma. Br. J. Ophthalmol. 71:618–622

Knierim R, Jack MK, 1975. Conjunctivitis due to *Thelazia californiensis*. Arch. Ophthalmol. 93:522–523

Kobayashi A, Katakura K, Hamada A, Suzuki T, Hataba Y, Tashiro N, Yoshida A, 1986. Human case of dracunculiasis in Japan. Am. J. Trop. Med. Hyg. 35: 159–161

Kosin E, Kosman ML, Depary AA, 1989. First case of human thelaziasis in Indonesia. Southeast Asian J. Trop. Med. Public Health 20:233–237

Kozlov DP, 1962. Developmental cycle of the nematode *Thelazia callipaeda*—a parasite in the eye of man and carnivorous mammals. Dokl. Akad. Nauk. USSR 142:732–733

Kurathong P, Boonprasan C, Kurathong S, 1979. An evanescent malignancy—resembling colonic mass: probably due to visceral gnathostomiasis. J. Med. Assoc. Thail. 62:512–515

Laohapand T, Sonakul D, Lolekha S, Dharamadach A, 1981. Gnathostomiasis of the colon simulating malignancy: a case report. J. Med. Assoc. Thail. 64:192–195

Lyons ET, Drudge JH, 1975. Occurrence of the eyeworm, *Thelazia lacrymalis*, in horses in Kentucky. J. Parasitol. 61:1122–1124

Mahanta J, Alger J, Bordoloi P, 1996. Eye infestation with *Thelazia* species. Indian J. Ophthalmol. 44:99–101

Martinez-Cruz JM, Bravo-Zamudio R, Aranda-Patraca A, Martinez-Maranon R, 1989. La gnathostomiasis en Mexico. Sal. Pub. Mex. 31:541–549

Mathur PPS, Dharker SR, Hiran S, Sardana V, 1981. Lumbar extradural compression by Guinea worm infestation. Surg. Neurol. 17:127–129

Mazariegos-Bonilla CA, 1987. Mieloencephalitis secundaria a *Gnathostoma spinigerum*. (Reporte del primer caso diagnosticado en Guatemala.) VIII Congreso Latinoamericano Parasitologia I Congreso Guatemalteco de Parasitologia y Medicina Tropical Guatemala, Guatemala Nov. 17–22, 1987, pp. 140

McLaughlin GE, Utsinger PD, Trakat WF, Resnick D, Moidel RA, 1984. Rheumatic syndromes secondary to guinea worm infestation: brief report. Arthritis Rheum. 27:694–697

Migasena P, Dhanaphumi S, Charoenlarp P, 1964. Urinary gnathostomiasis. J. Med. Assoc. Thail. 47:85–90

Mimori T, Korenaga M, Hirai H, Minematsu T, Tada I, Okamura R, 1991. *Thelazia callipaeda* infections in man in Kumamoto Prefecture, Japan. Kumamoto Med. J. 42:101–105

Miroshnichenko VA, Desiaterik MP, Novik AP, Gorbach AP, Papernova NI, 1988. A case of ocular thelaziasis in a 3-year-old child. Vestn. Oftalmol. 104:64

Miyazaki I, 1960. On the genus *Gnathostoma* and human

gnathostomiasis with special reference to Japan. Exp. Parasitol. 9:338–370

Miyazaki I, 1966. *Gnathostoma* and gnathostomiasis in Japan. In: Morishita K, Komiya Y, Matsubayashi H (eds), *Progress of Medical Parasitology in Japan*, Vol. 3. Tokyo: Meguro Parasitological Museum, pp. 529–586

Muller R, 1992. Guinea worm eradication: four more years to go. Parasitol. Today 8:387–390

Nagler A, Pollack S, Hassoun G, Kerner H, Barzilai D, Lengy J, 1983. Human pleuropulmonary gnathostomiasis: a case report from Israel. Israel J. Med. Sci. 19:834–837

Nawa Y, Imai JI, Ogata K, Otsuka K, 1989. The first record of a confirmed human case of *Gnathostoma doloresi* infection. J. Parasitol. 75:166–169

Nicolaides NJ, Musgrave J, McGuckin D, Moorhouse DE, 1977. Nematode larvae (Spirurida: Physalopteridae) causing infarction of the bowel in an infant. Pathology 9:129–135

Nitidandhaprabhas P, Hanchansin S, Vongsloesvidhya Y, 1975a. A case of expectoration of *Gnathostoma spinigerum* in Thailand. Am. J. Trop. Med. Hyg. 24:547–548

Nitidandhaprabhas P, Sirikarana A, Harnsomburana KA, 1975b. Human urinary gnathostomiasis: a case report from Thailand. Am. J. Trop. Med. Hyg. 24:49–51

Odaibo SK, Awogun IA, Oshagbemi K, 1986. Paraplegia complicating dracontiasis. J. R. Coll. Surg. 31:376–378

Ogata K, Imai JI, Nawa Y, 1988. Three confirmed and five suspected human cases of *Gnathostoma doloresi* infection found in Miyazaki Prefecture, Kyushu. Jpn. J. Parasitol. 37:358–364

Ogata K, Nawa Y, Akahane H, Diaz C, Lamothe-Argumedo R, Cruz-Reyes A, 1998. Short report: gnathostomiasis in Mexico. Am. J. Trop. Med. Hyg. 58:316–318

Okazaki A, Ida T, Muramatsu T, Shirai T, Nishiyama T, Araki T, 1993. Creeping disease due to larva of spiruroid nematoda. Int. J. Dermatol. 32:813–814

Ollague W, 1985. Gnathostomiasis (nodular migratory eosinophilic paniculitis). J. Am. Acad. Dermatol. 13:835–836

Ollague W, Eduardo Gomez L, Manuel Briones I, 1988. Infeccion natural de peces de agua dulce con el tercer estado larvario de *Gnathostoma spinigerum* y su dinamica de transmision al hombre. Primer reporte en Ecuador y America. Med. Cutan. Iber. Lat. Am. 16:291–294

Pages R, Gaud J, 1951. A propose de la filariose au Maroc. Un cas de parasitisme humain par gongylonemae. Maroc. Med. 30:584–585

Pelaez D, Perez-Reyes R, 1970. Gnatostomiasis humana en America. Rev. Lat. Am. Microbiol. 12:83–91

Pendse AK, Sharma AK, Mewara PC, 1987. *Dracunculus* orchitis: a case report. J. Trop. Med. Hyg. 90:153–154

Pendse AK, Soni BM, Omprakash R, Gupta SP, 1982. Testicular dracunculosis—a distinct clinical entity. Br. J. Urol. 54:56–58

Peries H, Cairncross S, 1997. Global eradication of Guinea worm. Parasitol. Today 13:431–437

Pinkus H, Fan J, Degiusti D, 1981. Creeping eruption due to

Gnathostoma spinigerum in a Taiwanese patient. Int. J. Dermatol. 20:46–49

Piyaratn P, Samranwetaya P, 1971. Pathology and pathogenesis of human gnathostomiasis. Chulalongkorn Med. J. 16:254–264

Prasansuk S, Hinchcliffe R, 1975. Gnathostomiasis. A case of otological interest. Arch. Otolaryngol. 101:254–258

Punyagupta S, Bunnag T, Juttijudata P, 1990. Eosinophilic meningitis in Thailand. Clinical and epidemiological characteristics of 162 patients with myeloencephalitis probably caused by *Gnathostoma spinigerum*. J. Neurol. Sci. 96:241–256

Punyagupta S, Juttijudata P, 1967. Gnathostomiasis in a case of eosinophilic myeloencephalitis. R. Thai. Army Med. J. 20:367–374

Punyagupta S, Limtrakul C, Vichipanthu P, Karuchancheta-nee C, Nye SW, 1968. Radiculomyeloencephalitis associated with eosinophilic pleocytosis. Report of nine cases. Am. J. Trop. Med. Hyg. 17:551–560

Radomyos P, Daengsvang S, 1987. A brief report on *Gnathostoma spinigerum* specimens obtained from human cases. Southeast Asian J. Trop. Med. Public Health 18:215–217

Ransom BH, 1923. A new case of *Gongylonema* from man. J. Parasitol. 9:244

Reddy CRRM, Valli VV, 1967. Extradural Guinea-worm abscess: report of two cases. Am. J. Trop. Med. Hyg. 16:23–25

Rossi-Espagnet A, Salera U, 1955. Infestazione da *Gongylonema pulchrum* nell'uomo. Riv. Parassitol. 16:221–224

Roussel L, 1987. Dracunculose lombaire. A propos d'un cas. Med. Trop. 47:89–90

Rysavy B, Sebek Z, Tenora F, 1969. The finding of *Gongylonema pulchrum* Molin, 1857 (Nematoda) in man. Folia Parasitol. 16:66

Sato H, Kamiya H, Hanada K, 1992. Five confirmed human cases of gnathostomiasis nipponica recently found in northern Japan. J. Parasitol. 78:1006–1010

Seal GN, Gupta AK, Das MK, 1969. Intra-ocular gnathostomiasis. J. All-India Ophthalmol. Soc. 17:109

Seguchi K, Matsuno M, Kataoka H, Kobayashi T, Maruyama H, Itoh H, Koono M, Nawa Y, 1995. A case report of colonic ileus due to eosinophilic nodular lesions caused by *Gnathostoma doloresi* infection. Am. J. Trop. Med. Hyg. 53:263–266

Sen K, Ghose N, 1945. Ocular gnathostomiasis. Br. J. Ophthalmol. 29:618–626

Sirikulchayanonta V, Chongchitnant N, 1979. Gnathostomisis, a possible etiologic agent of eosinophilic granuloma of the gastrointestinal tract. Am. J. Trop. Med. Hyg. 28:42–44

Sliwensky M, 1941. Drei Falle von *Gongylonema pulchrum* bei Erwachsenen in Bulgarien. Dtsch. Tropenmed. Z. 45:712–714

Srisawai P, Jongwutiwes S, Kulkumthorn M, 1988. Lingual gnathostomiasis: a case report. J. Med. Assoc. Thai. 71:285–288

Stiles CW, 1921a. A probable (third) case of *Gongylonema hominis* infection in man. US. Public Health Rep. 36:1177–1178

Stiles CW, 1921b. A third case of *Gongylonema* from man. J. Parasitol. 7:197

Stiles CW, Baker CE, 1928. A fifth case of *Gongylonema hominis* in man in the United States. JAMA 91:1891–1892

Stowens D, Simon G, 1981. Gnathostomiasis in Oneida County. NY. State J. Med. 81:409–410

Taniguchi Y, Ando K, 1992. Human gnathostomiasis: successful removal of *Gnathostoma hispidum*. Int. J. Dermatol. 31:175–177

Taniguchi T, Katsuhiko A, 1994. Creeping eruption due to larvae of the suborder Spirurina—A newly recognized causative parasite. Int. J. Dermatol. 33:279–281

Tansuphasiri P, 1974. Corneal perforation from *Gnathostoma spinigerum*. A case report [in Thai. English summary]. Siriraj Hosp. Gaz. 26:2111–2119

Tesjaroen S, Wongkongsawat T, Parichatikanond P, 1990. A breast mass caused by gnathostomiasis: brief report of a case. Southeast Asian J. Trop. Med. Public Health 21:151–153

Thomas LJ, 1952. *Gongylonema pulchrum*, a spirurid nematode infecting man in Illinois, USA. Proc. Helminthol. Soc. Wash. 19:124–126

Thuraisingam V, Peter Tan EA, Sandosham AA, 1969. A presumptive case of gnathostomiasis in Malaysia. Med. J. Malaya 24:107–111

Tudor C, Blair E, 1971. *Gnathostoma spinigerum*: an unusual cause of ocular nematodiasis in the Western Hemisphere. Am. J. Ophthalmol. 72:185–190

Verma AK, 1966. Ocular dracunculosis. J. Indian Med. Assoc. 47:188

Verma AK, 1968. Ocular dracontiasis. Int. Surg. 50:508–509

Vibulseth S, Leelarasamee A, 1980. A case of pulmonary gnathostomiasis. Siriraj Hosp. Gaz. 32:23–24

Visudhiphan P, Chiemchanya S, Somburanasim Ra, 1980. Causes of spontaneous subarachnoid hemorrhage in Thai infants and children. J. Neurosurg. 53:185–187

Waite CH, Gorrie R, 1935. A *Gongylonema* infestation in man. JAMA 105:23–24

Ward HB, 1916. *Gongylonema* in the role of a human parasite. J. Parasitol. 2:119–125

Watts SJ, 1987. Dracunculiasis in Africa in 1986: its geographic extent, incidence, and at-risk population. Am. J. Trop. Med. Hyg. 37:119–125

Weber G, MacHe K, 1973. Uber Hauterscheinungen bei *Gongylonema pulchrum* seine Erstbeobachtung in Deutschland beim Menschen. Hautarzt 24:286–288

Witemberg G, 1951. Some unusual observations on helminthiasis in Israel. Harefuah 41:178–180

Yospaiboon Y, Sithithavorn P, Maleewong V, Ukosanakarn U, Bhaibulaya M, 1989. Ocular thelaziasis in Thailand: a case report. J. Med. Assoc. Thai. 72:469–473

Young MD, Hayne I, 1953. *Gongylonema* infection in South Carolina. Report of a case. JAMA 151:40

Zaman V, Connor DH, Ahmed M, 1985. A dracunculosis case with unusual presentation from Pakistan. Short communication. Acta Trop. 42:195–196

19

SPIRURIDA—FILARIAE OF THE LYMPHATICS

The superfamily Filarioidea is one of the largest superfamilies of the order Spirurida, with genera and species inhabiting almost every tissue, organ system, and body cavity of vertebrates. One family, the Onchocercidae, contains all the genera with species parasitic in humans: *Wuchereria*, *Brugia*, *Onchocerca*, *Loa*, *Mansonella*, *Dirofilaria*, and *Meningonema*. Two biologic aspects of filariids are as follows: (*1*) their developmental life cycle, like that of most spiruriids, requires an invertebrate intermediate host, and (*2*) they produce a *microfilaria*, an intermediate stage (embryo) between the egg and the fully developed larva. Females lay microfilariae in the tissues or body fluids of the host. In some species, the microfilariae retain the egg membrane, which becomes an elongated envelope for them. In other species, the microfilariae break out and shed the membrane, resulting in *sheathed* or *unsheathed* microfilariae, respectively.

From the site of their release, microfilariae enter the general blood circulation or the skin, where they are ingested during the blood meal of a suitable arthropod intermediate host. Each species of filariid has its own specific vectors in which the microfilariae develop to third-stage infective larvae. The larvae eventually locate in the mouthparts of the arthropod, from which they enter the new host during its next blood meal. Development of the young filariids begins soon after they enter the new host. Eventually the worms migrate to their own specific tissue or organ system, where they reach maturity (Fig. 19–1).

Almost two dozen species of filariids have been recorded in humans at various times. For some of these filariids, humans are their only natural host; for others, both humans and animals are suitable natural hosts; still other filariids that occur naturally in animals may invade humans accidentally. This last group are the zoonotic filariids, which in humans usually do not attain full maturity (i.e., do not grow to adults and produce microfilariae). In this discussion, the filariae are organized according to the tissue or the organ system they inhabit in the final host. This approach is used for didactic purposes because it is useful for pathologists and diagnosticians. In this chapter the lymphatic filariae, *Wuchereria* and *Brugia*, are discussed. In Chapter 20 the filariae inhabiting subcutaneous tissues and body cavities—*Onchocerca*, *Loa*, *Mansonella*, and some species of *Dirofilaria*—are covered. In Chapter 21, the filariae of lungs, brain, eye, and other sites—*Dirofilaria*, *Meningonema*, and others—are discussed.

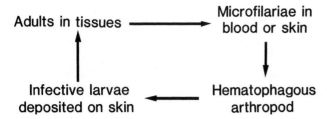

Fig. 19–1. Schematic representation of the general life cycle of filarial worms infecting man. Almost any tissue in the body can be parasitized by one or more species of filariids.

Wuchereria and *Brugia*— Lymphatic Folariasis

Wuchereria and *Brugia* are referred to as the *lymphatic filariae* because the diseases they produce occur mostly in the lymphatic system, resulting in elephantiasis. Elephantiasis is one of the most important infectious diseases in the tropics and subtropics because of the large number of individuals infected and because of the morbidity it produces in endemic areas. Species belonging to two genera, *Wuchereria* and *Brugia*, are responsible for elephantiasis; *Wuchereria* has only one species, *W. bancrofti*, which is highly specific for humans; no animal reservoirs are known. *Brugia* has several species, some of which are endemic in both animals and humans, for example *B. malayi* and *B. timori* (described by Partono et al. 1977). Several other species of *Brugia* are primarily enzootic (in animals) and produce zoonotic infections in humans. Since the diseases produced by *W. bancrofti*, *B. malayi*, and *B. timori* (Dennis et al. 1976; Partono et al. 1977) are generally similar both clinically and physiopathologically, they will be considered together in the following paragraphs, followed by a discussion of the zoonotic *Brugia* infections.

Morphology. *Wuchereria bancrofti*, *B. malayi*, and *B. timori* are small, filiform, and whitish in color, with delicate bodies that make them difficult to isolate from tissues for study. The female of *W. bancrofti* is 80 to 100 mm long by 240 to 300 μm wide, and the male is 40 mm long by 100 μm wide. The female of *B. malayi* is 43 to 55 mm long by 130 to 170 μm wide, and the male is 13 to 20 mm long by 70 to 80 μm wide. The female of *B. timori* is 30 mm long by 100 μm wide, and the male is 20 mm long by 70 μm wide (Beaver et al. 1984). The size of these worms is provided here only to give a general idea of their dimensions. The diame-

ter is especially important because it is helpful in identifying these worms in tissue sections. Other morphologic features that allow differentiation between the species are outside the scope of this discussion.

The microfilariae of *Wuchereria* and *Brugia* are sheathed (Figs. 19–2 and 19–3; *color plate* VIII A–B) and occur in blood (microfilaremia) in variable concentrations throughout the 24-hour period. *Wuchereria bancrofti* and *B. malayi* have two biologic variants. One variant produces microfilaremia that peaks between 10:00 P.M. and 2:00 A.M., with virtual disappearance of microfilariae during the rest of the day, a phenomenon termed *nocturnal periodicity*. The other variant produces a more or less continuous microfilaremia during the 24-hour period, with a slight increase at certain times of the day or night, for which the termed *subperiodic* is used. *Wuchereria bancrofti* is diurnal subperiodic in some areas of the Pacific and

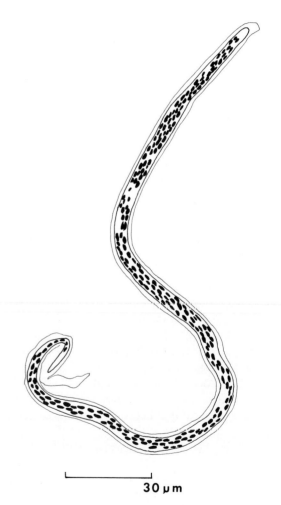

Fig. 19–2. *Wuchereria* bancrofti microfilaria, scale drawing from a thick blood smear made from Knott's concentration and stained with iron hematoxylin stain.

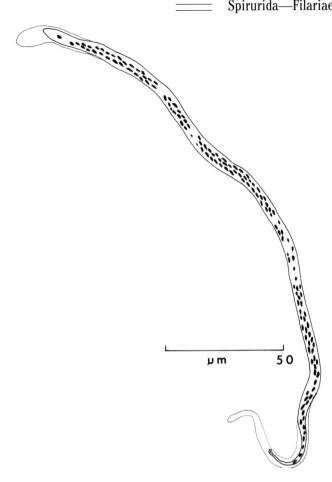

Fig. 19–3. *Brugia malayi* microfilaria, scale drawing from a thick blood smear made from a Knott's concentration and stained with iron hematoxylin stain.

nocturnal periodic elsewhere. The variant of *B. malayi* that occurs naturally in animals is nocturnal subperiodic, and the variant adapted to humans is nocturnal periodic. *Brugia timori* is nocturnal periodic. When the microfilariae are not in the circulatory system, they are lodged in the capillary bed of the lungs. The nocturnal periodicity of microfilariae has been extensively studied in both animals and humans. It was found to be related to differences in oxygen concentration in venous and arterial blood during resting and active periods. In addition, if the difference in venous arterial oxygen tension is less than 50 mm Hg, the microfilariae leave the lungs and enter the general circulation (Hawking et al. 1964).

Life Cycle. The life cycles of the lymphatic filariae have many similarities that allow some generalizations (Fig. 19–4). The vectors are several species of mosquitoes of the genera *Culex, Anopheles, Aedes,* and *Mansonia.*

Each endemic area of the world has different species of mosquitoes that serve as vectors. One common characteristic of the mosquitoes that serve as the main vectors is that they have a peak feeding period that coincides with the peak microfilaremia in the host. Once the mosquito ingests the microfilariae, their transformation into infective larvae begins. The microfilariae migrate to the thoracic muscles of the mosquito, where they remain until their transformation is completed; then they migrate to the mouthparts. The infective larvae remain in the mouthparts of the mosquito until they take their next blood meal; then they move to the skin and enter the host to mature into adults. In the final host, *W. bancrofti* requires approximately 1 year to develop from infective larvae to adults capable of producing microfilariae; *Brugia* takes about 2 months.

Geographic Distribution and Epidemiology. The geographic distribution of lymphatic filariae is shown in Figures 19–5 and 19–6. The prevalence of the infection is difficult to assess in spite of surveys made in every endemic area of the world. The problem is that surveys of microfilaremic individuals miss the amicrofilaremic ones, and assessments of elephantiasis miss the individuals with few symptoms. Whenever all these factors are assessed, the number of infected individuals is found to be greater than was previously estimated (Bundy et al. 1991; Kar, 1986; Katamine, 1966). The World Health Organization estimates that there are 2.7 billion persons living in countries where lymphatic filariasis is endemic; 1 billion of them are at risk of contracting the infection, and approximately 90 million are microfilaremic (WHO, 1984). In an autopsy study of the scrotal organs of 330 males over 10 years of age in Puerto Rico during the early 1960s, worms were found in 24%. The number of worms varied from one to seven, and they were located in the cord, the epididymis, or the testis; only 6% of the 191 worms studied were alive (Galindo et al. 1962). A survey of over 20,000 individuals living in many small communities in Thailand showed that 2.3% of them were microfilaremic and that elephantiasis occurred in 1.3%. The

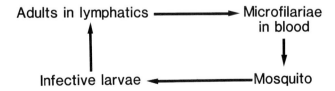

Fig. 19–4. *Wuchereria* and *Brugia,* schematic representation of the life cycle of lymphatic filariae.

area with the highest endemicity had an infection rate of 14%, which was considered moderate; the rate of microfilaremia was 11%, and that of elephantiasis was over 3% (Harinasuta et al. 1970).

Wuchereria bancrofti was introduced with the slave trade to some areas of South Carolina, Florida, and probably other southern states of the United States. The last known focus of endemicity was Charleston, South Carolina, where the last infected person was seen in 1930. The reasons for the disappearance of the infection have been widely discussed; the poor transmission capability of the local vector, *Culex quinquefasciatus*, is probably the main factor. The construction of a municipal sewage-water system, begun in 1890, probably helped by eliminating polluted domestic water, the preferred breeding place of the vector (Chernin, 1987).

Clinical Findings. The clinical manifestations of lymphatic filariasis vary, depending on the geographic area, the susceptibility of the infected person, and the duration of the infection. However, it is possible that the observed differences in the disease among geographic areas are distortions due to the methodology used to assess the infection, the disease, and the microfilaremia (Bundy et al. 1991). A few studies on the clinical manifestations produced by *B. malayi* have been carried out (Bonne et al. 1941; Dondero et al. 1972; Rao, 1945; Seo, 1978), showing that the morbidity (Lie, Sandosham, 1969) and distribution of lesions (Edeson, 1972) in *Brugia* infections are somewhat different from those of *Wuchereria* infections. Often the urogenital system is spared in *Brugia* infections (Dondero et al. 1971, 1972). It has been suggested that the difference in the distribution of the lesions corresponds to the anatomical distribution of the worms due to differences in the biting habits of the vectors (Wharton, 1962). In both *Wuchereria* and *Brugia* infections, the symptoms and the disease processes are modulated by the interaction between the parasite and the host. "The spectrum of disease pictures [varies] from one of severe clinical manifestations without microfilaremia, which is disadvantageous to both parasite and host, to one of asymptomatic microfilaremia, which is advantageous to the parasite and well tolerated by the host" (Beaver et al. 1984, p. 360). In addition to classical filariasis that results from the inflammatory reaction to the par-

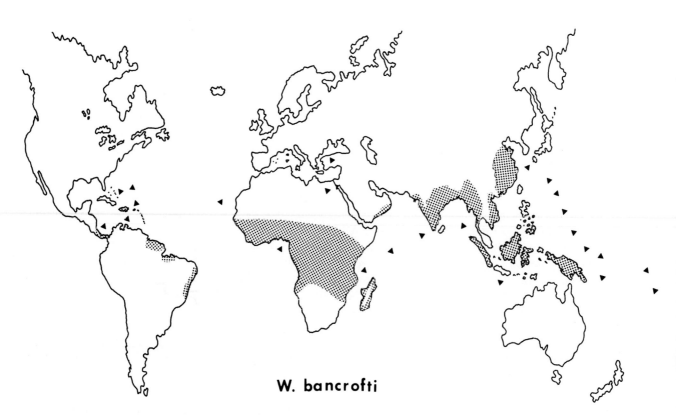

W. bancrofti

Fig. 19–5. Geographic distribution of lymphatic filariae. *Wuchereria bancrofti*. (Redrawn and printed with permission. In: WHO. 1984. Lymphatic Filariasis. Technical Report Series No. 702. Geneva: World Health Organization.)

asites in the lymphatics, leading to lymphadenitis, lymphangitis, lymphedema, and finally elephantiasis, two other diseases are recognized. One disease is an allergic hyperresponsiveness to dead microfilariae in the lungs, with marked inflammation leading to pulmonary manifestations, known as *tropical eosinophilia* (see below). The second disease is an inflammatory response to dead microfilariae in the lymph nodes and spleen resulting in their enlargement, known as the *Meyers-Kouwenaar syndrome* (see below). In addition, the acute and chronic phases of both diseases have distinct clinical manifestations.

Acute Infection. As stated, the prepatent period of the infection lasts for about 1 year from the time the infective larvae enter the skin and microfilariae appear in the circulation. In endemic areas the first infections occur at an early age, but they are seldom symptomatic. In some areas where bancroftian filariasis occurs, the bouts of adenolymphangitis begin at 6 years of age and

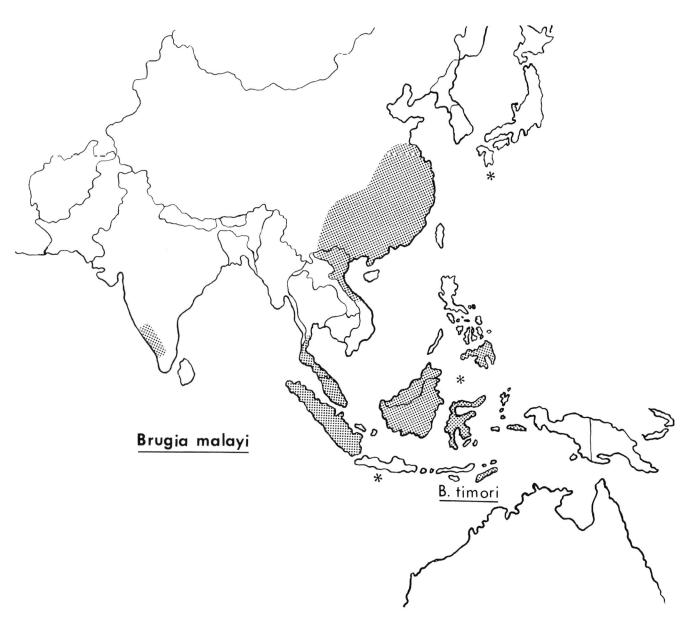

Fig. 19–6. Geographic distribution of lymphatic filariae. *Brugia malayi* and *B. timori*. (Redrawn and printed with permission. In: WHO. 1984. Lymphatic Filariasis. Technical Report Series No. 702. Geneva: World Health Organization.)

occur two or three times per year, becoming most intense by the age of 25. In brugian filariasis, the disease may manifest as early as 2 years of age. The acute symptoms of local adenolymphangitis in bancroftian and brugian filariasis are similar, and are usually associated with systemic symptoms of malaise and fever. The episodes of adenolymphangitis last for 3 to 15 days and resolve spontaneously. The lymphangitis is always retrograde, beginning in the axilla, elbows, or groin and descending slowly (Coggeshall, 1946). The lymph node enlargement is usually painless and occurs anywhere in the body; bancroftian filariasis in males may affect the lymphatics of the genitalia, leading to funiculitis, epididymitis, and orchitis. The spermatic cord is easily palpable and may become painful, without signs of an acute process; hydrocele commonly develops. Swelling of the axillary, breast, or arm lymph nodes (Rao, Maplestone, 1940) is sometimes the predominant presentation of brugian filariasis (WHO, 1984); genital involvement is observed less often (Rao, 1945; Seo, 1978). Finally, peripheral eosinophilia is not significant compared with that of uninfected members of the community (Dondero et al. 1971).

Filariasis without Microfilaremia. The clinical picture of filariasis without microfilaremia is seen primarily in persons from nonendemic locations who enter endemic areas and become infected. The initial acute symptoms of the disease in these individuals (immune virgins) occur sooner, manifesting long before the worms become adults and begin producing microfilariae (Beaver, 1970). The early symptoms in these patients are due to the tissue reaction to worm cuticles shed during molting and other worm secretions (Lie, Sandosham, 1969). The symptoms are variable; for example, of 62 servicemen who were exposed for 1 year and developed symptoms, there were genital manifestations in 47. Superficial lymphangitis and lymphadenitis of the extremities occurred in 13, involvement of the deep lymphatics in 1, and microfilaremia without symptoms in 1; one-fourth of all patients had multiple lesions (Hodge et al. 1945). Of the servicemen who lived under endemic conditions for 1 year, 85% developed signs and symptoms of filariasis (Behm, Hayman, 1946). Removal from the endemic area limits the disease due to lack of reinfection, but bouts of symptoms recur several times during a period of no more than 1 to 1½ years after the initial infection. Examination of peripheral blood for microfilariae is negative in the vast majority of cases, and complete resolution without sequelae is the rule (Beaver, 1970; Wartman, 1947). Removal and examination of the enlarged lymph nodes revealed the worms in 5 of 17 cases examined; most of the worms were dead (Wartman, 1944).

Chronic Infection. The chronic stage of the disease develops in some patients, while others may remain microfilaremic and asymptomatic for many years. The chronic disease usually develops 10 to 15 years later in persons exposed continuously to reinfection. The repeated bouts of adenolymphangitis damage the lymphatic vessels, causing retention of lymph that results in lymphedema, transient at first but becoming chronic and more pronounced as time passes. The extent of the damage is determined more accurately in vivo by lymphangiography (Tan et al. 1985). The chronic insult to the lymph nodes and the lymphatics results in sclerosis, fibrosis, and calcification of the lymph nodes, and the chronic accumulation of lymph leads to elephantiasis (*color plate* VIII *G–I*). Bancroftian filariasis may result in hydrocele and elephantiasis of the scrotum in some areas (*color plate* VIII *I*); elephantiasis of the leg, arm, penis, vulva, and breast are also seen. Compromise of the internal abdominal lymph nodes results in chyluria and microfilaruria. Brugian filariasis produces similar syndromes, often with less genital involvement and less disease (Rao, 1945). In certain endemic areas, some individuals have necrosis of the lymph nodes, abscess formation, and suppuration (Kar, 1986), sometimes with superimposed bacterial infections. Symptomatic lymphatic filariasis usually manifests with very low levels of microfilaremia. Asymptomatic individuals in endemic areas may have detectable microfilaremia, indicating that infection and disease do not necessarily occur together and that some special susceptibility is probably present in those who develop symptoms.

Immunity. The immunology of lymphatic filariasis has been studied in animal models, especially for species of *Brugia*, because cats and other animals are susceptible to the infection. Less work has been done both in humans and in infections with *Wuchereria*. The pioneer studies of Denham and coworkers in the 1970s concerning infections of cats with *B. pahangi* are of interest in understanding the immunopathology of the infection (Denham et al. 1972; Denham, McGreevy, 1977). Denham and coworkers infected cats up to 50 times with 50 larvae at 10-day intervals. All animals developed an infection with detectable microfilariae in the blood. As time went by, the animals were separated into two groups: one group remained microfilaremic throughout, while the other group suddenly became amicrofilaremic. In most cases, the microfilaremic animals were susceptible to challenge with the 50 infective larvae, though a few were resistant; however, all animals in this group had live worms in their lymphatics at necropsy.

The second group, the amicrofilaremic animals, responded in two ways to the infection: (1) some animals had live worms in the lymphatics and were resistant to all challenges with the 50 larvae (only 1% of infective larvae were recovered 1 day after inoculation versus up to 60% of infective larvae in control animals) and (2) other animals had no live worms. On challenge with infective larvae they were resistant, and if inoculated with microfilariae into their bloodstream, they showed a detectable microfilaremia for only 1 hour (control animals had detectable disease for up to 3 weeks) and developed an anaphylactic reaction (Denham, McGreevy, 1977). The resistance of the animals to challenge with the parasite was due to a specific acquired immunity elicited by all stages of the parasite. However, since cats infected with *B. pahangi* develop only transient lymphedema and never elephantiasis, it is not possible to determine whether the immune response in the animals modulates production of the lesions.

Lymphocyte transformation in the presence of antigens in vitro, using lymphocytes from infected patients, gave results that somewhat paralleled those in the cats. Lymphocytes from patients with elephantiasis alone (amicrofilaremic) reacted against adult worm antigen, while lymphocytes from none of the other patients with other forms of the disease did so. Normal subjects from the endemic area without the disease or microfilariae, plus one-half of those with disease and microfilariae, responded to microfilaria antigens. The majority of patients with microfilaremia did not respond to microfilaria antigens (Piessens et al. 1980a). Studies on the presence of antibodies against the sheath of *Brugia* microfilariae in these individuals showed that the presence of the antibodies (IgG and IgM) correlated with the absence of microfilariae in the blood. In addition, cell-mediated reaction to microfilariae antigens occurred in the absence of filarial antibodies, but no cellular reaction was seen in the presence of these antibodies (Piessens et al. 1980b).

Taken together, the findings of these studies indicate that in lymphatic filariasis a state of profound unresponsiveness or immunologic tolerance to adult worms and microfilaria exists in microfilaremic individuals who are asymptomatic (Maizels, Lawrence, 1991). This state of tolerance is not maintained by all individuals and over time it tends to break down (natural evolution of the infection), probably due to continuous reinfections that result in disease. This gradual breakdown of tolerance is demonstrated in epidemio-

logic studies in which the total prevalence of disease approximated the cumulative proportion of the population that had been microfilaremic in the past (Bundy et al. 1991). Therefore, at any given time in endemic areas, there are three groups of individuals: (1) those who are immune to the infection and the disease (no symptoms, no microfilariae); (2) those tolerant to the disease (no symptoms, but microfilariae present), moving with time and repeated reinfections to the next group; and (3) those with an abnormal immune response who have adenolymphangitis and are progressing to elephantiasis (Bundy et al. 1991; Maizels, Lawrence, 1991; Ottesen, 1984).

It has been suggested that the main forces driving the development of tolerance are the microfilariae, either in the active infection (Maizels et al. 1995) or in utero when the microfilariae of an infected mother cross the placenta and expose the fetus to microfilarial antigens (Eberhard et al. 1993b). Transplacental passage of microfilariae has been documented (Bloomfield et al. 1978; Brinkmann et al. 1976) and explains why children born to infected mothers are three times more likely to develop infection than those born to uninfected mothers (Lammie et al. 1991). The tolerance that develops to lymphatic filariasis is not total because production of antibodies (IgE and IgG4) continues (Kwan-Lim et al. 1990), indicating that the hyporesponsiveness is limited to the T helper 1 (Th1) cell subpopulation of T lymphocytes (Maizels et al. 1995; Maizels, Lawrence, 1991). And, as stated above, this tolerance is reversed by the progression of the infection, but also by treatment, and return of responsiveness results in disease, the mechanism of which is unknown. The IgG1, IgG2, and IgG3 isotypes of specific antibodies somehow appear to mediate the modulation of disease (Maizels et al. 1995).

Pathology. The histopathologic picture of bancroftian and brugian filariasis is essentially similar (Lie, Sandosham, 1969), is related to the presence of adult worms in the lymph channels and lymph nodes, and is identical regardless of the body site. Lymph nodes removed from patients with clinical filarial lymphadenitis are moderately to markedly enlarged, firm, and often fibrotic or with small areas of calcification. Adjacent lymph nodes may be matted, forming larger masses; on section, the node usually appears abnormal, and sometimes foci of macroscopic necrosis are visible. Lymph nodes from individuals with advanced disease are markedly fibrotic and calcified. The soft tissues affected by elephantiasis are firm and on section are whitish, with a wet appearance and multiple foci of adipose tissue.

Microscopically, the lymphatic channels and lymph nodes have variable amounts of inflammatory reaction, depending on the duration of the infection (Fig. 19–7 A–D, 19–8 A–D, and *color plate* VIII C–D). Nodes with well-preserved worms usually show parasites within distended subcapsular sinuses (Fig. 19–8 B). The node is hyperplastic, with abundant lymphocytes, plasma cells, and variable numbers of polymorphonuclear leukocytes, especially eosinophils (Fig. 19–9 B). Often the parasites are found in lymph channels outside the nodes, where eventually they provoke a chronic inflammatory reaction with formation of lymphoid aggregates and germinal centers similar to those of lymph nodes (Fig. 19–7 A–B).

Lymph nodes with dead worms (Fig. 19–8 C) are more common. They show necrosis and infiltration by polymorphonuclear cells, histiocytes, and granulomas with giant cells containing fragments of parasites (Fig. 19–7 D). Charcot-Leyden crystals and abundant eosinophils occur often. In lymph nodes from individuals living in endemic areas, worms in different stages of degeneration and calcification are sometimes found; in other areas, live worms are seen. This pattern indicates that reinfection is occurring continuously. Deposition of minerals with eventual calcification occurs in dead worms (Figs. 19–7 C–D and 19–8 D). These changes have often been observed in clinical material from human patients (Jungmann et al. 1991; Lichtenberg, 1957) and experimental animals with brugian filariasis. However, the early inflammatory reactions in humans, those beginning with arrival of young parasites in the lymphatics, have not been described. Nor is it known what factor or factors modulate the tissue response that results in elephantiasis in some patients, while others are unresponsive and develop a benign infection manifested only by microfilariae in their blood.

Other Sites. Thickening of the spermatic cord (funiculitis) is due to lymphangitis, lymphadenitis, and fibrosis of the lymphatics of the cord. Thickening of the tunica albuginea is usually due to inflammation, fibrosis, and formation of granulomas with multinucleated foreign body giant cells. In the breast, solitary nodules, usually lymphoid in nature, with dead, degenerating, or calcified worms are common in some areas (Lang et al. 1987; Yeuhan, Qun, 1981). Recovery of juvenile and adult *W. bancrofti* and *B. malayi* from the eye has been reported (Bhagwat et al. 1973; Wright et al. 1935). A *W. bancrofti* adult was identified in a branch of the pulmonary artery in an infarct-like lesion of the lung (see Fig. 21–7; Beaver, Cran, 1974), as were a *B. malayi* adult (Case Records of the Massachusetts General Hospital, 1974) and a *B. malayi*-like adult (Fig. 21–7; Beaver et al. 1971). Both brugias were alive in the branches of the pulmonary artery, eliciting an endarteritis that was probably the cause of the infarction; both patients had lived in India for many years. A glomerulonephritis due to deposition of soluble antigen–antibody complexes has been observed in some patients with *Wuchereria* infections (Ormerod et al. 1983; Waugh et al. 1980). In many cases, filariids have been recovered from the eyes of patients living in endemic areas. In most of these cases, identification of the worm was based on circumstantial evidence (see Chapter 21).

Microscopically, the soft tissues affected by elephantiasis show large amounts of collagenous tissues (fibroplasia) with interspersed islands of fat cells. A chronic mononuclear cell infiltrate occurs throughout in small foci, sometimes around small and medium-sized blood vessels (Fig. 19–9 A–B).

Diagnosis. The diagnosis of lymphatic filariasis is usually made on clinical grounds, especially in endemic areas. It should be kept in mind that lymphadenitis is nonspecific and that in populations that walk barefoot, this is a common condition of the lower extremities. Lymphedema and elephantiasis have etiologies other than filariasis, and these must be ruled out before a diagnosis of lymphatic filariasis is made. In areas of Africa, nonendemic elephantiasis (podoconiosis) is common (De Lalla et al. 1988). Lymphadenitis and some degree of lymphedema are also manifestations of *Onchocerca volvulus* in some patients (see Chapter 20).

Fig. 19–7. *Brugia malayi* **in a cat infected experimentally, sections stained with hematoxylin and eosin stain. A, Low-power view of a greatly dilated popliteal lymphatic channel, containing several *B. malayi* adults. Note the beginning of an inflammatory infiltrate surrounding the vessel, ×70. B, Higher magnification illustrating different cross sections of a male *Brugia* and the infiltrate composed mainly of mononuclear cells (lymphocytes and plasma cells) and eosinophils, ×180. C,** Older infection in another animal illustrating the usual fate of the parasite: death, disintegration, and calcification. Note that the parasites now appear to be located within a lymph node, the formation of which is the usual host response to the worm, ×55. *D,* Higher magnification showing a granuloma with a dead worm and calcification, ×220. (Preparations courtesy of A. Ewert, Ph.D., Department of Microbiology, University of Texas Medical Branch, Galveston, Texas.)

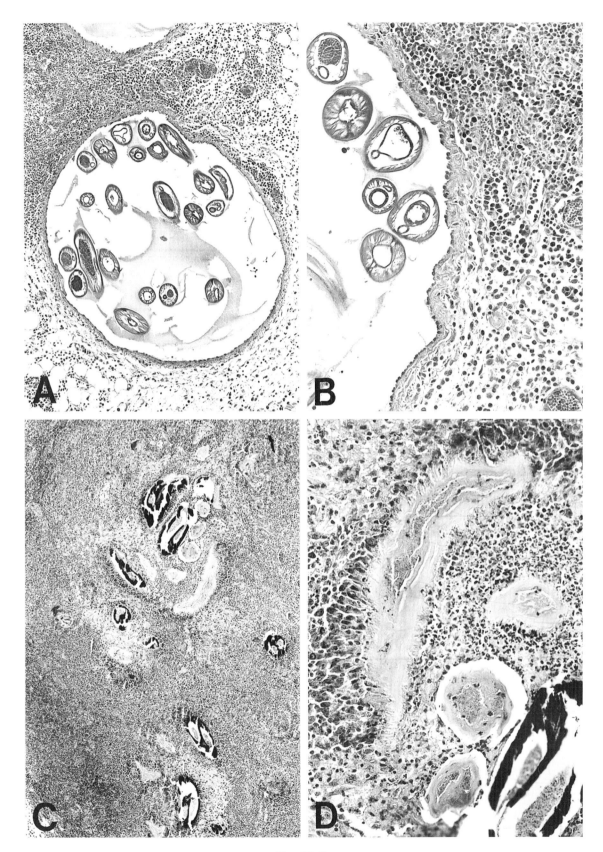

Fig. 19–7.

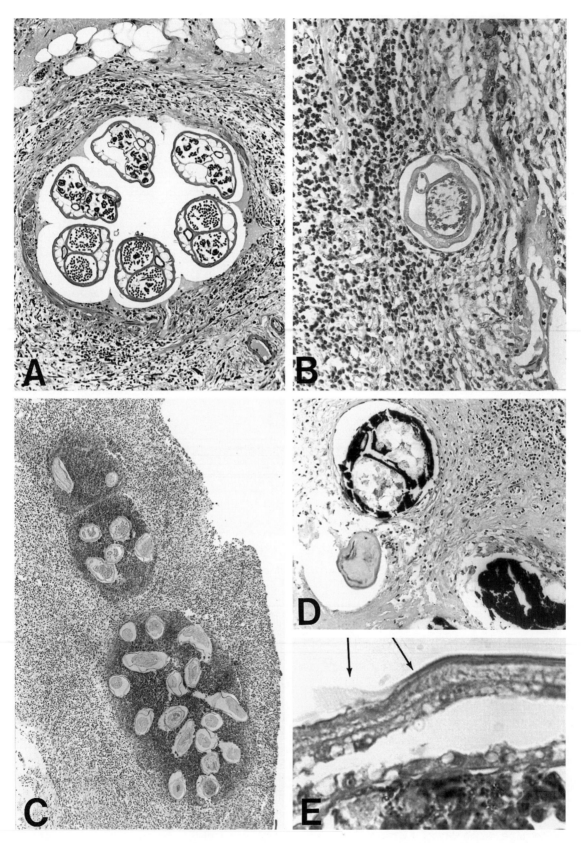

Fig. 19–8. *Wuchereria bancrofti* in humans, sections stained with hematoxylin and eosin stain. *A*, Low-power view of cross sections of a living adult female in the lymph channel of the epididymis, ×110. *B*, Male worm in a lymph node from another case, ×220. *C*, Dead worms in a lymph node, ×55. *D*, Calcified worms, ×140. *E*, Longitudinal section showing minute transverse striations of the cuticle (arrows), ×1,000.

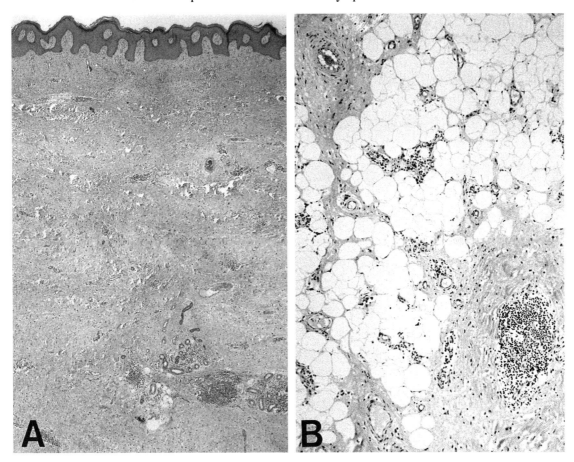

Fig. 19–9. *Wuchereria bancrofti*, histologic sections of tissues from patients with elephantiasis stained with hematoxylin and eosin stain. *A*, Low-power view of dermis from a patient with elephantiasis showing significant thickening, ×22. *B*, The subcutaneous tissue are composed of islands of adipose tissue among fibrous connective tissue and chronic inflammatory cells, ×70.

Individuals who contract lymphatic filariasis after visiting or living temporarily in endemic areas usually do not have detectable circulating microfilariae. In view of the benign course of the disease in these patients, a clinical diagnosis and follow-up may suffice.

Blood samples to search for the microfilariae of *Wuchereria* and *Brugia* should be collected between 10:00 P.M. and 2:00 A.M., when microfilaremia is highest. Thin and thick blood smears or smears from concentrated blood should be stained with Giemsa stain or periodic acid–Schiff hematoxylin stain for detailed study of the morphologic features (Figs. 19–2 and 19–3), the only basis for specific identification of the parasites (Eberhard, Lammie, 1991). Artifacts are often mistaken for microfilariae in blood, in cytology smears, and even in fine needle aspirates (Dey, Walker, 1994). Concentration following the procedure described by Knott is easily done: 2 ml of heparinized blood is mixed well with 10 ml of 2% nonbuffered formalin and centrifuged for a few minutes. The aqueous formalin lyses the red blood cells and fixes the microfilariae more or less in an uncoiled position. The supernatant is then discarded, and the sediment is used for direct examination. Both thick and thin smears should be stained. Other concentration techniques use membranes for filtration, such as Millipore and Nuclepore filters (Eberhard, Lammie, 1991). However, these techniques are more involved than Knott's procedure, which can be used even by the most modest routine clinical laboratory.

The microfilariae can also be found in other fluids, such as urine in cases of chyluria, vaginal and cervical smears (Leong, 1971), nipple secretions (Lahiri, 1975), hydrocele fluid (Vassilakos, Cox, 1974), and fine needle aspiration specimens (Swarup et al. 1990). This is because microfilariae are found not only in the blood, but also in the tissues.

In the clinical laboratory, several serologic tests have been used for diagnosis, mostly to detect antibody to filarial antigens and circulating antigens in the blood of infected individuals. The serologic methods have serious limitations because they lack specificity, and detection of circulating antigen is not very sensitive. More recently, a polymerase chain reaction for detection of circulating parasite DNA, which is useful in seroepidemiologic studies of *W. bancrofti*, has been developed (Zhong et al. 1996)

In tissues, the size of the parasite at midbody on cross sections is usually helpful in distinguishing *Wuchereria* from *Brugia*. The maximum diameter of the female of *Wuchereria* is about 300 μm. It has a cuticle less than 1 μm thick on average (Fig. 19–8 A–B), except over the lateral cords, where an inward expansion of about 3 μm forms a low ridge. There are three or four muscle cells per quadrant. The contractile portion is 12 to 15 μm in height, which is less than one-half of the cell substance (Fig. 19–10 A–B). The lateral cords are wide, slightly

taller at some levels than the contractile muscle, and occupy 40% of the circumference of the worm (Fig. 19–10 A). They are divided into two distinct sublateral bands with one small nucleus each per histologic section (Fig. 19–10 A–B). The esophagus measures up to 25 μm in the anterior muscular portion and up to 75 μm in the glandular portion. The intestine measures about 20 μm, with an empty lumen, and has eight to ten epithelial cells per section, with poorly defined cell limits (Fig. 19–8 A). The most prominent structures are the paired uteri, usually filled with eggs (Fig. 19–10 A), maturing microfilariae (Fig. 19–10 B), or fully developed microfilariae (Figs. 19–8 B and 19–7 A–B; Beaver, Cran, 1974; Franz, Buttner, 1986).

The female of *B. malayi* has a maximum diameter of approximately 170 μm, and that of the *B. timori* female is 80 μm. The cuticle is thick in relation to the diameter of the worm compared to *Wuchereria*. The size of the worm in cross sections and the relative thick-

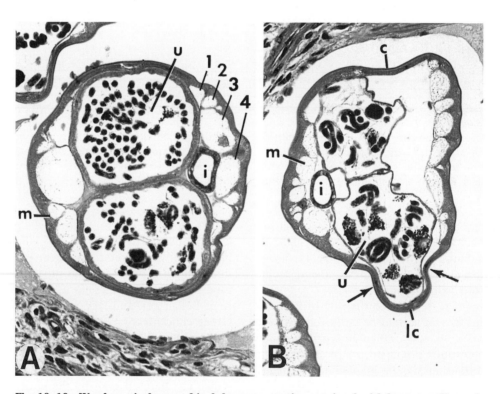

Fig. 19–10. *Wuchereria bancrofti* **adult worm, sections stained with hematoxylin and eosin stain. *A* and *B*, Cross sections of *W. bancrofti* at the midbody level. The two uteri (u) fill the cavity of the worm almost entirely. The uteri contain developing eggs in *A* and discernible microfilariae in *B*. The intestine (i) is about one-tenth the diameter of the worm at this level. The muscle cells (m), about four per quadrant (one to four), have a low contractile portion. The lateral cords (lc) are low and wide, with one or two nuclei per histologic section (arrows). The cuticle (c) is less than 1 μm thick. Both the thickness of the cuticle and the diameter in cross sections are the conspicuous features that allow the separation of *Wuchereria* and *Brugia*, ×385.**

ness of the cuticle are features that distinguish *Brugia* from *Wuchereria*. Other morphologic features of *Brugia* are similar to those of *Wuchereria*.

Tropical Eosinophilia

An intense peripheral eosinophilia was observed for many years in patients from areas where filariasis was endemic. The best clinical description of the condition referred to it as "a pseudo-tuberculous condition associated with eosinophilia" (Frimodt-Moller, Barton, 1940). Soon afterward, the term *tropical eosinophilia* (Shah, 1943) was used for the disease (Weingarten, 1943). The syndrome is produced by an abnormal host response, mainly in the lungs, to the microfilariae of *Wuchereria* and *Brugia* (Neva et al. 1975). The disease is therefore seen in endemic areas of these parasites, but the great majority of cases occur in India and in Southeast Asia in persons of Indian descent (Chaudhuri et al. 1956). Tropical eosinophilia also has been reported to a lesser extent from Indonesia (Danaraj, 1947), Africa (Sanjivi et al. 1952; Wilson, 1947), Egypt (Parsons-Smith, 1944; Stephan, 1946), Curaçao (Hartz, Van Der Sar, 1948), Brazil (Coutinho, 1956; Crandall et al. 1982), the Pacific Islands (Levin, 1956; Rifkin, Eberhard, 1946), Vietnam (Friess et al. 1953; Sullivan, 1970), British Guiana (Williams et al. 1960), and Puerto Rico (Diaz-Rivera et al. 1954). Sporadic cases have been described in Americans and Europeans after residing in one of the endemic areas (Appley, Grant, 1945; Casile, Floch, 1957; Hirst, McCann, 1945; Irwin, 1946). Three cases in American servicemen returning from the Pacific were referred to as *classical filariasis* (Coggeshall, 1946, p. 182). The condition was suspected to be filarial, because the patients were relieved by antifilarial therapy and usually had positive serologic tests against antigens of filarial worms. However, none of the patients with tropical eosinophilia had microfilaremia at any time, and adult filarial worms were never found in any area of the body. For these reasons, some authors felt that the name *occult filariasis* was more appropriate (Lie, 1962); still others used the term *eosinophilic lung* (Chakravarty, Roy, 1943; Danaraj, 1951).

Although the filarial nature of the condition was the accepted norm, the species of the worm responsible for the disease was debated because other species in animals were known to occur in the endemic areas of human filariasis. An animal filarial worm could explain the syndrome as a response to a parasite in an abnormal host; however, the predilection of the disease for persons of Indian extraction was not understood. Experimental infections in volunteers included *B. malayi* from a monkey, *B. pahangi* from a cat, and *B. malayi* from a human. In all volunteers, infections with these parasites were produced, with some features of tropical eosinophilia but not the full-blown syndrome (Buckley, 1958; Buckley, Wharton, 1961; Edeson et al. 1960). The best proof of the etiology of tropical eosinophilia was provided by the painstaking process of reviewing many histologic sections of pulmonary biopsy specimens from patients with the disease, finding the microfilariae, and recognizing the morphologic characteristics that allowed their identification (Danaraj et al. 1966).

Clinical Findings. The chief complaint is an insidious cough that rapidly becomes nocturnal and paroxysmal, lasting for periods ranging from several weeks to several months. The cough is dry or is accompanied by scant sputum and is frequently violent, producing vomiting; hemoptysis, if present, is minimal. These paroxysms occur for short periods interspersed with remissions, always returning in a few days or weeks (Ball, 1950; Danaraj, 1951). Each time the paroxysms return, they are more severe and last longer (eventually leading to dyspnea and orthopnea), resembling severe asthma and producing serious loss of sleep. Retrosternal chest pain aggravated by the cough is often present. Symptoms of tropical eosinophilia may first appear after 1 year of exposure to the infection (Dalrymple, 1955).

Physical examination reveals bronchitis, bronchiolitis, or asthma with dry, creaking, and medium to coarse crepitations at the bases. The patient's temperature varies between 35.7°C and 39.5°C. If fever is present, it lasts for about 1 week. Some patients may have adenopathies, with or without an enlarged spleen. Laboratory tests reveal eosinophilia of 2000 white blood cells, often over 10,000 per cubic millimeter. Chest radiograms show striations and mottling at the bases; serologic tests for filarial parasites are usually positive; microfilaremia is always absent.

Pathology. There are few reports on the microscopic appearance of the lungs in patients with tropical eosinophilia; most of them are based on pulmonary biopsy specimens because the disease is rarely fatal (Chaudhuri, Saha, 1961; Danaraj, 1959; Udwadia, Joshi, 1964; Viswanathan, 1947; Webb et al. 1960). On microscopic examination, the lung parenchyma has

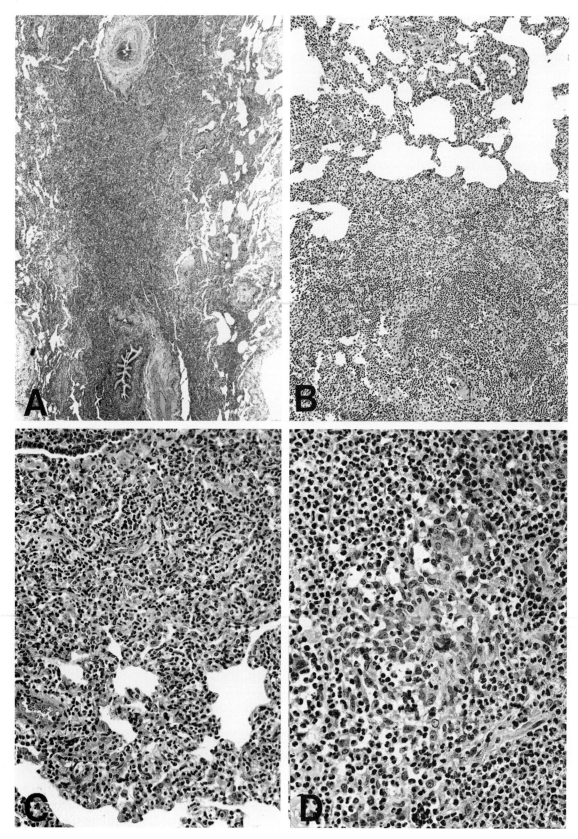

Fig. 19–11.

scattered areas of pneumonic infiltration (Fig. 19–11 A). The septae are thickened and congested, infiltrated by eosinophils, histiocytes, lymphocytes, and plasma cells (Fig. 19–11 B–C). The infiltrate extends to and fills the alveolar spaces, forming microabscesses composed of eosinophils (Fig. 19–11 B). In some areas there are poorly to well-formed granulomas, approximately 500 μm in diameter, with multinucleated giant cells interspersed with epithelioid cells, histiocytes, and fibroblasts (Fig. 19–11 D; Danaraj et al. 1966). In the center of some granulomas is an amorphous eosinophilic mass, which in experimental animals has been found to consist of periodic acid–Schiff–positive material deposited around a dead, degenerating microfilaria similar to the Hoeppli-Splendore phenomenon (Crandall et al. 1982). There are approximately five granulomas per square centimeter of histologic lung section, and each granuloma is 400 to 1600 μm in diameter (Danaraj et al. 1966).

The rest of the pulmonary parenchyma has various degrees of emphysema and atelectasis, other nonspecific inflammatory changes, and mild eosinophilic infiltration of the vessels. The smaller bronchi have a thick mucous exudate in the lumen and are surrounded by infiltration with eosinophils, but the lesions are located away from the bronchi, indicating that they do not represent a primary respiratory tract insult (bronchocentric). The lesions are usually located close to the pulmonary venules because the microfilariae are in the pulmonary capillary bed (Danaraj et al. 1966). Study of many sections of lung has revealed degenerating microfilariae of *Wuchereria* or *Brugia*; these microfilariae usually cannot be differentiated in tissue sections. Adult filarial parasites have not been recovered from patients with tropical eosinophilia.

Diagnosis. The diagnosis of tropical eosinophilia is usually made on clinical grounds. Microfilariae are not present in the circulation, and lung biopsy specimens are not necessary. Serologic tests for filariae are positive, and antifilarial therapy should improve the patient's condition.

Meyers-Kouwenaar Syndrome

Meyers-Kouwenaar syndrome consists of an enlargement of groups of lymph nodes and sometimes of the spleen, accompanied by high peripheral eosinophilia. The syndrome occurs exclusively in individuals living in endemic areas of lymphatic filariasis (Lie, Sandosham, 1969; Meyers, Kouwenaar, 1939). It is more prevalent in Southeast Asia, where *B. malayi* has higher endemicity, while tropical eosinophilia tends to occur where *W. bancrofti* is more prevalent. In India the condition is often seen in patients with tropical eosinophilia and is considered part of the clinical picture, but it also exists as an isolated entity (Dhayagude, 1945). In other areas, especially in Southeast Asia and the Pacific, enlargement of the lymph nodes and spleen is seen with or without tropical eosinophilia. Since the majority of patients do not have microfilariae in their circulation, and since adult worms are generally not found, the syndrome is considered another form of occult filariasis and is referred to as the *Meyers-Kouwenaar syndrome* (Beaver, 1970; Lie, 1962). The main groups of enlarged lymph nodes are the axilla, the inguinal, the cervical, and the epitrochlear lymph nodes, either singly or in any combination. Sometimes only one lymph node is enlarged. The nodes are painless, firm, sometimes movable, and soft, reaching a diameter of up to 5 cm. The lack of pain differentiates this adenopathy from that of classic filariasis, and the nodes do not suppurate.

Histologically, the lymph nodes are hyperplastic and show a benign lymphadenitis (Fig. 19–12 A) characterized by large numbers of eosinophils throughout the node (Fig. 19–12 B), forming microabscesses that eventually evolve to granulomas. The granulomas are in different stages of evolution, some with a dead mi-

---

Fig. 19–11. Tropical eosinophilia, sections of lung stained with hematoxylin and eosin stain. A, Low-power view of lung showing marked consolidation and infiltration by inflammatory cells. Note the medium-sized bronchus (bottom) and the blood vessel (top), neither of which is involved, ×28. B, Higher magnification showing a granuloma and a thickened septa, ×70. C, Higher magnification illustrating the nature of the infiltrate, consisting mainly of eosinophils and lymphocytes, ×178. D, Higher magnification of the granuloma showing histiocytes, eosinophils, and mononuclear cells, ×280. (Preparations courtesy of P.C. Beaver, Ph.D., School of Public Health and Tropical Medicine, Tulane University, New Orleans, Louisiana. Reported by: Danaraj, T.J., Pacheco, G., Shanmugaratnam, K., et al. 1966. The etiology and pathology of eosinophilic lung (tropical eosinophilia). Am. J. Trop. Med. Hyg. 15:183–189.)

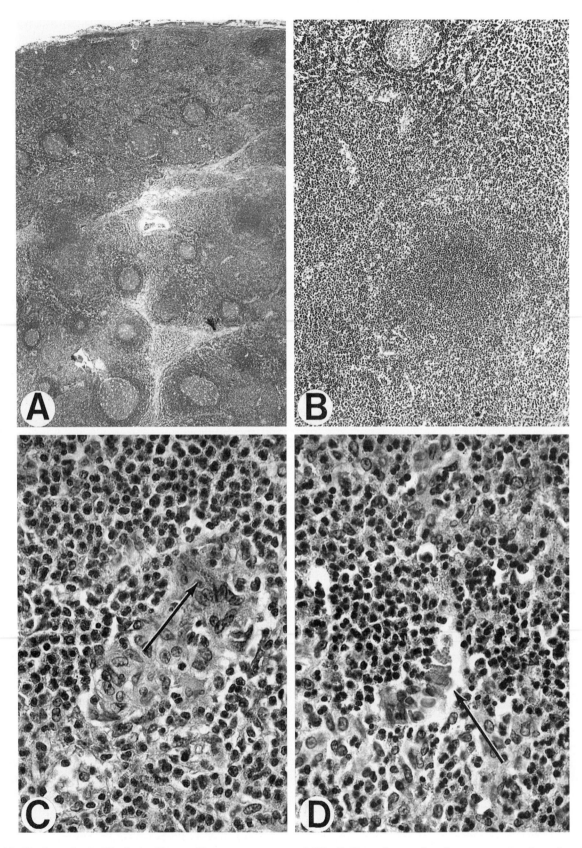

Fig. 19–12. Lymphatic filariasis, Meyers-Kouwenaar syndrome, sections stained with hematoxylin and eosin stain. *A*, Low-power view of a lymph node showing hyperplasia and microabscesses, ×9. *B*, Higher magnification showing a microabscess composed of eosinophils, ×75. *C*, Granuloma showing remnants of a microfilaria (arrow) phagocytized by a foreign body giant cell, ×340. *D*, Microabscess with an amorphous eosinophilic mass, the Meyers-Kouwenaar body, at the center (arrow), ×340.

crofilaria, others with a microfilaria in more advanced stages of degeneration (*color plate* VIII *E*). The final remnants of the microfilariae are an unrecognizable mass of eosinophilic, amorphous material similar to that seen in the lungs of patients with tropical eosinophilia (see above; Fig. 19–12 *C*). This amorphous material is referred to as the *Meyers-Kouwenaar body* (Fig. 19–12 *D* and *color plate* VIII *F*). Mature granulomas with foreign body giant cells are also seen (Bras, Lie, 1951; Crosnier et al. 1954; Friess et al. 1953).

Zoonotic *Brugia* Infection

Reports of infections with species of *Brugia* other than those occurring naturally in humans are now well known (Baird et al. 1986; Coolidge et al. 1979; Gutierrez, Petras, 1982; Orihel, Beaver, 1989). These cases of zoonotic *Brugia* have been found sporadically in several areas of the world but have been seen in greater numbers in the northeastern United States (Gutierrez, 1984; Harbut, Orihel, 1995). All known cases presented clinically as a benign lymphadenopathy that sometimes lasted for several months before the nodes became inflamed and painful. In one case, when the affected lymph node was removed, a histologic study found a living parasite in a patient who had a malignancy and was routinely checked when the enlarged, painless nodule was discovered (Gutierrez, Petras, 1982). In most other cases, the worm, always a sexually mature male or female, was dead and in the early or late stages of degeneration with morphologic characteristics of a *Brugia*. With the exception of an immune-suppressed infant in Oklahoma who presented with lymphedema and circulating microfilariae classified as *Brugia* (Simmons et al. 1984), none of these patients had microfilaremia.

The geographic location of the human cases in the United States is mainly the northeast (New Jersey, Massachusetts, Rhode Island, Ohio, Pennsylvania, and New York). However, cases have also been reported from Michigan (Eberhard et al. 1993a), Florida and California (Baird et al. 1986), Louisiana (Jung, Harris, 1960), and Oklahoma (Simmons et al. 1984). Infections outside the United States have been recorded in Colombia (Botero et al. 1965; Kozek et al. 1984), Ecuador, and Peru (Baird, Neafie, 1988). No adult worms have been retrieved in toto from humans, and all studies have been done in tissue sections. Two species of *Brugia*, perhaps three, are known to be indigenous in animals in the United States—*B. beaveri* in

raccoons (Ash, Little, 1964), *B. leporis* in wild rabbits (Eberhard, 1984), and a species of *Brugia* in a domestic cat in California (Beaver, Wong, 1988). *Brugia beaveri* is known only in the southeastern United States and *B. leporis* in the southeastern and northeastern areas; this writer has found it in 17% of wild rabbits examined in northeastern Ohio.

Pathology and Diagnosis. All lymph nodes are enlarged and nonadherent to the skin or deeper tissues. On section they appear hyperplastic, sometimes with necrotic areas. On microscopic examination, the salient features are the presence of the worm, with no reaction, eosinophilic granulomatous inflammation, or both. Intact, well-preserved worms are usually located in the subcapsular sinuses (Fig. 19–13 *A–D*; Gutierrez, Petras, 1982). The usual finding is a worm with different degrees of necrosis and degeneration (Coolidge et al. 1979), which sometimes makes its precise recognition and identification difficult (Fig. 18–14 *A–C*). There are foci of necrosis surrounded by abundant polymorphonuclear cells, especially eosinophils and histiocytes, and sometimes foreign body multinucleated giant cells are present. Some granulomas contain identifiable dead worms (Fig. 19–14 *A–C*), others only remnants seen as cuticular fragments (Fig. 19–14 *D*). One patient had a prominent monocytoid B-cell proliferation (Elenitoba-Johnson et al. 1996). In some sections, the distribution of the granulomas follows a subcapsular sinus. Sometimes the histologic picture only suggests a zoonotic *Brugia* (Fig. 19–15 *A–D*). The diagnostic characteristics of zoonotic *Brugia* in tissue sections are generally consistent with those of *B. malayi*, although minor differences have been described in the cuticular structure, the number of muscle cells, and the subcuticle (Orihel, Beaver, 1989). The diameter of the worm is the best distinguishing feature, being smaller than that of *B. malayi* (see above). The *Brugia* found in human lymph nodes in North America have a diameter of 50 to 120 μm for the female (average, 100 μm) and 35 to 55 μm for the male. The cuticle is about 1 μm thick, slightly more at the lateral cords; it is nonlayered and has minute transverse striae. The lateral cords are inconspicuous, and each cord occupies about 10% of the circumference of the worm. The most prominent feature is the paired uteri, sometimes filled with immature eggs, others appearing as empty tubes. There are usually three or four muscle cells per quadrant, with distinct contractile and cytoplasmic elements (Orihel, Beaver, 1989).

The species of *Brugia* found in animals in the United States have females with midbody diameters

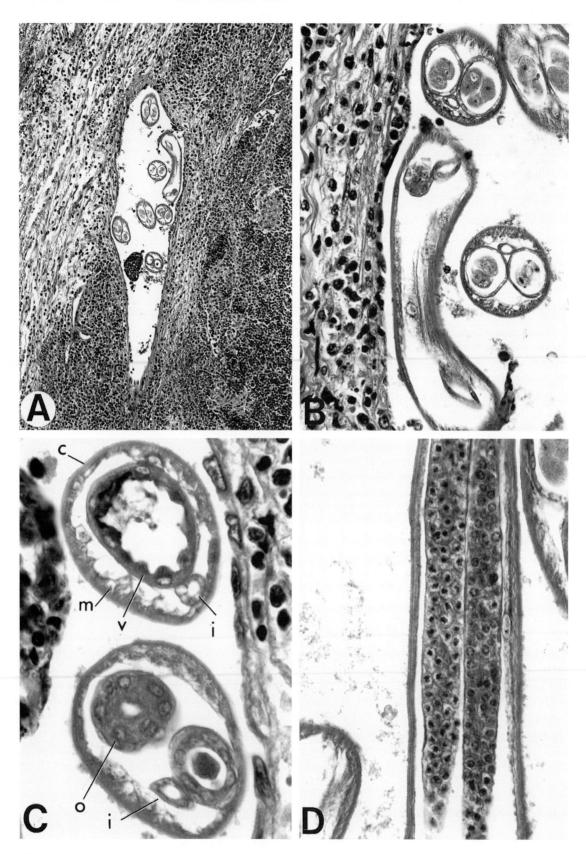

Fig. 19–13. Zoonotic *Brugia* in the United States, well-preserved parasite, sections stained with hematoxylin and eosin stain. *A*, Low-power view of an inguinal lymph node showing a subcapsular sinus with a well-preserved *Brugia* species, ×110. *B*, Higher magnification illustrating the morphology of the parasite on cross sections: two uteri with unfertilized ova, a smaller tube, the intestine and the thin cuticle (measuring less than 1 μm), and muscle cells, ×480. *C*, Higher magnification of two cross sections toward the anterior portion of the parasite showing the cuticle (c), muscle cells (m), intestine (i), oviduct (o), and vagina uterina (v), ×1,000. *D*, Longitudinal section showing the two uteri with ova, ×800. (Reported by Gutierrez, Y., and Petras, R.E. 1982. *Brugia* infection in northern Ohio. Am. J. Trop. Med. Hyg. 31:1128–1130.)

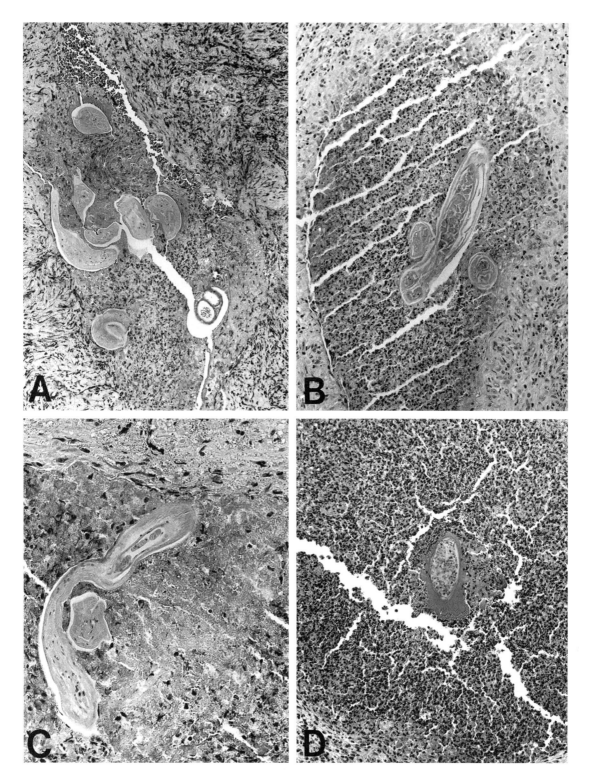

Fig. 19–14. Zoonotic *Brugia* in the United States, dead, disintegrating parasite, sections stained with hematoxylin and eosin stain. *A–C*, Different views of a granuloma with dead *Brugia* species in lymph nodes of a patient with a single hyperplastic lymph node. Note the effacement of the normal anatomy of the parasite, the necrotic tissue around the parasite, and the well-walled-off granuloma in *B*. The morphologic characteristics of the parasite still allow its identification as a *Brugia*, ×140. *D*, Higher magnification of another cross section of the worm from the same patient showing complete effacement of the internal anatomy; the cuticle appears to be greatly swollen, with an amorphous eosinophilic precipitate, ×280.

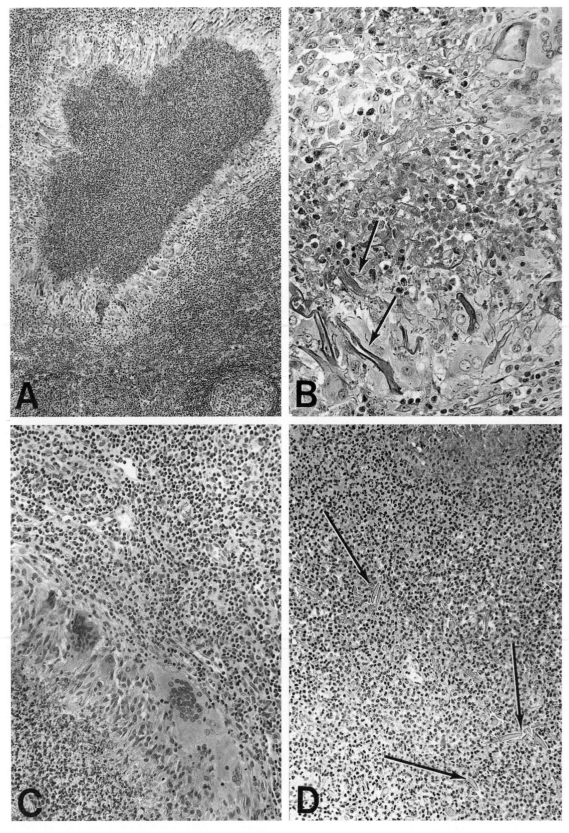

Fig. 19–15. Lymph node, granulomas without worms, zoonotic *Brugia* in the United States, sections stained with hematoxylin and eosin stain. *A*, Large, well-formed granuloma with many eosinophils and pseudopalisading histiocytes, ×70. *B*, Higher magnification of the granu- loma wall showing pseudoepithelioid histiocytes and gi- ant cells, with remnants of what appears to be the cuti- cle of the parasite (arrows), ×280. *C* and *D*, Illustration of the infiltrate showing many eosinophils and Charcot- Leyden crystals (arrows), ×180.

varing from 60 to 134 μm. *Brugia beaveri* is 94 μm (Ash, Little, 1964; Harbut, Orihel, 1995), *B. leporis* is 134 μm (Eberhard, 1984), and the species of *Brugia* found in a cat in California is 60 μm (Beaver, Wong, 1988). Based on the diameter alone, any of these species of *Brugia* could be responsible for the human infections reported in the United States. However, based on the known geographic distribution of enzootic *Brugia* in the United States, *B. leporis*, occurring in the northeastern and southeastern areas, is at present the most likely candidate (Eberhard et al. 1991). Other species of *Brugia* found in animals (and potentially zoonotic in humans) occur outside the United States. Their diameters are usually less than 190 μm, with the exception of *B. buckleyi* found in the heart and blood vessels of the Sri Lanka hare, the female of which may reach 350 μm in diameter (Dissanaike, Paramananthan, 1961).

References

Appley J, Grant GH, 1945. Tropical eosinophilia as seen in England. Lancet 1:812–813

Ash LR, Little MD, 1964. *Brugia beaveri* sp. n. (Nematoda: Filarioidea) from the raccoon (*Procyon lotor*) in Louisiana. J. Parasitol. 50:119–123

Baird JK, Alpert LI, Friedman R, Schraft WC, Connor DH, 1986. North American brugian filariasis: report of nine infections of humans. Am. J. Trop. Med. Hyg. 35:1205–1209

Baird JK, Neafie EC, 1988. South American brugian filariasis: report of a human infection acquired in Peru. Am. J. Trop. Med. Hyg. 39:185–188

Ball JD, 1950. Tropical pulmonary eosinophilia. Trans. R. Soc. Trop. Med. Hyg. 44:237–258

Beaver PC, 1970. Filariasis without microfilaremia. Am. J. Trop. Med. Hyg. 19:181–189

Beaver PC, Cran IR, 1974. *Wuchereria*-like filaria in an artery, associated with pulmonary infarction. Am. J. Trop. Med. Hyg. 23:869–876

Beaver PC, Fallon M, Smith GH, 1971. Pulmonary nodule caused by a living *Brugia malayi*-like filaria in an artery. Am. J. Trop. Med. Hyg. 20:661–666

Beaver PC, Jung RC, Cupp EW, 1984. *Clinical Parasitology*. Philadelphia: Lea & Febiger

Beaver PC, Wong MM, 1988. *Brugia* sp. from a domestic cat in California. Proc. Helminthol. Soc. Wash. 55:111–113

Behm CAW, Hayman JM, 1946. The course of filariasis after removal from an endemic area. Am. J. Med. Sci. 211:385–394

Bhagwat RD, Rao LK, Deodhar LP, 1973. Parasite in the anterior chamber of the eye. A case report. Indian J. Ophthalmol. 21:34–35

Bloomfield RD, Suarez JR, Malangit AC, 1978. Transpla-

cental transfer of bancroftian filariasis. J. Natl. Med. Assoc. 70:597–598

Bonne C, Lie KJ, Molenkamp WJJ, Mreyen FW, 1941. *Wuchereria malayi*, de macrofilaria behoorende bij de Microfilaria malayi (English summary). Ned. Tijdschr. Geneeskd. 81:1487–1501

Botero D, Restrepo A, Velez H, 1965. La filariasis humana en Colombia. Antioquia Med. 15:623–630

Bras G, Lie KJ, 1951. Histological findings in lymph nodes of patients with the Myers-Kouwenaar syndrome. Doc. Neerl. Indones. Morb. Trop. 3:289–294

Brinkmann UK, Kramer P, Presthus GT, Sawadogo B, 1976. Transmission in utero of microfilariae of *Onchocerca volvulus*. Bull. WHO 54:708–709

Buckley JJC, 1958. Occult filarial infections of animal origin as a cause of tropical pulmonary eosinophilia. E. Afr. Med. J. 35:493–500

Buckley JJC, Wharton RH, 1961. Anomalous results from an experimental infection of man with *Brugia malayi* (Brug, 1927). J. Helminthol. 35(Suppl):17–24

Bundy DAP, Grenfell BT, Rajagopalan PK, 1991. Immunoepidemiology of lymphatic filariasis: the relationship between infection and disease. Parasitol. Today 7:71–75

Case Records of the Massachusetts General Hospital, 1974. Resolving pulmonary densities and hemoptysis in a 27 year old woman. Case 26-1974. N. Engl. J. Med. 291:35–42

Casile M, Floch H, 1957. Sur l'eosinophilie tropicale. Bull. Soc. Pathol. Exot. 50:90–94

Chakravarty UN, Roy SC, 1943. A case of tropical eosinophilia? Indian Med. Gaz. 78:596–597

Chaudhuri RN, Chaudhuri MNR, Basu SP, 1956. Tropical eosinophilia: a follow-up study. Bull. Calcutta Sch. Trop. Med. 4:113

Chaudhuri RN, Saha TK, 1961. Histology of lung in tropical eosinophilia. Bull. Calcutta Sch. Trop. Med. 9:149–150

Chernin E, 1987. The disappearance of bancroftian filariasis from Charleston, South Carolina. Am. J. Trop. Med. Hyg. 37:111–114

Coggeshall LT, 1946. Filariasis in the serviceman: retrospect and prospect. JAMA 131:8–12

Coolidge C, Weller PF, Ramsey PG, Ottesen EA, Beaver PC, Von Lichtenberg FC, 1979. Zoonotic *Brugia* filariasis in New England. Ann. Intern. Med. 90:341–343

Coutinho A, 1956. Tropical eosinophilia: clinical, therapeutic and etiologic considerations. Experimental work. Ann. Intern. Med. 44:88–104

Crandall RB, McGreevy PB, Connor DH, Crandall CA, Neilson JT, McCall JW, 1982. The ferret (*Mustela putorius furo*) as an experimental host for *Brugia malayi* and *Brugia pahangi*. Am. J. Trop. Med. Hyg. 31:752–759

Crosnier R, Darbon A, Moras P, Laurens L, 1954. Nouvelles observations de filariose lymphatic a *W. malayi* chez des repatries d'Indochine. Bull. Soc. Pathol. Exot. 47:87–91

Dalrymple W, 1955. Tropical eosinophilia—report of two cases occurring more than a year after departure from India. N. Engl. J. Med. 252:585–586

Danaraj TJ, 1947. Eosinophilic lung. Med. J. Malaya 1:278–288

Danaraj TJ, 1951. Eosinophilic lung: A study of 150 cases seen in Singapore. Thesis, pp. 1–57

Danaraj TJ, 1959. Pathologic studies in eosinophilic lung (tropical eosinophilia). Arch. Pathol. 67:515–524

Danaraj TJ, Pacheco G, Shanmugaratnam K, Beaver PC, 1966. The etiology and pathology of eosinophilic lung (tropical eosinophilia). Am. J. Trop. Med. Hyg. 15:183–189

De Lalla F, Zanoni P, Lunetta Q, Moltrasio G, 1988. Endemic non-filarial elephantiasis in Iringa District, Tanzania: a study of 30 patients. Trans. R. Soc. Trop. Med. Hyg. 82:895–897

Denham DA, McGreevy PB, 1977. Brugian filariasis: epidemiological and experimental studies. Adv. Parasitol. 15:243–309

Denham DA, Ponnudurai T, Nelson GS, Rogers R, Guy F, 1972. Studies with *Brugia pahangi*—II. The effect of repeated infection on parasite levels in cats. Int. J. Parasitol. 2:401–407

Dennis DT, Partono F, Purnomo, Atmosoedjono S, Saroso JS, 1976. Timor filariasis: epidemiological and clinical features in a defined community. Am. J. Trop. Med. Hyg. 25:797–802

Dey P, Walker R, 1994. Correspondence. Microfilariae in a fine needle aspirate from a skin nodule. Acta Cytol. 38:114

Dhayagude RG, 1945. Microfilarial granuloma of the spleen. Arch. Pathol. 40:275–278

Diaz-Rivera RS, Ramos-Morales F, Cintron-Rivera AA, 1954. Infiltrative eosinophilia. Arch. Intern. Med. 94:102–121

Dissanaike AS, Paramananthan DC, 1961. On *Brugia* (*Brugiella* subgen. nov.) *buckleyi* n. sp., from the heart and blood vessels of the Ceylon hare. J. Helminthol. 35:209–221

Dondero TJ Jr, Mullin SW, Balasingam S, 1972. Early clinical manifestations in filariasis due to *Brugia malayi*: observations on experimental infections in man. Southeast Asian J. Trop. Med. Public Health 3:569–575

Dondero TJ Jr, Ramachandran CP, Yusoff OB, 1971. Filariasis due to *Brugia malayi* in West Malaysia Part I: clinical, laboratory, and parasitological aspects. Southeast Asian J. Trop. Med. Public Health 2:503–515

Eberhard ML, 1984. *Brugia leporis* sp. n. (Filarioidea: Onchocercidae) from rabbits (*Sylvilagus aquaticus, S. floridanus*) in Louisiana. J. Parasitol. 70:576–579

Eberhard ML, DeMeester LJ, Martin BW, Lammie PJ, 1993a. Zoonotic *Brugia* infection in western Michigan. Am. J. Surg. Pathol. 17:1058–1061

Eberhard ML, Hitch WL, NcNeeley DF, Lammie PJ, 1993b. Transplacental transmission of *Wuchereria bancrofti* in Haitian women. J. Parasitol. 79:62–66

Eberhard ML, Lammie PJ, 1991. Laboratory diagnosis of filariasis. Clin. Lab. Med. 11:977–1010

Eberhard ML, Telford SR, Spielman A, Telford I, Sam R, 1991. A *Brugia* species infecting rabbits in the northeastern United States. J. Parasitol. 77:796–798

Edeson JFB, 1972. Filariasis. Br. Med. Bull. 28:60–65

Edeson JFB, Wilson T, Wharton RH, Laing ABG, 1960. Experimental transmission of *Brugia malayi* and *Brugia pahangi* to man. Trans. R. Soc. Trop. Med. Hyg. 54:229–234

Elenitoba-Johnson KSJ, Eberhard ML, Dauphinais RM, Lammie PJ, Khorsand J, 1996. Zoonotic Brugian lymphadenitis: an unusual case with florid monocytoid B-cell proliferation. Am. J. Clin. Pathol. 105:384–387

Franz M, Buttner DW, 1986. Histology of adult *Brugia malayi*. Trop. Med. Parasitol. 37:282–285

Friess J, Pierrou M, Segalen J, 1953. Des certains formes cliniques de la filariose lymphatique (*W. malayi*); relations avec les eosinophilies traophicales. Bull. Soc. Pathol. Exot. 46:1037–1063

Frimodt-Moller C, Barton RM, 1940. A pseudo-tuberculous condition associated with eosinophilia. Indian Med. Gaz. 75:607–613

Galindo L, Von Lichtenberg F, Baldizon C, 1962. Bancroftian filariasis in Puerto Rico: infection pattern and tissue lesions. Am. J. Trop. Med. Hyg. 11:739–748

Gutierrez Y, 1984. Diagnostic features of zoonotic filariae in tissue sections. Hum. Pathol. 15:514–525

Gutierrez Y, Petras RE, 1982. *Brugia* infection in northern Ohio. Am. J. Trop. Med. Hyg. 31:1128–1130

Harbut CL, Orihel TC, 1995. *Brugia beaveri*: microscopic morphology in host tissues and observations on its life history. J. Parasitol. 81:239–243

Harinasuta C, Charoenlarp P, Sucharit S, Deesin T, Surathin K, Vutikes S, 1970. Studies on Malayan filariasis in Thailand. Southeast Asian J. Trop. Med. Public Health 1:29–39

Hartz PH, Van Der Sar A, 1948. Tropical eosinophilia in filariasis. Occurrence of radiating processes about microfilariae. Am. J. Clin. Pathol. 18:637–644

Hawking F, Adams WE, Worms MJ, 1964. The periodicity of microfilariae. VII. The effect of parasympathetic stimulants upon the distribution of microfilariae. Trans. R. Soc. Trop. Med. Hyg. 57:178–194

Hirst WR, McCann WJ, 1945. Tropical eosinophilia. Report of a case. U.S. Naval Med. Bull. 44:1277–1281

Hodge IG, Denhoff E, Vander Veer JB, 1945. Early filariasis (*Bancrofti*) in American soldiers. Am. J. Med. Sci. 210:207–223

Irwin JW, 1946. Tropical eosinophilia. Ann. Intern. Med. 25:329–339

Jung RC, Harris FH, 1960. Human filarial infection in Louisiana. Arch. Pathol. 69:371–373

Jungmann P, Figueredo-Silva J, Dreyer G, 1991. Bancroftian lymphadenopathy: a histopathologic study of fifty-eight cases from northeastern Brazil. Am. J. Trop. Med. Hyg. 45:325–331

Kar SK, 1986. Atypical features in lymphatic filariasis. Indian J. Med. Res. 84:270–274

Katamine D, 1966. On the clinical and pathological problems of filariasis. In: Morishita K, Komiya Y, Matsubayashi H (eds), *Progress of Medical Parasitology in Japan*, Vol. 3. Tokyo: Meguro Parasitological Museum, pp. 441–479

Kozek WJ, Reyes MA, Ehrman J, Garrido F, Nieto M, 1984. Enzootic *Brugia* infection in a two-year-old Colombian girl. Am. J. Trop. Med. Hyg. 33:65–69

Kwan-Lim GE, Forsyth KP, Maizels RM, 1990. Filarial-specific IgG4 response correlates with active *Wuchereria bancrofti* infection. J. Immunol. 145:4298–4305

Lahiri VL, 1975. Microfilariae in nipple secretion. Acta Cytol. 19:154

Lammie PJ, Hitch WL, Walker A, Hightower W, Eberhard ML, 1991. Maternal filarial infection as risk factor for infection in children. Lancet 337:1005–1006

Lang AP, Luchsinger IS, Rawling EG, 1987. Filariasis of the breast. Arch. Pathol. Lab. Med. 111:757–759

Leong ASY, 1971. *Brugia malayi* in a cervical smear. Am. J. Trop. Med. Hyg. 25:655–656

Levin JJ, 1956. Tropical eosinophilia (followed for seven years). Ann. Intern. Med. 44:1264 1269

Lichtenberg F, 1957. The early phase of endemic Bancroftian filariasis in the male; pathological study. Mt. Sinai J. Med. 26:983–1000

Lie KJ, 1962. Occult filariasis: its relationship with tropical pulmonary eosinophilia. Am. J. Trop. Med. Hyg. 11:646–652

Lie KJ, Sandosham AA, 1969. The pathology of classical filariasis due to *Wuchereria bancrofti* and *Brugia malayi* and a discussion of occult filariasis. In: Sandosham AA, Zaman V (eds), *Proceedings of Seminar on Filariasis and Immunology of Parasitic Infections and Laboratory Meeting*. Singapore: pp. 125–135

Maizels RM, Lawrence RA, 1991. Immunological tolerance: the key feature in human filariasis? Parasitol. Today 7:271–276

Maizels RM, Sartono E, Kurniawan A, Partono F, Selkirk ME, Yazdanbakhsh M, 1995. T-cell activation and the balance of antibody isotypes in human lymphatic filariasis. Parasitol. Today 11:50–56

Meyers FM, Kouwenaar W, 1939. Over hypereosinophilie en over een merkwaardigen vorm van filariasis. (Studies on hypereosinophilia and a remarkable form of filariasis. Ned. Tijdschr. Geneeskd. 79:853–873 [English summary on p. 872]

Neva FA, Kaplan AP, Pacheco G, Gray L, Danaraj TJ, 1975. Tropical eosinophilia. A human model of parasitic immunopathology, with observations on serum IgE levels before and after treatment. J. Allergy Clin. Immunol. 55:422–429

Orihel TC, Beaver PC, 1989. Zoonotic *Brugia* infections in North and South America. Am. J. Trop. Med. Hyg. 40:638–647

Ormerod AD, Petersen J, Hussey JK, Weir J, Edward N, 1983. Immune complex glomerulonephritis and chronic anaerobic urinary infection—complications of filariasis. Postgrad. Med. J. 59:730–733

Ottesen EA, 1984. Immunological aspects of lymphatic filariasis and onchocerciasis in man. Trans. R. Soc. Trop. Med. Hyg. 78:9–18

Parsons-Smith BG, 1944. Tropical eosinophilia. Lancet 1:433–434

Partono F, Purnomo, Dennis DT, Atmosoedjono S, Oemijati S, Cross JH, 1977. *Brugia timori* sp. n. (Nematoda: Filarioidea) from Flores Island, Indonesia. J. Parasitol. 63:540–546

Piessens WF, McGreevy PB, Piessens P, McGreevy M, Koiman I, Suliani-Saroso J, Dennis D, 1980a. Immune responses in human infections with *Brugia malayi*: specific cellular unresponsiveness to filarial antigens. J. Clin. Invest. 65:172

Piessens WF, McGreevy PB, Ratiwayanta S, McGreevy M, Piessens PW, Koiman I, Sulianti-Saroso J, Dennis D, 1980b. Immune responses in human infections with *Brugia malayi*: correlation of cellular and humoral reactions to microfilarial antigens with clinical status. Am. J. Trop. Med. Hyg. 29:563–570

Rao SS, 1945. Filarial infection in Dhamda (Drug District, C.P.) due to *Wuchereria malayi*. Indian J. Med. Res. 33:175–176

Rao SS, Maplestone PA, 1940. The adult of *Microfilaria malayi* Brug, 1927. Indian Med. Gaz. 75:159–160

Rifkin H, Eberhard TP, 1946. Pulmonary filariasis. Ann. Intern. Med. 25:324–329

Sanjivi KS, Friedmann HC, Thiruvengadam KV, 1952. ACTH in tropical eosinophilia. Lancet 2:590

Seo BS, 1978. Malayan filariasis in Korea. Korean J. Parasitol. 16:1–108

Shah RL, 1943. A case of pseudo-tuberculosis of the lungs with eosinophilia. Indian Med Gaz 78:597

Simmons CF Jr, Winter HS, Berde C, Schrater F, Humphrey GB, Rosen FS, Beaver PC, Weller PF, 1984. Zoonotic filariasis with lymphedema in an immunodeficient infant. N. Engl. J. Med. 310:1243–1245

Stephan E, 1946. Tropical eosinophilia in Egypt. Lancet 2:236

Sullivan TJ, 1970. Tropical eosinophilia in the Republic of South Vietnam. Am. J. Trop. Med. Hyg. 19:947–949

Swarup K, Samal N, Sharma SM, Mulay R, Patil VM, 1990. Fine needle aspiration cytology in the diagnosis of bancroftian filariasis. Trans. R. Soc. Trop. Med. Hyg. 84: 113

Tan TJ, Kosin E, Tan TH, 1985. Lymphographic abnormalities in patients with *Brugia malayi* filariasis and "idiopathic tropical eosinophilia." Lymphology 18:169–172

Udwadia FE, Joshi VV, 1964. A study of tropical eosinophilia. Thorax 19:548–554

Vassilakos P, Cox JN, 1974. Filariasis diagnosed by cytologic examination of hydrocele fluid. Acta Cytol. 18:62–64

Viswanathan R, 1947. Post-mortem appearance in tropical eosinophilia. Indian Med. Gaz. 82:49–50

Wartman WB, 1944. Lesions of the lymphatic system in early filariasis. Am. J. Trop. Med. 24:299–313

Wartman WB, 1947. Filariasis in American armed forces in World War II. Medicine 26:333–394

Waugh DA, Alexander JH, Ibels LS, 1980. Filarial chyluria associated glomerulonephritis and therapeutic considerations in the chyluric patient. Aust. N.Z. J. Med. 10: 559–562

Webb JKG, Job CK, Gault EW, 1960. Tropical eosinophilia. Demonstration of microfilariae in lung, liver and lymphnodes. Lancet 1:835–842

Weingarten RJ, 1943. Tropical eosinophilia. Lancet 1:103–105

Wharton RH, 1962. The biology of *Mansonia* mosquitoes in relation to the transmission of filariasis in Malaya. Inst. Med. Res. Bull. No. 11, pp. 1–113

WHO, 1984. Lymphatic filariasis. Technical Report Series 702. Geneva: WHO, 1–112

Williams FMW, Hamilton HF, Singh B, Herlinger R, 1960. Tropical eosinophilia in British Guiana—a preliminary report. West Indian Med. J. 9:149–155

Wilson HTH, 1947. Tropical eosinophilia in East Africa. Br. Med. J. 1:801–804

Wright RE, Iyer PVS, Pandit CG, 1935. Description of an adult filaria (male) removed from the anterior chamber of the eye of man. Indian J. Med. Res. 23:199–203

Yeuhan C, Qun X, 1981. Filarial granuloma of the female breast: a histopathological study of 131 cases. Am. J. Trop. Med. Hyg. 30:1206–1210

Zhong M, McCarthy J, Bierwert L, Lizotte-Waniewski M, Chanteau S, Nutman TB, Ottesen EA, Williams SA, 1996. A polymerase chain reaction assay for detection of the parasite *Wuchereria bancrofti* in human blood samples. Am. J. Trop. Med. Hyg. 54:357–363

20

SPIRURIDA—FILARIAE OF THE SUBCUTANEOUS TISSUES AND BODY CAVITIES

The filariids of the subcutaneous tissues and body cavities of humans are species of the genera *Onchocerca*, *Loa*, and *Mansonella*, which are natural parasites in humans, and of *Dirofilaria*, several species of which produce zoonotic infections. One species, *D. immitis*, occurs both in the skin as immature worms and in the pulmonary arteries (see Chapter 21). In human infections with *Dirofilaria* the worms generally do not attain maturity, and no infection becomes patent (i.e., no patients develop microfilaremia). The most important species of this group is *O. volvulus* because of the morbidity it produces in endemic areas. Infections with zoonotic *Onchocerca* have also been described.

Onchocerca—Onchocerciasis

The genus *Onchocerca* has one species found in humans, *O. volvulus*, and several other species that occur naturally in wild and domestic animals. Animals infected naturally with *O. volvulus* have been a spider monkey and a gorilla; experimentally, the chimpanzee is a good host (Duke, 1962). This makes *O. volvulus*

almost exclusively a parasite of humans. The main morphologic characteristic of the genus is the presence of external transverse ridges and internal striations in the cuticle. These characteristics are useful in identifying *Onchocerca* in longitudinal and oblique sections of the parasite in tissues. Biologically, *O. volvulus* is characterized by microfilariae that inhabit the skin and by having a fly as its intermediate host. The importance of *Onchocerca* as a pathogen lies in the capacity of the microfilariae to produce severe forms of dermititis and blindness due to their presence in the skin and their ability to invade the cornea and enter the eye.

Morphology and Life Cycle. The adult males of *O. volvulus* are 1.9 to 4.2 cm in length by 130 to 210 μm in diameter. The females are 33.5 to 50 cm in length by 270 to 400 μm in diameter. The worms are embedded in fibrous nodules and occasionally have been retrieved from tissues where they may be found free (Becker, 1950). At other times, they are extruded from abscesses as smaller fragments (Oomen, 1967); in these cases, they almost never reach the clinical laboratory or the operating room. The techniques available for isolating the worms from nodules used are mostly by par-

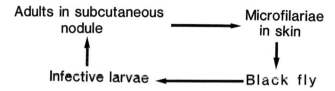

Fig. 20–1. *Onchocerca volvulus,* **schematic representation of the life cycle.**

asitologists in taxonomic studies. The nodules may contain several worms and appear to grow up to 5 cm in diameter due to the arrival of new worms at already formed nodules. The microanatomy of *Onchocerca* in cross sections is described below (see Diagnosis).

The life cycle of *Onchocerca* involves a biologic vector that belongs to the genus *Simulium,* commonly known as *black flies.* The main species are *S. damnosum* and *S. neavei* in Africa, *S. ochracecum* in Central America, *S. metallicum* in Venezuela, and *S. sanguineum* in Brazil. In the tissues, the adult worms produce microfilariae that move to the skin (Fig. 20–1); rarely, they occur in the circulating blood. The simuliids ingest microfilaria while feeding on their natural

hosts, and they develop to infective larvae that eventually are deposited on the skin of the new host during the fly's next blood meal. The larvae enter the skin and subcutaneous tissues and mature to adults in about 1 year. The host's response that produces the fibrous reaction around the adult worms, forming the onchocercoma (nodule), is slow, and the worms may lie free in the tissues for years (Nnochiri, 1966). It is estimated that the worms live in humans for up to 16 years (Roberts et al. 1967); the life span of the microfilariae of *O. volvulus* is estimated to be up to 30 months (WHO, 1976, 1987). The ecologic condition required for the development of *Simulium* is very specific: abundant clean running water found especially in rivers. For this reason, onchocerciasis occurs along rivers, hence the name of the disease, *river blindness.*

Geographic Distribution and Epidemiology. The geographic location of *O. volvulus* is tropical Africa in a territory extending from 15° north latitude to 12° south latitude (Fig. 20–2). The disease was apparently introduced into the American continent with the slave trade (Nelson, 1991). At present, it is found in relatively con-

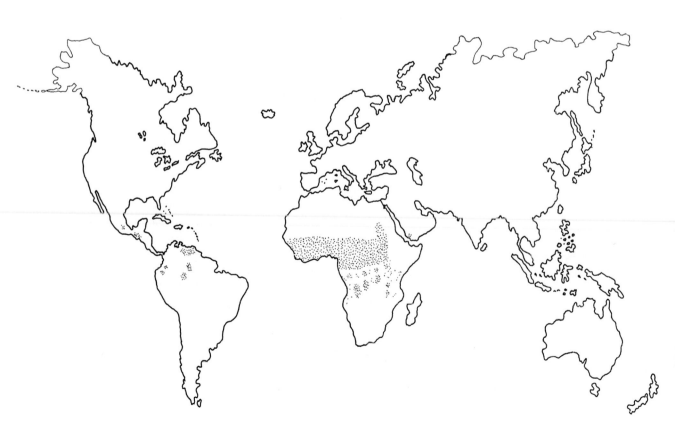

Fig. 20–2. *Onchocerca volvulus,* **geographic distribution (Adapted from: WHO, 1977. WHO Expert Committee on Onchocerciasis. Third Report. Technical Report Series No. 752. Geneva: World Health Organization.)**

fined foci in some parts of Guatemala, Mexico, Colombia, Venezuela, Ecuador, and Brazil (Fig. 20–2). It is estimated that at least 18 million individuals are infected with O. *volvulus*, of whom over 0.3 million are blind (WHO, 1987). Until recently, control campaigns against the disease were directed to mass removal of the nodules and control of the vector by chemical treatment of rivers, but mass treatment of infected individuals has now been found to be more effective. This focus on patients is due largely to the availability of ivermectin, a good, safe, and inexpensive drug introduced in 1987 (Remme, 1995).

Transmission of the infection varies in intensity in different geographic areas. The number of worms in a given individual depends on the level of transmission and the length of residence in endemic areas because the worms are acquired continuously. Continuous infectivity results in different loads of microfilariae in the skin of infected patients and in increased morbidity because morbidity is directly proportional to the number of microfilariae present; adult worms are of secondary clinical importance (Akogun et al. 1992; Nelson, 1970, 1991).

The nodules are often found in subcutaneous tissues, sometimes deep in the fascia or close to the periosteum, producing deep pain. In Central America, the nodules are usually located on the upper part of the body, with over half of them found on the head, one-fourth in the chest wall, and one-fourth at the pelvis or below. In Africa and Venezuela the nodules commonly occur around the pelvis, especially over the iliac crest, the greater trochanter of the femur, the coccyx, and the sacrum (Fig. 20–3 A). The body distribution of the nodules in African patients correlates with a greater concentration of microfilariae in the skin of the lower body (Kershaw et al. 1954). The differences in the location of the nodules in African and Central American patients are apparently related to the fly's propensity to bite the lower parts of the body in Africa and the higher parts in Central America. The ocular lesions in African patients also occur in those with the largest concentrations of microfilariae in the skin. This is because the microfilariae, which in this region are usually located in the lower half of the body, "spill" over to the upper part and the eye (Nelson, 1970).

Rates of prevalence vary with the geographic region and the assessment method used, that is, focusing on microfilariae, nodules, ocular lesions, or skin lesions. In an endemic area in Nigeria, 45% of the population had skin lesions attributed to the infection but only 32% had subcutaneous nodules (Akogun et al. 1992). West Sub-Saharan Africa had prevalences varying from 80% to 88% before control campaigns started

in the region. The percentage is now below 50% (Molyneux, Davies, 1997). In Ecuador, ocular morbidity is increasing among the infected population of Esmeraldas Province, correlated with an increase in the number of microfilariae per person over a 10-year period (Cooper et al. 1996). In addition, the Ecuadorian focus is spreading due to migration of infected individuals, and the percentage of infected persons rose from 27% in 1992 to 40% in 1996 (Guderian, Shelley, 1992).

Clinical Findings. The incubation period of onchocerciasis is not known; the prepatent period (from the time of infection to the appearance of microfilariae) is estimated to be between 12 and 15 months after infection (WHO, 1987). In general, no symptoms appear to be associated with the growing worms in the tissues, although some allergies have been described. The clinical incubation period is longer and more variable than the prepatent period and may last for several years. Asymptomatic carriers of the infection are found in endemic areas during epidemiologic surveys on close clinical examination of patients. In symptomatic individuals, the clinical and pathologic manifestations of onchocerciasis are produced by the presence of the onchocercomas but, more important, by the tissue reaction to dead microfilariae (Buck, 1974; Connor et al. 1983; Gibson, Connor, 1978; Gibson et al. 1980). The nodules are generally of secondary importance clinically, and in children less than 2 years of age they are usually absent in the presence of microfilaremia. When present, well-formed *Onchocerca* nodules are 1 to several centimeters in diameter, easily seen, and sometimes detected only with careful palpation because they occur deep in the soft tissues. The nodules are rounded or oval and sometimes are felt as hard, lobulated structures. The number of nodules per patient varies, and patients with 100 nodules have been reported. In hyperendemic areas of Africa, the usual number is 5 to 10 superficial nodules, plus 3 or 4 in the deeper tissues. Nodules containing live worms are painless and movable; those with calcified worms are stone hard. Nodules with dead worms may become painful and soft, and may form abscesses that often produce sinus tracks through which chronic suppuration drains into the skin. Dead worms or fragments of worms may be found in the pus. Apart from the poor aesthetic appearance due to the nodules, the pain they produce when located close to the bone, and the rare partially inflamed ones, no other morbidity is associated with them.

As stated above, the main signs and symptoms of onchocerciasis are due to the microfilariae in the tis-

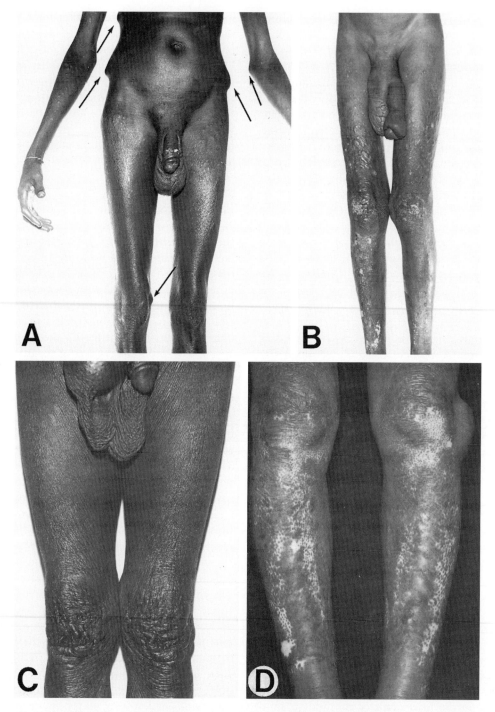

Fig. 20–3. *Onchocerca volvulus*, skin lesions. *A*, Subcutaneous nodules (arrows), Air Force Institute of Pathology (AFIP) negative No. 68-7638-3. *B*, Hypertrophic dermatitis, AFIP negative No. 68-7912-1. *C*, Atrophic dermatitis, AFIP negative No. 72-4500-A. *D*, Leopard skin, AFIP negative No. 72-17223.

sues, especially the collagenous connective tissue of the skin, the conjunctiva, the cornea, and other eye structures. The microfilariae of *Onchocerca* have the ability to enter and pass through collagenous connective tissues without producing an inflammatory reaction, but when they die, they elicit strong inflammatory changes with systemic, dermal, ocular, and lymphatic manifestations.

Systemic Disease. Manifestations of systemic disease have been described in patients with onchocerciasis, but the assessment of their importance is difficult and remains mostly anecdotal. Lower body weight among infected individuals compared with noninfected ones is common in endemic areas. Another condition that correlates with the geographic distribution of *O. volvulus* in Uganda is the *nakalanga syndrome* or *nakalanga dwarfism*. This disease consists of dwarfism, absence of secondary sexual characteristics, skeletal deformities, and mental retardation (Kipp et al. 1996). In hyperendemic areas, microfilariae of *Onchocerca* may occur in the peripheral blood and urine of one-third of infected individuals. Both microfilaremia and microfilaruria increase after treatment, when microfilariae are also found in the cerebrospinal fluid. Other fluids from which microfilariae have been recovered are tears, sputum, synovial fluid, hydrocele fluid, and vaginal secretions, as well as in the skin and cord blood of 3% of infants born to infected mothers. In other geographic areas, general symptoms of cachexia, dwarfism, and a high prevalence of epilepsy have been associated anecdotally with onchocerciasis (WHO, 1976, 1987). Peripheral eosinophilia may be present, especially in hyperreactive disease. In Cameroon, soluble antigen–antibody complexes have been associated with glomerulonephritis (Ngu et al. 1985).

Eye. The most important manifestations of onchocerciasis occur in the eye. The disease is a leading cause of blindness in endemic areas. Microfilariae reach the eye through the conjunctiva, entering the cornea and the anterior chamber; through the bloodstream; and through the sheets of the ciliary vessels and nerves at the posterior pole of the eye. Microfilariae in the eye occur in the cornea, the sclera, the vitreous, the anterior and posterior chambers, the entire uveal tract, the retina, and the optic nerve. In any of these locations live microfilariae are inert, but they eventually die, producing the inflammatory reaction that damages the ocular structures.

The clinical manifestations and the intensity of ocular onchocerciasis vary, depending on the geographic area. In Central America, blindness is relatively rare compared with Africa; and in hyperendemic areas of West Africa, the rate of blindness varies between the savanna (2% to 15%) and the rain forest (less than 2%). Microfilariae in the eye are easily seen in the anterior chamber and the cornea, especially during the early part of the disease. If the patient sits with the head between the knees for 2 minutes before the examination, the microfilariae concentrate at the center of the anterior chamber and are easier to find. With the slit lamp the microfilariae appear as small white worms that wiggle actively, sometimes attached to the epithelium of the posterior lens. In the cornea, live microfilariae are more difficult to detect and sometimes require special examination; dead microfilariae are easier to see as opaque, straightened worms, often forming the core of a punctate corneal opacity. The lesion progresses to "fluffy" or "snowflake" corneal opacities that vary in diameter.

The early changes in the cornea progress slowly over a period of several years to sclerosing keratitis, which starts as an arch from below and at the sides of the cornea, moving toward the center and eventually involving the entire cornea. The end-stage lesion can be seen at a distance as an opaque cornea. In the anterior uveal tract, the iritis and iridocyclitis produced by *Onchocerca* are very variable. In some patients with severe lesions, posterior synechiae of the iris produce deformities of the pupil, and extensive synechiae may close the pupil completely. Another lesion of the anterior uveal tract is glaucoma. In the choroid and the retina, a chorioretinitis that varies widely from patient to patient results in different clinical syndromes. The lesions are focal at first, but they extend to the entire retina, producing retinal pigment epithelial atrophy, chorioretinal atrophy, and subretinal fibrosis. Finally, lesions of the nerve consisting of neuritis and atrophy have been described (Rodger, 1977; WHO, 1976, 1987).

Skin. The most common manifestations of onchocerciasis are seen in the skin, and like the ocular lesions, the skin manifestations vary with the geographic area and the region studied. The early manifestations consist of pruritus and scratching with urticaria, intermittent at first but becoming permanent, sometimes producing insomnia and often with secondary inflammation due to scratching. The intensity of these symptoms usually correlates with the number of microfilariae in the skin. Continuous seeding of the skin with microfilariae over the years results in progressive gross and histologic changes that manifest clinically as dermatitis. The main types of dermatitis are *(1) hypertrophic*, with marked thickening of the squamous epithelium (Fig. 20–3 *B*); *(2) atrophic* with loss of connective tissue and a glossy, wrinkled appearance in severe cases (Fig. 19–3 *C*); *(3) leopard skin* or a late depigmentation phase consisting of areas of spotty depigmentation seen more commonly in the lower limbs (Fig. 20–3 *D*); *(4) craw craw* or *gale filarienne*, consisting of small intradermal papules that become small pustules that drain clear fluid or pus often containing microfilariae (Fig. 20–4 *A*) and producing intense pruritus; and *(5) sowda* ("black" in Arabic), seen in Yemen, a localized, usually unilateral, well-cir-

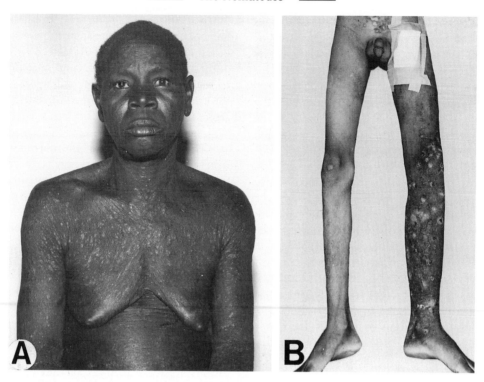

Fig. 20–4. *Onchocerca volvulus*, skin lesions. *A*, Craw-craw, AFIP negative No. 68-7835-6. *B*, Sowda, AFIP negative No. 72-17140.

cumscribed lesion in exposed parts of the body that produces intense itching (onchodermatitis) (Connor et al. 1983). Sowda is accompanied by papules, pustules, edema, pachydermia, and enlargement of local lymph nodes (Fig. 20–4 *B*; Abdel-Hameed et al. 1987). This lesion is somewhat similar to *erisipela de la costa* seen in Central America.

Lymph Nodes. Any group of superficial lymph nodes may be involved, but the ones most often affected are those draining any area of dermatitis. Discrete lymphadenopathy with lymphedema resembling that of lymphatic filariasis is often seen in patients with sowda; this lesion is curable (WHO, 1987). Elephantiasis of the genitalia due to onchocerciasis has been described in some parts of Africa (Buck, 1974; Gibson et al. 1980).

Manifestations during Treatment. Treatment of *Onchocerca* with certain drugs brings about a recrudescence of symptoms. This reaction is due to the large number of microfilariae mobilized from the skin into the blood and from the blood into different tissues and organs, producing circulatory collapse, shortness of breath, coughing, and vertigo. The number of mi-

crofilariae in patients undergoing treatment for *Onchocerca* infection may reach 300 per cubic millimeter.

Immunity. In many respects, the human immunologic response to *O. volvulus* parallels that of the lymphatic filariae. In a given endemic area where the population is continually exposed to the infection, three groups of individuals can be distinguished, depending on their response to the infection.

1. Immune individuals, defined as those who are not patent (do not have microfilariae) and are free of symptoms.
2. Tolerant individuals, those who, in spite of being patent, do not suffer the disease. In this group, there is a state of anergy with impaired cellular responses (T-helper 1, Th1) to specific parasite antigens. In addition, there is a predominant Th2-cell response, with increased circulating IgG and IgE, which are parasite specific. This immune hyporesponsiveness may explain the increased incidence of lepromatous leprosy in areas of *Onchocerca* hyperendemicity. The mechanism for the unresponsiveness to *Onchocerca* is not clear, but it is probably due to a de-

fect in the production of interleukin-2. The tolerance produced by *Onchocerca* is probably only partial and resides in a subset of the Th1 T-cell population. Moreover, as in lymphatic filariasis, this tolerance is unstable; it breaks down over time and moves these infected individuals into group 3, those with clinical manifestations and an inappropriate immune response. This breakdown of tolerance also explains the increased prevalence of disease in older age groups. It is thus the critical event that initiates the tissue lesions (disease).

3. Individuals with an inappropriate immune response who are infected show few or no microfilariae and suffer the disease. Most of the individuals in this group have the usual skin (onchodermatitis) and eye lesions, but some are hyperresponsive and develop classic sowda lesions. These persons with an inappropriate immune response have high levels of parasite-specific IgG and IgE, as well as a marked proliferative cellular immune response demonstrated in experimental in vitro and in vivo work. These hyperreactive patients also have intact cell-mediated immunity, as demonstrated by the production of delayed hypersensitivity on skin testing using adult *Onchocerca* antigens. In these patients, the main modulator of

the lesions is the enhanced Th2 cytokine response, which destroys the microfilariae in the tissues; eosinophils are the main effector cells. Eosinophils that degranulate in tissues release their cytotoxic proteins, including eosinophil major basic protein, eosinophil cationic protein, eosinophil peroxidase, and eosinophil-derived neurotoxin. These and other cytotoxic products, such as those produced by the degranulation of mast cells, are the direct cause of the tissue damage.

Pathology

Nodules. On gross examination, excised *Onchocerca* nodules are round to oval, hard, and grayish white, with strands of fibrous tissue attached to their surface (Fig. 20–5 *A*), sometimes matted and loosely adherent to skin and deep tissues but easy to separate. On section, the nodules have numerous 0.5 to 1.0 mm cavities, each with a section of the worm (Fig. 20–5 *B*) and sometimes with small fragments of the worm protruding from one or more of these cavities. Inflamed nodules have necrotic centers with characteristics of abscesses. Microscopically, the nodule appears as compact fibrous tissue with tightly coiled worms (Fig. 20–5 *C*) cut at numerous levels in cross, oblique, and

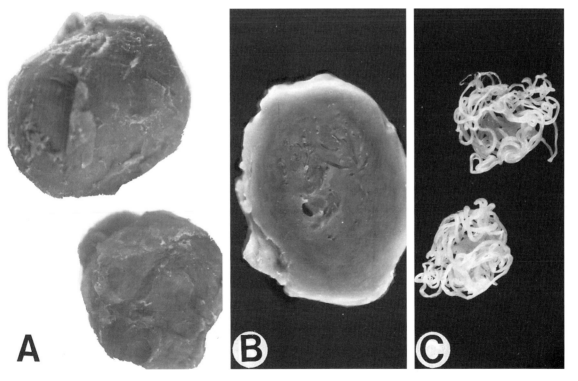

Fig. 20–5. *Onchocerca volvulus*, nodules. *A*, Gross appearance. *B*, Section showing cut portions of the parasite. *C*, Worms digested out of the nodules.

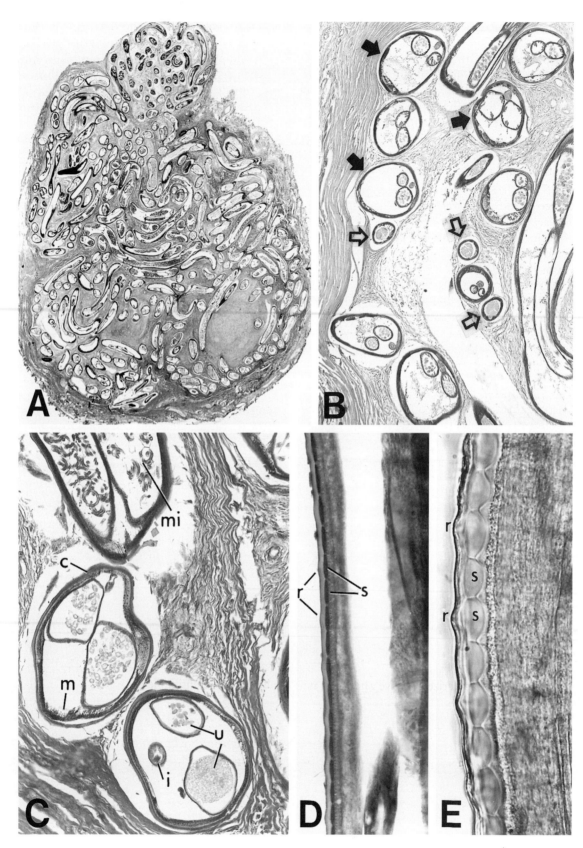

Fig. 20–6.

longitudinal sections (Fig. 20–6 *A–E*); microfilariae are often seen in the fibrous tissue. Usually there is no inflammatory reaction to live worms, but dead worms are surrounded by an abundant polymorphonuclear cell infiltrate, which often forms a large abscess (Fig. 20–7 *A–D*).

Eye. The gross appearance of the eye was discussed above. Microscopically, live and dead microfilariae are found in all layers and tissues of the eye (Paul, Zimmerman, 1970). The gross fluffy opacities in the cornea are microscopic foci of inflammatory cells around dead microfilariae; these lesions are more clearly seen in lightly infected children living in hyperendemic areas or in persons of any age in hypoendemic areas. The cornea sometimes contains large numbers of microfilariae that do not produce deleterious effects (Rodger, 1977; WHO, 1976). The repeated corneal insult results in sclerosing keratitis with permanent opacification due to chronic inflammation and fibrosis (*color plate* IX *A–B*). Other ocular tissues have similar inflammatory changes, with mononuclear and polymorphonuclear cells and occasional eosinophils. In the anterior chamber, common findings are iridocyclitis, with plasma cells and eosinophils infiltrating the iris and the ciliary body at first; later, fibrosis, necrosis, and synechiae develop. In the posterior chamber, important changes also leading to blindness are chorioretinitis and optic nerve atrophy. In the retina, there are degenerative changes in photoreceptors and ganglion cell layers, as well as destruction of capillaries with scar formation. The pigment epithelium shows disorganization and hyperplasia. In some patients, autoantibodies to retinal tissues have been found in the vitreous fluid (Chan et al. 1987).

Skin. In early stages of the infection the skin is normal, with live microfilariae in all layers, most numerous in the upper dermis, and with no inflammatory reaction. The chronic skin lesions of onchocerciasis are related to the number of microfilariae, the immune response, and the duration of the infection. Histologically, the disease is characterized by live and dead microfilariae. Dead microfilariae usually have eosinophils and eosinophilic material in close contact with their cuticle; degenerated microfilariae have pyknotic nuclei surrounded by histiocytes and eosinophils. Antigens released by microfilariae produce a reaction that damages connective tissue and vessels of the cutis. Collections of inflammatory cells, mainly lymphocytes, plasma cells, macrophages, mast cells, and variable numbers of eosinophils, are seen throughout the dermis, often around blood vessels. In the epidermis, changes such as hyperkeratosis, acanthosis, or focal parakeratosis are found, and in cases of craw-craw there are intraepidermal microabscesses filled with fluid and polymorphonuclear cells (Fig. 20–8 *B*). Hyper- or hypopigmentation may be present. In cases of atrophic dermatitis, there is usually loss of fibrous connective tissue in the dermis and thinning of the epidermis (Fig. 20–8 *A*). Patients with hypertrophic dermatitis have marked thickening of the epidermis and fibrosis of the dermis, sometimes with collagenization of the entire dermis (Fig. 20–8 *C–D*). Perivascular fibrosis, decreased skin appendages, and loss of elastic fibers may be seen. Russell-Movat stains show degeneration of dermal collagen.

In patients with sowda, intense inflammation of the involved area and a small number of microfilariae are found. These individuals have high eosinophilia and high levels of circulating antifilarial antibodies. Other changes are similar to those of hypertrophic dermatitis.

Lymph Nodes. The lymph nodes of individuals with *Onchocerca* infections in Africa have atrophy of lymphoid tissue, with fibrosis and scarring of up to 90% of the cross-section surface of the node. Microfilariae are present throughout, within both the fibrous connective tissue and the medullary portion. Some nodes contain macrophages in the sinusoids, with phagocytized melanin pigment and plasma cells (Connor et al. 1970; Gibson, Connor, 1978). Lymph nodes from patients with sowda have reactive hyperplasia, minimal fibrosis, and absent (Gibson, Connor, 1978) or small numbers of identifiable *O. volvulus* microfilariae (Abdel-Hameed et al. 1987).

◄

Fig. 20–6. ***Onchocerca volvulus*, microscopic appearance, *A–C*. Sections stained with hematoxylin and eosin stain. *A*, Low-power view of a nodule showing numerous sections of tightly coiled male and female parasites, ×8.7. *B*, Higher magnification showing the cross section of a female (solid arrows) and a male (open arrows), ×55. *C*, Detail of a female worm. Abbreviations: c, cuticle; m, mus-** cle; u, uteri; i, intestine; mi, microfilariae in the uterus, ×140. *D*, Cuticle, longitudinal section, trichrome stain. Note the cuticle with transverse ridges (r) and the striae (s), ×440. *E*, Cuticle, longitudinal optical section of a worm cleared in glycerol, unstained. The transverse ridges (r) are better appreciated, and the striae (s) are seen clearly in a pattern of two striae for each ridge, ×380.

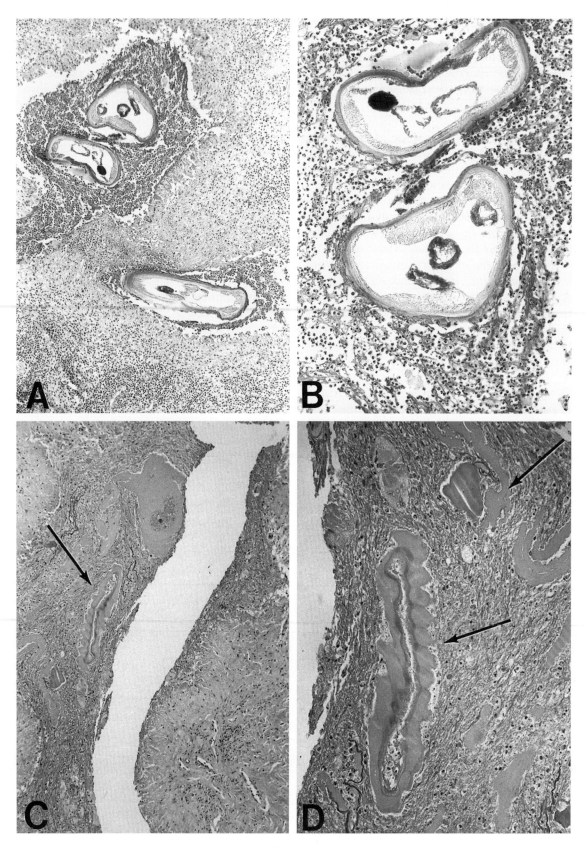

Fig. 20–7.

Diagnosis. The diagnosis of onchocerciasis is based on the clinical presentation and a history of living in or traveling to an endemic area, and is confirmed in the laboratory by finding microfilariae. Microfilariae found in skin snips (small, bloodless, superficial shavings of skin examined in distilled water or in stained preparations) have a typical morphology. In well-fixed stained preparations, the microfilariae of *O. volvulus* are 315 to 360 μm long by 6 μm wide, and the anterior and posterior ends are free of nuclei (Fig. 20–9 and *color plate* IX *D*; Eberhard et al. 1991). Microfilariae of *O. volvulus* have occasionally been found in peripheral blood, sputum, and urine. A polymerase chain reaction for detection of microfilariae DNA in skin snips is as accurate as the direct examination of samples for detection of the parasites (Fischer et al. 1996). Histologic examination of nodules revealing the worm also confirms the infection. In addition, the microfilariae can be found in other fluids, such as blood, urine, scrotal fluid (Gratama, 1970), tears, vaginal smears (Borges, 1971), and cerebrospinal fluid after the patient has been treated. Ocular lesions also are diagnosed clinically in endemic areas. Examination of the eye with the slit lamp in early infections reveals microfilariae in the cornea or the anterior chamber (see above).

In tissue specimens (nodules) recovered during biopsy or at autopsy, the adult worms are generally found in the nodules. In cross, oblique, and longitudinal sections of the parasite in tissues, the diagnosis is made on the basis of the morphologic characteristics (Ali-Khan, Meerovitch, 1973; Beaver et al. 1974; Neafie, 1972). The maximum diameter of the female in tissues is 350 μm, and that of the male is 125 μm (Fig. 20–6 *B*). In longitudinal sections, the cuticle is about 6 μm thick and appears two-layered, with distinct transverse or spiral ridges sometimes up to 4 μm in height. These ridges are located on the surface, regularly spaced at intervals ranging from 40 to 70 μm in longitudinal sections and less in oblique ones (Fig. 20–6 *D–E*). The ridges plus the outer half of the cuticle make up the outer layer of the cuticle, which is barely separated from the inner layer. The inner layer has the most conspicuous feature of *Onchocerca*; the striae, which run transversely. *Onchocerca volvulus* has two striae for each external ridge in the female (Fig. 20–6 *D–E* and *color plate* IX *C*). The striae stain deep red with Masson's trichrome stain. On cross sections, the cuticle has variable thickness, depending on the level of the section. If the section is between the ridges, it is 6 μm, but if the section includes the ridge, it is 10 μm (Fig. 20–10 *C*). Slightly oblique sections may contain both areas (the one between the ridge and the ridge itself), appearing uneven (Fig. 20–10 *C*). The muscle layer is 25 μm high, with a dorsal and a ventral portion that are often not well separated. The lateral cords, usually lower than the muscle bands, are faintly divided into sublateral bands. There are one or two lateral cord nuclei per histologic section, and each cord is about 7 μm in diameter. The intestine is relatively small, measuring 13 to 26 μm in transverse sections, usually with less than one nucleus per histologic section (Fig. 20–6 *B–C*). The sex organs are generally similar to those of other filariids (Beaver et al. 1974).

Zoonotic Onchocerciasis

Some *Onchocerca* infections were acquired in Europe (Azarova et al. 1965; Siegenthaler, Bugler, 1965), North America (Ali-Khan, Meerovitch, 1973; Beaver et al. 1974), and Japan (Beaver et al. 1989; Takaoka et al. 1996). Since these areas are not endemic for *O. volvulus*, the nature of these infections is zoonotic. All patients presented with subcutaneous nodules, in some cases in the wrist, which produce symptoms of carpal tunnel syndrome. The worms, studied in tissue sections of the nodules, are morphologically indistinguishable from *O. gutturosa* of cattle and *O. cervicalis* of horses. The differentiating feature, four striae per transverse ridge, is observed in longitudinal sections of the parasite (see above; Fig. 20–10 *A–E*; Beaver et al. 1974).

Fig. 20–7. *Onchocerca volvulus*, dead parasites in an inflamed nodule, sections stained with hematoxylin and eosin stain. *A* and *B*, Low- and high-power views of a nodule with a recently dead parasite showing marked inflammatory changes. Note that the parasite is beginning to show degenerative changes (internal organs and muscles appear granular) and that polymorphonuclear cells are attached to the cuticle, *A* ×55, *B* ×140. *C* and *D*, Nodule from another patient with a sinus track draining in the skin. Note that the remnants of the parasite's cuticle (arrows) are greatly swollen and not identifiable as *Onchocerca*. However, a presumptive diagnosis is supported by the fact that other nodules with live parasites were present elsewhere in the skin, *C* ×70, *D* ×180.

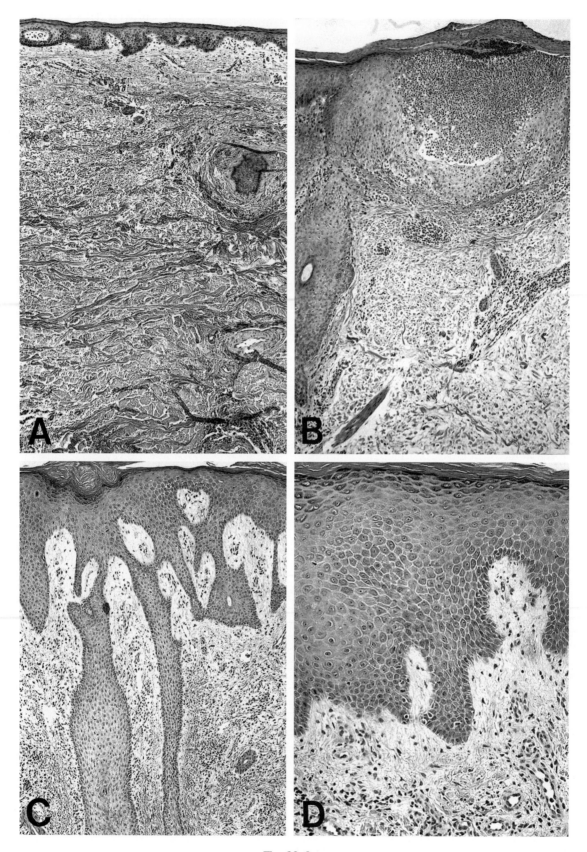

Fig. 20–8.

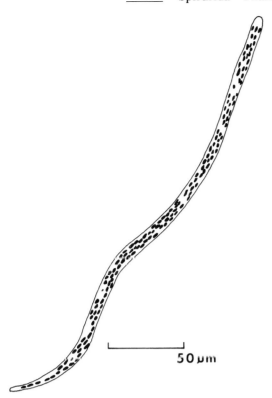

The worms are whitish, with the anterior end slightly tapered; the cuticule has small, irregularly distributed protuberances throughout most of the body (missing toward both the ends of the male) known as *bosses*. The posterior end of the male is curved ventrally and possesses alae similar to those of the dirofilariids (Fig. 20–18 *A*). The microfilariae found in blood are 250 to 300 μm long and contain a sheath (Fig. 20–11 and *color plate* IX *E*).

The life cycle of *Loa* is similar to that of other filariids (see above); the intermediate hosts are day-biting flies of the genus *Chrysops*, which makes *Loa* a filaria with diurnal periodicity that peaks at about 12 noon. Infections with *Loa* are sometimes diagnosed in Europeans, Americans, and other visitors to endemic areas (Bourgeade et al. 1989; Gibbs, 1979; Nutman et al. 1986). Most of these cases are reported in the literature and can now be counted in the low hundreds. They have added little to our understanding of the infection.

Fig. 20–9. *Onchocerca volvulus*, **drawing of a microfilaria from skin snips preparation, stained with Giemsa stain.**

Loa Loa—Loiasis

Loa loa is another subcutaneous filaria of humans, but unlike *Onchocerca*, it does not form nodules. Instead, the parasite migrates constantly in the subcutaneous tissues, sometimes under the conjunctiva, where it is easily seen, hence the name *eye worm*.

Morphology and Life Cycle. The adult females measure 40 to 70 mm long by 0.5 mm wide, and the males measure 30 to 35 mm long by 0.35 to 0.4 mm wide.

Geographic Distribution and Epidemiology. The geographic distribution of *Loa* corresponds to that of the rain forest of central and western Africa (Nelson, 1965), the only place where the main vectors of the infection, *C. silacea* and *C. dimidiata*, are known. In some areas, disease prevalence is up to 61% in children (Ogunba, 1971). Studies of loiasis in communities of Cameroon (Garcia et al. 1995) and the Democratic Republic of Congo (Noireau, Pichon, 1992) have shown that the number of infected individuals was stable throughout a longitudinal study period, indicating that loiasis is not a cumulative infection. Infected individuals in these areas can be either microfilaremic or amicrofilaremic. Their status does not change over time, also indicating that a possible genetic predisposition to the disease exists (Garcia et al. 1995).

Clinical Findings. As stated, the main characteristic of *Loa loa* is migration through the subcutaneous tissues,

◄

Fig. 20–8. *Onchocerca volvulus*, **histologic appearance of skin lesions, sections stained with hematoxylin and eosin stain.** *A*, **Low-power view of atrophic dermatitis showing thinning of the epidermis and dermis. AFIP preparation No. 378762, ×70.** *B*, **Section of an intraepidermal lesion from the individual with craw-craw. Note the microabscess within the squamous epithelium and the inflammatory infiltrate in the dermis. AFIP prepara-** tion No. 37861 2-C, ×70. *C* and *D*, **Hypertrophic dermatitis. Note the thickening and proliferation of the squamous epithelium and the inflammatory reaction in the dermis. AFIP preparation No. 377482.** *A, C* ×70; *D* ×140. **(Preparations courtesy of R.C. Neafie, M.S., Division of Geographic Pathology, Armed Forces Institute of Pathology, Washington, D.C.)**

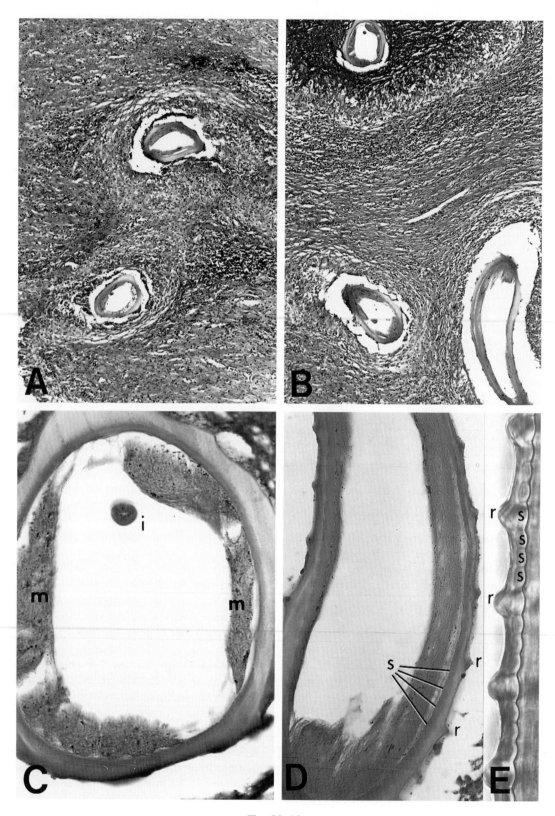

Fig. 20–10.

where the parasite may be seen and felt under the dermis, especially in areas where the skin is thin. The clinical manifestations of loiasis are variable and depend largely on previous experience of the host with the parasite. For example, in endemic areas of *Loa* the signs of infection are generally benign episodes of localized angioedema or *fugitive swellings* and the feeling of the worm migrating through the subcutis or the eye. These manifestations may occur many years after the infection is acquired, in one case 15 years after the individual left the endemic area (Oberg et al. 1987). In addition, a modest eosinophilia, a microfilaremia that peaks at about midday, and low antibody titers to filarial antigens are generally found. In a hyperendemic area in the Democratic Republic of Congo, a study of the infected individuals reported fugitive swellings in 51%, a history of worms in the eye in 70%, and episodes of subcutaneous migration of the worm during the past year in 11% (Noireau et al. 1990a).

Individuals from nonendemic areas who become infected have a more intense clinical course (*color plate IX E*), especially those with swellings and higher peripheral eosinophilia (Churchill et al. 1996). The swellings, known as *calabar swellings*, are pronounced, ill-defined indurations that form in the subcutaneous tissues. Allergic manifestations, which may be marked, consist of marked pruritus, urticarial swellings of the skin and mucous membranes, sometimes with fever, and high peripheral eosinophilia. Swellings pressing on peripheral nerves may produce weakness and loss of sensation in the innervated area (Sarkany, 1959). Microfilaremia is absent more often than not, but peripheral eosinophilia, increased IgE, and low filarial antibody titers are the rule (Nutman et al. 1986). Persons who traveled to or lived for a short period in endemic areas usually acquire a single worm that dies, eliciting the local inflammatory reaction and the swelling. In some cases, the worm is recovered in toto from the subcutaneous tissues while migrating or from the swollen

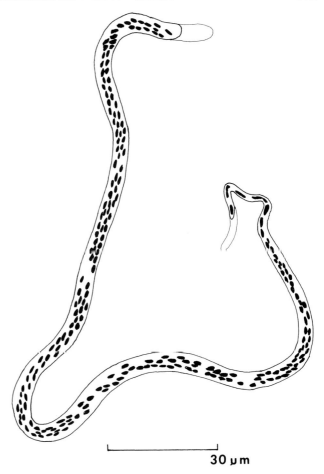

Fig. 20–11. *Loa loa* **microfilaria, thin blood smear stained with Wright stain.**

area; in others, it is found in biopsy specimens taken from the subcutaneous swelling (Charters et al. 1972). The inflammatory reaction to the worm is often moderate (Fig. 20–12 *A–B*), consisting mainly of eosinophils. Dead worms in the tissues may calcify (Le Guyadec et al. 1992; Novak, 1989).

Fig. 20–10. Zoonotic *Onchocerca* species in humans, section stained with hematoxylin and eosin stain. *A* and *B*, Two views of the microscopic appearance of a nodule removed from the wrist of a patient with carpal-tunnel syndrome. Note the cross sections of the parasite showing only the cuticle and somatic muscles, due to the artifactual loss of the sex organs in the cutting room, and the moderate to marked inflammatory infiltration, ×60. *C*, Cross section of a parasite showing the intestinal tube (i), the degenerating muscles (m), and the cuticle, which varies from thin (bottom) to rather thick (right and upper portions) due to oblique sectioning through the trans- verse ridge (thick portion), ×480. ***D*, Longitudinal section showing the transverse ridges (r) and, faintly, the striae (s). Note the four striae for each ridge, ×380. *E*, Cuticle of *O. gutturosa* from cattle, optical section of a whole worm cleared in glycerine. Note the similar pattern of four striae to one ridge, ×380. (*A–D*, preparations courtesy of P.C. Beaver, Ph.D., School of Public Health and Tropical Medicine, Tulane University, New Orleans, Louisiana. Reported by: Beaver, P.C., Horner, G.S., and Bibs, J.Z. 1974. Zoonotic onchocerciasis in a resident of Illinois and observations on the identification of *Onchocerca* species. Am. J. Trop. Med. Hyg. 23:595–607.)**

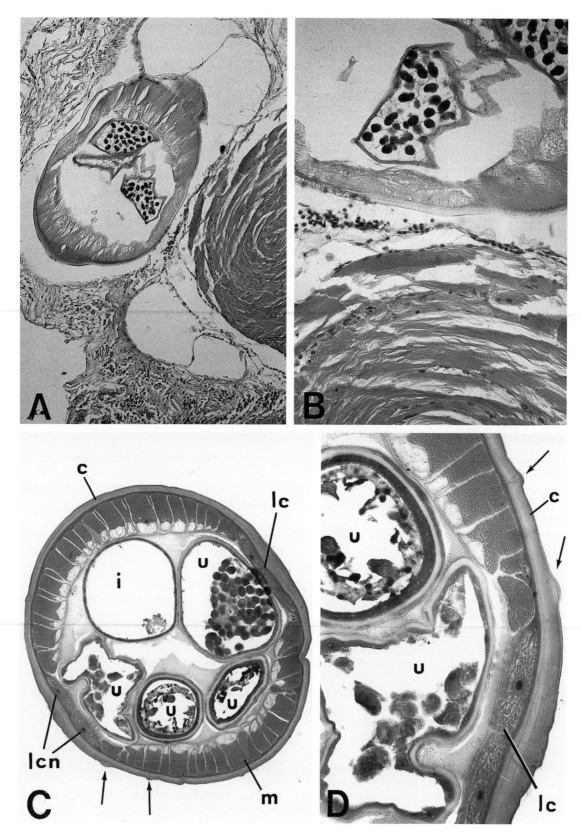

Fig. 20–12.

Other manifestations of loiasis have been described in some individuals, especially in the spleen, kidneys, eye, and joints. In the spleen, a lesion attributed to the microfilaria is a nodular fibrosis (Klotz, 1930) similar to that produced in primates infected experimentally with *Loa loa* (Orihel, Eberhard, 1985). In addition, the spleen shrinks. Lesions in the spleen of individuals who visited endemic areas a few years earlier, were interpreted as malignant lymphomas both clinically and on ultrasonograms (Burchard et al. 1996). In the kidneys, a membranous glomerulonephritis has been described in some patients, possibly due to deposition of soluble antigen–antibody complexes in the basement membrane (Abel et al. 1986; Katner et al. 1984; Pillay et al. 1973). In renal biopsy specimens the microfilaria has been found in the glomeruli, accompanied by an inflammatory reaction and mesangial proliferation (Abel et al. 1986). In addition to the migration of adult worms through the conjunctiva, other ocular manifestations are attributed to loiasis, mostly in Uganda, a country that is not considered endemic for the parasite (Poltera, 1973). These manifestations include yellow nodules in the bulbar conjunctiva, edema of the eyelids and face known as *bug-eye* or *bung eye*, and occasional proptosis of the eyelid (Nnochiri, 1972). These lesions are produced by adult worms many times smaller than *Loa*, probably *M. perstans* (see below and Chapter 21). In the joints, arthritis with joint effusions containing eosinophils and large numbers of microfilariae has been reported (Bouvet et al. 1977; Doury et al. 1983; Jaffres et al. 1983). And finally, a patient with a pleural effusion that contained many eosinophils and *Loa loa* microfilariae, with no known cause for the effusion, responded to antifilarial treatment (Klion et al. 1992).

Manifestations Produced by Treatment. The treatment of loiasis with diethylcarbamazine has produced adverse reactions in some patients due to the death of numerous microfilariae in the blood vessels and some organs. The condition is acute, developing soon after

treatment begins, and occurs mostly in patients with high microfilaremias. In a series of five cases, the lowest microfilaremia was 250 per milliliter and the highest was 28,700 per milliliter (Carme et al. 1991).

The main clinical symptoms are slight fever, fatigue, weakness of some muscle groups, and somnolence that may progress to encephalopathy with coma and death. If the patient develops encephalopathy and recovers, temporary or permanent neurologic sequelae may be observed (Carme et al. 1991; Stanley, Kell, 1982). The syndrome has been reported since diethylcarbamazine was introduced for the treatment of loiasis more than four decades ago (Bogaert et al. 1955; Kivits, 1952; Negesse et al. 1985; Toussaint, Danis, 1965). The pathophysiology of the condition has not been determined, but formation of intravascular platelet-fibrin thrombi around masses of microfilariae suggests that cerebral ischemia may result from mechanical blockage of the circulation (Fig. 20–13 *A–D*; Carme et al. 1991).

Embolized (masses of microfilariae in blood vessels) after treatment have been observed in the arteries of the retina, producing retinal edema (Toussaint, Danis, 1965), hemorrhages (Garin et al. 1975), and retinal ischemia (Corrigan, Hill, 1968). Similar ocular manifestations were also described in a patient who had not received treatment but who had 4500 microfilariae per milliliter (Renard et al. 1978). Soon after therapy with diethylcarbamazine, large concentrations of dead microfilariae were found in the liver sinusoids of another patient (Woodruff, 1951). In addition, in two patients, peripheral nerve damage, observed after treatment with the drug, was attributed to death, degeneration, and organization of adult *Loa* worms in tissues around the nerves (Schofield, 1955). Mass treatment with ivermectin for control of onchocerciasis in areas where coinfections with *Loa* are common has raised some concern because of the possibility of producing some of these adverse effects. Studies of large numbers of patients treated with ivermectin, for *Onchocerca* infection revealed that the

Fig. 20–12. *Loa loa* infection in a man, sections stained with hematoxylin and eosin stain. *A*, Low-power view of an adult female *Loa* in subcutaneous tissues of a patient in Australia with a calabar swelling, ×70. *B*, Higher magnification shows the parasite with a thick cuticle; bosses are not seen in this section. Note the scant inflammatory reaction, composed mainly of eosinophils, ×140. (Preparation courtesy of G.R.H. Kelsall, M.D., Western Australia, Australia. Reported by: Charters, A.D., Welborn, T.A., and Miller, P. 1972. Calabar swellings in immigrants in Western Australia. Med. J. Aust. 1:268–271.) *C*, Cross section of a female *Loa* demonstrates the anatomic features of the worm; intestine (i), uteri (u) with developing eggs, and cuticle (c); note the thickening at the level of the lateral cords (lc), the muscles (m), and the bosses (arrows), ×180. *D*, Higher magnification showing the smooth cuticle (c) with bosses (arrows); its layers are seen more clearly at the lateral cord (lc); lateral cord nuclei (lcn), ×450. (Adult worms courtesy of R.C. Lowry, Jr., Ph.D., Tulane University Delta Regional Primate Research Center, Covington, Louisiana.)

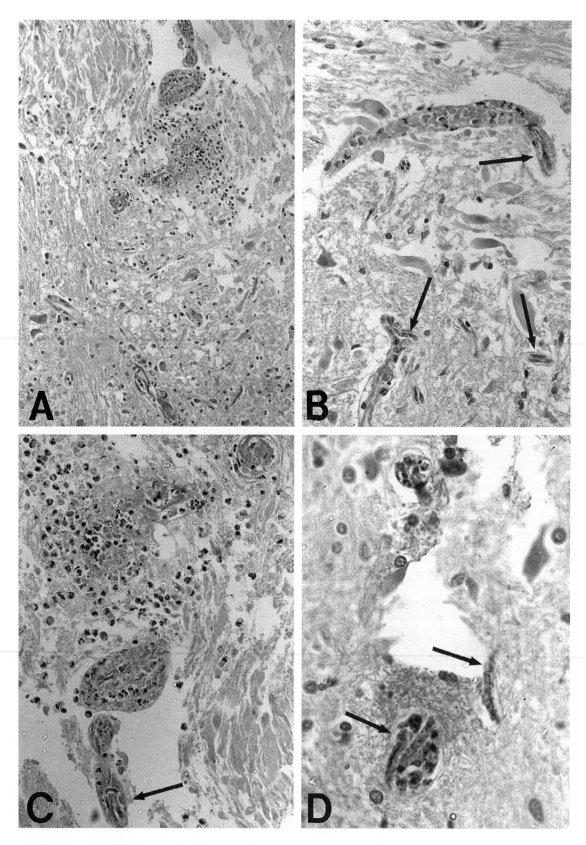

Fig 20–13. *Loa loa* microfilariae in the brain of a patient with encephalopathy due to an adverse reaction to drug treatment. Sections stained with hematoxylin and eosin stain. *A,* Low-power view showing a small area of necrosis and an infiltrate around small blood vessels, ×140. *B* and *C,* Medium-power magnification showing the vessels with sections of microfilariae (arrows), the necrosis, and the infiltrate, ×280. *D,* Higher magnification of capillaries filled with microfilariae (arrows), ×570.

drug produced only moderate complications in a small number of individuals with *Loa* infections (Chippaux et al. 1996; Ducorps et al. 1995). However, other studies revealed a small number of adverse reactions to ivermectin in patients with *Loa* coinfections (Gardon et al. 1997). For fear of adverse complications, some workers have used plasmapheresis to decrease the microfilarial load in peripheral blood before instituting treatment (Bouree et al. 1993; Brumpt et al. 1966; Chandenier et al. 1987). This has been done in spite of the fact that ivermectin is not active against *Loa loa*.

Immunity. Little is known about the immunity of humans to *Loa* infections. Most of the attention to this aspect of the disease is related to the presence and production of immunoglobulins (Goussard et al. 1984), especially IgE (King et al. 1990), because many of the manifestations of the infection are allergic. Serum IgE is elevated in most patients with naturally acquired loiasis, often accompanied by high titers of antifilarial antigens (Orlando et al. 1982). In a study of Gabonese children using a metabolic antigen of *Loa*, only maternal IgG was present at birth, which decreased during the first year of life when new synthesis began. The IgM antibody appeared at 6 months of age, probably due to a new infection. The percentage of children positive for specific IgM and IgE peaked between 2 and 3 years of age and then declined slightly. By age 5, the levels of these immunoglobulins comparable to those of the adult population. The children rarely had microfilaremia (Goussard et al. 1984). The role of antibodies in protecting against the infection or the disease has been studied in endemic areas where the population can be divided into one of three groups: (*1*) those who are resistant, with no symptoms or parasites, have specific circulating antibodies against the parasites; in this group, both adult parasite and microfilaria-specific anti-IgG1 and anti-IgG4 fractions are elevated (Akue et al. 1994; Akue et al. 1997; (*2*) those with circulating microfilariae that do not recognize specific *Loa* antigens (Egwang et al. 1988; Egwang et al. 1989); and (*3*) those who are infected with adult worms but without microfilariae.

Some immunity is provided by the antibodies because antibodies that recognize specific somatic antigens of the worm are present in the sera of the amicrofilaremic and resistant groups. Similar findings were obtained when microfilariae sheet antigens rather than somatic worm antigens were used (Pinder et al. 1992). The relationship between circulating microfilariae and disease was studied both in infected persons living in endemic areas and in infected persons from nonendemic

areas. Microfilaremia was found in 90% of individuals in one endemic area, of whom 16% had calabar swellings. In contrast, only 10% of infected individuals from nonendemic areas had microfilaremia, and swellings occurred in 95% of the cases (Klion et al. 1991).

Pathology. The microscopic changes seen in sections of biopsy specimens or in autopsy material from patients with loiasis are variable. In cases of calabar swellings, the sections show inflammation, as mentioned above, and sometimes the adult worm (see the description below). Worms may be found in the subcutaneous tissues, in deeper tissues, or even in abdominal organs such as the colonic wall and the testis, producing hydrocele (Negesse et al. 1985). Worms have also been recovered from the anterior chamber of the eye (Zue, 1985). The status of the worms is also variable. Some worms are alive, with little inflammation around them; others may be dead in abscesses, degenerated, or with evidence of calcification (Negesse et al. 1985). Calcified worms may be seen in radiograms of the extremities or other areas (Wilms et al. 1983). Calabar swellings may appear spontaneously or after treatment with diethylcarbamazine. In either case, the inflammatory reaction and the edema are attributed to antigens released by the adult worm, reaction to microfilariae around the worm, antigens unmasked by the drug, and other causes. Damage to the worm is best illustrated by the case of an infected physician who, on detecting the worm in his eyelid, fixed it with a suture for later removal; 2 hours after the suture immobilized the worm, an acute swelling began (Eveland et al. 1975). Changes described in the lymph nodes of patients with loiasis living in endemic areas, should be considered nonspecific. In one study, fibrosis of inguinal lymph nodes was attributed to the parasite without evaluation of lymph nodes from uninfected persons living in the same area (Paleologo et al. 1984). This evaluation of uninfected persons would have been ideal, since inguinal lymph nodes in barefoot individuals invariably show chronic inflammatory changes and fibrosis.

The most notable microscopic changes are produced by microfilariae in the capillaries of the central nervous system of patients dying of encephalopathy due to diethylcarbamazine treatment (Fig. 20–13 *A–D*). These changes are known because a few patients who died underwent autopsy (Kivits, 1952; Toussaint, Danis, 1965; Van Bogaert et al. 1955). In another autopsy, it was uncertain whether the patient had been treated with diethylcarbamazine (Negesse et al. 1985). Grossly, the brain and other organs were normal; microscopically, the remarkable finding was the microfilariae, enmeshed in thrombi, filling the blood vessels. Inflammation around the blood vessels was mild, and microfilariae were never present outside the vessels. The changes seen in the brain were also present in other viscera; and as mentioned, in one case it resulted in apparent thrombosis of the retinal arteries (Toussaint, Danis, 1965).

Diagnosis. The diagnosis of loiasis is made clinically, based on a history of exposure and on typical clinical symptoms. Microfilariae recovered in blood samples drawn around noontime are characteristic (Fig. 20–11 and *color plate* IX *F–G*); however, in individuals who acquire the infection while traveling in endemic areas, microfilariae are difficult to find. The sheath of *Loa* microfilariae is difficult to stain and as a rule is not seen in preparations stained with the usual stains for blood (*color plate* IX *F–G*). Microfilariae of *Loa* have been recovered from gastric juice (Whitaker et al. 1980); synovial fluid in cases of arthritis (Bouvet et al. 1977; Roussel et al. 1989); pleural (Klion et al. 1992) and ascitic effusions (Hautekeete et al. 1989); and gynecologic smears (Callihan et al. 1977; de Brux et al. 1983). Specific parasite DNA in circulating blood is demonstrable with the polymerase chain reaction (Toure et al. 1997).

On cross sections, the adult female measures up to 500 μm and the male up to 300 μm in diameter. The cuticle is smooth, layered, and up to 10 μm thick, which is one-half the thickness at the level of the lateral cords, where the layers are best seen (Fig. 20–12 *D*). On the external surface the cuticle has knob-like thickenings. The bosses are up to 6 μm high (Fig. 20–12 *C–D*); they lack the anterior and posterior ends of the male. The bosses, one of the most conspicuous features of *Loa loa*, are irregularly distributed, and sometimes they do not appear in a given section. Deeper, serial, or step sections often are necessary to demonstrate the cuticular bosses. There are approximately 14 muscle cells per quadrant, clearly divided into dorsal and ventral fields by the lateral cords (Fig. 20–12 *C–D*). The contractile portion is up to 40 μm high, with a small cell substance. Muscle cell nuclei are often seen. The lateral cords are one-tenth the circumference of the worm and approximately 15 μm tall (Fig. 20–12 *C–D*). They are clearly divided into two portions and have one to two nuclei per histologic section (Fig. 20–12 *C–D*). The intestine is variable in size and is sometimes up to one-third the diameter of the worm, especially in the anterior portion of the female. The intestinal wall is composed of flattened cells with small nuclei and an inconspicuous brush border (Fig. 20–12 *C*). The sexual organs are similar to those of other filariae.

Mansonella—Mansonelliasis

The genus *Mansonella* has several species infecting humans that are widely distributed in tropical America and Africa (Orihel, Eberhard, 1982). These organisms are normal dwellers of the subcutaneous tissues and body cavities and usually produce little or no symptomatology. The life cycle of *Mansonella* is the same as that of other filarial worms; the vectors are small gnats belonging to the genera *Culicoides* and *Simulium*.

Mansonella ozzardi—Mansonelliasis

Mansonella ozzardi is found in the body cavities and produces asymptomatic infections (McNeeley et al. 1989). The parasite occurs only in Latin America and especially in Amerindians living in remote areas ranging from northern Argentina through Bolivia, Peru, the Guianas, Colombia, Venezuela, Panama, and southern Mexico. In addition, it exists in the West Indies, Trinidad, Haiti, the Dominican Republic, Anguilla, Antigua, Guadeloupe, Dominica, Martinique, St. Lucia, and St Vincent. In some areas of Brazil the prevalence rate is up to 48% (Moraes et al. 1978), and in southern Colombia, in individuals over 12 years of age, the prevalence is 96% (Marinkelle, German, 1970). The vectors in these areas are probably several species of *Culicoides* and *Simulium*. The main vectors appear to be *C. furens* in Haiti (Lowrie, Raccurt, 1981), *C. phlebotomus* in Trinidad (Nathan, 1981), and probably several other species that are good hosts under laboratory conditions (Lowrie et al. 1982). In the Amazon region, *S. amazonicum* is the vector (Shelley, Shelley, 1976).

The diagnosis of *M. ozzardi* is made by identifying typical microfilariae, occurring in small numbers in blood, in samples taken at any time of the day (Fig. 20–14). Microfilariae of *M. ozzardi* have been found in histologic sections of skin (Ewert et al. 1981) and in skin snips (Nathan, 1979). This finding is important because on the American continent *M. ozzardi* microfilariae should be differentiated from microfilariae of *Onchocerca* in skin snips. In the United States, the parasite has been diagnosed in persons who have traveled

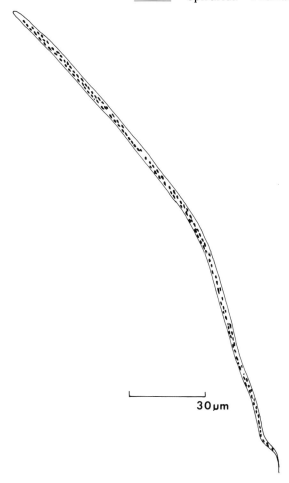

Fig. 20–14. *Mansonella ozzardi* **microfilaria, drawing at scale from a thick blood smear from Knott's concentration stained with iron hematoxylin stain.**

in endemic areas (Weller et al. 1978) and in Haitian refugees (Yangco et al. 1984).

Mansonella perstans—Mansonelliasis *perstans*

Mansonella perstans inhabits the peritoneal, pleural, and pericardial cavities of humans. Adult worms have also been recovered from mesenteric lymph nodes, pancreas, kidney, liver, and rectum (Baird et al. 1987). *Mansonella perstans* is found in the tropical areas of South America, especially Panama, Colombia, Venezuela, Surinam, Trinidad, and Brazil, extending to northern Argentina, (Beaver et al. 1984). In tropical Africa, the parasite exists in an extensive area including Sierra Leone, Ghana,

Nigeria, the Democratic Republic of Congo, Cameroon, Uganda, Tanzania, Zambia, Tunis, and Algeria. Its prevalence in individuals above 15 years of age in areas of the Democratic Republic of Congo is 65% (Zanetti, Lambrecht, 1948), and among pygmies it is up to 80% (Noireau et al. 1990b). The vector in some areas of Africa is *C. austeni*.

Most authorities believe that *M. perstans* produces asymptomatic infections in individuals living in endemic areas (Wiseman, 1967). However, nonspecific transient swellings and allergic manifestations have been described in such individuals (Baker et al. 1967). The condition known as *bung-eye* (see Chapter 21), or the Kampala eye worm, has also been attributed to *M. perstans* based on histologic studies of conjunctival nodules showing cross sections of worms (Baird et al. 1988). It has been suggested that the common peripheral eosinophilia observed in Central African natives is due to infections with *M. perstans*. The majority of symptomatic infections occur in nonnatives, who acquire the infection during temporary residence in endemic areas (Charters et al. 1972; Gelfand, Wessels, 1964; Petithory, Sang, 1965; Sondergaard, 1972; Stott, 1962). Central nervous system involvement has also been described (Dukes et al. 1968), but this is probably due to *Meningonema* rather than *M. perstans* (see Chapter 21). The diagnosis of mansonelliasis perstans is made by finding the typical microfilariae in blood, which measure about 200 μm in length (Fig. 20–15). These microfilariae are not strictly periodic, but their numbers are lower during the day, that is, they are subperiodic. The adults have been found in tissues once and have been described in cross sections (Baird et al. 1987). The finding of a microfilaria of *M. perstans* in aspirated follicular fluid in a patient undergoing in vitro fertilization is not surprising or unexpected; the microfilariae occur in all tissues (Goverde et al. 1996).

Mansonella streptocerca—Streptocerciasis

Mansonella streptocerca inhabits the subcutaneous tissues of humans and monkeys in central west Africa (Gardiner et al. 1979; Meyers et al. 1972; Neafie et al. 1975). The adult parasites are found 1.0 mm below the epidermis, tightly coiled (Fig. 20–16 *A–B*), and produce microfilariae that remain in the skin. The life cycle of *M. streptocerca* is similar to that of other filariids, and *C. grahamii* is likely the intermediate host (Duke, 1954).

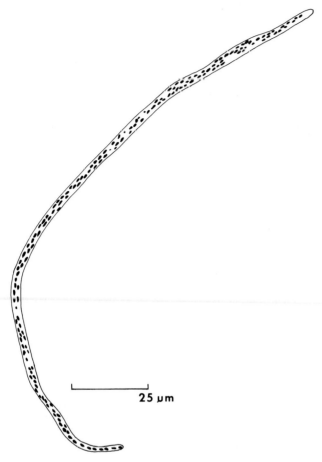

Fig. 20–15. *Mansonella perstans* microfilaria, drawing from a thick blood smear from Knott's concentration stained with Giemsa stain.

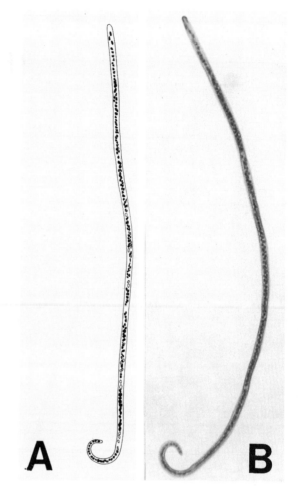

Fig. 20–16. *Mansonella streptocerca* microfilaria teased from skin snip. *A*, Drawing. *B*, Stained with iron hematoxylin, ×540. (In Faust, E.C., Beaver, P.C., and Jung R.C. 1975. Animal Agents and Vectors of Human disease, 4th ed. Philadephia: Lea & Febiger. Reproduced with permission).

The symptoms and signs of streptocerciasis appear mostly in the skin, producing hypopigmentation that is easily confused with leprosy; however, anesthesia is absent. Some patients have urticarial patches or slight pruritus, while others are asymptomatic (Meyers et al. 1972). Symptoms are more pronounced 24 hours after commencement of treatment, with papules 1.0 to 2.5 cm in diameter appearing on the skin of 80% of patients and pruritus with itching, especially over the papules, in 70%. Microfilariae are not found in blood

during or after treatment but are present in the skin (Meyers et al. 1972).

Skin biopsy specimens from individuals with streptocerciasis show slight acanthosis and edema in some cases and increased fibrous connective tissue with infiltration by lymphocytes, histiocytes, and eosinophils

Fig. 20–17. *Mansonella streptocerca* in human skin, sections stained with hematoxylin and eosin stain. *A,* Low-power view showing the location of the parasite within the dermis, ×55. *B,* Higher magnification shows the scanty inflammatory infiltrate below the epidermis and around the worm, ×140. *C* and *D,* Detail of the female worm show two uteri with microfilariae. Note the delicate, thin cuticle and the muscle cells. The inflam-

matory reaction around the worm followed drug treatment, ×350. (AFIP preparation No. 377582-B courtesy of W.M. Meyers, M.D., Ph.D., Division of Microbiology, Armed Forces Institute of Pathology, Washington, D.C. Reported by: Meyers, W.M., Connor, D.H., Harman, L.E., et al. 1972. Human streptocerciasis. A clinico-pathologic study of 40 Africans (Zairians) including identification of the adult filaria. Am. J. Trop. Med. Hyg. 21:528–545.)

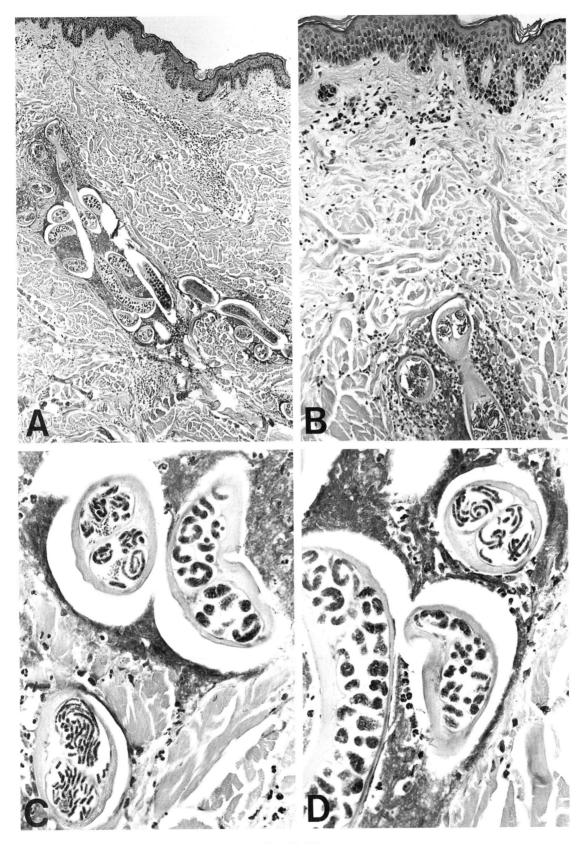

Fig. 20–17.

in other cases, usually within a matrix of acid mucopolysaccharide, around small dermal vessels (Fig. 20–17 A–B). Some of these changes are increased in posttreatment biopsy specimens (Fig. 20–17 A–B). Microfilariae are present, and if sections fall through the anterior and posterior portions, the characteristic morphology of the microfilariae allows differentiation from microfilariae of *O. volvulus*. Microfilariae in tissue sections do not have a sheath. The cephalic space (the distance from the anterior end to the first nucleus) is 3 to 5 μm long; the first four nuclei are oval, in shape and arranged in single file, followed by 7 to 10 rounded smaller nuclei, also in single file. The tail contains a column of 9 to 12 nuclei varying in shape, and the caudal space is about 1 μm long. The tail of the microfilaria is curved in a "shepherd's crook" configuration (Fig. 20–16 A–B). Microfilariae are present in all layers of the skin but are more numerous in the upper third, in the endothelium-lined spaces, probably the lymphatics (Meyers et al. 1972; Orihel, 1984). The microfilariae are 180 to 240 μm in length by 3 to 5 μm in width and have no sheath.

The most conspicuous feature of biopsy specimens from papules formed after treatment of patients with streptocerciasis is the presence of adult parasites. The worms appear to be coiled and surrounded by an inflammatory reaction (Fig. 20–17 A and C). Biopsy specimens from untreated individuals rarely demonstrate the adult worm, but if the worm is present, it is not coiled or surrounded by an inflammatory infiltrate (Meyers et al. 1972).

In cross sections, the female is 85 μm in the largest diameter; the cuticle is 1 to 2 μm thick and is smooth, without striations, and slightly thicker at the level of the lateral cords; the lateral cords are narrow and low, with round to elongated nuclei; the ventral and dorsal cords are inconspicuous. The muscle cells, about 10 per quadrant, have a prominent contractile portion with a barely evident sarcoplasm (Fig. 20–17 C–D). The intestinal tract is small, and the paired uteri fill the body cavity (Fig. 20–17 C–D; Meyers et al. 1977; Neafie et al. 1975).

Dirofilaria—Cutaneous Dirofilariasis

The genus *Dirofilaria* has many species in wild and domestic animals throughout the world; the males are characterized by a coiled posterior end, with highly developed caudal alae and numerous large papillae (Fig. 20–18 A–B). The size of the adult varies from a few centimeters to 35 cm in *D. immitis*. The females are usually larger than the males, and females from different species are often indistinguishable (Fig. 20–18 D). One characteristic of some of the subcutaneous *Dirofilaria* found in humans is the presence of longitudinal ridges on the cuticle, which are visible under the light microscope (Fig. 20–18 C–D).

The life cycle of *Dirofilaria* is the same as that of other filariids; the microfilariae, without sheaths, occur in the blood, and several species of mosquitoes, simuliids, and other blood-sucking arthropods are the usual intermediate hosts. Speciation of the genus *Dirofilaria* is outside the scope of this discussion (Anderson, 1952; Uni, 1978); instead, the characteristics in cross sections of *Dirofilaria* recovered from humans are discussed.

All species of *Dirofilaria* found in the subcutaneous tissues of humans are accidental zoonotic infections and occur in many parts of the world. Some of these filariids were reported as *D. conjunctiva* because in many cases the worms were located in the conjunctiva or other external eye structures Fig. 20–19). The known zoonotic *Dirofilaria* species found in subcutaneous tissues of humans are *D. repens*, *D. tenuis*, *D. ursi*-like, *D. striata*, and a species of *Dirofilaria* that is indistinguishable from *D. immitis*, also referred to as *D. immitis*-like (Gutierrez et al. 1996). The clinical manifestations of the infection and the morphologic appearance of the lesions produced by these dirofilariids in humans are similar.

Clinical Findings. The clinical manifestation of subcutaneous dirofilariasis is a 1 to 3 cm nodule anywhere in the body. The nodule is painless, with no signs of inflammation at first. If it is located in an area that causes concern, such as near the eye (Fig. 20–19), the conjunctiva, the genitals, or the breast, the person usually consults a physician. In these cases, opening the lesion often produces a living worm. A nodule in the breast is often removed because of the suspicion of malignancy (Ashford et al. 1989; Bennett et al. 1989; Frouge et al. 1992; Gutierrez, Paul, 1984; MacDougall et al. 1992). Worms have also been recovered from the peritoneal cavity of patients undergoing surgery (De Gentile et al. 1992; Delage et al. 1984). More often, medical attention is sought when the nodule grows larger or becomes painful, with signs of inflammation. In these cases, the lesion is usually removed and submitted for histologic examination. The painless nodule may remain for several months before becoming inflamed, or it may disappear and reappear in another location (Shenefelt et al. 1996). Rarely has a patient

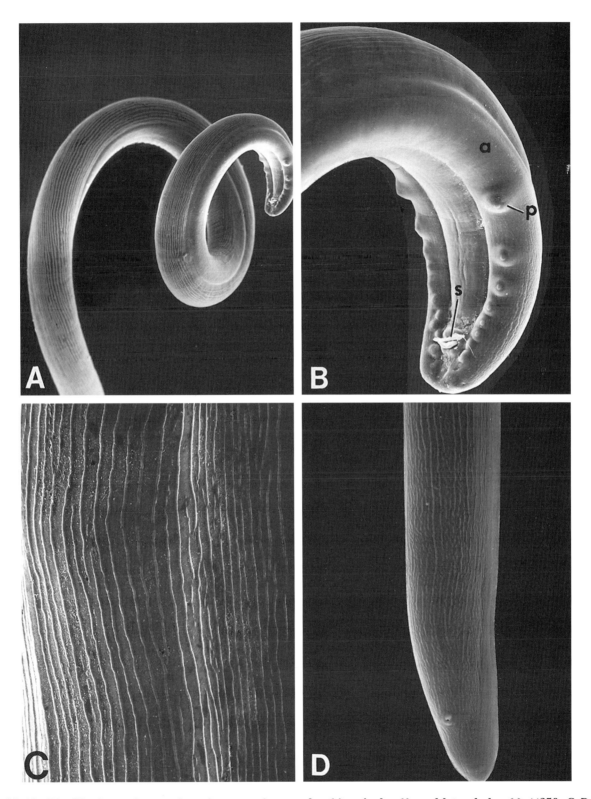

Fig. 20–18. *Dirofilaria ursi*, scanning electron micrographs illustrating general morphologic features of a *Dirofilaria*. *A*, Coiled posterior end of a male, ×60. *B*, Detail of the ventral posterior end of a male shows papil-lae (p), spicules (s), and lateral alae (a), ×250. *C*, Detail of the cuticle shows longitudinal ridges, ×200. *D*, Posterior end of a female. Note the anus at the posterior end, ×100.

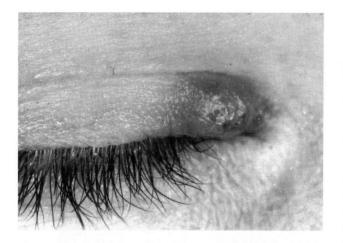

Fig. 20–19. *Dirofilaria tenuis* in eyelid. Note the small nodule in this man from Texas, the location of which (near the eye) is a reason to seek medical attention. (Courtesy of M.D. Little, Ph.D., Department of Tropical Medicine, School of Public Health and Tropical Medicine, Tulane University, New Orleans, Louisiana.)

presented with two or more nodules (Herzberg et al. 1995). A patient with an infection attributed to *D. repens*, acquired in Africa, presented twice with nodules, 10 months apart, as a result of a single infection. The worms were recovered and identified on both occasions (Orihel et al. 1997).

Pathology. The gross specimen is commonly labeled by the clinician as a cyst, infected cyst, ruptured cyst, subcutaneous nodule, abscess, or another lesion. The removed nodule is usually 1 to 2 cm in diameter and consists of indurated subcutaneous and fibroadipose tissue with no gross visible inflammation or necrosis. On section, the nodule may appear solid. It often has a necrotic center and sometimes shows a cavity filled with thick fluid. Microscopically, the nodule usually appears as an abscess in different stages of organization, composed of inflammatory cells and fibrous tissue (Figs. 20–21 *A* and 20–23 *A*). Early abscesses show

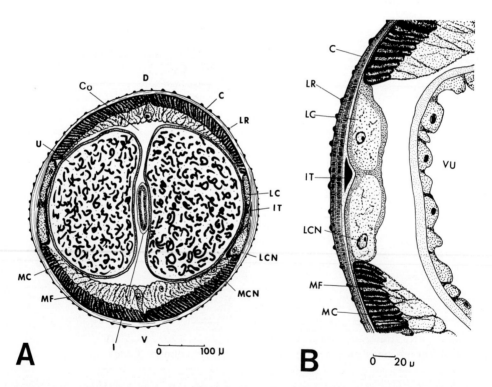

Fig. 20–20. *Dirofilaria.* Schematic representation of morphology on cross section. *A*, Cross section. *B*, Detail of the cuticle at the level of the lateral cords. Abbreviations: c, cuticle; co, pseudocoelom; d, dorsum; i, intestine; it, internal thickening of the cuticle; lc, lateral cords; lcn, lateral cord nucleus; lr, longitudinal ridge; mc, muscle cell; mcn, muscle cell nucleus; mf, muscle fibers; u, uterus; v, ventrum; vu, vagina uterina. (In: Gutierrez, Y. 1984. Diagnostic features of zoonotic filariae in tissue sections. Hum. Pathol. 15:514–525. Reproduced with permission.)

the worm either well preserved (Fig. 20–22 C) or in the early stages of degeneration (Fig. 20–22 B), with focal necrosis (Fig. 20–23 A), polymorphonuclear cells, some eosinophils, and fibrosis, growing into the surrounding adipose tissues. Advanced lesions have central necrosis and sometimes a cavity filled with debris and inflammatory cells. In all cases, the most conspicuous element is the worm in various stages of degeneration.

Microscopic Characteristics of Dirofilaria. On cross sections, most species of *Dirofilaria* have uniform general characteristics that distinguish them from other filarial worms (Gutierrez, 1984; Orihel, Beaver, 1965; Uni et al. 1980). The size of the parasite varies from 100 to 600 μm in diameter. The cuticle is thick, layered, and either smooth (Fig. 22–23 B and *color plate* X A) or with longitudinal ridges (Figs. 20–20 A–B, 20–21, 20–22, 20–23, and *color plate* X B–F) that on cross section are seen as rounded or sharply elevated structures, either crowded together or separated by well-defined intervals (Figs. 20–20 A–B and 20–23 B–C). The different layers of the cuticle are easily discernible, especially at the level of the lateral cords or on oblique sections (Figs. 20–20 A–B and 20–21 C). The outer two layers are composed of fibers running oblique to the body axis and perpendicular to each other, better appreciated on tangential sections (Fig. 20–23 D). The inner layer of the cuticle has a thickening, or ridge, at each of the two lateral aspects of the worm. These two ridges vary in size and shape, depending on the species, the body level at which the worm is sectioned, and the sex of the worm (Figs. 20–20 B, 20–21 C, 20–22 A and D), and 20–23 C). The internal ridges are located at the middle of each lateral cord and are seen as a triangular structure that protrudes internally. The muscle cells are numerous and well developed (Figs. 20–20 A–B, 20–21 D, and 20–22 D). The sexual organs of most *Dirofilaria* found in humans are immature (Fig. 20–22 D); mature worms are rarely found (Jung, Espenan, 1967; Pacheco, Schofield, 1968; Pampiglione et al. 1992). This general description permits identification of the genus *Dirofilaria* in most cases. The best-known species of *Dirofilaria* in humans have characteristics that allow specific identification; the less well known ones may permit only a presumptive or approximate identification, and some have not been possible to identify. The microanatomy of many of the known species of *Dirofilaria* has not been studied, and other species probably have not yet been named (Beaver et al. 1987).

The longitudinal ridges of *Dirofilaria* are an important morphologic characteristic that aids their identification, but they are often a source of confusion. The ridges are well defined in *D. repens*, *D. tenuis*, *D. ursi*, and *D. subdermata*; absent in *D. immitis* and *D. lutrae*; and poorly developed and irregular in *D. striata*. In reality, *D. immitis* has attenuated longitudinal ridges that are visualized only with the scanning electron microscope, and because they are extremely attenuated, they have been referred to as *longitudinal markings* (Uni, Takada, 1986). Longitudinal ridges have a distinct appearance that often eludes those who are unfamiliar with them. They vary with the species in question and are uniform throughout the entire surface, with small variations in spacing at the lateral aspects of the worm, where they are slightly closer to each other than in other areas. All longitudinal ridges have a convex apex that is sometimes sharp, as in *D. ursi*, and wide, in other species, such as *D. tenuis*. Dead worms in tissues allow eosinophils to attach to their cuticle and start the destruction (degeneration) of the worm. One of the first signs of this destruction is lysis of the cuticle, which occurs first at the site of attachment of each eosinophil or polymorphonuclear cell, creating a cavity. The process of lysis gives a scalloped appearance that in cross sections is often mistaken for ridges. Therefore, the recognition and evaluation of ridges is more difficult in degenerating specimens. To reemphasize, identification of *Dirofilaria* in tissue sections is based on the recognizable structures, the diameter of the worm, its location in the body, and the geographic area where the patient acquired the infection. The homing instinct of helminths is very powerful, and in both normal and abnormal hosts, the organ or tissue where they are found is often key in their identification.

Dirofilaria repens

Dirofilaria repens is the subcutaneous *Dirofilaria* of dogs and cats in Europe, Asia, and Africa. Many human infections with this parasite have been reported in the last 100 years, mostly from Italy (Pampiglione et al. 1995), Russia (Kovalev et al. 1971), France (Desportes, 1939; Desportes, 1940), and almost every European country. Cases have been reported in the Indian subcontinent (Dissanaike, 1971; Dissanaike et al. 1993), Southeast Asia (Le Van Hoa, Le Thi Ty, 1971), the Middle East (Gutierrez et al. 1995; Hira et al. 1994), Africa (Orihel et al. 1997), and other areas. The first descriptions of the worm referred to it as *D. conjunctiva* or *Loa extraocularis* (Skrjabin, 1917) because many of the infections were located in the conjunctiva, often producing conjunctivitis, or near the eye. Based

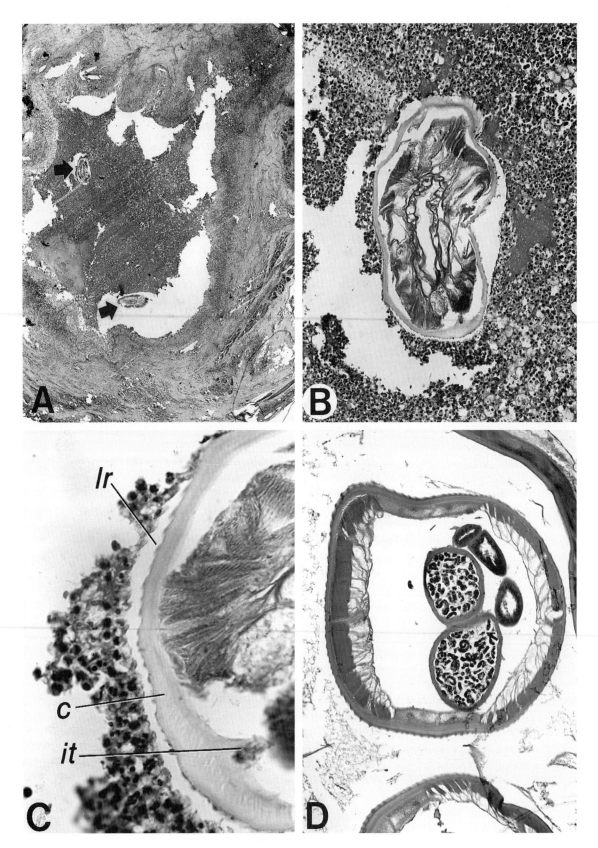

Fig. 20–21.

on the study of recovered male worms it was conclusively demonstrated that *D. repens* was the cause of the lesions (Ratnavale, Dissanaike, 1964; Skrjabin et al. 1930).

One morphologic characteristic of *D. repens* in cross sections is a diameter of 220 to 600 μm, over 300 μm in the great majority of cases (Fig. 20–21 *B–C* and *color plate* X *D*). In only one instance was the diameter recorded as 175 μm (MacLean et al. 1979). The longitudinal cuticular ridges total between 95 and 105 in each cross section at midbody (25 per quadrant). *Each ridge is separated from the others by a distance larger than the width of the ridge itself* (see Fig. 19–19 *B–D*; Kotkan, 1951; MacLean et al. 1979). In well-developed specimens, the distance between the ridges is about 12 μm (Fig. 20–21 *D*; Pinon et al. 1980). The lateral cords have two to five nuclei per histologic section (Fig. 20–21 *D*).

Dirofilaria tenuis

Human infections with *D. conjunctiva* began to be recognized around 1941 in the southeastern United States. The clinical characteristics of the lesions and of the worm were generally identical to those observed in Europe. In 1965, the reported cases of *D. conjunctiva* in the United States, plus several new ones, were extensively reviewed and were found to be identical to *D. tenuis*, a filariid from the subcutaneous tissues of the raccoon (*Procyon lotor*) (Orihel, Beaver, 1965). *Dirofilaria tenuis* has been found only in raccoons in the southeastern United States, in an area stretching from Florida to Texas and north to about Arkansas. About three-fourths of all *D. tenuis* infections have been reported from Florida, where the main vectors are the black salt marsh mosquitoes *Aedes taeniorhynchus* and *Anopheles quadrimaculatus*. Under experimental laboratory conditions, other species are also suitable hosts.

The prevalence of the infection in raccoons in endemic areas is variable. The rate of microfilaremia in these animals decreases from 45% in southern Florida to 21% in the central part of the state to 6% in the northern part (Isaza, Courtney, 1988); in Arkansas, only 1 of 30 raccoons examined was found to be infected (Richardson et al. 1992). The slow growth of the worm makes it possible for a traveler from nonendemic states to become infected and develop clinical manifestations months later at home (Gutierrez, Paul, 1984).

The distinguishing anatomic features of *D. tenuis* in tissue sections are a diameter ranging from 150 to 330 μm and longitudinal cuticular ridges (Fig. 20–22 *A–D* and *color plate* X *B*); living in or having visited the endemic area is also necessary for the diagnosis, given our present knowledge of the range of the species. The longitudinal ridges are *relatively low and rounded, with a wavy, broken, and branching pattern; the spaces between the ridges are narrower than the ridges themselves* (Fig. 20–22 *C–D*; Orihel, Beaver, 1965). Most parasites recovered from humans are mature or young adults; in two cases, the worms were fertilized females with developed microfilariae in the uteri (Jung, Espenan, 1967; Pacheco, Schofield, 1968).

Dirofilaria ursi-like

A number of infections with subcutaneous *Dirofilaria* in the northern United States and Canada are generally recognized as being produced by a species different from *D. tenuis*. The parasite appears to be one of two *Dirofilaria* with well-spaced cuticular longitudinal ridges that are endemic in the area. One is *D. ursi*, occurring in the perirenal fat and the mediastinum of bears (*Ursus americanus*); the other is *D. subdermata*, found in the subcutaneous tissues of porcupines (*Erethizon dorsatum*) (Beaver, Samuel, 1977; Meerovitch et al. 1976). After cross sections of adults of *D. subdermata* and *D. ursi*

Fig. 20–21. *Dirofilaria repens*, **sections stained with hematoxylin and eosin stain.** *A*, **Low-power view of a granuloma with a necrotic center containing two cross sections of parasites (arrows), ×16.** *B*, **Higher magnification shows the polymorphonuclear cell infiltrate and an oblique section of the parasite, ×150.** *C*, **Detail of a parasite showing the thick-layered cuticle (c), the internal thickening (it), and the longitudinal ridges (lr). Note the mass of polymorphonuclear cells against the worm's cuticle, which makes the morphology rather vague, ×600.** *D*, **Well-pre-** served *D. repens*, **cross section from an animal infected experimentally, ×150. (Preparations for *A–C* courtesy of A.S. Dissanaike, M.D., Department of Parasitology, Faculty of Medicine, Colombo, Sri Lanka. Preparation for *D* courtesy of M.M. Wong, Ph.D., Department of Veterinary Microbiology, University of California, Davis, California. *A–D* in: Gutierrez, Y. 1984. Diagnostic features of zoonotic filariae in tissue sections. Hum. Pathol., 15:514–525. Reproduced with permission.)**

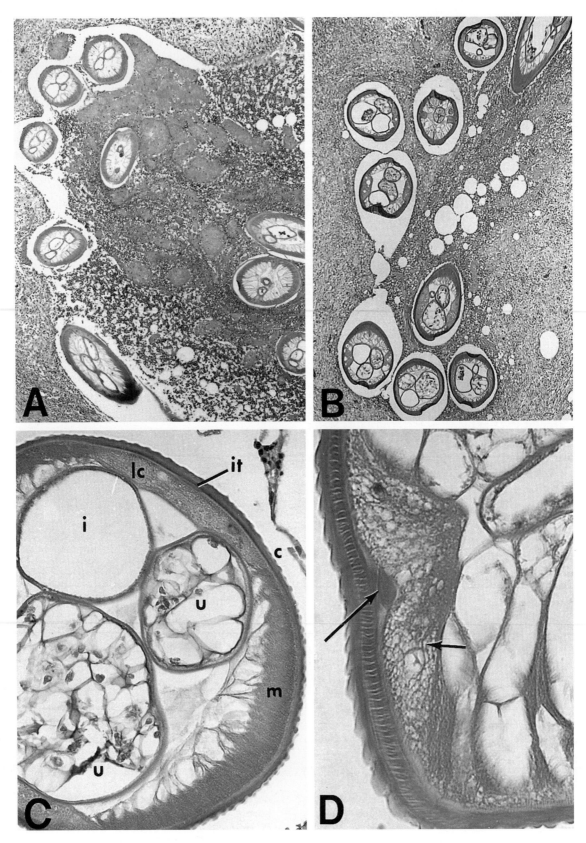

Fig. 20–22.

were studied, it was suggested that the reported human infections were probably *D. ursi* because the morphology of the worms in humans was similar to that of *D. ursi* (Gutierrez, 1983, 1984).

In a review of all reported cases of *D. ursi* or *D. subdermata* in the northern United States and Canada, it was concluded that the differences described in the adult worms were not easily applicable to the immature, necrotic worms found in humans (Beaver et al. 1987). However, the morphology of the individual longitudinal ridges of the filariids in humans most closely resembles the morphology of the ridges of *D. ursi*; thus, the term *D. ursi*-like was used for these worms (Beaver et al. 1987).

The worms are usually less than 200 µm in diameter (Fig. 20–23 A–D), with *tall, sharply crested, narrow ridges separated by a distance three to four times the width of the ridges themselves* (Fig. 20–23 B–C and *color plate* X C). Most worms are necrotic, but the morphology of the cuticle and the ridges is usually well preserved. All infections with *D. ursi*-like worms have been found in women, with the exception of the last case reported (and mistakenly referred to as *D. tenuis*) (Preshaw et al. 1993).

Dirofilaria Species (*immitis*-like)

There are several reports of infections with a subcutaneous *Dirofilaria* in the United States, characterized morphologically by a thick-layered, smooth cuticle resembling that of *D. immitis* (Billups et al. 1980; Blecka et al. 1978; Brumback et al. 1968; Gutierrez et al. 1996; Thomas et al. 1976). The location of the parasites is consistent with *D. immitis*, which after entering the body needs a period of about 3 months in the subcutaneous tissues for growth and maturation before locating in the pulmonary arteries (Orihel, 1961). In addition to the subcutaneous tissues, this *Dirofilaria* has also been found in the peritoneal cavity and the orbit (Fig. 20–24 B); on reported measurements, the diameter of the worms varied from 120 to 320 µm. Cuticular longitudinal ridges have been found only on the ventral posterior region of the male (a characteristic of *D. immitis*). The somatic muscle cells of the parasite are numerous and well developed, numbering about 20 per quadrant and resembling those of immature *D. immitis* (Billups et al. 1980). Because of these characteristics, the worm in question has been referred to as *D. immitis*-like (Fig. 20–24 B; Gutierrez et al. 1996).

In Japan, cases of subcutaneous *Dirofilaria* with morphology in tissue sections similar to that described above have been classified as *D. immitis* (Kaneda et al. 1980; Mimori et al. 1986). In other cases, worms recovered from the eye and studied in toto (see Chapter 21) have been conclusively identified as *D. immitis* (Dissanaike et al. 1977; Kerkezenov, 1962; Moorhouse, 1978).

Dirofilaria striata

Dirofilaria striata dwells in the deep tissues and muscle fascia of several species of wild cats on the American continent (Orihel, Ash, 1964). Only one human infection with *D. striata* is known, occurring in a 6-year-old boy living in Buncombe County, North Carolina (Orihel, Isbey, 1990). The anatomic characteristics of *D. striata* are small but conspicuous lateral alae, seen as low, rounded protrusions of the cuticle on both lateral aspects of the worm, and poorly developed, irregular cuticular longitudinal ridges (*color plate* X E–F) (Orihel, Isbey, 1990).

Other Subcutaneous Filarial Parasites

In addition to the above species, other subcutaneous zoonotic filariids, not fully classified or having features consistent with a species of *Dipetalonema* or *Dipetalonema*-like, have been described (Ando et al. 1985; Beaver, Orihel, 1965).

Fig. 20–22. *Dirofilaria tenuis* infection in humans, sections stained with hematoxylin and eosin stain. *A* and *B*, Low magnification of nodules shows a necrotic center with up to 10 sections of *D. tenuis*, ×46. *C*, Intermediate magnification shows some anatomical landmarks of the parasite: an attenuated internal thickening (it), cuticle with longitudinal ridges (c), the intestine (i), the two uteri (u), lateral cords (lc), and well-preserved muscles (m), ×350. *D*, Higher magnification demonstrating the layers of the cuticle, a prominent internal thickening (long arrow), the lateral cords (short arrow), and the longitudinal ridges. Note that the ridges in this species appear crowded next to each other; contrast with Figures 20–21 *D*, 20–18 *C*, and 20–23 *B* and *C*, ×721.

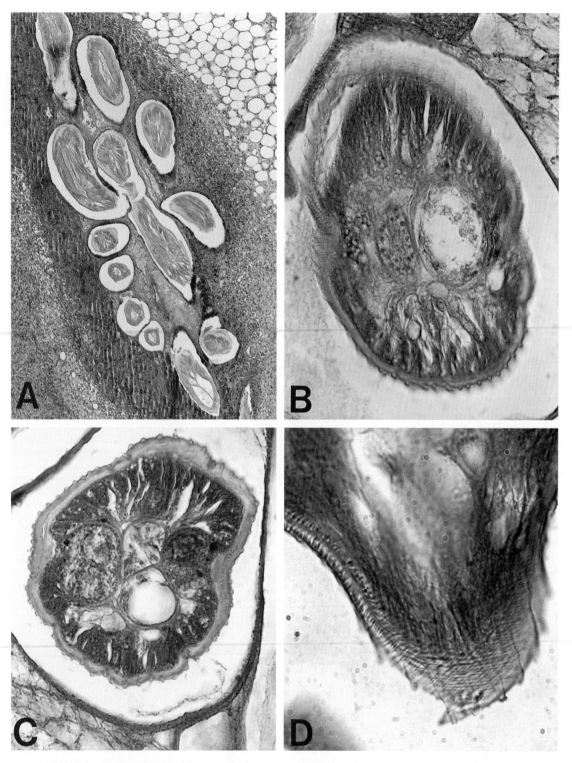

Fig. 20–23. *Dirofilaria ursi*-like species in a man, sections stained with hematoxylin and eosin stain. *A*, Low-power view of a granuloma with a necrotic center containing a degenerating worm, ×50. *B* and *C*, Two cross sections of the worm show details of the cuticle. Note the longitudinal ridges, and contrast their configuration with those of *D. tenuis* (Fig. 20–22) and *D. repens* (Fig. 20–21), ×600. *D*, Higher magnification of an oblique sec- tion showing the layers of the cuticle, composed of fibers running perpendicular to each other, ×1,150. (Preparation courtesy of H.M. Payan, M.D., Department of Pathology, Bell Memorial Hospital, Ishpeming, Michigan. (*C–D* in: Gutierrez, Y. 1984. Diagnostic features of zoonotic filariae in tissue sections. Hum. Pathol. 15:514–525. Reproduced with permission.)

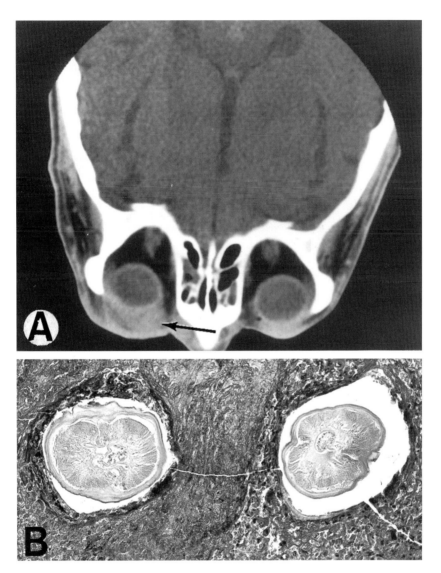

Fig. 20–24. *Dirofilaria immitis*-like species in a man from Indiana, sections stained with hematoxylin and eosin stain. *A*, Computed tomographic scan of the orbits of a patient with a soft tissue mass in the left one (arrow). *B*, Two sections of the worm, with characteristics similar to those of a *Dirofilaria*, as described in previous figures. Note, however, that the cuticle of this worm is smooth, with no longitudinal ridges, ×180. (Reported by Gutierrez, Y., Catallaer, M., and Wicker, D.L. 1996. Extrapulmonary *Dirofilaria immitis*-like infections in the Western Hemisphere. Am. J. Surg. Pathol. 20:299–305. Reproduced with permission.)

References

Abdel-Hameed AA, Noah MS, Schacher JF, Taher SA, 1987. Lymphadenitis in Sowda. Trop. Geogr. Med. 39:73–76

Abel L, Ioly V, Jeni P, Carbon C, Bussel A, 1986. Apheresis in the management of loiasis with high microfilariaemia and renal disease. Br. Med. J. Clin. Res. Ed. 292:24

Akogun OB, Akoh JI, Hellandendu H, 1992. Non-ocular clinical onchocerciasis in relation to skin microfilaria in the Taraba River Valley, Nigeria. J. Hyg. Epidemiol. Microbiol. Immunol. 36:368–383

Akue JP, Egwang TG, Devaney E, 1994. High levels of parasite-specific IgG4 in the absence of microfilaremia in *Loa loa* infection. Trop. Med. Parasitol. 45:246–248

Akue JP, Hommel M, Devaney E, 1997. High levels of parasite-specific IgG1 correlate with the amicrofilaremic state in *Loa loa* infection. J. Infect. Dis. 175:158–163

Ali-Khan, Z, Meerovitch E, 1973. The first reported case of a zoonotic *Onchocerca* sp in man. Abstracts, 48th Annual Meeting of the American Society of Parasitologists, Toronto, 29 June, p. 51

Anderson RC, 1952. Description and relationships of *Dirofilaria ursi*, Yamaguti 1941, and a review of the genus *Dirofilaria* Raillet and Henry, 1911. Trans. R. Can. Inst. 29:35–64

Ando K, Beaver PC, Soga T, Maehara T, Kitamura S, 1985. Zoonotic subcutaneous filaria of undetermined classification. Am. J. Trop. Med. Hyg. 34:1138–1141

Ashford RW, Dowse JA, Rogers WN, Powell DE, 1989. Correspondence. Dirofilariasis of the breast. Lancet 1:1198

Azarova NS, Miretsky OY, Sonin MD, 1965. The first instance of detection of nematode *Onchocerca* Diesing, 184 in a person in the USSR. Med. Parasitol. 34:156–158

Baird JK, Neafie RC, Connor DH, Lanoie L, 1988. Nodules in the conjunctiva, bung-eye, and bulge-eye in Africa caused by *Mansonella perstans*. Am. J. Trop. Med. Hyg. 38:553–557

Baird JK, Neafie RC, Lanoie L, Connor DH, 1987. Adult *Mansonella perstans* in the abdominal cavity in nine Africans. Am. J. Trop. Med. Hyg. 37:578–584

Baker NM, Baldachin BJ, Rachman I, Thomas JE, 1967. A study of eosinophilia and *A. perstans* infestation in African patients. Cent. Afr. J. Med. 13:23–31

Beaver PC, Horner GS, Bilos JZ, 1974. Zoonotic onchocercosis in a resident of Illinois and observations on the identification of *Onchocerca* species. Am. J. Trop. Med. Hyg. 23:595–607

Beaver PC, Jung RC, Cupp EW, 1984. *Clinical Parasitology*. Philadelphia: Lea & Febiger

Beaver PC, Orihel TC, 1965. Human infection with filariae of animals in the United States. Am. J. Trop. Med. Hyg. 14:1010–1029

Beaver PC, Samuel WM, 1977. Dirofilariasis in man in Canada. Am. J. Trop. Med. Hyg. 26:329–330

Beaver PC, Wolfson JS, Waldron MA, Swartz MN, Evans GW, Adler J, 1987. *Dirofilaria ursi*-like parasites acquired by humans in the northern United States and Canada: re-

port of two cases and brief review. Am. J. Trop. Med. Hyg. 37:357 362

Beaver PC, Yoshimura H, Takayasy S, Hashimoto H, Little MD, 1989. Zoonotic *Onchocerca* in a Japanese child. Am. J. Trop. Med. Hyg. 40:298–300

Becker CK, 1950. Filaires adultes (*Onchocerca volvulus*) libres dans les tissus. Ann. Soc. Belge Med. Trop. 30:9–10

Bennett IC, Furnival CM, Searle J, 1989. Dirofilariasis in Australia: unusual cause of a breast lump. Aust. N.Z. J Surg. 59:671–673

Billups J, Schenken JR, Beaver PC, 1980. Subcutaneous dirofilariasis in Nebraska. Arch. Pathol. Lab. Med. 104:11–13

Blecka LJ, Miller A, Graf EC, 1978. Human subcutaneous dirofilariasis in Illinois. JAMA 240:245–246

Bogaert LV, Dubois A, Janssens PG, Radermecker J, Tverdy G, Wanson M, 1955. Encephalitis in *Loa-loa* filariasis. J. Neurol. Neurosurg. Psychiatry 18:103–119

Borges RD, 1971. Findings of microfilarial larval stages in gynecologic smears. Acta Cytol. 15:476–478

Bouree P, Duedari N, Bisaro F, Norol F, 1993. Interet de la filariophorese dans le traitement de la filariose a *Loa loa*. Pathol. Biol. Paris 41:410–414

Bourgeade A, Nosny Y, Olivier Paufique M, Faugere B, 1989. A propos de 32 cas d'edemes localises recidivants au retour des tropiques. Bull. Soc. Pathol. Exot. 82:21–28

Bouvet JP, Therizol M, Auquier L, 1977. Microfilarial polyarthritis in a massive *Loa loa* infestation. A case report. Acta Trop. 34:281–284

Brumback GF, Morrison HM, Weatherly NF, 1968. Orbital infection with *Dirofilaria*. South. Med. J. 61:188, 192–188, 192

Brumpt LC, Pequignot H, L'hermitte F, Petithory J, Remy H, 1966. Loase avec microfilaremie elevee, encephalite therapeutique, traitement par exsanguino-transfusion. Bull. Mem. Soc. Med. Hop. Paris 117:1049–1058

Buck AA, 1974. *Onchocerciasis: Symptomatology, Pathology, Diagnosis*. Geneva, WHO

Burchard GD, Reimold JU, Burkle V, Kretschmer H, Vierbuchen M, Racz P, Lo Y, 1996. Splenectomy for suspected malignant lymphoma in two patients with loiasis. Clin. Infect. Dis. 23:979–982

Callihan TR, Oertel YC, Mendoza M, 1977. *Loa loa* in a gynecologic smear. Am. J. Trop. Med. Hyg. 26:572–573

Carme B, Boulesteix J, Boutes H, Puruehnce MF, 1991. Five cases of encephalitis during treatment of loiasis with diethylcarbamazine. Am. J. Trop. Med. Hyg. 44:684–690

Chan CC, Nussenblatt RB, Kim MK, Palestine AG, Awadzi K, Ottesen EA, 1987. Immunopathology of ocular onchocerciasis 2. Anti-retinal autoantibodies in serum and ocular fluids. Ophthalmology 94:439–443

Chandenier J, Pillier Loriette C, Datry A, Rosenhcim M, Danis M, Felix H, Nozais JP, Gentilini M, 1987. Interet de la cytapherese dans le traitement des loases a fortes microfilaremies. Resultats a propos de sept cas. Bull. Soc. Pathol. Exot. 80:624–633

Charters AD, Welborn TA, Miller P, 1972. Calabar swellings in immigrants in western Australia. Med. J. Aust. 1: 268–271

Chippaux JP, Boussinesq M, Gardon J, Gardon-Wendel N, Ernould JC, 1996. Severe adverse reaction risks during mass treatment with ivermectin in loiasis-endemic areas. Parasitol. Today 12:448–450

Churchill DR, Morris C, Fakoya A, Wright SG, Davidson RN, 1996. Clinical and laboratory features of patients with loiasis (*Loa loa* filariasis) in the U.K. J. Infect. 33:103–109

Connor DH, Gibson DW, Neafie RC, Merighi B, Buck AA, 1983. Sowda—onchocerciasis in North Yemen: a clinicopathologic study of 18 patients. Am. J. Trop. Med. Hyg. 32:123–137

Connor DH, Morrison NE, Kerdel-Vegas F, Berkoff HA, Johnson F, Tunnicliffe R, Failing FC, Hale LN, Lindquist K, 1970. Onchocerciasis: onchocercal dermatitis, lymphadenitis, and elephantiasis in the Ubangi territory. Hum. Pathol. 1:553–579

Cooper PJ, Proano R, Beltran C, Anselmi M, Guderian RH, 1996. Onchocerciasis in Ecuador: changes in prevalence of ocular lesions in *Onchocerca volvulus* infected individuals over the period 1980–1990. Mem. Inst. Oswaldo Cruz. 91:153–158

Corrigan MJ, Hill DW, 1968. Retinal artery occlusion in loiasis. Br. J. Ophthalmol. 52:477–480

de Brux JA, Baup HF, Kaeding H, 1983. Correspondence. *Loa loa* microfilariae in an endometrial smear. Acta Cytol. 27:547–549

De Gentile L, Cerez H, Francois H, Ronceray J, Chabasse D, 1992. Dirofilariose peritoneale de decouverte fortuite. Bull. Soc. Pathol. Exot. 85:171–173

Delage A, Baumel H, Deixonne B, Pignodel C, Lauraire MC, 1984. Dirofilariose intraperitoneale. Bull. Soc. Pathol. Exot. 77:678–685

Desportes C, 1939. *Filaria conjunctivae* Addario, 1885, parasite accidental de l'homme, est un *Dirofilaria*. Ann. Parasitol. Hum. Comp. 17:380–404

Desportes C, 1940. *Filaria conjunctivae* Addario, 1885, parasite accidental de l'homme, est un *Dirofilaria*. Suite et fin. Ann. Parasitol. Hum. Comp. 17:515–532

Dissanaike AS, 1971. Human infections with *Dirofilaria*, a filarial parasite of animals in Ceylon, with a brief review of recent cases. Ceylon Med. J. 16:91–99

Dissanaike AS, Premaratne UN, Hettiarachchi S, Weerasooriya M, Abeyewickreme W, Ismail MM, 1993. Human infection with *Dirofilaria* (*Nochtiella*) *repens* in Sri Lanka. Ceylon Med. J. 38:22–24

Dissanaike AS, Ramalingam S, Fong A, Pathmayokan S, Thomas V, Kan SP, 1977. Filaria in the vitreous of the eye of man in peninsular Malaysia. Am. J. Trop. Med. Hyg. 26:1143–1147

Doury P, Saliou P, Charmot G, 1983. Les epanchements articulaires a eosinophiles. A propos d'une observation. Semin. Hop. 59:1683–1685

Ducorps M, Gardon WN, Ranque S, Ndong W, Boussinesq M, Gardon J, Schneider D, Chippaux JP, 1995. Effets secondaires du traitement de la loase hypermicrofilaremique par l'ivermectine. Bull. Soc. Pathol. Exot. 88:105–112

Duke BOL, 1962. A standard method of assessing microfilarial densities in onchocerciasis surveys. Bull. WHO 27:629–632

Duke BOL, 1954. The uptake of the microfilariae of *Acanthocheilonema streptocerca* by *Culicoides grahamii*, and their subsequent development. Ann. Trop. Med. Parasitol. 48:416–420

Dukes DC, Gelfand M, Gadd KG, Clarke VdV, Goldsmid JM, 1968. Cerebral filariasis caused by *Acanthocheilonema perstans*. Cent. Afr. J. Med. 14:21–27

Eberhard ML, Telford SR, Spielman A, Telford I, Sam R, 1991. A *Brugia* species infecting rabbits in the northeastern United States. J. Parasitol. 77:796–798

Egwang TG, Akue JP, Dupont A, Pinder M, 1988. The identification and partial characterization of an immunodominant 29–31 kilodalton surface antigen expressed by adult worms of the human filaria *Loa loa*. Mol. Biochem. Parasitol 31:263–272

Egwang TG, Dupont A, Leclerc A, Akue JP, Pinder M, 1989. Differential recognition of *Loa loa* antigens by sera of human subjects from a loiasis endemic zone. Am. J. Trop. Med. Hyg. 41:664–673

Eveland LK, Yermakov V, Kenney M, 1975. *Loa loa* infection without microfilaraemia. Trans. R. Soc. Trop. Med. Hyg. 69:354–355

Ewert A, Smith JH, Corredor Arjona A, 1981. Microfilariae of *Mansonella ozzardi* in human skin biopsies. Am. J. Trop. Med. Hyg. 30:988–991

Fischer P, Rubaale T, Meredith SE, Buttner DW, 1996. Sensitivity of a polymerase chain reaction-based assay to detect *Onchocerca volvulus* DNA in skin biopsies. Parasitol. Res. 82:395–401

Frouge C, Vanel D, Tristant H, 1992. Correspondence. Dirofilariasis of the breast mimicking carcinoma on mammography. Am. J. Roentgenol. 159:220–221

Garcia A, Abel L, Cot M, Ranque S, Richard P, Boussinesq M, Chippaux JP, 1995. Longitudinal survey of *Loa loa* filariasis in southern Cameroon: long-term stability and factors influencing individual microfilarial status. Am. J. Trop. Med. Hyg. 52:370–375

Gardiner CH, Meyers WM, Lanoie LO, 1979. Recovery of intact male and female *Dipetalonema streptocerca* from man. Am. J. Trop. Med. Hyg. 28:49–52

Gardon J, Gardon WN, Demanga N, Kamgno J, Chippaux JP, Boussinesq M, 1997. Serious reactions after mass treatment of onchocerciasis with ivermectin in an area endemic for *Loa loa* infection. Lancet 350:18–22

Garin JP, Rougier J, Mojon M, 1975. Loase et uveite posterieure. A propos d'une observation. Acta Trop. 32:384–388

Gelfand M, Wessels P, 1964. *Acanthocheilonema perstans* in a European female. A discussion of the possible pathogenicity and a suggested new syndrome. Trans. R. Soc. Trop. Med. Hyg. 58:552–556

Gibbs RD, 1979. Loiasis: report of three cases and literature review. J. Natl. Med. Assoc. 71:853–854

Gibson DW, Connor DH, 1978. Onchocercal lymphadenitis: clinicopathologic study of 34 patients. Trans. R. Soc. Trop. Med. Hyg. 72:137–154

Gibson DW, Heggie C, Connor DH, 1980. Clinical and pathologic aspects of onchocerciasis. Path. Annu. 15: 195–240

Goussard B, Ivanoff B, Frost E, Garin Y, Bourderiou C, 1984. Age of appearance of IgG, IgM, and IgE antibodies specific for *Loa loa* in Gabonese children. Microbiol. Immunol. 28:787–792

Goverde AJ, Schats R, van Berlo PJ, Claessen FA, 1996. An unexpected guest in follicular fluid. Hum. Reprod. 11: 531–532

Gratama S, 1970. Microfilaria *bancrofti* and Microfilaria *volvulus* in hydrocele fluid and tissue sections: morphology and differential diagnosis. Trop. Geogr. Med. 22:459–471

Guderian RH, Shelley AJ, 1992. Onchocerciasis in Ecuador: the situation in 1989. Mem. Inst. Oswaldo Cruz 87: 405–415

Gutierrez Y, 1983. Diagnostic characteristics of *Dirofilaria subdermata* in cross sections. Can. J. Zool. 61:2097–2103

Gutierrez Y, 1984. Diagnostic features of zoonotic filariae in tissue sections. Hum. Pathol. 15:514–525

Gutierrez Y, Catallaer M, Wicker DL, 1996. Extrapulmonary *Dirofilaria immitis*-like infections in the Western Hemisphere. Am. J. Surg. Pathol. 20:299–305

Gutierrez Y, Misselevich I, Fradis M, Podoshin L, Boss JH, 1995. *Dirofilaria repens* in northern Israel. Am. J. Surg. Pathol. 19:1088–1091

Gutierrez Y, Paul GM, 1984. Breast nodule produced by *Dirofilaria tenuis*. Am. J. Surg. Pathol. 8:463–465

Hautekeete ML, Pailoux G, Marcellin P, Girard PM, Degott C, Benhamou JP, 1989. Correspondence. Presence of *Loa loa* microfilariae in ascitic fluid. J. Infect. Dis. 160: 559–560

Herzberg AJ, Boyd PR, Gutierrez Y, 1995. Subcutaneous dirofilariasis in Collier County, Florida. Am. J. Surg. Pathol. 19:934–939

Hira PR, Madda JP, Al-Shamali MA, Eberhard ML, 1994. Dirofilariasis in Kuwait: first report of human infection due to *Dirofilaria repens* in the Arabian Gulf. Am. J. Trop. Med. Hyg. 51:590–592

Isaza R, Courtney CH, 1988. Possible association between *Dirofilaria tenuis* infections in humans and its prevalence in raccoons in Florida. J. Parasitol. 74:189–190

Jaffres R, Simitzis Le Flohic AM, Chastel C, 1983. Arthrite filarienne a *Loa loa* avec microfilaires dans le liquide articulaire. Rev. Rhum. Mal. Osteoartic. 50:145–147

Jung RC, Espenan PH, 1967. A case of infection in man with *Dirofilaria*. Am. J. Trop. Med. Hyg. 16:172–174

Kaneda Y, Asami K, Kawai T, Sakuma M, 1980. A case of human infection wirth *Dirofilaria immitis* in the subcutaneous tissues. Jpn. J. Parasitol. 29:245–249

Katner H, Beyt BE Jr, Krotoski WA, 1984. Loiasis and renal failure. South. Med. J. 77:907–908

Kerkezenov N, 1962. Intra-ocular filariasis in Australia. Br. J. Ophthalmol. 46:607–615

Kershaw WE, Duke BO, Budden FH, 1954. Distribution of microfilariae of O. *volvulus* in the skin. Its relation to the skin changes and to eye lesions and blindness. Br. Med. J. 2:724–729

King CL, Ottesen EA, Nutman TB, 1990. Cytokine regulation of antigen-driven immunoglobulin production in filarial parasite infections in humans. J. Clin. Invest. 85: 1810–1815

Kipp W, Burnham G, Bamuhiiga J, Leichsenring M, 1996. The Nakalanga syndrome in Kabarole District, Western Uganda. Am. J. Trop. Med. Hyg. 54:80–83

Kivits M, 1952. Quatre cas d'encephalite mortelle avec invasion du liquide cephalo-rachidien par Microfilaria *Loa*. Ann. Soc. Belge Med. Trop. 32:235–242

Klion AD, Eisenstein EM, Smirniotopoulos TT, Neumann MP, Nutman TB, 1992. Pulmonary involvement in loiasis. Am. Rev. Respir. Dis. 145:961–963

Klion AD, Massougbodji A, Sadeler BC, Ottesen EA, Nutman TB, 1991. Loiasis in endemic and nonendemic populations: immunologically mediated differences in clinical presentation. J. Infect. Dis. 163:1318–1325

Klotz O, 1930. Nodular fibrosis of the spleen associated with *Filaria loa*. Am. J. Trop. Med. 10:57–64

Kotkan A, 1951. On a new case of human filariidosis in Hungary. Acta Vet. Acad. Sci. Hung. 1:69–79

Kovalev NE, Zueva VK, Mareich OI, 1971. Human dirofilariasis. [In Russian. English summary]. Med Parazitol. Mosk. 40:741–742

Le Guyadec T, Wolkenstein P, Ortoli JC, Ponties Leroux B, Beaulieu P, Millet P, 1992. Granulome a corps etranger sur la filaire *Loa loa* calcifiee. Ann. Dermatol. Venereol. 119:127–130

Le Van Hoa, Le Thi Ty, 1971. Etude comparative entre *Dirofilaria macacae*, Sandground 1933, parasite des primates et *Dirofilaria repens*, Raillet and Henry 1911, parasite des carnivores du Viet-Nam. Bull. Soc. Pathol. Exot. 64:347–360

Lowrie RC Jr, Orihel TC, Eberhard ML, 1982. *Culicoides variipennis*, a laboratory vector for the Amazon form of *Mansonella ozzardi*. Am. J. Trop. Med. Hyg. 31:166–167

Lowrie RC Jr, Raccurt C, 1981. *Mansonella ozzardi* in Haiti II. Arthropod vector studies. Am. J. Trop. Med. Hyg. 30:598–603

MacDougall LT, Magoon CC, Fritsche TR, 1992. *Dirofilaria repens* manifesting as a breast nodule. Diagnostic problems and epidemiologic considerations. Am. J. Clin. Pathol. 97:625–630

MacLean JD, Beaver PC, Michalek H, 1979. Subcutaneous dirofilariasis in Okinawa, Japan. Am. J. Trop. Med. Hyg. 28:45–48

Marinkelle CJ, German E, 1970. Mansonelliasis in the Comisaria del Vaupes of Colombia. Trop. Geogr. Med. 22: 101–111

McNeeley DF, Raccurt CP, Boncy J, Lowrie RCJ, 1989. Clinical evaluation of *Mansonella ozzardi* in Haiti. Trop. Med. Parasitol. 40:107–110

Meerovitch E, Faubert G, Groulx G, 1976. Zoonotic subcutaneous dirofilariasis in Quebec. Can. J Public Health 67:333–335

Meyers WM, Connor DH, Harman LE, Fleshman K, Moris R, Neafie RC, Conner DH, 1972. Human streptocerciasis. A clinico-pathologic study of 40 Africans (Zairians) including identification of the adult filaria. Am. J. Trop. Med. Hyg. 21:528–545

Meyers WM, Neafie RC, Moris R, Bourland J, 1977. Streptocerciasis: observation of adult male *Dipetalonema streptocerca* in man. Am. J. Trop. Med. Hyg. 26: 1153–1155

Mimori T, Tada I, Takeuchi T, 1986. *Dirofilaria* infection in the breast of a woman in Japan. Southeast Asian J. Trop. Med. Public Health 17:165–167

Molyneux DH, Davies JB, 1997. Onchocerciasis control: moving towards the millennium. Parasitol. Today 13: 418–425

Moorhouse DE, 1978. *Dirofilaria immitis*: a cause of human intra-ocular infection. Infection 6:192–193

Moraes MAP, Almeida MMR, Lovelace JK, Chaves GM, 1978. *Mansonella ozzardi* entre Indios Ticunas do Estado do Amazonas, Brasil. Bol. Sanit. Panam. 85:16–25

Nathan MB, 1979. A comparison of *Mansonella ozzardi* microfilaria densities in the blood and in skin snips from three areas of the body. Trans. R. Soc. Trop. Med. Hyg. 73:338–340

Nathan MB, 1981. Transmission of the human filarial parasite *Mansonella ozzardi* by *Culicoides phlebotomus* (Williston) (Diptera: Ceratopogonidae) in coastal north Trinidad. Bull. Entomol. Res. 71:97–105

Neafie RC, 1972. Morphology of *Onchocerca volvulus*. Am. J. Clin. Pathol. 57:574–586

Neafie RC, Connor DH, Meyers WM, 1975. *Dipetalonema streptocerca* (Macfie and Corson, 1922): description of the adult female. Am. J. Trop. Med. Hyg. 24:264–267

Negesse Y, Lanoie LO, Neafie RC, Connor DH, 1985. Loiasis: "Calabar" swellings and involvement of deep organs. Am. J. Trop. Med. Hyg. 34:537–546

Nelson GS, 1965. Filarial infections as zoonoses. J. Helminthol. 39:229–250

Nelson GS, 1970. Onchocerciasis. Adv. Parasitol 8:173–224

Nelson GS, 1991. Human onchocerciasis: notes on the history, the parasite and the life cycle. Ann. Trop. Med. Parasitol. 85:83–95

Ngu JL, Chatelanat F, Leke R, Ndumbe P, Youmbissi J, 1985. Nephropathy in Cameroon: evidence for filarial derived immune-complex pathogenesis in some cases. Clin. Nephrol. 24:128–134

Nnochiri E, 1966. Observations on onchocercal lesions seen in autopsy specimens in western Nigeria. Ann. Trop. Med. Parasitol. 58:89–93

Nnochiri E, 1972. The causal agent of the ocular syndrome of the "Kampala eye worm." E. Afr. Med. J. 49:198

Noireau F, Apembet JD, Nzoulani A, Carme B, 1990a. Clinical manifestations of loiasis in an endemic area in the Congo. Trop. Med. Parasitol. 41:37–39

Noireau F, Itoua A, Carme B, 1990b. Epidemiology of *Mansonella perstans* filariasis in the forest region of south Congo. Ann. Trop. Med. Parasitol. 84:251–254

Noireau F, Pichon G, 1992. Population dynamics of *Loa loa* and *Mansonella perstans* infections in individuals living in an endemic area of the Congo. Am. J. Trop. Med. Hyg. 46:672–676

Novak R, 1989. Calcifications in the breast in filaria loa infection. Acta Radiol. 30:507–508

Nutman TB, Miller KD, Mulligan M, Ottesen EA, 1986. *Loa loa* infection in temporary residents of endemic regions: recognition of a hyperresponsive syndrome with characteristic clinical manifestations. J. Infect. Dis. 154:10–18

Oberg MS, McGowen BA, Kleiman DA, 1987. Loiasis 15 years after exposure. Tex. Med. 83:36–37

Ogunba EO, 1971. Loiasis in Ijebu Division, West Nigeria. Trop. Geogr. Med. 23:194–200

Oomen AP, 1967. Onchocerciasis in the Kaffa province of Ethiopia. Trop. Geogr. Med. 19:231–246

Orihel TC, 1961. Morphology of the larval stages of *Dirofilaria immitis* in the dog. J. Parasitol. 47:251–262

Orihel TC, 1984. The tail of the *Mansonella streptocerca* microfilaria. Am. J. Trop. Med. Hyg. 33:1278

Orihel TC, Ash LR, 1964. Occurrence of *Dirofilaria striata* in the bobcat (*Lynx rufus*) in Louisiana with observations on its larval development. J. Parasitol. 50:590–591

Orihel TC, Beaver PC, 1965. Morphology and relationship of *Dirofilaria tenuis* and *Dirofilaria conjunctivae*. Am. J. Trop. Med. Hyg. 14:1030–1043

Orihel TC, Eberhard ML, 1982. *Mansonella ozzardi*: a redescription with comments on its taxonomic relationships. Am. J. Trop. Med. Hyg. 31:1142–1147

Orihel TC, Eberhard ML, 1985. *Loa loa*: development and course of patency in experimentally-infected primates. Trop. Med. Parasitol. 36:215–224

Orihel TC, Helentjaris D, Alger J, 1997. Subcutaneous dirofilariasis: single inoculum, multiple worms. Am. J. Trop. Med. Hyg. 56:452–455

Orihel TC, Isbey EKJ, 1990. *Dirofilaria striata* infection in a North Carolina child. Am. J. Trop. Med. Hyg. 42:124–126

Orlando G, Galli M, Lazzarin A, Serino G, Inzoli C, Calello G, Almaviva M, 1982. Humoral immune responses in human loaiasis. Boll. Inst. Siroter. Milan 61:258–261

Pacheco G, Schofield HLJ, 1968. *Dirofilaria tenuis* containing microfilariae in man. Am. J. Trop. Med. Hyg. 17:180–182

Paleologo FP, Neafie RC, Connor DH, 1984. Lymphadenitis caused by *Loa loa*. Am. J. Trop. Med. Hyg. 33:395–402

Pampiglione S, Azzaro S, Bonjiorno J, Fioravanti ML, Garavelli PL, La Valle S, 1995. La dirofilariosi oculare umana in Italia: Descrizione de 6 nuovi casi. Revisione della casistica Italiana. Ann. Ottalmol. Clin. Ocul. 71:257–277

Pampiglione S, Schmid C, Montaperto C, 1992. Dirofilariasi umana: retrovamento di femmina gravida di *Dirofilaria repens* in nodulo sottocutaneo. Pathologica 84:77–81

Paul EV, Zimmerman LE, 1970. Some observations on the ocular pathology of onchocerciasis. Hum. Pathol. 1:581

Petithory J, Sang HT, 1965. Symptomatologie de la filariose a *Dipetalonema perstans*. Bull. Soc. Pathol. Exot. 58:496–501

Pillay VK, Kirch E, Kurtzman NA, 1973. Glomerulopathy associated with filarial loiasis. JAMA 225:179

Pinder M, Leclerc A, Everaere S, 1992. Antibody-dependent cell-mediated immune reactions to *Loa loa* microfilariae in amicrofilaraemic subjects. Parasite Immunol. 14:541–556

Pinon JM, Dousset H, Ologoudou L, Sulahian A, Adnet JJ, 1980. Dirofilariasis of the breast in France. Am. J. Trop. Med. Hyg. 29:1018–1019

Poltera AA, 1973. The histopathology of ocular loiasis in Uganda. Trans. R. Soc. Trop. Med. Hyg. 67:819–829

Preshaw LE, Konkal PJ, Proctor EM, 1993. Conjunctival dirofilariasis in British Columbia. Can. J Ophthalmol. 28:343–345

Ratnavale WD, Dissanaike AS, 1964. On the second case of human infection with Dirofilaria (Nochtiella) repens from Ceylon. J. Helminthol. 38:287–290

Remme JHF, 1995. The African programme for onchocerciasis control: preparing to launch. Parasitol. Today 11:403–406

Renard G, Morand L, Lacombe E, Offret G, 1978. Un cas de retinopathie filarienne. J. Fr. Ophtalmol. 1:41–46

Richardson DJ, Owen WB, Snyder DE, 1992. Helminth parasites of the raccoon (Procyon lotor) from north-central Arkansas. J. Parasitol. 78:163–166

Roberts JM, Neumann E, Gockel CW, Highton RB, 1967. Onchocerciasis in Kenya 9, 11 and 18 years after elimination of the vector. Bull. WHO 37:195–212

Rodger FC, 1977. *Onchocerciasis in Zaire: A New Approach to the Problem of River Blindness.* Oxford: Pergamon Press

Roussel F, Roussel C, Brasseur P, Gourmelen O, Le Loet X, 1989. Aseptic knee effusion with Loa loa microfilariae in the articular fluid. Acta Cytol. 33:281–283

Sarkany L, 1959. Loiasis with involvement of peripheral nerves. Trans. St. Johns Hosp. Dermatol. Soc. 42:49–51

Schofield FD, 1955. Two cases of loiasis with peripheral nerve involvement. Trans. R. Soc. Trop. Med. Hyg. 49:588–589

Shelley AJ, Shelley A, 1976. Further evidence for the transmission of Mansonella ozzardi by Simulium amazonicum in Brazil. Ann. Trop. Med. Parasitol. 70:213–217

Shenefelt PD, Esperanza L, Lynn A, 1996. Elusive migratory subcutaneous dirofilariasis. J. Am. Acad. Dermatol. 35:260–262

Siegenthaler R, Bugler R, 1965. Paraarticulares Nematodengranulom (einheimische Onchocerca). Schweiz. Med. Wochenschr. 95:1102–1104

Skrjabin KI, 1917. *Loa extraocularis* nov. sp. parasite nouveau de l'oeil de l'homme. C.R. Soc. Biol. Paris 80:759–762

Skrjabin KI, Al'Tgauzen A, Shul'man ES, 1930. First case of *Dirofilaria repens* from man. Trop. Med. Vet. Mosk. 8:9–11

Sondergaard J, 1972. Filariasis caused by Acanthocheilonema perstans. Arch. Dermatol. 106:547–548

Stanley SL Jr, Kell O, 1982. Ascending paralysis associated with diethylcarbamazine treatment of Loa loa infection. Trop. Doc. 12:16–19

Stott G, 1962. Pathogenicity of Acanthocheilonema perstans. J. Trop. Med. Hyg. 65:230–232

Takaoka H, Bain O, Tajimi S, Kashima K, Nakayama I, Korenaga M, Aoki C, Otsuka Y, 1996. Second case of zoonotic Onchocerca infection in a resident of Oita in Japan. Parasite 3:179–182

Thomas D, Older J, Kandawalla NM, Torczynski E, 1976. The Dirofilaria parasite in the orbit. Am. J. Ophthalmol. 82:931–933

Toure FS, Bain O, Nerrienet E, Millet P, Wahl G, Toure Y, Doumbo O, Nicolas L, Georges AJ, McReynolds LA, Egwang TG, 1997. Detection of Loa loa–specific DNA in blood from occult-infected individuals. Exp. Parasitol. 86:163–170

Toussaint D, Danis P, 1965. Retinopathy in generalized Loa loa filariasis. A clinicopathological study. Arch. Ophthalmol. 74:470–476

Uni S, 1978. Scanning electron microscopic study of Dirofilaria species (Filarioidea Nematoda) of Japan and a review of the genus Dirofilaria. J. Osaka City Med. Cent. 27:439–458

Uni S, Kimata I, Takada S, 1980. Cross-section morphology of Dirofilaria ursi in comparison with D. immitis. Jpn. J. Parasitol. 29:489–497

Uni S, Takada S, 1986. The longitudinal cuticular markings of Dirofilaria immitis adult worm. Jpn. J. Parasitol. 35:191–199

Van Bogaert L, Dubois A, Janssens PG, Radermecker J, Tverdy G, Wanson M, 1955. Encephalitis in Loa-loa filariasis. J. Neurol. Neurosurg. Psychiatry 18:103–119

Weller PF, Simon HB, Parkhurst BH, Medrek TF, 1978. Tourism-acquired Mansonella ozzardi microfilaremia in a regular blood donor. JAMA 240:858–859

Whitaker D, Reed WD, Shilkin KB, 1980. A case of filariasis diagnosed on gastric cytology. Pathology. 12:483–486

WHO, 1976. Epidemiology of onchocerciasis: report of a WHO Expert Committee. Technical Report Series No. 597 1–94. Geneva: WHO

WHO, 1987. Expert Committee on Onchocerciasis: Third Report. World Health Organization Technical Report Series No. 572. Geneva: WHO

Wilms G, Tschibwabwa Ntumba E, Nijssens M, Baert AL, 1983. Calcified Loa-loa infestations. J. Belge Radiol. 66:133–136

Wiseman RA, 1967. *Acanthocheilonema perstans.* A cause of significant eosinophilia in the tropics: Comments on its pathogenicity. Trans. R. Soc. Trop. Med. Hyg. 61:667–673

Woodruff AW, 1951. Destruction of microfilariae of Loa loa in the liver in loiasis treated with banocide (Hetrazan). Trans. R. Soc. Trop. Med. Hyg. 44:479–480

Yangco BG, Vincent AL, Vickery AC, Nayar JK, Sauerman DM, 1984. A survey of filariasis among refugees in south Florida. Am. J. Trop. Med. Hyg. 33:246–251

Zanetti V, Lambrecht FL, 1948. Notes sur la malaria indigene au Nepoko. Ann. Soc. Belge Med. Trop. 28:355–370

Zue NC, 1985. Filariose endo-oculaire a propos d'un cas de filaire Loa loa dans la chambre anterieure. Bull. Soc. Ophtalmol. Fr. 85:237–238

21

SPIRURIDA—FILARIAE OF THE LUNGS, BRAIN, AND EYES

The adults of *Dirofilaria immitis* occur in the pulmonary arteries of dogs, their natural hosts, and ectopically in other blood vessels. The adults of *Meningonema peruzzi* are parasites of the brain stem of primates and humans. In addition, both immature and adult filarial worms of humans and animals can occur in the eye of humans. The filariae in these locations are the subject of this chapter. The manifestations and the lesions produced by microfilariae of lymphatic filariae in the lungs (tropical eosinophilia, Chapter 19), the brain (*Loa loa*, Chapter 20), and the eye (*Onchocerca volvulus*, Chapter 20) have already been discussed.

Filariae of Lungs: *Dirofilaria immitis*—Pulmonary Dirofilariasis

Immature filariae in pulmonary nodules resected because of a clinical diagnosis of carcinoma, mainly in the United States, were reported during the 1940s and 1950s. The review of these cases determined that *D. immitis*, the dog heartworm, is the agent responsible for the infection (Beaver, Orihel, 1965).

Morphology. In the dog, the natural host, the adult female *D. immitis* is up to 31 cm in length and the male is up to 18 cm in length; the diameter of both sexes is about 1 mm. The cuticle of *D. immitis* is smooth and has no longitudinal ridges, except for the posterior ventral aspect of the male. However, very attenuated longitudinal ridges, referred to as *cuticular markings* and seen only in scanning electron micrographs, have been described (Uni, Takada, 1986). The parasites in humans are smaller than those in dogs because humans are not natural hosts and full growth is not attained. The general appearance of a *Dirofilaria* in cross sections was discussed in Chapter 20. Below, under Diagnosis, particular characteristics of *D. immitis* are outlined.

Life Cycle and Biology. The life cycle of *D. immitis* is similar to that of other filarial worms (Fig. 21–1). The adult parasites live in the right side of the heart and in pulmonary arteries in wild and domestic animals, most of which belong to the family Canidae. The microfilariae ingested during a blood meal taken by mosquitoes of the genera *Aedes*, *Anopheles*, *Culex*, and others develop into infective larvae. These larvae are

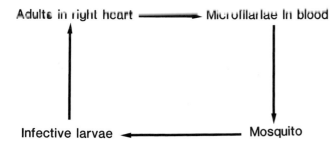

Adults in right heart ────────► Microfilariae in blood

Infective larvae ◄──────── Mosquito

Fig. 21–1. *Dirofilaria immitis,* schematic representation of life the cycle.

Pulmonary dirofilariasis occurs twice as often in men as in women. The average age at presentation varies from 28 to 77 years; 66% of patients are in the 40- to 59-year age group. About 60% are asymptomatic. A pulmonary *coin lesion* found on a routine chest x-ray film is usually diagnosed as a malignancy that requires surgical exploration and removal. In retrospect, a few patients have complained of chest discomfort, malaise, low-grade fever, cough, and occasionally hemoptysis. Some patients have slight eosinophilia (Dayal, Neafie, 1975).

deposited on the skin by the mosquito during feeding. They gain access to the subcutaneous tissues, where they grow to 3 cm in approximately 90 days before locating in the right side of the heart (Fig. 21–2 *A–B*; Orihel, 1961). Infections in humans are accidental zoonoses; they have been recognized only since the 1960s.

Geographic Distribution. *Dirofilaria immitis* is a common parasite of dogs in the tropical and subtropical areas of the world (Fig. 21–3). In the continental United States, *D. immitis* occurs in every state, but the South, the eastern seaboard, and the Mississippi and Ohio River basins have the highest enzooticity. Most human infections recognized in the United States are found in these areas (Ciferri, 1981, 1982). Outside the United States, the infection occurs in humans in every place where the worm is endemic. When recognized, it is often reported in the literature (Fabbretti et al. 1990; Monchy et al. 1993; Pampiglione et al. 1994). Serologic surveys for specific antibodies to *D. immitis* antigens in an endemic area of Spain revealed positivity of over 9% in the general population (Simon et al. 1991). The seroprevalence in Puerto Rico was 2.6% (Villanueva, Rodriguez Perez, 1993). In Australian aborigines it was 21% compared with 2% to 6% in Caucasians (Welch, Dobson, 1974).

Clinical Findings. Pulmonary dirofilariasis is a relatively uncommon infection, but since reports of single cases or clusters of small numbers of cases are not warranted, there are many more cases than reported. One report of eight cases (Neafie, Piggott, 1971) and several reviews of the literature account for most of the published cases of pulmonary dirofilariasis (Asimacopoulos et al. 1992; Ciferri, 1982; Dayal, Neafie, 1975; de Brux et al. 1983; Ro et al. 1989).

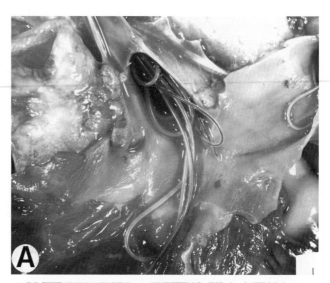

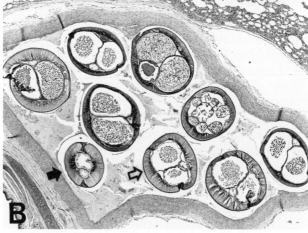

Fig. 21–2. *Dirofilaria immitis* in a dog. *A,* Right ventricle and pulmonary arteries showing several adult parasites. *B,* Microscopic section of a pulmonary artery stained with hematoxylin and eosin stain, with several sections of a female and one section of a male (solid arrow). Note the smooth cuticle (open arrow), strong muscle mass, and paired uteri with eggs and developing microfilariae, ×21.

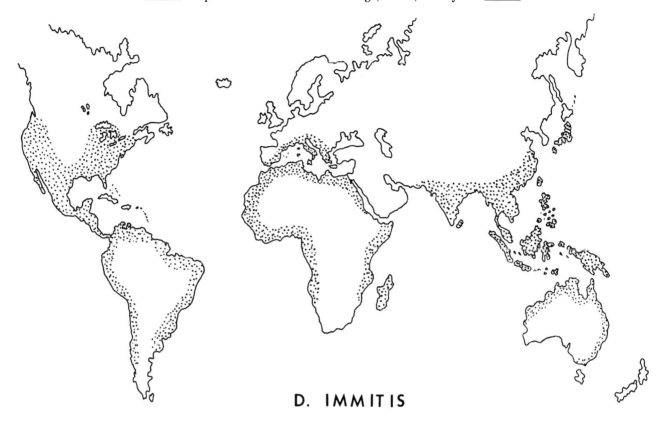

D. IMMITIS

Fig. 21–3. *Dirofilaria immitis*, geographic distribution in natural hosts.

Pathology. The lesions removed from patients with pulmonary dirofilariasis have a uniform appearance. They consist of a generous portion of lung to be used for diagnosis on frozen sections (Fig. 21–4 *A*). Palpation of the lung segment reveals a hard nodule at the center. On section, the nodule is up to 4 cm in diameter and is well circumscribed if the lesion is old; new lesions have ill-defined borders. Well-circumscribed lesions are firm, have a uniformly yellowish necrotic appearance, and are surrounded by normal lung parenchyma (Fig. 21–4 *A*). Ill-defined lesions tend to be less necrotic, are whitish, and seem to infiltrate the surrounding lung parenchyma.

Microscopically, the lesion is a recent (Fig. 21–4 *B*), organizing (Fig. 21–4 *C*), or organized pulmonary infarct (Fig. 21–4 *D*). Sections through the center of the nodule usually show a small to medium-sized branch of the pulmonary artery. The artery is sometimes difficult to see because it is necrotic, but staining of the section with elastic stain reveals it. Within the lumen of the artery is a thrombus in different stages of organization, with one or several cross sections and oblique sections of the worm. Depending on the degree of organization, the artery and the parasite may be dif-

ficult to recognize. Recent lesions have relatively well preserved worms and are necrotic; various degrees of degeneration and calcification are seen in older lesions (Fig. 21–5 *A–D*).

Early lesions consist of a marked inflammatory reaction that at the periphery has an arteritis involving adjacent branches of the occluded vessel (Fig. 21–6 *B*). Often this reaction is granulomatous, with abundant histiocytes, foreign body giant cells, eosinophils, lymphocytes, and plasma cells (Fig. 21–6 *C–D*). The degree of tissue eosinophilia is variable and sometimes resembles a hypersensitivity pneumonitis (Jung-Legg, Legg, 1983). The vasculitis varies from moderate to extensive. The process in these cases appears to be both interstitial and alveolar (Fig. 21–6 *A*), probably due to the centrifugal leakage of antigens from the disintegrating worm. These lesions need careful examination and differentiation from limited Wegener's granulomatosis and other forms of angiitis. Older lesions are typically well-circumscribed, organized infarcts (Fig. 21–4 *C–D*). Over the long term, the lesion probably becomes a burned-out collagenous nodule or a calcified granuloma that is sometimes found at autopsy.

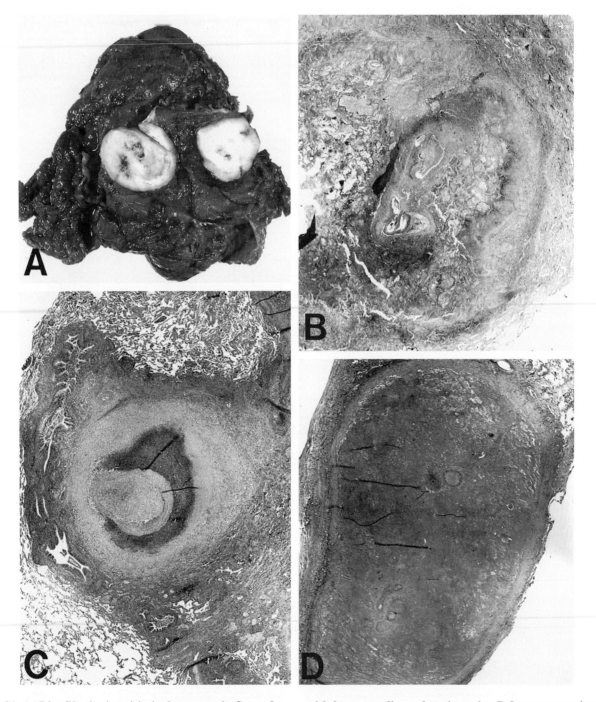

Fig. 21–4. *Dirofilaria immitis* in humans. *A*, Gross lesion in a lung segment removed from a patient diagnosed with lung cancer. Note the well-circumscribed lesion and the necrotic appearance. *B–D*. Microscopic appearance of three different lesions in sections stained with hematoxylin and eosin stain. *B*, Low-power view of a recent infarct produced by *D. immitis*. Note the ill-defined borders of the lesion, ×9. *C*, Slightly older lesion showing organization, ×16. *D*, Well-organized lesion with well-defined borders, ×9.

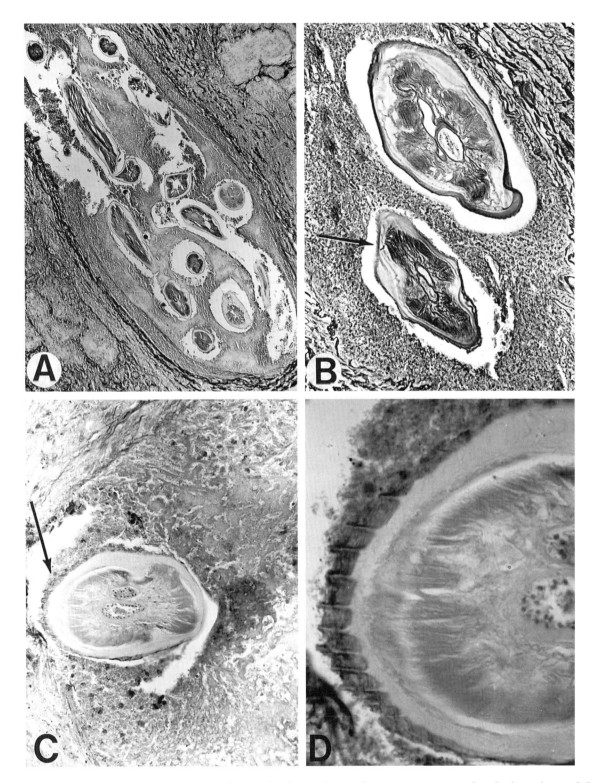

Fig. 21–5. *Dirofilaria immitis* in humans, sections stained with hematoxylin and eosin stain. *A*, Low-power view of a medium-sized pulmonary artery with 13 sections of the worm, ×50. *B*, Higher magnification of a parasite from another individual showing two sections of a male. Note the muscle layer separated from the cuticle due to necrosis and that the muscles fill most of the worm's cavity. Two tubes at the center correspond to the intestine and the gonad. Cuticular longitudinal ridges in the ventral surface of the posterior end of the male are visible (arrow), ×150. *C*, Higher magnification of a section through the posterior end of a male showing similar characteristics (arrow), ×225. *D*, Same worm illustrating the ventral aspect of the body with longitudinal ridges, ×600.

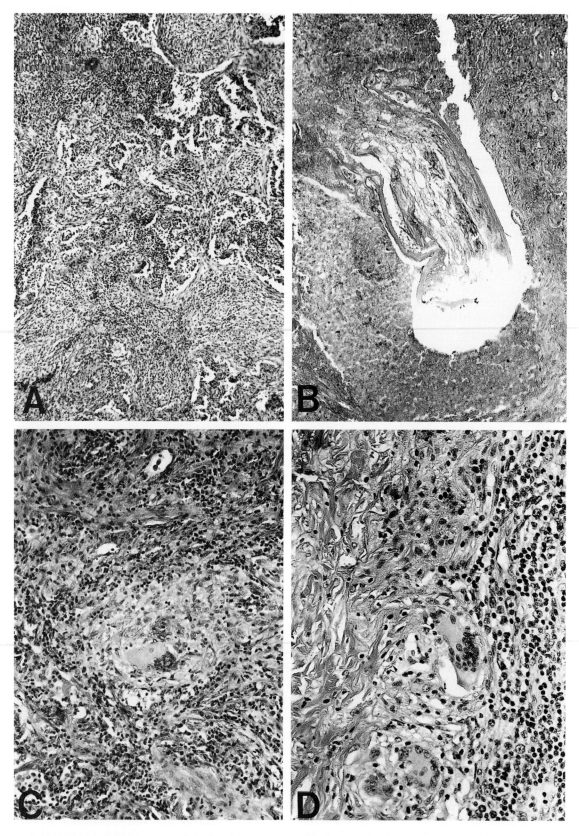

Fig. 21–6. *Dirofilaria immitis* in a human. Microscopic appearance of a recent infarct caused by *Dirofilaria*, same case shown in Figure 21–4 *B*, sections stained with hematoxylin and eosin stain. *A*, Low-power view showing inflammatory infiltration of the alveoli and early organization, ×58. *B*, Higher magnification of necrotic *Dirofilaria* in a pulmonary artery close to the lesion shown in *A*, ×146. *C*, Granulomatous inflammation with foreign body giant cells and numerous mononuclear and polymorphonuclear cells, especially eosinophils, ×146. *D*, Higher magnification showing the infiltrating cells, ×230.

Diagnosis. The basis for the identification of *D. immitis* in tissue sections is its morphologic appearance; the general morphologic characteristics of the genus *Dirofilaria* on cross section are discussed in Chapter 20. The diameter of *D. immitis* in cross sections of human tissues is 140 to 200 μm in males and up to 300 μm in females. The cuticle is smooth (Fig. 21–5 *B*) and has no longitudinal ridges, except at the posterior ventral aspect of the male (Fig. 21–5 *B–C*). The female genital tract is single in the anterior part of the body and double in the rest of the worm. In one case, developing microfilariae in the female uteri were reported (Anonymous, 1983). In the absence of the worm, a definitive diagnosis is not possible, but the histologic picture may suggest pulmonary dirofilariasis. In at least one case, the diagnosis of *D. immitis* was based on material recovered with fine needle aspiration (Hawkins et al. 1985).

Other filariids occur in the branches of the pulmonary arteries of humans. A species of *Brugia* (Fig. 21–7 *A–B*; Beaver et al. 1971; Case Records of the Massachusetts General Hospital, 1974) and *Wuchereria*-like (Fig. 21–8 *A–B*; Beaver, Cran, 1974) worms occurred in individuals who came from or had been in India. In these cases, the parasites produced pulmonary nodules (infarcts) similar to those due to *D. immitis*, except that the *Brugia* and *Wuchereria* worms were alive, resulting in thrombus formation. In addition, *D. repens* (see Chapter 20) has been described in cases of pulmonary dirofilariasis (Pampiglione et al. 1984, 1991).

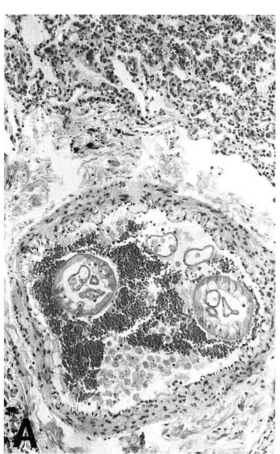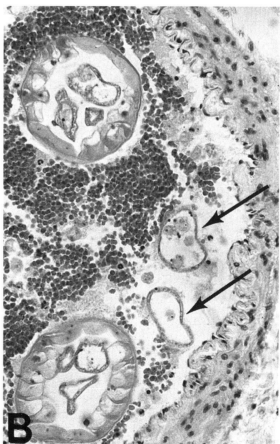

Fig. 21–7. *Brugia malayi* in human lung, preparations stained with hematoxylin and eosin stain. *A*, Low-power view of a medium-sized pulmonary artery with two cross sections of the parasite, ×140. *B*, Higher magnification showing the morphology of the parasite. Two sections of the uterus of the worm are seen in the lumen of the artery (arrows) due to artifact during cutting in the surgical room, ×180. (Preparation courtesy of M.D. Little, Ph.D., School of Public Health and Tropical Medicine, Tulane University, New Orleans, Louisiana. Reported by: Beaver, P.C., Fallon, M., and Smith, G.H. 1971. Pulmonary nodule caused by a living *Brugia malayi*-like in an artery. Am. J. Trop. Med. Hyg. 20:661–666.)

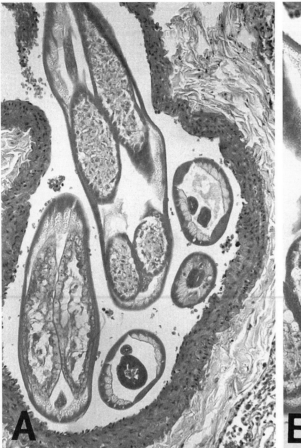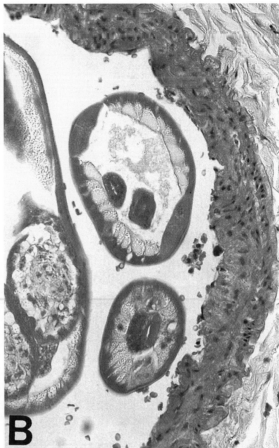

Fig. 21–8. *Wuchereria bancrofti* in human lung, preparation stained with hematoxylin and eosin stain. *A,* Low-power view of a medium-sized pulmonary artery with two cross sections of the parasite, ×140. Note the size of the worm, and compare it with the size of *B. malayi* in Figure 21–7 *A,* with the same magnification. *B,* Higher magnification showing the morphology of the parasite. (Preparation courtesy of M.D. Little, Ph.D., School of Public Health and Tropical Medicine, Tulane University, New Orleans, Louisiana. Reported by: Beaver, P.C., and Cran, I.R. 1974. *Wuchereria*-like filaria in an artery, associated with pulmonary infarction. Am. J. Trop. Med. Hyg. 23:869–876.)

Extrapulmonary D. Immitis. In its natural hosts, *D. immitis* usually enters the arterial circulation and embolizes to a peripheral vessel (ectopic location), often producing serious clinical manifestations. The worms enter the arterial rather than the venous circulation during migration to the heart or by passing from the right to the left side of the heart through a patent foramen ovale (Gutierrez et al. 1996). In many cases, *D. immitis* has been reported in ectopic locations in dogs, including the cerebral arteries, producing infarcts (Kotani et al. 1975; Patton, Garner, 1970); the femoral arteries, producing paresis or muscle necrosis (Cooley et al. 1987; Slonka et al. 1977); and the epidural spaces, producing tetraparesis and paraparesis (Blass et al. 1989; Shires et al. 1982). In all of these cases, the worm was recovered from the site mentioned and was conclusively identified.

Adults of *D. immitis* in humans found in several cases at autopsy were located in the right side of the heart and the pulmonary arteries, their natural location (De Magalhaes, 1887; Faust et al. 1941; Takeuchi et al. 1981). An adult worm was also located ectopically in a portocaval shunt (Fig. 21–9; Goldstein, Smith, 1985), possibly because of postmortem migration. In addition to these well-documented cases, other premature reports of ectopic *D. immitis*, based on positive serologic tests in patients with obscure symptoms and peripheral eosinophilia, have been published. In one report, the sera from patients with eosinophilic meningitis of unknown etiology were positive by immunofluorescence for *D. immitis* antigen and produced an Arthus reaction in guinea pigs (Dobson, Welch, 1974). Another patient with hemoptysis,

1986). These cases are considered ectopic locations of *D. immitis* in humans (Gutierrez et al. 1996). It is expected that additional cases will be found and documented by recovery, identification, and description of the worm.

Filariae of Brain

Manifestations of organic brain symptoms or psychologic symptoms in patients with microfilariae resembling those of *M. perstans* are known in some endemic areas of the parasite. A patient described by Chambon (1933) had both African trypanosomes and *M. perstans* microfilariae in cerebrospinal fluid, as well as peripheral blood and central nervous system symptoms that were attributed to the flagellate. Other cases with central nervous system symptoms and microfilariae resembling *D. perstans* in the spinal fluid (Dukes et al. 1968) are different. In these patients, microfilariae were found only in the cerebrospinal fluid, the brain symptoms were mild, and all patients recovered after a few days. Study of the microfilariae in the spinal fluid of these patients led Orihel (1973) to suggest that the filarial species producing the syndrome was *M. peruzzi* (Orihel, Esslinger, 1973), not *D. perstans*. Recently, a case of asymptomatic infection with *Meningonema*, with recovery of the parasite from the spinal fluid, was described in Cameroon (Boussinesq et al. 1995). *Meningonema* is a parasite of the subarachnoid spaces of the brain stem of African monkeys, with microfilariae in blood and cerebrospinal fluid (Fig. 21–10 A–B). The microfilariae of *M. peruzzi* superficially resemble those of *M. perstans*, but they have a sheath, in addition to other morphologic characteristics that allow their separate classification (Orihel, 1973).

Filariae of the Eye

In both endemic and nonendemic areas for human filariasis, adult filariids are recovered from time to time from various ocular (Beaver, 1989) and extraocular structures. Intraocular worms are located in the anterior and posterior chambers and sometimes in the iris, areas that allow surgical recovery of the worm. Less often, worms are retrieved from the retina. In these cases the diagnosis is more difficult and is often presumptive, based on observations of the worm in the

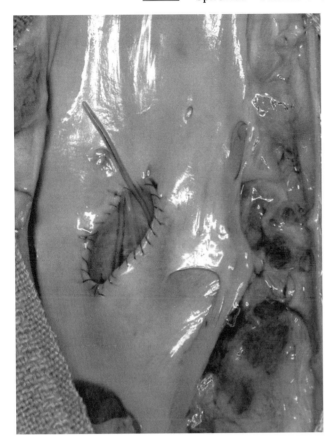

Fig. 21–9. *Dirofilaria immitis* **adult in a man from Florida. Female in a portocaval shunt. (Courtesy of J.D. Goldstein, M.D., Department of Pathology, University Hospital of Jacksonville, Jacksonville, Florida. Reported by: Goldstein, J.D., and Smith, D.R. 1985.** *Dirofilaria immitis* **in a portocaval shunt. Hum. Pathol. 16:1172–1173. Reproduced with permission.)**

meningeal irritation, peripheral eosinophilia, and pain radiating down her arms and back was diagnosed and treated for dirofilariasis based on a positive serologic test (Feldman, Holden, 1974). In a third report, a patient with spinal fluid eosinophilia was diagnosed as having *D. immitis* infection (Kuberski, 1979). In none of these cases was the worm recovered, identified, and described, and they should not be considered cases of dirofilariasis.

In two cases, a *Dirofilaria* worm was located ectopically in peripheral arteries of humans. One was found in an artery of a finger of a man in Brazil whose symptoms resembled those of Raynaud syndrome (identified as *D. spectans*; Freitas, Mayall, 1953). The other occurred in a digital artery of a man in Costa Rica (indistinguishable from *D. immitis*) (Beaver et al.

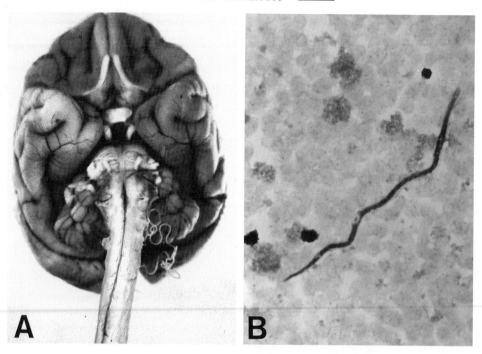

Fig. 21–10. *Meningonema peruzzi* in the *Talopian* monkey. *A*, Gross picture of brain showing the adult parasites in the meninges. *B*, Microfilaria of *M. peruzzi* in a thick blood film stained with Giemsa stain; the sheath is not seen, ×550. (Photographs courtesy of T.C. Orihel, Ph.D., School of Public Health and Tropical Medicine, Tulane University, New Orleans, Louisiana. In: Orihel, T.C. 1973. Cerebral filiariasis in Rhodesia—A zoonotic infection. Am. J. Trop Med. Hyg. 22:596–599. Reproduced with permission.)

retina, on photographs of the worm, and on photographs of the infected area. In a review of 56 cases of human intraocular filariasis found in the literature (Beaver, 1989), 6 cases were artifacts and in 8 cases there was a motile worm that was not a filaria. The rest of the cases had a motile filaria or filaria-like worm, but only in six of them was the worm recovered, identified, and described. In three cases a species of *Dipetalonema* was found, all from Oregon in the United States (Beaver et al. 1980; Burns et al. 1975; Samples et al. 1988). Of the other three, one was a species of *Loaina* (Botero et al. 1984), one was *Dirofilaria* (Vodovozov et al. 1973), and one was *Wuchereria* (Joseph, Raju, 1980). *Wuchereria* is a parasite of humans; the others are parasites of animals and thus are zoonotic.

In extraocular tissues, the worms are more commonly located in the conjunctiva, followed by other adnexa. Filarial worms (and other parasites) in the conjunctiva are often removed for study in toto or are found in tissue sections of biopsy specimens. The best example of a filaria in the conjunctiva is *L. loa* (eye-worm), as well as the zoonotic filariae *D. tenuis* and

D. repens (see Chapter 20). These filariids are usually visible with the naked eye because of their large size and often are recovered for study. Filariids not visible with the naked eye are usually studied in histologic sections of biopsy specimens.

The conjunctival lesion known as *bung-eye*, *bulge-eye*, or *Kampala worm*, seen commonly in Uganda, has long been attributed to a filarial infection (Owen, Hennessey, 1932). These lesions produce ocular syndromes consisting of one or more small yellow nodules in the bulbar conjunctiva, edema of the eyelids and face, and occasionally proptosis. Tissue sections of these nodules usually show a small, necrotic filariid measuring 50 to 100 μm that is difficult to identify, but is considered by some to be *Loa* (Poltera, 1973). Beaver and coworkers (1984) suggested that the parasite producing bung-eye is a species of *Mansonella* or *Dipetalonema*, probably the latter. The worm was later identified as *M. perstans* (Baird et al. 1988). However, since bung-eye is not known to occur in other areas where *M. perstans* is endemic, the identification of the species must be confirmed by the study of worms recovered in toto.

As stated above, other intraocular filariids have been reported in the literature. In one case, the parasite was not identified (Kerkezenov, 1962). In another case, it was called *D. immitis*, but the parasite was not described (Moorhouse, 1978). Both cases were more consistent with a species of *Loaina* based on the length/width ratio of the worm (Beaver, 1989).

References

Anonymous, 1983. Human dirofilariasis. Report on the Symposium on Human Dirofilariasis, Bay Pines Veterans Administration Medical Center, St. Petersburg, Sept. 22, 1988. Norden News Topics Vet. Med. 58:4–8

Asimacopoulos PJ, Katras A, Christie B, 1992. Pulmonary dirofilariasis. The largest single-hospital experience. Chest 102:851–855

Baird JK, Neafie RC, Connor DH, Lanoie L, 1988. Nodules in the conjunctiva, bung-eye, and bulge-eye in Africa caused by *Mansonella perstans*. Am. J. Trop. Med. Hyg. 38:553–557

Beaver PC, 1989. Intraocular filariasis: a brief review. Am. J. Trop. Med. Hyg. 40:40–45

Beaver PC, Brenes R, Ardon J, 1986. *Dirofilaria* from the index finger of a man in Costa Rica. Am. J. Trop. Med. Hyg. 35:988–990

Beaver PC, Cran IR, 1974. *Wuchereria*-like filaria in an artery, associated with pulmonary infarction. Am. J. Trop. Med. Hyg. 23:869–876

Beaver PC, Fallon M, Smith GH, 1971. Pulmonary nodule caused by a living *Brugia malayi*-like filaria in an artery. Am. J. Trop. Med. Hyg. 20:661–666

Beaver PC, Jung RC, Cupp EW, 1984. *Clinical Parasitology*. Philadelphia: Lea & Febiger

Beaver PC, Meyer EA, Jarroll EL, Rosenquist RC, 1980. *Dipetalonema* from the eye of a man in Oregon, U.S.A. A case report. Am. J. Trop. Med. Hyg. 29:369–372

Beaver PC, Orihel TC, 1965. Human infection with filariae of animals in the United States. Am. J. Trop. Med. Hyg. 14:1010–1029

Blass CE, Holmes RA, Neer TM, 1989. Recurring tetraparesis attributable to a heartworm in the epidural space of a dog. JAVMA 194:787–788

Botero D, Aguledo LM, Uribe FJ, Esslinger JH, Beaver PC, 1984. Intraocular filaria, a *Loaina* species, from man in Colombia. Am. J. Trop. Med. Hyg. 33:578–582

Boussinesq M, Bain O, Chabaud AG, Gardon WN, Kamgno J, Chippaux JP, 1995. A new zoonosis of the cerebrospinal fluid of man probably caused by *Meningonema peruzzii*, a filaria of the central nervous system of Cercopithecidae. Parasite 2:173–176

Burns RP, Helzerman R, Patrick M, Gerhardt N, Beaver PC, 1975. Intraocular filariasis (a motion picture). Trans. Am. Acad. Ophthalmol. Otolaryngol. 79:745–748

Case Records of the Massachusetts General Hospital, 1974.

Resolving pulmonary densities and hemoptysis in a 27 year old woman. Case 26-1974. N. Engl. J. Med. 291:35–42

Chambon M, 1933. Presence de microfilaires dans le liquide cephalorachidien d'un trypanosome avance. Bull. Soc. Pathol. Exot. 26:613–614

Ciferri F, 1981. Human pulmonary dirofilariasis in the West. West. J. Med. 134:158–162

Ciferri F, 1982. Human pulmonary dirofilariasis in the United States: a critical review. Am. J. Trop. Med. Hyg. 31:302–308

Cooley AJ, Clemmons RM, Gross TL, 1987. Heartworm disease manifested by encephalomyelitis and myositis in a dog. JAVMA 190:431–432

Dayal Y, Neafie RC, 1975. Human pulmonary dirofilariasis. A case report and review of the literature. Am. Rev. Respir. Dis. 112:437–443

de Brux JA, Baup HF, Kaeding II, 1983. Correspondence. *Loa loa* microfilariae in an endometrial smear. Acta Cytol. 27:547–549

De Magalhaes PS, 1887. Descripcao de uma especie de filarias encontradas no coracao humano preudida de uma contribucao para o estudo defilariose de Wucherer e do respectivo parasito adulto a *Filaria bancrofti* (Cobbold) ou *Filaria sanguinis hominis* (Lewis). Rev. Cursos Prat. Theor. Fac. Med. Rio de J. 3:129–216

Dobson C, Welch JS, 1974. Dirofilariasis as a cause of eosinophilic meningitis in man diagnosed by immunofluorescence and Arthus hypersensitivity. Trans. R. Soc. Trop. Med. Hyg. 68:223–228

Dukes DC, Gelfand M, Gadd KG, Clarke V de V, Goldsmid JM, 1968. Cerebral filariasis caused by *Acanthocheilonema perstans*. Cent. Afr. J. Med. 14:21–27

Fabbretti G, Fedeli F, Alessi A, Boaron M, Salpietro V, Brisigotti M, 1990. Human pulmonary dirofilariasis: report of a new European case. Histol. Histopathol. 5:311–313

Faust EC, Thomas EP, Jones J, 1941. Discovery of human heartworm infection in New Orleans. J. Parasitol. 27:115–122

Feldman RG, Holden MJ, 1974. Meningeal irritation, hemoptysis, and eosinophilia—a case of human dirofilariasis? JAMA 228:1018–1019

Freitas JFT de, Mayall Rd, 1953. Fenomeno de Raynaud na mao esquerda, provocado por *Dirofilaria spectans*. Rev. Bras. Med. 10:463–467

Goldstein JD, Smith DR, 1985. *Dirofilaria immitis* in a portacaval shunt. Hum. Pathol. 16:1172–1173

Gutierrez Y, Catallaer M, Wicker DL, 1996. Extrapulmonary *Dirofilaria immitis*-like infections in the Western Hemisphere. Am. J. Surg. Pathol. 20:299–305

Hawkins AG, Hsiu JG, Smith RM, Stitik FP, Siddiky MA, Edwards OE, 1985. Pulmonary dirofilariasis diagnosed by fine needle aspiration biopsy. A case report. Acta Cytol. 29:19–22

Joseph A, Raju NSD, 1980. Immature stage of *Wuchereria bancrofti* in the human eye. Indian J. Ophthalmol. 28:89–90

Jung-Legg Y, Legg MA, 1983. Pulmonary granulomas. In: Ioachim HL (ed), *Pathology of Granulomas*. New York: Raven Press, pp. 223–256

Kerkezenov N, 1962. Intra-ocular filariasis in Australia. Br. J. Ophthalmol. 46:607–615

Kotani T, Tomimura T, Ogura M, Yoshida II, Mochizuki II, 1975. Cerebral infarction caused by *Dirofilaria immitis* in three dogs. Nippon. Juigaku. Zasshi. 37:379–390

Kuberski T, 1979. Eosinophils in the cerebrospinal fluid. Ann. Intern. Med. 91:70–75

Monchy D, Levenes H, Guegan H, Poey C, Dubourdieu D, 1993. Dirofilariose pulmonaire. Med. Trop. 53:366–371

Moorhouse DE, 1978. *Dirofilaria immitis*: a cause of human intra-ocular infection. Infection 6:192–193

Neafie RC, Piggott J, 1971. Human pulmonary dirofilariasis. Arch. Pathol. 92:342–349

Orihel TC, 1961. Morphology of the larval stages of *Dirofilaria immitis* in the dog. J. Parasitol. 47:251–262

Orihel TC, 1973. Cerebral filariasis in Rhodesia—a zoonotic infection? Am. J. Trop. Med. Hyg. 22:596–599

Orihel TC, Esslinger JH, 1973. *Meningonema peruzzii* gen. et sp. n. (Nematoda: Filarioidea) from the central nervous system of African monkeys. J. Parasitol. 59: 437–441

Owen HB, Hennessey RSF, 1932. A note in some ocular manifestations of helminthic origin in natives in Uganda. Trans. R. Soc. Trop. Med. Hyg. 25:267–273

Pampiglione S, Candiani G, Del Maschio O, Pagan V, 1991. Dirofilariasi polmonare nell' uomo. Un terzo caso in Italia. Pathologica 83:21–27

Pampiglione S, Del Maschio O, Pagan V, Rivasi F, 1994. Pulmonary dirofilariasis in man: a new Italian case. Review of the European literature. Parasite 1:379–385

Pampiglione S, Rivasi F, Canestri Trotti G, 1984. Dirofilariosi polmonare umana: un cas in Italia. Pathologica 76:565–572

Patton CS, Garner FM, 1970. Cerebral infarction caused by heartworms (*Dirofilaria immitis*) in a dog. JAVMA 156:600–605

Poltera AA, 1973. The histopathology of ocular loiasis in Uganda. Trans. R. Soc. Trop. Med. Hyg. 67:819–829

Ro JY, Tsakalakis PJ, White VA, Luna MA, Chang Tung EG, Green L, Cribbett L, Ayala AG, 1989. Pulmonary dirofilariasis: the great imitator of primary or metastatic lung tumor. A clinicopathologic analysis of seven cases and a review of the literature. Hum. Pathol. 20:69–76

Samples JR, Fraunfelder FT, Swan KC, Beaver PC, Rashad AL, Rosenquist R, 1988. A technique for removal of filariasis of the anterior chamber. Ophthalmic Surg. 19:124–127

Shires PK, Turnwald GH, Qualls CW, King GK, 1982. Epidural dirofilariasis causing paraparesis in a dog. JAVMA 180:1340–1343

Simon F, Muro A, Cordero M, Martin J, 1991. A seroepidemiologic survey of human dirofilariosis in western Spain. Trop. Med. Parasitol. 42:106–108

Slonka GF, Castleman W, Krum S, 1977. Adult heartworms in arteries and veins of a dog. JAVMA 170:717–719

Takeuchi T, Asami K, Kobayashi S, Masuda M, Tanabe M, Miura S, Asakawa M, Murai T, 1981. *Dirofilaria immitis* infection in man: report of a case of the infection in heart and inferior vena cava from Japan. Am. J. Trop. Med. Hyg. 30:966–969

Uni S, Takada S, 1986. The longitudinal cuticular markings of *Dirofilaria immitis* adult worm. Jpn. J. Parasitol. 35:191–199

Villanueva EJ, Rodriguez Perez J, 1993. Immunodiagnosis of human dirofilariasis in Puerto Rico. Am. J. Trop. Med. Hyg. 48:536–541

Vodovozov AM, Jarulin GR, Djakonowa SW, 1973. *Dirofilaria* in the human vitreous body. Ophthalmologica 166:88–93

Welch JS, Dobson C, 1974. The prevalence of antibodies to *Dirofilaria immitis* in aboriginal and Caucasian Australians. Trans. R. Soc. Trop. Med. Hyg. 68:466–472

22

TRICHINELLOIDEA AND DIOCTOPHYMATOIDEA

The order Enoplida, comprising aphasmid nematodes (see the introduction to Part II), has two superfamilies, Trichinelloidea and Dioctophymatoidea. In addition to the characteristics of the order, outlined in the introduction to Part II, the females of this group have a single genital organ: one ovary, continuing with the oviduct, the uterus, and the vagina. In members of Trichinelloidea the esophagus (stichosome) consists of a capillary tube surrounded by gland-like cells, the stichocytes, and there are eggs with mucous plugs at either end. The Dioctophymatoidea have a cylindrical, muscular esophagus.

Trichinelloidea has two families: Trichuridae and Trichinellidae. The former consists of the genera *Trichuris*, *Aonchotheca*, *Calodium*, *Eucoleus* (included previously in the genus *Capillaria*), and *Anatrichosoma*. The latter has one genus, *Trichinella*, with several species in humans. These six genera have species that are important in human and veterinary medicine. Species of *Trichuris* and *Trichinella* are well-known human parasites, while the capillariids and *Anatrichosoma* are parasites of animals that sometimes produce zoonotic infections in humans. Most infections produced by these parasites occur sporadically, but *Aonchotheca philippinensis* (= *Capillaria philippinensis*) sometimes results in epidemics.

The Dioctophymatoidea are all parasites of animals; species of two genera, *Dioctophyme* and *Eustrongylides*, are also found rarely in humans. *Dioctophyme renale* occurs in humans in its adult form (Beaver et al. 1984a), and a species of *Eustrongylides* occurs in its larval stage.

Trichuris trichiura— Trichuriasis or Trichocephaliasis

Trichuris is one of the most commonly found and widely distributed intestinal nematodes, producing morbidity especially in children. The parasite was known for many years, but only in the 1950s was its pathogenic role in humans conclusively demonstrated. *Trichuris* is a soil-transmitted helminth that, like *Ascaris*, affects mostly children of low socioeconomic status.

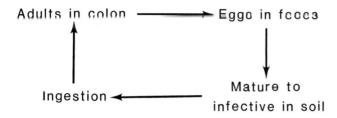

Adults in colon ——————→ Eggs in feces

Ingestion ←—————— Mature to infective in soil

Fig. 22–1. *Trichuris trichiura*, schematic representation of the life cycle.

Morphology. *Trichuris trichiura* is commonly known as *whipworm* because of its characteristic gross appearance. The adult worm is generally up to 4.5 cm in length, and more than half of its body is thin, filiform, and occupied only by the esophagus. The males have a ventrally curved posterior end, often showing two copulatory spicules. The females have a gently tapered, straight posterior end. In gross specimens of colon with *Trichuris*, the thicker posterior portion of the worm protrudes from the mucosa and is free in the lumen. The anterior filiform end of the parasite is threaded in the superficial cells, firmly attached to the mucosa. If pulled, the worm may break easily. The microanatomy of the worm is discussed below under Diagnosis.

Life Cycle. As stated, *T. trichiura* inhabits the colon, mainly the cecum, but also extends to the rectum, when large numbers of worms are present. The eggs laid by the worm pass with the feces into the environment, where they mature in appropriate soil in about 3 to 5 weeks, depending on climatic conditions. Ingested infective eggs hatch in the small intestine, releasing larvae that travel to the colon and enter the superficial epithelium (Fig. 22–1). As the parasite grows, the posterior end protrudes into the lumen while the anterior end remains in the mucosa, in the same location for the rest of the worm's life (Fig. 22–2 *A–B*; Beer, 1973).

Geographic Distribution and Epidemiology. *Trichuris trichiura* occurs in warm, wet parts of tropical areas and,

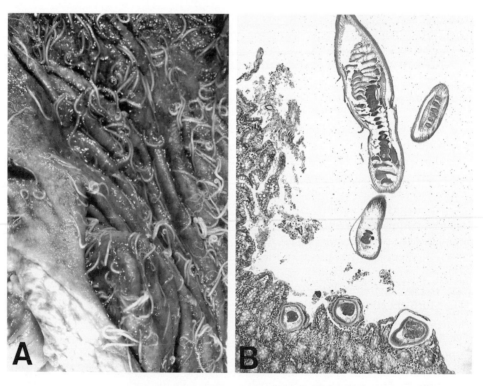

Fig. 22–2. *Trichuris trichiura*, gross and microscopic lesions. *A*, Parasites in the colon of a heavily infected child. *B*, Section of colon stained with hematoxylin and eosin stain showing the parasites threaded in the superficial cell layer of the colon and protruding into the lumen, ×47. (In: Gutierrez, Y., and Smith, J. H. 1996. Metazoan Diseases. In: Damjanov, I., and Linder, J. (eds.), *Anderson's Pathology*, 10th ed. Mosby, New York. Reproduced with permission.)

to a lesser extent, in subtropical areas. As stated, it infects especially children, although *Trichuris* tends to occur more often in school children than in toddlers. In most places the prevalence of *Trichuris* often parallels that of *Ascaris* (Bundy, 1986; Cooper et al. 1986); in some tropical populations the prevalence is over 90% (WHO, 1981). A study in Colombia reported a prevalence of 50%; one-half of the patients had symptoms and one-fifth had diarrhea. In Poland, with a prevalence of 36%, only 5% of the patients had symptoms and none had diarrhea (WHO, 1980). In the United States, *Trichuris* occurs mainly in the southeastern part of the country. Many species of *Trichuris* other than *T. trichiura* occur in wild and domestic animals; *T. vulpis*, the whipworm of dogs, occasionally produces human infections in the intestine (Kagei et al. 1986; Kenney, Yermakov, 1980). Two reports of visceral larva migrans produced by *T. vulpis* exist in the literature. In one, the diagnosis rested on immunoelectrophoretic studies of sera from two patients with eosinophilia (Sakano et al. 1980; Singh et al. 1993). The other report was based on sections of a worm found in the lung, the photographs of which do not support the identification of *T. vulpis*. Because the worm lacks a migratory phase in its final host and does not reach the tissues, it cannot produce visceral larva migrans. *Trichuris suis* of pigs, a species almost indistinguishable morphologically from *T. trichiura*, produced infections experimentally in humans (Beer, 1976). A *Trichuris* found in the wild monkey (*Macaca fuscata*) in Japan, identical to *T. trichiura*, was successfully transmitted experimentally to human volunteers (Horii, Usui, 1985).

Clinical Findings. The clinical symptoms of trichuriasis are directly related to the number of worms in the intestine (Bundy, 1986; Jung, Beaver, 1951), the nutritional status of the host (Gilman et al. 1983), and the duration of the infection. Normally, a small number of worms do not produce symptoms, but a large number, especially in children, result in colitis (Gilman et al. 1976; Jung, Beaver, 1951).

Infections with a moderate number of *Trichuris* worms produce nonspecific complaints of right lower quadrant pain, indigestion, weight loss, and constipation. Infections with a large number of worms produce prolonged diarrhea with blood-streaked stools, abdominal pain, and weight loss (Jung, Beaver, 1951). In some patients there is anemia due to blood loss and poor nutrition; sometimes there is peripheral eosinophilia of less than 15% (Jung, Jelliffe, 1952). If the disease is prolonged because of lack of treatment, growth retardation, weight loss, and anemia become

more manifest and clubbing of the fingers may develop (Bowie et al. 1978; Gilman et al. 1983; Kamath, 1973). In heavy trichuriasis with colitis and proctitis, rectal prolapse may develop, especially in undernourished young children. On examination, the prolapsed rectum usually has numerous *Trichuris* worms attached to the mucosa, a sign of the intensity of the infection. Children with more than 20,000 eggs per gram of feces may develop severe diarrhea or even dysentery (WHO, 1981) that is indistinguishable clinically from amebic colitis or other forms of colitis (Gilman et al. 1976). Comparison of children with *Trichuris* dysentery and with *Entamoeba histolytica* dysentery shows that trichuriasis lasts longer, results in more hospitalizations, and produces a higher percentage of rectal prolapse than amebiasis (Gilman et al. 1976). In addition, children with trichuriasis have a greater than expected tendency to develop amebic infection (Jung, Beaver, 1951; Gilman et al. 1983), probably because the damaged mucosa permits amebic colonization more easily. A single *Trichuris* worm in an elderly Japanese woman, found during a colonoscopy performed because of abdominal pain, *was not* responsible for the patient's symptoms, as the report claimed (Yoshida et al. 1996). This report and many others as such in the literature, are only examples of misinterpretation of facts.

The clinical laboratory tests in trichuriasis with low and moderate worm burdens are usually not helpful, except for revealing the presence of eggs in the stools and, rarely, low-level eosinophilia. Colonic endoscopy may reveal some worms in the mucosa, and double-contrast barium enemas may show small S-shaped filling defects (Davis et al. 1986). In heavy infections, microcytic hypochromic anemia with a mean hemoglobin level of 5.4 g/dl, peripheral eosinophilia, hypoalbuminemia, and hyperglobulinemia are common findings. In addition, the stools have large numbers of eggs, eosinophils, and Charcot-Leyden crystals (Kamath, 1973).

The mechanism by which *Trichuris* produces symptoms in humans not known. The parasite, buried in the superficial mucosa, stimulates the production of syncytium-like epithelial cells that form a tunnel with the roof made of atrophic epithelium; there is no other apparent damage. Attachment of the worms is probably caused by the action of a pore-forming protein found in the secretory/excretory products of the worm (Drake et al. 1994). The large number of eosinophils in the stools suggests an allergic reaction to the worms, but this remains unproven. Some patients with trichuriasis may have anemia, possibly due to blood loss produced by the parasite. Studies of histologic sections of colon from patients with heavy infections do not support this

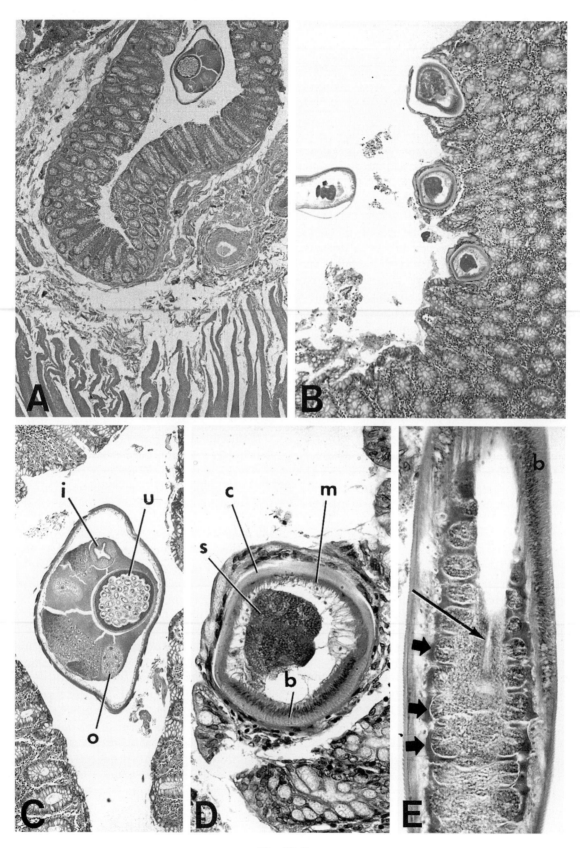

Fig. 22–3.

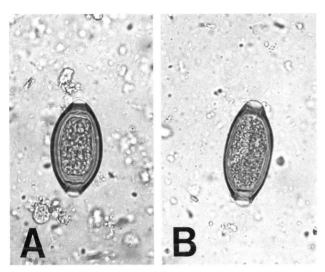

Fig. 22–4. *A, B,* **Trichuris trichiura eggs, unstained, ×540.**

idea. The parasites in the colon are found in tunnels in the superficial layer of enterocytes; they are not located near capillaries or smaller vessels of any significance to produce bleeding. In addition, controlled studies have established that the anemia seen in whipworm infections is due to poor nutrition of the host (Greenberg, Cline, 1979; Lotero et al. 1974).

Pathology. The colonic mucosa in clinically evident whipworm infections is hyperemic, edematous, friable, and bleeds easily with minimal trauma during sigmoidoscopy. Small mucosal lacerations are usually present, but the most characteristic finding is the large number of worms (Jung, Jelliffe, 1952). Most cases of trichuriasis with light to moderate worm burdens have few microscopic alterations of the mucosa, mainly edema and infiltration by plasma cells, lymphocytes, and rare polymorphonuclear eosinophils (Hartz, 1953). In heavy infections, microscopic mucosal damage is also minimal, and the epithelial cells forming the roof of the tunnel where the parasite is buried show atrophy. Infiltration by inflammatory cells, edema, and hyperemia of the mucosa are more pronounced. The main finding is the parasite within the mucosa (Figs. 22–2 *B* and 22–3 *B, C,* and *D*), cut at different levels, with the posterior end in the lumen (Fig. 22–3 *A–B*).

Reports of suppurative anal cryptitis (Feigen, 1987), as well as colonic obstruction and perforation (Fishman, Perrone, 1984) in individuals with *Trichuris* infection, are concomitant occurrences rather than a direct result of the infection.

Diagnosis. The clinical diagnosis of whipworm infection is easy, especially in a child with typical symptoms and rectal prolapse with worms attached to the mucosa. In other cases, the diagnosis is made in the clinical laboratory by finding the eggs in the stools. These eggs measure 50 to 54 × 22 to 23 μm and have the characteristic mucous plugs at either end (Fig. 22–4). Patients undergoing treatment, especially with thiabendazole, have eggs in their stools with somewhat distorted characteristics and often larger than normal (Correa et al. 1980; Little, 1968; Vanhaelen Lindhout, Smit, 1971).

The worms are occasionally found in histologic sections of colon or appendix. Identification of the parasite in these cases may be unimportant clinically, but it may be desirable for assessment of other lesions in the colon. Sections of the parasites are within the superficial layers of the mucosa and in the lumen; those within the mucosa show the esophagus. The diameter of the worm is approximately 100 to 150 μm, and the cuticle is 8 to 12 μm thick. The cuticle of *Trichuris* has a characteristic structure known as the *bacillary band*; it consists of cuticular pores, each with a hypodermal gland cell (Fig. 22–3 *C–D*). The bacillary band of *Trichuris* is more than twice as thick as the rest of the cuticle and extends the length of the esophagus. In the anterior esophagus, the band is narrow; in the posterior esophagus, it comprises up to one-half of the worm's circumference. Sections closer to the mouth opening of the worm show the muscular esophagus. Posterior to the muscular esophagus is the glandular esophagus made of a gland-like stichosome (Fig. 22–3 *D–E*) composed of a row of cells (stichocytes) with a

Fig. 22–3. *Trichuris trichiura* **in human colon, sections stained with hematoxylin and eosin stain.** *A,* **Low-power view of colon showing a cross section through the posterior of an adult female in the lumen, ×28.** *B,* **Low-power view of intestinal mucosa with three sections through the anterior portion of the worm, ×70.** *C,* **Cross section through the posterior part of the female illustrating the** uterus with eggs (u), intestine (i), and ovary (o), ×70. *D,* **Higher magnification of the esophageal portion showing the cuticle (c), the muscle layer (m), the bacillary band (b), and the stichocytes (s); note their glandular character, ×280.** *E,* **Slightly oblique section through the esophagus (stichosome) (short arrows) showing the esophageal lumen (long arrow); note the bacillary band (b), ×280.**

capillary esophageal lumen (Fig. 22–3 E). Sections of the worm located in the lumen (Fig. 22–3 A–D) may also show the esophagus, but most of them correspond to the posterior half of the body, which is 0.5 mm in diameter. These sections reveal the intestine and the single genital tube in the females, with the uterus usually filled with eggs (Fig. 22–3 A–C). The male worms have an intestine and a genital tract, also seen as two tubular structures.

The Capillariids: *Aonchotheca, Calodium,* and *Eucoleus*

The genus formerly called *Capillaria* contained many species parasitic in the intestine, lower and upper respiratory tracts, liver, and other organs of animals. Because the genus was so large, the newer classification that divides *Capillaria* into 16 different genera has been adopted. Of these genera, three have species important to humans (Moravec et al. 1987): *Aonchotheca, Calodium,* and *Eucoleus.* Humans are accidental host of several species of these genera, some of which produce morbidity and mortality, sometimes in epidemic proportions. The life cycle of most capillariids is direct, with infection resulting from ingestion of infective eggs with food or water; other species have intermediate hosts. The eggs of capillariids superficially resemble those of *Trichuris.* They have two mucous plugs, and the outer shell of the egg in some species is ornate, often with minute pits or striations (Figs. 22–7 and 22–10 D). The species of capillariids important in human medicine are *Aonchotheca philippinensis* in the intestine, *Calodium hepaticum* in the liver, and *Eucoleus aerophilus* in the lung.

*Aonchotheca (= Capillaria) philippinensis—*Intestinal Aonchotheciasis

Aonchotheca philippinensis was recovered in 1962 from a man from Ilocos Norte, the Philippines, who suffered from recurrent ascitis, emaciation, and cachexia. Later, the parasite was recovered from patients during an epidemic of obscure, often fatal gastrointestinal disease in Ilocos Sur (Chitwood et al. 1964, 1968).

Morphology and Life Cycle. The adults of *A. philippinensis* live buried in the epithelial cells of the lower duodenum, jejunum, and ileum in a manner similar to that of *Trichinella* and *Trichuris.* The females are 2.5 to 4.3 mm in length, and the males are 2.3 to 3.2 mm in length. The anterior portion of the body of the worm is slightly slender and contains the esophagus; the posterior portion contains the intestine and the genital tract.

The life cycle of *A. philippinensis* is partially known; it appears to involve small freshwater fish as intermediate hosts (Fig. 22–5). On ingestion of raw fish with infective larvae, the parasites become free in the small intestine and enter the mucosa, where they grow into adults. After mating, the females lay larvae, which rapidly mature to infective stages in the intestine and reenter the mucosa to grow into adults (internal autoinfection) (Cross et al. 1972). Other females produce eggs that are evacuated with the feces to become infective in fresh or brackish water in about 2 weeks (Bhaibulaya et al. 1979). After embryonated eggs are ingested by freshwater fish, they hatch in the intestine; the larvae develop into infective stages in about 3 weeks. Fish become infective and, when fed to experimental animals, produce the infection with adults in the intestine (Cross, 1990). The natural host of *C. philippinensis* remains unknown; humans are the only hosts infected naturally. Under experimental conditions, some species of fish-eating birds support the infection (Bhaibulaya et al. 1979), but whether birds are the natural definitive hosts of *A. philippinensis* requires further study. Only once was a single male of *A. philippinensis* recovered from a naturally infected bird (Cross, Basaca-Sevilla, 1991).

Geographic Distribution and Epidemiology. *Aonchotheca philippinensis* is found in areas other than the Philippines, mainly in Thailand (Bhaibulaya et al., 1977; Pradatsundarasar et al. 1973), Taiwan (Chen et al. 1989), Japan (Nawa et al. 1988), Indonesia (Bangs

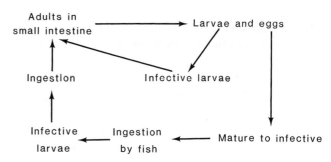

Fig. 22–5. *Aonchoteca philippinensis,* **schematic representation of the life cycle.**

et al. 1994), Korea (Hong et al. 1994), India (Kang et al. 1994), Iran (Hoghooghi-Rad et al. 1987), Egypt (Youssef et al. 1989), Morocco (Mugarza Hernandez et al. 1995), and Colombia (Dronda et al. 1993).

Clinical Findings. Intestinal aonchotheciasis occurs mainly in men 20 to 50 years old. The infection usually causes watery diarrhea that does not respond to customary therapy and develops into a sprue-like syndrome with weight loss due to fat, vitamin, protein, and carbohydrate malabsorption (Dauz et al. 1967; Watten et al. 1972). Sometimes the infection results in abdominal pain, anorexia, and slight fever. On physical examination, the patient appears emaciated, dehydrated, and weak. Laboratory tests, which are mostly normal, sometimes show a slight increase in white blood cells, eosinophilia, and low albumin levels. Stool examination demonstrates *Aonchotheca* eggs, and sometimes larvae and adult worms (Cabrera et al. 1967). Radiographs of the small intestine reveal inflammatory disease. Untreated infections are invariably fatal.

Pathology. At autopsy the intestinal tract is often grossly normal, but hyperemia, thickening of the wall with atrophy of the mucosa, and superficial erosions are sometimes observed (Canlas et al. 1967; Fresh et al. 1972). Microscopically, the most striking feature is the presence of numerous adult worms and larvae buried in the mucosa, sometimes without but often with an overt inflammatory reaction (Fig. 22–6 A–D). The mucosa may have some flattening of the villi, with reduced thickness (Fig. 22–6 B), dilated crypts, cellular debris, and inflammatory cells (Fig. 22–6 A–B). In some cases, metaplastic changes in the epithelial cells and moderate to marked infiltration of the mucosa by plasma cells, lymphocytes, macrophages, and a few eosinophils are found (Fig. 22–6 A–C).

Diagnosis. In endemic areas, intestinal aonchotheciasis is diagnosed clinically by physicians acquainted with the disease. It is confirmed in the laboratory by examination of stool samples, which reveal eggs 36 to 45 μm in length by about 21 μm in width (Fig. 22–7 A–B), larvae, and sometimes adult parasites.

In histologic sections of small intestine, the parasites are found in the mucosa, buried in a manner similar to that of *Trichinella* (Fig. 22–6 A). The maximum diameter of the female is 47 μm and that of the male is 28 μm. The cuticle is 1 μm thick, with inconspicuous bacillary bands. Sections through the posterior esophagus contain the stichosome (Fig. 22–6 C). The muscle layer is delicate, with a contractile portion twice as thick as the cuticle. The lateral bacillary bands are difficult to distinguish and have about two nuclei per histologic section. In some sections the intestine is one-third to one-fourth the diameter of the worm and is composed of several cuboidal cells (Fig. 22–6 E). The genital tract consists of a single tube; the uterus contains developing eggs (Fig. 22–6 D and F) and sometimes larvae (Fig. 22–6 E).

Calodium hepaticum (*Capillaria hepatica*)— Hepatic Calodiasis

Calodium hepaticum is a worldwide parasite found in the liver of rats, squirrels, prairie dogs, monkeys, and other animals. The females are approximately 52 mm long by 110 μm wide; the males are smaller. The worms have two lateral bacillary bands that extend the entire length of the body. A third bacillary band, narrower and less conspicuous, is present in the ventral aspect of the female (Wright, 1961). The adult worms live in the liver parenchyma, where the female lays its eggs; both the adults and the eggs in the liver elicit granuloma formation and marked fibrosis indistinguishable from those of cirrhosis (parasitic cirrhosis) in infected animals. The adults are eventually destroyed by the inflammatory process, but the eggs remain in the tissues until a predator ingests the infected animal. Digestion of the liver by the predator frees the eggs, which pass with the feces to mature in appropriate soil in a few weeks. In addition, heavily infected animals with extensive hepatic lesions excrete eggs in their feces (Chieffi et al. 1981). Ingestion of infective eggs, either by the appropriate final host or accidentally by humans, produces the infection. Once swallowed, the eggs hatch in the small intestine and free larvae that migrate via the portal system to the liver, where they grow into adults and start oviposition in about 4 weeks (Fig. 22–8).

Known human infections with *C. hepaticum* are few. The reported cases have occurred in the continental United States, Hawaii, England, India, Turkey, Nigeria, South Africa, Mexico, Brazil, Italy, Switzerland, Germany, Korea, Japan, and Czechoslovakia. Most infections occur in small children (Calle, 1961) because the parasite is a soil-transmitted helminth. Infections in adults are extremely rare and have occurred in persons living under deplorable sanitary conditions

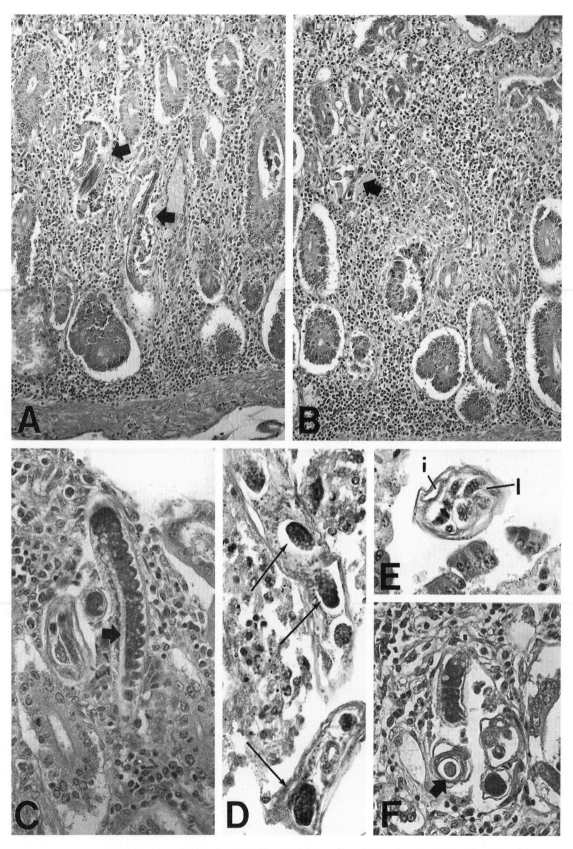

Fig. 22–6.

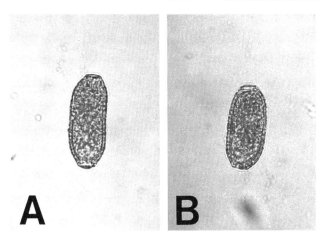

Fig. 22–7. *A*, *B*, *Aonchoteca philippinensis* eggs in human stools, unstained, ×495. (Sample courtesy of J.H. Cross, Ph.D., Department of Preventive Medicine and Biometry, Uniformed Services University, Bethesda, Maryland.)

(Attah et al. 1983; Sumner, Tinsley, 1967). Asymptomatic infections in adults discovered in autopsy material are known in Europe; these infections consisted of isolated small nodules (granulomas) found incidentally at autopsy (Slais, 1974). On occasion, eggs of capillariids are found in the stools of patients, a situation referred to as *spurious infection*, produced by the ingestion of liver or other viscera of parasitized animals (Bergner et al. 1973; McQuown, 1950). If the eggs persist in the stools for several days in the absence of ingestion of meat, the sputum needs careful examination for eggs. If the exam is positive, pulmonary eucoliasis requires attention (see below).

Clinical Findings. The clinical manifestations of *C. hepaticum* are variable. At first, symptoms of acute or subacute hepatitis occur, but later, a picture similar to that of visceral larva migrans, especially in children, may develop (see Chapter 17). The liver is tender and enlarged, often 2 to 3 cm below the costal margin (this

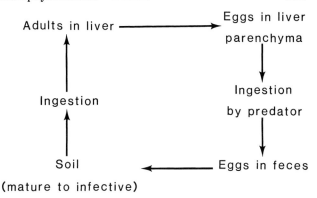

(mature to infective)

Fig. 22–8. *Calodium hepaticum*, schematic representation of the life cycle.

finding should alert the astute clinician to search for a cause other than *Toxocara* for the disease because *Toxocara* never enlarges the liver this much). Other findings are anorexia and weight loss. The only positive laboratory test result is high peripheral eosinophilia, in some cases 94% (Attah et al. 1983).

Pathology. In acute hepatic calodiasis the liver is enlarged and soft; in chronic infections it is hard due to fibrosis, which is sometimes severe (Attah et al. 1983). Microscopically, acute cases have numerous areas of focal liver parenchyma destruction and granulomas (Fig. 22–9 *A–C* and *color plate* X *G–H*) consisting of large numbers of mononuclear cells and eosinophils. In the early stages, only immature worms without eggs are found (Fig. 22–9 *D–F*), misleading pathologists into diagnosing *Toxocara*, which is easily ruled out by its smaller diameter. In more advanced cases, adult worms and eggs are scattered throughout the liver parenchyma, producing a granulomatous inflammation (Fig. 22–10 *A–D*). As oviposition continues, the granulomas with eggs coalesce to form a mass of eggs separated only by thin bundles of fibrous connective tissue infiltrated by lymphocytes and polymorphonuclear cells, especially eosinophils (Fig. 22–10 *D*). Similar in-

Fig. 22–6. *Aonchoteca philippinensis* in human intestine, sections stained with hematoxylin and eosin stain. *A* and *B*, Low-power views illustrating the parasites deep in the crypts (arrows) and the inflammatory infiltrate consisting mostly of mononuclear and polymorphonuclear cells. Note the distortion of the mucosa and the flattening of the villi, ×140. *C*, Higher magnification of an oblique section through the esophagus showing the stichosome with the lumen (arrow), ×350. *D*, Higher

magnification of a longitudinal section of two females with developing eggs in the uterus (arrows), ×450. *E*, Cross section of the posterior aspect of a female showing larvae in the uterus (l) and the intestine (i), ×350. *F*, Another mucosal crypt with a female with an egg on cross section (arrow), ×450. (Preparation courtesy of J.H. Cross, Ph.D., Department of Preventive Medicine and Biometry, Uniformed Services University, Bethesda, Maryland.)

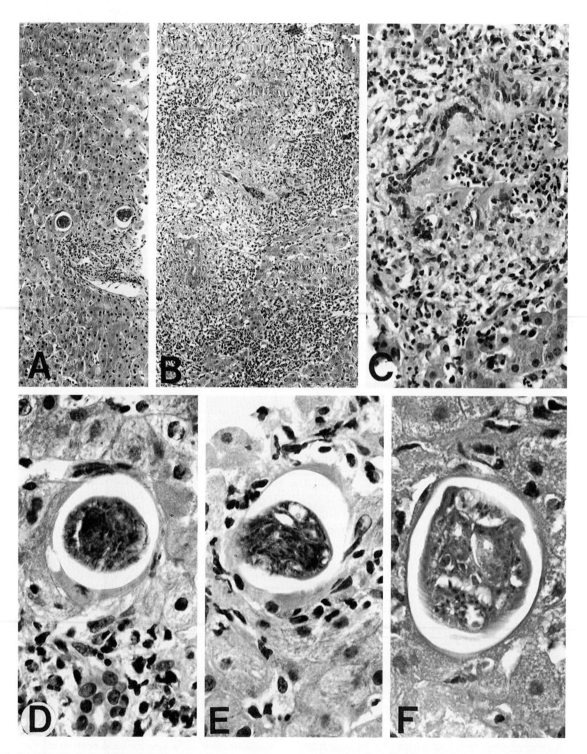

Fig. 22–9. *Calodlum hepaticum* in human liver, early infection, sections stained with hematoxylin and eosin stain. *A* and *B*, Low-power view of a liver biopsy specimen showing a young adult and marked tissue necrosis with infiltration, especially by eosinophils, ×80. *C*, Higher magnification of a granuloma corresponding to the track left by a migrating *C. hepaticum* in the liver, ×300. *D–F*, Higher magnification of the parasite cut at three different levels. A stichocyte is seen in *D* and *E*, ×560. (Preparation courtesy of G. Jacobs, M.D., Institute of Pathology, Case Western Reserve University, Cleveland, Ohio. The patient is a 2-year-old girl from Johannesburg, South Africa.)

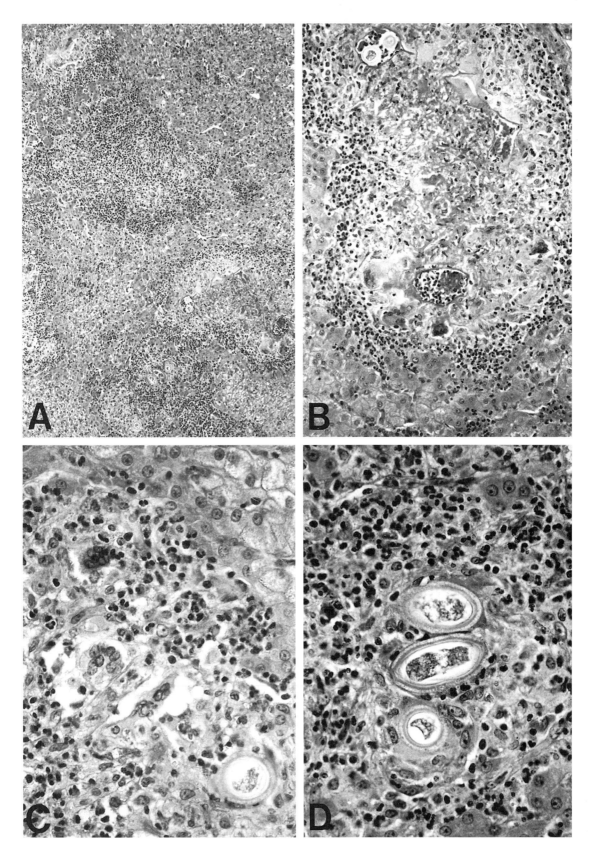

Fig. 22–10. *Calodium hepaticum* in human liver, older infection, sections stained with hematoxylin and eosin stain. *A*, Low-power view of liver with multiple granulomas, ×70. *B*, Medium magnification showing a large granuloma with necrosis and remnants of cuticle; two eggs are seen at the top, ×180. *C* and *D*, Higher magni- fication showing granulomas with eggs; note the mixed inflammatory infiltrate with abundant eosinophils, ×450. (Preparation courtesy of V.M. Arean, M.D., Department of Pathology, Saint Anthony's Hospital, St. Petersburg, Florida.)

flammatory changes occur around the adult worms, and as the infection progresses, the eggs become more numerous and the fibrosis more abundant. Some eggs are surrounded by multinucleated giant cells and are destroyed, as are adult worms, which eventually disappear. The infected adults found at autopsy (see above) had a single parasite producing a nodule that on microscopy demonstrated an adult *Calodium* in different stages of organization, disintegration, and calcification (Slais, 1973).

Diagnosis. Hepatic calodiasis is diagnosed on the basis of liver biopsy specimens or postmortem material. *Calodium hepaticus* eggs in the stools indicate spurious parasitism rather than a true liver infection. In liver biopsy specimens taken early in the infection, the characteristic finding is immature parasites (Fig. 22–9 D–F);

later, adult worms (Fig. 22–11 A), numerous eggs (Fig. 22–11 B), and extensive liver fibrosis (Fig. 22–11 B) appear. In tissue sections, the eggs measure 48 to 62 × 28 to 37 µm and have a radially striated, thick outer shell with two polar plugs (Fig. 22–10 C–D). Sections of the worms vary in diameter, depending on the degree of maturation. Adult females are usually up to 130 µm and males are up to 50 µm in diameter (Fig. 22–11 A). The cuticle is 1 µm thick and has two wide bacillary bands, each occupying one-fifth of the circumference, dividing the muscle layer into two separate areas. The third bacillary band in the ventral aspect of the female is inconspicuous. The muscles are 4 to 6 µm tall; the coelomatic cavity sometimes appears to be wide open. The single uterus contains eggs in different stages of maturation. The intestine stains darkly with hematoxylin and eosin stain, is about one-fourth to one-fifth the diameter of the gonad, and has numerous cuboidal

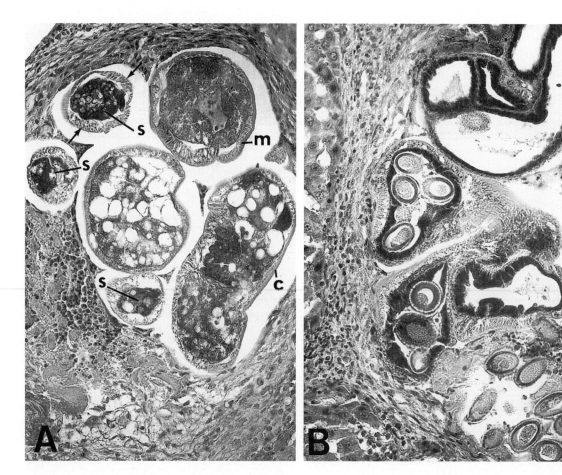

Fig. 22–11. *Calodium hepaticum,* adult worm in the liver of rat, sections stained with hematoxylin and eosin stain. *A* and *B,* Sections of granulomas containing adult *C. hepaticum* and eggs. Note the thin cuticle (c), the weak muscle layer (m), the stichosome (s) seen in several sections, and the lateral bacillary bands (arrows); eggs in *B* are within the uterus of what appears to be a degenerating worm, ×220.

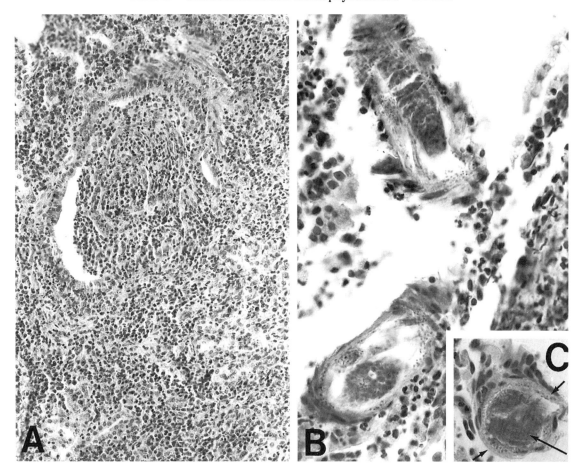

Fig. 22–12. *Eucoleus aerophilus* in human lung, sections stained with hematoxylin and eosin stain. *A,* Low-power view of lung illustrating the inflammatory reaction with involvement of a small bronchus, ×180. *B,* Higher magnification showing oblique sections of the worm and the infiltrate, composed mostly of eosinophils, ×450. *C,* Cross section of worm buried in bronchial epithelium. The stichocyte (long arrow) and the bacillary bands (short arrows) are evident, ×450. (Preparation courtesy of P.C. Beaver, Ph.D., Department of Tropical Medicine, School of Tropical Medicine and Public Health, Tulane University, New Orleans, Louisiana. Reported by: Aftandelians, R., Raafat, F., Taffazoli, M., et al. 1977. Pulmonary capillariasis in a child in Iran. Am. J. Trop. Med. Hyg. 26:64–71.)

cells with many nuclei per histologic section and an inconspicuous brush border. Sections through the esophagus show the stichocytes.

Eucoleus aerophilus—Pulmonary Eucoleiasis

Eucoleus aerophilus is a worldwide parasite of wild carnivores. The adults live buried under the mucosa of the upper and lower respiratory tracts of their natural hosts. The females are 20 mm long by 105 μm wide, and the males are 18 mm long by 70 μm wide. The eggs laid in the respiratory mucosa eventually move with the mucus to the epiglottis, are swallowed and evacuated in the feces, embryonate in soil, and gain access to the new host with contaminated food or water. Human infections are zoonoses reported from Russia, Morocco, and Iran.

Clinical Findings. All cases of pulmonary eucoleiasis in the former Soviet Union have occurred in adults with acute tracheobronchitis, dyspnea, and a painful dry cough; in a few cases, when sputum was produced, it was red-tinged. Some individuals had fever of up to 39°C, and others complained of asthma attacks (Skrjabin et al. 1957).

In children, the infection occurred once in Morocco and once in Iran, producing severe dyspnea, increased respiration, cough, and expectoration. Abnormal laboratory test results were leukocytosis and slight to moderate eosinophilia. On physical examination the children had hepatomegaly and were cyanotic, with fine moist rales over both lungs. Chest radiograms showed an infiltrate with a reticulogranular pattern in both lung fields, which progressed to a honeycomb pattern at the bases.

Pathology and Diagnosis. There has been only one study of a biopsy specimen in pulmonary eucoleiasis (Aftandelians et al. 1977). The specimen showed numerous granulomatous lesions less than 0.5 mm in diameter, with foreign body multinucleated giant cells containing the parasite. Outside the granulomas, there was an inflammatory infiltrate with lymphocytes, plasma cells, eosinophils, and fibrin deposition. The granulomas were located mainly within the bronchiolar wall, producing marked destruction of the airways (Fig. 22–12 A). The parasite was identified in tissue sections (Fig. 22–12 B–C).

Anatrichosoma—Anatrichosomiasis

The anatrichosomes are poorly studied parasites that inhabit the superficial skin and mucosa or underlying tissues of animals (Fig. 22–13). *Anatrichosoma cynamolgi* and *A. cutaneum* live in the nasal mucosa and the skin of Old World primates (Orihel, 1970; Swift et al. 1922).

Two infections with *A. cynamolgi* are known in humans. One occurred in a Vietnamese man who presented with cutaneous and mucosal lesions consisting of superficial tunnels in the right hand, the scrotum, and the right foot. The lesions were visible with the naked eye. Those in the hand and the scrotum measured about 3 cm in length, and intense itching was felt at the end of the tunnel. The infection had been contracted 2 months previously, after a parachute jump in which the patient fell into a briar patch and had multiple scratches that became secondarily infected a few days later. The patient received treatment for his infection, which resolved; 2 weeks later, the skin tracks appeared. Worms removed from the end of the skin tracks were identified and described (Le-Van-Hoa et al. 1963). The second patient was a 43-year-old Japanese man from Osaka City. The patient presented with "linear redness on the middle finger of the left hand and on the right ankle, which thereafter advanced in a zigzag manner about 5 to 10 mm a day, causing severe

pruritus." Each of the skin tracks had a female worm at the end; both worms were removed and described (Morishita, Tanei 1960).

Trichinella spiralis, T. pseudospiralis, T. nativa, T. nelsoni, and T. britovi— Trichinosis or Trichinelliasis

The genus *Trichinella*, with only one species, *T. spiralis*, remained unchanged for many years until 1972, when other species were described. Because the morphologic characteristics of all species of *Trichinella* are almost identical, some investigators have proposed referring to these species as *siblings*, *subspecies*, or *races* of *T. spiralis*. One of these, *T. pseudospiralis*, has

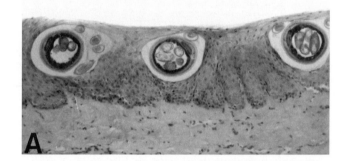
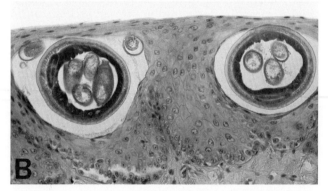

Fig. 22–13. *Anatrichosoma* species in squamous epithelium, preparation stained with hematoxylin and eosin stain. *A*, Low-power view of the parasite threaded in the epithelial layer in a tunnel where it laid the eggs. Note the lack of inflammatory reaction, ×100. *B*, Higher magnification. (Preparation courtesy of M.D. Little, Ph.D., Department of Tropical Medicine, School of Tropical Medicine and Public Health, Tulane University, New Orleans, Louisiana.)

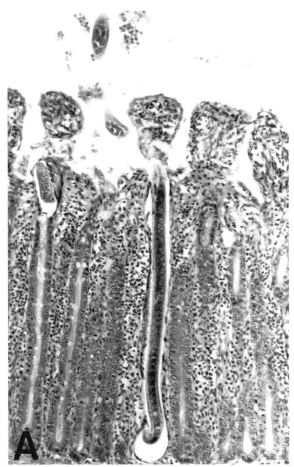
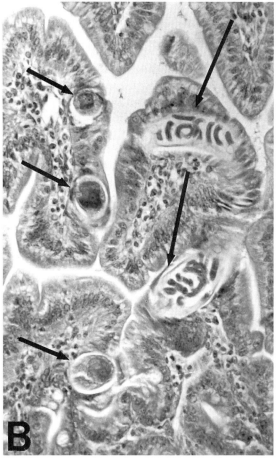

Fig. 22–14. *Trichinella* in the intestine of a rat, section stained with hematoxylin and eosin stain, *A*, Low-power view showing the adult parasite buried in the mucosa, ×140. *B*, Higher magnification showing sections of a female clearly threaded in the epithelial cells (short ar- rows), with the uterus filled with larvae (long arrows), ×280. (Preparation courtesy of M.D. Little, Ph.D., Department of Tropical Medicine, School of Tropical Medicine and Public Health, Tulane University, New Orleans, Louisiana.)

smaller larvae and adults than *T. spiralis*, and are not encapsulated in the muscles; in addition, it is the only easily identified species. Other species (*T. nativa, T. nelsoni,* and *T. britovi*) are identified on the basis of their biologic, biochemical, epidemiologic, and immunologic characteristics (Pozio et al. 1992). Because *T. pseudospiralis* infects primates, Pawlowski and Ruitenberg (1978) predicted that humans should be infected with this species; however, human infections occur with all five species.

In a report of a patient infected with *T. pseudospiralis*, the parasite was identified morphologically (Andrews et al. 1993, 1994). Subsequent work using the polymerase chain reaction conclusively showed that the DNA of the human *T. pseudospiralis* is identical to that of a stock isolate from animals (Andrews et al. 1995). In outbreaks of trichinelliasis in southern Italy,

the parasite isolated from humans was *T. britovi* (Pozio et al. 1993). All species of *Trichinella* occur widely in both wild and domestic animals, some in both. *Trichinella* produces a dual infection in its host in which the adults inhabit the gastrointestinal tract and the larval stages inhabit the skeletal muscles.

Morphology and Life Cycle. The adult *T. spiralis* is minute; the females are no more than 2.2 mm long by 90 μm wide, and the males are 1.2 mm long by 60 μm wide. The anterior end of the worm is delicate, and the posterior end is slightly thicker. The adult trichina inhabits the duodenum and jejunum, living intracellularly within the superficial enterocytes in a fashion similar to that of *Trichuris* (Fig. 22–14; Gardiner, 1976). The parasites do not damage or destroy the epithelial host cell (Wright, 1979). After insemination the female develops eggs, which mature within the uterus and produce larvae that are laid by the females, and travel, mostly through the hepatic and portal vessels (Wang, Bell, 1986), to the skeletal musculature. Larviposition by the females probably lasts no longer than 4 weeks, because by this time the inflammatory reaction around the adult worms dislodges the adult parasites from the mucosa into the lumen, which are lost in the feces. While in circulation, the larvae may enter the brain, heart, and cerebrospinal fluid, but eventually they relocate inside the skeletal muscles, grow and develop to the infective stage, and encapsulate (see below). Once the larvae encapsulate, they are ready to infect another host that happens to ingest them with the muscles. Once in the stomach, the cysts are freed from the muscles. The larvae began excystation either there or in the duodenum. Freed larvae enter the mucosa, where they grow into adults by the second day of infection and begin mating as early as 30 hours postinfection (Fig. 22–15; Beaver et al. 1984a).

Once the larvae arrive in the skeletal muscles, they enter the cells and become the largest intracellular organism known. The larva does not kill the muscle cell, as do most other parasites except viruses, but is modified to maintain its development and meet its needs throughout its natural life. This kind of adaptation is remarkable because the myocyte becomes a highly specialized, anatomically independent unit, a nurse cell for the parasite (Despomier, 1990).

Geographic Distribution and Epidemiology. *Trichinella spiralis* and *T. pseudospiralis* are cosmopolitan organisms that occur mainly in the temperate zones, and to a lesser extent, in other areas. *Trichinella nativa* occurs in the arctic and subarctic regions. *Trichinella nelsoni* occurs in tropical Africa and *T. britovi* in the temperate zone of the Palearctic region (Europe, Africa north of the Sahara, northern Arabia, and northern and central Asia) (Pozio

et al. 1992). In Europe, both *T. spiralis* and *T. britovi* occur (Pozio, 1998). In nature, *Trichinella* has been isolated from species of animals, both wild and domestic, representative of all orders except the Insectivora (Despomier, 1990). Most *Trichinella* species are not resistant to freezing conditions, with the exception of *T. nativa*, which is highly resistant, and *T. britovi*, which has low to moderate resistance. The prevalence of *Trichinella* infection is declining, but it is still important in eastern European countries and the former Soviet Union. In the United States, trichinosis has declined steadily in spite of a lack of control programs (Most, 1965). A study of over 3200 pigs sacrificed in the north central states (Minnesota, Wisconsin, Iowa, South Dakota, and North Dakota) did not reveal a single infection. Samples from over 400 wild animals showed only two with *Trichinella* (Stromberg, Prouty, 1987). In the early 1940s, approximately 450 cases of trichinosis were reported yearly to the Centers for Disease Control in the United States. This figure has decreased steadily to fewer than 100 cases more recently (Bailey et al. 1987). Cases of trichinelliasis usually occur in small clusters, and at least one-third of those acquired in the United States are due to consumption of meat from wild animals such as bears (Clark et al. 1972) and walruses (Margolis et al. 1979). One recent outbreak in Idaho was due to consumption of cougar jerky (CDC, 1996; Dworkin et al. 1996). A case due to ingestion of commercially purchased pork (Graves et al. 1996), as well as an outbreak (McAuley et al. 1992), occurred among Southeast Asian immigrants. This indicates that commercially available pork in the United States is still contaminated and that only education of the public is responsible for the small number of cases seen. Three outbreaks occurred in France due to consumption of horse meat imported from the United States (Ancelle et al. 1985; Dupouy et al. 1994; Laurichesse et al. 1997). Outbreaks are not rare in Spain due to ingestion of raw or poorly cooked pork (Tiberio et al. 1995, 1997).

Clinical Findings. The clinical manifestations of trichinelliasis vary with the sibling species producing the infection. *Trichinella spiralis* has the highest degree of virulence, while *T. britovi* and *T. nelsoni* are moderately virulent. The virulence of *T. pseudospiralis* and *T. nativa* for humans is not known. In addition to the character of the sibling species, the severity of the disease varies with the number of larvae ingested. The most common manifestations of trichinosis correspond, first, to the intestinal phase and, second, to the muscular phase of development of the parasite. Other organs are infected by a large number of parasites, and the brain and the heart are often involved. Patients re-

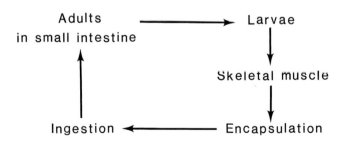

Fig. 22–15. *Trichinella*, **schematic representation of the life cycle.**

covering from the infection have no demonstrable sequelae (Harms et al. 1993). A skin rash has been observed in patients of three epidemics in Japan (Hanada et al. 1987).

Intestine. Intestinal symptoms begin soon after ingestion of infected meat. A few larvae usually produce an asymptomatic infection, but larger numbers of larvae result in malaise, vomiting, diarrhea, nausea, and abdominal cramps. The symptoms often occur simultaneously in several members of a family or in a group of friends who acquire the infection after eating the same infected food. Larger groups of individuals may become infected after consuming infected food during celebrations and other social gatherings. In either case the clinical diagnosis is often food poisoning, but astute clinicians may reach a diagnosis quickly by examining any remains of the infective meal, when available.

Skeletal Muscles. Invasion of muscles by the larvae produces symptoms of acute myositis that begin after the intestinal symptoms subside. Fever, muscle aches, and edema of the face (sometimes periorbital) and hands are common manifestations. Generalized weakness, weakness of the most compromised muscle groups, and high peripheral eosinophilia are often present. Respiratory muscle involvement results in respiratory failure (Brashear et al. 1971). The myositis progresses steadily, and difficulties in eye movement, breathing, chewing, and swallowing may develop. The fever lasts for approximately 10 days, occasionally longer, and in fatal cases it may reach 40°C. Vital organs such as the heart and the central nervous system may be involved, resulting in death.

Heart. The clinical manifestations of *Trichinella* myocarditis usually begin during the second or third week of infection, mainly with tachycardia, hypotension, elevated venous pressure, and edema. In some cases, there are electrocardiographic abnormalities suggestive of myocardial damage, especially during epidemics. A review of 1039 published cases of trichinosis showed 20% with electrocardiographic abnormalities. These consisted of T-wave changes in 53%, low QRS voltage in 15%, aberrant conduction in 14%, and prolonged P-R interval in 10% (Metzler et al. 1972). In a 20-year-old man, the myocardial involvement was consistent electrocardiographically with an anterior myocardial infarct (Kirschberg, 1972). Some individuals may have residual electrocardiographic changes even after 3 months. Death is due mainly to myocarditis and less often due to arrhythmia.

Central Nervous System. Involvement of the central nervous system usually begins during the third week of infection, as other symptoms begin to disappear. Signs of encephalitis with psychotic changes, delirium, disorientation, headache, hyperreflexia, and amnesia may be present. Sometimes there are signs of meningitis simulating a viral or bacterial illness. The cerebrospinal fluid is mostly normal, though sometimes under high pressure, and may contain eosinophils and, rarely, larvae. Focal neurologic involvement may be seen, as well as electroencephalographic alterations (Barr, 1966). In computed tomograms, multifocal hypodense lesions that enhanced with contrast were thought to be due to hypoxia and infarction caused by the parasite in one case (Ellrodt et al. 1987). In another case, brain infarcts attributed to the parasite resulted in the death of the patient (Gay et al. 1982). However, the brain lesions in these two cases were probably not produced by the parasite, in spite of the fact that the patients had trichinosis; the larvae of *Trichinella* are far too small to produce gross lesions in the brain. Laboratory tests are not helpful, making the clinical diagnosis very difficult (Ryczak et al. 1987).

Immunity. The immune response to *Trichinella* has been studied extensively, especially in relation to the expulsion phase of the worms from the intestine. However, most studies have involved animals, mainly rats, because of the ease with which the cycle is maintained in the laboratory. It is well known that after the infection is acquired, the adult worms are expelled from the intestine in a few days, coinciding with an intense inflammatory response in the intestine. Animals that become infected and are subsequently challenged have an accelerated inflammatory response, and the worms are expelled quickly. One can view this phenomenon as protective to both the host and the parasite. The host has an initial infection that produces a finite number of larvae that encapsulate because the worms are expelled from the intestine. The parasite has a limited time to produce its progeny; the number of progeny produced usually do not kill the host, and thus the cycle continues. In addition, the host becomes "immune" not to the reinfection, but to the maturation of worms, which on a second infection are expelled before they begin producing larvae.

The encapsulated larvae in the muscle mass have a slow attrition rate because they are eliminated, possibly due to the host's immune response. A granulomatous response around some larvae has been observed in humans, resulting in destruction of the larvae. A decrease in larval burdens has been seen in humans several decades after the initial infection.

The mechanism for worm expulsion from the intestine was known to be related to host immunity because of cell transfer experiments. It was also known to be cell mediated, and previously it was believed to be the result of mediated hypersensitivity, with the eosinophil being the main effector cell. More recent studies showed that effector T cells in the intestine were the main mediators of the immune response in rats. Today there is a better understanding of the expulsion mechanism of *Trichinella* from the gut, mediated by the CD4[+] T lymphocyte. During the primary infection, the CD4[+] T cell mediates a weak response characterized by a T helper 1 (Th1) cell cytokine profile (interferon gamma, tumor necrosis factor alpha) and mast cell differentiating activity. In addition, a strong Th2 T-cell cytokine response occurs, producing an increase in interleukin 10 (IL-10), IL-5, and IL-4. The cytokine IL-5 increases the eosinophil population in the mucosa, and IL-4, which is also produced by mast cells, increases the immunoglobulin E (IgE) observed in the infection. The Th2 cytokine response is responsible for the strong immunity in *T. spiralis* infections and in other intestinal and extraintestinal infections with helminths.

Pathology. The main pathologic abnormalities produced by *Trichinella* adults occur in the small intestine, and those caused by larvae appear in the skeletal muscles, brain, and heart. A case of chronic endometritis attributed to encapsulated larvae of *Trichinella* is a mistaken identification of artifacts (Hernandez et al. 1995, Figs. 1 and 2).

Small Intestine. The lesion in the duodenal and jejunal mucosa depends on the number of worms. Grossly, the intestine appears normal or slightly edematous, without visible parasites. Microscopically, animals infected with large numbers of larvae have an interstitial inflammatory reaction, mostly with lymphocytes, polymorphonuclear cells, eosinophils, and petechial hemorrhages. Adult worms are found within the mucosal epithelium in tunnels similar to those produced by *Trichuris* (see above). In sections of biopsy specimens from infected individuals, the only changes observed were focal infiltration with mononuclear cells and eosinophils; special stains showed a slight increase in mast cells.

Skeletal Muscles. In the skeletal muscles, lesions appear soon after arrival and penetration of larvae in the muscle fibers. At first, the fiber shows basophilic degeneration, edema, and a slight increase in size, and the nuclei become enlarged (Fig. 22–16 A–D). As the larva matures, the muscle cell begins to shrink, and there are alterations in the position of the muscle cell nuclei and replacement of the cell cytoplasm by an eosinophilic network of fibers (Fig. 22–16 B). By the fifth week, the parasite is fully developed and encapsulated. Formation of a wall around the larva is complete in about 3 months (Fig. 22–17 C–D), and the remaining muscle cell forms a scar. The capsule containing the coiled parasite is homogeneous, translucent, and hyaline, with no structural details; it appears to have a double contour, with its poles slightly extended (Fig. 22–17 C). During encapsulation, there is an inflammatory reaction (myositis) characterized by involvement of single muscle fibers, with degeneration and infiltration by polymorphonuclear cells, mainly eosinophils, lymphocytes, and a few histiocytes (Fig. 22–17 A–B). The myositis subsides as the larvae encapsulate and all infiltrating cells resolve (Fig. 22–17 D). The long-term fate of the larvae is death and eventual calcification (Fig. 22–18 A–B; Beck, Beverley-Burton, 1968).

Heart. Grossly, the heart may be normal. Sometimes it has endocardial petechial hemorrhages. In other cases, there may be mural thrombi that occasionally are massive (Andy et al. 1977). In cases of full-blown myocarditis the heart is enlarged, flabby, and pale, with approximately 100 ml of fluid in the pericardial cavity (Gould, 1970). In some patients large pericardial effusions occur, but these are unusual. Microscopically, the heart shows myocarditis with focal areas of necrosis and infiltration by numerous eosinophils, lymphocytes, macrophages, and histiocytes (Fig. 22–19 A–D). Larvae of *Trichinella* are rarely found in the heart, and they never encapsulate. The mechanism for the production of myocardial damage by *Trichinella* infections is not known. The endocardial lesions with mural thrombi, frequently seen, probably relate to the hypereosinophilia because similar lesions are common in other conditions with high peripheral eosinophilia. In 94% of all deaths in *Trichinella* infections, myocarditis is the cause (Andy et al. 1977).

Central Nervous System. At autopsy, patients with *Trichinella* infection involving the central nervous system show a grossly hyperemic brain, sometimes with a slight meningeal exudate and, rarely, with edema and herniation. Microscopically, there are small areas of necrosis with a cellular infiltrate. Glial nodules composed of glial cells, lymphocytes, neutrophils, and many eosinophils are common, and the meninges sometimes have an abundant eosinophilic infiltrate. The larvae are difficult to demonstrate, but if present, they are found

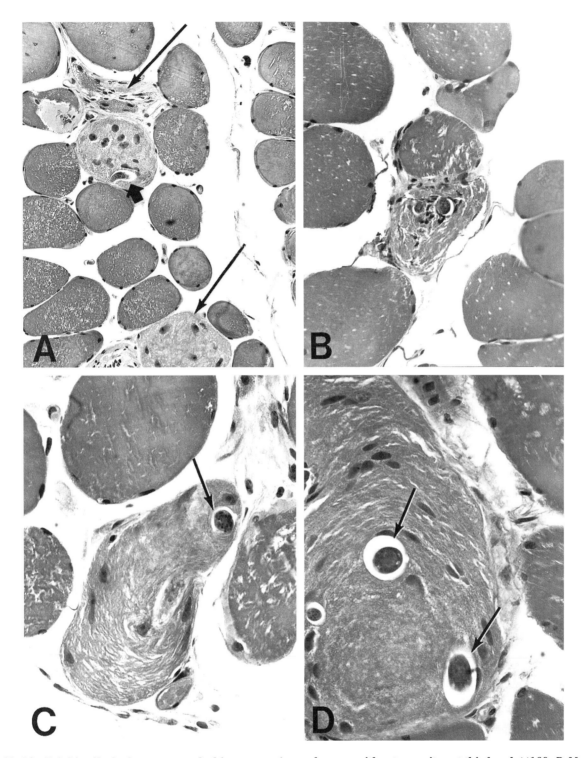

Fig. 22–16. *Trichinella* in human muscle biopsy specimen 3 weeks after infection, sections stained with hematoxylin and eosin stain. *A*, Low-power view showing a muscle cell with a young larva (short arrow). Note the light-staining properties of the cell cytoplasm and the displacement of the muscle fiber nuclei toward the center. Neighboring cells (long arrows) show similar changes without parasites at this level, ×160. *B*, Medium magnification showing slightly more advanced changes and two sections of the larva, ×250. *C* and *D*, Higher magnification illustrating the fibrillar degeneration of the cell cytoplasm and the parasites (arrows). Note the lack of inflammatory reaction in all of these sections because invasion of muscle fibers is too recent, ×400.

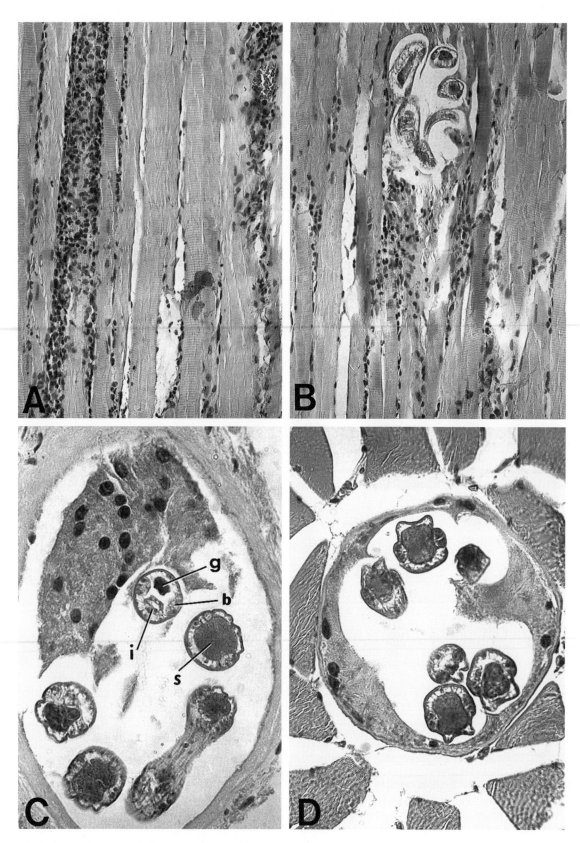

Fig. 22–17. *Trichinella* in human muscle, hematoxylin and eosin stain. *A* and *B*. Five weeks after infection. *A*, Longitudinal section of deltoid muscle showing marked myositis involving single muscle fibers. Note the marked cytoplasmic degeneration and the abundant infiltrate, ×180. *B*, Another section showing the larva beginning encapsulation, ×180. *C* and *D*. Older infection. *C*, Lon- gitudinal section of a pseudocyst containing an infective larva within a multinucleated matrix. Stichocyte (s), intestine (i), gonad (g), bacillary band (b), ×450, *D*, Cross section of a pseudocyst with similar morphologic characteristics. Note the lack of inflammatory reaction in this phase of the infection, ×450.

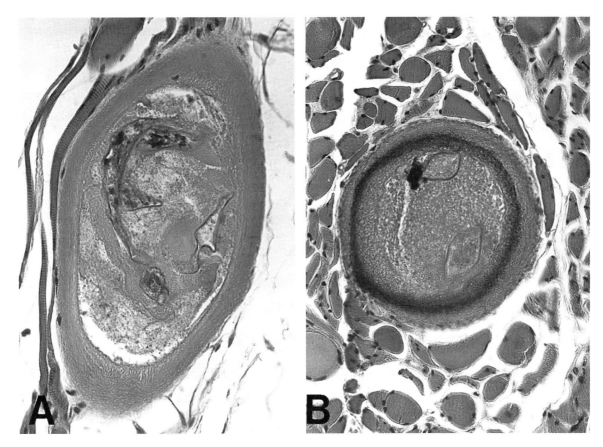

Fig. 22–18. *Trichinella* in human muscle, hematoxylin and eosin stain. Longitudinal (*A*) and transverse (*B*) sections of a *Trichinella* pseudocyst undergoing calcification, ×280.

within the areas of inflammation. Often the diagnosis can be made only by examination of skeletal muscles.

Diagnosis. The clinical diagnosis of trichinosis rests on the clinical history of the patient and the presenting symptoms and signs. Cases that occur in clusters must be distinguished from outbreaks of food poisoning. The most widely recommended laboratory test is the muscle biopsy; however, in one study biopsy specimens taken 6 weeks after the initial symptoms appeared were positive in only 56% (Au et al. 1983). In addition, sections of muscle biopsy specimens taken during the migratory phase of the parasite are sometimes difficult to interpret because the larvae are not encapsulated. The same is true for infections with *T. pseudospiralis*, a parasite that does not form cysts in the muscles. The enzyme-linked immunosorbent assay, and other serologic tests such as radioimmunoassay and indirect hemagglutination tests, are available. The enzyme-linked immunosorbent assay appears to have excellent specificity and sensitivity (Au et al. 1983).

Muscle biopsy specimens received fresh should be cut and a portion used for a pressed preparation: 0.5 cc of muscle or less is pressed firmly between two glass

slides and examined under the microscope with low power. Encapsulated larvae are detected easily (Fig. 22–20), but nonencapsulated ones are difficult to see. In tissue sections of muscle, the microscopic changes of myositis with abundant eosinophils suggest infection with *Trichinella* and other nematodes (see the discussion of myositis caused by *Ancylostoma* larvae in Chapter 14). The worms are identified on the basis of their morphologic characteristics or determinations of specific DNA (Rodriguez et al. 1995).

Larvae of *Trichinella* recently located in a muscle fiber are nonencapsulated, loosely coiled, and measure 13 to 15 μm in diameter (Fig. 22–16 *B–D*). Encapsulated, tightly coiled parasites are up to 35 μm in diameter and are contained within a multinucleated matrix (Fig. 22–17 *C–D*). The entire pseudocyst measures 350 × 200 μm, and the capsule is 15 μm thick. The cuticle and the muscle layer of the larva are 4 μm thick (Fig. 22–17 *C–D*); the lateral bacillary bands are slightly taller than the muscle layer and have two or three discrete cells (Fig. 22–17 *C*). Cross sections through the esophagus show the stichocytes, cells consisting of a large mass of cytoplasm, that stain darkly with hematoxylin and eosin stain; the lumen of the capillary-like esophagus is often inconspicuous. The sex

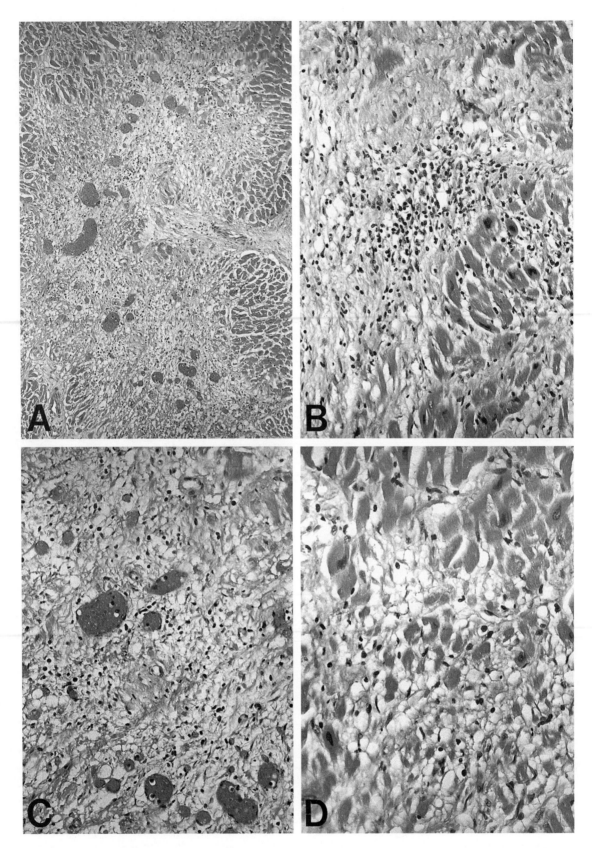

Fig. 22–19. *Trichinella*. Human heart 6 weeks after infection, sections stained with hematoxylin and eosin stain. *A*, Low-power view of myocardium showing extensive microscopic necrosis, ×70. *B* and *C*, Higher magnification illustrating focal myocarditis, organization of necrotic areas, and infiltration mostly by mononuclear cells and eosinophils, ×180. *D*, Higher magnification of another area showing scant infiltration, ×280. (Preparation courtesy of P.C. Beaver, Ph.D., Department of Tropical Medicine, School of Tropical Medicine and Public Health, Tulane University, New Orleans, Louisiana.)

organs are composed of small aggregates of cells (Fig. 22–17 C), and the intestine is an open tube composed of six to eight cells (Fig. 22–17 C).

Dioctophyme renale

Dioctophyme renale is a large nematode of worldwide distribution in mammals that usually inhabit one of the two kidneys. The female can grow up to 100 cm long by 1.2 cm wide and the male up to 20 cm long by 0.6 cm wide. The eggs evacuated with the urine develop to the infective stage in about 4 weeks. Embryonated eggs are ingested by oligochaetes (related to earthworms but aquatic), where they develop into infective larvae. Infection in animals occurs by ingestion of oligochaetes with infective larvae. Fish and other aquatic animals may also ingest infected oligochaetes and act as transport hosts, passing on the infection to the suitable host by carnivorism.

Over a dozen authentic reports of *D. renale* infections in humans exist in the literature. In most cases the parasite has been found at autopsy or has passed through the urethra (Lisboa, 1945). In one case, the worm was recovered from an abscess communicating with the kidney; in other cases, it was diagnosed by recovery of typical eggs in the urine (Hanjani et al. 1968). At least two reports of *D. renale* infection in humans (Fernando, 1983; Sun et al. 1986) were the result of misdiagnoses. The nature of the alleged worm and its eggs in the kidney, were mineral deposits known as *Liesegang rings* (Seige et al. 1988; Tuur et al. 1987). Another common mistaken identification of adult *Dioctophyme* is an *Ascaris* worm in the kidney. The most recent records of *Dioctophyme* in humans are of a larva in the subcutaneous tissues (Fig. 22–21 A–D; Beaver, Khamboonruang, 1984; Beaver, Theis, 1979; Gutierrez et al. 1989).

Eustrongylides

The adult stages of *Eustrongylides* occur in the mucosa of the esophagus, proventriculus, or intestine of birds, and the larval stages occur in the connective tissues and body cavity of freshwater fish, amphibians, and reptiles. Human infections described in the United States occur in persons with a history of eating raw fish. In one instance, three fishermen presented with abdomi-

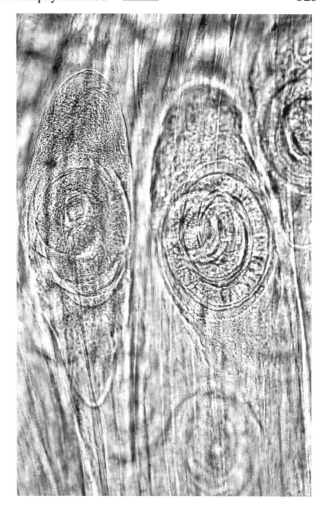

Fig. 22–20. *Trichinella* **in muscle of rat 12 weeks after infection, pressed preparation, unstained. Note the shape of the pseudocyst with tapering ends, ×198.**

nal pain after eating live bait minnows, two of whom required surgery. One patient had a perforated cecum; nearby, two worms measuring 1 to 2 mm in diameter by 8 to 12 cm in length were found (Guerin et al. 1982; Gunby, 1996). Another patient had symptoms of appendicitis; in one case, as a grossly normal appendix was removed, a 4.2 cm long worm was found in the peritoneal cavity (Wittner et al. 1989). In another case, two worms measuring 5.5 and 5.9 cm were recovered from the abdominal cavity of a 17-year-old boy who had developed an acute abdomen due to intestinal perforation after swallowing live minnows (Eberhard et al. 1989). Still another case is that of a patient who expectorated the larva, but a report was not published; the worm is now deposited in the National Helminthological Collection (Abram, Lichtenfels, 1974). In all of

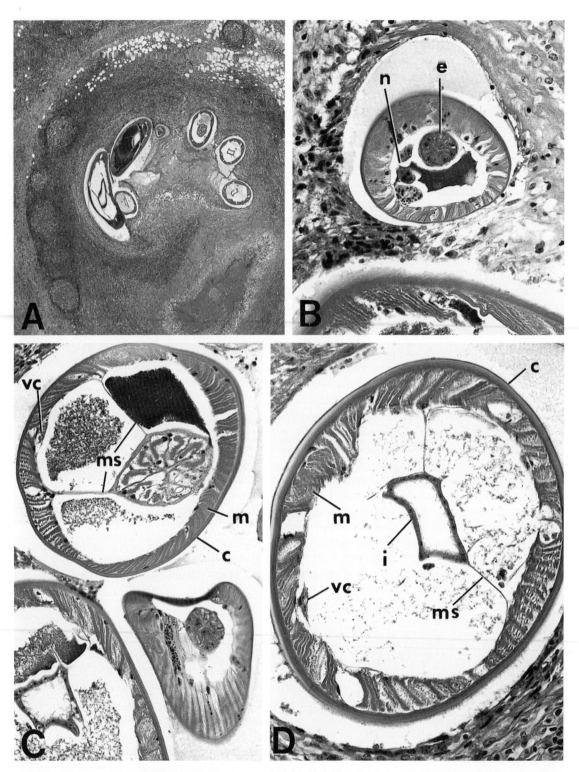

Fig. 22–21. *Dioctophyme* larva in subcutaneous tissues of a woman in Ohio, hematoxylin and eosin stain. *A*, Low-power view of a granuloma showing several cross sections of the larva, ×22. *B*, Higher magnification of a section through the esophagus (e) and nerve ring (n), ×280. *C*, Section through the anterior muscular esophagus (bottom) and posterior glandular eosphagus (top). Note the cuticle (c), the muscle layer (m), the ventral cord composed of numerous small nuclei (vc), the mesenteries (ms), and the darkly stained granular material in the coelom, ×180. *D*, Section through the middle portion of the worm showing structures similar to those in *C* and the intestine composed of many small cuboidal cells, ×280. (In Gutierrez, Y., Cohen, M., and Machicao, C.N. 1989. *Dictophyme*-like larva in the subcutaneous tissues of a woman in Ohio. Am. J. Surg. Pathol. 13:800–802. Reproduced with permission.)

these cases, the recovered worms were strongly red tinted and were identified as larvae of a species of *Eustrongylides*. The microanatomy of *Eustrongylides* and *Dioctophyme* larvae is rather similar, except for the size: 10 cm in *Eustrongylides* and 10 mm in *Dioctophyme* (Panesar, Beaver, 1979).

References

Abram JB, Lichtenfels JR, 1974. Larval *Eustrongylides* sp. (Nematoda: Dioctophymatoidea) from otter, *Lutra canadensis*, in Maryland. Proc. Helminthol. Soc. Wash. 41:253 253

Aftandelians R, Raafat F, Taffazoli M, Beaver PC, 1977. Pulmonary capillariasis in a child in Iran. Am. J. Trop. Med. Hyg. 26:64–71

Ancelle T, Dupouy-Camet J, Heyer F, Faurant C, Lapierre J, 1985. Outbreak of trichinosis due to horse meat in the Paris area. Lancet 2:660

Andrews JRH, Ainsworth R, Abernethy D, 1993. Correspondence. *Trichinella pseudospiralis* in man. Lancet 342:298–299

Andrews JRH, Ainsworth R, Abernethy D, 1994. *Trichinella pseudospiralis* in humans: description of a case and its treatment. Trans. R. Soc. Trop. Med. Hyg. 88:200–203

Andrews JRH, Bandi C, Pozio E, Gomez Morales MA, Ainsworth R, Abernethy D, 1995. Identification of *Trichenella pseudospiralis* from a human case using random amplified polymorphic DNA. Am. J. Trop. Med. Hyg. 53:185–188

Andy JJ, O'Connell JP, Daddarlo RC, Roberts WC, 1977. Trichinosis causing extensive ventricular mural endocarditis with superimposed thrombosis. Evidence that severe eosinophilia damages endocardium. Am. J. Med. 63:824–829

Attah EB, Nagarajan S, Obineche EN, Gera SC, 1983. Hepatic capillariasis. Am. J. Clin. Pathol. 79:127–130

Au AC, Ko RC, Simon JW, 1983. Study of acute trichinosis in Ghurkas: specificity and sensitivity of enzyme-linked immunosorbent assays for IgM and IgE antibodies to *Trichinella* larval antigens in diagnosis. Trans. R. Soc. Trop. Med. Hyg. 77:412–415

Bailey TM, Schantz PM, CDC, 1987. Trichinosis surveillance, 1985. Morb. Mort. Weekly Rep. 36:1–5

Bangs MJ, Purnomo, Andersen EM, 1994. A case of capillariasis in a highland community of Irian Jaya, Indonesia. Ann. Trop. Med. Parasitol. 88:685–687

Barr R, 1966. Human trichinosis: report of four cases, with emphasis on central nervous system involvement and a survey of 500 consecutive autopsies at the Ottawa Civic Hospital. Can. Med. Assoc. J. 95:912–917

Beaver PC, Jung RC, Cupp EW, 1984. *Clinical Parasitology*. Philadelphia: Lea & Febiger

Beaver PC, Khamboonruang C, 1984. *Dioctophyma*-like larval nematode in a subcutaneous nodule from man in

northern Thailand. Am. J. Trop. Med. Hyg. 33:1032–1034

Beaver PC, Theis JH, 1979. Dioctophymatid larval nematode in a subcutaneous nodule from man in California. Am. J. Trop. Med. Hyg. 28:206–212

Beck JW, Beverley-Burton M, 1968. The pathology of *Trichuris*, *Capillaria* and *Trichinella* infections. Helminthol. Abst. 37:1–26

Beer RJ, 1973. Studies on the biology of the life-cycle of *Trichuris suis* Schrank, 1788. Semin. Respir. Infect. 67:253–262

Beer RJ, 1976. The relationship between *Trichuris trichiura* (Linnaeus 1758) of man and *Trichuris suis* (Schrank 1788) of the pig. Res. Vet. Sci. 20:47–54

Bergner JF Jr, McCroddan DM, Khaw OK, Devlin J, McCroddan DM, 1973. A team approach to a disease survey on an aboriginal island (Orchid Island, Taiwan). I. Protozoa and helminth parasites of the Yami aborigines. Chinese J. Microbiol. 6:164–172

Bhaibulaya M, Benjapong W, Noeypatimanond S, 1977. Infection of *Capillaria philippinensis* in man from Phetchabun Province, northern Thailand: a report of the fifth case. J. Med. Assoc. Thail. 60:507–509

Bhaibulaya M, Indra-Ngarm S, Ananthapruti M, 1979. Freshwater fishes of Thailand as experimental intermediate hosts for *Capillaria philippinensis*. Int. J. Parasitol. 9:105–108

Bowie MD, Morison A, Ireland JD, Duys PJ, 1978. Clubbing and whipworm infestation. Arch. Dis. Child. 53:411–413

Brashear RE, Martin RR, Glover JL, 1971. Trichinosis and respiratory failure. Am. Rev. Respir. Dis. 104:245–248

Bundy DA, 1986. Epidemiological aspects of *Trichuris* and trichuriasis in Caribbean communities. Trans. R. Soc. Trop. Med. Hyg. 80:706–718

Cabrera BD, Canlas B Jr, Dauz U, 1967. Human intestinal capillariasis. III. Parasitological features and management. Acta Med. Philipp. 4:92–103

Calle S, 1961. Parasitism by *Capillaria hepatica*. Helvet. Paediatr. Acta 648–655

Canlas BD Jr, Cabrera BD, Dauz U, 1967. Human intestinal capillariasis. II. Pathological features. Acta Med. Philipp. 4:84–91

CDC, 1996. Outbreak of trichinellosis associated with eating cougar jerky—Idaho, 1995. Morb. Mort. Weekly Rep. 45:205–206

Chen CY, Hsieh WC, Lin JT, Liu MC, 1989. Intestinal capillariasis: report of a case. Taiwan I Hsueh Hui Tsa Chih. J. Formosan Med. Assoc. 88:617–620

Chieffi PP, Mangini ACS, Grispino DMA, Dias Pacheco MA, 1981. *Capillaria hepatica* (Bancroft, 1893) em murideas capturados no municipio de Sao Paulo, Brasil. Rev. Inst. Med. Trop. Sao Paulo 23:143–146

Chitwood MB, Velasquez C, Salazar NP, 1964. Physiological changes in a species of *Capillaria* (Trichuroidea) causing a fatal case of human intestinal capillariasis. In: Carradetti A (ed), *Proceedings of the First International Congress of Parasitology* Vol. 2 (1st ed, 1966). Oxford: Pergamon Press, pp. 797–798

Chitwood MB, Velasquez C, Salazar NG, 1968. *Capillaria philippinensis* sp. n. (Nematoda: Trichinellida), from the intestine of man in the Philippines. J. Parasitol. 54: 368–371

Clark PS, Brownsberger KM, Saslow AR, Kagan IG, Noble GR, Maynard JE, 1972. Bear meat trichinosis. Epidemiologic, serologic, and clinical observations from two Alaskan outbreaks. Ann. Intern. Med. 76:951–956

Cooper ES, Bundy DAP, Henry FJ, 1986. Chronic dysentery, stunting, and whipworm infestation. Lancet 2:280–281

Correa LL, Yamanaka MT, Correa M, Silfa M, Silva R, 1980. Ocorrencia de ovos grandes de *Trichuris trichiura* em fezes humanas. Rev. Inst. Adolfo Lutz Sao Paulo 40: 59–64

Cross JH, 1990. Intestinal capillariasis. Parasitol. Today 6:26–28

Cross JH, Banzon T, Clarke MD, Basaca-Servilla V, Watten RH, Dizon JJ, 1972. Studies on the experimental transmission of *Capillaria philippinensis* in monkeys. Trans. R. Soc. Trop. Med. Hyg. 66:819–827

Cross JH, Basaca-Sevilla V, 1991. Capillariasis *philippinensis*: a fish-borne parasitic zoonosis. Southeast Asian J. Trop. Med. Public Health 22(Suppl):153–157

Dauz U, Cabrera BD, Canlas B Jr, 1967. Human intestinal capillariasis. I. Clinical features. Acta Med. Philipp. 4:72–83

Davis M, Matteson A, Williams WC, 1986. Correspondence. Radiographic and endoscopic findings in human whipworm infection (*Trichuris trichiura*). J. Clin. Gastroenterol. 8:700–701

Despommier DD, 1990. *Trichinella spiralis*: the worm that would be virus. Parasitol. Today 6:193–196

Drake L, Korchev Y, Bashford L, Djamgoz M, Wakelin D, Ashall F, Bundy D, 1994. The major secreted product of the whipworm, *Trichuris*, is a pore-forming protein. Proc. R. Soc. Lond. B. Biol. Sci. 257:255–261

Dronda F, Chaves F, Sanz A, Lopez-Velez R, 1993. Human intestinal capillariasis in an area of nonendemicity: case report and review. Clin. Infect. Dis. 17:909–912

Dupouy CJ, Soule C, Ancelle T, 1994. Recent news on trichinellosis: another outbreak due to horsemeat consumption in France in 1993. Parasite 1:99–103

Dworkin MS, Gamble HR, Zarlenga DS, Tennican PO, 1996. Outbreak of trichinellosis associated with eating cougar jerky. J. Infect. Dis. 174:663–666

Eberhard ML, Hurwitz H, Sun AM, Coletta D, 1989. Intestinal perforation caused by larval *Eustrongylides* (Nematoda: Dioctophymatoid) in New Jersey. Am. J. Trop. Med. Hyg. 40:648–650

Ellrodt A, Halfon P, Le Bras P, Halimi P, Bouree P, Desi M, Caquet R, 1987. Multifocal central nervous system lesions in three patients with trichinosis. Arch. Neurol. 44:432–434

Feigen GM, 1987. Suppurative anal cryptitis associated with *Trichuris trichiura*. Dis. Colon Rectum 30:620–622

Fernando SSE, 1983. The giant kidney worm (*Dioctophyma renale*) infection in man in Australia. Am. J. Surg. Pathol. 7:281–284

Fishman JA, Perrone TL, 1984. Colonic obstruction and perforation due to *Trichuris trichiura*. Am. J. Med. 77: 154–156

Fresh JW, Cross JH, Reyes V, Whalen GE, Uylangco CV, Dizon JJ, 1972. Necropsy findings in intestinal capillariasis. Am. J. Trop. Med. Hyg. 21:169–173

Gardiner CH, 1976. Habitat and reproductive behavior of *Trichinella spiralis*. J. Parasitol. 62:865–870

Gay T, Pankey GA, Beckman EN, Washington P, Bell KA, 1982. Fatal CNS trichinosis. JAMA 247:1024–1025

Gilman RH, Chong YH, Davis C, Greenberg B, Virik HK, Dixon HB, 1983. The adverse consequences of heavy *Trichuris* infection. Trans. R. Soc. Trop. Med. Hyg. 77: 432–438

Gilman RH, Davis C, Fitzgerald F, 1976. Heavy *Trichuris* infection and amoebic dysentery in Orang Asli children. A comparison of the two diseases. Trans. R. Soc. Trop. Med. Hyg. 70:313–316

Gould SE, 1970. *Trichinosis in Man and Animals*. Springfield, Ill.: Charles C. Thomas

Graves T, Harkess J, Crutcher JM, 1996. Case report: locally acquired trichinosis in an immigrant from Southeast Asia. J Okla. State Med. Assoc. 89:402–404

Greenberg ER, Cline BL, 1979. Is trichuriasis associated with iron deficiency anemia? Am. J. Trop. Med. Hyg. 28:770–772

Guerin PF, Marapudi S, McGrail L, Moravec CL, Schiller E, Hopf EW, Thompson R, Lin FYC, Israel E, Bier JW, Jackson GJ, 1982. Intestinal perforation caused by larval *Eustrongylides*—Maryland. Morb. Mort. Weekly Rep. 31:383–384, 389

Gunby P, 1996. One worm in the minnow equals too many in the gut, JAMA 248:163

Gutierrez Y, Cohen M, Machicao CN, 1989. *Dioctophyme* larva in the subcutaneous tissues of a woman in Ohio. Am. J. Surg. Pathol. 13:800–802

Hanada K, Hashimoto I, Yamaguchi T, Ezaki Y, 1987. Cutaneous changes in trichinellosis seen in Japan. J. Dermatol. 14:586–589

Hanjani AA, Sadighian A, Nikakhtar B, Arfaa F, 1968. The first report of human infection with *Dioctophyma renale* in Iran. Trans. R. Soc. Trop. Med. Hyg. 62:647–648

Harms G, Binz P, Feldmeier H, Zwingenberger K, Schleehauf D, Dewes W, Kress-Hermesdorf I, Klindworth C, Bienzle U, 1993. Trichinosis: a prospective controlled study of patients ten years after acute infection. Clin. Infect. Dis. 17:637–643

Hartz PH, 1953. Histopathology of the colon in massive trichocephaliasis of children. Doc. Med. Geogr. Trop. 5:303–313

Hernandez M, Ramos ME, Diaz GD, 1995. Endometritis cronica por *Trichinella spiralis*. Presentacion de un caso. Ginecol. Obstet. Mex. 63:109–111

Hoghooghi-Rad N, Maraghi S, Narenj-Zadeh A, 1987. *Capillaria philippinensis* infection in Khoozestan Province, Iran: case report. Am. J. Trop. Med. Hyg. 37:135–137

Hong ST, Kim YT, Choe G, Min YI, Cho SH, Kim JK, Kook J, Chai JY, Lee SH, 1994. Two cases of intestinal capillariasis in Korea. Korean J. Parasitol. 32:43–48

Horii Y, Usui M, 1985. Experimental transmission of *Trichuris* ova from monkeys to man. Trans. R. Soc. Trop. Med. Hyg. 79:423

Jung RC, Beaver PC, 1951. Clinical observations on *Trichocephalus trichiurus* (whipworm) infestation in children. Pediatrics 8:548–557

Jung RC, Jelliffe DB, 1952. The clinical picture and treatment of whipworm infection. West. African Med. J. 1:3–7

Kagei N, Hayashi S, Kato K, 1986. Human cases of infection with canine whipworms, *Trichuris vulpis* (Froelich, 1789), in Japan. Jpn. J. Med. Sci. Biol. 39:177–184

Kamath KR, 1973. Severe infection with *Trichuris trichiura* in Malaysian children. A clinical study of 30 cases treated with stilbazium iodide. Am. J. Trop. Med. Hyg. 22:600–605

Kang G, Mathan M, Ramakrishna BS, Mathai E, Sarada V, 1994. Human intestinal capillariasis: first report from India. Trans. R. Soc. Trop. Med. Hyg. 88:204

Kenney M, Yermakov V, 1980. Infection of man with *Trichuris vulpis*, the whipworm of dogs. Am. J. Trop. Med. Hyg. 29:1205–1208

Kirschberg GJ, 1972. Trichinosis presenting as acute myocardial infarction. Can. Med. Assoc. J. 106:898–899

Laurichesse H, Cambon M, Perre D, Ancelle T, Mora M, Hubert B, Beytout J, Rey M, 1997. Outbreak of trichinosis in France associated with eating horse meat. Commun. Dis. Rep. CDR Rev. 7:R69–R73

Le-Van-Hoa, Duong-Hong-Mo, Nguyen-Luu-Vien, 1963. Premier cas de capillariose cutanée humaine. Bull. Soc. Pathol. Exot. 56:121–126

Lisboa A, 1945. Estrongilose renal humana. Brasil Med. 59:101–102

Little MD, 1968. A strain of *Trichuris trichiura* having large eggs. Program of the 43rd annual meeting of the American Society of Parasitologists, June 16–21, 1968, Madison, Wisconsin.

Lotero H, Tripathy K, Bolanos O, 1974. Gastrointestinal blood loss in *Trichuris* infection. Am. J. Trop. Med. Hyg. 23:1203–1204

Margolis HS, Middaugh JP, Burgess RD, 1979. Arctic trichinosis: two Alaskan outbreaks from walrus meat. J. Infect. Dis. 139:102–105

McAuley JB, Michelson MK, Hightower AW, Engeran S, Wintermeyer LA, Schantz PM, 1992. A trichinosis outbreak among Southeast Asian refugees. Am. J. Epidemiol. 135:1404–1410

McQuown AL, 1950. *Capillaria hepatica*: a report of genuine and spurious cases. Am. J. Trop. Med. 30:761–767

Metzler MH, Sahgal KK, Wolff GS, 1972. Second degree atrioventricular block in acute trichinosis. Am. J. Dis. Child. 124:598–601

Moravec F, Prokopic J, Shlikas AV, 1987. The biology of nematodes of the family capillariidae Neveu-Lemaire, 1936. Folia Parasitol. 34:39–56

Morishita K, Tani T, 1960. A case of *Capillaria* infection causing cutaneous creeping eruption. J. Parasitol. 46:79–83

Most H, 1965. Trichinellosis in the United States. JAMA 193:871–873

Mugarza Hernandez MD, Gimbel Moral LF, Rodriguez Garcia MD, Asensio Martin MJ, 1995. Correspondencia. Diarrea por *Capillaria philippinensis*. Med. Clin. 105:677

Nawa Y, Imai JI, Abe T, Kisanuki H, Tsuda K, 1988. A case report of intestinal capillariasis—the second case found in Japan. Jpn. J. Parasitol. 37:113–118

Orihel TC, 1970. Anatrichosomiasis in African monkeys. J. Parasitol. 56:982–985

Panesar TS, Beaver PC, 1979. Morphology of the advanced-stage larva of *Eustrongylides wenrichi* Canavan 1929, occurring encapsulated in the tissues of *Amphiuma* in Louisiana. J. Parasitol. 65:96–104

Pawlowski ZS, Ruitenberg EJ, 1978. Is *Trichinella pseudospiralis* likely to be a human pathogen? Lancet 1:1357

Pozio E, 1998. Trichinellosis in the European Union: epidemiology, ecology and economic impact. Parasitol. Today 14:35–38

Pozio E, La Rosa G, Murrell KD, Lichtenfeis JR, 1992. Taxonomic revision of the genus *Trichinella*. J. Parasitol. 78:654–659

Pozio E, Varese P, Morales MAG, Croppo GP, Pelliccia D, Bruschi F, 1993. Comparison of human trichinellosis caused by *Trichinella spiralis* and by *Trichinella britovi*. Am. J. Trop. Med. Hyg. 48:568–575

Pradatsundarasar A, Pecharanond K, Chintanawongs C, Ungthavorn P, 1973. The first case of intestinal capillariasis in Thailand. Southeast Asian J. Trop. Med. Public Health 4:131–134

Rodriguez E, Nieto J, Rodriguez M, Garate T, 1995. Use of random amplified polymorphic DNA for detection of *Trichinella britovi* outbreaks in Spain. Clin. Infect. Dis. 21:1521–1522

Ryczak M, Sorber WA, Kandora TF, Camp CJ, Rose FB, 1987. Difficulties in diagnosing *Trichinella* encephalitis. Am. J. Trop. Med. Hyg. 36:573–575

Sakano T, Hamamoto K, Kobayashi Y, Sakata Y, Tsuji M, Usui T, 1980. Visceral larva migrans caused by *Trichuris vulpis*. Arch. Dis. Child. 55:631–633

Singh S, Samantaray JC, Singh N, Das GB, Verma IC, 1993. *Trichuris vulpis* infection in an Indian tribal population. J. Parasitol. 79:457–458

Skrjabin KI, Shikhobalova NP, Orlov IV, 1957. *Essentials of Nematology. VI. Trichocephalidae and Capillariidae of Animals and Man and the Diseases caused by Them.* Moscow: Academy of Sciences of USSR

Slais J, 1973. The finding and identification of solitary *Capillaria hepatica* (Bancroft, 1893) in man from Europe. Folia Parasitol. 20:149–151

Slais J, 1974. Notes on the differentiation of *Capillaria hepatica* and visceral larva migrans. Folia Parasitol. 21:95

Sneige N, Dekmezian RH, Silva EG, Cartwright J Jr, Ayala AG, 1988. Pseudoparasitic Liesegang structures in perirenal hemorrhagic cysts. Am. J. Clin. Pathol. 89:148–153

Stromberg BE, Prouty SM, 1987. Prevalence of trichinellosis in the north United States. Proc. Helminthol. Soc. Wash. 54:231–232

Sumner D, Tinsley EGF, 1967. Encephalopathy due to visceral larva migrans. J. Neurol. Neurosurg. Psychiatry 30:580–584

Sun T, Turnbull A, Lieberman PH, Sternberg SS, 1986. Giant kidney worm (*Dioctophyma renale*) infection mimicking retroperitoneal neoplasm. Am. J. Surg. Pathol. 10:508–512

Swift HF, Boots RH, Miller CP, 1922. A cutaneous nematode infection in monkeys. J. Exp. Med. 35:599–620

Tiberio G, Lanzas G, Galarza MI, Sanchez J, Quilez I, Martinez AV, 1995. An outbreak of trichinosis in Navarra, Spain. Am. J. Trop. Med. Hyg. 53:241–242

Tiberio G, Rivero M, Lanzas G, Redin D, Ardanaz E, Fernandez C, Martinez AV, 1997. Triquinelosis: estudio de dos brotes en Navarra. Enferm. Infecc. Microbiol. Clin. 15:151–153

Tuur SM, Nelson AM, Gibson DW, Neafie RC, Johnson FB, Mostofi FK, Connor DH, 1987. Liesegang rings in tissue. How to distinguish Liesegang rings from the giant kidney worm, *Dioctophyma renale*. Am. J. Surg. Pathol. 11:598–605

Vanhaelen Lindhout E, Smit AM, 1971. Abnormally shaped eggs of *Trichuris trichiura* after thiabendazole treatment. Trop. Geogr. Med. 23:381–384

Wang CH, Bell RG, 1986. *Trichinella spiralis*: newborn larval migration route in rats reexamined. Exp. Parasitol. 61:76–85

Watten RH, Beckner WM, Cross JH, Gunning JJ, Jarimillo J, 1972. Clinical studies on capillariasis *philippinensis*. Trans. R. Soc. Trop. Med. Hyg. 66:828–834

Wittner M, Turner JW, Jacquette G, Ash RL, Salgo MP, Tanowitz HB, 1989. Eustrongyliasis—a parasitic infection acquired by eating sushi. N. Engl. J. Med. 320:1124–1126

WHO, 1980. Scientific working group. Parasite-related diarrhoeas. Bull. WHO 58:819–830

WHO, 1981. Intestinal protozoan and helminthic infections. Technical Report Series No 666 1–150 Geneva: WHO

Wright KA, 1961. Observations in the life cycle of *Capillaria hepatica* (Bancroft, 1893) with a description of the adult. Can. J. Zool. 38:167–182

Wright KA, 1979. *Trichinella spiralis*: an intracellular parasite in the intestinal phase. J. Parasitol. 65:441–445

Yoshida M, Kutsumi H, Ogawa M, Soga T, Nishimura K, Tomita S, Kawabata K, Kinoshita Y, Chiba T, Fujimoto S, 1996. A case of *Trichuris trichiura* infection diagnosed by colonoscopy. Am. J. Gastroenterol. 91:161–162

Youssef FG, Mikhail EM, Mansour NS, 1989. Intestinal capillariasis in Egypt: a case report. Am. J. Trop. Med. Hyg. 40:195–196

Part III

The Trematodes

The trematodes and the tapeworms, which belong to the phylum Platyhelminthes are commonly known as *flatworms*. Their characteristics include a body generally flattened dorsoventrally, organs usually bilateral and symmetric, and lack of a body cavity. The body of the parasite consists of the usual organs of helminths, surrounded by the tegument, with the space in between filled with lax or spongy mesenchymatous tissue. In general, all flatworms are hermaphrodites (with a few exceptions), and their life cycles are usually indirect, requiring one or more intermediate hosts. The platyhelminths are adapted to a parasitic existence and are found in all species of animals; they are subdivided into two groups: the Trematoda and the Cestoda.

Adult trematodes occur in all tissues and organs of their hosts, in contrast to the adult tapeworms, which are almost exclusively parasites of the gastrointestinal tract. Trematodes are composed of a single-unit body; tapeworms are composed of a chain of units or segments (see the introduction to Part IV). The trematodes of importance in human medicine are characterized by the presence of two *suckers* (see below) and therefore are placed in a group known as the Digenea, or *digenetic trematodes*, and commonly known as *flukes*. Flukes are multicellular animals with a leaf-like general appearance and complicated life cycles that involve a gastropod (snail) as a first intermediate host, in which several larval stages develop. Most trematodes require two or more hosts to complete their life cycle.

Adult

The adult stage of trematodes varies in size from less than 1 mm to several centimeters in length (Fig. 19–1 *A–B*). The conspicuous external structures are the suckers or *acetabula*, one located at the mouth opening, called the *oral sucker*, and the other located posteriorly along the median line and known as the *ventral sucker* or *acetabulum*. The acetabulum is a blind pouch located on the ventral surface of the worm, and both suckers serve to attach the worm to the organ they inhabit. The anterior end of the worm is referred to as the *cephalic* end (Fig. III–1 *A–B* and *color plate* XIII *F*).

Tegument

The surface of adult trematodes consists of a *tegument* composed of a *cytoplasmic syncytium* of cells that cover the entire worm. This cytoplasmic syncytium consists of extensions of the cytoplasm of the tegumental cells located in the mesenchyme just beneath the muscle cells (Fig. III–2). In some digenetic trematodes the tegument is covered with spines; the size, shape, and distribution of these spines are used for taxonomic purposes.

Musculature

The muscular system of trematodes consists of smooth muscle cells forming both suckers, the muscle cells of the tegument, and the muscles of other organs. The muscle fibers of the tegument are oriented in circular, oblique, and longitudinal bundles and, as stated above, are located between the surface syncytium of the tegumental cells and the cytoplasmic body of the cells (Fig. III–2).

Digestive System

All trematodes have a digestive system, often called the *cecum*, composed of an opening in the cephalic end, the *oral cavity*, surrounded by the oral sucker. Next

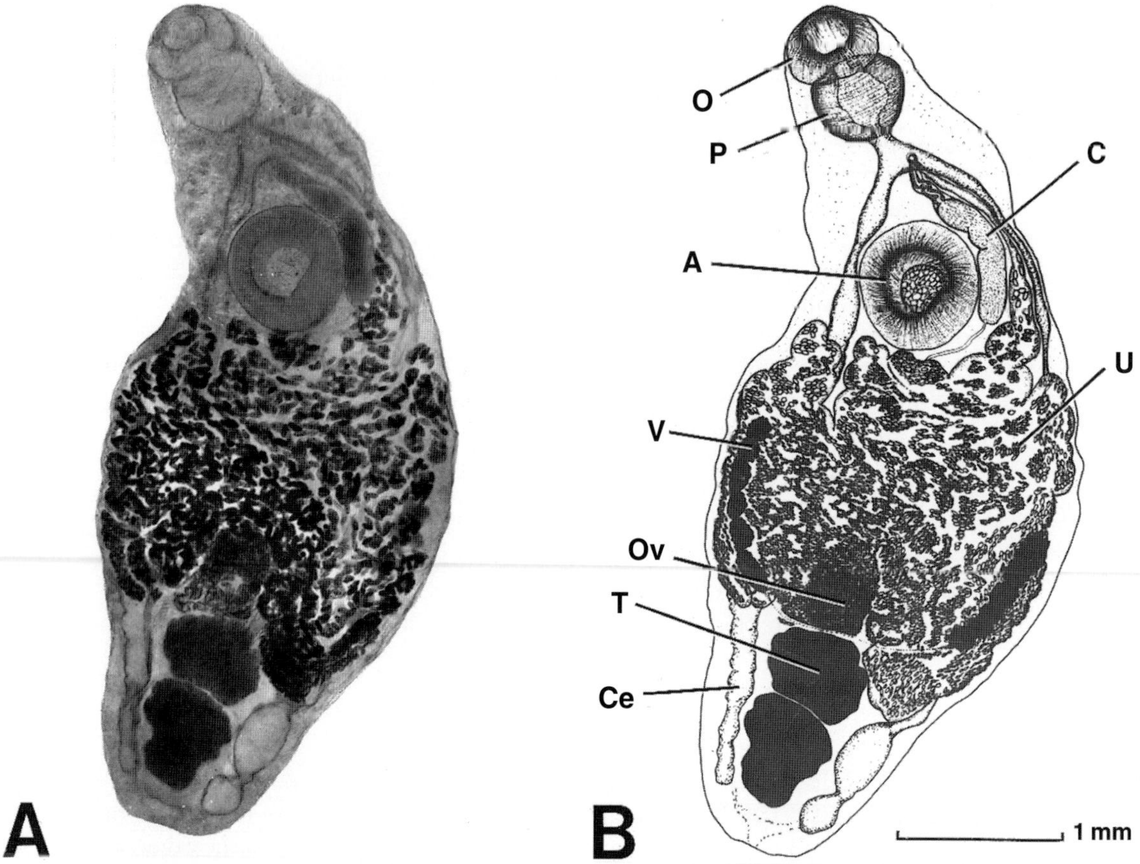

Fig. III–1. Trematode anatomy and general organization. *Philophthalmus* species removed from the eye of a person. *A*, Acetic alum-carmine stain showing the organs, ×22. *B*, Drawing of the same specimen illustrating the main structures needed for identification in these sections. Abbreviations: A, acetabulum; C, cirrus pouch; Ce, cecum; O, oral sucker; Ov, ovary; P, pharynx; T, testis; U, uterus; V, vitelaria. (In: Gutierrez, Y., Grossniklaus, H.E., and Annable, W.C. 1987. Human conjunctivitis caused by the bird parasite *Philophthalmus*. Am. J. Ophthalmol. 104:417–419. Reproduced with permission.)

to the oral cavity is the *prepharynx*, followed by the *pharynx* and the *esophagus*, which divides into two *ceca* (Fig. III–1). The point of bifurcation of the digestive system of trematodes that are parasitic in humans occurs at the level of the acetabulum. In some species the cecum is highly branched, for example in *Fasciola hepatica* and *F. gigantica*, but in all trematodes the cecum ends in blind pouches without opening to the outside (Figs. III–1 *A–B*). There is no anus in trematodes. The digestive system is a conspicuous organ; recognition of this organ is helpful in identifying these trematodes in tissue sections (Figs. III–3 *A–B*).

Genital System

The genital system and its microscopic anatomy are complicated. In general, it is not necessary to know all the structures and their relationships to diagnose the presence of trematodes in tissue sections. The most conspicuous structures of the genital system are (*1*) the *uterus*, usually recognized in sections as several pockets filled with eggs characteristic of the particular species, genus, or group (Fig. III–3 *B*); (*2*) the *vitelline glands* or *vitelaria*, composed of numerous aggregations of glandular acini located symmetrically in the lateral fields of the worm (Figs. III–3 *A* and III–10

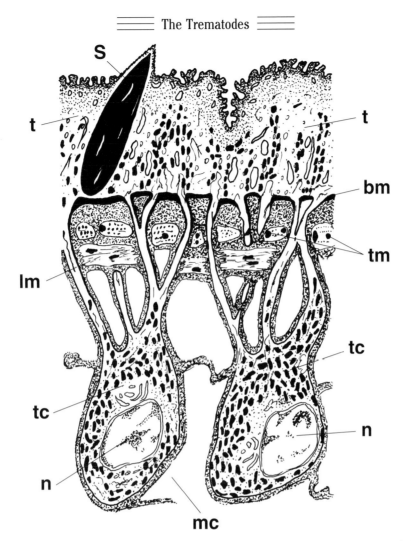

Fig. III–2. Trematode. Schematic of the ultrastructure of the tegument of *Fasciola hepatica*. Note the tegument (t) is an extension of the tegument cells below. The spine is covered with the cell membrane, making it intracytoplasmic. The cytoplasmic nature of the tegument of trematodes suggests that it is capable of absorption, and this has been confirmed in several groups. Abbreviations: bm, basement membrane; lm, longitudinal muscle; mc, cytoplasm of mesenchymal cell; n, nucleus of mesenchymal cell; s, spine; t, tegument; tc, tegumental cell; tm, transverse muscle. (Redrawn from: Threadgold, L.T. 1963. The tegument and associated structures of *Fasciola hepatica*. Q. J. Microscop. Sci. 104:505–512. Reproduced with permission.)

C); and (3) a single testis or, more commonly, a pair of testes, which may or may not be branched (Fig. 24–13 *B*). In general, all trematodes are hermaphrodites (both sexes occur in the same worm), except for the schistosomes, which have separate males and females (*color plate* XI *A* and Fig. 23–11 *B*). The sexual organs are located on the ventral aspect of the worm (Fig. 24–4 *B*), and the vitelline glands are located on the dorsal aspect (Figs. III–3 *A* and 24–4 *B*).

Nervous and Excretory Systems

The nervous and excretory systems of trematodes have little value for their classification in tissue sections. In some trematodes, the *excretory bladder* is conspicu-

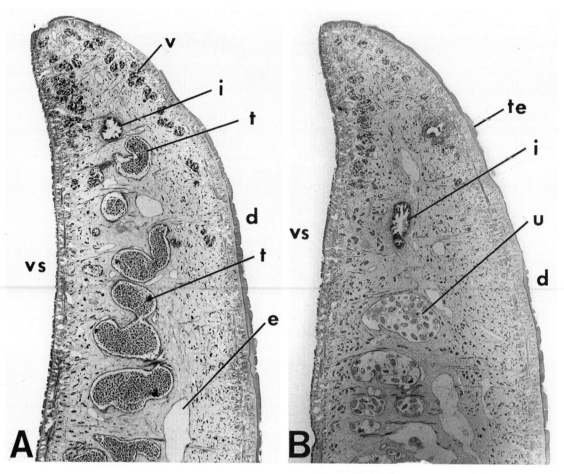

Fig. III–3. Trematode. Cross section of *Fasciolopsis buski* at two levels illustrating some structures, section stained with hematoxylin and eosin stain. *A*, Section at the level of the branched testes, ×22. *B*, More anterior section at the level of the uterus, ×22. Compare this with Figure 25–4, which depicts the entire worm. Shown here is only one-half of the entire cross section. Abbreviations: d, dorsal surface; e, excretory channel; i, intestine or ceca; t, testis; te, tegument; u, uterus with eggs; v, vitelaria; vs, ventral surface.

ous and is seen as a large, empty space in cross sections (Figs. 28–10 *D* and 24–13 *A*). Trematodes do not have calcareous corpuscles in their mesenchyme, an important feature that distinguishes them from cestodes (see Chapter 25).

Life Cycles

The life cycles of trematodes are complicated and require one or more intermediate hosts, the first of which is a *snail*. Thus, the term *snail-transmitted infections* is applied to the diseases produced by trematodes. The second intermediate host varies with the group in question, consisting of different species of aquatic animals and plants and terrestrial animals.

When either embryonated or nonembryonated eggs are evacuated in feces, urine, sputum, or other secretions of the definitive host, the eggs reach the environment and, in most cases, water. In water, the eggs may be ingested by the snail, the intermediate host, or they may hatch and produce a larva (the miracidium) that swims and enters the snail on its own. In either case, the larvae gain access to the tissues of the gastropod and multiply, producing several generations of larval stages, the last of which is known as *cercariae*. Cercariae leave the snail and swim freely for a short time. If they are cercariae of any of the species of *Schistosoma*, they penetrate the skin of their natural definitive hosts, migrate in the tissues, and grow into adults (see Chapter 24). If they are cercariae of *Fasciola* or *Fasciolopsis*, they encyst (form *metacercariae*) on aquatic vegetation; on ingestion by the definitive host, the metacercariae develop into adults. Cercariae of *Clonorchis*, *Opistorchis*, and other genera gain access to fish, and those of *Paragonimus* gain access to crabs and crayfish. In all of these instances, the metacercariae, or infective stages, form in the tissues of these intermediate hosts, and after they are ingested by the natural definitive hosts of the parasite, they develop into adult trematodes. In other species, the cercariae enter their intermediate hosts and do not encyst, remaining as *mesocercariae*, larvae that migrate through the tissues of the intermediate hosts. Moreover, if hosts other than their definitive hosts ingest these mesocercariae, they migrate from the intestine to the tissues and remain unchanged. Thus, mesocercariae undergo paratenism and may have many paratenic hosts that aid in transmission of the parasite (see Chapter 17).

The development of adult trematodes involves a series of changes that begin when the cercariae (schistosomes), or in other species the encysted or nonencysted mesocercariae, reach their natural definitive hosts. Migration to their habitat in the host (biliary ducts, lungs, intestine, blood vessels) and rapid growth of the parasite occur simultaneously. In some groups (*Schistosoma*), the young parasites begin covering their tegument with host proteins to evade the host's immunologic system (see Chapter 25). In others, the parasites encapsulate in the tissues (*Paragonimus*) and become more or less isolated inside a fibrous capsule produced by the host. The longevity of most species of trematodes of humans is not known, but in some cases *Schistosoma* infections have lasted for over four decades.

Geographic Distribution

Trematodes occur worldwide in all species of vertebrates. Their distribution is generally restricted by the geographic range of the mollusks' natural intermediate hosts. The distribution of trematodes that produce human infections is restricted not only by the range of the snails, but also by different customs and tastes related to food preparation and consumption. In general, most trematode infections in humans occur as sporadic cases or are limited to small geographic foci where transmission to humans is common. Some, trematodes, such as the flukes of the biliary system (*Clonorchis* and *Opistorchis*), occur in a wide geographic area, and large proportions of the population are infected. In many cases, both humans and animals are good hosts for a given trematode species; in others, humans are the sole natural host. The schistosomes have a wide geographic range in the tropical and temperate zones. This range is increasing because irrigation of land for agricultural purposes produces artificial breeding habitats for the snails' natural intermediate hosts. The human schistosomes produce great morbidity and mortality in millions of infected individuals.

Classification

The zoological classification of the class Trematoda is difficult because there is little agreement on the major groups. Most authorities on the subject usually list the families (about 24) and the groups, which are divided into subfamilies, genera, and species. A description of the morphologic characteristics of each family, and how the various families are distinguished from each other, is outside the scope of this discussion. As stated, the subclass Digenea contains all the families, genera, and species of trematodes that are parasitic in humans. The following abbreviated clas sification given here is for the trematodes of human interest. It should serve as a guide to understand the relationships of the organisms discussed in the following chapters. Readers who are interested in the subject should consult the monumental work of E. Malek (*Snail-transmitted Parasitic Diseases*, 2 volumes, CRC Press, 1980).

Family: Schistosmatidae

(See Chapter 23)

Family: Paragonimidae

Genus: Paragonimus (lung). *P. westermani, P. heterotremus, P. africanus, P. uterobilateralis, P. kellicotti, P. mexicanus, P. pulmonalis, P. amazonicus, P. caliensis*

Family: Nanophyetidae

Genus: *Nanophyetus* (intestine). *N. salmincola*

Family: Troglotrematidae

Genus: *Troglotrema* (lung). *Troglotrema* spp.

Family: Achillurbainiidae

Genus: *Achillurbainia* (= *Poikilorchis*) (nasal sinuses, tissues, skin). *A. recondita, A. nouveli*

Family: Opistorchiidae

Genus: *Opistorchis* (bile ducts). *O. felineus, O. viverrini*

Genus: *Clonorchis* (bile ducts). *C. sinensis*

Genus: *Amphimerus* (bile ducts). *A. pseudophelineus*

Genus: *Metorchis* (bile ducts). *M. conjunctus*

Family: Heterophyidae

Subfamily: Heterophyinae

Genus: *Heterophyes* (intestine). *H. heterophyes, H. nocens, H. continua*

Genus: *Haplorchis* (intestine). *H. taichui, H. yokogawai, H. calderoni, H. vanissima, H. pumilio*

Genus: *Stellantchasmus* (intestine). *S. falcatus*

Genus: *Centrocestus* (= *Stamnosoma*) (intestine). *C. armatum, C. formosanus, C. asadai*

Genus: *Cryptocotyle* (intestine). *C.* (= *Tocotrema*) *lingua*

Genus: Pygidiopsis (intestine). *P. summa*

Subfamily: Metagoniminae

Genus: *Metagonimus* (intestine). *M. yokogawai, M. takahashii*

Family: Fasciolidae

Genus: *Fasciola* (bile ducts). *F. hepatica, F. gigantica*

Genus: *Fasciolopsis* (intestine). *F. buski*

Family: Paramphistomatidae

    Genus: *Gastrodiscoides* (intestine). *G. hominis*

    Genus: *Watsonius* (intestine). *W. watsoni*

Family: Dicrocoeliidae

    Genus: *Dicrocoelium* (bile ducts). *D. dendriticum, D. hospes*

    Genus: *Eurythrema* (pancreatic ducts, rarely bile ducts). *E. pancreaticum*

Family: Echinostomatidae

    Subfamily: Echinostamatinae

        Genus: *Echinostoma* (intestine). *E. lidoense, E. malayanum, E. ilocanum, E. revolutum, E. hortense, E. machrorchis, E. cinetorchis*

        Genus: *Echynoparyphium* (intestine). *E. recurvatum*

        Genus: *Euparyphium* (intestine). *E. melis*

        Genus: *Hypoderaeum* (intestine). *H. conoideum*

        Genus: *Paryphostomum* (intestine). *P. sufrartyfex* (= *Artyfechinostomum sufrartyfex*), *P. mehri*

    Subfamily: Echinochasminae

        Genus: *Echinochasmus* (intestine). *E. perfoliatus*

    Subfamily: Himasthlinae

        Genus: *Himastla* (intestine). *H. muehlensi*

Family: Psilostomatidae

    Genus: *Psilorchis* (intestine). *P. hominis*

Family: Cathaemasiidae

    Genus: *Cathaemasia* (intestine). *C. cabrerai*

Family: Philophthalmidae

    Genus: *Philophthalmus* (eye). *Philophthalmus* spp.

Family: Plagiorchiidae

    Genus: *Plagiorchis* (intestine). *P. muris, P. javanensis*

Family: Prostogonimidae

    Genus: *Prosthogonimus* (oriduct and bursa of fabricii). *P. putschowskii*

Family: Microphallidae

    Genus: *Spelotrema* (intestine). *S. brevicaeca* (= *Heterophyes brevicaeca*)

    Genus: *Gymnophalloides* (intestine). *G. seoi*

Family: Lecithodendriidae

    Genus: *Phaneropsoulus* (intestine). *P. bonnei*

    Genus: *Prosthodendrium* (intestine). *P. molenkampi*

Family: Diplostomatidae

Genus: *Neodiplostomum* (= *Fibricola*) (intestine). *N. seoulense*

Genus: *Alaria* (intestine in animals; tissues in humans). *A. marcinae*, *A. americana*

Family: Clinostomastidae

Genus: *Clinostomun* (intestine). *Clinostomum* spp.

In the following chapters, the trematodes are divided in accordance with the organ system they affect: blood vessels (Chapter 23), biliary and pancreatic infections (Chapter 24), and pulmonary, intestinal, eye, and trematode larval infections (Chapter 25).

23

TREMATODES OF THE BLOOD VESSELS—SCHISTOSOMES

The schistosomes are trematodes that inhabit the blood vessels of humans and animals and produce *schistosomiasis* or *bilharziasis*, the general terms applied to the infection. Schistosomiasis is one of the most important parasitic diseases in the world because of the number of individuals affected and the morbidity and mortality produced. The disease usually occurs in persons living in poor socioeconomic conditions in tropical and subtropical areas.

The classification of the schistosomes is rather complicated if all species that produce zoonotic infections, especially schistosomal dermatitis in humans, are included. In general, all the species of importance to human medicine belong to the family Schistosomatidae. This family is divided into several subfamilies, genera, and species, the relationship of which is summarized, for the sake of completeness, as follows:

Family: Schistosomatidae

   Subfamily: Schistosomatinae

      Genus: *Schistosoma* (producing schistosomiasis)

         Species: *S. mansoni, S. haematobium, S. japonicum, S. mekongi, S. bovis, S. mattheei, S. mar-*
grebowiei, S. leiperi, S. rodhaini, S. incognitum, and *S. intercalatum*

      Genus: *Heterobilharzia* (one species, producing dermatitis)

      Genus: *Ornithobilharzia* (two species producing dermatitis)

      Genus: *Australobilharzia* (two species producing dermatitis)

   Subfamily: Bilharziellinae

      Genus: *Bilharziella* (one species producing dermatitis)

      Genus: *Trichobilharzia* (six species producing dermatitis)

   Subfamily: Gigantobilharziinae

      Genus: *Gigantobilharzia* (five species producing dermatitis)

   Subfamily: Dendritobilharziinae

      Genus: *Dendritobilharzia* (one species producing dermatitis)

Zoologically, the family Schistosomatidae is characterized by species with two separate sexes and ceca that join at the posterior end to form a single slender limb that terminates near the posterior extremity of the worm. In addition, in most species, the body of the male is wide laterally and rolled upon itself, forming the gynecophorous canal where the female is located. The genus *Schistosoma* includes the species generally associated with human infections: *S. mansoni, S. haematobium,* and *S. japonicum.* Two other species, *S. mekongi* and *S. malayensis,* are known in humans only on the basis of their eggs found in tissues and stools; the adult parasites have not been recovered from humans. The other species of *Schistosoma* listed above are zoonotic and produce human infections, especially in Africa. The remaining genera listed above have species that occur naturally in birds. The infective stages of these species may invade the skin of humans to produce schistosomal dermatitis, a disease that occurs worldwide (Beaver et al. 1984; Malek, 1980).

Morphology. Adult schistosomes are slender and slightly curved ventrally; on superficial examination, they resemble roundworms (*color plate* XI *A*). The males of the schistosomes are up to 20 mm in length and the females are up to 26 mm in length, depending on the species. The male has a gynecophorous canal formed by the folding of the lateral aspects of its body toward the ventral midline. This occurs during the early development of the worm. Soon afterward, the female locates inside this canal and remains there for the rest of the natural life of the worm (*color plate* XI *A*; Figs. 23–1 and 23–21 *A–B*). This peculiar arrangement results in the unique configuration of the worms in cross sections; the male appears as a tight C, with the female at the center of the C (Figs. 23–6 *A* and 23–25 *A*).

The two suckers of the male are prominent, especially the ventral one, which protrudes from the body of the worm. The tegument of *S. japonicum* is rather smooth, with no integumentary tuberculations (Fig. 23–27 *A–B*); *S. haematobium* has numerous minute tuberculations (Fig. 23–11 *B*); and *S. mansoni* has tuberculations that are more conspicuous. Other anatomic characteristics allow the human schistosomes to be distinguished from each other, but they are outside the scope of this discussion.

Life Cycle and Biology. The life cycles of the human schistosomes are similar (Fig. 23–1). The adult worms are located in the venules of the portal system of the colonic wall and in the venules of the urinary bladder

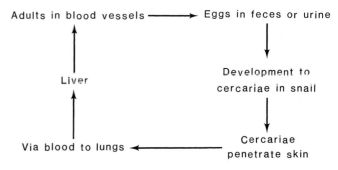

Fig. 23–1. *Schistosoma,* **schematic representation of the life cycle.**

wall. The females lay their eggs in venules that are smaller than those in which they are located. They do so by moving down into the venules, which are about 60 to 80 μm in diameter, and distending them considerably. After the female retracts, the deposited eggs (which are larger than the venule) become firmly anchored when the venule returns to its original size. The eggs then begin the process of extrusion into the lumen of the viscus. After breaking through the tissues, the fully embryonated eggs are passed to the environment with either feces or urine. If the eggs reach fresh water, a larva known as the *miracidium* leaves the egg through its operculum to swim and find a suitable snail. On entering the snail, the miracidium begins to develop through several other larval stages that finally form *cercariae.* The cercariae are the infective stages that leave the snail and swim for a few hours; if they find an appropriate definitive host, they enter it through the skin. Once in the new host, the young cercariae transform into *schistosomula* (immature worms) that travel through the circulatory system to the lungs and then to the liver. In the liver, a maturation phase follows, after which the males and females form pairs that migrate once more via the portal system to the venules in the large intestine or urinary bladder to begin oviposition.

The aspect of the life cycle of schistosomes dealing with extrusion of eggs from the tissues into the lumen of the viscera requires some elaboration. The adult parasites within the vessels produce no inflammatory reaction because early in their development, the worms incorporate host proteins into their tegument. These host proteins make the worm immunologically unrecognizable as non-self (Smithers et al. 1969), a fact that may account for the longevity of schistosomes in humans, sometimes for up to 47 years (Hall, Kehoe, 1970). In contrast, the eggs are strongly immunogenic and elicit an inflammatory reaction that initially consists of a microabscess that allows movement of the egg through the tissues into the lumen of the viscera. This reaction appears to be a CD4$^+$ T lymphocyte–dependent immune response because individuals coinfected with human immune deficiency virus (HIV) excrete eggs in lesser numbers that are directly proportional to their CD4$^+$ T lymphocyte number (Karanja et al. 1997). Some of the eggs remain trapped in the wall of the viscus, producing a granulomatous inflammation. Others, taken with the blood flow of the portal vein, lodge in the liver and sometimes in other organs (traveling via portocaval anastomoses), where they form granulomas. *The granuloma formation elicited by the eggs in the different viscera is the cause of all the clinical and pathologic manifestations of schistosomiasis.* The granulomas formed around the eggs have cell populations that produce a lymphokine, *fibroblast stimulating factor-1*, that promotes fibrosis (scarring) of the liver and other organs in schistosomal infections.

Geographic Distribution and Epidemiology. Schistosomiasis is found in certain tropical and subtropical areas of the world (Fig. 23–2). *Schistosoma mansoni* oc-

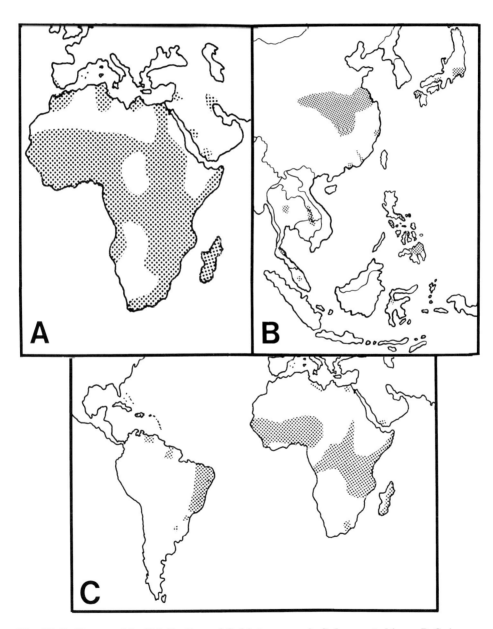

Fig. 23–2. Geographic distribution of *Schistosoma. A, S. haematobium, B, S. japonicum, C, S. mansoni*, geographic distribution.

curs widely in Africa; in the Western Hemisphere it occurs in northeastern Brazil and Dutch Guiana and focally in Venezuela and some Caribbean islands, such as Antigua, Guadeloupe, Martinique, Santa Lucia, and Puerto Rico. Recent surveys in Puerto Rico revealed a prevalence of less than 1% in areas of previously known endemicity; moreover, the main snail vector, *Biomphalaria glabrata*, has disappeared (Giboda et al. 1997). *Schistosoma japonicum* occurs in China, Japan, and the Philippines. *Schistosoma haematobium* is widely distributed in Africa and the Middle East, with foci in southern Portugal and Cyprus; the disease was recently introduced to Jordan (Saliba et al. 1997). *Schistosoma mekongi* is indigenous in northern Thailand, Laos, and northern Cambodia. Data on the prevalence of human schistosomiasis exist only for isolated areas or countries. The global prevalence in 1947 was estimated at about 147 million persons. These estimates included only the first three schistosomes mentioned above, since *S. mekongi* was undescribed at the time. Today the estimate is 200 million cases worldwide, making schistosomiasis one of the most important parasitic infections of humankind (WHO, 1980). This increase in the number of cases occurred in spite of many control efforts and in spite of the fact that the disease has been eradicated from places in Asia, South America, North Africa, and the Middle East (Savioli et al. 1997). The infection occurs in 74 developing nations. In 1993 the World Health Organization estimated that in these countries, between 500 to 600 million persons are at risk of contracting the infection.

Schistosomes are snail-transmitted infections acquired by immersion in water containing infective stages, the cercariae. *Schistosoma haematobium* occurs exclusively in humans; there is no animal reservoir. *Schistosoma mansoni* is almost exclusively a human parasite, with sporadic cases of natural infections in primates. *Schistosoma japonicum* occurs in both humans and animals throughout the endemic areas. *Schistosoma mekongi* has been found mostly in dogs, the probable natural reservoirs (Sornmani et al. 1980). There are many species of snail intermediate hosts of schistosomes, depending on the geographic area. *Schistosoma haematobium* uses mostly species of *Bulinus*; *S. mansoni* uses *Biomphalaria* and *Tropicorbis*; *S. japonicum* uses *Oncomelania*; and *S. mekongi* uses *Lithoglyphopsis*.

Immunity. Most of the immunologic work in schistosomiasis has been done in experimental animals; very little work has been done in humans with the infection. In earlier work, much attention was devoted to the mechanism of granuloma formation and the modulation of the disease (see below). The seminal observation that adult schistosomes are immunologically inert (Smithers et al. 1969) led to the idea that the young schistosomula entering the skin and traveling to the lungs and the liver are the targets for protective immunity (McLaren, 1989). This idea was reinforced by the finding that 3-hour-old schistosomula were killed in vitro by several immunologic mechanisms (McLaren, 1989). Later studies demonstrated that in both normal and immune mice, the infecting schistosomula of *S. mansoni* were eliminated in the lungs (Dean, Mangold, 1992). Moreover, in immune animals, elimination of the parasite occurred earlier and continued for a longer period than in nonimmune ones (Dean, Mangold, 1992). The inflammatory process elicited by the schistosomula in the lungs of experimentally infected animals consists of T cells of the helper (Th) subset. In vaccination experiments, immune animals depleted of their CD4$^+$ T lymphocytes during skin migration of the schistosomula greatly reduced the expression of their immunity (McLaren, 1989). Macrophages activated by schistosome antigens in in vitro systems kill the parasites, a reaction apparently mediated by gamma interferon.

Once the parasites grow into adults and begin laying eggs in the tissues, the formation of granulomas is the main manifestation of the infection. The morphologic variations in granulomas and their basic composition are discussed below under Pathology. The immune modulation of granuloma formation and its consequences for the host are examined in the following paragraphs. As explained below, the granulomas formed by *S. mansoni* are large and are mediated by a cell-mediated immune response to the parasite (see below). The mechanism for this is now better understood; it is mediated by a Th2 T-cell response, as demonstrated in experimental animals. The large granulomas of *S. mansoni* can be considerably decreased in size by antibodies against interleukin-4 (IL-4), one of the main cytokines produced by Th2 cells. By the same token, antibodies against IL-2 (one of the cytokines of Th1 cells, whose main function is to promote the growth of T cells) also inhibit the production of granulomas. The destruction of Th2 cells in infected animals decreases the size of the granulomas, but more important, it reduces hepatic fibrosis as well. A great deal of other work on the same lines of cytokine manipulation in experimentally infected animals has produced responses, as expected, for their functions. Th2 cells also modulate the granulomas produced by *S. japonicum*. Differences in the effect that various cytokines have in infected mice, compared with those in *S. mansoni*, are probably due to the normally reduced size of the granulomas produced by *S. japonicum*. However, how these cytokine systems operate in natural human *Schistosomia mansoni* infections is not known.

Some data on the immunity of schistosomiasis in humans were collected in field studies of individuals with *S. haematobium* and *S. mansoni* infections. After treatment, both the rate and the intensity of reinfection under natural conditions were reduced, indicating the presence of an acquired immunity that limited the infection and its morbidity. This immunity is evident only after many years of exposure, and it is acquired earlier in areas where higher levels of infection occur (Hagan, 1992).

Clinical Findings. The clinical manifestations of schistosomiasis begin on the skin, where the parasites penetrate, causing local allergic symptoms and signs consisting of wheals, urticarial rash, and edema. Generalized allergic manifestations follow, with involvement of several mucosae and fever lasting for up to 4 weeks. In some patients there is a slight increase in body temperature and a headache; peripheral eosinophilia is present in all patients. A history of exposure to the infection is obtained from most patients, but careful questioning is required since the incubation period varies from 2 to 8 weeks. These symptoms correlate with the tissue migration of the worms and subside as soon as the worms reach the intestine or the urinary bladder, when the chronic phase of the disease begins. The above symptoms and signs are known as *Katayama syndrome*. This syndrome was first described in Japan, in infections with *S. japonicum*, but later was recognized in all species. In South Africa, and probably in many other places, the syndrome often occurs in children (Walt, 1954).

In the chronic phase of the infection many organ systems are involved, depending on the duration of the infection, the occurrence of the parasite at ectopic locations, the species, the number of worms, and the susceptibility of the host. As stated above, most symptoms of the chronic phase are due to the eggs and the granulomatous inflammation they elicit rather than to the adult worms. Asymptomatic infections are common in most areas; for example, in Puerto Rico, up to 60% of infected individuals are asymptomatic. The main organs involved are considered separately in the following sections.

Intestine. Schistosoma mansoni and *S. japonicum* involve mainly the large intestine, producing symptoms that depend on the species and the strain of the parasite because there are geographic differences (Warren,

1978). *Schistosoma haematobium* involves the rectum in 70% of the cases; the colon and appendix are affected less often. Between the 4th and 12th weeks of infection, the acute symptoms are diarrhea, sometimes dysenteric; fever; abdominal pain; anorexia; weight loss; and enlargement and tenderness of the liver and spleen. Laboratory tests show marked leukocytosis, peripheral eosinophilia, and *Schistosoma* eggs in the stools. These symptoms subside and the infection becomes chronic, with return of the liver to its normal size and decreased blood eosinophilia, leukopenia, and anemia. In the absence of reinfections the disease becomes quiescent for years, with constant elimination of eggs in the feces or a slow decline in the number of eggs. The decrease in eggs is due to their being trapped in the colonic wall and diverted into the liver and other organs. The gastrointestinal symptoms in the final stages of the infection are mostly chronic diarrhea, but dysentery with colonic ulcerations may also develop, especially in *S. japonicum* infections.

Hepatosplenic Syndrome. Involvement of the liver and spleen during the chronic phase of schistosomiasis is silent at first. However, portal hypertension develops with enlargement of the liver and spleen, as well as ascites, collateral circulation (seen on the abdominal wall as the medusa head), and esophageal varices. Loss of liver function, weight loss, hypoalbuminemia, and low levels of clotting factors are common manifestations of the terminal phase; rupture of esophageal varices with gastrointestinal hemorrhage is a possible lethal complication. The hepatosplenic syndrome is more common in *S. japonicum* infections, less frequent in *S. mansoni*, and rare in *S. haematobium*.

Urinary System. The manifestations of urinary schistosomiasis are related to the number of worms (Smith, Christie, 1986) and begin soon after the flukes locate in the pelvic organs and start oviposition. For practical purposes, all urinary symptoms are seen in infections produced by *S. haematobium* because of its distribution in the venules of the lower urinary tract, including the distal ureters, urinary bladder, lower rectum, and genital organs. Other species of *Schistosoma* may produce similar symptoms, but these are rare. Early symptoms, usually found in children and young adults, are microscopic bleeding at first and blood-tinted urine later. Glomerular function is not impaired, but some tubular dysfunction is found in 7% of patients and excretory urograms show abnormalities in 43% (Cooppan et al. 1987). As the infection becomes chronic, difficult urination, urine retention with dilatation of the bladder, and bouts of urinary tract infections sometimes leading to renal failure are common (Zahran, Badr, 1980). The chronic uropathy of schistosomiasis occurs with a 9:1 male:female ratio, and the average age of presentation with fully developed disease is 37 years (Smith et al. 1977a). The chronic urinary symptoms occur in up to 42% of infected individuals, depending on the geographic area. The most common complaint is renal colic (occurring in 85% of patients), equally divided between the right and left kidneys or occurring bilaterally. Dysuria occur in 57%, hematuria in 35%, pyuria in 28%, urinary frequency in 25%, suprapubic pain in 17%, and passage of urinary tissue in 8% (Smith et al. 1977a).

The chronic obstructive uropathy of urinary schistosomiasis is best demonstrated on roentgenograms or with other imaging techniques that show constrictions with dilatation of the ureters, the pelvices, and the caliceal system (Fig. 23–3 A; Oyediran, 1979). Often the calcification of the urinary bladder appears on routine radiograms of the pelvis (Fig. 23–3 B). Finally, squamous cell carcinoma of the urinary bladder may develop in some infected individuals (Bhagwandeen, 1976).

Schistosomal Glomerulonephritis. Soluble antigen–antibody complexes may develop in patients with schistosomiasis; as expected, these complexes may deposit in the glomerular membrane, producing glomerulonephritis (Andrade, Rocha, 1979). Most patients with this condition are young adults, more often men than women, usually with advanced schistosomiasis. In addition, these patients may have nephrotic syndrome, proteinuria, and high blood pressure. All patients come from endemic areas and almost invariably have eggs in their stools. Sections of kidney biopsy specimens demonstrate the diffuse glomerulonephritis, and electron micrographs reveal the basement membrane deposits of antigen–antibody complexes (Andrade, Rocha, 1979).

In experimental animal models, the antigen responsible for the renal lesions was a polysaccharide probably derived from the worms' gut; however, other worm or egg antigens could not be excluded (Houba, 1979).

Lungs. Embolization of large numbers of eggs into the capillary bed of the lungs produces pulmonary schistosomiasis with manifestations of pulmonary hypertension, congestive heart failure, precordial pain, syncope, hemoptysis, and chronic cyanosis, with clubbing of the fingers in advanced cases. It is estimated that these complications occur in less than 5% of infected individuals and that the disease is more often seen in

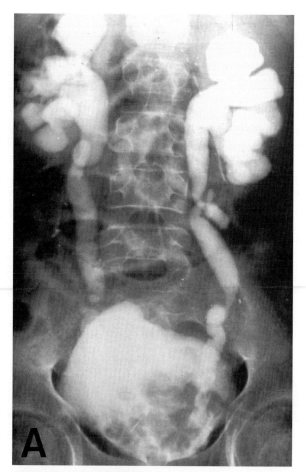

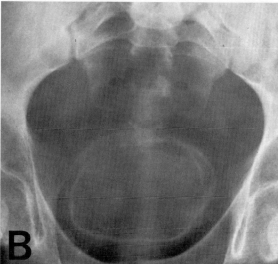

Fig. 23–3. *Schistosoma haematobium*, x-ray film of individuals with uropathy. *A*, Urogram showing dilation of ureters, renal pelvices, and caliceal system due to obstruction in the lower portion. Note the filling defects in the urinary bladder corresponding to a tumor. *B*, Calcification of the urinary bladder. (Courtesy of J.H. Smith, M.D., Department of Pathology and Laboratory Medicine, College of Medicine, Texas A & M University, College Station, Texas.)

S. mansoni infections (Morris, Knauer, 1997). Moreover, fibrosis of the liver and portal hypertension are both necessary for the development of pulmonary symptoms. Physical examination reveals signs of congestive heart failure on the right side of the heart. Chest x-ray films show enlargement of the right ventricle, with congestion of the pulmonary arteries and sometimes a characteristic fine, diffuse, mottling similar to that of miliary tuberculosis. Electrocardiograms show right cardiac hypertrophy.

Central Nervous System. Involvement of the central nervous system is infrequent, but it is an important complication of ectopic adult worms in the brain and spinal cord. Cerebral schistosomiasis occurs more often in *S. japonicum* infections, less often with *S. mansoni*, and rarely with *S. haematobium* (Marcial-Rojas, Fiol, 1963). The usual presentation includes epilepsy, a brain mass, aphasia, amnesia, and other less specific signs and symptoms such as dizziness, reduced vision, headache, or sensory disturbances. It appears that only 12 histologically confirmed cases of cerebral schistosomiasis have been reported since 1984 (Pittella, 1997). The spinal cord is more commonly involved in *S. haematobium* and *S. mansoni* infections and is rarely affected in *S. japonicum* infections (Case Records of the Massachusetts General Hospital, 1996a; Marcial-Rojas, Fiol, 1963). The presentation is that of a myelopathy developing either rapidly (Queiroz et al. 1979) or slowly over a long period. Low back pain is sometimes followed by rapid progressive paraparesis, with sensory loss and sphincter incontinence (Case Records of the Massachusetts General Hospital, 1985, 1996b; Dominguez, Borges, 1962; Lechtenberg, Vaida, 1977; Razdan et al. 1997). The clinical diagnosis is almost always based on circumstantial evidence because only when the patient dies is tissue available for histologic diagnosis. An enzyme-linked immunosorbent assay of cerebrospinal fluid is helpful in making the diagnosis (Pammenter et al. 1996), but like all tests based on detection of antibodies, it does not confirm the infection.

Genital Involvement. Schistosomes may involve both the female and male genital organs, more often in *S. haematobium* infections than in *S. mansoni* or *S. japonicum* infections (Wright et al. 1982). In women, the vulva may have papules, warts, plaques, or nodules, which grow rapidly and bleed easily; these lesions are produced by eggs deposited by the worms under the epidermis. In the vagina, there are polyps, plaques, granulomatous lesions, and ulcerations. The involved cervix is irregularly shaped and eroded, bleeds easily, and often has a granulomatous inflammation forming plaques (Wright et al. 1982). *Schistosoma* eggs are found in vaginal and cervical smears stained with Papanicolaou stain (*color plate* XI *H–I*).

In men, the prostate, seminal vesicles, cord, epididymis, and testis are often involved. The symptoms are usually mild and consist of hemospermia, hydrocele, and enlargement and thickening of the cords; the eggs of the parasite are recovered in the sperm (Gelfand et al. 1970). Infections with *S. haematobium*, *S. intercalatum*, and *S. mansoni* have manifested with hematospermia, also with eggs in the semen (Corachan et al. 1994).

Skin. The skin is one of the most common sites of ectopic schistosomiasis, but this picture may represent a distortion due to the accessibility of the lesions for diagnosis. However, ectopic skin lesions produced by the schistosomes are difficult to diagnose clinically, and biopsy specimens are always required for confirmation. The skin lesions present clinically as red, itchy papules (Fig. 23–4) measuring up to 1 cm in diameter or as small nodules anywhere in the body. Sometimes these lesions appear after a few weeks of exposure to the infection, in which case peripheral eosinophilia develops (Farrell et al. 1996). The most common sites of the lesions are the lower torso and the pelvis; these areas are more commonly involved in infections with *S. mansoni* and *S. haematobium* (Obasi, 1986). A history of living in or having visited an endemic area is necessary for the clinical diagnosis. Ectopic skin lesions in schistosomiasis are due to oviposition by the adult female in a vessel that irrigates the affected area of the skin. These lesions should not be confused with schistosomal dermatitis produced by the cercariae in the epidermis (see below). In *S. haematobium*, the genital skin, especially in women, is commonly affected. A combination of left-sided forehead dermatitis and ocular lesions (chorioretinitis) with visual symptoms was described in a patient apparently 4 months after exposure to the infection (Milligan, Burns, 1988).

Other Sites. Ectopic locations of *Schistosoma* occur in any organ system of the body. Appendices removed at surgery frequently have large numbers of *Schistosoma* eggs, often calcified and sometimes seen on x-ray films (Edington et al. 1975; Fataar, Satyanath, 1986). One patient who underwent esophageal resection for Chagas'-related disease had numerous granulomas with *S. mansoni* eggs in the wall of the resected esophagus (Gagliardi et al. 1997).

Pathology. The pathologic changes due to acute and chronic schistosomiasis result from deposition of eggs

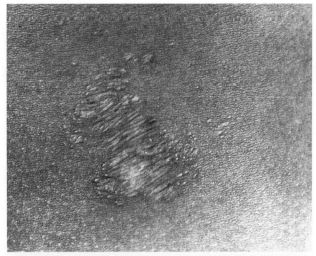

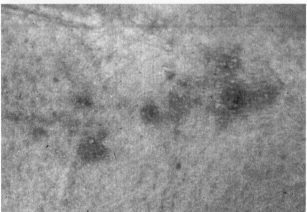

Fig. 23–4. *Schistosoma mansoni*, ectopic lesions in skin. *A*, Regressing lesion in the left abdominal wall. *B*, Erythematous pigmented papules in the axilla. (In: Convit, J., and Reyes, O. 1973. Ectopic skin lesions produced by *Schistosoma mansoni*. Am. J. Trop. Med. Hyg. 22:482–484. Reproduced with permission.)

in the tissues, and from the granulomatous reaction and fibrosis produced by the host. Much attention has been devoted to the dynamics of granuloma formation produced by *Schistosoma* eggs in experimental animals, but there is little or no information about similar processes in humans.

A brief overview of some of the biologic aspects of granulomas provoked in experimental animals by *Schistosoma* eggs is of interest here. Formation of granulomas around *S. mansoni* and *S. haematobium* eggs is an immunologic reaction of the delayed hypersensitivity type. This immunologic reaction occurs because granuloma formation is specific; it is accelerated after previous exposure to eggs (sensitization); and the specificity of this sensitization is transferred by cells, not by serum (Warren et al. 1967). In contrast, granulomas

produced by *S. japonicum* appear to be influenced by serum factors, one of which is an antiidiotypic antibody (Olds, Kresina, 1985). The dynamics of granuloma formation in *S. mansoni* and *S. haematobium* are similar: in unsensitized animals the granulomas reach their maximum size at about 16 days, while in homologously sensitized ones, they peak at about 8 days. In *S. japonicum* the cellular reaction around the eggs begins as early as 24 hours after they are laid; the mature granulomas are small, and no sensitization occurs after previous exposure (Warren, Domingo, 1970a, 1970b). Granuloma formation results in the destruction of the eggs; this occurs earliest in *S. japonicum*, followed by *S. haematobium* and *S. mansoni* (Warren, Domingo, 1970b). The size of the granulomas produced by different species of *Schistosoma* has been investigated frequently in animals; it appears to correlate with some observations in humans (Warren, Domingo, 1970b). However, one should bear in mind that the size of the granulomas varies even with the strain of mice used (Cheever et al. 1987) and probably, varies even more with the animal species infected. The tissue fibrosis responsible for the hepatosplenic form and for other changes in schistosomiasis appears to result from modulation by factors such as active molecules and the worm burden. Active molecules that stimulate fibrosis have been isolated from both the egg and the cells forming the granuloma (Wyler, 1983), and heavy worm burdens in mice significantly decrease the fibrosis (Cheever et al. 1987). The extent to which other factors influence the formation of egg granulomas or fibrosis in schistosomiasis is not known. In addition, it is doubtful whether the density-dependent modulation factors in mice can be applied to human infections. The reason is that, in a mouse, one pair of *Schistosoma* worms probably produces an infection that is at the upper limit of heavy infections in humans (Cheever, 1969).

In humans, there are also differences in the size of granulomas produced by the three species of *Schistosoma* (Winslow, 1967). *Schistosoma mansoni* produces large granulomas, usually spaced in the tissues, and the eggs have little tendency to calcify. The granulomas of *S. haematobium* and *S. japonicum* are smaller and occur in large masses, and the eggs tend to calcify more often (Winslow, 1967). Degradation and eventual reduction in the number of eggs in tissues occur in all species of schistosomes. Tissue destruction seems to be the main mechanism for egg reduction in *S. mansoni* infections (Cheever, Anderson, 1971). In *S. haematobium* infection, eggs are eliminated by both destruction and elimination of calcified eggs (Smith et al. 1974; Smith, Von Lichtenberg, 1976).

Intestine. The majority of individuals infected with *Schistosoma* have no gross abnormalities in the intestine. In *S. mansoni* infections, about 16% of patients have lesions such as sandy patches and inflammatory polyps, mostly in the rectum. Sandy patches are thickenings of the colonic wall composed of fibrous tissue containing large numbers of eggs, granulomas, and an atrophic overlying mucosa. Inflammatory polyps (Fig. 23–5) are rounded elevations of the mucosa produced by large masses of eggs. The polyps are present in one-half of patients with sandy patches (Elwi, 1967). In *S. mansoni* infections, polyps are more common in Egypt (Dimmette et al. 1956) and are infrequent in Brazil (Andrade, Cheever, 1967). Both sandy patches and inflammatory polyps occur in infections with *S. japonicum* (Hamrick et al. 1950) and, less frequently, in infections with *S. haematobium* (Bhagwandeen, 1976). Patients with *S. japonicum* colitis and dysentery show mild to severe degrees of dysplastic changes; these changes are premalignant lesions (Chen et al. 1981).

Microscopically, most lesions are alike. They consist of granulomas in different stages of evolution, with variable amounts of fibrosis in the mucosa and sub-

mucosa. Adult worms are sometimes seen in histologic sections (Fig. 23–6 A). Early granulomas with intact, viable eggs consist exclusively of polymorphonuclear cells, many of which are eosinophils (microabscesses) responsible for extrusion of eggs through the tissues into the intestinal lumen (Fig. 23–6 B). Older granulomas have eggs in different stages of destruction and calcification (Fig. 23–7 A–D), as well as epithelioid cells, multinucleated foreign body giant cells, lymphocytes, and polymorphonuclear cells, some of which are eosinophils. Different amounts of fibrosis accompany these granulomas; fibrosis is more abundant in areas of sandy patches where eggs and granulomas are numerous. Under the microscope, inflammatory polyps are seen as rounded masses of eggs in the submucosa surrounded by fibrosis and overlaid by a thin, atrophic mucosa.

Appendices removed at surgery or during autopsy of individuals infected with *S. haematobium* have eggs in 37% of the cases, less often in *S. mansoni* infections (Edington et al. 1975). Sometimes the eggs are found in large numbers and frequently they are calcified, but they appear to play no role in appendicitis (*color plate XI D–E*; Edington et al. 1975; Gelfand, 1967).

Urinary Tract. As stated above, most of the changes in the urinary system are due to *S. haematobium*. In experimental animals, a large number of *S. haematobium* cercariae given in a single dose produce an infection, with worms located in the lower urinary tract. The same number of cercariae given in several smaller doses at different time intervals result in worms evenly distributed throughout the pelvic organs and the lower colon (Sadun et al. 1970). The females of *S. haematobium* lay their eggs in large numbers at a time. This is why the eggs of *S. haematobium* in tissues are found near each other in large masses. It is also the reason that *S. haematobium* forms granulomas that are intermediate in size and cell composition between those of *S. mansoni* and *S. japonicum* (Von Lichtenberg et al. 1971).

The gross and microscopic changes of urinary schistosomiasis resemble those in the intestine (*color plate XI F*). About 31% of infected persons have a normal urinary bladder (Elwi, 1967). The rest have different lesions that occur either alone or combined, the most common of which are described below (Von Lichtenberg et al. 1971).

Polypoid patches. These sharply delineated lesions are resilient, round or lobulated, more often sessile than pedunculated, and covered with a granular reddish mucosa with petechial hemorrhages. They occur with decreasing frequency in the fundus and in the posterior

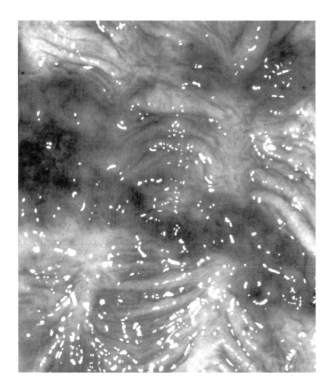

Fig. 23–5. ***Schistosoma haematobium***, **inflammatory polyps of the sigmoid colon. (Courtesy of J.H. Smith, M.D., Department of Pathology and Laboratory Medicine, College of Medicine, Texas A & M University, College Station, Texas.)**

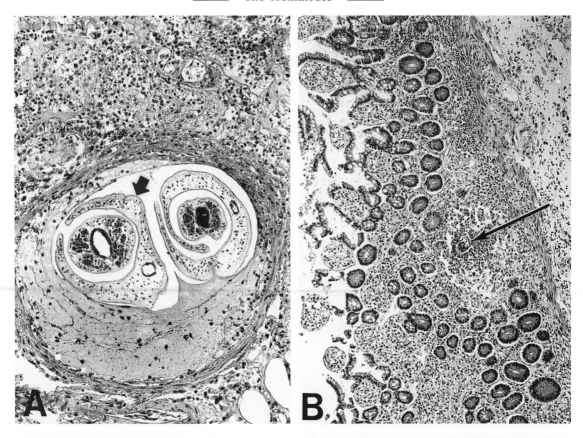

Fig. 23–6. *Schistosoma mansoni* in human colon, sections stained with hematoxylin and eosin stain. *A,* Medium-power view of two cross sections of a pair of worms in a medium-sized vessel. Note the male (arrow) with the female in the gynecophorous canal, ×70. *B,* The colonic mucosa with a microabscess (immature granuloma) contains an egg (arrow) being extruded into the lumen, ×120.

and lateral walls of the bladder. Some polyps attain a large size and on gross examination can be confused with tumors. Microscopically, polypoid patches are active lesions composed of granulation tissue infiltrated by lymphocytes, plasma cells, eosinophils, and histiocytes. Numerous granulomas with immature and mature eggs occur from the base of the epithelium down. Some microscopic abscesses, containing mainly eosinophils and Charcot-Leyden crystals, are present; a few calcified eggs may be seen (Fig. 23–9 *A–B;* Smith et al. 1977b).

Sandy patches. These patches are slightly elevated, with irregular borders. They are covered with a finely granular epithelium that has a characteristic rough, sandy surface at touch and a gritty consistency on section. In severe infections, the sandy patches coalesce to produce a thick, fibrous, often calcified bladder (*color plate* XII *A*). Ulcerations occur less frequently. Fibrosis of the urinary bladder neck results in urinary retention, and around the ureteral opening

ings, fibrosis leads to hydroureter and hydronephrosis (*color plate* XII *B–C*), more often on the left side (Elwi, 1967; Smith et al. 1977a; Von Lichtenberg et al. 1971). Involvement of one or both ureters can occur at any level and produce obstruction (Fig. 23–8 *A–B*). Microscopically, the sandy patches are either active or inactive. Active sandy patches contain many closely packed eggs (Fig. 23–9 *A*), one-half of which are calcified, within small granulomas, as well as a minimal cell reaction. Fibrosis separates groups of eggs. There is infiltration, mainly by lymphocytes and a few eosinophils, and the changes on the overlying epithelium are proliferative. Inactive sandy patches contain mostly calcified eggs, with little or no inflammatory reaction and abundant fibrosis (Fig. 23–10 *A* and *D*).

Residual fibrosis. This lesion consists of collagenized fibrous tissue with a few eggs deep in the submucosa. The inflammatory changes are minimal or absent. They resemble the fibrous nodules produced by

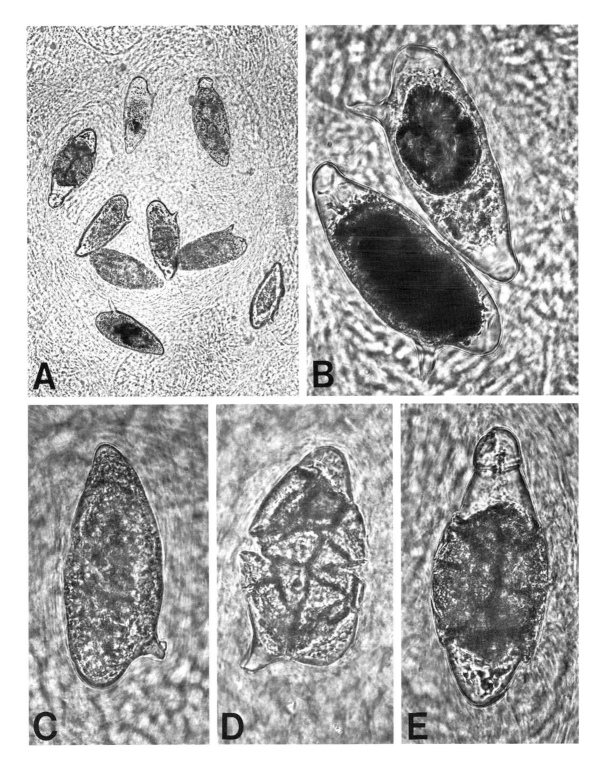

Fig. 23–7. *Schistosoma mansoni* eggs in mucosa of colon, pressed preparation, unstained. *A*, Low-power view illustrates several calcified eggs within granulomas, ×140. *B*, Two eggs with calcified miracidia, ×450. *C–E*, Different stages of calcification distorting the eggs. Note that the eggs are artifactually fractured in *D* and *E*, ×450. (Preparation courtesy of F.H. Shipkey, M.D., Department of Pathology, College of Medicine, King Saud University, Riyadh, Saudi Arabia.)

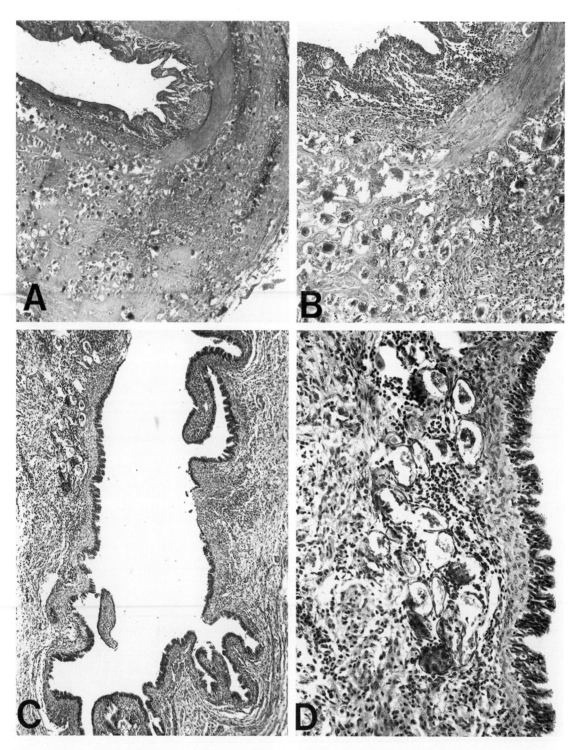

Fig. 23–8. *Schistosoma haematobium* in the ureter and *S. japonicum* in the fallopian tube, sections stained with hematoxylin and eosin stain. *A* and *B*, Low- and medium-power magnification of a ureter from a man with obstructive uropathy due to *S. haematobium* infection. Note the significant thickening and fibrosis of the ureteral wall and the large number of eggs. *A*, ×28; *B*, ×70. *C* and *D*, Medium- and high-power magnification of a fallopian tube of a woman infected with *S. japonicum*. Note the eggs, some of which are calcified, the inflammatory reaction, and the small granulomas, *C*, ×55; *D*, ×180.

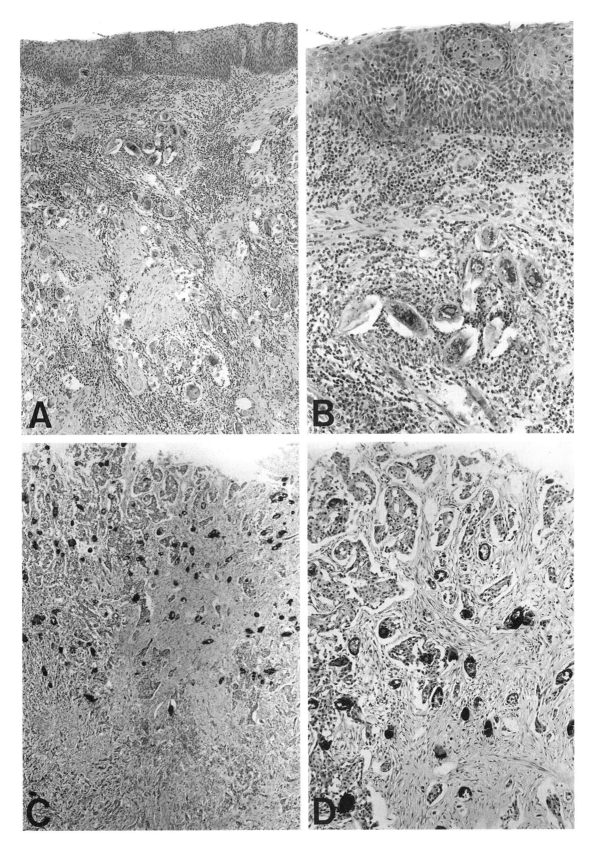

Fig. 23–9. *Schistosoma haematobium* in urinary bladder, sections stained with hematoxylin and eosin stain. A. Low-power view of a sandy patch showing squamous metaplasia of the epithelium, relatively large numbers of eggs within granulomas (some of which appear calcified), and inflammatory infiltration, ×55. B, Higher magnification illustrating the same changes and the infiltrate composed of mononuclear cells and eosinophils, ×140. C, Squamous cell carcinoma of urinary bladder with numerous calcified eggs, ×28. D, Higher magnification shows the tumor and the eggs, ×70.

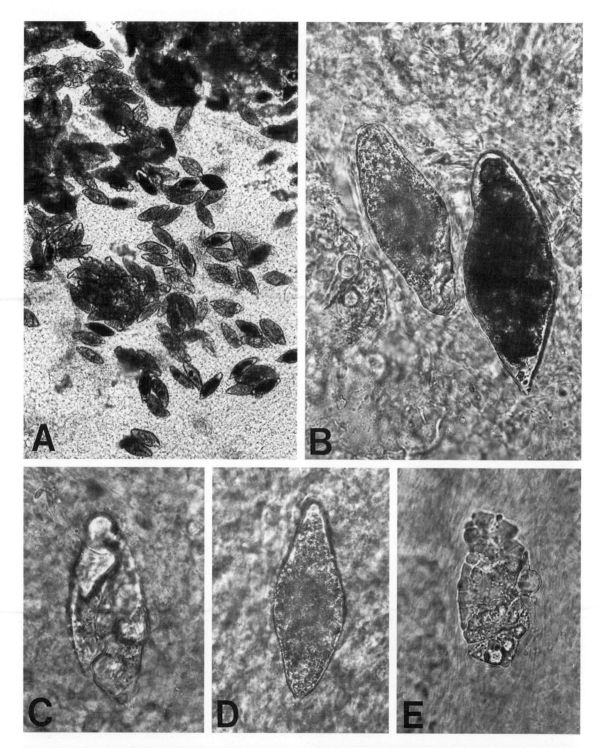

Fig. 23–10. *Schistosoma haematobium*, pressed preparation of mucosal biopsy specimen, unstained. *A*, Low-power view of a large number of calcified eggs, ×70. *B*, Eggs with calcified miracidia, ×450. *C–E*, Calcified eggs showing significant distortion due to calcium deposition, ×450. (Preparation courtesy of F.H. Shipkey, M.D., Department of Pathology, College of Medicine, King Saud University, Riyadh, Saudi Arabia.)

ectopic worms in the mesentery and lymph nodes (see below; Von Lichtenberg et al. 1971).

The uroepithelial changes associated with chronic urinary schistosomiasis are Brum's nests, cystitis cystica, cystitis glandularis, squamous metaplasia (Fig. 23–9 A–B), and leukoplakia, all of which are preneoplastic lesions. These changes are nonspecific and are observed equally often in common bacterial infections or other irritations, because of the metaplastic potential of the urothelium.

Genital Involvement. In men, schistosomal lesions in the cord, epididymis, prostate gland, seminal vesicles, and testis appear grossly as fibrosis and thickening; in rare cases, the lesions simulate a tumor. Studies of digested tissues at autopsy show that the number of eggs per gram is greater in the urinary bladder, followed by the seminal vesicles and the prostate (Edington et al. 1975; Gelfand et al. 1970).

In women, the most important lesions are found in the cervix and vagina, consisting mainly of polyps, sandy patches, and fibrosis (see above) that are recognized on gross and digital examinations. The colposcope may detect dysplastic changes and may reveal the granulomatous appearance of the lesion; petechial bleeding occurs often. Other lesions found in the uterus, fallopian tubes, and ovaries are nodules or fibrous thickenings. Vulvar lesions consist of masses of variable size, or of marked thickening of the skin; histologically, these lesions are similar to those at other sites (Mawad et al. 1992).

Microscopically, all lesions show eggs under the epithelium, usually in large aggregates (Figs. 23–8 C–D and 23–11 A–D; *color plate* XI G) and often calcified; occasionally, adult parasites are observed in dilated venules (Fig. 23–11 A–B). The granulomas and the inflammatory infiltrate (see Fig. 24–14 C–D) are as described above; similar lesions occur in any tissue section from the male or female genital organs (Fig. 23–12 A–B). The schistosome most commonly found in genital lesions is S. haematobium. However, lesions are also produced by S. mansoni (Edington et al. 1975; Gelfand et al. 1970, 1971), S. japonicum, and the zoonotic species. The epithelial surface of the endocervix may have changes of squamous metaplasia or dysplasia, and the cervix and vagina may have dysplastic changes. In lesions of the female genital tract, the eggs of the parasite are seen in cytologic specimens stained with Papanicolaou stain (*color plate* XI H–I and Fig. 23–13 A–C). In lesions of the male genital tract, the eggs are found in the semen.

Hepatosplenic Syndrome. The hepatosplenic form of schistosomiasis represents the end stage of the disease and is most commonly found in infections with S. mansoni and S. japonicum. In Egypt it is frequently found in the north, where both S. haematobium and S. mansoni occur, but it is rare in the south, where only S. haematobium is endemic (Mousa et al. 1967). The hepatosplenic lesions in schistosomiasis are grossly and histologically similar throughout most endemic areas (DePaola, Winslow, 1967).

The gross appearance of the liver and the spleen varies, depending on the evolution of the disease (*color plate* XI B–C). The average weight of the liver is 1550 g (range, 900 to 3700 g; Andrade et al. 1962). The left lobe is usually enlarged disproportionately, and often the external and cut surfaces have numerous nodules 1 cm or more in diameter, resembling a macronodular or postnecrotic cirrhosis (*color plate* XI C). The liver is firm, brownish, and hard, with fibrosis distributed in the periportal areas, a condition referred to as Symmer's pipe steam fibrosis. In advanced cases, rare regenerating nodules may be present, especially in the subcapsular zone. The spleen is normal in size and consistency or is moderately enlarged; however, it may weigh over 1000 g. Ascites, in variable proportions, is present in all patients with portal hypertension.

Microscopically, fibrous tissue fills the portal spaces of the liver, forming fibrous bands of variable width, with infiltration by lymphocytes, plasma cells, and a few neutrophils (Fig. 23–14 A–B). *Schistosoma* eggs in the tissues occur in variable numbers, are at different stages of degeneration and calcification, and sometimes obstruct small branches of the portal vein. In larger vessels, embolized dead worms produce obstruction and larger granulomas. Signs of remote phlebosclerosis may be seen by recanalization of organized thrombi accompanied by large areas of parenchymal damage. Moreover, if repeated gastrointestinal bleeding due to esophageal varices occurs, focal postnecrotic changes grossly resembling postnecrotic cirrhosis may develop in the liver (Andrade et al. 1962). The hepatocellular lesions of patients with schistosomiasis are probably aggravated by poor nutrition (DeWitt et al. 1964).

Lung. Pulmonary schistosomiasis usually develops in the hepatosplenic form due to embolization and lodging of large numbers of eggs in the lung. In a study in Upper Egypt, 58% of patients with pulmonary schistosomiasis were infected with S. haematobium and 31% with S. mansoni; 11% had mixed infections (Shaw, Ghareeb, 1938). Moreover, 33% had pulmonary lesions, but only in 2% were these lesions the

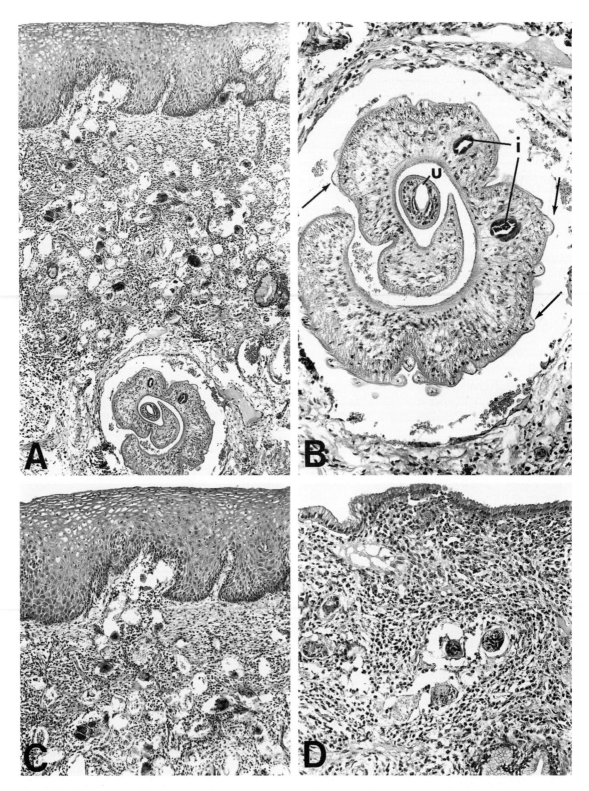

Fig. 23–11. *Schistosoma haematobium* in cervix, hematoxylin and eosin stain. *A*, Low-power view of endocervix shows multiple granulomas with eggs, an inflammatory infiltrate, and a pair of *Schistosoma* worms in a blood vessel, ×55. *B*, Higher magnification illustrates the worms. The tegument has widely spaced tubercles (arrows); the intestine (ceca) (i) is seen clearly in the male, and in the female the ceca are next to the uterus (u), ×140. *C*, Close-up view shows granulomas and some calcified eggs, ×70. *D*, The endocervix with granulomas, eggs, and the inflammatory infiltrate, ×140.

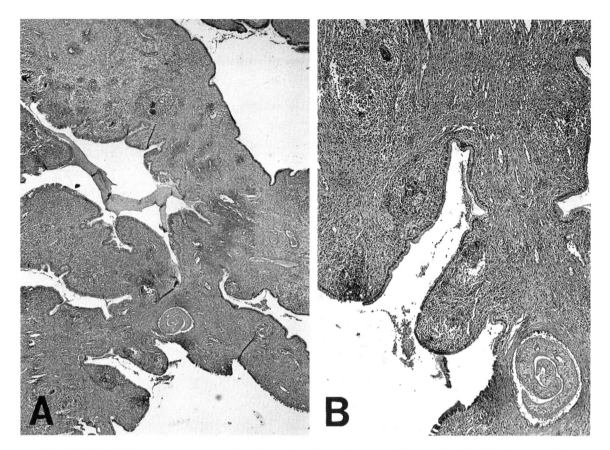

Fig. 23–12. *Schistosoma mansoni*, polyp of endometrium, sections stained with hematoxylin and eosin stain. *A*, Low-power view of the polypoid mass, ×22. *B*, Higher magnification shows a male schistosome, ×55.

immediate cause of death. Pulmonary vascular lesions of clinical significance occur more often in *S. mansoni* infections (Shaw, Ghareeb, 1938).

Grossly, the lungs generally have a normal appearance and consistency. On section, numerous small white granulomas measuring 0.5 mm in diameter are seen. The large branches of the pulmonary artery have atheromatous plaques, and the right side of the heart shows dilation and hypertrophy. Microscopically, both in arterioles 50 to 100 μm in diameter and in the lung

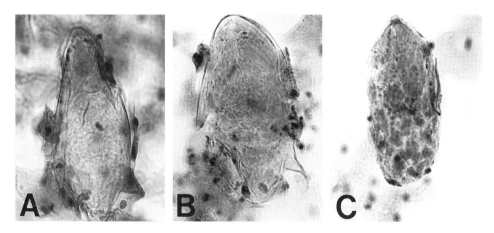

Fig. 23–13. *Schistosoma mansoni* in a vaginal smear stained with Papanicolaou stain. *A* and *B*, Distorted and fractured eggs with the characteristic lateral spine. *C*, Miracidium without a shell, all ×450.

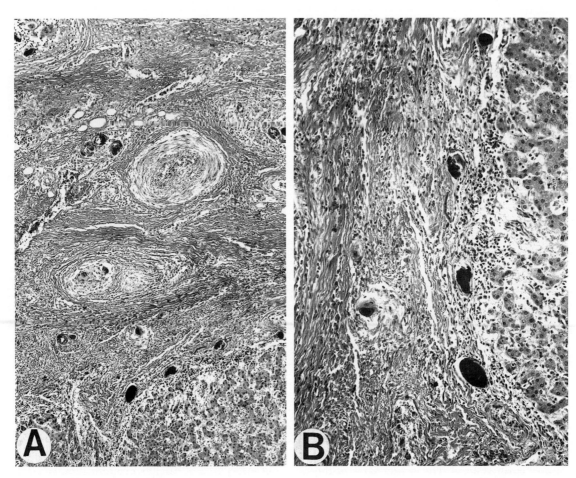

Fig. 23–14. *Schistosoma japonicum* in human liver, sections stained with hematoxylin and eosin stain. *A,* Low magnification shows the marked fibrosis with some granulomas and calcified eggs, ×70. *B,* Higher magnification shows some calcified eggs and a scant mononuclear cell infiltrate, ×140.

parenchyma, there are granulomas that contain either eggs or their calcified remnants (Fig. 23–15 *A*). Granulomas in the parenchyma are probably the result of vessel rupture, with extrusion of the eggs to surrounding alveolar tissues. On average, the granulomas are 250 to 375 μm in diameter; they are composed of foreign body giant cells, mononuclear cells, and eosinophils (see Fig. 23–15 *B*). In addition to the granulomas, there are microthrombi in the pulmonary arterioles and often a necrotizing arteritis near the embolized egg, but more commonly, the arteritis is seen in the absence of ova. The arteriolar changes consist of thickening of the intima with narrowing of the lumen, sometimes associated with edema and deposition of amorphous periodic acid–Schiff–positive material, mainly fibrin (Sadigursky, Andrade, 1982). Small arteries and arterioles have medial hypertrophy and hyalinization (Andrade, Andrade, 1970). Massive embolization of eggs produces dilation of arterioles and their collaterals, with arteriolitis, arteritis, and pulmonary hypertension because of blockage of many vessels; plexiform lesions develop (Fig. 23–16 *A–B*). Plex-

iform or angiomatoid lesions appear as dilated arterioles and veins; some of them have organized thrombi surrounded by fibrous tissue that may contain few or no granulomas. Embolization of adult worms producing larger granulomas also occurs, more often in advanced hepatosplenic disease.

Central Nervous System. The presence of *Schistosoma* eggs in brain tissue from persons with advanced hepatosplenic disease is well documented. These eggs travel in the general circulation and form only scattered microscopic granulomas and focal lesions, mainly arteritis and aneurysmal dilation of small vessels (Pittella, 1985). In most cases, these findings are incidental and have no clinical manifestations.

The clinically important central nervous system lesions are due to adult worms in vessels that lay eggs that lodge in a small area of brain tissue, the meninges, or the spinal cord. Grossly, the brain and the spinal cord are normal in appearance and consistency. Microscopically, recent lesions have eggs, granulomas and coagulative necrosis (Fig. 23–17 *A–D*). Older lesions

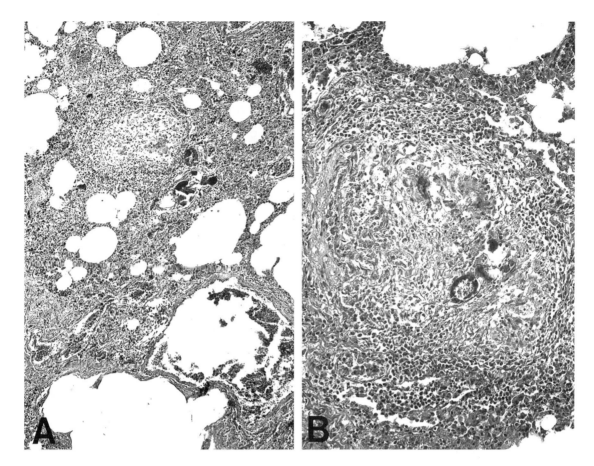

Fig. 23–15. *Schistosoma japonicum*, human lung, sections stained with hematoxylin and eosin stain. *A*, Low-power view illustrating granulomas in the pulmonary parenchyma and calcified eggs, ×70. *B*, Higher magnification of one granuloma, ×140.

have well-formed granulomas, and in *S. haematobiun* and *S. japonicum* infections the eggs are seen in masses (Fig. 23–18 *A–D*). Infiltration by mononuclear and polymorphonuclear cells is variable; astrocytes and gitter cells may be present (Fig. 23–17 *C–D*). Close to the lesion, there is a leptomeningitis with moderate infiltration by lymphocytes and plasma cells (Fig. 23–17 *B*). The ova are usually in different stages of calcification and degeneration; some egg remnants phagocytized by macrophages and giant cells may be seen (Fig. 23–17 *D*). The adult parasites are occasionally seen inside a vessel near the lesion. More commonly, older lesions in the brain are fibrotic. Special stains reveal a loss of myelin (Marcial-Rojas, Fiol, 1963; Pittella, 1985). In one case, the eggs were recovered in imprints made from a biopsy specimen submitted for frozen sections (Fig. 23–18 *D*).

Skin. The skin lesions of ectopic schistosomiasis consist of a granulomatous inflammation of the dermis caused by the eggs of the parasite (Fig. 23–4). Finding and identifying the eggs is necessary for proper diagnosis. The granulomas usually have a marked lymphocytic and plasmacytic infiltrate and may occur deep in the subcutaneous tissues (Fig. 23–19 *A–B*).

Other Sites. *Schistosoma* lesions may occur in almost every organ of the body, usually due to the ectopic location of adult worms that lay eggs in a circumscribed area. In the abdominal cavity the adults may die, forming nodules that are usually recovered during surgery or at autopsy (Fig. 23–20 *A–B*). The nodules are 1 to 2 cm in diameter, hard, and gritty. Microscopically, they are composed of masses of fibrous tissue, sometimes collagenized, and granulomas with eggs in different stages of degeneration and calcification. The name sometimes applied to these lesions is *schistosomatoma* or *bilharzioma*; microscopically, they often consist of remnants of a lymph node (Fig. 23–21 *A–B*). In one patient, numerous bilharziomas in the abdominal cavity presented with marked colonic obstruction that clinically simulated an advanced lymphoma (Elmasalme et al. 1997).

Schistosomes and Cancer. The cause–effect association between schistosomiasis and carcinomas of the

563

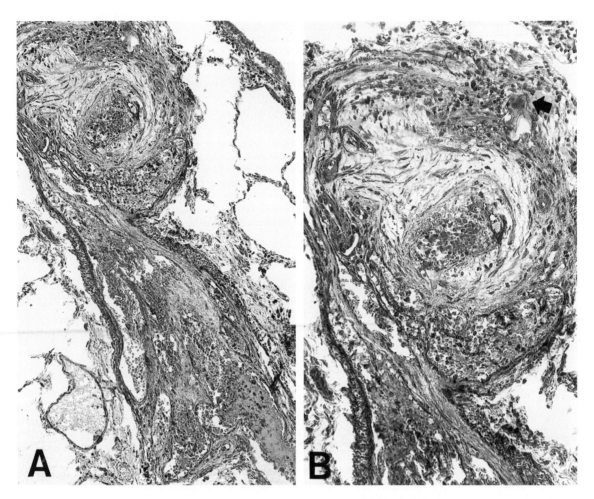

Fig. 23–16. *Schistosoma mansoni* in lung with pulmonary hypertension, sections stained with hematoxylin and eosin stain. *A*, Medium magnification showing a plexiform lesion characteristic of advanced pulmonary hypertension, ×140. *B*, Higher magnification shows detail of a vessel with thickening of the wall. Note the granuloma with a *Schistosoma* egg (arrow). (Preparation courtesy of R. Falzoni, M.D., Department of Pathology, Hospital das Clinicas da Faculdade de Medicina da Universidade de São Paulo, São Paulo, Brazil.)

colon and the urinary system is a debated issue. In Egypt, up to 35% of patients with a resected adenocarcinoma of the colon were infected with *S. mansoni*, and in many of these patients there were eggs within the tumor (Fig. 23–22 *A–B*). However, in a study of the tumors and other colonic lesions associated with the parasite, no cause–effect relationship between the parasite and the tumor was found (Dimmette et al. 1956). In China, studies of colonic lesions from patients with advanced schistosomiasis, colitis, and dysen-

tery revealed many premalignant colonic lesions (Chen et al. 1981).

Squamous cell carcinoma of the urinary bladder is the most common tumor of the urothelium in some endemic areas of urinary schistosomiasis; in contrast, transitional cell carcinoma is rare (Kitinya et al. 1986). It is found in 9% of cases of schistosomiasis, and it occurs at a younger age (fourth and fifth decades) than squamous cell carcinomas in nonendemic areas (seventh and eighth decades) (Fig. 23–9 *C–D*; Mostafa et

Fig. 23–17. *Schistosoma mansoni* in spinal cord, section stained with hematoxylin and eosin stain. *A*, Low-power view of spinal cord shows focal areas of destruction and the inflammatory infiltrate, ×22. *B*, Higher magnification illustrating the necrosis, inflammation, and meningitis (top), ×70. *C*, Higher magnification show-

ing granulomas with marked necrosis and eggs in different stages of disintegration. Note the inflammatory reaction, ×140. *D*, Detail illustrating disintegrating eggs, ×220. (Preparation courtesy of J.E. Gonzales, M.D., Instituto Anatomopatologico, Universidad Central de Venezuela, Caracas, Venezuela.)

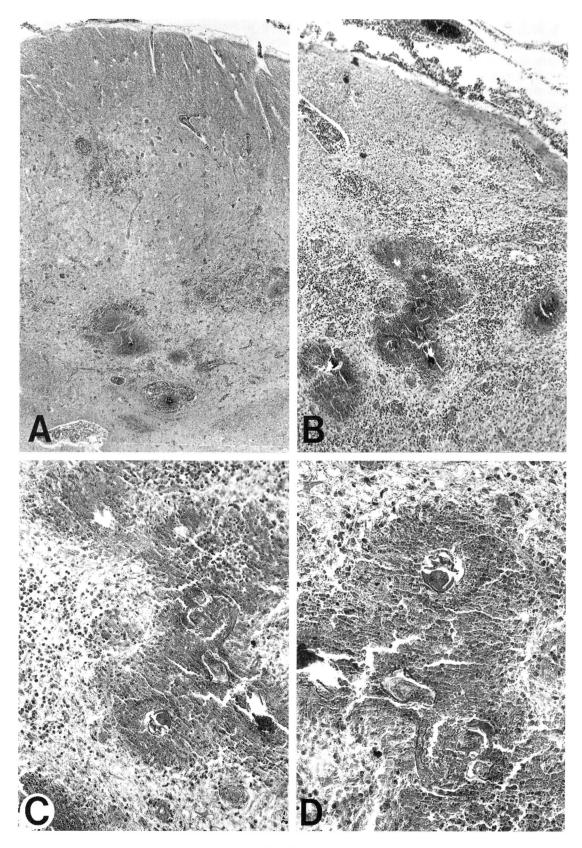

Fig. 23–17.

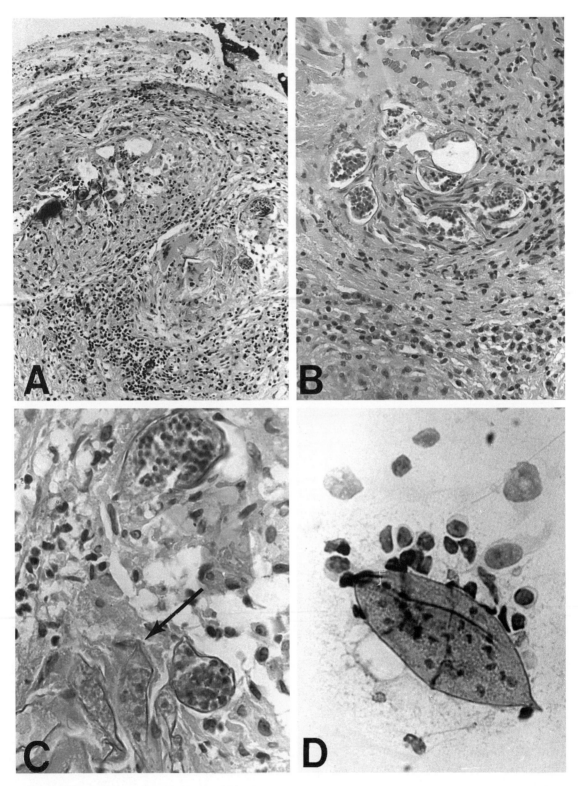

Fig. 23–18. *Schistosoma haematobium* in spinal cord. *A–C*. Sections stained with hematoxylin and eosin stain. *A*, Low-power view of inflammatory reaction and granulomas, ×140. *B*, Higher magnification shows several eggs within a large granuloma, ×280. *C*, Detail of eggs showing the terminal spine (arrow), ×570. *D*, Typical egg in an imprint of a biopsy specimen submitted for frozen sections, ×570. (Courtesy of C. Lobo, M.D., Servicio de Patologia, Hospital Aranzazu, San Sebastian, Universidad del Pais Vasco, Spain.)

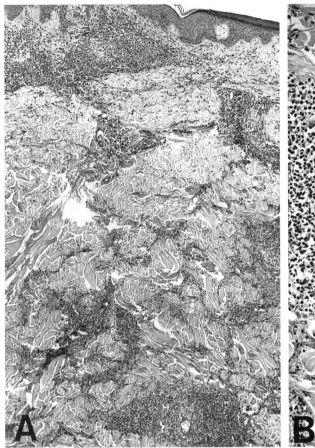 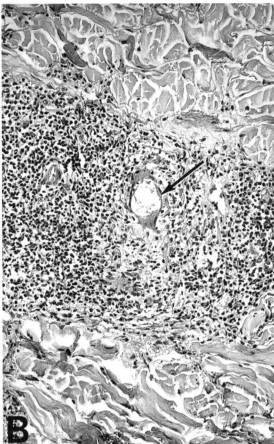

Fig. 23–19. *Schistosoma mansoni* ectopic in human skin, section stained with hematoxylin and eosin stain. *A*, Low-power view of skin shows a granulomatous inflammation of the dermis, ×55. *B*, Higher magnification shows a disintegrating egg of *S. mansoni* in a granuloma (arrow). Note that the inflammatory reaction consists predominantly of mononuclear cells and a few eosinophils, ×180.

al. 1995). The male:female patient ratio is 4:1 (Mostafa et al. 1995). The tumor is located in the lateral, posterior, and anterior walls, vault, and trigone in decreasing frequency (Elem, Purohit, 1983; Elwi, 1967). An association between the parasite and the tumor was first noted in Egypt, where both diseases occur commonly. However, because the tumor did not occur in other endemic areas for *S. haematobium*, the cause–effect relationship between parasite and tumor was an open question (Anthony, 1974). More recent evidence has conclusively linked the tumor to the parasite (Thomas et al. 1990), but probably not as the sole cause. The parasite is probably a promoting agent, causing altered conditions in the urinary bladder, such as urinary retention, that are conducive to the development of the tumor by concentrating carcinogens (Bhagwandeen, 1976). The most important carcinogens are nitrates, nitrites, and *N*-nitroso compounds formed

endogenously by nitrate-reducing bacteria, causing secondary infections in individuals with schistosomiasis (Mostafa et al. 1995).

Diagnosis. Schistosomiasis is diagnosed on the basis of the clinical manifestations and the history of exposure to the infection. Infected individuals in the United States are usually immigrants from endemic areas. In rare cases, the infection is found in former visitors to endemic areas because acquisition of the disease requires contact with water contaminated with cercariae. Military personnel are more likely to become infected. Ultrasonography of the liver for the diagnosis and for assessment of the hepatic and splenic lesions is an excellent method and correlates with the clinical status of the patient (Abdel-Wahab et al. 1992; Hatz et al. 1992; Yazdanpanah et al. 1997). Ultrasound evaluation of the

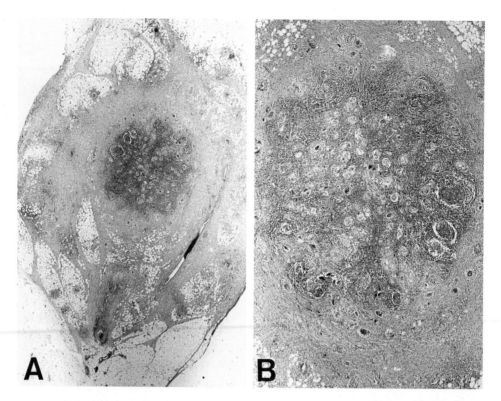

Fig. 23–20. *Schistosoma haematobium* in an omental nodule, section stained with hematoxylin and eosin stain. *A*, Low-power view shows the fibrosis and an inflammatory reaction infiltrating the surrounding fibroadipose tissue, ×10. *B*, Slightly higher magnification shows the granulomatous nature of the inflammation. Barely discernible are groups of calcified eggs, ×19.

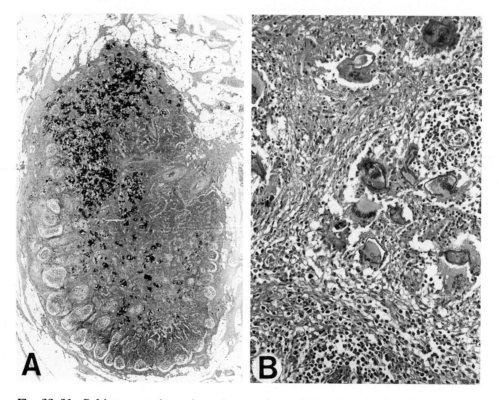

Fig. 23–21. *Schistosoma japonicum* in a peritoneal lymph node, hematoxylin and eosin stain. *A*, Low-power view showing the node with large masses of calcified eggs, ×8. *B*, Higher magnification illustrates granulomas and degenerating eggs, ×153.

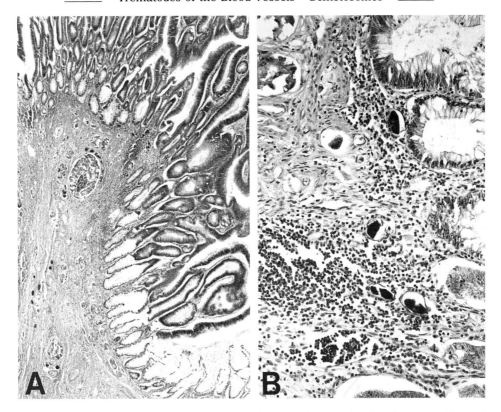

Fig. 23–22. *Schistosoma japonicum* and adenocarcinoma of colon, hematoxylin and eosin stain. *A*, Low-power view of a tumor and many scattered, calcified eggs in the submucosa, ×24. *B*, Higher magnification illustrates the calcified eggs, the slight granulomatous inflammation, and the mononuclear cell infiltrate, ×119. (Preparation courtesy of K.T. Tham, M.D., Hong Kong.)

urinary bladder in patients with *S. haematobium* allows the severity of the infection to be measured (Medhat et al. 1997).

The infection is usually confirmed in the clinical laboratory based on the recovery of eggs with typical morphology in wet preparations made directly from stools (Figs. 23–23, 23–24, and 23–25) and urine samples (Fig. 23–26). Concentration of these samples by one of several methods is also recommended to increase the yield of positive samples. Sometimes the eggs are found in cytologic smears (Berry, 1971; *color plate* XI *H–I* and Fig. 23–13 *A–C*) or in pressed preparations of colonic biopsy specimens (Figs. 23–7 *A–E* and 24–10 *A–E*). Pressed preparations done in the surgical cutting room require unfixed tissues. A portion (the size of a grain of rice) of the submitted biopsy specimens of colon, urinary bladder, cervix, and other tissues is taken and placed on a glass slide. Another slide is placed on top and is firmly pressed until the tissue covers about 1 cm².

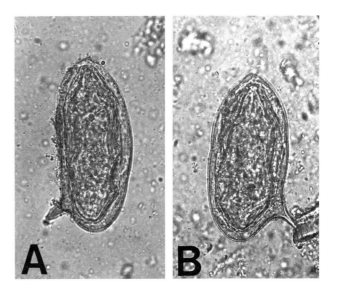

Fig. 23–23. *A* and *B*, *Schistosoma mansoni* eggs in human stools, unstained, ×504.

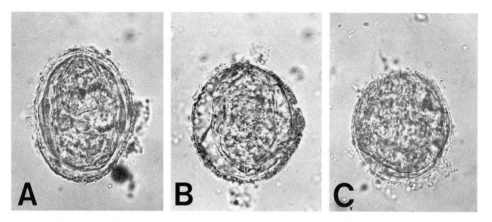

Fig. 23–24. *A–C, Schistosoma japonicum* eggs in human stools, unstained, ×383.

The preparation is inmediately examined directly under the microscope. These pressed preparations can be fixed on the slide after examination, and later dehydrated, clarified, and mounted to be archived as permanent slides. All *Schistosoma* eggs found by any of these methods need careful measurement, because identification of the species sometimes rests on the size of the eggs. The eggs of *S. mansoni* measure 114 to 175 × 45 to 68 μm (Fig. 23–23 *A–B*); those of *S. haematobium* are 112 to 170 × 40 to 70 μm (Fig. 23–26 *A–B*); those of *S. japonicum* are 70 to 100 × 50 to 65 μm (Fig. 23–24 *A–C*); and those of *S. mekongi* are subspherical, measuring 40 by 45 μm (Fig. 23–25 *A–B*). The sizes of the eggs of the zoonotic schistosomes are given below.

The diagnosis of schistosomiasis in tissues generally rests on finding the eggs in sections stained with hematoxylin and eosin stain; rarely, it depends on finding adult parasites. The eggs in tissues are usually in different stages of degeneration and calcification, are seen in granulomas, and can be found in almost any tissue. Eggs in tissues are also identified on the basis of their size and their morphologic characteristics. The terminal spine of *S. haematobium* and the lateral spine of *S. mansoni* must be visualized for proper identification. This often requires careful examination of many individual eggs or serial sections to find a typical spine. Fixation and processing usually distort the shell of the egg, resulting in the formation of artifacts that often resemble a spine. The eggs of *S. haematobium* are acid-

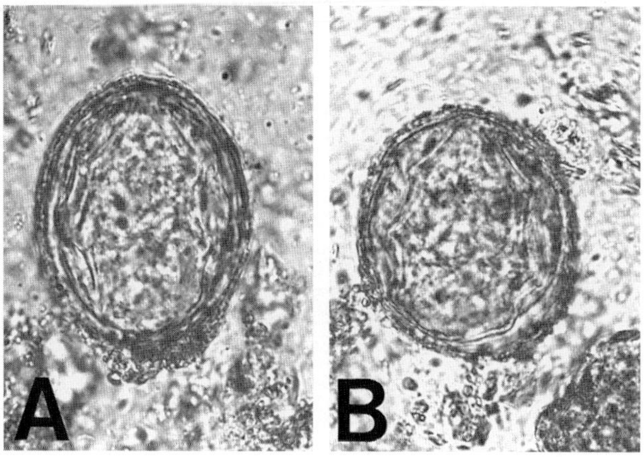

Fig. 23–25. *A* and *B, Schistosoma mekongi* eggs in human stools, unstained, ×504.

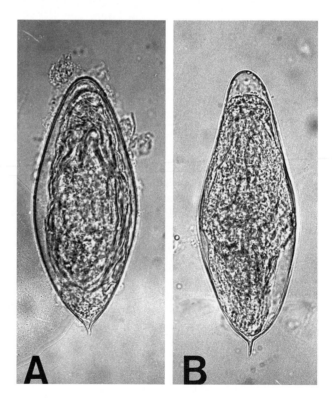

Fig. 23–26. *A* and *B, Schistosoma haematobium* eggs in human urine, unstained, ×495.

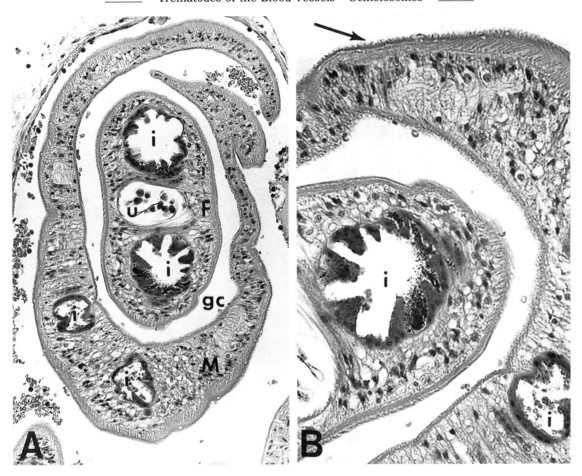

Fig. 23–27. *Schistosoma japonicum*, adults in mesenteric veins of a mouse infected experimentally, section stained with hematoxylin and eosin stain. *A*, Cross section of a male (m) and a female (f) in the gynecophorous canal (gc). Intestine (i); uterus (u) with eggs, ×220. *B*, Higher magnification illustrating the tegument (arrow), ×450.

fast negative if stained by a modified Ziehl-Nielsen technique. The eggs of *S. mansoni* and *S. japonicum*, are acid-fast positive. In some cases, this feature helps to differentiate the eggs of *S. mansoni* from those of *S. haematobium* in tissues from persons in endemic areas where the distribution of both species overlaps. In tissues, markedly calcified eggs are classically dark blue or black when stained with hematoxylin and eosin stain; sometimes they are difficult to recognize (Fig. 23–22 *B*). Decalcification of the eggs reveals their morphology, mainly the multinucleated miracidium, allowing their identification (Cheever, 1986). Decalcification of tissues can be done either before processing or during processing and embedding. Histologic sections are deparaffinized before processing for staining and are treated with 1 N HCl to remove the minerals. If the sections are overstained with hematoxylin, they will lose their calcium when destained in acid-alcohol (Cheever, 1986).

Adult worms in tissue sections are recognized because of their typical trematode tegument and morphol-

ogy (Fig. 23–6 *A*; see the introduction to Part III). On cross sections, the male appears as a tight C with the female at the center (Fig. 23–6 *A*). The tegument of *S. mansoni* males has multiple sensory papillae covered with minute spines on the dorsal aspect of the body (Fig. 23–6 *A*). *Schistosoma haematobium* has minute integumentary tuberculations (Fig. 23–11 *A*), and *S. japonicum* has minute acuminate spines (Fig. 23–27 *B*).

Zoonotic Patent Schistosomiasis

Several species of schistosomes from animals produce zoonotic infections in humans in different areas of the world. In general, the number of reported cases involving each of these species, with a few exceptions, is very small. These schistosomes are usually grouped by the shape of their eggs and are referred to as the *haematobium complex*, the *mansoni complex*, and the *japon-*

icum complex (Malek, 1980). One important aspect of these infections is that in most of them a specific diagnosis is possible based on the morphology and measurements of the eggs recovered in the stools or urine. The followng outline of these parasites provides the salient characteristics of each.

The *haematobium* Complex

As stated, the characteristic of this group is the presence of a terminal spine in the eggs; because of the large number of species in the group and the number of human infections, this group is the most important. The members of the complex will now be discussed:

Schistosoma bovis. This is a parasite of cattle, sheep, goats, horses, and camels, found in parts of northern Africa, southern Europe, and Southeast Asia. Human infections of the urinary tract and intestine have been reported from Uganda, South Africa, Egypt, Sudan, the Republic of Niger, Kenya, Senegal, and Rhodesia. The eggs of *S. bovis* measure 208 by 55 μm (Alves, 1949).

Schistosoma mattheei. This species infects cattle, sheep, and goats in an area south of the normal geographic range of *S. bovis*, but especially in South Africa and Rhodesia. Infections of the intestine and the urinary system occur in humans in Zambia (Hira, 1975) and Rhodesia. The eggs of *S. mattheei* measure 200 by 64 μm (Alves, 1949). In at least one patient, *S. mattheei* produced spinal cord lesions (Fripp, Joubert, 1991).

Schistosoma intercalatum. This species occurs in the Democratic Republic of Congo, Gabon, Cameroon, Chad, Uganda (Odongo-Aginya et al. 1994), the Central African Republic (Bouree, 1979), and equatorial Guinea (Corachan et al. 1987). In a survey in some communities, a prevalence of 32% was found (Anonymous, 1989). Human infections occur exclusively in the intestinal tract, and several hundred cases are known in the Democratic Republic of Congo, Gabon, Cameroon, and the Central African Republic. The eggs measure 140 to 240 $\times$ 50 to 85 μm.

Schistosoma incognitum. This species inhabits dogs and pigs in India and rodents in Thailand, Java, and In-

donesia. On at least two occasions, the eggs of *S. incognitum* were found in human stools of patients from India. The eggs measure 97 to 148 $\times$ 45 to 81 μm.

Schistosoma leiperi (= *S. spindale*). This species occurs in many herbivore species, including cattle and antelopes in Zambia and South Africa. Eggs of this species were once found in the urine of humans in South Africa. The eggs measure 210 to 305 $\times$ 38 to 65 μm.

The *mansoni* Complex

Besides *S. mansoni*, only one other species, *S. rodhaini*, occurs in this group. It is a parasite of rodents in the Democratic Republic of Congo. Human infections reported from that country cause intestinal schistosomiasis. The parasite also occurs in Uganda and Kenya. The eggs of *S. rodhaini* are polymorphic, with a lateral or terminal spine. An infection with laterally spined eggs similar to those of *S. mansoni* was reported from northern Thailand (Attawibool et al. 1983).

The *japonicum* Complex

Other than *S. japonicum* and *S. mekongi* (Voge et al. 1978), two other species have been placed in this group. However, there are also reports of human infections with other schistosomes in this group that have not been speciated.

Schistosoma margrebowiei. This species occurs in cattle and sheep in South Africa. It has eggs similar to those of *S. japonicum* and was reported in the stools of humans in South Africa. Some authors believe that it is identical with *S. japonicum* (Malek, 1980).

Schistosoma malayensis. This species has been reported in rodents in peninsular Malaysia (Greer et al. 1988) and in humans based on the appearance of the eggs in biopsy specimens (Murugasu et al. 1978) and autopsy material (Shekhar, 1991). The eggs of *S. malayensis* have a size range that falls between those of *japonicum* and *mekongi* (52 to 90 μm [average, 67 μm] by 33 to 62 μm [average, 54 μm]).

Schistosome Dermatitis or Cercarial Dermatitis

At least 7 genera (see above) of schistosomes, mostly parasites of birds, have about 18 species that occasionally enter the skin of humans and produce local reactions; however, they never attain patency (grow into adults) (Cort, 1950). In addition, the human and zoonotic schistosomes can produce the disease (Biocca, 1960; Carta, 1953; Cassagne, Discamps, 1977). This infection, known as *schistosome dermatitis*, *cercarial dermatitis*, or *swimmer's itch*, is acquired during immersion in fresh or brackish water. Cercarial dermatitis occurs in many areas of the tropical and temperate zones, sometimes in outbreaks (CDC, 1992). Each place where the infection is prevalent has one or two species of causative schistosomes. For example, in selected places on the North American continent, the disease is widely distributed in the northern United States and the provinces of Canada. In Michigan, Wisconsin, Minnesota, and Manitoba, the agent is *Trichobilharzia stagnicolae*; in Washington state, the species are *T. physellae* and *T. ocellata*. In Canada the disease is caused by *Gigantobilharzia huronensis*. In Japan the agent is *G. sturniae*; in China and Taiwan, *Ornithobilharzia odhneri*; and in Australia, *Australobilharzia variglandis*. In Europe, *T. ocellata*, *T. szidati*, and *Bilharziella polonica* are the main species responsible for the infection.

Clinical Findings. The symptoms and signs of schistosome dermatitis are due to repeated exposure to the infection and sensitization to the parasite. Initial exposures do not produce symptoms, but later there is usually a prickling or itching sensation that lasts for 1 hour. A macula about 1 to 2 mm in diameter develops at the site of penetration of each cercaria; some maculas disappear within a few hours, but others persist for longer periods. Sometimes diffuse erythema or urticarial rash occurs instead of macules. Ten to 15 hours later, these lesions progress to discrete papules measuring 3 to 5 mm in diameter that produce intense pruritus (*color plate* XI *J*). The papules are indurated and surrounded by erythema; edema is related to the amount of scratching. The papules usually disappear in about 1 week; some may become vesicles that rupture easily during scratching. If secondary infections occur, the vesicles may become pustules. The disease is self-limiting and generally benign.

Pathology and Diagnosis. The lesions produced by the cercariae responsible for schistosome dermatitis are short intraepidermal burrows where the parasite is destroyed (Brackett, 1940). The burrow contains the cercaria, which soon dies and degenerates, producing an inflammatory reaction of mononuclear cells at first. The infiltrate then changes to a polymorphonuclear one consisting mostly of eosinophils as soon as the parasite dies; later, macrophages appear (Brackett, 1940). The histologic changes in the dermis are more pronounced in individuals with previous sensitization (MacFarlane, 1949). A relationship between the cercaria of *S. mansoni* in tissues and the release of histamine has been observed; however, histamine release stops when the cercariae are transformed into schistosomula (Catto et al. 1980). This observation may explain the symptoms and lesions produced by cercariae of animal schistosomes, which do not progress beyond this stage in humans. The diagnosis of schistosome dermatitis is based on the clinical presentation and a history of exposure to the infection.

References

Abdel-Wahab M, Farid E, Gamal F, Afaf EB, Yaser A, Strickland GT, 1992. Grading of hepatic schistosomiasis by the use of ultrasonography. Am. J. Trop. Med. Hyg. 46:403–408

Alves W, 1949. The eggs of *Schistosoma bovis*, *S. mattheei* and *S. haematobium*. J. Helminthol. 23:127–134

Andrade ZA, Andrade SG, 1970. Pathogenesis of schistosomal pulmonary arteritis. Am. J. Trop. Med. Hyg. 19:305–310

Andrade ZA, Cheever AW, 1967. Clinical and pathological aspects of schistosomiasis in Brazil. In: Mostofi FK (ed), *Bilharziasis*. New York: Springer-Verlag, pp. 157–166

Andrade ZA, Rocha H, 1979. Schistosomal glomerulopathy. Kidney Int. 16:23–29

Andrade ZA, Santana S, Rubin E, 1962. Hepatic changes in advanced schistosomiasis. Gastroenterology 42:393–400

Anonymous, 1989. *Schistosoma intercalatum*. Parasitol. Today 5:273

Anthony PP, 1974. Carcinoma of the urinary tract and urinary retention in Uganda. Br. J. Urol. 46:201–208

Attawibool S, Bunnag T, Thirachandra S, Sinthuprama K, Sornmani S, 1983. *Schistosoma mansoni*-like infection in Phayao Province, northern Thailand. Southeast Asian J. Trop. Med. Public Health 4:463–466

Beaver PC, Jung RC, Cupp EW, 1984. *Clinical Parasitology*. Philadelphia: Lea & Febiger

Berry A, 1971. Evidence of gynecologic bilharziasis in cytologic material: a morphologic study for cytologists in particular. Acta Cytol. 15:482–498

Bhagwandeen SB, 1976. Schistosomiasis and carcinoma of the bladder in Zambia. S. Afr. Med. J. 50:1616–1620

Biocca E, 1960. Osservazioni sulla morfologia e biologia del ceppo sardo di *Schistosoma bovis* e sulla dermatite umana da esso provocata. Parassitologia 2:47–54

Bouree P, 1979. *Schistosoma intercalatum*: criteres epidemiologiques de differenciation. Med. Mal. Infect. 9:397–406

Brackett A, 1940. Pathology of schistosome dermatitis. Arch. Dermatol. Syphilogr. 42:410–418

Carta A, 1953. Dermatite papulare da cercarie di *Schistosoma bovis* nell'uomo. Bol. Soc. Ital. Biol. Sper. 29:1936–1938

Case Records of the Massachusetts General Hospital, 1985. Case 21-1985. N. Engl. J. Med. 312:1376–1383

Case Records of the Massachusetts General Hospital, 1996a. Case 39-1996. N. Engl. J. Med. 335:1906–1914

Case Records of the Massachusetts General Hospital, 1996b. Case 4-1996. N. Engl. J. Med. 334:382–389

Cassagne JP, Discamps G, 1977. A propos d'un cas de complication hepatique d'une bilharziose a *Schistosoma intercalatum*. Med. Trop. 37:87–89

Catto BA, Lewis FA, Ottesen EA, 1980. *Cercaria*-induced histamine release: a factor in the pathogenesis of schistosome dermatitis? Am. J. Trop. Med. Hyg. 29:886–889

CDC, 1992. Cercarial dermatitis outbreak at a state park—Delaware, 1991. Morb. Mort. Weekly Rep. 41:225–228

Cheever AW, 1969. Quantitative comparison of the intensity of *Schistosoma mansoni* infections in man and experimental animals. Trans. R. Soc. Trop. Med. Hyg. 63:781–795

Cheever AW, 1986. Decalcification of schistosome eggs during staining of tissue sections: a potential source of diagnostic error. Am. J. Trop. Med. Hyg. 35:959–961

Cheever AW, Anderson LA, 1971. Rate of destruction of *Schistosoma mansoni* eggs in the tissues of mice. Am. J. Trop. Med. Hyg. 20:62–68

Cheever AW, Duvall RH, Hallack TA Jr, Minker RG, Malley JD, Malley KG, 1987. Variation of hepatic fibrosis and granuloma size among mouse strains infected with *Schistosoma mansoni*. Am. J. Trop. Med. Hyg. 37:85–97

Chen MC, Chuang CY, Wang FP, Chang PY, Chen YJ, Tang YC, Chou SC, 1981. Colorectal cancer and schistosomiasis. Lancet 1:971–973

Cooppan RM, Naidoo K, Jialal I, 1987. Renal function in urinary schistosomiasis in the Natal province of South Africa. Am. J. Trop. Med. Hyg. 37:556–561

Corachan M, Mas R, Palacin A, Romero R, Mondelo F, Pujol J, 1987. Autochthonous case of *Schistosoma intercalatum* from equatorial Guinea. Am. J. Trop. Med. Hyg. 36:343–344

Corachan M, Valls ME, Gascon J, Almeda J, Vilana R, 1994. Hematospermia: a new etiology of clinical interest. Am. J. Trop. Med. Hyg. 50:580–584

Cort WW, 1950. Studies on schistosome dermatitis. XI. Status of knowledge after more than twenty years. Am. J. Hyg. 52:251–307

Dean DA, Mangold BL, 1992. Evidence that both normal and immune elimination of *Schistosoma mansoni* take place at the lung stage of migration prior to parasite death. Am. J. Trop. Med. Hyg. 47:238–248

DePaola D, Winslow DJ, 1967. Geographic pathology of schistosomiasis *mansoni*. Studies of liver injury. In: Mostofi FK (ed), *Bilharziasis*. International Academy of Pathology. Special Monograph. New York: Springer-Verlag, pp. 212–229

DeWitt WB, Oliver-Gonzalez J, Medina E, 1964. Effects of improving the nutrition of malnourished people infected with *Schistosoma mansoni*. Am. J. Trop. Med. Hyg. 13:25–35

Dimmette RM, Elwi AM, Sproat HF, 1956. Relationship of schistosomiasis to polyposis and adenocarcinoma of large intestine. Am. J. Clin. Pathol. 26:266–276

Dominguez A, Borges J, 1962. La mielitis producida por el *Schistosoma mansoni*. Arch. Venez. Patol. Trop. Parasitol. Med. 4:129–141

Edington GM, Nnwabuebo I, Junaid TA, 1975. The pathology of schistosomiasis in Ibadan, Nigeria with special reference to the appendix, brain, pancreas and genital organs. Trans. R. Soc. Trop. Med. Hyg. 69:153–162

Elem B, Purohit R, 1983. Carcinoma of the urinary bladder in Zambia. A quantitative estimation of *Schistosoma haematobium* infection. Br. J. Urol. 55:275–278

Elmasalme FN, Raheem MA, Badawy A, Zuberi SR, Matbouli SA, 1997. Rectosigmoid bilharzioma causing intestinal obstruction. J. Pediatr. Surg. 32:631–633

Elwi AM, 1967. Pathological aspects of bilharziasis in Egypt. In: Mostofi FK (ed), *Bilharziasis*. International Academy of Pathology. Special Monograph. New York: Springer-Verlag, pp. 39–44

Farrell AM, Woodrow D, Bryceson AD, Bunker CB, Cream JJ, 1996. Ectopic cutaneous schistosomiasis: extragenital involvement with progressive upward spread. Br. J. Dermatol. 135:110–112

Fataar S, Satyanath S, 1986. The radiographic evaluation of appendiceal calcification due to schistosomiasis. Am. J. Trop. Med. Hyg. 35:1157–1162

Fripp PJ, Joubert J, 1991. Occurrence of *Schistosoma mattheei*-like eggs in a spinal cord lesion. Trans. R. Soc. Trop. Med. Hyg. 85:230

Gagliardi D, Corsi PR, Eckley CA, Marigo C, Fava J, 1997. Esophageal schistosomiasis in a patient with megaesophagus. Dis. Esophagus 10:71–73

Gelfand M, 1967. Some remarkds on the cliinical and pathological aspects of schistosomiasis in Central Africa. In: Mostofi FK (ed), *Bilharziasis*. International Academy of Pathology. Special Monograph. New York: Springer-Verlag, pp. 104–114

Gelfand M, Ross CMD, Blair DM, Castle WM, Weber MC, 1970. Schistosomiasis of the male pelvic organs: severity of infection as determined by digestion of tissue and histologic methods in 300 cadavers. Am. J. Trop. Med. Hyg. 19:779–784

Gelfand M, Ross MD, Blair DM, Weber MC, 1971. Distribution and extent of schistosomiasis in female pelvic organs, with special reference to the genital tracts, as determined at autopsy. Am. J. Trop. Med. Hyg. 20:846–849

Giboda M, Malek EA, Correa R, 1997. Human schistosomiasis in Puerto Rico: reduced prevalence rate and absence of *Biomphalaria glabrata*. Am. J. Trop. Med. Hyg. 57:564–568

Greer GJ, Yang CKO, Yong HS, 1988. *Schistosoma malayensis* n. sp.: a *Schistosoma japonicum*-complex schistosome from peninsular Malaysia. J. Parasitol. 74:471–480

Hagan P, 1992. Reinfection, exposure and immunity in human schistosomiasis. Parasitol. Today 7:2–16

Hall SC, Kehoe EL, 1970. Prolonged survival of *Schistosoma japonicum*. California Med. 113:75–77

Hamrick LW, Cleve EA, Carson RP, 1950. Chronic schistosomiasis japonica: diagnosis by rectal biopsy with description of sigmoidoscopic abnormalities. Am. J. Med. Sci. 220:393–399

Hatz C, Jenkins JM, Ali QM, Abdel-Wahab MF, Cerri GG, Tanner M, 1992. A review of the literature on the use of ultrasonography in schistosomiasis with special reference to its use in field studies. 2. *Schistosoma mansoni*. Acta Trop. 51:15–28

Hira PR, 1975. Observations on *Schistosoma mattheei* Veglia and Le Roux, 1929 infections in man in Zambia. Ann. Soc. Belge Med. Trop. 55:633–642

Houba V, 1979. Experimental renal disease due to schistosomiasis. Kidney Int. 16:30–43

Karanja DM, Colley DG, Nahlen BL, Ouma JH, Secor WE, 1997. Studies on schistosomiasis in western Kenya: I. Evidence for immune-facilitated excretion of schistosome eggs from patients with *Schistosoma mansoni* and human immunodeficiency virus coinfections. Am. J. Trop. Med. Hyg. 56:515–521

Kitinya JN, Lauren PA, Eshleman LJ, Paljarvi L, Tanaka K, 1986. The incidence of squamous and transitional cell carcinomas of the urinary bladder in northern Tanzania in areas of high and low levels of endemic *Schistosoma haematobium* infection. Trans. R. Soc. Trop. Med. Hyg. 80:935–939

Lechtenberg R, Vaida GA, 1977. Schistosomiasis of the spinal cord. Neurology 27:55–59

MacFarlane WV, 1949. Schistosome dermatitis in New Zealand. Part II. Pathology and immunology of cercarial lesions. Am. J. Hyg. 50:152–167

Malek EA, 1980. *Snail-transmitted Parasitic Diseases*. Vols. I and II. Boca Raton, Fla.: CRC Press

Marcial-Rojas RA, Fiol RF, 1963. Neurologic complications of schistosomiasis: review of the literature and report of two cases of transverse myelitis due to *S. mansoni*. Ann. Intern. Med. 59:215–130

Mawad NM, Hassanein OM, Mahmoud OM, Taylor MG, 1992. Schistosomal vulval granuloma in a 12 years old Sudanese girl. Trans. R. Soc. Trop. Med. Hyg. 86:644

McLaren DJ, 1989. Will the real target of immunity to schistosomiasis please stand up? Parasitol. Today 5:279–282

Medhat A, Zarzour A, Nafeh M, Shata T, Sweifie Y, Attia M, Helmy A, Shehata M, Zaki S, Mikhail N, Ibrahim S,

King C, Strickland GT, 1997. Evaluation of an ultrasonographic score for urinary bladder morbidity in *Schistosoma haematobium* infection. Am. J. Trop. Med. Hyg. 57:16–19

Milligan A, Burns DA, 1988. Ectopic cutaneous schistosomiasis and schistosomal ocular inflammatory disease. Br. J. Dermatol. 119:793–798

Morris W, Knauer CM, 1997. Cardiopulmonary manifestations of schistosomiasis. Semin. Respir. Infect. 12:159–170

Mostafa MH, Badawi AF, O'Connor PJ, 1995. Bladder cancer associated with schistosomiasis. Parasitol. Today 11:87–89

Mousa AH, Ata AA, El Rooby A, 1967. Clincio-pathological aspects of hepatosplenic bilharziasis. In: Mostofi FK (ed), *Bilharziasis*. International Academy of Pathology. Special Monograph. New York: Springer-Verlag, pp. 15–29

Murugasu R, Wang F, Dissanaike AS, 1978. *Schistosoma japonicum*-type infection in Malaysiaùreport of the first living case. Trans. R. Soc. Trop. Med. Hyg. 72:389–391

Obasi OE, 1986. Cutaneous schistosomiasis in Nigeria. an update. Br. J. Dermatol. 114:597–602

Odongo-Aginya EI, Mueller A, Loroni-Lakwo T, Ndugwa CM, Southgate VR, Schweigmann U, Seitz HM, Doehring-Schwerdtfeger E, 1994. Evidence for the occurrence of *Schistosoma intercalatum* at Albert Nile in northern Uganda. Am. J. Trop. Med. Hyg. 50:723–726

Olds GR, Kresina TF, 1985. Network interactions in *Schistosoma japonicum* infection: identification and characterization of a serologically distinct immunoregulatory auto-antiidiotypic antibody population. J. Clin. Invest. 76:2338–2347

Oyediran ABOO, 1979. Renal disease due to schistosomiasis of the lower urinary tract. Kidney Int. 16:15–22

Pammenter MD, Haribhai HC, Epstein SR, Rossouw EJ, Bhigjee AI, Bill PLA, 1996. The value of immunological approaches to the diagnosis of schistosomal myelopathy. Am. J. Trop. Med. Hyg. 44:329–335

Pittella JEH, 1985. Vascular changes in cerebral schistosomiasis *mansoni*: a histopathological study of fifteen cases. Am. J. Trop. Med. Hyg. 34:898–902

Pittella JEH, 1997. Neuroschistosomiasis. Brain Pathol. 7:649–662

Queiroz L de S, Nucci A, Facure NO, Facure JJ, 1979. Massive spinal cord necrosis in schistosomiasis. Arch. Neurol. 36:517–519

Razdan S, Vlachiotis JD, Edelstein RA, Krane RJ, Siroky MB, 1997. Schistosomal myelopathy as a cause of neurogenic bladder dysfunction. Urology. 49:777–780

Sadigursky M, Andrade ZA, 1982. Pulmonary changes in schistosomal cor pulmonale. Am. J. Trop. Med. Hyg. 31:779–784

Sadun EH, Lichtenberg FV, Cheever AW, Erickson DG, Hickman RL, 1970. Experimental infection with *Schistosoma haematobium* in chimpanzees. Parasitologic, clinical, serologic, and pathological observations. Am. J. Trop. Med. Hyg. 19:427–458

Saliba EK, Tawfiq MR, Kharabsheh S, Rahamneh J, 1997. Urinary schistosomiasis contracted from an irrigation pool in Ramah, the southern Jordan Valley, Jordan. Am. J. Trop. Med. Hyg. 57:158–161

Savioli L, Renganathan E, Montresor A, Davis A, Behbehani K, 1997. Control of schistosomiasis—a global picture. Parasitol. Today 13:444–448

Shaw AFB, Ghareeb AA, 1938. The pathogenesis of pulmonary schistosomiasis in Egypt with special reference to Ayerza's disease. J. Pathol. Bacteriol. 46:401–429

Shekhar KC, 1991. *Schistosoma malayensis*: the biologic, clinical, and pathologic features in man and experimental animals. Prog. Clin. Parasitol. 2:145–178

Smith JH, Christie JD, 1986. The pathobiology of *Schistosoma haematobium* infection in humans. Hum. Pathol. 17:333–345

Smith JH, Kamel IA, Elwi A, von Lictenberg F, 1974. A quantitative postmortem analysis of urinary schistosomiasis in Egypt I. Pathology and pathogensis. Am. J. Trop. Med. Hyg. 23:1054–1071

Smith JH, Kelada AS, Khalil A, Torky AH, 1977a. Surgical pathology of schistosomal obstructive uropathy: a clinicopathologic correlation. Am. J. Trop. Med. Hyg. 26:96–108

Smith JH, Torky H, Kelada AS, Farid Z, 1977b. Schistosomal polyposis of the urinary bladder. Am. J. Trop. Med. Hyg. 26:85–88

Smith JH, Von Lichtenberg F, 1976. Tissue degradation of calcific *Schistosoma haematobium* eggs. Am. J. Trop. Med. Hyg. 25:595–601

Smithers SR, Terry RJ, Hockley DJ, 1969. Host antigens in schistosomiasis. Proc. R. Soc. 171:483–494

Sornmani S, Kitikoon V, Thirachantra S, Harinasuta C, 1980. Epidemiology of Mekong schistosomiasis. In: Bruce JSS (ed), *The Mekong Schistosome*. Malacol. Rev. (Suppl 2):9–18

Thomas JE, Bassett MT, Sigola LB, Taylor P, 1990. Relationship between bladder cancer incidence, *Schistosoma haematobium* infection, and geographical region in Zimbabwe. Trans. R. Soc. Trop. Med. Hyg. 84:551–553

Voge M, Bruckner D, Bruce JI, 1978. *Schistosoma mekongi* sp. n. from man and animals, compared with four geographic strains of *Schistosoma japonicum*. J. Parasitol. 64:577–584

Von Lichtenberg F, Edington GM, Nwabuebo I, Taylor JR,

Smith JH, 1971. Pathologic effects of schistosomiasis in Ibadan, western state of Nigeria. II. Pathogenesis of lesions of the bladder and ureters. Am. J. Trop. Med. Hyg. 20:244–254

Walt F, 1954. The Katayama syndrome. S. Afr. Med. J. 28:89–92

Warren KS, 1978. The pathology, pathobiology and pathogenesis of schistosomiasis. Nature 273:609–612

Warren KS, Domingo EO, 1970a. *Schistosoma mansoni*: Stage specificity of granuloma formation around eggs after exposure to irradiated cercariae, unisexual infections, or dead worms. Exp. Parasitol. 27:60–66

Warren KS, Domingo EO, 1970b. Granuloma formation around *Schistosoma mansoni*, *S. haematobium* and *S. japonicum* eggs. Size and rate of development cellular composition, cross-sensitivity and rate of egg destruction. Am. J. Trop. Med. Hyg. 19:292–304

Warren KS, Domingo EO, Cowan RBT, 1967. Granuloma formation around schistosome eggs as a manifestation of delayed hypersensitivity. Am. J. Pathol. 51:735–756

WHO, 1980. Scientific working group. Parasite-related diarrhoeas. Bull. WHO 58:819–830

Winslow DJ, 1967. Histopathology of schistosomiasis. In: Mostofi FK (ed), *Bilharziasis*. International Academy of Pathology. Special Monograph. New York: Springer-Verlag, pp. 230–241

Wright ED, Chiphangwi J, Hutt MSR, 1982. Schistosomiasis of the female genital tract. A histopathological study of 176 cases from Malawi. Trans. R. Soc. Trop. Med. Hyg. 76:822–829

Wyler DJ, 1983. Regulation of fibroblast functions by products of schistosomal egg granulomas: potential role in the pathogenesis of hepatic fibrosis. In: *Cytopathology of Parasitic Disease*. Ciba Foundation Symposium 99. London: Pitman Books Ltd., pp. 190–206

Yazdanpanah Y, Thomas AK, Kardorff R, Talla I, Seydou S, Niang M, Stelma FF, Decam C, Rogerie F, Gryseels B, Capron A, Doehring E, 1997. Organometric investigations of the spleen and liver by ultrasound in *Schistosoma mansoni* endemic and nonendemic villages in Senegal. Am. J. Trop. Med. Hyg. 57:245–249

Zahran MM, Badr MM, 1980. Study of bilharzial uropathy by means of Hippuran I131 extended renography. Am. J. Trop. Med. Hyg. 29:576–581

24

BILIARY AND PANCREATIC TREMATODES

The trematodes of the biliary and pancreatic ducts of humans belong to three families: Fasciolidae, Opistorchiidae, and Dicrocoeliidae. Fasciolidae includes *Fasciola hepatica*, which is endemic worldwide, producing important morbidity in certain geographic areas, and *F. gigantica*, with a more restricted distribution. The members of Opistorchiidae are widely distributed, producing a large number of infections but generally with low morbidity. Finally, the members of Dicrocoeliidae have species that usually occur in humans as sporadic zoonotic infections. All species in these families have two intermediate hosts. The first is a snail; the second, varying with the group, consists of either plants, fish, or arthropods (Beaver et al. 1984; Malek, 1980). The accompanying classification of these trematodes is provided only for general information. It follows Malek's (1980) classification, showing only the genera and the species of human importance.

Most of the genera and species of these three families are parasites of the gallbladder, the biliary ducts, and the pancreatic excretory ducts. Members of the family Fasciolidae occur naturally in herbivorous mammals, especially cattle, sheep, goats, and humans; those of the Dicrocoeliidae are parasites of both mammals and birds; and those of the Opistorchiidae occur nat-

Family: Fasciolidae
    Genus: *Fasciola. F. hepatica* and *F. gigantica*

Family: Opistorchiidae
    Genus: *Clonorchis. C. sinensis*
    Genus: *Opistorchis. O. felineus* and *O. viverrini*
    Genus: *Amphimerus. A. pseudofelineus*
    Genus: *Metorchis. M. conjunctus*

Family: Dicrocoeliidae
    Genus: *Dicrocoelium. D. dendriticum* and *D. hospes*
    Genus: *Eurythrema. E. pancreaticum*

urally in several classes of vertebrates, including humans. Since humans use as food many of the animal species that these trematodes inhabit, individuals sometimes ingest parasites with the cooked or raw viscera. In these cases, the digestion of the viscera with the parasites frees the eggs from the tissues, and they pass in the feces, where they are sometimes found in the stools. When this occurs, the result is a spurious parasitism, or pseudoparasitism, which requires careful investigation before making a definitive diagnosis (see below).

Fasciola—Fascioliasis

The trematodes causing fascioliasis have been known for 120 years and occur in almost every place in the world where cattle and sheep are raised. In some areas these parasites are endemic in humans, in whom they sometimes produce outbreaks. Infections in humans are important because of the morbidity they produce, manifested clearly as chronic cholangitis. In general, two species are known: *F. hepatica*, the more common one, and *F. gigantica*.

Morphology. The genus *Fasciola* is characterized by a highly branched ceca (Fig. 24–1 *A*), which allows the parasites to be easily identified in tissue sections (Figs. 24–4 *B* and 24–6 *B*). *Fasciola hepatica* measures up to 4.0 cm in length by 1.3 cm in width and 0.1 cm in thickness; it is a relatively slender, delicate worm with a cephalic cone resting on two shoulders. *Fasciola gigantica* measures up to 7.0 cm long by 1.1 cm wide and 0.1 cm in thickness; see Fig. 23–1 *B*). On superficial examination, the adult worms of these two species look similar, but they have morphologic differences other than their size. In general, *F. hepatica* is wider, with wider shoulders and a larger cephalic cone; in addition, the ceca are less branched than those of *F. gigantica* (Malek, 1980). The two suckers are more or less similar in size, and the ventral sucker (acetabulum) is located at the base of the cephalic cone.

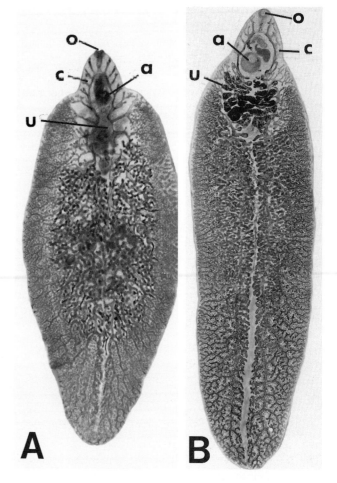

Fig. 24–1. *Fasciola* adults, acetic-alum carmine stain. *A*, *F. hepatica*, ×4. *B*, *F. gigantica*, ×2.8. Abbreviations: o, oral sucker; a, acetabulum; c, branched ceca (intestine); u, uterus. Note that the highly branched ceca make the ovary and testes difficult to recognize in these black-and-white pictures.

Life Cycle. The parasites are located within the biliary ducts, where they deposit eggs that measure 130 to 150 × 63 to 90 μm (*F. hepatica*) and 160 to 190 × 70 to 90 μm (*F. gigantica*). The eggs are passed with the bile into the intestine and with the feces to the outside environment, where they embryonate in fresh water to produce miracidia, which enter an appropriate snail, the first intermediate host. After development through several larval stages in the snail, the cercariae develop and exit the snail to encyst in aquatic vegetation that, on ingestion, releases the infective stages in the intestine. The young larvae penetrate the intestinal wall and pass into the peritoneal cavity, where they migrate toward the liver. On reaching the liver, the larvae enter Glisson's capsule and migrate through the parenchyma until they find the appropriate bile duct, where they attain maturity (Fig. 24–2; Malek, 1980). Because of the migratory pathway followed by *Fasciola* in their final host, ectopic locations of these parasites are the most important factor for the anatomic pathologist. Immature stages and adults of *Fasciola* potentially occur in every organ system, but the subcutaneous tissue is most commonly affected. In experimental infections of animals, the prepatent period (from infection to appearance of eggs in the stools) was 8 weeks, and the patent period was about 40 weeks (DeLeon et al. 1981).

Geographic Distribution and Epidemiology. *Fasciola hepatica* has a worldwide distribution in cattle, sheep,

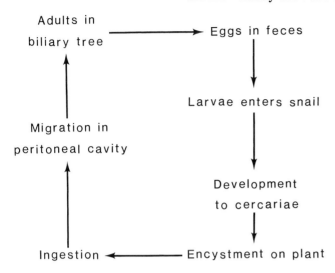

Adults in
biliary tree → Eggs in feces

↓

Larvae enters snail

↓

Development
to cercariae

↓

Migration in
peritoneal cavity

Ingestion ← Encystment on plant

Fig. 24–2. *Fasciola*, **schematic representation of the life cycle.**

goats, other animals, and humans. *Fasciola gigantica* is more restricted and occurs in Africa, certain areas of the Middle East, India, Southeast Asia, and Hawaii, where it is a parasite mainly in cattle, sheep, goats, and water buffaloes. Human infections caused by *F. gigantica* occur in the endemic areas, producing identical clinical and pathologic manifestations. Fascioliasis is endemic in humans mainly in Central and South America, Europe, the Middle East, North and South Africa, and Hawaii. The infection is particularly important in France, Spain (the Basque region, Navarra, and Rioja; Garcia-Rodriguez et al. 1985), Puerto Rico, Cuba, Brazil, Bolivia (the Altiplano) (Esteban et al. 1997a), and other Latin American countries where the disease is not rare. Outbreaks have occurred in the United Kingdom (Facey, Marsden, 1960; Hunt, 1972) and recently in Bolivia (Bjorland et al. 1995). Clusters of cases in families have also been reported (Bechtel et al. 1992), and one case acquired in the continental United States is known (Norton, Monroe, 1961). More often, the cases seen in the United States are imported (Price et al. 1993), but autochthonous cases are common in Hawaii (Alicata, 1953; Stemmermann, 1953) and Puerto Rico (Anibal et al. 1978; Bendezu et al. 1982). The infection in humans is acquired mostly by the ingestion of raw watercress nuts (Alicata, Bonnet, 1955; Amaral, Busetti, 1979). The snail species that acts as the first intermediate host of *Fasciola* varies with the locality, but most of these snails belong to the genus *Lymnaea*; in the Caribbean and the southern United States, the main hosts are species of *Fossaria* (Malek, 1980).

No reliable data on the worldwide prevalence of fascioliasis exist. A stool survey in a community of the Bolivian Altiplano showed a general prevalence of 67%; the rate was 75% in children and 42% in adults (Esteban et al. 1997b). In another community of the Altiplano, 28% of the children were infected (Esteban et al. 1997a). In the Nile Delta of Egypt, a coprologic survey showed a prevalence of over 7% (Farag et al. 1979). A serologic survey in Chile demonstrated that in three provinces examined, the prevalence was less than 1%, which corresponded to about 2000 cases in the population surveyed (Apt et al. 1993). In recent years the number of cases in known endemic areas has increased, but whether this increase is the result of better diagnostic techniques or a true increase in prevalence is not known.

Clinical Findings. The main symptoms and signs of fascioliasis involve the gastrointestinal system, specifically the biliary system. In some individuals the onset of the acute disease is sudden, with acute chest, epigastric, or right hypochondrial pain often radiating to the right scapular area and occasionally to the iliac fossa. Fever of 39°C to 41°C with considerable sweating and weight loss are often present (de Gorgolas et al. 1992). In children, fever and abdominal pain are the main symptoms (el Shabrawi et al. 1997). These symptoms vary in duration, sometimes lasting for several days. In other patients, the same symptoms have a more insidious onset, progressing slowly until they become full blown. Allergic manifestations, consisting mostly of urticarial rash (Rodriguez-Barreras et al. 1986), pruritus, weals with dermatographia, and asthma, are present in most cases. Anorexia, fatigue, and weight loss often occur. In chronic cases, which sometimes last for several years, the symptoms are more nonspecific and are related to the abdomen and the biliary tree. Obstructive biliary symptoms with fluctuant jaundice may be apparent, especially in critically ill individuals (Banna et al. 1979; Bannerman, Manzur, 1986; Cosme et al. 1979). Profuse bleeding due to ulceration of the bile duct has been reported (Acuna-Soto, Braun-Roth, 1987; Bannerman, Manzur, 1986).

Physical examination reveals an enlarged and tender liver, exquisite epigastric pain, and sometimes a positive Murphy's sign (Arjona et al. 1995). Moderate splenomegaly is present in some patients. In some cases, the obstructing fluke has been removed from the distal common bile duct during endoscopy (Danilewitz et al. 1996). Laboratory tests are positive for leukocytosis up to 41,500 with eosinophilia up to 81%, but there is no correlation between the symptoms and peripheral blood eosinophilia. Examination of stools or aspirated duodenal contents reveals the characteristic *Fasciola* eggs in less than 50% of cases (Arenas et al. 1948). Computed tomography of the liver shows multiple low-density nodules that tend to decrease in size (Pagola Serrano et al. 1987; Takeyama et al. 1986). Radiograms of the biliary tree, especially with percutaneous cholangiography (Condomines et al. 1985), ultrasonography (Eisencher, Sauget, 1980), and endoscopic retrograde cholecystopancreatography, may demonstrate the parasites in the biliary tree (Alvarez et al. 1994; Tombazzi et al. 1994; Wong et al. 1985; Fig. 24–3). Endoscopic retrograde cholecystopancreatography is recommended for follow-up of patients under

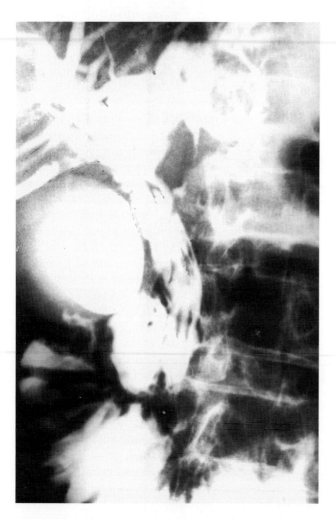

Fig. 24–3. *Fasciola hepatica*, endoscopic retrograde cholangiopancreatogram. Note the marked dilatation of the common bile duct and the filling defects with a "lanceolated" shape (arrows). (Courtesy of J.I. Arenas, M.D., Servicio de Gastroenterologia, Hospital Aranzazu San Sebastian, Universidad del Pais Vasco, Spain.)

treatment (Dias et al. 1996), and endoscopic sphincterotomy allows balloon extraction of the worms for treatment (El-Newihi HM et al. 1995). Computed tomograms and magnetic resonance imaging studies of the liver usually reveal the abscesses and the migratory tracts of the worms (Han et al. 1993, 1996). Laparoscopic examination of the liver shows white and yellow areas with necrotic tracks (Anton-Aranda et al. 1985; Moreto, Barron, 1980).

The ectopic locations of *Fasciola* have no uniform clinical presentation because they vary with the site and the affected organ. Specific diagnosis is based on examination of biopsy or surgical specimens and, rarely, on examination of autopsy material that demonstrates the worm. The most common location, as stated before, is the subcutis, and the clinical presentation consists of a nodule with or without signs of inflammation. The diagnosis of pulmonary migration of the worms is often based on the clinical picture. If the pulmonary symptoms occur in conjunction with the demonstration of the worm in the liver or other places, or the eggs in the stools, they are more credible (Alcoaba-Leza et al. 1973). In these patients there are either pulmonary infiltrates, pleural effusions, pneumothorax, or a combination of the three (Alcoaba-Leza et al. 1973; Crinquette et al. 1965). The worms have been passed by patients in the urine (Catchpole, Snow, 1952), sneezed up, and coughed up (Stemmermann, 1953).

Pathology. The pathologic changes produced by *Fasciola* infection in humans resemble to some extent those observed in their natural definitive hosts. In animals experimentally infected, there is a phase of acute hepatitis produced by the migration of young flukes through the parenchyma. The worms locate first in small bile ducts and later in larger ones where they attain full growth. Eosinophilia is high, especially during the migration of the parasites, and falls to within normal limits after the worms locate in the biliary tree. In chronic infections, the worms result in marked fibrosis of the biliary ducts (Fig. 24–4 *A*), as well as proliferation of the biliary duct epithelium (Fig. 24–4 *B–D*). This proliferation is due to the worm's secretion of proline, an amino acid (Modavi, Isseroff, 1984; Wolf-Spengler, Isseroff, 1983).

In humans, most gross descriptions of the liver in *Fasciola* infections are based on observations during laparoscopy or exploratory laparotomy. The early liver lesions are not well known, but as the infection progresses, small, hemorrhagic, sometimes track-like areas develop (Aguirre-Errasti et al. 1978). The adult para-

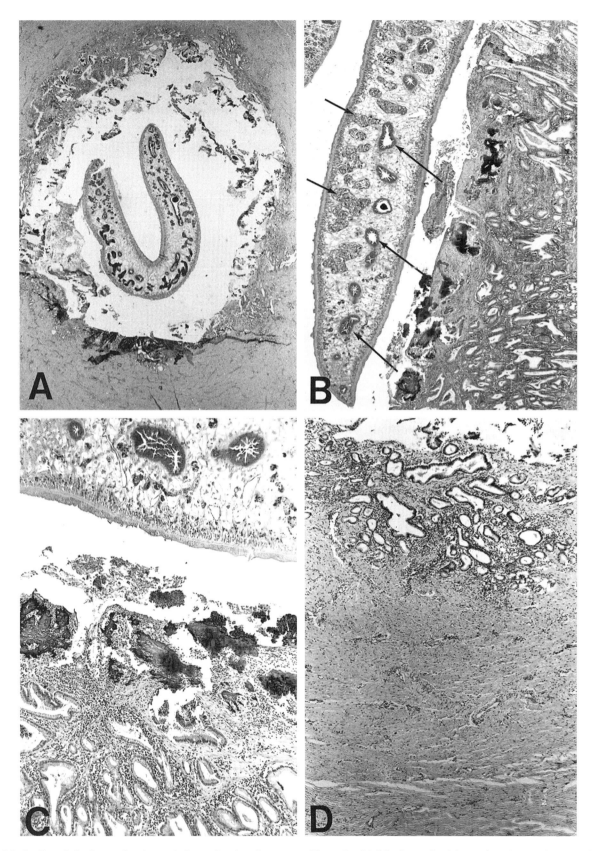

Fig. 24–4. *Fasciola hepatica* in an infected animal, sections stained with hematoxylin and eosin stain. *A*, Low-power view of a bile duct with an adult parasite. Note the fibrosis of the duct wall, ×11. *B*, Higher magnification showing a portion of the parasite and the adenomatous proliferation of the bile duct epithelium. Note the highly branched intestine (cecum) toward the ventral aspect of the worm (long arrows) and the testis in the dorsal aspect (short arrows), ×22. *C* and *D*, Higher magnification illustrates the parasite in *C*, the epithelial proliferation in *C* and *D*, and the duct fibrosis in *D*, ×55.

sites commonly form abscesses, with necrosis of the bile duct and involvement of the adjacent liver parenchyma. The eggs trapped in the wall of the abscess or the parenchyma often produce a granulomatous inflammation. The abscesses, if numerous, result in cholangitis with abscess formation and enlargement of the liver, which grossly shows multiple yellow nodules 0.5 to 1.5 cm in diameter. The nodules may be seen on the surface and sometimes have been mistaken for metastatic tumor (Acosta-Ferreira et al. 1979; Anton-Aranda et al. 1985). On cut section, the abscesses often occur throughout the entire parenchyma; sometimes the flukes can be recovered from these abscesses or from the bile ducts (Acosta-Ferreira et al. 1979). Abscesses on the diaphragmatic surface of the liver can rupture into the pleural cavity, producing an effusion that is difficult to treat (Alicata, 1953).

Microscopic examination reveals track-like lesions consisting of granulomas produced by eggs lost in the parenchyma (Fig. 24–5 C) and abscesses, sometimes with *Fasciola* eggs (Fig. 24–5 A–B). Some abscesses are believed to originate in a bile duct because they are partially lined with epithelium (Fig. 24–5 B); they produce obstruction manifested by the adjacent bile duct proliferation (Fig. 24–5 D). Older lesions are organized and fibrotic (Fig. 24–5 A) and may contain *Fasciola* eggs in well-formed granulomas or in the liver parenchyma. Charcot-Leyden crystals and infiltration by polymorphonuclear cells, especially eosinophils, are common in early lesions (Fig. 24–5 B), changing later to polymorphonuclear cells and many histiocytes and lymphocytes. As the lesions become older, fibrosis and calcification with a predominantly lymphocytic and plasmacytic infiltration develop (Acosta-Ferreira et al. 1979; Aguirre-Errasti et al. 1978; Anton-Aranda et al. 1985; Echevarrieta et al. 1982). Another microscopic change in the gallbladder is infiltration of the wall by eosinophils.

Ectopic Locations. *Fasciola* has often been described in tissues and organs other than the liver, more commonly the subcutaneous tissues. Other organs and sites affected are the inner ear, producing otitis media (Alicata, 1953); the lung (Alcoaba-Leza et al. 1973; Atias,

Fernandez, 1965; Crinquette et al. 1965); the brain (Aguirre-Errasti et al. 1981; Catchpole, Snow, 1952); the intestinal wall (Park et al. 1984; Fig. 24–6 A–D) and the stomach (Catchpole, Snow, 1952); the urinary system (Catchpole, Snow, 1952); the pancreas (Imai et al. 1974; Stemmermann, 1953); the epididymis (Aguirre-Errasti et al. 1981); the peripheral veins (Catchpole, Snow, 1952) and the portal vein (Duval, 1842); the spleen (Rao, Choudary, 1979); the lymph nodes (Arjona et al. 1995); the eye, producing inflammatory changes that require enucleation (Cho et al. 1994); and the skeletal muscles (Hoffmann, Guerra, 1923). The pathologic manifestations are those of an abscess, usually with the parasite and sometimes with eggs in the tissues.

Diagnosis. *Fasciola* infection is diagnosed on clinical grounds, especially in endemic areas. Liver and bile duct imaging techniques may show suggestive patterns of liver lesions; images of worms in the bile tree are diagnostic (Fig. 24–3). Laparoscopy and exploratory laparotomy often show the typical gross lesions; biopsy specimens may show eggs, adult worms, or changes suggestive of the infection. Often the diagnosis is made by recovery of adult worms from a removed gallbladder or from the bile ducts during biliary surgery. *Fasciola hepatica* eggs (Fig. 24–7 A–B) are usually not recovered from the stools and are found in only about 40% of duodenal aspirates (Arenas et al. 1948). All individuals with *Fasciola* eggs in their stools should be reexamined 3 days after abstention from consumption of liver and other meat products; spurious parasitism should always be ruled out (see above). The enzyme-linked immunosorbent assay has been used to detect antibodies against excretory-secretory products of the parasite as antigens (Hillyer et al. 1992). With this assay, the diagnosis appears specific enough to differentiate *Fasciola* from other trematode infections (Espino et al. 1987). The enzyme-linked immunosorbent assay, using cathepsin L1 secreted by juvenile parasites as an antigen to detect specific immunoglobulin G4 (IgG4) antibodies, has been found highly reliable for diagnosis. However, the availability of cathepsin L1 is limited

Fig. 24–5. *Fasciola hepatica* in human liver, sections stained with hematoxylin and eosin stain. *A,* Low-power view of a large granuloma with a necrotic center containing eggs (arrows) and a fibrous wall. Note the inflammatory infiltrate, ×55. *B,* Higher magnification of a bile duct partially destroyed by necrosis extending beyond its wall. Two nonviable *Fasciola* eggs are seen within the necrotic debris, ×140. *C,* Liver parenchyma showing a granuloma, fibrosis, and an intense inflammatory reaction, ×55. *D,* Medium-sized bile duct showing epithelial proliferation and fibrosis, ×55. (Preparations courtesy of A. Gastaminza, M.D., Hospital Provincial de Guipuzcoa, San Sebastian, Spain.)

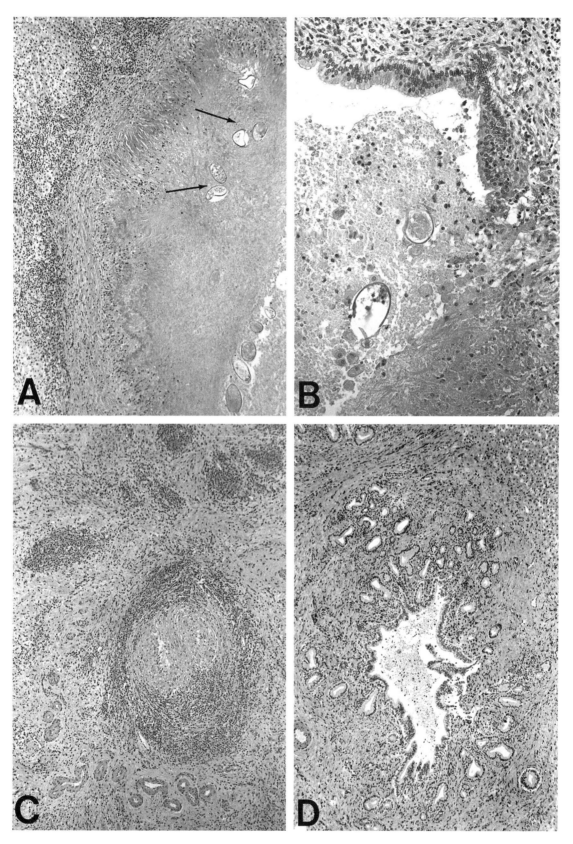

Fig. 24–5.

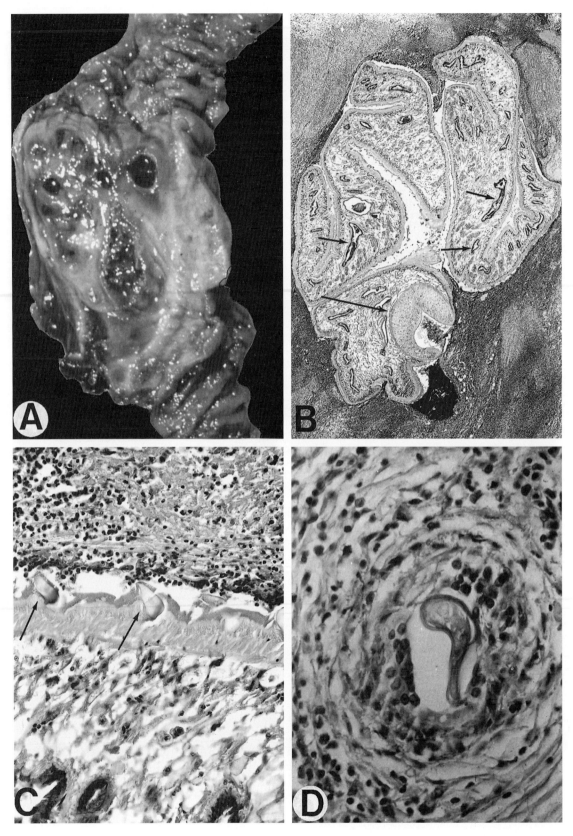

Fig. 24–6.

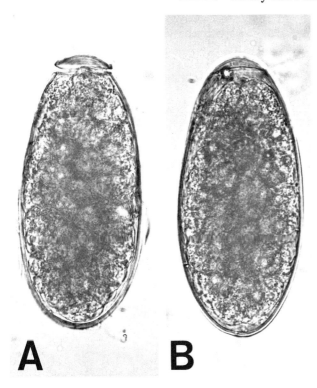

Fig. 24–7. *A* and *B*, *Fasciola hepatica* eggs, unstained, ×495.

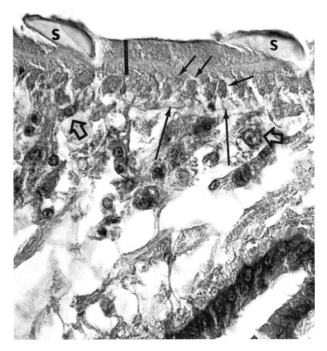

Fig. 24–8. *Fasciola hepatica* tegument, hematoxylin and eosin stain. The tegument of *Fasciola* is similar to that of other trematodes. The outer zone (vertical bar) is composed of a continuous cytoplasmic layer consisting of cytoplasmic extensions from cells located below in the mesenchyme of the worm (open arrow). These cells extend portions of their cytoplasm through the muscle layer of the worm (longitudinal muscles, long arrows; circular and oblique muscles, short arrows) to form the outer zone. The spines (s) of the worm are covered by cell membrane and thus are intracellular, ×495. (See Fig. III–2.)

at present (O'Neill et al. 1998). Serology, imaging techniques, and the response to specific treatment were considered diagnostic in one case (Hauser, Bynum, 1984).

In histologic sections of liver, the diagnosis is based on characteristic lesions, adults, and eggs. In ectopic locations, the diagnosis is based on finding the adult parasite and identifying it morphologically. *Fasciola hepatica* and *F. gigantica* are indistinguishable in tissue sections, and only the generic term *Fasciola* should be used when reporting the identity of the worm (Figs. 24–4 *A–B* and 24–6 *B*).

On histologic sections, *Fasciola* has all the characteristics of a trematode. The tegument of the worm (the most exterior aspect) is composed of several regions (Fig. 24–8). The exterior surface consists of a continu-

ous layer of cytoplasm that corresponds to a distal cytoplasmic extension of cells located deeper in the mesenchyme. This layer varies in thickness up to 60 μm and contains spines that are slightly longer than the thickness of the outer layer of the tegument. The spines are cover by the cell membrane and thus are intracellular (Fig. 24–8). Below the outer layer of the cuticle are longitudinal and circular muscle fibers, and below

Fig. 24–6. *Fasciola*, ectopic location in the wall of the cecum of a Korean woman, with a clinical diagnosis of colonic carcinoma before resection. *A*, Cecal mass with numerous abscess-like cavities corresponding to the migratory path of the worm. *B–D*. Histologic sections stained with hematoxylin and eosin stain. *B*, Oblique section showing several cuts of a single twisted parasite appearing as three separate worms. Note the highly branched intestine (short arrows), the acetabulum (long arrow), and the mesenchymal tissue filling the worm's body, ×16. *C*, Higher magnification of tegument illustrating the body spines (arrows), ×200. *D*, A granuloma within the cecal wall produced by an egg, indicating that the worm was a mature adult, ×350. (In: Park, C.I., Kim, H., Ro, J.Y., et al. 1984. Human ectopic fascioliasis in the cecum. Am. J. Surg. Pathol. 8:73–77. Reproduced with permission.)

those are the bodies of the cells that make up the outer tegument (Fig. 24–8).

The internal organs are contained within a lax mesenchyme that fills the entire worm. The uterus containing eggs in mature worms, the testes, the ovaries, the vitelline glands, and the ceca are structures found in histologic sections of the worm, depending on the plane of sectioning. The most prominent structure of *Fasciola* in cross section is the branched ceca (Figs. 24–4 B and 24–6 B), which is seen in almost all cuts of the parasite. The uterus containing eggs is the second most important structure because it allows study and measurements of the eggs, but the uterus is seen infrequently because it is confined to a small region of the worm.

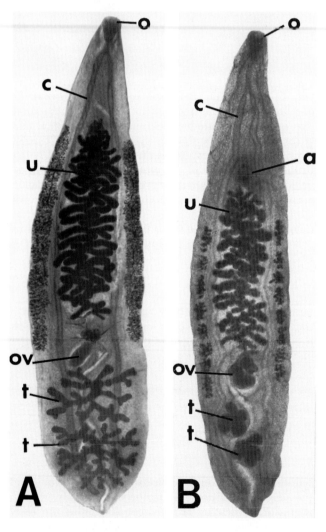

Fig. 24–9. *Clonorchis sinensis* and *Opistorchis viverrini*, adults. A, *C. sinensis*, ×11. B, *O. viverrini*, ×12. Abbreviations: o, oral sucker; a, acetabulum; c, ceca (intestine); t, testes; ov, ovary; u, uterus.

Clonorchis, Opistorchis, and *Amphimerus*—Clonorchiasis, Opistorchiasis, and Amphimeriasis

The family Opistorchiidae (see above) has several genera and species that occur naturally in the bile ducts of fish-eating mammals. Two genera, *Clonorchis* and *Opistorchis*, have species widely distributed in humans and animals because the parasites have low host specificity. One species of the genus *Amphimerus* (*A. pseudophelineus*) occurs in a restricted area of Ecuador, where it was originally described in humans as *Opistorchis guayaquilensis* (Rodriguez-M et al. 1949). The fourth genus, *Metorchis*, also has one species, *M. conjunctus*, reported in humans in Canada (Babbott et al. 1961; Eaton, 1975). The second intermediate host of these species is usually a freshwater fish.

Morphology. The members of the family Opistorchiidae parasitizing humans have a delicate appearance. They are elongated worms that vary in size, depending on their stage of development and the species in question. The largest member of the group is *C. sinensis*, which is up to 25 mm long by 5 mm wide by less than 0.1 mm thick (Fig. 24–9 A and *color plate* XII D). *Amphimerus pseudofelineus* (*color plate* XII H) is approximately one-half the size of *Clonorchis*, and *O. viverrini* is even smaller (Fig. 24–9 B and *color plate* XII F). The eggs of *Clonorchis* vary from 25 to 35 × 12 to 19 μm (Fig. 24–10 A–B), and because of their size, they may be distinguishable from those of *O. viverrini* (16 by 28 μm). The eggs of *O. felineus* (11 by 30 μm) are close in size to those of *O. viverrini*,

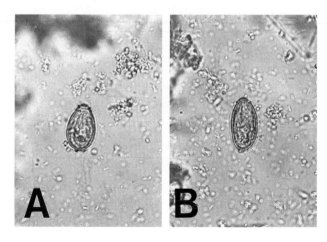

Fig. 24–10. A, B, *Clonorchis-Opistorchis* eggs in human stools, unstained, ×495.

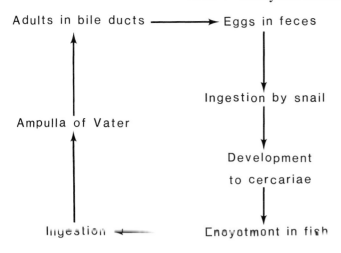

Adults in bile ducts ⟶ Eggs in feces

Ampulla of Vater

Ingestion by snail

Development
to cercariae

Ingestion ⟵ Encystment in fish

Fig. 24–11. *Opistorchiis,* **schematic representation of the life cycle.**

making their differentiation impossible. The eggs of *A. pseudofelineus* are 17 by 35 μm, a size similar to that of *Opistorchis,* but because its geographic distribution is unique so far, it is speciated for clinical purposes on this basis.

Life Cycle. The adult parasites in the biliary ducts lay fully embryonated eggs that pass with the bile into the duodenum and to the outside with the feces. The eggs are ingested by the snails, the first intermediate host, where they hatch. After developing through several larval stages, they produce cercariae that are released by the snail. The cercariae swim to find the fish that act as the second intermediate host and enter through the underside of the fish scales to encyst in the muscles. Ingestion of the fish, either raw or partially cooked, frees the encysted larvae in the stomach and duodenum,

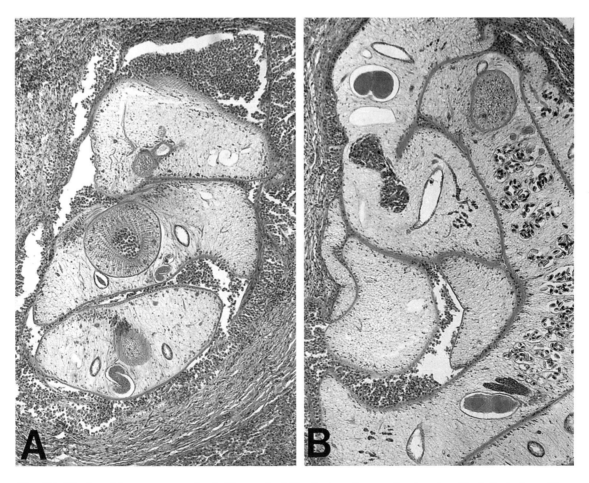

Fig. 24–12. *Amphimerus pseudophelineus* **in bile ducts of an animal naturally infected, section stained with hematoxylin and eosin stain.** *A* **and** *B,* **Parasites within the bile ducts and thickening of the duct wall, ×44.**

where they enter the common bile duct through the ampulla of Vater, migrate to the biliary tree, and grow to adults (Fig. 24–11).

Geographic Distribution and Epidemiology. *Clonorchis sinensis*, the best known of these parasites, is widely distributed in dogs, cats, and humans in China, Taiwan, Japan, Korea, and Vietnam. *Opistorchis felineus* infects humans in southern, central, and eastern Europe, Russia, Turkey, Ukraine, and western Siberia. *Opistorchis viverrini* is endemic in Southeast Asia, especially northern Thailand, Laos, the Mekong Valley, Malaya, Malaysia, and probably other Southeast Asian countries. *Amphimerus pseudofelineus* (= *O. guayaquilensis*) is found in the American continent in cats, dogs (Fig. 24–12), and humans in a small focus in Ecuador. The snails, important intermediate hosts in human transmission, vary across the endemic areas. The species of *Parafossarulus* and *Alocinma* are the vectors of *C. sinensis*. The genus *Bithynia* has the species that act as intermediate hosts for *O. felineus*, and *O. viverrini*.

In endemic areas of *Clonorchis* and *Opistorchis*, rates of human infection are variable. Some places in Japan, China, and Taiwan have prevalence rates of up to 50% with *C. sinensis* infections; in Korea the rate is up to 21% (Seo et al. 1981). In some villages of Russia, *O. felineus* infection rates can reach 65%. In northern Thailand, infections with *O. viverrini* are up to 90% (Sadun, 1955, 1957; Upatham et al. 1982, 1984, 1985). Prevalence rates are even higher among rural dwellers (Kurathong et al. 1987). *Amphimerus pseudofelineus* has been found in up to 32% of individuals in an Ecuadorian village.

Clinical Findings. The clinical manifestations of *Clonorchis* and *Opistorchis* infections vary with the species and the number of worms present at one time. The infection is most prevalent in the 25- to 60-year age group. Acute infection with *Clonorchis* has been described both in Europeans with no previous contact with the parasite (Koenigstein, 1949) and in Chinese in Hong Kong (McFadzean, Yeung, 1965). The initial symptoms in the Europeans are general malaise, fever of up to 40°C, slight jaundice, enlargement and tenderness of the liver, and peripheral eosinophilia of 10% to 88%. The Chinese subjects with previous infections had epigastric pain, fever, and vomiting. Three to 4 weeks later, all infected individuals had *Clonorchis* eggs in their stools. Other laboratory tests, especially biliary tree imaging (ultrasound scans, cholangiograms, and endoscopic retrograde cholangiograms) may demonstrate the worms (Choi et al. 1984) and often biliary

obstruction (Fig. 24–13). Peritoneal endoscopy shows the marked inflammation of the biliary tree (Hitanant et al. 1987); endoscopic biliary lavage has been used to remove the worms, biliary mud, and stones (Navab et al. 1984).

The chronic infection is apparently asymptomatic. In controlled studies of individuals infected with *Clonorchis* living in the United States (without reinfection), no chronic symptoms could be attributed to the parasite even in those with large numbers of eggs in their stools (Markell, 1966; Strauss, 1962). However, the overall morbidity of these infections has not been fully evaluated. Ultrasonographic studies of individuals living in endemic areas, showed that most of them, with mild to moderate infections with *O. viverrini*, developed chronic inflammation of the biliary tree; these changes reverted after treatment (Pungpak et al.

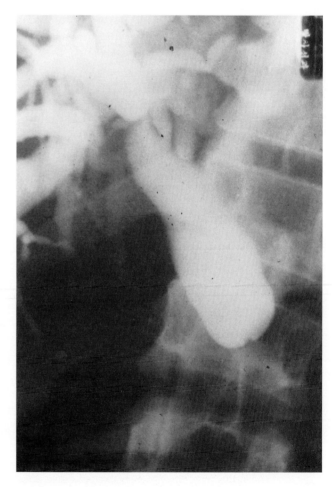

Fig. 24–13. *Clonorchis sinensis*, **cholangiogram of a heavily infected individual. Note the marked distention of the bile passages due to obstruction. (Courtesy of H. Kim, M.D., Department of Pathology, Yonsei University Medical College, Seoul, South Korea.)**

1997). Apparent complications of the chronic infection are pancreatitis produced by obstruction of the lower common bile duct (Choi, Wong, 1984) and recurrent pyogenic cholangitis (Sun, 1984).

The acute and chronic manifestations in persons infected with O. *felineus* and O. *viverrini* (Harinasuta, Vajrasthira, 1960) are similar to those produced by *Clonorchis*. A study of a population in Thailand infected with O. *viverrini* revealed a relationship between worm burden (eggs per gram of stools) and a few nonspecific symptoms (Upatham et al. 1982). For practical purposes, chronic infections are asymptomatic, and the only laboratory abnormality, other than the eggs in the stools, is a statistically significant increase in serum IgE (Woolf et al. 1984).

Pathology. The pathologic changes in *Clonorchis* and *Opistorchis* infections are similar, as demonstrated in large series of autopsies. Grossly, the liver is enlarged and slightly heavier than normal. Early in the infection, or in individuals with low worm burdens, the liver appears normal. Sectioning reveals thickening of small, medium-sized, and large bile ducts due to fibrosis and epithelial proliferation, usually in ducts near the free edge of the liver and especially in the left lobe. Some bile ducts, mainly those that are 3 to 6 mm in diameter, are dilated and tortuous, but if they are dissected, these changes usually are not found to extend beyond 5 cm in length. The parenchyma adjacent to compromised bile ducts is normal; the ducts contain worms, thick inspissated bile, and stones, producing biliary obstruction. Similar changes occur in the common bile duct and gallbladder (Hou, 1955). Some individuals have a primary liver tumor that is often not manifested clinically (Hou, 1956; Koompirochana et al. 1978; Sonakul et al. 1978). Abscesses are present only in a small number of cases. The flukes are also recovered from the pancreatic duct, especially if the liver is massively infected; dilatation of the pancreatic ducts is the main abnormality (Chan, Teoh, 1967).

The main microscopic changes are an adenomatous proliferation of the bile duct epithelium (Figs. 24–14 *A* and 24–15 *A* and *C*; *color plate* XII *E* and *G*) and marked fibrosis of the wall of the bile ducts (Fig. 24–14 *B–C*). At this stage, slight inflammatory changes composed of mononuclear cells and a few polymorphonuclear cells, mainly eosinophils, are present (Fig. 24–15 *C–D*). A conspicuous feature is the presence of adult parasites within the duct's lumen (Fig. 24–15 *A–C*), often well preserved, sometimes dead and in various stages of degeneration (Fig. 24–15 *C*). The eggs, often found, are within thick, inspissated bile. The gallbladder shows similar microscopic changes (Fig. 24–15 *A*).

Relationship to Cholangiocarcinoma. The cause–effect relationship between *Clonorchis* and *Opistorchis* infections and cholangiocarcinoma (Fig. 24–14 *D*) was suspected for a long time (Hou, 1956). In recent decades, different studies in endemic areas have confirmed this relationship (Flavell, 1981). Case-controlled studies of patients support this association (Kurathong et al. 1985). Another study of 15,641 autopsies showed 154 with O. *viverrini* infection; of these, 85 (55%) had carcinoma of the liver, 67 (44%) of which were cholangiocarcinoma (Koompirochana et al. 1978). More recently, with the use of ultrasound, a correlation between abnormalities consistent with early tumors and the intensity of the infection was demonstrated (Elkins et al. 1990, 1996; Haswell-Elkins et al. 1992). Ultrasonographic studies of patients with O. *viverrini* infections detected abnormalities consistent with early cholangiocarcinoma in 8 of 87 patients (Elkins et al. 1990). The tumors occur in men two to three times more often than in women (Elkins et al. 1996).

Diagnosis. The clinical diagnosis of *Clonorchis* and *Opistorchis* infection is usually confirmed by the recovery of eggs in the stools (Fig. 24–10). However, the species are difficult to separate on the basis of the size or morphology of the eggs alone (see above). Duodenal aspirates and biliary lavage fluid may reveal the eggs (Fig. 24–16 *A–B*), as well as small fragments of crushed gallstones from surgical or autopsy material examined directly under the microscope (Min et al. 1977). Other forms of diagnosis include an enzyme-linked immunosorbent assay for O. *viverrini* (Sirisinha et al. 1991).

The adult parasites are sometimes found during biliary surgery and are often submitted as separate specimens. In the surgical cutting room, the adults are recovered from gallbladder specimens and in the autopsy room from the bile ducts of liver specimens. In either case, the worms should not be submitted for histologic sections. Instead, they should be submitted to the clinical laboratory for staining, mounting, and examination in toto (Fig. 24–9 *A–B*).

In tissue sections of liver, the worms are located in the lumen of the thickened, fibrosed bile duct (Fig. 24–14 *A–C*); sometimes they are dead and undergoing degeneration (Fig. 24–15 *C*); eggs may be present in the bile plugs. The morphologic characteristics are those of a trematode, and some sections show the uterus with the typical eggs. The morphologic characteristics and the size of the worms are diagnostic, and sections through the testis differentiate *Clonorchis* (branched testis) from the other species with a more lobated testis (*color plate* XII *E* and *G*; Fig. 24–14 *A–B*). Gallstones and stones in the biliary tree can be used for histologic sections. These sec-

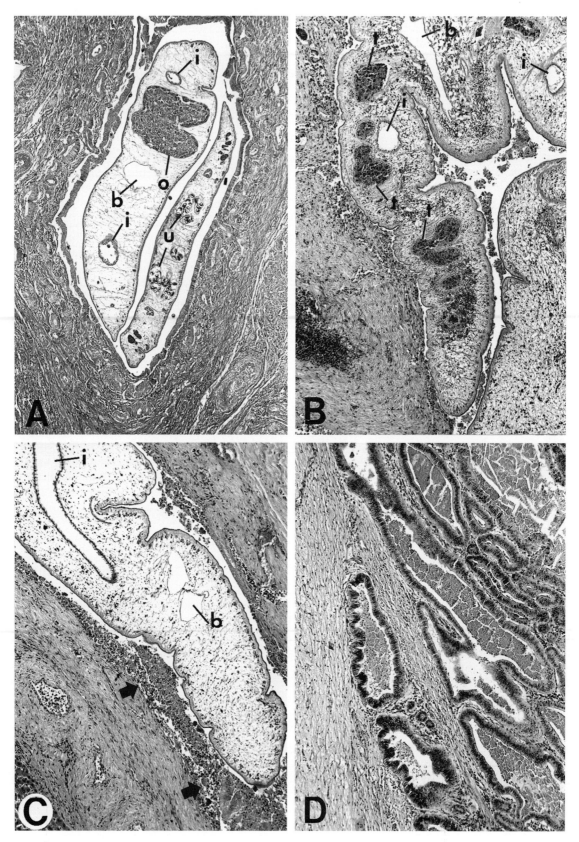

Fig. 24–14. *Clonorchis-Opistorchis* in human liver, sections stained with hematoxylin and eosin stain. *A*, Low-power view shows two sections, probably of one worm in a bile duct with significant epithelial proliferation. Abbreviations: i, intestine; o, ovary; u, uterus with eggs; b, excretory bladder, ×55. *B* and *C*, Other sections illustrating the marked ductal fibrosis and similar anatomic landmarks plus several sections of the highly branched testes (t). Note the biliary mud (arrows), ×70. *D*, Cholangiocarcinoma in a Chinese patient heavily infected with *C. sinensis*, ×55.

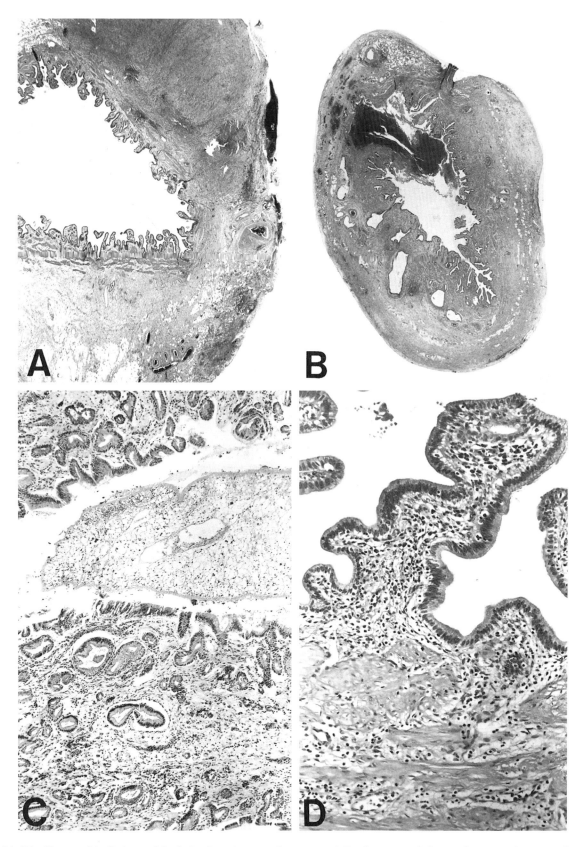

Fig. 24–15. *Clonorchis-Opistorchis* infection in an elderly Chinese man who had acute biliary symptoms, sections stained with hematoxylin and eosin stain. *A*, Low-power view of a portion of gallbladder shows marked fibrosis of the wall, ×8.7. *B*, Cross section of common bile duct illustrating similar changes, ×12. *C*, Section of common bile duct containing a degenerating parasite. Note the bile duct proliferation, ×55. *D*, Higher magnification of gallbladder showing inflammatory infiltrates in the submucosa, most of which are eosinophils, ×140. (Preparation courtesy of H. McCorkle, M.D., Department of Pathology, Fairview General Hospital, Cleveland, Ohio.)

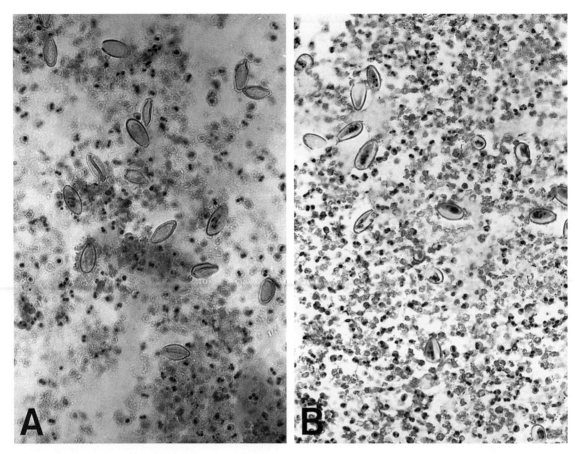

Fig. 24–16. *Clonorchis sinensis* eggs in biliary mud obtained with fine needle aspiration from enlarged common bile duct of the patient in Figure 24–12. Note also the inflammatory cells indicating that there was a superimposed bacterial cholangitis. *A*, Sections of the cell block stained with hematoxylin and eosin stain, ×238. *B*, Smear of biliary mud, Papanicolaou stain, ×238. (Preparations courtesy of H. Kim, M.D., Department of Pathology, Yonsei University Medical College, Seoul, South Korea.)

tions, if stained with hematoxylin and eosin stain, reveal the eggs or vestiges of the parasites (Min et al. 1977).

Dicrocoelium—Dicrocoeliasis

There are at least two species of *Dicrocoelium*, *D. dendriticum* and *D. hospes*, in the biliary passages of cattle and sheep and sporadically in humans. *Dicrocoelium dendriticum* (*color plate* XII *I*) occurs throughout Europe, eastern Russia, Turkey, Turkmenistan, Siberia, India, Syria, the Philippines, and southern China. On the American continent, it exists in Nova Scotia, Quebec, British Columbia, Colombia, and Brazil. *Dicrocoelium hospes* occurs mainly in central and western Africa (King, 1971).

The life cycle of *Dicrocoelium* involves a terrestrial snail; species belonging to several genera are the first intermediate hosts. The snail sheds the cercariae in the mucus and the second host, an ant, usually of the genus *Formica*, ingests them. Within the ant, the cercariae become infective for the final host. Human infections occur by the accidental ingestion of ants with vegetables and fruits. These infections are usually sporadic and occur as isolated cases. Spurious infections resulting from the ingestion of animal liver with the parasite are more common (see above; Bengtsson et al. 1968; Carney et al. 1977; Wolfe, 1966).

There are few accounts of clinical manifestations of *Dicrocoelium* in humans. These reports usually describe nonspecific gastrointestinal symptoms and peripheral eosinophilia. Most true infections have occurred in France (Cavier, Leger, 1967; Mandoul et al. 1966; Vermeil et al. 1964). One case reported in the

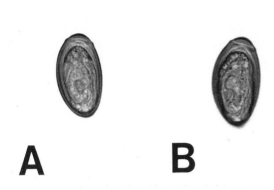

Fig. 24–17. *A, B, Dicrocoelium dendriticum* **eggs in human stools, unstained, ×495.**

U.S. (Drabick et al. 1988) was based on incomplete data and should be disregarded (Bada, 1988). Other cases have been reported from Lagos (Harmon, Oyerinde, 1976), Korea (Im, Koh, 1971), Ghana (Odei, 1966), Nigeria (Roche, 1948), and Germany (Scheid et al. 1950).

The pathologic changes resulting from *Dicrocoelium* inection in humans are not known. One case, in which liver sections were available for study, revealed fibrous thickening of the bile duct wall (Roche, 1948). The diagnosis is confirmed by the examination of stools, where the eggs should be present for several days, after the patient abstains from eating liver and liver products (Fig. 24–17 A–B).

Eurythrema pancreaticum— Eurythremiasis

The other dicrocoelid flukes are parasites of domestic and wild mammals, including primates. The species of human importance is *Eurythrema pancreaticum*, a parasite of the pancreatic ducts, sometimes found in the biliary system of pigs, goats, cattle, and buffaloes. This parasite is found in China, Japan, India, the Philippines, the Malay Archipelago, Brazil, and other countries in South America. The life cycle of *Eurythrema* involves a terrestrial snail of the genus *Bradybaena* and a grasshopper as the second intermediate host.

The proven human infections, by identification of the worms of *Eurythrema*, are few: two in China (Tang,

Tang, 1977) and three in Japan (Ishii et al. 1983; Takaoka et al. 1983). However, several other cases observed earlier, referred to as *Clonorchis* infections of the pancreatic ducts and studied on tissue sections, are probably eurythremiasis (Galliard et al. 1936; Galliard, Guyet-Rousset, 1961).

References

Acosta-Ferreira W, Vercelli-Retta J, Falconi LM, 1979. *Fasciola hepatica* human infection. Histopathological study ot sixteen cases. Virchows Arch. Pathol. Anat. 383:319–327

Acuna-Soto R, Braun-Roth G, 1987. Bleeding ulcer in the common bile duct due to *Fasciola hepatica.* Am. J. Gastroenterol. 82:560–562

Aguirre-Errasti C, Merino-Angulo J, Flores-Torres M, De Los Rios A, 1981. Formas desusuales de infestacion por *Fasciola hepatica*. Report de dos casos. Med. Clin. 76: 125–128

Aguirre-Errasti C, Valerdi-Alvarez E, Pastor-Rodriguez A, De-La-Riva-Aguinaco C, Alvarez-Blanco A, Flores-Torre M, Martinez-Ortiz-De-Zarate JM, De-Los-Rios-Saiz-De-La-Maza A, Merino-Angulo J, 1978. *Fasciola hepatica*. Estudio de siete pacientes. Med. Clin. 71:14–20

Alcoaba-Lcza M, Lopcz-Lopcz C, Lopcz-Nicolas S, 1973. Distomatosis por *Fasciola hepatica*. Manifestaciones pleuropulmonares. Med. Clin. 60:119–123

Alicata JE, 1953. Human fascioliasis in the Hawaiian Islands. Hawaii Med. J. 12:196–201

Alicata JE, Bonnet DD, 1955. A study of watercress as a possible source of human infection with the common liver fluke of cattle. Station Progress Notes. Hawaii Agricultural Experiment Station, No. 107.

Alvarez M, Basterra G, Moreto M, Enciso C, Zabaleta S, Diaz-de OR, 1994. Colestasis por *Fasciola hepatica*. Rev. Esp. Enferm. Dig. 86:915–917

Amaral ADF, Busetti ET, 1979. Fasciolose hepatica humana no Brasil. Rev. Inst. Med. Trop. Sao Paulo 21:141–145

Anibal A, Ronald A, Rodolfo C, Geovanni D, Eduardo I, Silvia M, Jorge AM, Leon T, Alvaro U, 1978. Fasciolasis humana en Costa Rica como causa de hepatitis granulomatosa eosinofilica. Acta Med. Costar. 21: 239–245

Anton-Aranda E, Garcia-Carasusan M, Celador-Almaraz A, Cia-Lecumberri M, Uribarrena-Echevarria R, Rivero-Puente A, 1985. Fascioliasis hepatica. Revision de 5 casos. Rev. Clin. Espanola 176:54–57

Apt W, Aguilera X, Vega F, Alcaino H, Zulantay I, Apt P, Gonzalez V, Retamal C, Rodriguez J, Sandoval J, 1993. Prevalencia de fascioliasis en humanos, caballos, cerdos y conejos silvestres, en tres provincias de Chile. Bol. Oficina. Sanit. Panam. 115:405–414

Arenas R, Espinosa A, Padron E, Andreu RM, 1948. Fascioliasis hepatica con caracter de brote epidemico. Rev. Kuba Med. Trop. Parasitol. 4:92–97

Arjona R, Riancho JA, Aguado JM, Salesa R, Gonzalez MJ, 1995. Fascioliasis in developed countries: a review of classic and aberrant forms of the disease. Medicine 74:13–23

Atias A, Fernandez C, 1965. Un caso de fasciolasis distomatosis hepatica con posible localizacion en pulmon. Bol. Chil. Parasitol. 20:47–49

Babbott FL, Frye WW, Gordon JE, 1961. Intestinal parasites of man in arctic Greenland. Am. J. Trop. Med. Hyg. 10:185–190

Bada JL, 1988. Correspondence. Dicroceliasis: a fluke diagnosis or a false infection? JAMA 259:2998–2999

Banna P, Gulisano G, Musco A, Sagglo A, Privitera G, 1979. Ostruzione della via biliare principale da *Fasciola hepatica*. Prima osservazione in Sicilia. Minerva Med. 71:2555–2564

Bannerman C, Manzur AY, 1986. Fluctuating jaundice and intestinal bleeding in a 6-year-old girl with fascioliasis. Trop. Geogr. Med. 38:429–431

Beaver PC, Jung RC, Cupp EW, 1984. *Clinical Parasitology*. Philadelphia: Lea & Febiger

Bechtel U, Feucht HE, Held E, Vogl T, Nothdurft HD, 1992. *Fasciola hepatica*—Infektion einer Familie. Diagnostik und Therapie. Dtsch. Med. Wochenschr. 117:978–982

Bendezu P, Frame A, Hillyer GV, 1982. Human fascioliasis in Corozal, Puerto Rico. J. Parasitol. 68:297–299

Bengtsson E, Hassler L, Holtenius P, Nordbring F, Thoren G, 1968. Infestation with *Dicrocoelium dendriticum*—the small liver fluke—in animals and human individuals in Sweden. Acta Pathol. Microbiol. Scand. 74:85–92

Bjorland J, Bryan RT, Strauss W, Hillyer GV, McAuley JB, 1995. An outbreak of acute fascioliasis among Aymara Indians in the Bolivian Altiplano. Clin. Infect. Dis. 21:1228–1233

Carney WP, Van Peenen PFD, See R, Hagelstein E, Lima B, Hageletein E, 1977. Parasites of man in remote areas of central and south Sulawesi, Indonesia. Southeast Asian J. Trop. Med. Public Health 8:380–389

Catchpole BN, Snow D, 1952. Human ectopic fascioliasis. Lancet 2:711–712

Cavier R, Leger N, 1967. A propos d'un cas de distomatose a *Dicrocoelium dendriticum* chez l'homme. Bull. Soc. Pathol. Exot. 60:425–433

Chan PH, Teoh TB, 1967. The pathology of *Clonorchis sinensis* infestation of the pancreas. J. Pathol. Bacteriol. 93:185–189

Cho SY, Yang HN, Kong Y, Kim JC, Shin KW, Koo BS, 1994. Intraocular fascioliasis: a case report. Am. J. Trop. Med. Hyg. 50:349–353

Choi TK, Wong J, 1984. Severe acute pancreatitis caused by parasites in the common bile duct. J. Trop. Med. Hyg. 87:211–214

Choi TK, Wong KP, Wong J, 1984. Cholangiographic appearance in clonorchiasis. Br. J. Radiol. 57:681–684

Condomines J, Rene-Espinet JM, Espinos-Perez JC, Vilardell F, 1985. Percutaneous cholangiography in the diagnosis of hepatic fascioliasis. Am. J. Gastroenterol. 80:384–386

Cosme A, Marcos JM, Galvany A, Arriola JA, Bengoechea MG, Alzate LF, Diago A, 1979. Obstruccion del coledoco por *Fasciola hepatica*. Med. Clin. 73:438–442

Crinquette J, Beaquet R, Vialin B, 1965. Les manifestations respiratoires au cours de la distomatose a *Fasciola hepatica*. J. Fr. Med. Chir. Thorac. 19:259

Danilewitz M, Kotfila R, Jensen P, 1996. Endoscopic diagnosis and management of *Fasciola hepatica* causing biliary obstruction. Am. J. Gastroenterol. 91:2620–2621

de Gorgolas M, Torres R, Verdejo C, Garay J, Robledo A, Ponte MC, Fernandez GM, 1992. Infestacion por *Fasciola hepatica*. Biopatologia y nuevos aspectos diagnosticos y terapeuticos. Enferm. Infecc. Microbiol. Clin. 10:514–519

DeLeon D, Quinones R, Hillyer GV, 1981. The prepatent and patent periods of *Fasciola hepatica* in cattle in Puerto Rico. J. Parasitol. 67:734–735

Dias LM, Silva R, Viana HL, Palhinhas M, Viana RL, 1996. Biliary fascioliasis: diagnosis, treatment and follow-up by ERCP. Gastrointest. Endosc. 43:616–620

Drabick JJ, Egan JE, Brown SL, Vick RG, Sandman BM, Neafie RC, 1988. Dicroceliasis (Lancet fluke disease) in an HIV seropostive man. JAMA 259:567–568

Duval M, 1842. Note sur un cas de presence du distome hepatique (douve du foie) dans la veine-porte chez l'homme. Gaz. Med. Paris 10:769–772

Eaton RDP, 1975. Metorchiasis—a Canadian zoonosis. Epidemiol. Bull. 19:62–68

Echevarrieta J, Palacios M, Kutz M, Garde JA, 1982. Microabcesos hepaticos por *Fasciola*. Presentacion de un caso. Anales 17:61–64

Eisencher A, Sauget Y, 1980. Aspect ultrasonore des ascaridioses et distomatoses des voies biliaires. J. Radiol. 61:319–322

El-Newihi HM, Waked IA, Mihas AA, 1995. Biliary complications of *Fasciola hepatica*: the role of endoscopic retrograde cholangiography in management. J. Clin. Gastroenterol. 21:309–311

el Shabrawi M, el Karaksy H, Okasha S, el Hennawy A, 1997. Human fascioliasis: clinical features and diagnostic difficulties in Egyptian children. J. Trop. Pediatr. 43:162–166

Elkins DB, Haswell-Elkins MR, Mairiang E, Mairiang P, Sithithaworn P, Kaaewkes S, Bhudhisawasdi V, Uttravichien T, 1990. A high frequency of hepatobiliary disease and suspected cholangiocarcinoma associated with heavy *Opisthorchis viverrini* infection in a small community in northeast Thailand. Trans. R. Soc. Trop. Med. Hyg. 84:715–719

Elkins DB, Mairiang E, Sithithaworn P, Mairiang J, Chaiyakum J, Chamadol N, Loapaiboon V, Haswell-Elkins MR, 1996. Cross-sectional patterns of hepatobiliary abnormalities and possible precursor conditions of cholangiocarcinoma associated with *Opisthorchis viverrini* infection in humans. Am. J. Trop. Med. Hyg. 55:295–301

Espino AM, Dumenigo BE, Fernandez R, Finlay CM, 1987. Immunodiagnosis of human fascioliasis by enzyme-linked immunosorbent assay using excretory-secretory products. Am. J. Trop. Med. Hyg. 37:605–608

Esteban JG, Flores A, Aguirre C, Strauss W, Angles R, Mas CS, 1997a. Presence of very high prevalence and intensity of infection with *Fasciola hepatica* among Aymara children from the northern Bolivian Altiplano. Acta Trop. 66:1–14

Esteban JG, Flores A, Angles R, Strauss W, Aguirre C, Mas CS, 1997b. A population-based coprological study of human fascioliasis in a hyperendemic area of the Bolivian Altiplano. Trop. Med. Int. Health 2:695–699

Facey RV, Marsden PD, 1960. Fasciolasis in man: an outbreak in Hampshire. Br. Med. J. 2:619–625

Farag HF, Barakat RMR, Ragab M, Omar E, 1979. A focus of human fascioliasis in the Nile Delta, Egypt. J. Trop. Med. Hyg. 82:188–190

Flavell DJ, 1981. Liver fluke infection as an aetiological factor in bile-duct carcinoma of man. Trans. R. Soc. Trop. Med. Hyg. 75:814–824

Galliard H, Guyet-Rousset P, 1961. Etude comparative de la distomatose pancreatique chez l'homme et les bovides. Ann. Parasitol. Hum. Comp. 36:5–68

Galliard H, Phan-Huy-Quat, Dang-Van-Ngu, 1936. Le troisieme cas de distomatose pancreatique a *Clonorchis sinensis* observe au Tonkin. Bull. Soc. Med. Chirur. Indochine 4:1–5

Garcia-Rodriguez JA, Martin Sanchez AM, Fernandez Gorostarzu JM, Gaarcia Luis EJ, 1985. Fascioliasis in Spain: a review of the literature and personal observations. Eur. J. Epidemiol. 1:121–126

Han JK, Choi BI, Cho JM, Chung KB, Han MC, Kim CW, 1993. Radiological findings of human fascioliasis. Abdom. Imaging 18:261–264

Han JK, Han D, Choi BI, Han MC, 1996. MR findings in human fascioliasis. Trop. Med. Int. Health 1:367–372

Harinasuta C, Vajrasthira S, 1960. Opisthorchiasis in Thailand. Ann. Trop. Med. Parasitol. 54:100

Harmon WM, Oyerinde JPO, 1976. *Dicrocoelium* infection in Lagos. Niger. Med. J. 6:404–406

Haswell-Elkins MR, Sithithaworn P, Elkins D, 1992. *Opisthorchis viverrini* and cholangiocarcinoma in northeast Thailand. Parasitol. Today 8:86–89

Hauser SC, Bynum TE, 1984. Abnormalities on ERCP in a case of human fascioliasis. Gastrointest. Endosc. 30: 80–82

Hillyer GV, Soler-de GM, Rodriguez PJ, Bjorland J, Silva-de LM, Ramirez GS, Bryan RT, 1992. Use of the Falcon assay screening test—enzyme-linked immunosorbent assay (FAST-ELISA) and the enzyme-linked immunoelectrotransfer blot (EITB) to determine the prevalence of human fascioliasis in the Bolivian Altiplano. Am. J. Trop. Med. Hyg. 46:603–609

Hitanant S, Trong DTN, Damrongsak C, Chinapak O, Boonyapisit S, Plengvanit U, Viranuvatti V, 1987. Peritoneoscopic findings in 203 patients with *Opisthorchis viverrini* infection. Gastrointest. Endosc. 33:18–20

Hoffmann WH, Guerra A, 1923. Distoma hepatico originando un absceso muscular. Rev. Med. Ciruj. Habana 28:558–561

Hou PC, 1955. The pathology of *Clonorchis sinensis* infestation of the liver. J. Pathol. Bacteriol. 70:53–68

Hou PC, 1956. The relationship between primary carcinoma of the liver and infestation with *Clonorchis sinensis*. J. Pathol. Bacteriol. 72:239–246

Hunt AT, 1972. The Tidenham epidemic: forty cases of liver fluke infestation. Community Med. 128:211–212

Im KI, Koh TY, 1971. One case of Dicrocoeliidae infection. Korean J. Parasitol. 9:58–60

Imai J, Abe H, Hurakami F, 1974. A human case of heterotopic parasitism of liver fluke (*Fasciola* sp). Trop. Med. 16:21–26

Ishii Y, Koga M, Fufjino T, Higo H, Ishibashi J, Oka K, Saito S, 1983. Human infection with the pancreas fluke, *Eurytrema pancreaticum*. Am. J. Trop. Med. Hyg. 32:1019–1022

King EVJ, 1971. Human infection with *Dicrocoelium hospes* in Sierra Leone. J. Parasitol. 57:989

Koenigstein RP, 1949. Observations on the epidemiology of infections with *Clonorchis sinensis*. Trans. R. Soc. Trop. Med. Hyg. 42:503–506

Koompirochana C, Sonakul D, Chinda K, Stitnimankarn T, 1978. Opisthorchiasis: a clinicopathologic study of 154 autopsy cases. Southeast Asian J. Trop. Med. Public Health 9:60–64

Kurathong S, Lerdverasirikul P, Wongpaitoon V, Pramoolsinsap C, Kanjanapitak A, Varavithya W, Phoapradit P, Bunyaratvej S, Suchart Upatham E, Brockelman WY, 1985. *Opisthorchis viverrini* infection and cholangiocarcinoma. A prospective, case-controlled study. Gastroenterology 89:156

Kurathong S, Lerdverasirikul P, Wongpaitoon V, Pramoolsinsap C, Suchart Upatham E, 1987. *Opisthorchis viverrini* infection in rural and urban communities in northeast Thailand. Trans. R. Soc. Trop. Med. Hyg. 81:411–414

Malek EA, 1980. *Snail-transmitted Parasitic Diseases*. Vols. I and II., Boca Raton, Fla.: CRC Press

Mandoul R, Demartial L, Pestre M, Moulinier C, 1966. La distomase hepato-biliare a petit douve (a propos d'un nouveau cas). J. Med. Bordeaux 143:685–700

Markell EK, 1966. Laboratory findings in chronic clonorchiasis. Am. J. Trop. Med. Hyg. 15:510–515

McFadzean AJS, Yeung RTT, 1965. Hypogylcaemia in suppurative pancholangiitis due to *Clonorchis sinensis*. Trans. R. Soc. Trop. Med. Hyg. 59:179–185

Min DY, Soh CT, Hwang KC, Kim BJ, Kang KS, 1977. Parasitological examination of gallstones. Yonsei Rep. Trop. Med. 8:57–63

Modavi S, Isseroff H, 1984. *Fasciola hepatica*: collagen deposition and other histopathology in the rat host's bile duct caused by the parasite and by proline infusion. Exp. Parasitol. 58:239–244

Moreto M, Barron J, 1980. The laparoscopic diagnosis of the liver fasciliasis. Gastrointest. Endosc. 26:147–149

Navab F, Diner WC, Westbrook KC, Kumpuris DD, Uthman EO, 1984. Endoscopic biliary lavage in a case of *Clonorchis sinensis*. Gastrointest. Endosc. 30:292–294

Norton RA, Monroe L, 1961. Infection by *Fasciola hepatica* acquired in California. Gastroenterology 41:46–48

O'Neill SM, Parkinson M, Strauss W, Angeles R, Dalton JP,

1998. Immunodiagnosis of *fasciola hepatica* infection (Fascioliasis) in a human population in the Bolivian Altiplano using purified cathepsin ʟ cysteine proteinase. Am. J. Trop. Med. Hyg. 58:417–423

Odei MA, 1966. A note on dicrococliasis and *Fasciola gigantica* infection in livestock in northern Ghana, with a record of spurious and genuine *Dicrocoelium hospes* infections in man. Ann. Trop. Med. Parasitol. 60:215–218

Pagola Serrano MA, Vega A, Ortega E, Gonzalez A, 1987. Computed tomography of hepatic fascioliasis. J. Comput. Assist. Tomogr. 11:269–272

Park C II, Ro JY, Kin H, Gutierrez Y, 1984. Human ectopic fascioliasis in the cecum. Am. J. Surg. Pathol. 8:73–77

Price TA, Tuazon CU, Simon GL, 1993. Fascioliasis: case reports and review. Clin. Infect. Dis. 17:426–430

Pungpak S, Viravan C, Radomyos B, Chalermrut K, Yemput C, Plooksawasdi W, Ho M, Harinasuta T, Bunnag D, 1997. *Opisthorchis viverrini* infection in Thailand: studies on the morbidity of the infection and resolution following praziquantel treatment. Am. J. Trop. Med. Hyg. 56:311–314

Rao MR, Choudary C, 1979. An aberrant location of *Fasciola gigantica* in spleen and lung of Indian buffaloes (*Bubalus bubalis*) and pathological study. Indian Vet. J. 56:890–891

Roche PJL, 1948. Human dicrocoeliasis in Nigeria. Trans. R. Soc. Trop. Med. Hyg. 41:819–820

Rodriguez-Barreras ME, Diaz-Hernandez A, Marinez-Rodriguez R, Millan-Marcelo JC, Ruiz-Perez A, Perez-Avila J, 1986. Urticaria y *Fasciola hepatica*. Re. Cub. Med. Trop. 38:305–310

Rodriguez-M JD, Gomez-Lince LF, Montalvan-C JA, 1949. El *Opisthorchis guayaguilensis* (Una nueva especie de *Opisthorchis* encontrada en la Ecuador). Rev. Ecuator. Hig. Med. Trop. 6:11–24

Sadun EH, 1955. Studies on *Opisthorchis viverrini* in Thailand. Am. J. Hyg. 62:81–115

Sadun EH, 1957. Fasciolopsiasis and opisthorchiasis as helminthic components of tropical public health. Am. J. Trop. Med. Hyg. 6:416–422

Scheid G, Mendheim H, Amenda R, 1950. Die Lanzettegelinfektion (Dicrocoeliasis) beim Menschen nebst Mitteilung eines neuen Falles. Z. Tropenmed. Parasitol. 2:142–150

Seo BS, Lee SH, Cho SY, Chai JY, Hong ST, 1981. An epidemiologic study on clonorchiasis and metagonimiasis in riverside areas in Korea. Korean J. Parasitol. 19:137–150

Sirisinha S, Chawengkirttikul R, Sermswan R, Amornpant S, Mongkolsuk S, Panyim S, 1991. Detection of *Opisthorchis viverrini* by monoclonal antibody-based ELISA and DNA hybridization. Am. J. Trop. Med. Hyg. 44:140–145

Sonakul D, Koompirochana C, Chinda K, Stitnimakarn T, 1978. Hepatic carcinoma with opisthorchiasis. Southeast Asian J. Trop. Med. Public Health 9:215–219

Stemmermann GN, 1953. Human infestation with *Fasciola gigantica*. Am. J. Pathol. 29:731–753

Strauss WG, 1962. Clinical manifestations of clonorchiasis. A controlled study of 105 cases. Am. J. Trop. Med. Hyg. 11:525–830

Sun T, 1984. Pathology and immunology of *Clonorchis sinensis* infection of the liver. Ann. Clin. Lab. Sci. 14:208–215

Takaoka H, Mochizuki Y, Hirao E, Iyota N, Matsunagas K, Funiokas T, 1983. A human case of erytremiasis: demonstration of adult pancreatic fluke, *Eurytrema pancreaticum* (Janson, 1889) in resected pancreas. Jpn. J. Parasitol. 32:501–508

Takeyama N, Okumura N, Sakai Y, Kamma O, Shima Y, Endo K, Hayakawa T, 1986. Computed tomography findings of hepatic lesions in human fascioliasis: report of two cases. Am. J. Gastroenterol. 81:1078–1081

Tang Z, Tang C, 1977. The biology and epidemiology of *Eurytrema coelomaticum* (Giard et Billet, 1892) and *Eurytrema pancreaticum* (Janson, 1889) in cattle and sheep in China. Acta Zool. Sinica 23:267–283

Tombazzi C, Abdul HS, Lecuna V, Contreras R, Marquez D, 1994. Colangiopancreatografia retrograda endoscopica en fasciolasis hepatica. GEN 48:278–280

Upatham ES, Brockelman WY, Viyanant V, Lee P, Kaengraeng R, Prayoonwiwat B, 1985. Incidence of endemic *Opisthorchis viverrini* infection in a village in northeast Thailand. Am. J. Trop. Med. Hyg. 34:903–906

Upatham ES, Viyanant V, Kurathong S, Brockelman WY, Menaruchi A, Saowakontha S, Intarakhao C, Vajrasthira S, Warren KS, 1982. Morbidity in relation to intensity of infection in opisthorchiasis *viverrini*: study of a community in Khon Kaen, Thailand. Am. J. Trop. Med. Hyg. 31:1156–1163

Upatham ES, Viyanant V, Kurathong S, Rojborwonwitaya J, Brockelman WY, Ardsungnoen S, Lee P, Vajrasthira S, 1984. Relationship between prevalence and intensity of *Opisthorchis viverrini* infection and clinical symptoms and signs in a rural community in northeast Thailand. Bull. WHO 62:451–461

Vermeil C, Le Cloitre ML, Beaupere J, Rehel H, 1964. Un nouveau cas de distomatose humaine a *Dicrocoelium dendriticum*. A propos des distomatoses humaines observees a Nantes. Bull. Soc. Pathol. Exot. 57:946–949

Wolf-Spengler ML, Isseroff H, 1983. Fascioliasis: bile duct collagen induced by proline from the worm. J. Parasitol. 69:290–294

Wolfe MS, 1966. Spurious infection with *Dicrocoelium hospes* in Ghana. Am. J. Trop. Med. Hyg. 15:180–182

Wong RKH, Peura DA, Mutter ML, Heit HA, Birns MT, Johnson LF, 1985. Hemobilia and liver flukes in a patient from Thailand. Gastroenterology 88:1958–1963

Woolf A, Green J, Levine JA, Estevez EG, Weatfierly N, Rosenberg E, Frothincham T, 1984. A clinical study of Laotian refugees infected with *Clonorchis sinensis* or *Opisthorchis viverrini*. Am. J. Trop. Med. Hyg. 33:1279–1280

25

INTESTINAL, PULMONARY, EYE, AND OTHER TREMATODES

Many species of trematodes in the intestinal tract of humans have been described; pulmonary infections with several species of *Paragonimus* also occur in many places. Ocular and disseminated infections due to trematodes are more rare. The majority of these infections, if not all, are zoonotic and have a restricted geographic distribution, mostly because of the food preferences of the populations involved. Often these infections consist of single cases or small clusters of cases that occur with low frequency in certain areas. Because of the morphologic similarities between the eggs of many of these trematodes, the diagnosis is often made at the generic level, for example species of heterophyids and echinostomes. Specific identification requires the adult worms, which are recovered during autopsies, in surgical specimens, or after treatment of patients. The classification of trematodes provided in the introduction to Part III and according to the organ system where they occur is followed here in discussing these infections.

Intestinal Trematodes

Over three dozen species of trematodes in the intestinal tract of humans have been described. Most of the zoologic groups to which these species belong have a worldwide distribution in animals, and in most cases they are transmitted by consumption of uncooked or poorly cooked freshwater fish. The number of infections in humans and the geographic distribution are limited by culinary and feeding customs rather than by the parasite. Most trematodes have low host specificity, and they use several definitive hosts to complete their life cycles.

Nanophyetus (= *Troglotrema*) *salmincola*—Nanophyetiasis

Nanophyetus salmincola (= *Troglotrema salmincola*) is a parasite of wild and domestic dogs in eastern Siberia and the Pacific Northwest of the United States. Human infections with *Nanophyetus* have been known for a long time, especially in eastern Siberia, where prevalence rates of up to 98% occur (Filimonova, 1963). In the United States, human infections have been recognized in the State of Washington (Eastburn et al. 1987). *Nanophyetus* in dogs results in an infection known as *salmon poisoning*. It is produced by a rickettsia, *Neorickettsia helmintheca*, which is transmitted by the trematode (Milleman, Knapp, 1970). In this case, the worm replaces the arthropod vector of the rickettsia. Human infections with *N. helmintheca* are not known but are likely to occur (Beaver et al. 1984).

The life cycle of *Nanophyetus* is similar to that of other intestinal trematodes. The second intermediate hosts are fish, especially salmon, where cercariae encyst and become infectious to humans and dogs. The patients in the United States had symptoms similar to those described in Russia. Some individuals are asymptomatic, but most of them experience diarrhea, nausea, vomiting, weight loss, fatigue, anorexia, and blood eosinophilia of up to 43%. The diagnosis is difficult clinically, but the presence of typical eggs in the stools is confirmatory (Fig. 25–1). Often there is a history of recent consumption of raw, smoked, or partially cooked salmon in most people with symptoms when they are asked. Only 1 of the 10 patients studied in the United States had fever, indicating the possibility of *Neorickettsia* infection, but the diagnosis was not pursued (Eastburn et al. 1987). In some cases, symptoms can last for several months before they resolve spontaneously.

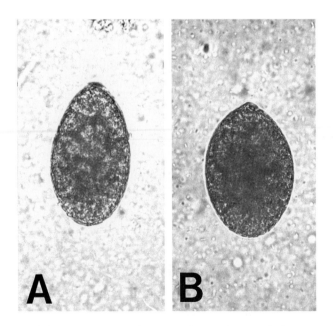

Fig. 25–1. *A, B, Nanophyetus salmincola* **eggs in human stools, unstained, ×495. (Stool sample courtesy of T.R. Fritsche, M.D., Department of Laboratory Medicine, University of Washington, Seattle, Washington.)**

Heterophyes heterophyes and Related Heterophyids—Heterophydiasis

The family Heterophyidae comprises two subfamilies with seven genera and many species of related organisms (see the classification scheme in the introduction to Part III) found in fish-eating mammals (*color plate* XIII *A* and *C*). Of these, two species are important: *H. heterophyes* and *Metagonimus yokogawai*, producing heterophydiasis and metagonimiasis, gastrointestinal diseases that on rare occasions have produced symptoms in other organs due to ectopic locations of the worms. The prevalence of *Heterophyes* infections in humans is not known because the eggs are similar to those of other heterophyids. In addition, the true prevalence of metagonimiasis is masked because the eggs of *Metagonimus* resemble those of *Clonorchis* and *Opistorchis*, making the diagnosis impossible. Moreover, the clinical manifestations produced by the heterophyids and by *Metagonimus* are identical. The heterophyids are small trematodes (*color plate* XIII *A, C,* and *D*) that live buried in the mucosa of the small intestine (Fig. 25–2 *A–B*), where some species may produce up to 1500 eggs per worm each day. *Heterophyes heterophyes* is a species widely distributed, occurring in the Nile Delta, Israel, Turkey, China, Japan, Taiwan, the Philippines, the Balkan countries, and West Africa. *Heterophyes nocens* is known in Japan and Korea (Chai et al. 1994, 1997), and *H. continua* is found in Korea (Hong et al. 1996). *Metagonimus yokogawai* is common in Japan, China, Siberia, the Balkan countries, and the pacific provinces of Russia.

The other genera and species of heterophyids are widely distributed. Species of *Haplorchis* (*H. taichui, H. yokogawai, H. calderoni, H. vanissima,* and *H. pumilio*) are endemic in Southeast Asia. *Stellantchasmus falcatus* occurs in the Philippines, Japan, Korea, Israel, and Hawaii (Alicata, Schattenburg, 1938). *Cryptocotyle lingua* exists in northern Europe and in North America, especially Canada. *Stamnosoma* occurs in Southeast Asia and *Pygidiopsis summa* in the Black Sea. Infections in humans with species of these genera occur as small clusters or as single cases, found mostly where they are investigated.

Heterophyes heterophyes is 1.0 to 1.5 mm in length by 0.3 to 0.4 mm in width; *M. yokogawai* is about 1.4 by 0.6 mm. The eggs of *H. heterophyes* are 28 to 30 × 15 to 17 μm; those of *M. yokogawai* are 27 to 28 × 16 to 17 μm (Beaver et al. 1984; Malek, 1980). The adults are delicate worms with their bodies covered by spines, a feature seen clearly in sections of the worm in tissues (Fig. 25–2). In the intestine, the worms lay

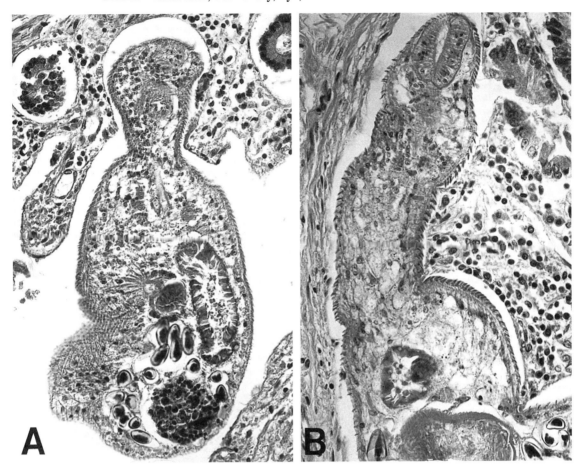

Fig. 25–2. Heterophyid in small intestinal mucosa of a man, hematoxylin and eosin stain. *A*, Adult parasite buried in a crypt of the small intestine. Note eggs in the uterus at the posterior end of the worm, ×240. *B*, Higher magnification of another worm showing oral sucker and numerous minute spines covering the tegument, ×300. (Preparation courtesy of J.H. Cross, Ph.D., Department of Preventive Medicine and Biometry, Uniformed Services University, Bethesda, Maryland.)

fully embryonated eggs that, after evacuation with the feces, reach fresh water, where they are ingested by the appropriate snails. In the snail, the eggs develop through several generations of larvae to produce cercariae that leave the snail and encyst in several species of fish. Ingestion of uncooked fish with the cysts produces the infection in animals and humans (Fig. 25–3).

Clinical Findings, Pathology, and Diagnosis. Infections with small numbers of heterophyids are usually asymptomatic, but heavy worm burdens may result in diarrhea, colicky pain, and stools with large amounts of mucus. At the site of attachment in the crypts of the small intestine, the worms produce ulcerations and inflammation characterized by a mononuclear and polymorphonuclear cell infiltrate consisting mainly of

eosinophils. Some worms are buried deep in the crypts, close to large lymphatics and blood vessels, resulting in the passage of either the worms, the eggs, or both into the general circulation, followed by their location in distant organs. In some infections with *Stellantchasmus falcatus*, the worm produced a segmental ileitis that required surgical resection (Tantachamrum, Kliks, 1978). In experimental infections of humans with *M. yokogawai*, the early manifestations of the infection consisted of dyspepsia and acute allergic symptoms (Zubov et al. 1970).

Ectopic Locations. Eggs of several species of heterophyid trematodes have been found in the brain, spinal cord, liver, and heart of patients with clinical manifestations related to these organs. In the brain, the adult parasites and their eggs were located in a cystic lesion

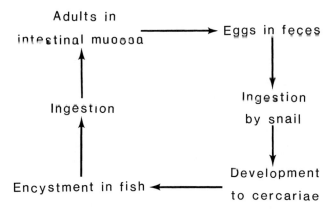

Fig. 25–3. *Heterophyes heterophyes*, schematic representation of the life cycle.

(Collomb, Bert, 1957; Collomb et al. 1960; Gallais et al. 1955). In other organs, there were only eggs eliciting a granulomatous inflammation (Africa et al. 1936). Eggs were also found in the heart valves of patients dying of congestive heart failure (Africa et al. 1935a, 1935b, 1937). The eggs of *Haplorchis pumilio* were recovered from the spinal cord of a patient with manifestations of transverse myelitis, with loss of motor and sensory function (Africa et al. 1937). In these ectopic locations, the eggs of heterophyids provoked a granulomatous inflammation that correlated with the symptoms observed. In all cases in which only the eggs were found in a specific site in the tissues, the worm was either not found or was destroyed by the tissue reaction. Of interest is that mice infected experimentally with *M. yokogawai* showed worms deep in the submucosa when the mice were artificially immune suppressed with steroids (Chai et al. 1995). A case of pulmonary involvement by *Heterophyes* is not convincing because neither the worms nor the eggs were demonstrated in the lungs; it should be disregarded (Gomaa, 1962).

The clinical diagnosis of heterophyids is difficult and usually rests on examination of the stools in the clinical laboratory. The eggs in the stools can be identified only to the generic level, based on their morphologic characteristics and their size; the species is impossible to determine without the adult worms.

Fasciolopsis buski—Fasciolopsiasis

Fasciolopsis buski, discovered over 150 years ago in the duodenum of a sailor in England, is the largest trematode found in the intestine of humans. The adult worms are up to 7.5 cm long, 2 cm wide, and 0.3 cm thick. The body is oval and fleshy, with one sucker on the cephalic end and the acetabulum located slightly

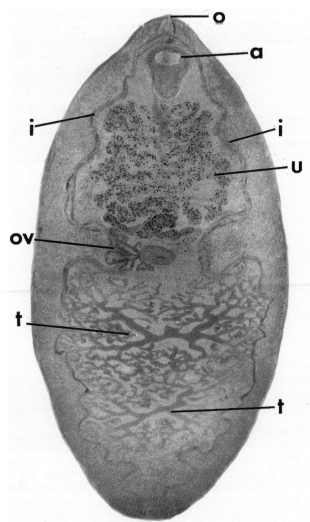

Fig. 25–4. *Fasciolopsis buski* adult, stained with acetic-alum carmine, ×3.1. Abbreviations: o, oral sucker; a, acetabulum; i, intestine (ceca); u, uterus; t, testes; ov, ovary.

posteriorly on the ventral surface. The acetabulum serves to attach the worm to the small intestinal mucosa (Fig. 25–4; *color plate* XII *B* and *G*), and the tegument is covered with numerous spines. Grossly, *F. buski* can be differentiated from *Fasciola* by the size of the worm, the lack of an anterior cone, and the ceca without branches.

Biology and Life Cycle. *Fasciolopsis* parasites inhabit the lumen of the small intestine, where they lay eggs that pass with the feces into the environment. After reaching fresh water, the eggs develop larval stages that leave the egg to enter the first intermediate host, a suitable species of snail. Development in the snail results in the production of numerous free-swimming cercariae

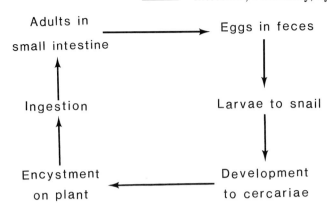

Fig. 25–5. *Fasciolopsis buski*, schematic representation of the life cycle.

that encyst on the surface of aquatic plants; ingestion of the plant with the cysts produces the infection (Fig. 25–5). While the parasites are usually restricted to the small intestine, in heavy infections they may parasitize the colon.

Geographic Distribution and Epidemiology. *Fasciolopsis* is a common parasite of both pigs and humans in Southeast Asia, mainly south China, Taiwan, Vietnam, Thailand (Manning, Ratanarat, 1970), Bangladesh, Assam, Borneo, and Sumatra. In Bangladesh, the parasite was apparently introduced with the massive migration of people from Bihar and Assam in 1948 (Gilman et al. 1982). The overall prevalence of the infection is unknown, but rates of up to 39% have been reported in school children near Dacca, Bangladesh (Muttalib, Islam, 1975). The role of pigs in the epidemiology of human fascioliasis is not clear because, in some areas with high prevalence of the parasite in pigs, the infection in humans is very low (Galliard, Ngu, 1947).

Clinical Findings, Pathology, and Diagnosis. The symptoms of fasciolopsiasis appear to result from trauma of the intestinal mucosa produced by the parasites and their metabolic products. The infection is more common in the 4- to 13-year age group, in whom a small to moderate number of worms are asymptomatic (Plaut et al. 1969; Rahman et al. 1981). Individuals with heavy worm burdens may develop intestinal obstruction due to the large size of the parasites. Others have diarrhea and epigastric pain, on occasion simulating a peptic ulcer, and massive infections may be fatal (Sadun, Maiphoom, 1953). Long-standing heavy infections result in chronic diarrhea, as well as electrolyte and protein imbalances that result in

anasarca, ascites, and generalized weakness. The stools are usually fluid, with undigested food but without blood or mucus (Daengsvang, Mangalasmaya, 1941). A study of older children and adults with mild to moderate infections showed no impairment of intestinal absorption (Jaroonvesama et al. 1986).

The intestinal mucosa of individuals infected with *Fasciolopsis* is usually normal (Jaroonvesama et al. 1986; Viranuvatti et al. 1953). However, some individuals have inflammation and petechial bleeding at the point of attachment of the worm, a lesion seen often in infected pigs (Kau, Wu, 1938). The clinical diagnosis of fasciolopsiasis is confirmed in the clinical laboratory by finding the typical operculated eggs, measuring up to 140 by 85 μm, in the stools (Fig. 25–6 A–B).

Paramphistoma—Paramphistomiasis

The paramphistomes comprise a large number of trematode species with a worldwide distribution that parasitize the stomach and intestine mostly of ruminants, but also of humans, primates, and in some cases birds. The classification of these organisms is difficult; several proposed schemes divide the group into several families or subfamilies (Malek, 1980). There are two species of paramphistomes in humans: *Gastrodiscoides hominis* and *Watsonius watsoni*. *Gastrodiscoides hominis* measures about 5 mm when fixed; its body is almost circular, with a prominent cone at the apical portion of the worm. One characteristic of the worm is the presence of an acetabulum at the posterior end, occupying about one-third the length of the body. *Watsonius watsoni* has a pyriform body 8 to 10 mm in length by 4 to 5 mm wide; the eggs are 120 to 130 × 75 to 80 μm.

Gastrodiscoides occurs in a wide area, but human infections have been found only in India (Assam, Bengal, Bihar, and Orissa), the Philippines, Kazakhstan, and Vietnam. *Watsonius* occurs rarely in humans, especially in Africa, where the parasite is found naturally in monkeys and baboons; it also occurs in animals in eastern Asia. The infection in humans has produced severe toxic diarrhea in some cases (Malek, 1980).

Echinostoma—Echinostomiasis

The echinostomes, one of the largest groups of intestinal trematodes in humans, belong to three subfamilies of the family Echinostomatidae (see the introduction to

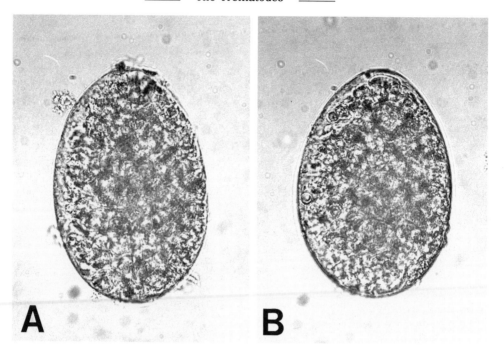

Fig. 25–6. *A, B, Fasciolopsis buski* eggs in human stools, unstained, ×450.

Part III for classification). Seven genera contain about 14 different species widely distributed throughout the world. The main morphologic characteristic of the family is the presence of a head collar, with a single or double row of spines, surrounding the oral sucker. In the main natural hosts, of the echinostomes, birds and mammals, the parasites live in the intestine, sometimes producing important morbidity. One biologic characteristic of the echinostomes is that the first intermediate hosts are snails and the second intermediate hosts are either snails or bivalves, depending on the species. Infections in humans and animals are due to consumption of raw snails or bivalves. In Indonesia infection with *E. lidoense* was common, but it has now disappeared because of changing food habits of the population living near Lake Lindu (Carney et al. 1980; Malek, 1980).

Rates of infection with echinostomes reported in the 1930s and 1940s around Lake Lindu were up to 96% in some populations (Sandground, Bonne, 1940). *Echinostoma hortense* was present in 10% of a population surveyed in Korea (Son et al. 1994). In northern Thailand, 53% of a population sample, had eggs of *Hypoderaeum conoideum* in their feces (Yokogawa et al. 1965). In the Philippines, the prevalence of *E. ilocanum* gradually fell from 48% in the late 1960s to 4% in the early 1980s after mass treatment (Cross, Basaca-Sevilla, 1986). Species of *Echinostoma* occur in humans mostly in Southeast Asia and Japan.

Echynoparyphium recurvatum exists in Japan and Egypt. *Euparyphium melis* occurs in Romania and China and *Hypoderaeum conoideum* in Thailand. Species of *Paryphostomum* occur in India, *Echinochasmus* in Japan, and *Himastla muehlensi* in Germany.

The clinical consequences of the infection in humans are negligible. In experimental infections with *E. hortense*, the prepatent period was 6 to 8 weeks. Abdominal pain developed 3 to 5 weeks postinfection and continued for several days; blood eosinophilia was slightly increased (Yoshida et al. 1976). Cases with epigastric pain and hematemesis due to duodenal ulcerations produced by *E. hortense* are known (Chai et al. 1994).

The diagnosis of echinostomiasis is confirmed by finding the typical eggs in the stools, some species of which have characteristic sizes. The eggs of *E. ilocanum* are 88 to 111 μm in length by 53 to 74 μm in width; those of *E. malayanum* are 120 to 130 × 80 to 90 μm; those of *E. revolutum* are 90 to 126 × 59 to 71 μm; and those of *E. lidoense* are 92 to 124 × 65 to 76 μm (Malek, 1980)

Other Intestinal Trematodes

The list of other intestinal trematodes is long. As stated before, the identification of these organisms rests on recovery of the adult worms at autopsy or after treatment. Most of the species in the following genera produce infections in low numbers; these infections are diagnosed sporadically in communities where there usually is an interest in the parasites. The families, genera, and species are as follows: Psilostomatidae (*Psilorchis hominis*), one case known, in Japan; Plagiorchiidae (*Plagiorchis muris* and *P. javanensis*) in the Philippines and Java; Prostogonimidae (*Prosthogonimus putschowskii*), with one case in Indonesia; Microphallidae (*Spelotrema brevicaeca* and *Gymnophalloides seoi*; *color plate* XII *E*), reported in the Philippines and Korea; Lecithodendriidae (*Phaneropsoulus bonnei* and *Prosthodendrium molenkampi*), found in Indonesia and Thailand; and Diplostomatidae (*Neodiplostomum* [= *Fibricola*] *seoulense*; *color plate* XIII *D*), found in Korea.

Pulmonary Trematodes

There are several genera and species of trematodes that are parasites in the lungs of animals, but *Paragonimus* is the only one in humans. It produces the disease known as *paragonimiasis*, *pulmonary distomiasis*, or *endemic hemoptysis*. Another species of the family Clinostomatidae (*Clinostomum complanatum*; Fig. 25–7 *A–B*), which parasitizes the pharynx of birds that eat fish, has been recorded in the pharynx of humans. Most cases are from Japan (Hirai et al. 1987; Kamo et al. 1962; Sakaguchi et al. 1966; Yamashita, 1938; Yoshimura et al. 1991), but recently, one was described in Korea (Chung et al. 1995).

Paragonimus—Paragonimiasis

Paragonimiasis is a disease of the tropics and to a lesser extent of the subtropics, with most cases occurring in the Far East. Endemic foci are also found in West Africa, Peru, Ecuador, and Central America. In these endemic areas, about 8 and possibly 10 species of *Paragonimus* infect humans, mostly in low numbers or as single cases, because the disease is zoonotic, with life

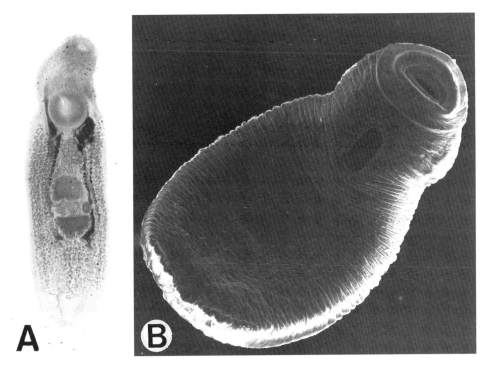

Fig. 25–7. *Clinostoma complanatum*, adult worms. *A*, Adult stained with acetic-alum carmine stain, ×4.5. (In: Chung, D.I. 1995. Demonstration of the second intermediate host of *Clinostomum complanatum* in Korea. Korean J. Parasitol. 33:305–311. Reproduced with permission.) *B*, Scanning electron micrograph, ×5. (Photographs courtesy of Dong-Il Chung, M.D., Department of Parasitology, Kyunpook National University, School of Medicine, Taegu, Korea.)

cycles occurring in wild animals. Of all these species, *P. westermani*, the first species described in humans over 100 years ago, is the best known and the one described in most textbooks. The infection is acquired by consuming raw freshwater crabs and crayfish, the natural second intermediate hosts. Assessments of prevalence are spotty at best and are available only for some small communities; worldwide estimates indicate that the number of cases is probably several million, but the true numbers are unknown.

Morphology. The worms measure up to 13 mm long, 6 mm wide, and 5 mm thick. The tegument is covered with minute scale-like spines, the distribution and shape of which are of taxonomic value. Fresh worms are ovoid and fleshy, with a small oral sucker and an acetabulum. The internal anatomy of the worm is similar to that of other trematodes (*color plate* XIII *H*). The worms have nonbranched ceca, and both the ovary and the two testes are deeply lobated. A large excretory bladder is present, seen in tissue sections as a wide, empty space.

Life Cycle and Biology. The adult worms live in pairs or triplets (Fig. 25–10 *B*), encapsulated in the lung parenchyma by a dense fibrous capsule. The encapsulated worms lay eggs that pass through a small hole between the capsule and the respiratory tree, where they move upward with the mucus and are either expectorated or evacuated in the feces. In fresh water, the eggs embryonate, hatch, and release larvae that enter the snails, the first intermediate hosts. The development in the snail goes through different larval stages that end with production of numerous cercariae. The cercariae leave the snail to gain access to the freshwater crustaceans, the second intermediate hosts, where they encyst and become metacercariae. After the metacercariae are ingested with uncooked crayfish or crabmeat, digestion frees the larvae from their cysts in the intestine. Once freed, the larvae enter the intestinal wall and pass to the peritoneal cavity, where the worms migrate, travel through the diaphragm), gain access to the thoracic cavity, enter the lung parenchyma, and reach maturity (Fig. 25–8).

In unsuitable definitive hosts, the metacercariae of *Paragonimus* migrate to the muscles rather than the lungs, where they encyst. The unsuitable host becomes a paratenic host and the larvae remain infective until, by predation, they reach the appropriate host to complete their development (Miyazaki, Habe, 1975, 1976). This indicates that human infections may result from

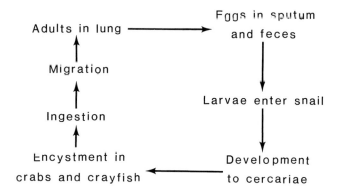

Fig. 25–8. *Paragonimus*, **schematic representation of the life cycle.**

ingestion of raw or partially cooked meat of animals, as well as crustaceans.

Two species of *P. westermani* and *P. pulmonalis* have some important biologic characteristics related to the pathophysiology of the disease they produce (Miyazaki et al. 1981b). *Paragonimus westermani*, like all other paragonimids, requires encapsulation of two or three worms in the same place for cross-copulation and insemination. One worm, in spite of being hermaphroditic, cannot inseminate itself (Miyazaki et al. 1981a). Thus, when they are single, the parasites do not encapsulate. Instead, they migrate extensively in the thoracic cavity to find a mate, producing much damage and inflammation, especially pleuritis and pleural effusions in the host (Miyazaki, 1982). *Paragonimus pulmonalis* does not require another worm for insemination; it is parthenogenetic. Once in the host, a single parasite readily causes the formation of a nodule in the lung parenchyma (Miyazaki et al. 1981a).

Geographic Distribution and Epidemiology. Infections with *Paragonimus* exist in many countries, both in humans and in animals. In humans, the parasites are not often recovered for study; thus, the exact species infecting a given patient usually remains unknown. In contrast, animal experiments usually permit the recovery of worms for taxonomic studies, increasing our knowledge of the worms, their geographic distribution, and their taxonomic relationships. However, the systematics of the genus *Paragonimus* is extremely difficult to determine, and there is no consensus as to the number of species or subspecies in the genus. In addition, the names proposed today are changed, fused, or disregarded with ease soon after they are proposed.

With these limitations in mind, it appears that the species infecting humans are *P. westermani* in India, Sri

Lanka, Thailand, Malaysia, Indonesia, the Philippines, China, Russia, and Japan. *Paragonimus pulmonalis* occurs in Japan, Korea, and Taiwan; *P. heterotremus* is the most important species in humans in Thailand, Laos, and Sri Lanka (Miyazaki, 1974). *Paragonimus Africanus* occurs in Cameroon, Nigeria, the Democratic Republic of Congo, equatorial Guinea, and Gabon, and *P. uterobilateralis* in Nigeria, Liberia (Sachs et al. 1986), and Gabon (Sachs et al. 1983). *Paragonimus mexicanus* exists in Ecuador, Peru, Panama, Costa Rica, Guatemala, and Mexico. A focus of *Paragonimus* species occurs in Vietnam (Queuche et al. 1997). Many other species occur in animals, and reports of human infections with these species are expected.

As to the prevalence of paragonimiasis in endemic areas, few data are available because surveys are usually limited to small communities. One survey in Leyte, the Philippines, showed about 14% of the population to be infected (Cabrera, Fevidal, 1974), a figure rather similar to the rates found in areas of Japan (Katamine et al. 1964). *Paragonimus africanus* in endemic areas of Cameroon occurred in about 5% of the population, with children having the heaviest rates of infection (Kum, Nchinda, 1982), and *P. uterobilateralis* occurred in Nigeria in 5% to 10% (Nwokolo, 1974). Also in Nigeria, an outbreak of paragonimiasis occurred during the civil war of 1967–1970 because the displaced community consumed large numbers of uncooked crabs (Nwokolo, 1972).

In the United States, cases of paragonimiasis occur mostly in Southeast Asian refugees (CDC, 1981; Johnson et al. 1982). A few autochthonous cases in the United States are probably due to *P. kellicotti*, the lung fluke of mink, opossums, and other wild animals (Abend, 1910; Fehleisen, Cooper, 1910; Mariano et al. 1986; Spitalny et al. 1982). The cases reported in Canada (Beland et al. 1969) are based on erroneous interpretation of artifacts in the clinical samples (Beaver et al. 1984).

Clinical Findings. The clinical symptoms of paragonimiasis are nonspecific and often follow a chronic benign course; some patients are asymptomatic. The majority of cases occur in the 10- to 25-year age group, and the severity of symptoms usually increases with age (Sadun, Buck, 1960). A chronic cough with blood-tinged sputum is the most common and most remarkable symptom, but in spite of the chronicity of the infection, the patient's health is relatively unimpaired. Peripheral eosinophilia ranges between 20% and 25%, and in heavy infections chest pain, dyspnea, and night sweats occur. Pleural effusion is sometimes found, with

marked leukocytosis and high eosinophilia (Romeo, Pollock, 1986; Singcharoen, Silprasert, 1987). Chest radiography and other imaging techniques show patchy infiltration, and sometimes calcification or cavities (Fig. 25–9; Singcharoen, Silprasert, 1987). Computed tomography is more effective in delineating and locating the lesions, as well as in tracing the migratory path of the worms (Im et al. 1992). Often the clinical diagnosis is pulmonary tuberculosis (Singh et al. 1986). In Japan, some patients presented with marked pleural effusions, high peripheral eosinophilia, and repeated spontaneous pneumothorax (Kobayashi et al. 1975). Sonograms of pleural effusions have demonstrated the eggs as small, hyperechoic foci (Uchida et al. 1995). Soon after treatment, some patients have expectorated the dead worms (Vanijanonta et al. 1981).

One aspect of paragonimiasis is its tendency to occur in ectopic locations such as the brain, abdominal cavity, subcutaneous tissues, heart, and, to a lesser extent, other organs, producing unusual clinical manifestations.

In the brain, *Paragonimus* produces mostly focal symptoms consistent with Jacksonian epilepsy (Higashi et al. 1971), hemianopsia, and gait disturbances (Toy-

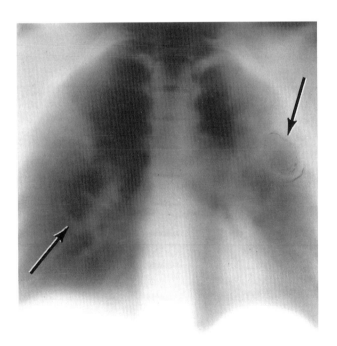

Fig. 25–9. *Paragonimus*, **tomogram of the chest of an infected individual. Note the typical cavitated lesions (arrows). (Courtesy of J.M. Stinson, M.D., Division of Pulmonary Diseases, Meharry Medical College, Nashville, Tennessee. In: Jackson, C.G., Talley, P.A., and Stinson, J.M. 1980. Bilateral pulmonary fibro-cavitary disease and eosinophilia. J. Natl. Med. Assoc. 72:411–412.)**

onaga et al. 1992), but the infection can simulate other syndromes like meningitis, paralysis, or mental retardation. It can also result in fatal cerebral hemorrhages (Brenes Madrigal et al. 1982). In the brain, the most characteristic radiologic finding is calcification; other studies may reveal an intracranial mass, or enlargement and deformity of the ventricles (Higashi et al. 1971). In the abdominal cavity the infection may mimic a malignant tumor, and if several worms are present, it may simulate a malignant tumor with metastases (Abe, Kitsuki, 1956). In the subcutaneous tissues and other organs, paragonimiasis usually manifests as an abscess that eventually organizes and calcifies (Oh, 1978).

Pathology. The pathologic manifestations of paragonimiasis vary with the number of worms, the susceptibility of the host, the duration of the infection, and, to some extent, the species of *Paragonimus*. Death rarely occurs during the acute phase; thus, most histopathologic reports deal with long-standing infections. Most pulmonary lesions produced by *Paragonimus* are best classified grossly as abscesses consisting of grayish-white nodules varying from 1.5 to 5.0 cm in diameter (Diaconita, Goldis, 1964; Yokogawa, 1965). On section, the nodules have a necrotic center, lined with a thick fibrous tissue wall, irregularly infiltrating the surrounding tissue. Early in the infection, the nodules contain two and sometimes three worms (Fig. 25–10 A–B); in long-standing infections in which the worms are resorbed, the nodules appear empty (Fig. 25–11 A) or filled with fluid or necrotic material. Some abscesses seem to originate from a bronchus, producing marked atelectasis of the surrounding pulmonary parenchyma. In a study of 16 patients, the abscesses were located, in decreasing order of frequency, in the right upper, right middle, right lower, and left lower lobes (Yokogawa, 1965).

The microscopic picture depends on the age of the lesion. Recent lesions contain parasites with abundant mononuclear and polymorphonuclear cell infiltrates, especially eosinophils, and little or no fibrosis (Fig.

25–10 D–E). Older lesions are more organized, have more fibrosis and a chronic infiltrate, and often do not contain parasites (Fig. III–11 A–B). Sometimes there is calcification (Fig. 25–12 A). *Paragonimus* eggs are the hallmark of the lesion and are numerous on the internal surface of the fibrous capsule, its wall, and the surrounding parenchyma (Fig. 25–11 B–D). The content of the lesion is variable; sometimes there is necrotic debris and Charcot-Leyden crystals, with various degrees of calcification. A marked granulomatous inflammation produced by eggs trapped in the surrounding pulmonary parenchyma is often seen (Fig. 25–11 C–D).

Ectopic Locations. The adult worms and their eggs, or the eggs alone, are sometimes found in organs other than the lungs. The organs most affected are the brain, where considerable morbidity is produced, and the abdominal cavity.

Brain. Immature *Paragonimus* migrate to the brain through the foramina at the base of the skull (more than likely the jugular vein foramen), which explains why cerebral paragonimiasis is more common in the posterior brain. In one case, an adult worm was found in the bridging veins leading to the lateral sinus (Kim, Walker, 1961). Because *Paragonimus* appears to develop only in the lung parenchyma (Yokogawa, 1965), it has been suggested that mature worms located in the brain originate in the lung. In support of this idea are the observations that all cases of cerebral paragonimiasis produce pulmonary lesions and that, experimentally, cerebral paragonimiasis has been produced only by implantation of adult worms in the brain (Oh, 1978). If this is true, worms found in other ectopic locations must also originate in the lungs, probably at very early stages of development.

Grossly, paragonimiasis in the central nervous system consists of focal lesions ranging from an acute abscess to an organized fibrous nodule to an area of calcification. The worms, especially in children, also produce extensive cerebral hemorrhages (Brenes Madrigal et al. 1982). Microscopically, these lesions

Fig. 25–10. *Paragonimus westermani* experimental infection in dog. *A and B.* Gross lesions. *A,* External surface of the left lung showing three nodules. *B,* Section through a nodule showing two encapsulated worms. *C–E.* Sections stained with hematoxylin and eosin stain. *C,* High magnification of the worm's tegument (t) illustrating the spines (s) in the tegument, the vitelline glands (v), and the mesenchymal cell nuclei (n), ×280. *D,* Low-power view of a worm beginning to encapsulate. Note the lack of a fibrous capsule and the significant inflammatory reaction forming the wall, indicating that the lesion is a recent one. The worm, cut tangentially, shows several sections of intestine (I); the central excretory bladder (b); the vitelline glands (v); the uterus with the immature eggs (u); and the mesenchyme filling the worm's body (p), ×9. *E,* Higher magnification illustrating the inflammatory reaction around the worm (seen at the top), composed mainly of mononuclear and polymorphonuclear cells. Numerous eggs are seen at the bottom, ×70. (Specimen courtesy of R.E. Kuntz, Ph.D., San Antonio Research Foundation, San Antonio, Texas.)

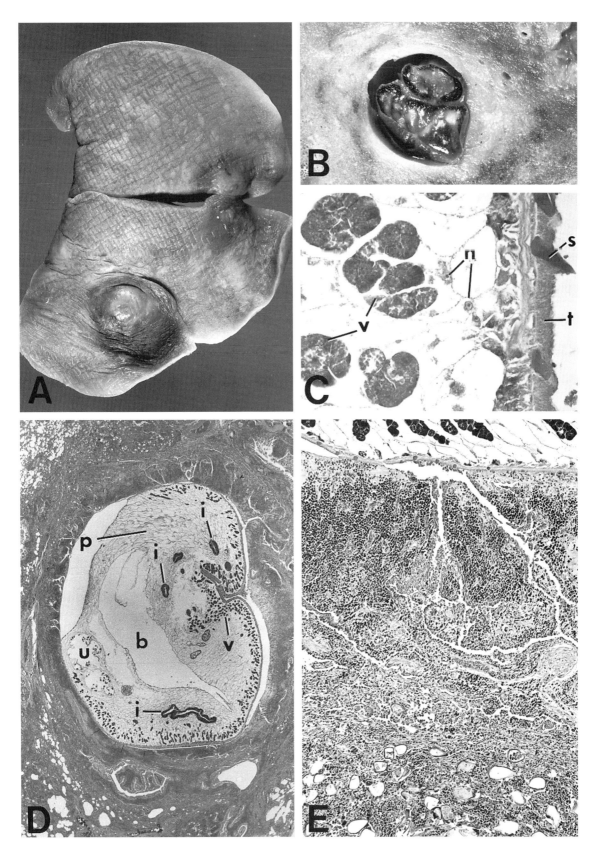

Fig. 25–10.

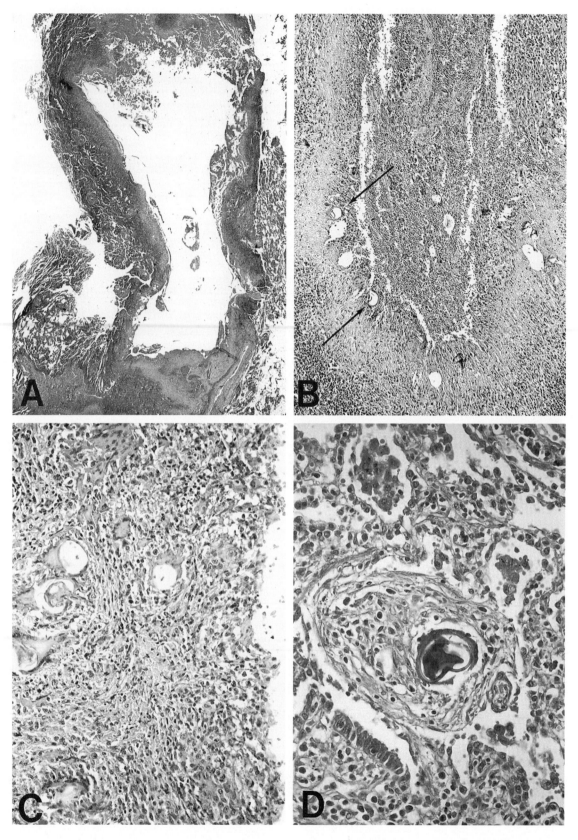

Fig. 25–11. *Paragonimus* in human lung, sections stained with hematoxylin and eosin stain. *A*, Low-power view of an empty nodule composed only of a fibrotic capsule in the lung of an individual with a long-standing infection, ×12. *B*, Aspect of another lesion showing the fibrous capsule and the lumen filled with debris. Note the presence of some eggs (arrows) in the inner aspect of the capsule, ×70. *C* and *D*, Medium- and higher-power magnification illustrating the granulomatous inflammation produced by the eggs. *C*, ×180; *D*, ×450. (Preparation courtesy of J.Y. Ro, M.D., Department of Pathology, M.D. Anderson Cancer Center, Houston, Texas.)

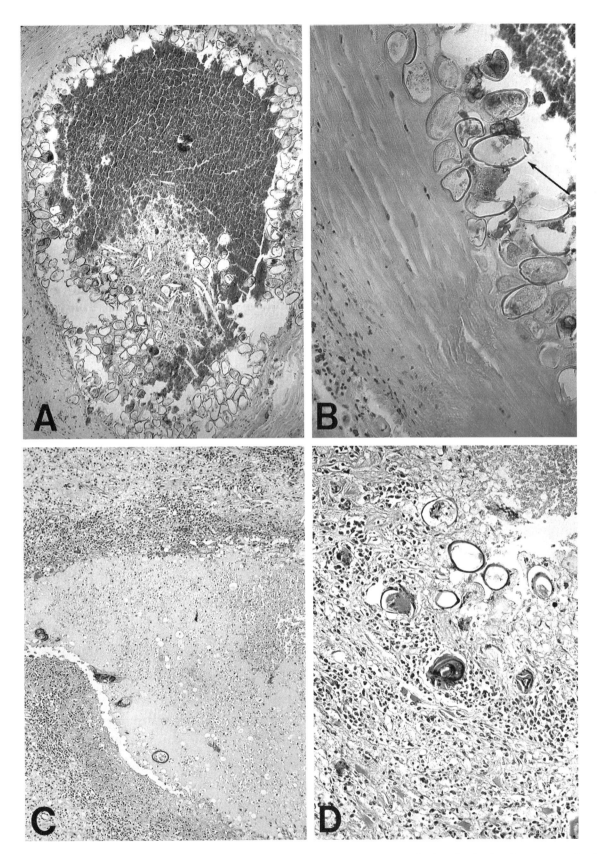

Fig. 25–12. *Paragonimus* in human brain, sections stained with hematoxylin and eosin stain. *A*, Old, calcified lesion with a thick, fibrous capsule containing numerous eggs and amorphous calcium deposits (darkly stained), cholesterol crystals, and other debris, ×55. *B*, Higher magnification showing the fibrous wall and the eggs inside; one egg (arrow) has the typical morphology of a *Paragonimus* egg with a visible operculum, ×180.

C, A more recent lesion in the brain composed of a fibrous capsule and an abundant infiltrate consisting of inflammatory cells. The center of the lesion is filled with necrotic debris, ×55. *D*, Higher magnification of the same lesion showing the inflammatory reaction and numerous eggs, ×140. (Preparation for *A* and *B* courtesy of J.Y. Ro, M.D., Department of Pathology, M.D. Anderson Cancer Center, Houston, Texas.)

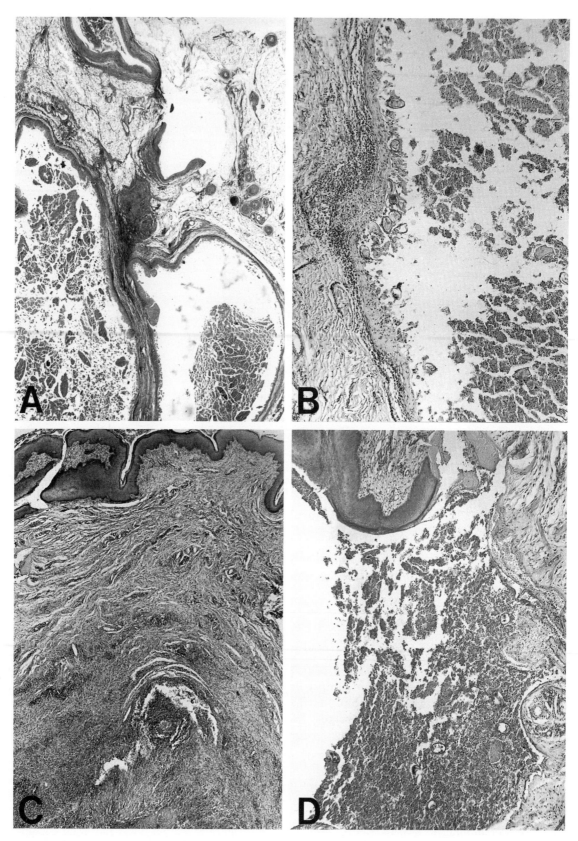

Fig. 25–13. *Paragonimus* lesions in omentum and skin, sections stained with hematoxylin and eosin stain. *A*, Low-power view of a calcified lesion in the omentum, ×9. *B*, Higher magnification showing the wall with numerous eggs and calcified debris, ×55. *C*, Low-power view of a section of skin showing the lesion in the dermis and subcutaneous tissues, ×22. *D*, Higher magnification of the lesion ulcerating to the skin surface, with necrotic material and many eggs, ×55. (Preparations courtesy of J.Y. Ro, M.D., Department of Pathology, M.D. Anderson Cancer Center, Houston, Texas.)

are similar to those found elsewhere, with destruction of tissue (Fig. 25–12 C), and numerous eggs provoking granuloma formation, mostly at the periphery of the necrotic area (Fig. 25–12 D). The eventual healing results in fibrous scars with degenerated eggs followed by calcification (Fig. 25–12 A–B). One case of cysticercus racemosus of the spine was misidentified as paragonimiasis (Moller et al. 1995).

Other ectopic locations of *Paragonimus* also produce nodules that measure 2 to 4 cm in diameter. These nodules are found in the abdominal cavity (Fig. 25–13 A–B), skin (Fig. 25–13 C–C), heart, and other organs. The histologic hallmark of the lesion is the presence of eggs that are identical morphologically to *Paragonimus* eggs. Otherwise, the nodules have histologic characteristics similar to those described above, and undergo identical changes of necrosis, organization, and calcification.

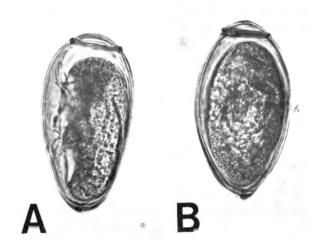

Fig. 25–14. A, B, Paragonimus westermani eggs in human stools, unstained, ×495.

Diagnosis. Paragonimiasis is difficult to diagnose clinically, even in endemic areas, and the clinical laboratory diagnostician must confirm the diagnosis by finding the eggs in sputum or stool samples. In some cases, the eggs are located in the pleural fluid of patients with effusions (Linford, Nguyen, 1994). *Paragonimus* eggs are operculated, measure 80 to 118 μm long by 48 to 60 μm wide (Fig. 25–14), and have a golden brown shell. Identification of the species of *Paragonimus* based on the morphologic characteristics of the eggs alone is not possible; adult worms are required. However, in Africa, where there are only two known species in humans, the size of their eggs allows them to be distinguished. *Paragonimus africanus eggs* measure 70 to 113 μm long by 42 to 57 μm wide, and those of *P. uterobilateralis* measure 62 to 73 μm long by 38 to 50 μm wide (Petavy et al. 1981). In tissue sections the diagnosis rests on the morphologic characteristics of the adult parasite and more commonly on the morphology and size of the eggs. In tissues, only a generic diagnosis is possible because sections of adults do not allow specific classification. Worms recovered at autopsy or in surgical specimens require proper handling in the clinical laboratory for their identification in toto.

In tissue sections *Paragonimus* is seen as a large worm with a tegument similar to that of other trematodes (see the Introduction to Part III and Fig. 20–2). The tegument has numerous spines, which differ in morphology depending on the level of the section (Fig. 25–10 C). The tegument of adult worms is up to 40 μm thick. The longitudinal, oblique, and circular muscle layers appear well defined; their combined thickness is about the same as that of the tegument (Fig. 25–10 C). The mesenchyme is composed of large, clear cells, few of which have a small nucleus, which is evi-

dent in all sections examined (Fig. 25–10 C). The sexual organs of the parasite are visible or not, depending on the level and the angle of the section. The vitelline glands are below the dorsal surface of the worm, extending to the sides and slightly to the ventral surface (Fig. 25–10 C–D). Some sections show the excretory bladder of the worm as an empty space (Fig. 25–10 D). The eggs have been recovered in fine needle aspirates of pulmonary lesions (Rangdaeng et al. 1992).

The eggs found in tissues require proper measurements, and their size range should fall within the range of *Paragonimus* eggs. A search for longitudinally cut eggs is necessary to observe the typical morphology of the egg and its operculum (Fig. 25–12 B). In some cases, eggs of other trematodes in human tissues may be mistaken for *Paragonimus* eggs. Infections with *Achillurbainia* (= *Poikilorchis*) in tissues produce nodules and abscesses in humans that are easily mistaken for an ectopic *Paragonimus* infection because of the resemblance of their eggs (see below).

Achillurbainia (= *Poikilorchis*)— Achillurbainiasis

Achillurbainia (= *Poikilorchis*) is a genus of the family Achillurbainiidae found in the respiratory sinuses and subcutaneous tissues of animals. The genus *Poikilorchis* was proposed for worms found in a retroauricular abscess of a man in the Democratic Republic of Congo, but the morphologic differences for its separation from *Achillurbainia* are minute. For this reason, some au-

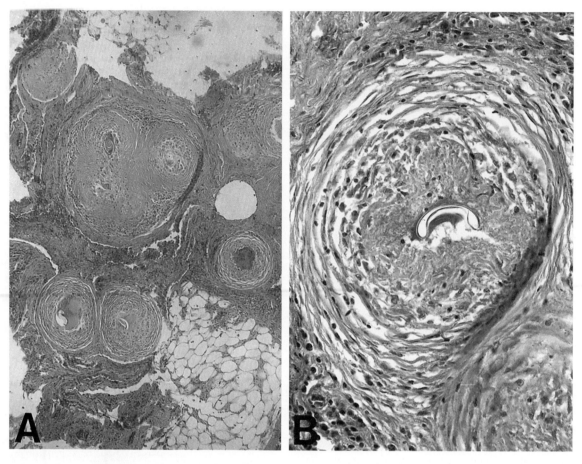

Fig. 25–15. *Achillurbainia* in human peritoneal cavity, section stained with hematoxylin and eosin stain. *A,* Low-power view of granulomas in omentum, ×44. *B,* Detail of a granuloma with an egg, ×235. (Preparation courtesy of M.D. Little, Ph.D., Department of Tropical Medicine, School of Public Health and Tropical Medicine, Tulane University, New Orleans, Louisiana. Reported by: Beaver, P.C., Duron, R.A., and Little, M.D. 1977. Trematode eggs in the peritoneal cavity of a man in Honduras. Am. J. Trop. Med. Hyg. 26:684–687.)

thorities believe that the two genera are the same (Beaver et al., 1977a; R.P. Dolfus, 1966; personal communication to P.C. Beaver, 1977). For simplicity, in this book the two genera are consider identical and, because of priority, are described under the name *Achillurbainia*.

The known human cases of achillurbainiasis in the Old World include one from China (Chen, 1965), four from the Democratic Republic of Congo (Fain, Vandepitte, 1957a, 1957b; Vandepitte et al. 1957), two from Malaysia (Lie et al. 1962; Wong, Lie, 1965), one from Guinea (Loubiere et al. 1977), four from Nigeria (Oyediran et al. 1975; Yarwood, Elmes, 1943), and one from Thailand (Tesjaroen et al. 1989). The cases in the New World are from Honduras (Fig. 25–19 *A–B*; Beaver et al. 1977a; Duron, 1965) and possibly Venezuela (Salas et al. 1973). A report from Taiwan of *P. westermani* in the omentum identified on the basis of the morphology of the eggs in tissue sections appears to fit *Achillurbainia* (Lee et al. 1997).

The main characteristic of the cases in the Old World is the location of the lesion, described as retroauricular in most, mastoid in one case, and left side of the neck in one. In the two cases in the New World, the parasites were located in the peritoneal cavity. One worm recovered from one African patient was identified as a new genus and species, *Poikilorchis congolenses*, and one worm from the patient in Thailand was identified as *A. nouveli*. No worms were recovered from the patients on the American continent, but in one, the suggested species was *A. recondita*. Both species of are known in animals in both the Old World (*A. nouveli*) and the New World (*A. recondita*).

The most common finding in cases of achillurbainiasis is the eggs in tissues (Fig. 25–15 *A–B*). These eggs generally measure 65 to 70 × 34 to 40 μm, and their configuration is different from that of *Paragonimus* eggs. In *Achillurbainia*, the operculum is flattened and does not rest on a shoulder, as it does in *Paragonimus* eggs (Beaver et al. 1984).

Eye

Philophthalmus—Philophthalmiasis

Philophthalmus is a genus of trematodes containing many species with a worldwide distribution, occurring in the nictitating membrane of domestic and wild birds. Human infections with *Philophthalmus* reported in the literature include two from Sri Lanka (Dissanaike, Bilimoria, 1958; Kalthoff et al. 1981), and one each from Yugoslavia (Markovic, 1939), Japan (Mimori et al. 1982), and the United States (Gutierrez et al. 1987).

In all five cases, the ophthalmologist found the worms in the eye and retrieved them for examination. All were described as a species of *Philophthalmus*. Two immature worms and one mature worm were on the conjunctival surface, producing conjunctivitis. The other two worms, found in the subconjunctiva, required surgical removal; both patients also presented with conjunctivitis accompanied by a foreign body sensation. Identification of the worms was based on their morphology (*color plate* XIII *F* and Fig. III–1). Mature worms have a uterus with characteristic eggs, each bearing a mature miracidium with two eyespots.

Infection with Trematode Larvae

There are a few reports of human infections with a trematode larva in the tissues of humans. A 29-year-old woman living in Ontario, Canada, had a trematode larva in the retina; laser treatment destroyed it in situ. No conclusive identification of the parasite was possible, except to say that because the worm did not encyst in the retina, it probably was a mesocercaria. (A mesocercaria is a stage between the cercaria and the metacercaria; it is found in tissues of animals other than the natural hosts. In these hosts, on penetration, the cercaria grows considerably and remains in the tissues until, by predation, it reaches the natural host and develops to an adult in the intestine.) It was also sug-

gested that the ocular infection in this woman occurred during handling and preparation of frogs for cooking (Shea et al. 1973). In this case, the mesocercaria of *Alaria americana*, which occurs naturally in frogs, the intermediate hosts, would be a good candidate for the infection. The cook's fingers probably transported a mesocercaria in the frog's flesh accidentally to the conjunctiva.

A second generalized infection with the mesocercaria of *A. americana* was reported in a 24-year-old man from Ontario (Fig. 25–16; Fernandes et al. 1976; Freeman et al. 1976). (*Alaria americana* is an intesti-

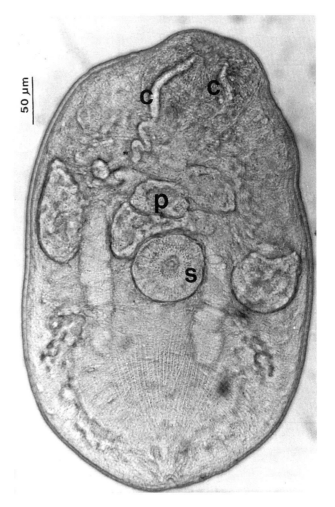

Fig. 25–16. *Alaria americana* **recovered from the lungs of a man in Ontario, Canada. Whole mount, unstained; bar represent 50 m. Penetration glands (p); acetabulum or ventral sucker (s) with several rows of small spines; ceca (c). (In: Freeman, R.S., Stuart, F.P., Cullen, J.B., et al. 1976. Fatal human infection with mesocercaria of the trematode** *Alaria americana.* **Am. J. Trop. Med. Hyg. 25:803–807. Reproduced with permission.)**

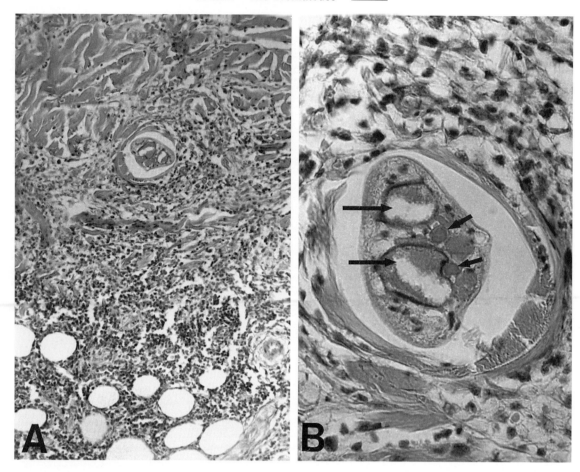

Fig. 25–17. *Alaria* in human skin, section stained with hematoxylin and eosin stain. *A,* Low-power view showing the parasite and the intense inflammatory reaction, ×140. *B.* Higher magnification of the parasite. The two large structures (arrows) are gland cells and next to them are the two ceca (short arrows), ×570. (Preparation courtesy of M.D. Little, Ph.D., Department of Tropical Medicine, School of Public Health and Tropical Medicine, Tulane University, New Orleans, Louisiana. Reported by: Beaver, P.C., Little, M.D., Tucker, C.F., et al. 1977. Mesocerearia in the skin of a man in Louisiana. Am. J. Trop. Med. Hyg. 26:422–426.)

nal fluke of foxes and dogs, and frogs are its natural intermediate hosts.) In this patient, the parasites were found in most tissues and organs examined (*color plate XIV A–C*). In a third case, small nodules in the subcutaneous tissues of a patient in Louisiana, the United States, contained parasites identified as a species of *Alaria* (Fig. 25–17 A–B; Beaver et al. 1977b). Further study of numerous serial histologic sections of one nodule permitted the reconstruction of the parasite and its identification as *A. marcianae* (Shoop, Corkum, 1983). A fourth patient, also in the United States, presented with a subcutaneous nodule; the parasite was identified in tissue sections as a mesocercarial species of *Alaria* or *Strigea* (Kramer et al. 1996).

References

Abe T, Kitsuki T, 1956. A case of abdominal paragonimiasis erroneously diagnosed as one of gastric cancer. Fukuoka Acta Med. 47:959–962

Abend L, 1910. Uber Hemoptysis parasitaria. Deutsche Archiv. Klin. Med. 100:501–511

Africa CM, Garcia EY, Leon W de, 1935a. Intestinal heterophyidiasis with cardiac involvement. A contribution to the etiology of heart failure. Philip. J. Public Health 2:1–35

Africa CM, Garcia EY, Leon W de, 1935b. Intestinal heterophyidiasis with cardiac involvement: a contribution to the etiology of heart failure. J. Philipp. Isl. Med. Assoc. 15:358–361

Africa CM, Leon W de, Garcia EY, 1936. Heterophyidiasis: III: ova associated with fatal hemorrhage in the right basal ganglia of the brain. J. Philipp. Isl. Med. Assoc. 16:22–26

Africa CM, Leon W de, Garcia EY, 1937. Heterophyidiasis: VI. Two more cases of heart failure associated with the presence of eggs in sclerosed valves. J. Philipp. Isl. Med. Assoc. 17:605–609

Alicata JE, Schattenburg OL, 1938. A case of intestinal heterophyidiasis of man in Hawaii. JAMA 110:1100–1101

Beaver PC, Duron RA, Little MD, 1977a. Trematode eggs in the peritoneal cavity of man in Honduras. Am. J. Trop. Med. Hyg. 26:684–687

Beaver PC, Jung RC, Cupp EW, 1984. *Clinical Parasitology*. Philadelphia: Lea & Febiger

Beaver PC, Little MD, Tucker CF, Reed RJ, 1977b. Mesocercaria in the skin of man in Louisiana. Am. J. Trop. Med. Hyg. 26:422–426

Beland JE, Boone J, Donevan RE, Manckiewicz E, 1969. Paragonimiasis (the lung fluke). Report of four cases. Am. Rev. Respir. Dis. 99:261–271

Brenes Madrigal RR, Rodriguez-Ortiz B, Vargas-Solano G, Ocampo-Obando EM, Ruiz-Sotela PJ, 1982. Cerebral hemorrhagic lesions produced by *Paragonimus mexicanus*. Report of three cases in Costa Rica. Am. J. Trop. Med. Hyg. 31:522–526

Cabrera BD, Fevidal PM, 1974. Studies on *Paragonimus* and paragonimiasis in the Philippines. Southeast Asian J. Trop. Med. Public Health 5:39–45

Carney WP, Sudomo M, Purnomo, 1980. Echinostomiasis: a disease that disappeared. Trop. Geogr. Med. 32:101–105

CDC, 1981. Paragonimiasis in Hmong refugees—Minnesota. Morb. Mort. Weekly Rep. 30:176, 181–182

Chai JY, Hong ST, Lee SH, Lee GC, Min YI, 1994. A case of echinostomiasis with ulcerative lesions in the duodenum. Korean J. Parasitol. 32:201–204

Chai JY, Kim IM, Seo M, Guk SM, Kim JL, Sohn WM, Lee SH, 1997. A new endemic focus of *Heterophyes nocens*, *Pygidiopsis summa*, and other intestinal flukes in a coastal area of Muan-gun, Chollanam-do. Korean J. Parasitol. 35:233–238

Chai JY, Kim J, Lee SH, 1995. Invasion of *Metagonimus yokogawai* into the submucosal layer of the small intestine of immunosuppressed mice. Korean J. Parasitol. 33:313–320

Chai JY, Nam HK, Kook J, Lee SH, 1994. The first discovery of an endemic focus of *Heterophyes nocens* (Heterophyidae) infection in Korea. Korean J. Parasitol. 32:157–161

Chen HT, 1965. *Paragonimus*, *Pagumogonimus* and a *Paragonimus*-like trematode in man. Chinese Med. J. 84:781–791

Chung DI, Moon CH, Kong HH, Choi DW, Lim DK, 1995. The first human case of *Clinostomum complanatum* (Trematoda: Clinostomidae) infection in Korea. Korean J. Parasitol. 33:219–223

Collomb H, Bert J, 1957. Distomatose cerebrale avec kystes parasitaires generalises. Rev. Neurol. 97:501–506

Collomb H, Deschiens R, Demarchi J, 1960. Sur deux cas de distomatose cerebrale a *Heterophyes heterophyes*. Bull. Soc. Pathol. Exot. 53:144–147

Cross JH, Basaca-Sevilla V, 1986. Studies on *Echinostoma ilocanum* in the Philippines. Southeast Asian J. Trop. Med. Public Health 17:23–27

Daengsvang S, Mangalasmaya M, 1941. A record of some cases of human infestation with *Fasciolopsis buskii* occurring in Thailand. Ann. Trop. Med. Parasitol. 35:43–44

Diaconita G, Goldis G, 1964. Investigations on pathomorphology and pathogenesis of pulmonary paragonimiasis. Acta Tubercul. Scand. 44:51–75

Dissanaike AS, Bilimoria DP, 1958. On an infection of a human eye with *Philophthalmus* sp. in Ceylon. J. Helminthol. 32:115–118

Duron MRA, 1965. Granulomatosis omento-mesenterico parasitaria. Reporte de un caso. Rev. Med. Hondur. 33:3–6

Eastburn RL, Fritsche TR, Terhune CA Jr, 1987. Human intestinal infection with *Nanophyetus salmincola* from salmonid fishes. Am. J. Trop. Med. Hyg. 36:586–591

Fain A, Vandepitte J, 1957a. Correspondence. A new trematode *Poikilorchis congolensis* n. g. n. sp., living in subcutaneous retroauricular cysts in man from the Belgian Congo. Nature 179:740

Fain A, Vandepitte J, 1957b. Description du nouveau distome vivant dans des kystes ou abees retroauriculaires chez l'homme au Congo Belge. Ann. Soc. Belge Med. Trop. 37:251–258

Fehleisen F, Cooper CM, 1910. Paragonimiasis or parasitic hemoptysis (report of an imported case in California). JAMA 54:697–699

Fernandes BJ, Cooper JD, Cullen JB, Freeman RS, Ritchie AC, Scott AA, Stuart PP, 1976. Systemic infection with *Alaria americana* (Trematoda). Can. Med. Assoc. J. 115:1111–1114

Filimonova LV, 1963. Life-cycle of the trematode *Nanophyetus schikhobalowi*. Trudy Gelminthol. Lab. 13:347–357

Freeman RS, Stuart P, Cullen J, Ritchie A, Mildon A, Fernandez B, 1976. A fatal infection with mesocercariae of *Alaria americana* (Trematoda). Trans. Am. Microbiol. Soc. 95:268

Gallais P, Paillas P, Collomb P, Luigi DM, Demarchi J, Deschiens R, 1955. Etude anatomo-pathologique d'un kyste parasitaire cerebral observe chez l'homme. Bull. Soc. Pathol. Exot. 48:830–832

Galliard H, Ngu DV, 1947. Recherces sur la specifite parasitaire de *Fasciolopsis buski*. Ann. Parasitol. Hum. Comp. 22:16–23

Gilman RH, Mondal G, Maksud M, Alam K, Rutherford E, Gilman JB, Khan MU, 1982. Endemic focus of *Fasciolopis buski* infection in Bangladesh. Am. J. Trop. Med. Hyg. 31:796–802

Gomaa T, 1962. Pulmonary complications of *Heterophyes* infestation. J. Egypt. Med. Assoc. 45:317–322

Gutierrez Y, Grossniklaus HE, Annable WL, 1987. Human conjunctivitis caused by the bird parasite *Philophthalmus*. Am. J. Ophthalmol. 104:417–419

Higashi K, Aoki H, Tatebayashi K, Morioka M, Sakata Y, 1971. Cerebral paragonimiasis. J. Neurosurg. 34:515–527

Hirai H, Ooiso H, Kifune T, Kiyota T, Sakaguchi Y, 1987. *Clinostomum complanatum* infection in posterior wall of the pharynx of a human. Jpn. J. Parasitol. 36:142–144

Hong SJ, Chung CK, Lee DH, Woo HC, 1996. One human case of natural infection by *Heterophyopsis continua* and three other species of intestinal trematodes. Korean J. Parasitol. 34:87–90

Im JG, Whang HY, Kim WS, Han MC, Shim YS, Cho SY, 1992. Pleuropulmonary paragonimiasis: radiologic findings in 71 patients. Am. J. Roentgenol. 159:39–43

Jaroonvesama N, Charoenlarp K, Areekul S, 1986. Intestinal absorption studies in *Fasciolopsis buski* infection. Southeast Asian J. Trop. Med. Public Health 17:587–590

Johnson JR, Falk A, Iber C, Davies S, 1982. Paragonimiasis in the United States. A report of nine cases in Hmong immigrants. Chest 82:168–171

Kalthoff H, Janitschke K, Mravak S, Schopp W, Werner H, 1981. Ein ausgereifter Saugwurm der Gattung *Philophthalmus* unter der Bindehaut des Menschen. Klin. Monatsbl. Augenheilk. 179:373–375

Kamo H, Ogino K, Hatsushika R, 1962. A unique infection with *Clinostomum* sp., a small trematode causing acute laryngitis. Yonago Acta Med. 6:37–40

Katamine D, Murakami F, Yoshimura O, Imai J, Yamamoto T, Ishii Y, 1964. Epidemiological survey on paragonimiasis in Kamitsushima-cho, Nagasaki Prefecture and Sumotomura, Kumamoto Prefecture, with particular reference to chest X-ray findings of the residents in endemic areas. Endemic Dis. Bull. Nagasaki Univ. 6:100–108

Kau LS, Wu K, 1938. Pathological findings among pigs experimentally infected with *Fasciolopsis buskii*. Ann. Trop. Med. Parasitol. 32:133–136

Kim SK, Walker AE, 1961. Cerebral paragonimiasis. Acta Psychiatr. Neurol. Scand. 36(Suppl):153

Kobayashi A, Suzuki S, Horiuchi K, Yokogawa M, Araki K, 1975. Four human cases of paragonimiasis *miyazakii*. Jikeikai Med. J. 22:127–135

Kramer MH, Eberhard ML, Blankenberg TA, 1996. Respiratory symptoms and subcutaneous granuloma caused by mesocercariae: a case report. Am. J. Trop. Med. Hyg. 55:447–448

Kum PN, Nchinda TC, 1982. Pulmonary paragonimiasis in Cameroon. Trans. R. Soc. Trop. Med. Hyg. 76:768–772

Lee SC, Jwo SC, Hwang KP, Lee N, Shieh WB, 1997. Discovery of encysted *Paragonimus westermani* eggs in the omentum of an asymptomatic elderly woman. Am. J. Trop. Med. Hyg. 57:615–618

Lie KJ, Williams HI, Miyazaki I, Wong SK, 1962. A subcutaneous retro-auricular abscess in a Dyak boy in Sarawak, probably caused by a trematode of the genus *Poikilorchis*, Fain and Vandepitte, 1957. Med. J. Malaya 17:37–40

Linford RA, Nguyen GK, 1994. Correspondence. *Paragonimus westermani* ova in pleural effusion. Diagn. Cytopathol. 11:95–96

Loubiere R, Doucet J, Ehouman A, Nozais JP, Guhi G, 1977. Premier cas de distomatose retro-auriculaire depiste chez un guineen. Nouv. Presse Med. 6:1771

Malek EA, 1980. *Snail-transmitted Parasitic Diseases*. Vols. I and II., Boca Raton, Fla.: CRC Press

Manning GS, Ratanarat C, 1970. *Fasciolopsis buski* (Lankester, 1857) in Thailand. Am. J. Trop. Med. Hyg. 19:613–619

Mariano EG, Borja SR, Vruno MJU, 1986. A human infection with *Paragonimus kellicotti* (lung fluke) in the United States. Am. J. Clin. Pathol. 86:685–687

Markovic A, 1939. Der erste Fall von Philophthalmose beim Menschen. Arch. Ophthalmol. 140:515–526

Milleman RE, Knapp SE, 1970. Biology of *Nanophyetus salmincola* and "salmon poisoning" disease. Adv. Parasitol. 8:1–41

Mimori T, Hiral H, Kifune T, Inada K, 1982. *Philophthalmus* sp. (Trematoda) in a human eye. Am. J. Trop. Med. Hyg. 31:859–861

Miyazaki I, 1974. Lung flukes in the world. Morphology and life cycle history. In: *A Symposium on Epidemiology of Parasitic Diseases*. Tokyo: International Medical Foundation of Japan, pp. 101–135

Miyazaki I, 1982. A review of *Paragonimus pulmonalis* (Baelz, 1880) Miyazaki, 1978, the lung fluke of medical importance. Med. Bull. Fukuoka Univ. 9:221–232

Miyazaki I, Habe S, 1975. A new mode of human infection with *Paragonimus westermani*. Yonsei Rep. Trop. Med. 6:76

Miyazaki I, Habe S, 1976. A newly recognized mode of human infection with the lung fluke, *Paragonimus westermani* (Kerbert 1878). J. Parasitol. 62:646–648

Miyazaki I, Habe S, Terasaki K, 1981a. On the pairing of adult lung flukes. Med. Bull. Fukuoka Univ. 8:159–167

Miyazaki I, Terasaki K, Habe S, 1981b. Comparison of single-worm infection to cats between *Paragonimus westermani* and *P. pulmonalis*. Med. Bull. Fukuoka Univ. 8:405–416

Moller A, Settnes OP, Jensen NO, Kruse LC, 1995. A case of cerebral paragonimiasis in Denmark. Case report. APMIS 103:604–606

Muttalib MA, Islam N, 1975. *Fasciolopsis buski* in Bangladesh—a pilot study. J. Trop. Med. Hyg. 78:135–137

Nwokolo C, 1972. Endemic paragonimiasis in eastern Nigeria. Clinical features and epidemiology of the recent outbreak following the Nigerian Civil War. Trop. Geogr. Med. 24:138–147

Nwokolo C, 1974. Endemic paragonimiasis in Africa. Bull. WHO 50:569–571

Oh SJ, 1978. Paragonimiasis in the central nervous system. In: Vinken PJ, Bruin OW (eds), *Handbook of Clinical Neurology. Infections of the Nervous System*, Vol. 35, Part III. Amsterdam, New York, and Oxford: North Holland Pub. Co., pp. 243–266

Oyediran ABOO, Fajemisin AA, Abioyi AA, Lagundoye SB, Olugbile AOB, Abioye AA, 1975. Infection of the mastoid bone with a *Paragonimus*-like trematode. Am. J. Trop. Med. Hyg. 24:268–273

Petavy AF, Cambon M, Demeocq F, Dechelotte P, 1981. Un cas Gabonais de paragonimose chez un enfant. Bull. Soc. Pathol. Exot. 74:193–197

Plaut AG, Kampanart-Sanyakorn C, Manning GS, 1969. A clinical study of *Fasciolopsis buski* infection in Thailand. Trans. R. Soc. Trop. Med. Hyg. 63:470–478

Queuche F, Cao VV, Le DII, 1997. Un foyer de paragonimose au Viet Nam. Sante 7:155–159

Rahman KM, Idris MD, Azad Khan AK, 1981. A study on fasciolopsiasis in Bangladesh. J. Trop. Med. Hyg. 84:81–86

Rangdaeng S, Alpert LC, Khiyami A, Cottingham K, Ramzy I, 1992. Pulmonary paragonimiasis. Report of a case with diagnosis by fine needle aspiration cytology. Acta Cytol. 36:31–36

Romeo DP, Pollock JJ, 1986. Pulmonary paragonimiasis: diagnostic value of pleural fluid analysis. South. Med. J. 79:241–243

Sachs R, Albiez H, Voelker J, 1986. Prevalence of *Paragonimus uterobilateralis* infection in children in a Liberian village. Trans. R. Soc. Trop. Med. Hyg. 80:800–801

Sachs R, Kern P, Voelker J, 1983. Le *Paragonimus uterobilateralis* comme cause de trois cas de paragonimose humaine au Gabon. Tropenmed. Parasit. 34:105–108

Sadun EH, Buck AA, 1960. Paragonimiasis in South Korea—immunodiagnostic, epidemiologic, clinical, roentgenologic and therapeutic studies. Am. J. Trop. Med. Hyg. 9:562–599

Sadun EH, Maiphoom C, 1953. Studies on the epidemiology of the human intestinal fluke, *Fasciolopsis buski* (Lankester) in central Thailand. Am. J. Trop. Med. Hyg. 2:1070–1084

Sakaguchi Y, Yamamoto T, Yamada N, 1966. *Clinostomum* sp. from the larynx of a man. Endem. Dis. Bull. Nagasaki Univ. 8:40–44

Salas LAR, Duran E, Morrell JR, 1973. Localizacion ectopica de *Paragonimus* sp. Braun 1899 (Trematoda: Troglotrematidae). Arch. Venezol. Med. Trop. Parasitol. Med. 5:365–374

Sandground JH, Bonne C, 1940. *Echinostoma lindoensis* n. sp. a new parasite of man in the Celebes with an account of its life history and epidemiology. Am. J. Trop. Med. 20:511–532

Shea M, Maberley AL, Walters J, Freeman RS, Fallis AM, 1973. Intraretinal larval trematode. Trans. Am. Acad. Ophthalmol. Otol. 77:784–791

Shoop WL, Corkum KC, 1983. Migration of *Alaria marcianae* (Trematoda) in domestic cats. J. Parasitol. 69:912–917

Singcharoen T, Silprasert W, 1987. CT findings in pulmonary paragonimiasis. J. Comput. Assist. Tomogr. 11:1101–1102

Singh TS, Mutum SS, Razaque MA, 1986. Pulmonary paragonimiasis: clinical features, diagnosis and treatment of 39 cases in Manipur. Trans. R. Soc. Trop. Med. Hyg. 80:967–971

Son WY, Huh S, Lee SU, Woo HC, Hong SJ, 1994. Intestinal trematode infections in the villagers in Koje-myon, Kochang-gun, Kyongsangnam-do, Korea. Korean J. Parasitol. 32:149–155

Spitalny KC, Senft AW, Meglio FD, 1982. Treatment of pulmonary paragonimiasis with a new broad spectrum antihelminthic, praziquantel. J. Pediatr. 101:144–146

Tantachamrum T, Kliks M, 1978. Heterophyid infection in human ileum: report of three cases. Southeast Asian J. Trop. Med. Public Health 9:228–231

Tesjaroen S, Ngaoten P, Lertlaituan P, 1989. The first report of *Achillurbaenia nouveli* Dellfus, 1939 in Thailand. Siriraj Hosp. Gaz. 41:500–503

Toyonaga S, Kurisaka M, Mori K, Suzuki N, 1992. Cerebral paragonimiasis—report of five cases. Neurol. Med Chir. Tokyo. 32:157–162

Uchida K, Sekiguchi S, Doi Y, Yamazaki H, 1995. Pulmonary paragonimiasis with pleural effusion containing *Paragonimus* ova: sonographical appearance of pleural effusion. Intern. Med. 34:1178–1180

Vandepitte J, Job A, Delaisse J, Tabarny MJ, 1957. Quatre cas d'abces retro-auriculaires chez des Congolais, produit par un nouveau distome. Ann. Soc. Belge Med. Trop. 37:309–315

Vanijanonta S, Radomyos P, Bunnag D, Harinasuta T, 1981. Pulmonary paragonimiasis with expectoration of worms: a case report. Southeast Asian J. Trop. Med. Public Health 12:104–110

Viranuvatti V, Stitnimankarn T, Tansurat P, 1953. A fatal case of infection with *Fasciolopsis buskii* in Thailand. Ann. Trop. Med. Parasitol. 47:132–133

Wong SK, Lie KJ, 1965. Another periauricular abscess from Sarawak, probably caused by a trematode of the genus *Poikilorchis*, Fain and Vandepitte. Med. J. Malaya 19:229–230

Yamashita J, 1938. *Clinostomum complanatum*, a trematode parasite new to man. Ann. Zool. Jpn. 17:563–566

Yarwood GR, Elmes BGT, 1943. *Paragonimus* cyst in a West African native. Trans. R. Soc. Trop. Med. Hyg. 36:347–351

Yokogawa M, 1965. *Paragonimus* and paragonimiasis. In: Dawes E. (ed), *Advances in Parasitology*. London and New York: Academic Press, Vol. 3, pp. 99–157

Yokogawa M, Harinasuta C, Charoenlarp P, 1965. *Hypoderaeum conoideum* (Bloch, 1872) Dietz, 1909, a common intestinal fluke in man in northeast Thailand. Jpn. J. Parasitol. 14:148–153

Yoshida Y, Arizono N, Uemoto K, Shimada Y, Shiota K, 1976. Experimental human infection with *Echinostoma hortense* Asada, 1926. Jpn. J. Parasitol. 25(Suppl 2):61

Yoshimura K, Ishigooka S, Satoh I, Kamegai S, 1991. *Clinostomum complanatum* from the pharynx of a woman in Akita, Japan. A case report. Jpn. J. Parasitol. 40:99–101

Zubov NA, Drozdov VN, Chernova AS, 1970. Clinical picture and pathology of metagonimiasis. Med. Parazitol. 39:392–394

Part IV

The Cestodes

Cestodes are metazoan organisms consisting of a chain of segments with the general appearance of a ribbon, each segment usually containing a set of male and female sexual organs. Cestodes are known commonly as *tapeworms*, probably a direct translation of the German word *bandwurm*, in vogue during the early 19th century. Two stages of the tapeworm life cycle are important for the anatomic pathologist: the adult and the larva.

Adult Worms

Most adult tapeworms parasitize the gastrointestinal tracts of animals and humans. Their size varies from a few millimeters to 10 m, and in general, they have complicated life cycles that involve two or more hosts. The body of an adult cestode is known as the *strobila*, which with few exceptions consists of a series of segments known as *proglottids* (Fig. IV–1, and *color plate* XV E). The worm grows in the *neck*, an area near the scolex, by a process known as *strobilation*, or formation of new proglottids. As a new proglottid begins differentiating from the growth area,

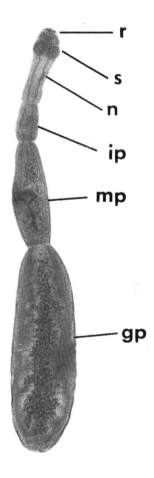

Fig. IV–1. *Echinococcus granulosus*, adult worm, aceto-alum carmine stain. This small tapeworm, found in the intestine of dogs, illustrates the general morphology of an adult cestode: rostellum (r) with hooklets; suckers (s); neck (n), the area where strobilation (formation of a new proglottis) occurs; immature proglottid (ip); mature proglottid (mp); gravid proglottid (gp). Note the uterus filled with eggs, ×35.

it displaces the next one (previously formed) toward the posterior end. The slow displacement of proglottids from the anterior end toward the posterior end allows sufficient time for differentiation and maturation of the sexual organs in each proglottid. Thus, in general, proglottids close to the anterior end of the worm are *immature*, those in the middle are *mature*, and those in the posterior are *gravid*.

The anterior end of a tapeworm is the *scolex*, with structures by which the worm attaches to the intestinal mucosa. The scolex is also of taxonomic value. Depending on whether the scolex has four suckers or two longitudinal grooves (*bothria*), the tapeworms important in human medicine belong to either the order Cyclophyllidea or the order Pseudophyllidea, respectively. Tapeworms belonging to the Cyclophyllidea may have, in addition to the four suckers, a *rostellum* armed with spines or hooks, usually arranged in two or more circular rows; the number and size of these spines or hooks are of taxonomic value (Fig. IV–2).

The morphology of the gravid proglottids is important to the pathologist because the diagnosis of tapeworm infections in the laboratory often rests on recognition of the proglottid or portions of the worm's strobila retrieved from the feces. In general, the gravid proglottid varies in size and shape, depending on the species, but it always has a uterus filled with eggs, which often allows identification of the

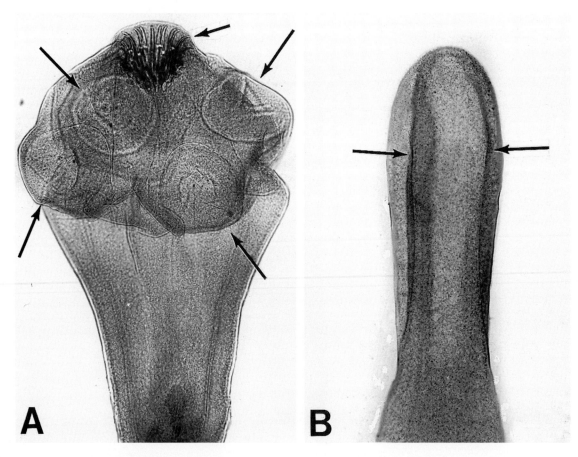

A

B

Fig. IV–2. Scolices of cyclophyllidean and pseudophyllidean tapeworms. A, *Taenia solium*, scolex, aceto-alum carmine stain. The rostellum is invaginated, and only the hooklets are seen (short arrow). The four suckers are easily seen (long arrows), ×70. B, *Spirometra*, scolex, **hematoxylin stain. Note the two bothria (arrows), ×70. (Preparation for B courtesy of M.D. Little, Ph.D., School of Public Health and Tropical Medicine, Tulane University, New Orleans, Louisiana.)**

genus and sometimes the species (Fig. IV–3). Most human tapeworms parasitize the gastrointestinal tract, producing few or no symptoms. There are many species of human tapeworms, some with worldwide distribution, others restricted to certain geographic areas. Some intestinal tapeworms occur sporadically as zoonotic infections acquired by consumption of exotic food or accidentally by consumption of contaminated food. Most of these tapeworms are well known, and are discussed in standard books on parasitology and in textbooks dealing with clinical laboratory diagnosis. The larval stages of tapeworms are tissue dwellers, and humans are host to a variety of them. Some of these larvae produce marked morbidity and mortality, and thus often fall within the realm of the anatomic pathologist. The larval stages of cestodes occurring in humans are the subject of the next two chapters.

The Tegument. The tegument of cestodes has some similarities to that of the trematodes in terms of structure and organization (see the introduction to Part III). On light microscopy, the tegument has an *outer layer* of variable thickness that consists of a homogeneous acellular layer that stains deeply eosinophilically. The outer layer corresponds to a cytoplasmic syncytium of gland cells located below it and forming the *inner* layer. These cells have a relatively large nucleus, and their function is to secret the outer layer. In electron micrographs, the outer surface of the acellular layer has microtriches similar to the brush border of the intestine of animals. These microtriches absorb the nutrients for the parasite, since cestodes do not have a digestive system. In the Cyclophyllidea, the adults have two layers of muscle fibrils (Fig. IV–12 *E*), one longitudinal and the other transverse, dividing the body of the worm into medullary and cortical areas. These layers of muscle fibrils are the main muscle system of the Cyclophyllidea, which in addition have smaller bundles of muscle fibrils that run dorsoventrally. In the Pseudophyllidea, the longitudinal muscles are scattered throughout the body of the parasite. These anatomic landmarks are important in the diagnosis of larval stages and sometimes are the only elements that allow proper diagnosis.

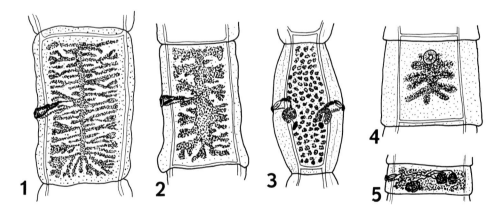

Fig. IV–3. Schematic representation of gravid proglottids of some common intestinal tapeworms of humans: *1, Taenia saginata. 2, Taenia solium* (note the number of branches of the uterus in each. *Taenia saginata* has over 16 branches and *T. solium* fewer than 14 on either side). *3, Dipylidium caninum. 4, Diphyllobothrium. 5, Hymenolepis.* Not at scale. (From: Smith, J.W. and Gutierrez, Y. 1991. Medical parasitology. In: J.B. Henry (ed.), *Todd, Sanford, Davidsohn Clinical Diagnosis and Management by Laboratory Methods.* 18th ed. Philadelphia: W.B. Saunders, p. 1201. Reproduced with permission.)

Larvae

In general, the cestodes have *indirect* life cycles that include one, two, or even three obligatory intermediate hosts. A few have *direct* life cycles; one of them, *Hymenolepis nana*, a parasite of humans, has both direct and indirect types of development (Fig. IV–4). As stated, with rare exceptions, all adult cestodes parasitize the intestinal tracts of vertebrates. Eggs or gravid proglottids containing the eggs pass with the feces into the environment, where they are picked up by the appropriate intermediate hosts. Once in the intestine the eggs hatch, freeing the embryo, which moves toward the intestinal wall, enters it, and migrates through the circulation to the appropriate tissues, where it develops into an infective larva. In the case of arthropods, the second intermediate hosts, the embryo usually migrates to the general cavity of the arthropod, where it develops into an infective larva. In their intermediate hosts, larvae grow in different tissues and produce diseases in accordance with the organ involved, the structures affected, and the rate of growth of the parasite. These cestode larvae have unique morphologic characteristics that allow their identification to the group level, to the genus level, and sometimes to the species level.

When humans ingest the eggs of certain tapeworms, the larvae develop and behave as if humans are the intermediate hosts. However, in these instances, humans are *terminal* hosts, since it is the exception rather than the rule that humans become food for the final hosts of the parasite. The cestode larvae that infect humans are important in medicine because they produce diseases, some of which are major health problems. In addition, the tapeworm larvae that occur in livestock result in great economic losses and thus are of veterinary importance. The main cestode larvae occurring in humans and their morphologic characteristics will now be discussed.

Cysticercus

Several morphologic variations of *Cysticercus*, referred to as *bladder worms*, are in general the larval stages of some species of *Taenia*. *Cysticercus cellulosae*, the larva of *T. solium*, and *C. bovis*, the larva of *T. saginata*, are the best-known species in human medicine. On gross examination, these two cyticerci are similar. They consist of an ovoid, delicate cyst, usually less than 1.0 cm in the largest dimension, formed by a delicate, translucent membrane filled with clear fluid and a scolex invaginated inside the cyst (Fig. IV–5 *A* and *color plate* XIV *D–E*). The size of the invaginated scolex and its neck together is approximately one-fourth to one-fifth the diameter of the cysticercus and appears as a grain of rice attached to the inner

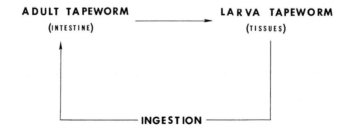

Fig. IV–4. General schematic representation of the life cycle of a tapeworm. Note that the larval stage of some tapeworms may require only one or sometimes more than one intermediate host.

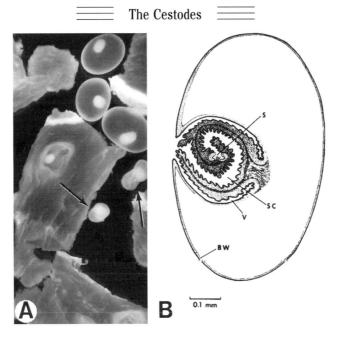

Fig. IV–5. *Cysticercus. A*, Gross photograph of cysticerci in muscle and isolated from muscle to illustrate their general morphology. Note the three intact cysticerci (top), with bladder filled with a fluid and the scolex tightly invaginated. Two other cysticerci (arrows) have ruptured bladder walls, and the walls are tightly contracted around the scolex (histologically, this will be seen as the cysticercus in Fig. 26–6 *B*), ×2. *B*, Schematic representation of the histologic section of a cysticercus showing all structures aligned in an ideal plane. Abbreviations: bw, bladder wall; v, vestibule; sc, spiral canal; s, scolex with suckers and hooklets.

wall of the cyst. In good tissue sections the cysticercus is characteristic and shows the cyst membrane and the inverted scolex within the cyst (Fig. IV–5 *B*). The main difference between *C. cellulosae* and *C. bovis* is that the former has a rostellum with two rows of hooklets; however, since the rostellum and the hooklets are rather small, they are difficult to demonstrate in histologic sections. The lack of a rostellum with hooklets in a few tissue sections prevents distinction of these cysticerci.

Another *Cysticercus, C. longicollis*, is the larval stage of *T. crassiceps* of the red fox and is commonly found in rodents in North America (*color plate* XV *A*). This larva reproduces asexually in the intermediate host by exogenous and sometimes endogenous budding at the pole opposite to the scolex. Budding stalks grow a new scolex, which in turn buds to produce another scolex (Fig. IV–6). The scolices have a rostellum with hooks, which permits a specific diagnosis based on their size; *C. longicollis* occurs in humans (see Chapter 26).

A special form of cysticercus found in humans is *Cysticercus racemosus* (*color plate* XV *B*), a proliferating larva that either has either no scolex or a degenerated scolex. *Cysticercus racemosus* is an abnormal developmental form of *C. cellulosae* of *T. solium* (see Chapter 26).

Cysticercoid

The cysticercoid is the larval stage of several tapeworms occurring in humans, such as *Hymenolepis* (*H. diminuta* and *H. nana*), and *Dipylidium caninum*. The cysticercoid has a double-walled bladder that encloses the invaginated scolex and has a short tail. It is possible to find this larva in the small intestine of humans infected with *H. nana*, undergoing a direct type of development, but it has not yet been re-

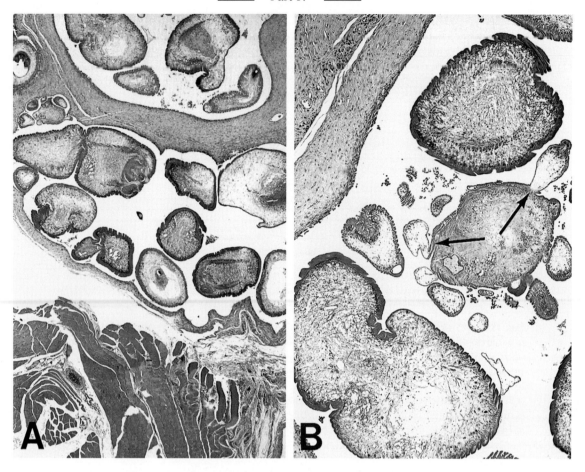

Fig. IV–6. *Taenia crassiceps*, cysticercus in animal, section stained with hematoxylin and eosin stain. *A,* Low-power view of larvae on the thoracic wall of woodchuck. Note the large cystic spaces with numerous cysticerci, ×22. *B,* Higher-power magnification showing the larvae, some with buds (arrows), ×55. (Specimen courtesy of D. Bowman, Ph.D., Department of Microbiology, Immunology and Parasitology, New York State College of Veterinary Medicine, Ithaca, New York.)

ported. In experimentally immune-suppressed hosts, the cysticercoid of *H. nana* proliferates in all tissues and organs, and at least two instances of this type of infection appear to have occurred in humans (see Chapter 26, Fig. 26–24).

Hydatid Cyst

The hydatid cyst, also known as the *Echinococcus* cyst, is a structure of variable shape, composition, and size. Commonly, hydatid cysts are round or oval, but they may assume the shape of the organ or space in which they grow. Growth may occasionally be infiltrative, and some hydat cysts may metastasize to distant organs. The basic structure of a hydatid cyst consists of several membranes. The innermost, or *germinal*, membrane is one or two cells thick; from this membrane, all larvae in the cyst proliferate. Cell proliferation is seen as a thickening that eventually results in the formation of a *protoscolex* (Fig. IV–7). The protoscolex may develop within a vesicle of a germinating membrane from which other protoscolices grow to form a *brood capsule* containing several protoscolices (larvae; Fig. IV–8 *A–B*). These brood capsules may rupture, and the larvae may drop into the fluid (*hydatid sand*); other brood capsules remain attached to the germinal membrane or form *daughter cysts* (smaller cysts inside the cyst). Outside the germinal membrane is the *acellular* or *laminated membrane* secreted by the parasite (Fig. IV–8 *A–B*). Surrounding the cyst is a fibrous capsule, a reaction of the host to the cyst (Fig. IV–8 *A*). Some hydatid cysts are composed of a single chamber (*unilocular*); others have several separate chambers (*multilocular, multivesicular,* or *polycystic*; Fig. IV–9). These different types of cysts correlate with the species responsible for the infection.

Coenurus

The coenurus is the larva of certain species of *Taenia*. It is a cyst several centimeters in diameter, filled with clear fluid and sometimes with hundreds of scolices on its inner surface, each similar in size and gross appearance to the scolex of a cysticercus (Fig. IV–10). Some coenuri grow by external and internal budding, forming extensions of the cyst into surrounding tissues.

Sparganum

The sparganum, also known as the *plerocercoid*, is the larval stage of certain genera of Pseudophyllidea, *Diphyllobothrium* and *Spirometra*. A well-preserved spar-

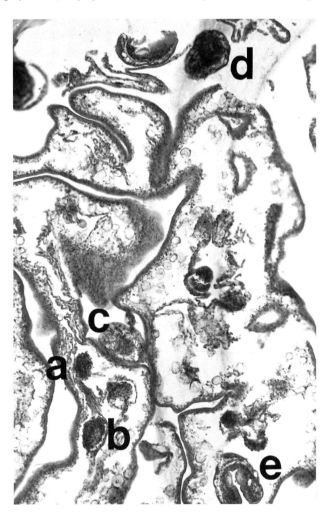

Fig. IV–7. *Echinococcus granulosus*, section of a collapsed germinal membrane showing several stages in the development of protoscolices, stained with hematoxylin and eosin. The protoscolex begins as an anlage of proliferative cells (a) that grows (b) to form the larva (c–e), ×151.

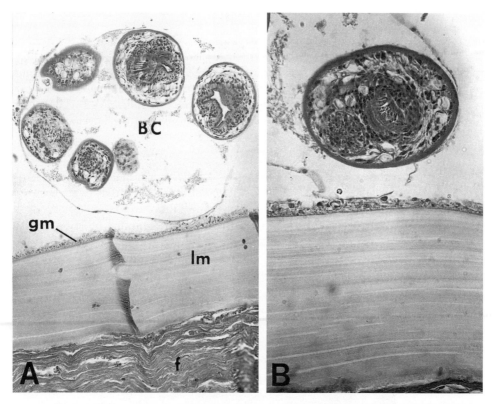

Fig. IV–8. *Echinococcus granulosus*, hydatid cyst, hematoxylin and eosin stain. *A*, High-power view of the cyst wall illustrating the fibrous capsule (f), laminated membrane (lm), germinal membrane (gm), and one brood capsule (BC) with five protoscolices, ×187. *B*, Higher magnification showing the laminated membrane, germinal membrane, and one protoscolex, ×383.

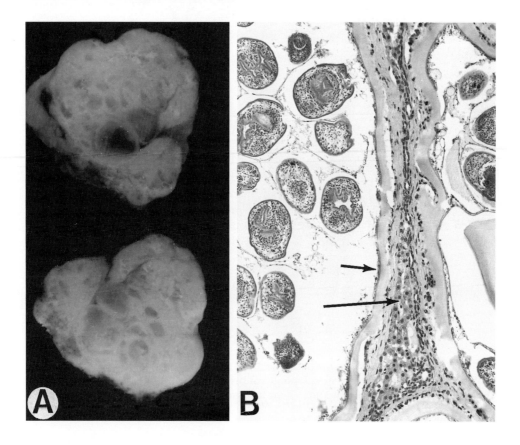

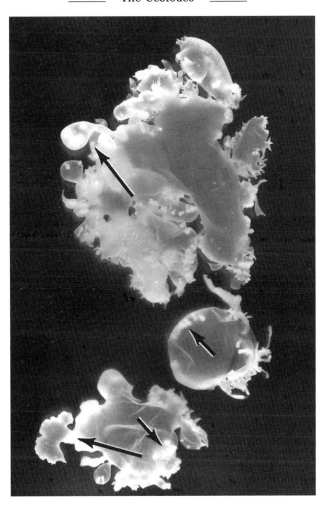

Fig. IV–10. *Coenurus* cyst from the subcutaneous tissues of a baboon. Note the exogenous growth of the bladder (long arrows) and the protoscolices (short arrows). (Specimen courtesy of R.F. Kuntz, Ph.D., Medical Research Foundation, San Antonio, Texas.)

ganum superficially resembles a roundworm. It is up to 20 cm in length by 3 mm wide and is white or creamy in color, with an inconspicuous scolex containing two sucking grooves (bothrids) at the anterior end (Fig. IV–11 *A*). Close examination reveals the flatfish character of the body, especially if it is well fixed (Fig. IV–11 *C–D*). Microscopically, a typical cestode tegument covers the sparganum. The body is filled with mesenchyme with well-defined excretory canals and scattered longitudinal muscle fibers. On cross sections, the muscle fibers are seen as large, irregular cells with minute nuclei (Fig. IV–11 *B*).

Fig. IV–9. *Echinococcus multilocularis* from a cotton rat infected experimentally. *A*, Gross picture of a hepatic cyst. Note the alveolar character, ×2. *B*, Hematoxylin and eosin stain. Medium-power view of a cyst showing some remnants of liver parenchyma (long arrow) between two cystic cavities. Note the thickness of the acellular (laminated) membrane in relation to the thickness of the germinal membrane (short arrow). Several brood capsules with protoscolices are seen, ×125. (Specimen courtesy of F.L. Andersen, Ph.D., Brigham Young University, Provo, Utah.)

Tetrathyridium

The tetrathyridium or plerocercus, is the second larval stage of species belonging to the genus *Mesocestoides* (*color plate* XIV *F–G*). Tetrathyridia are found in the body cavities and tissues of reptiles, birds, and small mammals, where they usually occur in large numbers. Tetrathyridia are likely to multiply asexually under abnormal conditions, as has been demonstrated with isolates maintained in the laboratory by serial intraperitoneal passage of the larvae. It has been suggested that these larvae may produce human infections (see Chapter 26).

Geographic Distribution and Epidemiology

Tapeworm infections in humans are worldwide in distribution. In some locations, these infections are major health problems. For example, hydatid cysts produce infections in areas of North America, the Middle East, Europe, Asia, Australia, New Zealand, and Argentina. However, tapeworm infections usually are of low endemicity, and most occur as sporadic cases. The many cestodes producing zoonotic infections occur either as adult worms in the intestine or as larval stages in the tissues. Because most of these infections occur very seldom, it is difficult for the clinician and the pathologist to become familiar with their diagnostic features.

An adult tapeworm is acquired by ingesting the larva that inhabits the tissues of an animal commonly ingested as food. Beef, pork, and fish are some of the main source of tapeworms such as *T. saginata*, *T. solium*, and *D. latum*, respectively. On

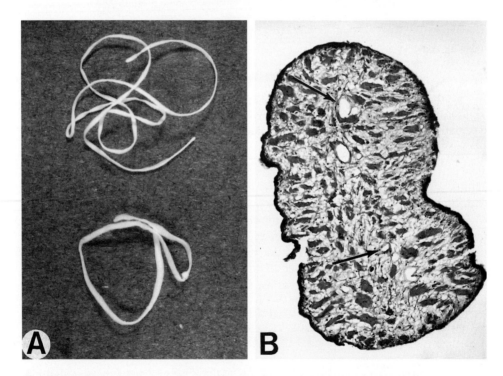

Fig. IV–11. *Sparganum. A*, Gross picture of two spargana recovered from the subcutaneous tissues of a raccoon. *B*, Cross section of the larva from the case in Figure 26–19. Note the excretory channels (arrows) and the numerous muscle cells cut transversely. This *Sparganum* was alive at the time it was recovered; thus the tissues are well fixed and preserved. Section stained with hematoxylin and eosin stain, ×118.

occasion, ingestion of exotic raw animal viscera or meat results in infections with unusual tapeworms such as *Mesocestoides*. In other cases, accidental ingestion of arthropod intermediate hosts with the cysticercoid larva produces infections with *Dipylidium caninum* and *Hymenolepis diminuta*.

Larval stages such as the cysticercus, hydatid cyst, coenurus, and sparganum are generally acquired by ingestion of food or water contaminated with human and animal feces containing the eggs of one of these tapeworms. *Sparganum* larvae also may be acquired by ingestion of raw meat with the larva because sparganum uses many animals, including pigs, as paratenic hosts. In these cases, the larva may be transferred directly from one animal to another or to humans; in the new host the larva remains unchanged (see Paratenesis, Chapter 17).

Infections with Adult Tapeworms

In the clinical laboratory, infections with intestinal tapeworms are diagnosed by examination of stool samples and identification of the eggs. Only on rare occasions does the anatomic pathologist have to identify tapeworms histologically; the best example is a proglottid lodged in the appendix (Fig. IV–12 *A–D*). More frequently, the proglottids or larger portions of the strobila passed in the stools are brought for examination to the surgical desk. In these cases, the pathologist should recognize the specimen as a proglottid, or as part of the strobila of a tapeworm, and refer the specimen to the clinical laboratory. Neither the proglottid nor the worm is to be submitted for histologic sectioning. For practical purposes, a tapeworm species cannot be identified in histologic sections.

In rare cases, a surgically removed appendix contains a tapeworm proglottid in the lumen. Some of these cases have been associated with appendicitis, and the parasite is identified on the basis of its morphologic characteristics (Fig. IV–12 *A* to *D*). As noted, speciation in sections is not possible. The size, the type of eggs in the uterus, and other characteristics usually indicate the major group: *Taenia*, *Diphyllobothrium*, or another genus. This finding indicates that the person has the adult worm in the intestine. A diagnosis can be made by examination of the stools.

Classification

The classification of tapeworms is difficult because of the large number of species that exist and our lack of knowledge about many of their life cycles. A simplified classification of the cestodes of human importance is as follows:

Subclass: Cestoda
    Order: Pseudophyllidea
        Family: Diphyllobothriidae
            Genus: *Diphyllobothrium. D. latum,* * *D. pacificum,* * *D. cordatum,* * *D. ursi,* * *D. dendriticum,* * *D. lanceolatum,* * *D. dalliae,* * *D. yanagoensis* *
            Genus: *Diplonogoporus. D. grandis,* * *D. brauni* *
            Genus: *Ligula. L. intestinalis* *
            Genus: *Spirometra. S. mansoni,*† *S. mansonoides,*† *S. houghtoni,* * *S. erinacei* *
    Order: Cyclophyllidea

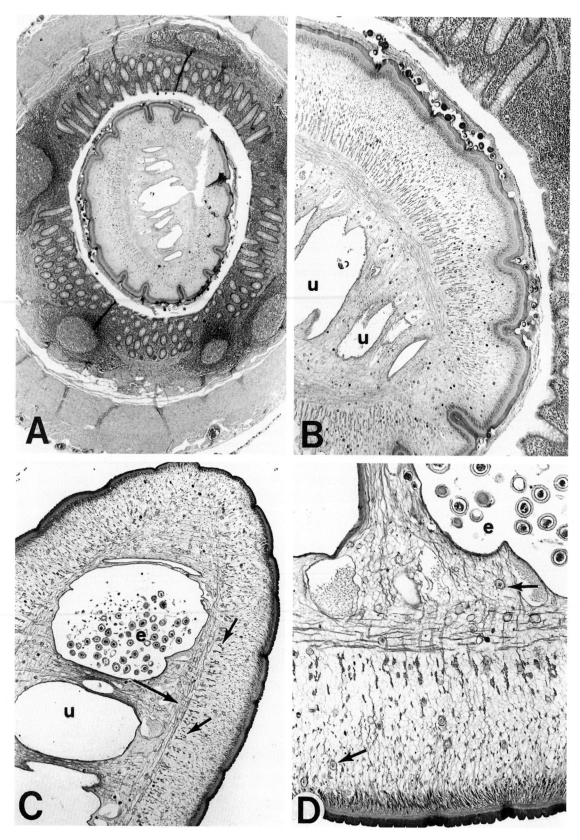

Fig. IV–12.

Family: Anaplocephalidae

    Genus: *Bertiella. B. studeri,** *B. mucronata**

Family: Davaineidae

    Genus: *Raillietina. R. celebensis,** *R. demerariensis**

Family: Linstowiidae

    Genus: *Inermicapsifer. I. Madagascariensis**

Family: Mesocestoidea

    Genus: *Mesocestoides. M. variabilis**

Family: Dilepidae

    Genus: *Dipylidium. D. caninum**

Family: Hymenolepididae

    Genus: *Hymenolepis. H. nana,** *H. diminuta**

Family: Taenidae

    Genus: *Taenia. T. solium,**† *T. saginata,** *T. asiatica,** *T. longihamatus,** *Taeniformis,*† *T. crassiceps,*† *T. multiceps,*† *T. serialis,*† *T. brauni,*† *T. glomerata*†

    Genus: *Echinococcus. E. granulosus,*† *E. multilocularis,*† *E. vogeli,*† *E. oligarthrus*†

The asterisks indicate the species that inhabit the intestinal tract, and the dagger indicates those that occur in the tissues of humans as larval stages. The Pseudophyllidea are characterized by a scolex with two bothria or grooves (sucking organs), one on the ventral aspect and the other on the dorsal aspect (Fig. IV–2 *B*). The strobila of species found in humans has central genital pores on the ventral surface; most of these species belong to the family Diphyllobothriidae. Four genera have species parasitic in humans: *Diphyllobothrium, Diplogonoporus, Ligula,* and *Spirometra*. All have species that occur as adult worms in the gastrointestinal tract. *Spirometra* also has some species with larval stages in the tissues, producing sparganosis.

The Cyclophyllidea have scolices with four suckers, and some have a *rostellum* (Fig. IV–2 *A*), a structure located at the apex of the scolex, protruding anteriorly as a dome or a finger, which may be either fixed or retractable (Fig. IV–1). In most species, the rostellum has thorn-like spines distributed in one or more circular rows which sometimes cover the entire rostellum. The size and distribution of these spines (hooks) are of taxonomic value (Fig. IV–2 *A*). A distinctly flattened body, simple suckers, and nonoperculate eggs are some of the characteristics of the important genera in human medicine. Some species of *Taenia* and *Echinococcus* have larval stages that occur in humans; all the other species are parasites of the intestinal tract.

◄

Fig. IV–12. *Taenia* species cross section. *A* and *B*. Adult in appendix, section stained with hematoxylin and eosin stain. *A*, Low-power view of appendix with a cross section of a proglottid filling the lumen, ×22. *B*, Higher magnification shows the uterine cavity (u). Many *Taenia* eggs are seen in the lumen of the appendix, ×55. *C* and *D*. Cross section of *Taenia* illustrates similar morphology. *C*, Medium magnification showing the uterus with typical *Taenia* eggs (e), the transverse muscle layer (long arrow), and the longitudinal muscles (short arrows) on cross section, ×55. *D*, Higher magnification illustrates same features and the calcareous corpuscles (arrows). Note the tegument of the parasite, ×140.

26

CYSTICERCOSIS, COENUROSIS, SPARGANOSIS, AND PROLIFERATING CESTODE LARVAE

As stated in the introduction to Part IV, the larval stages of certain tapeworms such as cysticercus, coenurus, hydatid, and sparganum occur in humans, where they often behave as they do in their natural intermediate hosts. These infections are by definition zoonotic. In certain geographic areas, some of them produce important morbidity and mortality. In addition to the four larval stages mentioned, other cestode larvae occur rarely in humans, and aberrant forms of cysticercus and sparganum occur in both immune-competent and immune-suppressed individuals. The recognition of cestode larvae in tissues is important for the anatomic pathologist because this is the basis for diagnosing these infections specifically. In this chapter, we will study the cysticercus, coenurus, sparganum, and proliferating cestode larvae; the hydatid larvae are covered in Chapter 27.

Taenia solium—Cysticercosis

Various species of *Taenia* are parasites of the human intestine (see introduction to Part IV). The two most widely known are *T. saginata* and *T. solium*, also referred to as the *beef* and *pork tapeworms*, respectively, because these animals are their intermediate hosts. A characteristic of *T. solium* is that its larval stage, the cysticercus, in addition to developing naturally in pigs, also develops in humans, producing cysticercosis.

Life Cycle and Morphology. *Taenia solium* inhabits exclusively the small intestine of humans; no other animal is known to be a suitable host under either natural or experimental conditions. In the small intestine the parasite lives in the lumen, with its scolex anchored to the mucosa and its body folded back and forth several times. The scolex measures about 1 mm, and has four suckers and a rostellum with two rows of hooklets (Fig. 26–2). Although there is usually only one worm in the intestine, on occasion several—and, rarely, many—worms are present. The strobila of an adult *T. solium* varies between 2 and 7 mm in length. The proglottids are immature in the anterior portion, mature in the middle, and gravid in the posterior portion. Immature proglottids are wider than they are long, mature ones are approximately square, and gravid ones are longer than they are wide. A gravid proglottid is

635

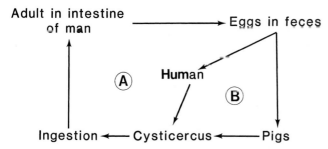

Fig. 26 1. *Taenia solium*, schematic representation of the life cycle. *A*, General cycle (human–pig–human) resulting in the maintenance of the parasite in nature; *B*, resulting in cysticercosis in humans.

about 1.5 to 2.0 cm in length by 0.6 to 0.9 cm in width. Immature proglottids have poorly formed sexual organs, and mature ones have well-developed sexual organs and are in the process of forming eggs and storing them in the uterus. Gravid proglottids have a uterus that is highly branched and filled with eggs that expand to produce atrophy of the sex organs of the worm. The number of branches of the uterus has some taxonomic value for the human *Taenia*, being about 7 to 13 (usually 9) in *T. solium* and 15 to 20 (usually 18) in *T. saginata*. The last proglottid of the strobila breaks off regularly, rupturing the anterior wall of the proglottid and the uterine cavity, allowing expulsion of the eggs into the feces. This process is aided by the contractions of the muscles of the proglottid and is the reason why many proglottids recovered from the stools do not have eggs.

The eggs of *T. solium* are almost spherical, measuring 31 to 43 μm in diameter. They are pale to brown in color and cannot be distinguished from the eggs of *T. saginata*. Once the eggs are evacuated with the feces to the environment, they are ingested by pigs that feed on food or water contaminated with them. In the small intestine, the embryos hatch from the eggs, penetrate the mucosa, gain access to blood vessels, and travel via the circulation to various tissues, where they differentiate into infective larvae, the cysticerci. Ingestion of raw pork with cysticerci produces the infection with the adult *T. solium* in humans (Fig. 26–1). This infection is mostly asymptomatic. It is diagnosed in the clinical laboratory by finding the typical *Taenia* eggs (Fig. 26–2) or proglottids in stools (Fig. 26–3; Beaver et al. 1984).

Geographic Distribution and Epidemiology. As stated, the *T. solium* infection is acquired through the consumption of raw or poorly cooked pork containing the cysticerci. The *Cysticercus* infection results from the ingestion of *T. solium* eggs with food or water contaminated with human excreta; thus, cysticercosis is common in individuals who harbor the adult tapeworm because they often infect themselves. The fecal-oral route of infection from one's own feces in individuals with adult *T. solium*, is known as *external autoinfection*. This route distinguishes this form of infection from regurgitation of proglottids from the intestine into the stomach during episodes of violent vomiting, freeing the eggs and resulting in *internal autoinfection*. From this discussion it can be surmised that the majority of patients with cysticercosis have the parasite in the intestine, that a large number of others have a history of close contact with a person who harbors the parasite, and that in the rest the source of infection remains undetermined. The infection in pigs is variable through-

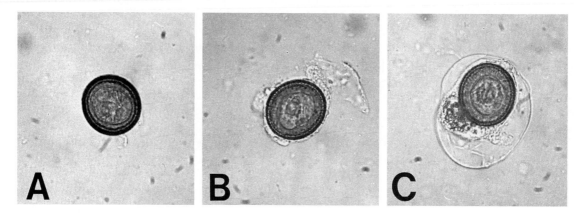

Fig. 26–2. *Taenia* species eggs. *A–C*. Eggs taken from a fixed proglottid, unstained. Note that the egg in *C* still has the outer envelope, ×450.

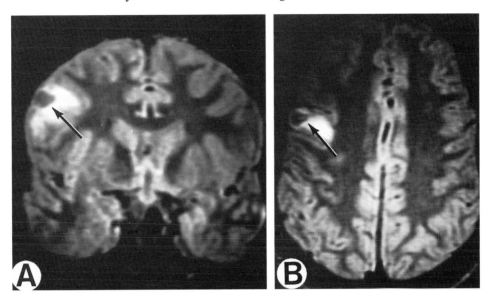

Fig. 26–3. Cysticercosis. Magnetic resonance imaging. *A,* Coronal view showing a lesion in the left parietal area. The cyst (arrow) is surrounded by a dense inflammatory reaction. *B,* Horizontal view showing the same lesion. Note the cyst, with the scolex (very faint) of the parasite at the center (arrow). (Courtesy of Z. Wszolek, M.D., Section of Neurology, University of Nebraska Medical Center, Omaha, Nebraska.)

out the endemic areas—for example, 3% in Brazil and 1% to 4% in other Latin American countries (Schenone, Letonja, 1974). In another study, the range for five Central American countries was between 2% and 3% (Acha, Aguilar, 1964), and in Iran less than 1% of sacrificed pigs had the infection (Afshar, 1967). In recent years, the disease was introduced into West Guinea with infected pigs. It produced an epidemic of cysticercosis that manifested first by an inordinate number of burns (the infected patients had seizures and fell into open fires) (Gajdusek, 1978; Subianto et al. 1978).

Infections with the adult *T. solium* are common in places where undercooked pork is consumed regularly, such as Mexico and other Latin American countries, north China, India, Pakistan, and Manchuria. In Europe, it occurs among the Slavic peoples. In a sample of 1500 individuals from a village in Mexico, 0.3% had *Taenia* eggs in the stools, 6% had a previous history of tapeworm, and 11% were seropositive to *T. solium* antigen (Sarti et al. 1992). In four Guatemalan communities, the mean prevalence of *T. solium* was about 3%, and women were more likely to be infected than men; the rate of infection increased until the end of the fourth decade and declined thereafter (Allan et al. 1996).

Cysticercosis occurs in places endemic for the adult *T. solium,* for which humans are the sole definitive hosts. The incidence of cysticercosis is declining in most places, especially in Central Europe, but is still prevalent in China, India, Mexico, and other Latin American countries, where both pigs and humans are infected at various rates (see above). Prevalence rates depend on the population under study: hospital patients, hospital-autopsied patients, children, adults, or others. A realistic figure for Santiago, Chile, is 28 cases per 100,000 forensic autopsies (Schenone et al. 1973). A study of autopsies in Mexico City revealed that 3.5% of the patients had cysticerci, one-half of which were incidental findings (Briceno et al. 1961). In the United States, infections with *T. solium* and cysticercosis were once present and then almost disappeared, but they are now becoming prevalent again. Both *T. solium* and cysticercosis are common among Mexican and Latin American immigrants (Sorvillo et al. 1992). Cysticercosis is being diagnosed more frequently in Americans who never traveled outside the country (Kruskal et al. 1993; Richards et al. 1985). However, up to now, there has been no recent case of autochthonous infection with the adult *T. solium* in Americans.

Clinical Findings. By definition, cysticercosis is a benign infection of the subcutaneous tissues, the intermuscular fascia, the muscles, and other organs. Every site in the body where these tissues occur is a suitable environment for growth and development of the larval stage of *T. solium*. In the subcutaneous tissue the cysts are often felt on light palpation of the skin, and in the mucosa of the mouth, especially under the tongue, the cysts are often seen. Clinically, cysticerci within the tongue may simulate a tumor (Puppin et al. 1993). Cysticerci in the conjunctiva or in the eyelid are also visible and sometimes may break, releasing the larva and curing the patient (Raina et al. 1996; Sapunar et al. 1982). The cysts are asymptomatic, and may remain so for a long time and finally disappear quietly; rarely, they calcify. Either of these outcomes is natural for cysticerci in tissues. In rare cases, the cyst becomes inflamed and manifests as a growing tense area with redness, edema, and pain. Depending on the site of the body where the lesion occurs, the physician is consulted. This happens more often for lesions in the mouth (Puppin et al. 1993), breast (Alagaratnam et al. 1988; Kunkel, Hawksley, 1987), and sexual organs. Inflammation of the cyst signifies the death of the parasite, with leakage of antigens and a cellular response of the body.

In rare cases, massive cysticercosis produced a myopathy with an increase in muscle mass (Chopra et al. 1986; Rao et al. 1972; Venkataraman, Vijayan, 1983). In other cases, the infection produced a carotid artery occlusion (McCormick et al. 1983). There are also descriptions of patients with solitary or multiple pulmonary nodules (Scholtz, Mentis, 1987; Walts et al. 1995), a laryngeal nodule (Tami et al. 1987), or nodules in the tongue (Webb et al. 1986). An individual with numerous calcified cysticerci in the soft tissues also had multiple infarcts and necrosis of bone, lesions attributed to the infection; there was no proof of bone invasion by the parasite (Lenczner, Wollin, 1958). A report of scrotal cysticercosis has an accompanying photomicrograph of a section containing the parasite, but it is a nematode rather than a cysticercus (Andrews, Mason, 1987). An intrasellar cysticercus presented as a pituitary tumor in a patient from Central America (Prosser et al. 1978).

Cysticerci in the heart are invariably a postmortem finding (Fig. 26–11 *A*; Saxena et al. 1972). The cysts are located in the pericardium, myocardium, or endocardium. In some reports, up to 15 cysticerci have been recovered, but in no case have symptoms been attributed to their presence (Marquez-Monter et al. 1963; Menon, Veliath, 1940). Other locations found at autopsy are the aorta, mesentery, small intestinal mucosa, thyroid (Leelachaikul, Chuahirun, 1977), pancreas, peritoneum, and retroperitoneum (Briceno et al. 1961).

Parasites located in the central nervous system and the eye sometimes produce more than usual morbidity and mortality, which makes the infection of paramount

importance in clinical medicine. Thus, in addition to the unusual presentations listed above, two main forms of cysticercosis are important: neurocysticercosis and ophthalmocysticercosis.

Neurocysticercosis. The clinical presentation of neurocysticercosis is variable and has no characteristic symptom or sign; the frequency of symptoms and signs differs in various series. After the embryo of *T. solium* reaches the brain or other tissues, the larva grows slowly and may take several weeks to attain its normal size. Once full grown, the cysticercus lies dormant, without producing symptoms, sometimes for years. Similarly to what occurs in other organs, the symptoms in the brain arise only after the cysticercus dies, producing an inflammatory reaction. Therefore, the incubation period of neurocysticercosis varies from a few months to 30 years, but most patients develop symptoms within 7 years. This pattern of development does not preclude the occurrence of cysticercosis in infants (Binstock et al. 1987). Neurocysticercosis affects both sexes equally; the age range is commonly 19 to 35 years, with 75% of all affected patients being under 40. In approximately 30% of humans with neurocysticercosis, there is usually no clinically detectable cysticercus outside the central nervous system.

The symptoms of neurocysticercosis are variable (Pittella, 1997), but often they are related to increased intracranial pressure: severe headaches, nausea, and vomiting in up to 98% of cases. Patients with large numbers of cysts may have cysticercus encephalitis produced by the inflammation of many cysts near the meninges; this form of the disease appears to affect young women more than any other group (Rangel et al. 1987). Cysticerci in the ventricular system may result in obstructive hydrocephalus and death due to brain stem compression (Keane, 1984). Seizures occurred in up to 40% of patients in some series (Earnest et al. 1987; Loo, Braude, 1982) and in up to 92% in one series (Dixon, Smithers, 1934). A realistic figure is probably just over 50% (Sotelo et al. 1985). The seizures are generalized, focal, Jacksonian, or any combination of these forms. The signs also correlate with increased intracranial pressure: papilledema, changes in mental status (disorientation, agitation, lethargy, obtundation, dementia, and confusion), cranial nerve palsies (mostly affecting cranial nerve IV), and hyperreflexia. Hydrocephalus secondary to arachnoiditis produced by cysticercosis is a complication in some individuals, resulting in a 50% mortality rate within 2 years after diagnosis and cerebrospinal fluid shunting (Sotelo, Marin, 1987). Most patients who survive recover, although a few remain in an unsatisfactory condition (Sotelo et al. 1985). Other signs and symptoms are variable and less frequent (Sotelo et al. 1985). In some cases, clear manifestations of encephalitis have been described, especially in women with numerous cysts in the brain tissue (Rangel et al. 1987). At least one case of *Acanthamoeba* encephalitis mimicked neurocysticercosis (Matson et al. 1988). Symptoms related to the spinal cord are rare and manifest with paraplegia, paraparesis, sphincter dysfunction, and pain, which signifies involvement of the cord (Holtzman et al. 1986; Sharma et al. 1987). In other patients, there is sensory loss and meningeal irritation simulating a spinal cord tumor (Akiguchi et al. 1979; Colli et al. 1994).

The following is important information needed in elucidating the clinical history of the patient with suspected neurocysticercosis: (*1*) the travel history if the individual is under evaluation in an area nonendemic for *T. solium*; (*2*) a history of tapeworm infection or the presence of proglottids or segments of the worm in the feces; (*3*) the presence of subcutaneous nodules, as assessed by careful palpation of the entire body; and (*4*) a history of headaches, seizures, or parasitism with a tapeworm in any family member, which must be determined by exhaustive interrogation of the patient and his or her relatives. Stool examination for the presence of *Taenia* eggs is necessary in the patient and all members of the family. The incidence of subcutaneous nodules in patients with neurocysticercosis is higher in China, Southeast Asia, and Africa than in other areas. In the American continent, at least one study showed that this condition occurs in less than 1% of cases (Cruz et al. 1994).

Laboratory tests are usually not helpful. Low or moderate peripheral eosinophilia occurs in 15% of cases. The cerebrospinal fluid is increased in pressure. There is elevated protein, low glucose, and pleocytosis in 80% of cases and moderate spinal fluid eosinophilia in 10% to 20% of cases. In some instances, the lymphocytes in the spinal fluid are highly variable in level and show atypia suggestive of a lymphoma (Wilber et al. 1980). Most serologic tests have a low positivity rate and are nonspecific because the antibodies cross-react with those elicited by other parasitic infections. However, high antibody titers are suggestive of infection (Earnest et al. 1987), and they are best interpreted in conjunction with imaging studies (Vinken et al. 1994). Testing of both serum and cerebrospinal fluid for antibodies enhances the sensitivity of the test, but often the added morbidity of a lumbar puncture in a patient with intracranial pressure does not justify the procedure. Tests based on a species-specific antigen from *T. solium* used in an enzyme-linked immunoelectrotransfer blot were reported to be very specific for

diagnosis (Richards, Schantz, 1991; Vinken et al. 1994). In other similar studies, the test was less specific but the antigen used was different, which precludes comparisons (Diaz et al. 1992).

The most important means of diagnosis at present are the techniques that image the brain. Conventional radiograms, angiography, neuroencephalography, and ventriculography provided only limited information about neurocysticercosis, usually an indirect signal about a cyst or a nodule. The most reliable information produced by these techniques concerned calcified cysticerci. Computed tomography (CT) scanning was a significant advance, though sometimes the scans are difficult to interpret because cysticercosis resembles other conditions. Live cysticerci are isodense because they are inert, and contrast studies do not enhance them. The most reliable images for diagnosis are those revealing multiple cystic lesions, a vesicle with a scolex, and lesions in different stages of evolution (Arriagada et al. 1997). CT scans do not show lesions in 10% of the cases and only signs of hydrocephalus in another 20%; discrimination of the location of lesions is difficult, as are the lesions in the ventricles and cisterns (Arriagada et al. 1997). Magnetic resonance imaging (MRI) is superior to CT because it permits localization of the lesions, defines more clearly the presence of the scolex, and reveals more precisely the stage of evolution of the lesion and the type of cysticercus present (Arriagada et al. 1997). For example, it is excellent for demonstrating cysts in the ventricular system; cysticerci in the cortex, both alive and dead; and racemosus-type cysticerci (Lotz et al. 1988). For this reason, MRI has become the method of choice for diagnosing neurocysticercosis (Fig. 26–3). Since the lesion and the cysticercus change as they evolve, the images they produce appear different, depending on the stage of evolution; thus interpretation of these images can be difficult (Earnest et al. 1987; Lotz et al. 1988). Often the single enhancing lesion on CT is indistinguishable from a tumor (Del Brutto, Quintero, 1995; Silver et al. 1996). Specific therapy, if given soon after the lesion is found, may produce resolution of the lesion, clarifying the diagnosis (Del Brutto, 1995). In the majority of radiologic images of the central nervous system, the lesion produced by a cysticercus is less than 2 cm in the largest dimension (Rajshekhar, Chandy, 1994). Larger cysts, sometimes up to one-third the diameter of the brain, have been documented (Berman et al. 1991).

Ophthalmocysticercosis. The embryo of *T. solium* invades the eye through the optic artery. The cysticercus develops in the subretinal space (Fig. 26–9 *A*), or more commonly in the vitreous, or grows attached to the retina. Other, less frequent locations in the eye include the anterior chamber and the intraretinal area. The ocular location of cysticercus is not unusual; the cases observed in the State of Sao Paulo, Brazil totaled 299 during a 10-year period (Almeida, Oliveira, 1971). The clinical presentation is almost invariably unilateral reduction in visual acuity to a greater or lesser extent, depending on the exact location of the cysticercus (Welsh et al. 1987). The parasite is usually seen on routine ophthalmologic examination; treatment consists of resection, depending on its location (Arciniegas, Gutierrez, 1988). If the parasite dies, the inflammatory reaction usually produces blindness in that eye. The cysts may also occur in the eye adnexa—for example, the conjunctiva, the eyelid, the lacrimal duct, and the orbit (Sen, 1980)

Pathology. The gross and histologic picture of cysticercosis is always related to the evolution of the parasite and the tissue reaction around it (Chi, Chi, 1978). The growth of a cysticercus is slow, produces a minimal inflammatory reaction, and in some tissues elicits formation by the host of a thin, fibrous capsule around it (Figs. 26–7 *A* and 26–12 *C*). Once fully grown, the parasite remains alive for several months to many years, depending on its location, the type of host, and probably other unknown factors. The life span of *Cysticercus cellulosae* in humans is unknown.

When a cysticercus dies in the tissues, it may follow one of several pathways; some of these pathways are probably related to the tissue or organ where the cysticercus is located. Commonly, after the cyst dies, it is slowly invaded by inflammatory cells and macrophages; finally, it is replaced by fibrous tissue, with complete resorption of the parasite. Often the dead parasite calcifies (Fig. 26–4), a process observed in up to 57% of cases of inactive cysticercosis of the central nervous system (Sotelo et al. 1985). In either case, there usually are no clinical symptoms at any time, though calcified cysterci may serve as a focus for Jacksonian seizures. The most important set of events occurs when the dead cysticercus provokes an inflammatory reaction, probably due to leakage of parasitic antigens into surrounding tissues. This inflammatory reaction may be more common around cysticerci located in tissues that do not form a fibrous capsule around them, such as the central nervous system and the eye. This conclusion is supported by the fact that in the central nervous system and in the eye, cysticerci commonly produce a marked inflammatory reaction, whereas those in other organs and tissues do so less frequently.

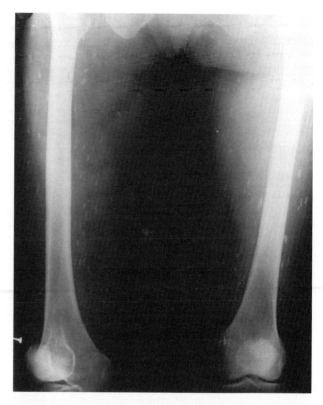

Fig. 26–4. *Cysticercus*, **plain x-ray film of the thigh muscles of a woman with numerous calcified cysticerci.**

Neurocysticercosis. The gross appearance of the brains of individuals dying with cysticercosis is variable. The number of cysts varies from a few to several hundreds. They are located in all areas of the central nervous system, from the meninges to the basal nuclei. The cysticerci may be apparent on the surface of the brain (Fig. 26–5 *C*), but more often they are seen better on coronal section (Fig. 26–5 *A–B*). Occasionally, the cysts are found in the ventricular spaces growing from the ependymal lining.

At least one-half of central nervous system cysticerci discovered at autopsy are incidental findings, usually in the absence of known symptoms (Briceno et al. 1961). The cysts are usually less than 1 cm in diameter and most of them appear viable, but some may be calcified. The cysts are easily shelled out intact from their cavity in the brain tissue and have all the characteristics of a viable cysticercus (Fig. 26–5 *A*). The cavity is often smooth, without evidence of inflammation (Fig. 26–5 *A–B*), although sometimes it may have minimal inflammatory changes (Fig. 26–8 *A*).

Specimens surgically removed from the central nervous system of individuals with a diagnosis of cysticercosis usually consist of a brain tissue fragment mea

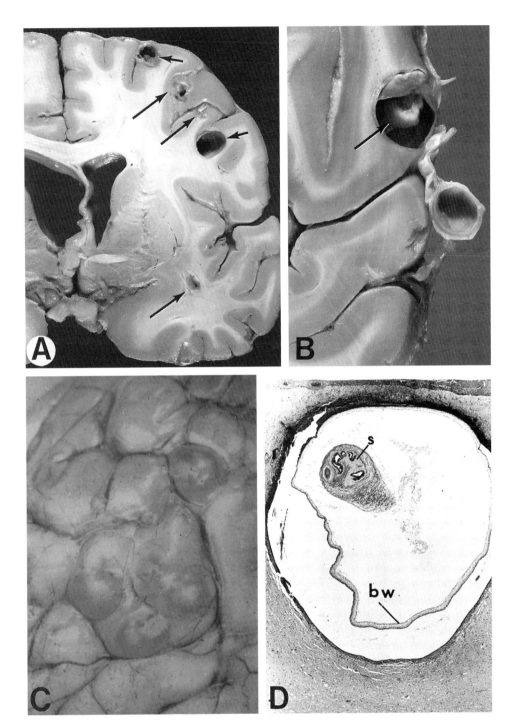

Fig. 26–5. *Cysticercus* in the central nervous system. *A–C.* Gross appearance. *A,* Coronal section of brain from an individual with neurocysticercosis. Two cysts (short arrows) do not show any inflammatory reaction. Portions of three other cysts (long arrows) show necrosis around the cyst. *B,* Higher magnification illustrating two cysts. One has the scolex at the center (arrow); the other, located in the meninges, is empty because the parasite fell off during sectioning. *C,* Gross appearance of cysticerci on the surface of the brain. *D,* Microscopic section stained with hematoxylin and eosin stain. Low-power view of a viable cysticercus illustrating the bladder wall (bw), the invaginated scolex (s), and the scant inflammatory reaction around the cyst, ×19.

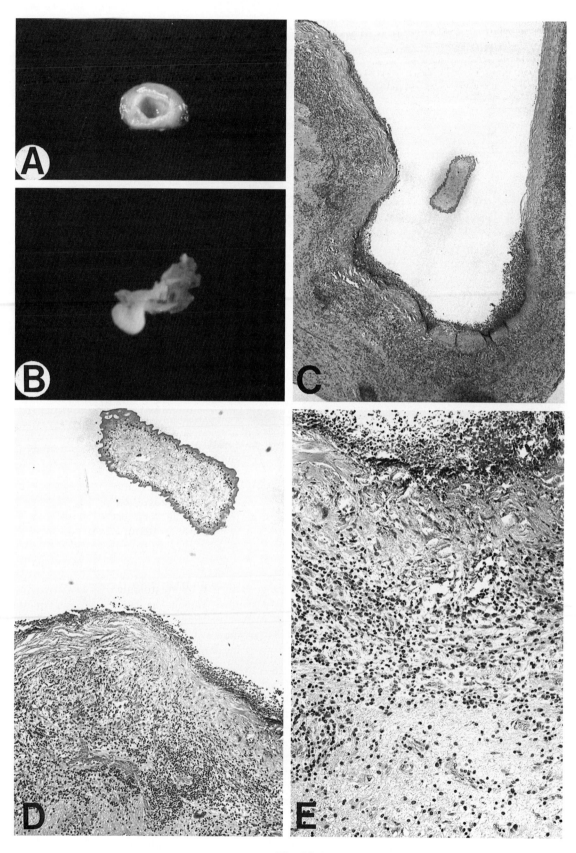

Fig. 26–6.

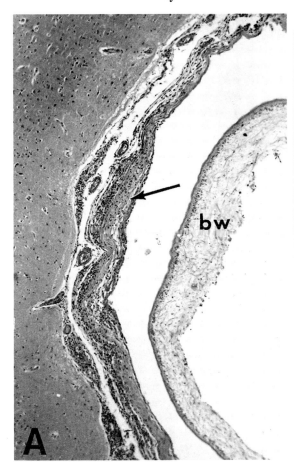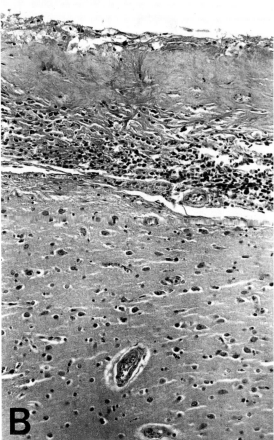

Fig. 26–7. *Cysticercus* in the central nervous system, section stained with hematoxylin and eosin stain. *A,* Medium-power view of a portion of a viable cysticercus in brain illustrating the intact bladder wall (bw), the fibrous reaction (capsule) (arrow) produced by the host, and the mild, mostly lymphocytic, inflammatory reaction, ×67. *B,* Higher magnification showing the fibrous capsule (top), the inflammatory cells (center), and the normal brain tissue (bottom), ×144.

suring 1.5 to 2.0 cm (Fig. 26–6 *A*). On section, there usually is a cavity filled with thick fluid (pus), which often contains a white, amorphous fragment of tissue corresponding to the bladder wall and scolex of the cysticercus (Fig. 26–6 *B*). This tissue fragment is often unrecognized as the parasite and is either discarded or

not submitted for histologic examination; in these cases, the nature of the lesion remains undiagnosed even with microscopic examination.

Microscopically, asymptomatic cysticerci in the central nervous system appear viable (Figs. 26–5 *D* and 26–7 *A*) and cause little or no inflammation (Fig 26–7

◄——

Fig. 26–6. *Cysticercus* in the central nervous system. *A* and *B*. Gross appearance. *A,* Close-up of a removed brain "lesion," bisected in the surgical pathology cutting room, illustrating the central cavity filled with semifluid necrotic material, ×2. *B,* Necrotic cysticercus found in the cavity. Note the rounded portion at the bottom corresponding to the scolex and neck and the delicate attached bladder wall, ×4. (Photographs courtesy of H.F. McCorkle, M.D., Department of Pathology, Fairview General Hospital, Cleveland, Ohio.) *C–E.* Microscopic appearance of a simi-

lar case, sections stained with hematoxylin and eosin stain. *C,* Low-power view of a portion of the nodule illustrating the central cavity and a small fragment of the parasite. Note the fibrous layer lining the cavity and the marked inflammatory reaction, ×28. *D,* Higher magnification showing the wall and the fragment of the cysticercus, ×70. *E,* The wall of the nodule showing the acute and chronic inflammatory reaction, ×140. (From G. Woods, M.D., Department of Pathology, University of Nebraska Medical Center, Omaha, Nebraska.)

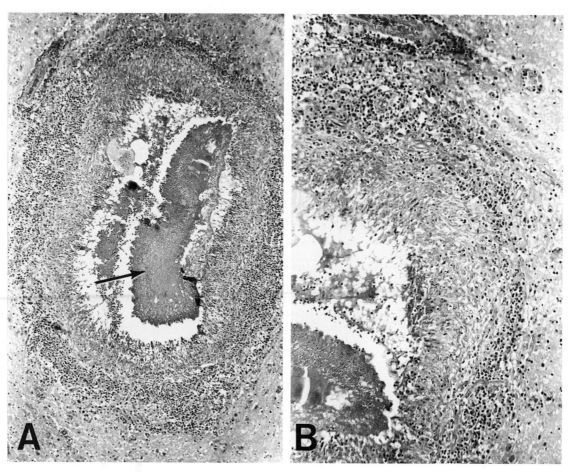

Fig. 26–8. *Cysticercus* in the central nervous system, section stained with hematoxylin and eosin stain. *A*, Medium-power view of a degenerated cysticercus in an individual who died with hundreds of cysticerci in the brain. Note the relatively small size of this lesion, the moderate inflammatory infiltrate, and the necrotic remnants of a cysticercus at the center (arrow). Iden-tification of the cysticercus is impossible on this spec-imen, but many viable and degenerating cysticerci throughout the brain support the diagnosis. Cysticerci like this one in the brain may resolve, producing a mod-erate inflammatory reaction without symptoms, ×67. *B*, Higher magnification illustrating similar features, ×115.

B). Other cysticerci are calcified or undergoing calcifi-cation or degeneration, with a minimal or moderate in-flammatory reaction (Fig. 26–8 *A–B*). Those that pro-duce symptoms are resected and often are submitted to the surgical pathologist, who usually finds that these specimens have a marked inflammatory reaction with granulation tissue around the dead cysticercus. The cen-tral cavity, with (Fig. 26–6 *C*) or without the parasite, is surrounded by necrotic tissue and by a marked poly-morphonuclear cell infiltrate consisting mostly of eosinophils, lymphocytes, and plasma cells (Fig. 26–6 *E*). Fibrous tissue with abundant histiocytes may be

Fig. 26–9. *Cysticercus* in the eye. *A*, Gross photograph of a cysticercus in the retina. Note the bladder with the invaginated scolex at the center. (Courtesy of F. Gutier-rez, M.D., Retina Department, Clinica Barraquer, Escuela Superior de Oftalmologia, Instituto Barraquer de Amer-ica, Bogota, Colombia.) *B–D*. Section stained with hema-toxylin and eosin stain. *B*, Low-power view of an eye with a cysticercus at the posterior pole (arrow). Note the marked inflammatory reaction, ×4.3. *C*, Medium-power magnification illustrating the scolex of the cysticercus (arrow), ×8.7. *D*, Higher magnification showing the de-generated cysticercus neck, with numerous calcareous corpuscles (arrows), ×280. (Preparation courtesy of H.E. Grossniklaus, Department of Ophthalmology and Pathol-ogy, University Hospitals of Cleveland and Case West-ern Reserve University, Cleveland, Ohio.)

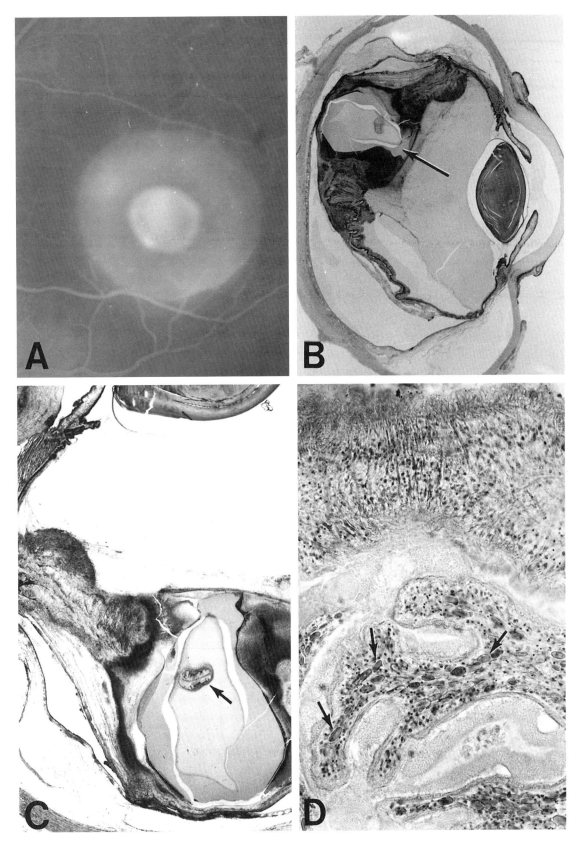

Fig. 26–9.

present, walling off the entire abscess. Sections of the parasite, either inside the cyst or by themselves (Fig. 26–6 C–D), are necessary for proper diagnosis (see below).

Ophthalmocysticercosis. A cysticercus removed from the eye appears grossly as a small, ivory white, collapsed cyst and histologically is often well preserved. If the entire eye is removed, it usually contains a dead cysticercus surrounded by a marked inflammatory infiltrate; the normal architecture of the eye has been destroyed (Fig. 26–9 B–D).

Other Organs. The gross and microscopic appearance of cysticerci is similar, regardless of the tissue or organ from which they are removed (Figs. 26–10 A and 26–11 A–D). The parasites are either well-preserved, dead, disintegrating, or calcified.

Diagnosis. Neurocysticercosis is diagnosed clinically based on the patient's history, symptoms, and signs. Often, the diagnosis is made by exclusion of other central nervous system diseases. Serologic tests are often not helpful, but if positive they are highly suggestive, especially if both serum and cerebrospinal fluid are positive. The enzyme-linked immunosorbent assay is used in some laboratories, and an enzyme-linked immunoelectrotransfer blot has been used in epidemiologic work (Jafri et al. 1998). The newer imaging techniques, such as CT and MRI, are the diagnostic methods of choice (Fig. 26–3; Earnest et al. 1987; Lotz et al. 1988; see above). Diagnosis of ocular cysticercosis is based on fundoscopic examination and recognition of the cysticercus subretinally, intravitreally, or in any other location in the eye. Cysticercosis of the intermuscular and subcutaneous tissues is diagnosed by careful palpation of the skin or, if the cysticerci are calcified, by x-rays of the thigh muscles (Fig. 26–4).

Histologically, the diagnosis is based on recognition of the cysticercus in the removed lesion and, increasingly, in fine needle aspiration biopsy specimens (Arora et al. 1994). However, one should remember that often a markedly degenerated cysticercus or a small fragment of it, which is available for diagnosis, may be unrecognizable or indistinguishable from other tapeworm larvae. The morphologic aspects of the cestode tissue discussed below are even more important in cases where fine needle aspirates are available for diagnosis (Kamal, Grover, 1995; Kung et al. 1989).

The anatomic pathologist usually receives a viable cysticercus when it is removed from the oral mucosa, breast, conjunctiva, or subcutaneous tissues. These cys-

ticerci are easily removed, and their presence in most of these sites usually arouses some concern in the patient. The specimen is often diagnosed clinically as a nodule, cyst, sebaceous cyst, or congenital cyst. The cysticercus may be found within fibroadipose connective tissue, or may have been shelled out intact (*color plate* XIV D–E), or is broken and collapsed (Figs. 26–9 A and 26–12 A–D). Histologically, there is little inflammatory reaction in the surrounding tissues (Fig. 26–12 A and C). The parasite stains well and all cellular elements are well preserved, without edema or inflammatory cells attached (Fig. IV–12 A–D). Sections through a cysticercus are often baffling to those who are not acquainted with their microscopic appearance (see the introduction to Part IV). Sometimes the histologic section includes the fibrous wall; the cyst membrane, either fully distended or, more often, collapsed against the scolex; and a well-oriented scolex (Fig. 26–12 A and D). More often, only small portions of either the cyst membrane or the scolex, or both, appear in the section (Fig. 26–6 C–D). In all cases, the typical histologic characteristics of cestode tissue must be recognized, even if a cysticercus with a scolex is not clearly evident (Fig. 26–6 C–D).

The bladder wall, the scolex, and the neck of viable *T. solium cysticerci* have a typical histological appearance (Figs. 26–13 and 26–14 A–B; Slais, 1970). The bladder wall is up to 80 μm thick, with a wart-like appearance (Fig. 26–13 A–B). It is composed of several layers; the outer layer consists of microvilli or barely visible hair-like processes measuring up to 6 μm in height (Fig. 26–13 B). The dense layer supporting the microvilli is about 1 μm thick and stains well with silver stain. This layer is a cytoplasmic extension of the tegument cells located below (Fig. 26–13 B) that are represented by dark-staining nuclei with no apparent cell cytoplasm. The muscle fibers between the nuclei have a loose arrangement and appear as rather thin bundles in well-distended bladder walls and slightly thicker bundles in collapsed bladder walls (Fig. 26–13 B). The rest of the bladder wall is composed of loose connective tissue and fibers with excretory ducts (Fig. 26–13 A–B). The internal side of the bladder wall appears irregular, is often covered with granular material, and appears to be broken (Fig. 26–13 A).

The scolex is solid, is filled with mesenchymatous tissue, and is characterized by a tegument similar to the one in the neck; suckers, a rostellum, and hooks may be evident (Fig. 26–12 B and D). The suckers appear as round (Fig. 26–15 A–B), as oval, or as a C-shaped mass of smooth muscle cells, depending on the plane of sectioning (Fig. 26–12 B and D). The rostellum is a tissue mass containing the hooks; on histologic sections

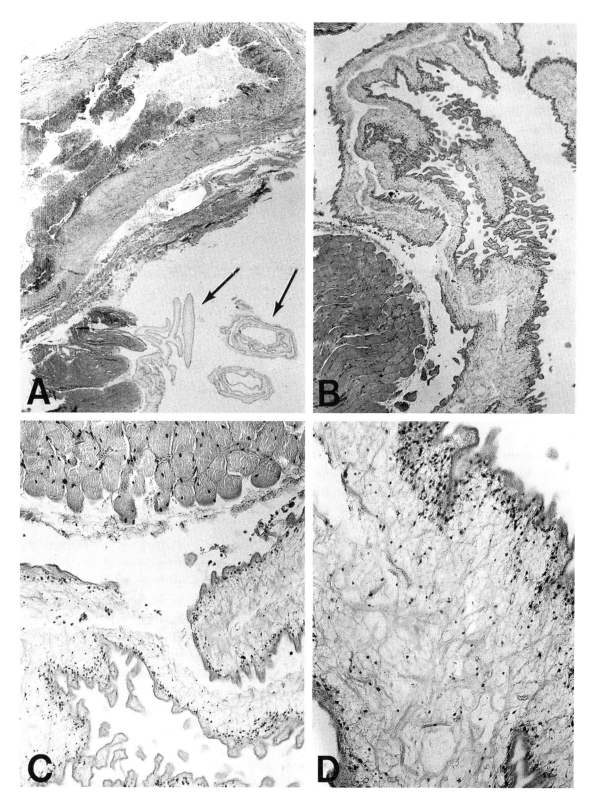

Fig. 26–10. *Cysticercus* in intermuscular tissues, example of a degenerated worm, section stained with hematoxylin and eosin stain. *A*, Low-power view showing the granuloma removed from the back of a 23-year-old woman with an inflammatory nodule. The fibrous wall around the cavity filled with necrotic tissue is seen at the top. The fragments of the bladder wall of the cysticercus is seen at the bottom (arrows), ×9. *B*, Medium-power view of the bladder wall. Note the tegument, the general cestode tissue, and the lack of longitudinal mesenchymal muscles, which distinguishes a cysticercus from a sparganum (see Fig. 26–19), ×55. *C*, Higher magnification showing the typical bladder wall of the parasite, ×140. *D*, Even higher magnification illustrating the beginning of degeneration. Note the attenuation of the worm tissues, ×220.

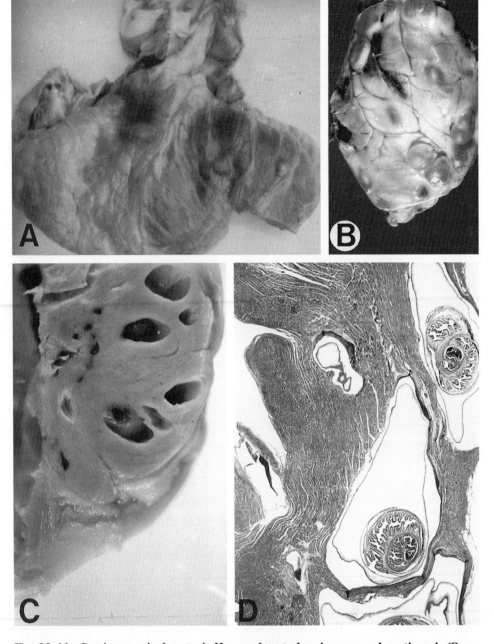

Fig. 26–11. *Cysticercus* in heart. *A*, Human heart showing several cysticerci. (Courtesy of E. Gall, M.D., Department of Pathology, University of Cincinnati School of Medicine, Cincinnati, Ohio.) *B–D.* Cysticerci in the heart of a pig. *B*, Cysticerci on the pericardium and *C* in the myocardium. *D*, Microscopic appearance, section stained with hematoxylin and eosin stain. Note the four viable cysticerci, which did not provoke an inflammatory reaction, ×7.6.

Fig. 26–12. *Cysticercus* in humans. Examples of viable cysticerci recovered from anatomic locations where the cyst is easily seen or palpated, sections stained with hematoxylin and eosin stain. *A* and *B*. Sublingual cysticerci. *A*, Low-power view showing the host fibrous capsule (long arrows), the invaginated scolex (s), and the bladder wall collapsed and contracted against the scolex (short arrows), ×11.5. *B*, Higher magnification illustrating the scolex, with a sucker (s) and the rostellum (r). Note the collapsed and contracted bladder wall membrane (short arrows), ×36. *C*, Cysticercus from the breast illustrating similar features, ×22. *D*, Cysticercus from the lip. Only the scolex and neck showing the spiral canal are seen here in a longitudinal section; most of the bladder wall was lost, ×2. (Preparation for *A*, *B*, and *D* courtesy of H. Estrada, M.D., Departamento de Patologia, Escuela de Medicina, Universidad de Caldas, Manizales, Colombia.)

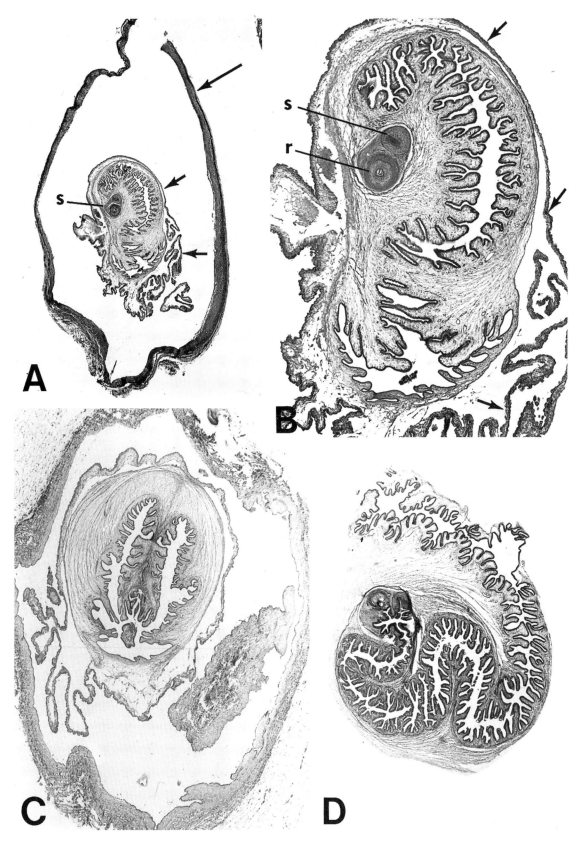

Fig. 26–12.

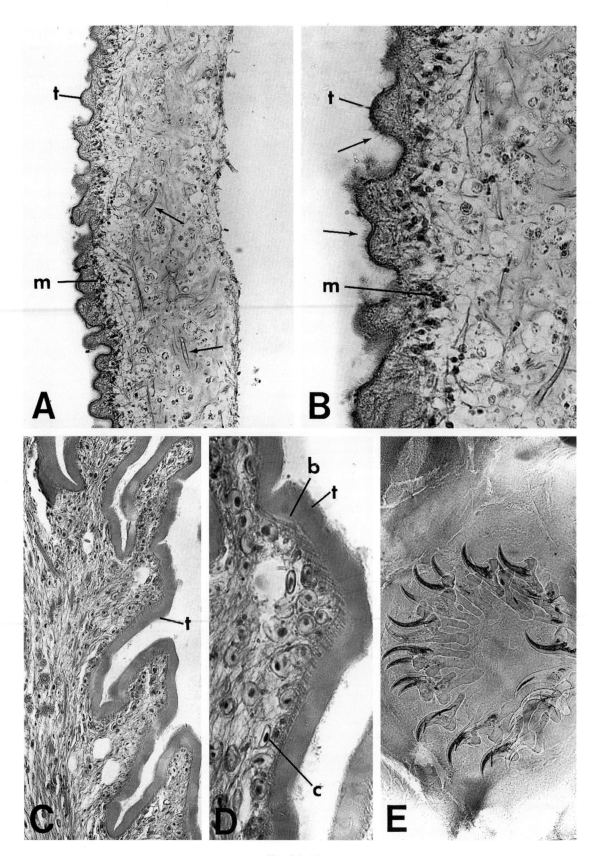

Fig. 26–13.

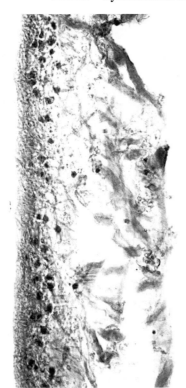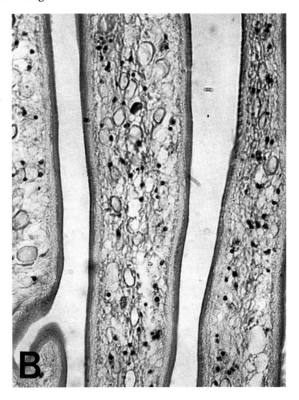

Fig. 26–14. *Cysticercus*. **Microscopic anatomy and diagnostic features of a degenerating cysticercus, hematoxylin and eosin stain. *A*, The bladder wall showing degeneration, with effacement of its normal architecture. Note the tegument, which is not clearly delineated, and the mesenchyme reduced to some fibers and pyknotic nuclei, ×450. *B*, The region of the neck appearing greatly thinned out. The calcareous corpuscles are preserved, ×450.**

the hooks are cut on different planes, but on squash preparations they are seen in their entirety (Fig. 26–13 *E*). The rest of the mesenchyme is composed of lax fibers and connective tissue with numerous excretory channels and calcareous corpuscles.

The scolex and the neck are both covered with a tegument that has a thick external layer without microvilli (Fig. 26–13 *C–D*). It measures between 10 to 15 μm in maximum thickness and stains deep red with hematoxylin and eosin stain. This layer is also a cytoplasmic extension of the tegumental cells below and

has numerous primary and secondary folds (Fig. 26–12 *A–D*), which are responsible for many unusual histologic appearances due to the plane of sectioning. The basal layer under the tegument is sometimes a thin, clear zone of irregular thickness. Below the basal layer, the muscle fibers are tightly arranged, traversing at right angles and seen better in tangential sections (Fig. 26–13 *D*). Beneath the muscle fibers are the nuclei of the tegumental cells (Fig. 26–13 *D*). The rest of the body is filled by the mesenchyme, with lax connective tissue and calcareous corpuscles (Fig. 26–13 *C–D*). The

Fig. 26–13. *Cysticercus*. **Microscopic anatomy and diagnostic features of a viable cysticercus in the brain, hematoxylin and eosin stain. *A* and *B*. The bladder wall. *A*, Wall of a cysticercus bladder showing the thin tegument (t), the muscles (m), and the mesenchyme with excretory ducts (arrows), ×180. *B*, Higher magnification showing** similar structures and the microvilli (arrows), ×450. *C* and *D*, Neck region showing the thick tegument (t) characteristic of the neck and the calcareous corpuscles (c). Under the tegument is the basal layer (b), ×280. *E*, Squash preparation of *T. solium* scolex showing the hooks arranged in two rows, ×140.

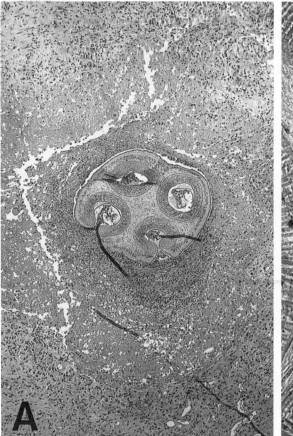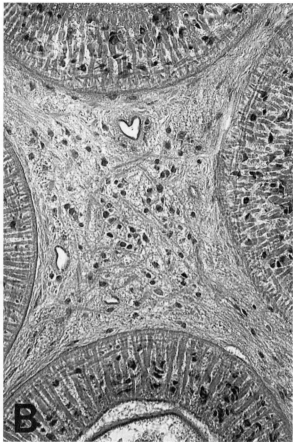

Fig. 26–15. *Cysticercus* in a brain biopsy specimen, section stained with hematoxylin and eosin stain. *A*, Low magnification showing a transverse section of the parasite through the top of the scolex; the four suckers are visible. Note the marked necrotic tissue around the worm and the inflammatory reaction. This section demonstrates that the parasite was probably evaginated from the cyst, a known occurrence in cysticerci of *T. solium*, ×55. *B*, Higher magnification showing the site of implantation of at least three hooklets (empty spaces), ×450.

calcareous corpuscles measure less than 15 μm, are round or oval, and consist of concentric layers of calcium, thus staining positive with van Kossa stain. The function of the calcareous corpuscles is not known; they dissolve easily in acid fixatives or acid hematoxylin and are one of the most important histologic markers of cestode tissue (larva or adult). Therefore, if the calcareous corpuscles are absent from tissues that otherwise appear to be cestode tissues, one should investigate whether the tissue was exposed to acid reagents.

Dead cysticerci are identified on the basis of similar histologic characteristics; all stages of degeneration, disintegration, and calcification may be found. When marked necrosis or full resorption has occurred, it may be impossible to make a diagnosis. Calcareous corpuscles and/or hooklets may be the only recognizable structures of the cestode. In these cases, the marked inflammation around both the parasite and the host tissues is evident (Fig. 26–9 *C–D*). Polymorphonuclear cells predominate in recently dead specimens, and polymorphonuclear leukocytes with lymphocytes and macrophages predominate in those dead for longer periods (Fig. 26–11 *A–B*). Granulation tissue and fibrosis with a mixed inflammatory reaction are present in specimens undergoing further degeneration; Charcot-Leyden crystals may also be found.

Other Cysticerci

Cysticerci from two other species of tapeworm, *T. saginata* (*C. bovis*) and *T. crassiceps* (*C. longicollis*), occur in humans; the cases are few and sporadic. The reports of these cases will now be discussed.

Cysticercus bovis. The larva of *T. saginata*, or beef tapeworm, is *C. bovis*, of which there are reports in humans (De Rivas, 1937; Fontan, 1919); because of the rarity of these cases and the lack of strict criteria for identification of the parasite, these reports are doubtful. The identification of *C. bovis* was based on the absence of a rostellum with hooklets, a feature difficult to appreciate in tissue sections. The best way to identify this cysticercus is by studying the whole specimen after clearing and mounting it in toto. In addition to the absence of the rostellum and hooklets, other histologic differences between *C. bovis* and *C. cellulosae* have been described (Slais, 1970), but they need confirmation. Another consideration in these cases is the possibility of an abnormal *C. cellulosae* that lacks a rostellum with hooklets.

Cysticercus longicollis. *Taenia crassiceps* is a natural parasite of the intestine of foxes and other canines; the larval stage, *C. longicollis*, occurs in various rodents that serve as intermediate hosts (*color plate* XV A). This cysticercus is another asexually proliferating larva of a cestode. *Taenia crassiceps* is found mainly in Europe, the North American continent (especially Alaska and Canada), and other places. Infections in humans with *C. longicollis* have occurred in the United States, Canada, and Europe. In the United States, a subretinal proliferating *C. longicollis* was removed from a 38-year-old woman (Chuck et al. 1997). In Canada, a 17-year-old girl living in rural Ontario presented with markedly decreased vision in her right eye. Examination revealed a yellowish cystic mass in the eye, which was removed and identified as *C. longicollis* (Freeman et al. 1973; Shea et al. 1973). In Europe, three cases of infection in patients with acquired immune deficiency syndrome (AIDS) have been reported. A 33-year-old man with AIDS presented with a subcutaneous paravertebral infiltrate resembling a hematoma that spread over a period of several weeks to cover the entire back. Bleeding in the tissues occurred due to a deficiency of clotting factor V and a fall in Quick values to less than 10%. Twenty-two days after admission to the hospital the mass ruptured spontaneously, with evacuation of a large number of 2 to 3 mm cysts identified as *C. longicollis* (Klinker et al. 1992). The second case in a man with AIDS was described in France. The patient developed a tumor in his right arm and forearm, which on ultrasound examination was revealed as a cystic mass. Removal of the mass revealed the parasites, which were classified conclusively based on characteristics of the hooklets (François et al. 1998). The third patient, also seen in France, developed a tumor on his left arm,

which grew and extended to the thorax in about 2 months. Excision of the mass revealed the 2 by 4 mm vesicles, which were identified as cysticerci of *T. crassiceps* (Chernette et al. 1995).

Another case in Germany, in an otherwise healthy 15-year-old girl, involved a small, apparently immature cysticercus removed from the anterior chamber of the eye. The parasite could not be identified, but a positive serologic test for *T. crassiceps* was the basis for its classification; for this reason, the identity of the parasite should remain doubtful (Arocker et al. 1992). The identification of *C. longicollis* is based on the size of the rostellar hooklets and on the parasite's asexual reproduction by exogenous and occasionally endogenous budding, usually at the opposite side of the scolex (Fig. 26–7 A–B). The large hooklets of *C. longicollis* are approximately 176 μm (range, 170 to 187 μm) in length; the small ones are about 132 μm long (range, 128 to 141 μm; Freeman et al. 1973).

Coenurus—Coenurosis

Coenurosis is an infection caused by the larvae of certain species of *Taenia* that previously were placed in a separate genus, *Multiceps*. The adult stages of these tapeworms are common parasites of the intestinal tracts of wild and domestic dogs, and their larval stages occur in several animals, including humans. In general terms, the life cycle of the species of *Taenia* producing coenurosis is similar to that of *T. solium* and *T. saginata*, but their larva is a *Coenurus* (Fig. 26–16). The great majority of cases of coenurosis (65%) are found in Europe and Africa; the infection is rare in the Western Hemisphere (Templeton, 1968, 1971). Most cases

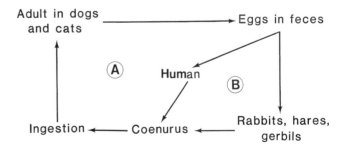

Fig. 26–16. *Coenurus*. Schematic representation of *Taenia* species producing coenurosis in humans: (a) general life cycle; (b) the infection in humans caused by ingestion of eggs in dog, or cat feces.

involve the subcutaneous tissues and the muscles; however, 70% of the cases in nontropical regions occur in the central nervous system (Orihel et al. 1970).

The main species of *Taenia* responsible for coenurosis in humans and their general geographic distribution are as follows: (*1*) *Taenia multiceps* is found in France (Duplay et al. 1955), Africa (Kaminsky et al. 1978; Manschot, 1976), England (Clapham, 1941), Brazil (Correa et al. 1962), and the United States (Barlow, Church, 1969; Hermos et al. 1970; Johnstone, Jones, 1950). The intermediate hosts include sheep, goats, cattle, horses, and antelopes, in which the larva (coenurus) develops in various tissues, commonly in the brain. (*2*) *Taenia serialis* is found in Canada and the United States. Rabbits, hares, and rodents are the intermediate hosts, in which the larva develops in the subcutaneous tissues and the intramuscular connective fascia (Kurtycz et al. 1983). (*3*) *Taenia brauni* occurs in North Africa, Ruanda (Fain, 1956; Vanderick et al. 1964), and the Democratic Republic of Congo. Gerbils are the intermediate hosts, in which the larva inhabits the subcutaneous tissues and other organs (Fain et al. 1956). (*4*) *Taenia glomerata* occurs in Nigeria and the Democratic Republic of Congo. It also has gerbils as intermediate hosts in the muscles, but the definitive host is not known (Beaver et al. 1984; Turner, Leiper, 1919).

Clinical Findings, Pathology, and Diagnosis. The clinical manifestations of coenurosis are variable and depend on the location of the cyst. Approximately five dozen cases have been reported in humans, with the cysts occurring, in decreasing order of frequency, in the brain, the subcutaneous or intermuscular tissues, the eye, and the spinal cord (Landells, 1949).

The symptoms and signs in the central nervous system usually consist of intracranial pressure with headache and papilledema, among others. The clinical diagnosis is difficult, but imaging techniques may reveal a cyst or a cystic mass, often located in one of the ventricles or the subarachnoid spaces (Pau et al. 1987). Cysts may also occur in the spinal cord (Buckley, 1947);

in either case, the lesion is usually recognized after removal and study of the cyst.

In the eye, the coenurus cyst is usually located in the posterior chamber, causing decreased vision (Boase, 1956; Epstein et al. 1959; Ibechukwu, Onwukeme, 1991; Williams, Templeton, 1971), or in the orbit (Manschot, 1976). In the subcutaneous and intermuscular tissues, the lesion presents as a mass, which is sometimes painful. In both cases, surgical removal of the parasite usually produces a well-preserved specimen (Kurtycz et al. 1983).

The diagnosis of coenurus is based on the gross and microscopic morphologic appearance of the cyst. It is a white, translucent structure varying from 2 to 10 cm in the largest dimension, filled with clear, watery fluid or a collapsed membrane with many protoscolices on its internal surface. The cysts from subcutaneous tissues are often unilocular. Those from the central nervous system are frequently multilocular, sometimes with multiple irregular vesicles and with a grape-like appearance. Viable cysts have many (often hundreds) protoscolices. The bladder of the coenurus has budding-off daughter bladders, either internally (Fig. 26–17 A–D), floating in the cystic fluid, or externally, attached by stalks.

The speciation of a coenurus based on its gross appearance is almost impossible. However, a unilocular coenurus in the brain, eye, or subcutaneous tissues, with protoscolices distributed in groups, is probably the larva of *T. multiceps*. Coenuri recovered from subcutaneous tissues (never from the central nervous system) of patients in tropical Africa probably belong to *T. brauni* (Beaver et al., 1984). Cases of coenurosis in the North American continent are probably due to *T. serialis*.

The speciation of a coenurus based on its microscopic appearance is difficult. A large tapeworm cyst with several protoscolices in the section is unquestionably a species of coenurus (Fig. 26–17 C–D). However, speciation is based on the number and size of rostellar hooklets (Clapham, Peters, 1941), a characteristic that should be carefully evaluated by individuals acquainted with the taxonomy of cestodes.

Fig. 26–17. *Coenurus.* *A*, Gross photograph of a *Coenurus* removed from the subcutaneous tissues of a primate. (Courtesy of R. Kuntz, Ph.D., San Antonio Medical Research Foundation, San Antonio, Texas.) *B–D.* Sections stained with hematoxylin and eosin stain of coenuri recovered from a man. *B*, Low-power view of a *Coenurus* recovered from the subcutaneous tissues of a child in Africa. The cyst had numerous protoscolices attached to the bladder wall, ×22. *C* and *D*, *Coenurus* recovered from the skeletal muscle of a 62-year-old woman from Texas, *C* ×22, *D* ×55. (Preparations courtesy of P.C. Beaver, Ph.D., School of Public Health and Tropical Medicine, Tulane University, New Orleans, Louisiana. Case for *C* and *D* reported by: Orihel, T.C., Gonzales, F., and Beaver, P.C. 1970. *Coenurus* from the neck of a Texas woman. Am. J. Trop. Med. Hyg. 19:255–257.)

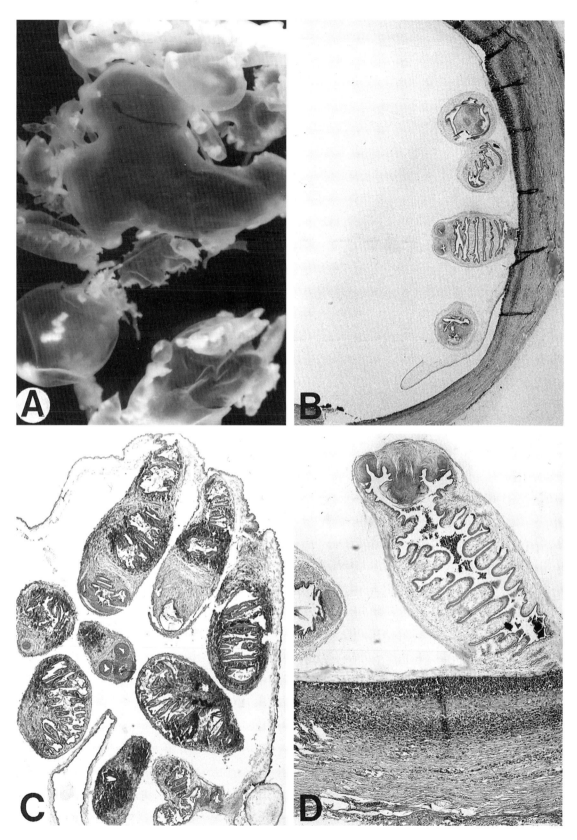

Fig. 26–17.

Spirometra—Sparganosis

Certain species of pseudophyllidian tapeworms have a sparganum or plerocercoid as their larval stage, which develops in many natural intermediate hosts and sometimes in humans (see the introduction to Part IV). The sparganum is a solid larva composed of a scolex with bothrids (two longitudinal groves), rather than suckers, and has an unsegmented strobila 20 to 30 cm in length. Specimens measuring 40 and 70 cm in length are recorded in the literature (Kittiponghansa et al. 1988). The sparganum occurs in the subcutaneous tissues and muscles of the many animals that serve as intermediate hosts.

Life Cycle. The species of tapeworms responsible for human sparganosis belong to the genus *Spirometra*, which has a life cycle similar to that of *Diphyllobothrium*; both genera have species that parasitize the intestines of humans and animals. *Spirometra* species are usually parasites of wild and domestic dogs and cats. The eggs laid by the parasite in the intestine are evacuated in the feces, and in fresh water they become infective. Many species of arthropods belonging to the genus *Cyclops* (copepod) ingest the infective eggs and serve as the first intermediate hosts. In the copepod, a larva known as the *procercoid* develops in the general cavity of the arthropod. After infected *Cyclops* are ingested by vertebrates such as frogs, snakes, and some

mammals, the second intermediate hosts, the procercoid larva is released and migrates through the intestinal wall to the tissues, where it grows into a *plerocercoid* or sparganum larva. When dogs or cats, the final hosts, ingest any of these second intermediate hosts, the sparganum develops into an adult *Spirometra* in the intestine (Fig. 26–18; Mueller, 1974). In general, the spargana of *Diphyllobothrium* are adapted to develop in cold-blooded animals, while the spargana of *Spirometra* are adapted to both cold-blooded and warm-blooded animals. The consensus is that the spargana of *Spirometra* produce sparganosis in humans, a fact that is probably related to their capacity to develop in warm-blooded animals. The spargana of *Diphyllobothrium* do not produce sparganosis in humans.

The genus *Spirometra* is difficult to speciate because there are substantial variations in morphology, even within a single worm (Iwata, 1972). Nevertheless, several species of *Spirometra* are mentioned in the literature: *S. mansoni*, *S. mansonoides*, *S. erinacei*, *S. ranarum*, *S. decipiens*, *S. houghtoni*, and others; these species are parasites of dogs and cats in different parts of the world. Infections in humans with adult *Spirometra* worms have been reported, for example *S. houghtoni* in China (Faust et al. 1929) and *S. erinacei* in Japan (Suzuki et al. 1982). *Spirometra mansonoides* is the only species known in the Western Hemisphere, and its larval stage is probably the agent of human sparganosis in this area. The other species are common in the Eastern Hemisphere, mostly in Asia and sporadically in other places, and produce human

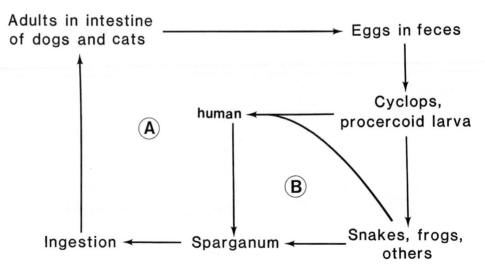

Fig. 26–18. *Spirometra*, **schematic representation of the life cycle. (*A*), The natural cycle between definitive and intermediate hosts. (*B*), The human infection resulting in sparganosis.**

sparganosis. However, in most experiments in which a sparganum recovered from humans was fed to cats, the adult worm recovered from the cats was a *S. ranarum* (Bonne, 1942). In the United States, some cases of sparganosis occur in an area southeast of a line between Texas and New York State. In the rest of the country, fewer cases have been found (Sanson, Bode, 1972).

Human sparganum infections occur in different ways; probably the most common method is drinking water contaminated with *Cyclops* harboring the procercoid larva. The procercoid larva in *Cyclops* is freed in the intestine, enters the intestinal wall, and migrates to the tissues, where it develops into the plerocercoid or sparganum. The second type of infection occurs by ingestion of undercooked meat containing some of the natural intermediate hosts (Corkum, 1966). In these cases, the plerocercoid larva (sparganum) released in the intestine loses the strobila and the scolex migrates through the intestinal wall to the tissues, where it grows back to its full length. A third possibile route of infection involves direct passage of the larva (sparganum) from animal flesh applied to the eye or vagina as a medicinal poultice, a common practice in some areas of Asia (Zhong et al. 1983). The last two situations involve the passage to and continuation of the same larval stage in another host, which is paratenesis (see Chapter 17). It has been suggested that the infections in the United States are probably acquired by ingestion of uncooked pork, a known paratenic host for the sparganum (Corkum, 1966).

Clinical Findings. The clinical manifestations of sparganosis are multiple and depend on the organ or tissue involved. For practical purposes, every tissue and organ system may be parasitized, but the subcutaneous tissues are most commonly affected. In the subcutaneous tissues, the lesion may be a nodule 1 to 2 cm in diameter that may persist for months or years without causing pain but that may become painful at any time. Other patients complain of migratory nodules that come and go, sometimes for several years (7 years in one patient; Araki et al. 1976). In these cases, the nodule may disappear, to reappear later at a distant location. Pain and inflammation of the nodule indicate that the worm is dead. A granulomatous mastitis due to the larva was found in a 64-year-old woman (Moreira et al. 1997).

Central Nervous System. In the central nervous system, the sparganum larva produces extensive damage and morbidity because of its large size and its propensity for migration (*color plate* XV *C–D*). The disease

is rare and most of the reported cases are from Southeast Asia, the largest series (34 cases) occurring in South Korea (Chang et al. 1992). Three cases reported in the United States all involved immigrants (Anders et al. 1984; Fan, Pezeshkopur, 1986; Holodniy et al. 1991). In the Korean study, 89% of the patients lived in a rural area; 75% had a history of ingesting raw frogs or snakes; and 84% presented with seizures, 59% with hemiparesis, and 56% with headaches (Chang et al. 1992). The disease involved the cerebral hemispheres, especially the frontoparietal lobes; in some cases, it extended to the basal ganglia and, rarely, to the cerebellum. In some patients, the disease manifests as a massive cerebral hemorrhage (Chamadol et al. 1992). The clinical diagnosis is based mainly on CT scans, which show areas of hypodensity and ventricular dilation in 88% of cases, irregular or nodular enhancing lesions in 88%, and small, punctate areas of calcification in 76%. These three findings on CT scans together appear to be a reliable basis for a clinical diagnosis of the disease and occur in 62% of the cases (Chang et al. 1992). Changes in the lesion observed on CT scans suggest that the worm is alive and migrating within the brain. However, these scans do not reveal whether the worm is dead (Chang et al. 1992). Another diagnostic and therapeutic modality is the stereotactic method for locating lesions in the brain, sometimes with recovery of the intact parasite (Tsai et al. 1993).

The male:female ratio of the disease is 4:1 to 5:1. Any age group can be affected, but the great majority of cases occur in 20- to 50-year-old individuals (Chang et al. 1992; Cho et al. 1975). Spinal cord infection is rare. It presents with symptoms of urinary incontinence, back pain, and numbness and weakness of the lower extremities (Fung et al. 1989).

Ocular Sparganosis. This is a relatively common condition in some areas of Southeast Asia, especially Vietnam and China, which may result in blindness (Zhong et al. 1983). The disease is associated with the custom, mostly in China, of applying poultices of frog muscles on the eye for medicinal purposes. The parasite in the frog's muscle migrates into the conjunctiva and enters the orbit (Joyeux et al. 1944); rarely, it enters the eye (Sen et al. 1989). In the orbital tissues, the larva is located in the posterior pole, producing inflammation that results in exophthalmia and lagophthalmia, which in turn cause ulceration of the cornea. Intense pain, irritation, excessive lacrimation, and marked swelling of the eyelids are some of the clinical manifestations of ocular sparganosis. In addition, the larva can enter the eye via the mouth. A conjunctival location of the larva, forming a nodule, has also been recorded (Jones, 1962; Kıttıponghansa et al. 1988).

Sparganosis of Other Organs. In other organs, the parasite may also produce inflammatory changes. For example, it may occur in the wall of the intestine, simulating a neoplastic growth (Bonne, Lie, 1940; Min et al. 1976a) or causing intestinal obstruction (Cho et al. 1987) or perforation (Min et al. 1976b). It may produce nodules in the breast (Kimura et al. 1967; Yamane et al. 1975), the scrotum (Ishii, Ikejiri, 1959; Park et al. 1964), and the epididymis (Nam, Kim, 1968). In the ureter, it may produce calculi (Kim, Kim, 1970) and cystitis in the urinary bladder (Oh et al. 1993). The parasite was recovered from the abdominal cavity of a patient undergoing surgery for an unrelated problem (Khamboonruang et al. 1974; Kron et al. 1991). In most of these cases, sparganosis presents as an inflamed nodule; peripheral eosinophilia is rare. Sparganum larvae have also been recovered from the right heart and right lung, where they produce infarction (Bonne, 1930, 1942).

Pathology and Diagnosis. The gross changes of sparganosis are similar to those of other helminths in tissues. Living parasites elicit little or no inflammatory reaction (Fig. 26–19 A–D), but dead ones provoke marked inflammation (Figs. 26–20 A–B, 26–21 A–D, and 26–22 A–D). Nodules with viable organisms consist of fibroadipose tissue with the larva at the center, a picture that is rather consistent, regardless of the organ involved (Fig. 26–20 A; Chi et al. 1980). The larva, which is easily recovered, is ivory white, measuring up to 40 cm long by 3 mm wide; it is unsegmented (Figs. IV–10 A and 26–19 A) and has a rudimentary scolex with bothrids at the anterior end. Nodules with a dead larva have the characteristics of an abscess filled with necrotic material (Fig. 26–20 A), but the parasite is often still recognizable based on its morphologic characteristics (Figs. 26–19 to 26–22).

On microscopic examination, the larva has the characteristic histology of a pseudophyllidian tapeworm: a tegument, a cellular subtegument, and lax mesenchymatous tissues with numerous large, longitudinal muscle cells and large excretory canals (Figs. 26–10 B; 26–19 B–D; 26–21 B and D). The bundles of muscle fibers are located throughout the body and are identified easily on cross sections (Figs. 26–10 B and 26–19 B) and longitudinal sections (Figs. 26–19 C and 26–22 C). Calcareous corpuscles are also evident (Figs. 26–19 B and D and 26–21 D; see above). The muscles of spargana, as described, contrast well with those of the Cyclophyllidea, which have longitudinal and circular mus-

cles at the center clearly dividing the body of the worm into the medullary and cortical fields (Fig. IV–11 C–D).

Proliferating Cestode Larvae

Under *normal* conditions, members of the Pseudophyllidea undergo asexual proliferation as part of their life cycle, which is characterized by the formation of *similar, cephalic (fertile)* larvae. One example is C. *longicollis* of T. *crassiceps*, which has been described in humans (see above). Under *abnormal* circumstances, members of both the Cyclophyllidea and the Pseudophyllidea may still undergo asexual proliferation, but because it is abnormal, it is characterized by the production of *dissimilar, acephalic, (sterile)* larvae. Examples of abnormal proliferating Cyclophyllidea are (1) the *racemose* type of cysticercus; (2) undifferentiated larvae consistent with *Hymenolepis* larvae; and (3) some *undifferentiated cestode larvae* with characteristics of a Pseudophyllidea but impossible to speciate at present. A fourth example that could be included in this list is the cyst of *Echinococcus multilocularis* in humans (see Chapter 27). There is only one example of an abnormally proliferating Pseudophyllidea, referred to as *Sparganum proliferum.* The reasons why these cestode larvae undergo abnormal proliferation are not understood, but since it does not provide an advantage for the parasite's survival, it must be an abnormal development. The behavior of these larvae sometimes resembles that of a malignant tumor that proliferates and metastasizes in the host, often resulting in its demise. We will examine each of these larvae individually and provide information useful for their diagnosis.

Cysticercus racemosus

Cysticercus racemosus is an abnormal proliferating cestode larva (*color plate* XV B). It is several centimeters in diameter and consists of multiple interconnected vesicles made of a thin, translucent membrane that grows by budding to produce a structure resembling a bunch of grapes (*color plate* XV B; Beaver et al. 1984). The cyst generally lacks a scolex; if it is present, it is in various stages of degeneration. In addition, it is always located in the ventricular system, the cysterna magna, the cerebellopontine angle, or the subarachnoid spaces. Cysts also occur in the subarachnoid space of the spinal canal (Cabieses et al. 1959; Rocca, Neira, 1980). In most cases, the parasite grows from the brain tissue into the adjacent space (Fig. 26–23 A–D; Ali-

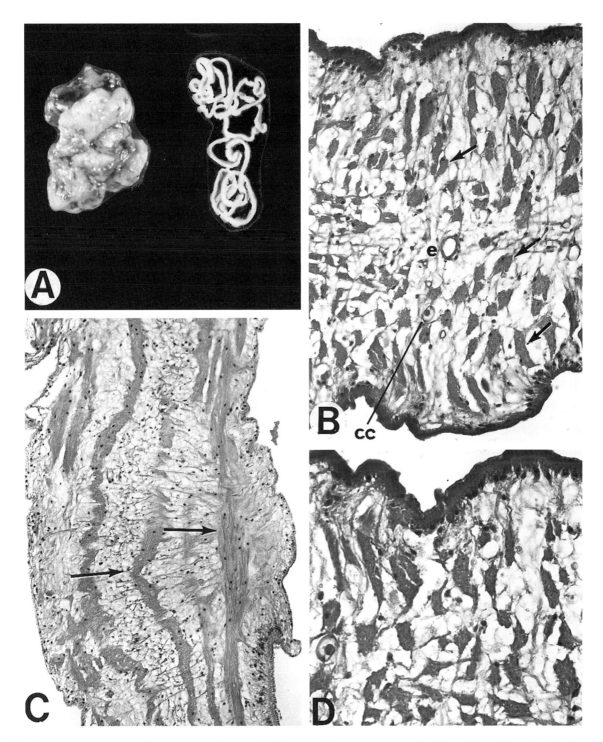

Fig. 26–19. *Sparganum* in subcutaneous tissues, viable. *A*, Nodule removed from the inguinal area (left) and the worm dissected from it (right). *B–D.* Sections stained with hematoxylin and eosin stain. *B*, Cross section of *Sparganum* showing the longitudinal muscles scattered throughout the entire body (arrows). Excretory canal (e); calcareous corpuscle (cc), ×280. *C*, Longitudinal section illustrating the muscles (arrows), ×180. *D*, Higher magnification of the cross section showing the typical cestode tegument, ×450. (Gross photograph courtesy of G.S. Hall, Ph.D., Department of Microbiology, The Cleveland Clinic Educational Foundation, Cleveland, Ohio.)

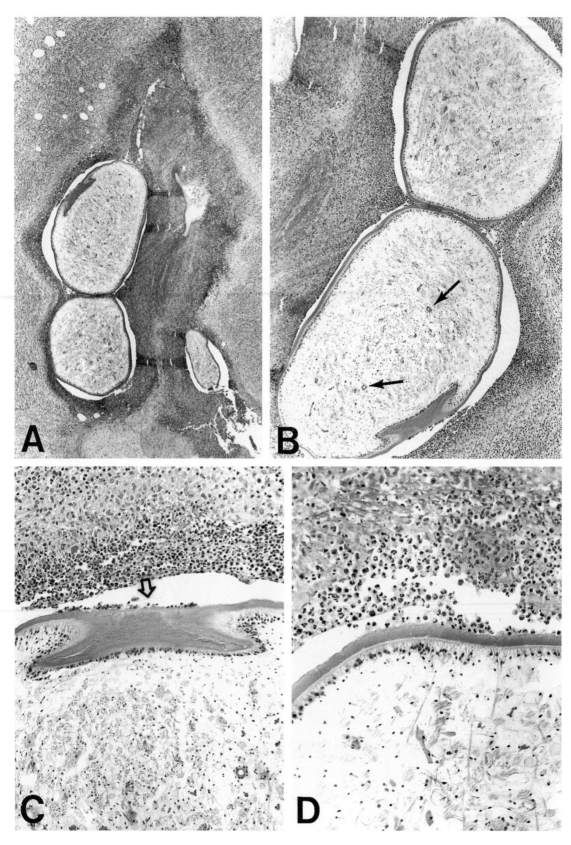

Fig. 26–20.

Khan et al. 1981; Baily, Levy, 1989; Jung et al. 1981; Ortega, Torres, 1991). It may sometimes extend into the cervical canal through the foramen magna (Bickerstaff et al. 1952, 1956). CT and MRI are the best modes for determining the location of the cyst, its extension, and the number of vesicles (Fig. 26–23 *A*; Rodacki et al. 1989).

It is generally believed that the racemose type of cysticercus is an aberrant larva of *T. solium* that begins as a normal cysticercus, grows close to the brain's surface, and erodes through the brain tissue to protrude into the adjacent space. This abnormal growth of the parasite probably occurs because of the lack of surrounding tissue that limits its growth; for example, hydatid larvae do not develop when the fibrous wall around the cyst fails to develop. In support of the belief that *T. solium* is the parent of the racemose cysticercus is that it is found almost exclusively in endemic areas of cysticercosis. In addition, when a degenerating or degenerated scolex is found, it is morphologically consistent with *C. cellulosae*. Further, some patients with the racemose type also have *C. cellulosae* in the brain or other organs (Briceno et al. 1961). Finally, intermediate stages between normal and racemose cysticercus are sometimes found (Rabiela Cervantes et al. 1985, 1989).

Large, sterile tapeworm cysts, with or without external proliferating buds recovered from the brains of humans, may correspond to cysts of *T. multiceps*, *T. serialis*, or an unknown species (Jung et al. 1981). In experimental infections with eggs of *T. serialis*, immune-suppressed mice developed sterile cysts in the subcutaneous tissues identical to those of *C. racemosus* in the brain (Lachberg et al. 1990). Large cysts in the brain tissue with a degenerating scolex identified as that of *T. solium* and lacking proliferating buds or vesicles have been identified as *C. cellulosae* (Berman et al. 1991). At least one known large, proliferating, sterile cyst, indistinguishable from racemose cysticerci, was found within the brain substance, not in a brain space (Ortega, Torres, 1991). A cyst in skeletal muscles

(Zavala-Velazquez et al. 1984) and another in bone (Rey et al. 1969), reported as *C. racemosus* outside the central nervous system, are not such by definition. More than likely, they correspond to a species of *Coenurus*. Morphologic differences between the bladder membrane of *C. cellulosae* of *T. solium* and the bladder membrane of *Coenurus cerebralis* of *T. multiceps* have been described. These differences are found mainly in the subtegumental muscles, excretory system, and microvilli (Slais, 1970), but they require wider confirmation (Jung et al. 1981).

Undifferentiated *Hymenolepis*-like Larva

An undifferentiated cestode larva occurred in a 58-year-old man with Hodgkin's disease from Pennsylvania. Autopsy revealed parasitic cysts up to 1 mm in diameter in all deep organs examined (Fig. 26–24 *A–B*; Connor et al. 1976). A similar infection occurred in a 44-year-old man from San Francisco with AIDS that presented with a febrile illness. On examination, the patient was found to have an 8 by 10 cm periumbilical mass, which on CT scans occupied the para-aortic, para-caval, and mesentery areas, and appeared to be lobulated and heterogeneous (Santamaria-Fries et al. 1996).

The morphologic characteristics of the parasite in both cases have marked similarities. The cysts are visible only under the microscope and are limited by a tegument consistent with that of a cestode with numerous microtriches. The earliest forms, judging by the size of the parasite, have a small cavity or none at all, but a cavity begins forming early and appears to be filled with fluid. Some cysts show an invaginated anlage of proliferating cells that are probably the beginning of a protoscolex; the parasites are in a very early stage of differentiation (Fig. 26–24). The first

---

Fig. 26–20. *Sparganum* in subcutaneous tissues, degenerating, section stained with hematoxylin and eosin stain. The specimen corresponds to a nodule on the left thigh of a 30-year-old woman. The nodule was noticed 2 years earlier but recently had grown slightly and had become painful. *A*, Low-power view of a section of a subcutaneous abscess containing three cross sections of a sparganum, ×28. *B*, Medium-power magnification showing the parasite, pale staining due to degeneration. Note the two excretory channels (arrows), ×55. *C*, Higher magnification of a section through the scolex showing part of a bothrid (open arrow), ×140. *D*, Even higher magnification illustrating the type of infiltrate, composed mainly of polymorphonuclear cells. Note the polymorphonuclear cells attached to the worm tegument, ×220. (From M.A. Pedraza, M.D., Department of Pathology, The Community Hospital of Springfield, Springfield, Ohio.)

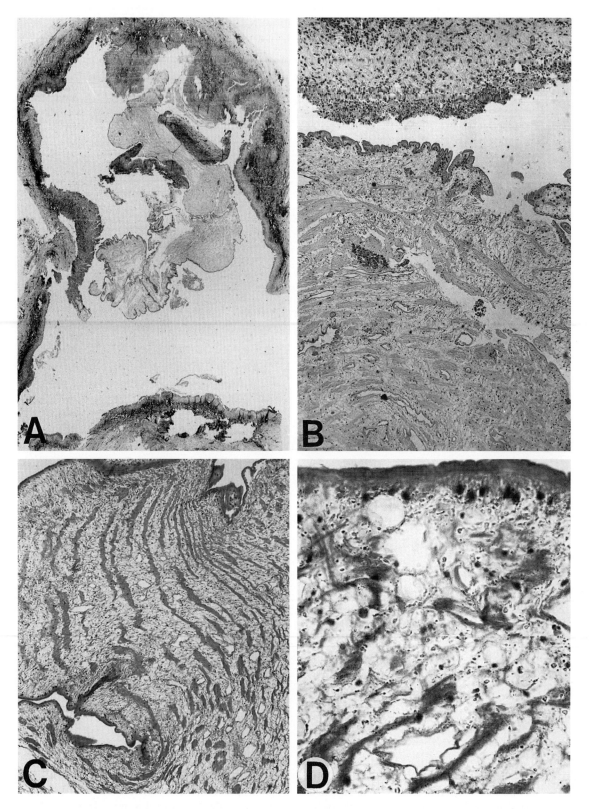

Fig. 26–21. *Sparganum*, another case with a worm in a greater state of disintegration, section stained with hematoxylin and eosin. *A*, Low-power of the nodule showing the fibrous wall surrounding the parasite, ×9.

B, Detail of the worm; notice that the muscles are swollen and stain faintly, ×70. *C* and *D*, From another case showing similar structures, *C* ×70, *D* ×450.

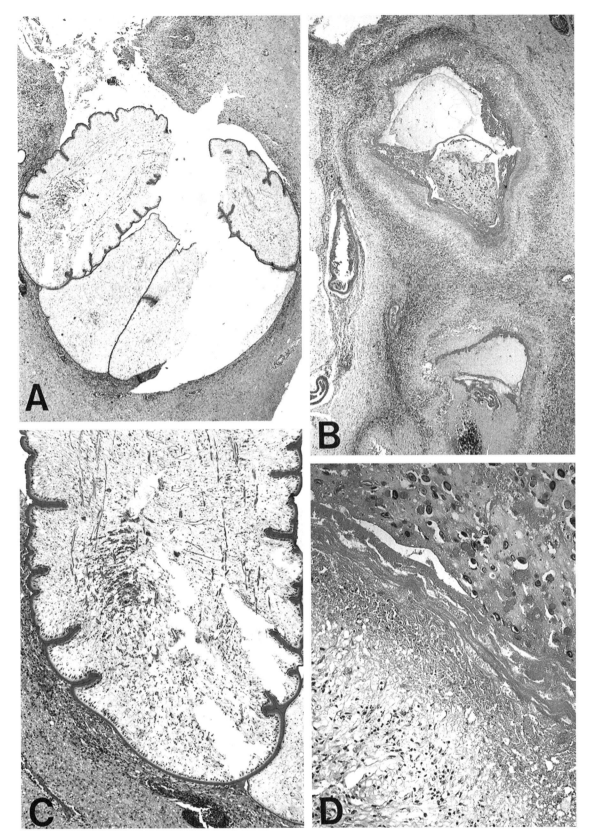

Fig. 26–22. *Sparganum* in human brain, sections stained with hematoxylin and eosin stain. *A,* Low-power view of brain showing four sections of a degenerating sparganum. Note the very faint longitudinal muscles, ×22. *B,* Another area of the brain showing two granulomas with remnants of the parasite. The worm dies and degenerates at different rates; thus, there are areas where it is still recognizable and areas where it is almost completely degenerated, ×22. *C,* Higher magnification illustrating the longitudinal muscles, ×55. *D,* The edge of a granuloma showing the calcareous corpuscles (top), the only remnants of the worm, ×140. (Preparation courtesy of C.H. Tse, M.D., Division of Pathology, Queen Elizabeth Hospital, Hong Kong. Reported by: Chan, S.T., Tse, C.H., Chan, Y.S. et al.). 1987. Sparganosis of the brain. Report of two cases. J. Neurosurg. 67:931–934.)

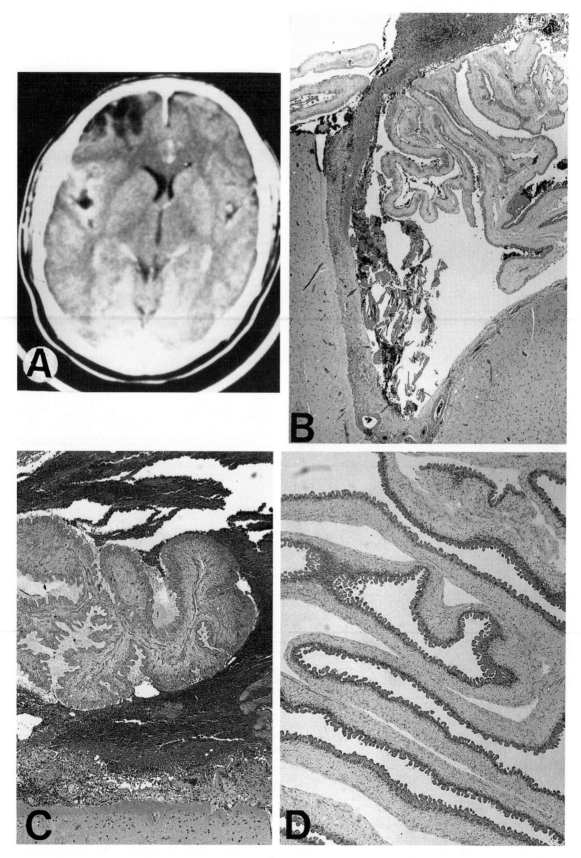

Fig. 26–23. *Cysticercus racemosus* removed from the temporal lobe. *A*, Computed tomogram showing the extent of the lesion. *B–D*, Sections stained with hematoxylin and eosin stain. *B*, Low-power view illustrating the parasite within the brain substance growing to the meninges (note part of the cyst wall at the top on the meninges), ×22. *C*, Higher magnification illustrating the typical budding of the bladder wall, ×55. *D*, Another aspect of the bladder wall, ×55.

case of this infection, in the 58-year-old man, was described as an aberrant *Sparganum proliferum* (Connor et al. 1976). Morphologically, however, the larva is similar to larvae of *H. nana* in experimental infections of mice deprived of their T cells. Moreover, the biologic behavior of the parasite in mice is identical to that in human patients, consisting mainly of dissemination to the internal organs (Beaver, Rolon, 1981; Lucas et al. 1979, 1980). In the patient with AIDS, the parasite was studied by rDNA sequencing analysis, which revealed that phylogenetically it was closest to *H. diminuta*. However, DNA of *H. nana* was not used in the analysis (Santamaria-Fries et al. 1996).

Undifferentiated Cestode Larvae

The third type of proliferative undifferentiated tapeworm larva belonging to the Cyclophyllidea and producing disseminated infections in humans is too abnormal and difficult to classify at present. These larvae grow by budding, resulting in small, motile masses of cestode tissue less than 1.0 cm in size, sometimes with slightly longer branching, ribbon-like forms without a grossly appreciable bladder. On microscopic examination, these larvae do not have parenchymal muscle bundles; some may have a small bladder or lacuna and dilated excretory channels (spaces lined with a membrane; Fig. 26–25 A–D). The

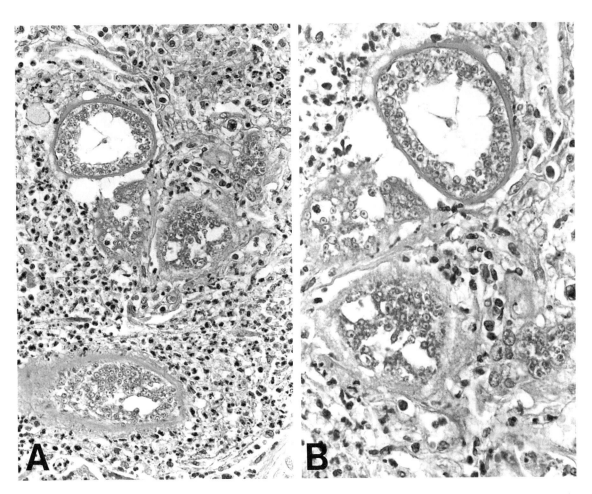

Fig. 26–24. Tapeworm larvae, undifferentiated, sections stained with hematoxylin and eosin stain. *A,* **Medium-power magnification showing several round structures corresponding to a metazoan organism. The structures show an early cystic formation similar to that observed in the early development of a cysticercoid of *Hymenolepis* or a proliferating cysticercus of *Taenia*, ×238.** *B,* **Higher magnification illustrating similar features, ×383. (AFIP specimen No. 1301994. Reported by Connor, D.H., Sparks, A.K., Strano, A.J., et al. 1976. Disseminated parasitosis in an immunosuppressed patient. Possibly a mutated sparganum. Arch Pathol. Lab Med. 100:65–68.)**

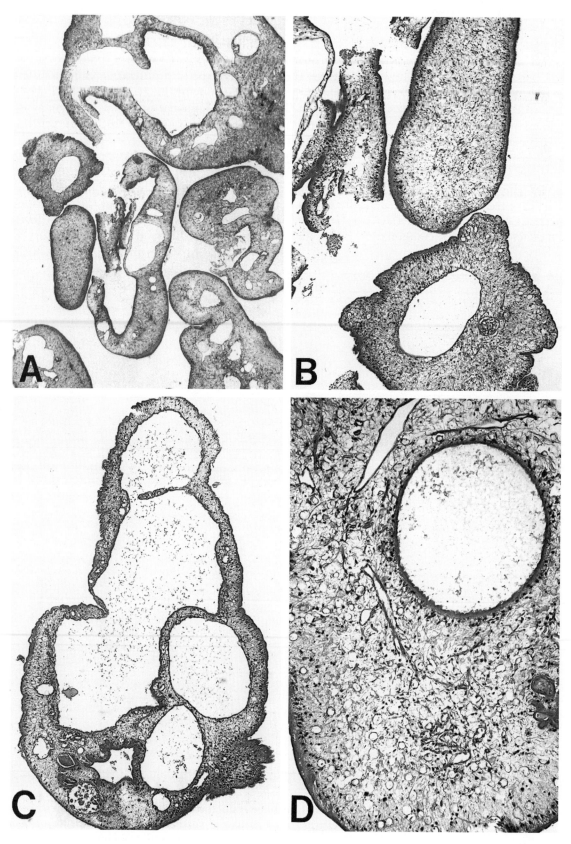

Fig. 26–25. Proliferating cestode larvae in spinal cord of a man, sections stained with hematoxylin & eosin. *A*, Low-power view of proliferating cestode larvae, ×24. *B* and *C*, Medium-power view showing the larvae, sometimes solid (top, *B*) but mostly with abnormally dilated channels, ×60. *D*, Higher-power magnification typical cestode tissue with tegument and calcareous corpuscles, ×187. (Preparation courtesy of H-C Lui, M.D., Department of Pathology, National Yang-ming Medical College, Taipei, Taiwan. Reported by: Lo, Y.-K., Chao, D., Yan, S.-H., et al. 1987. Spinal cord proliferative sparganosis in Taiwan: a case report. Neurosurgery 21:235–238.)

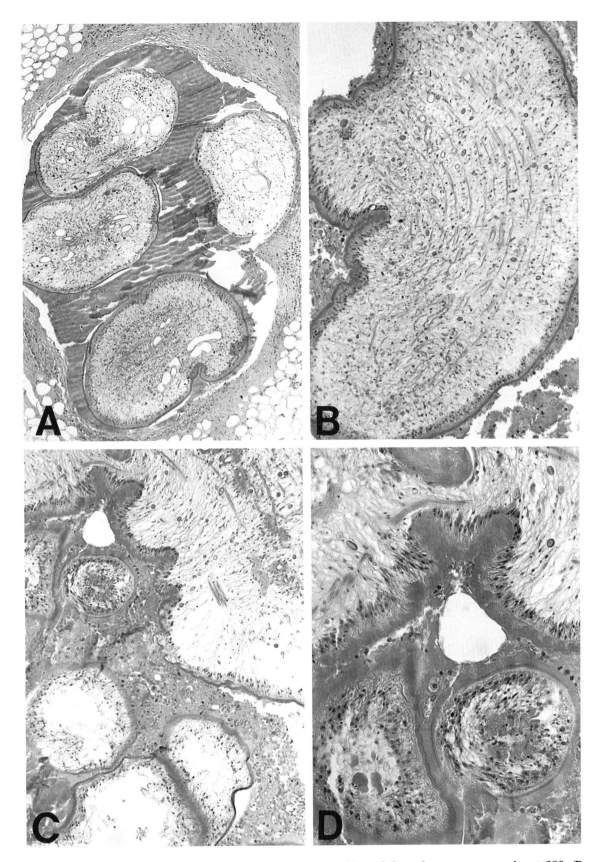

Fig. 26–26. *Sparganum proliferum* in human tissues, sections stained with hematoxylin and eosin stain. *A*, Low-power view of four parasites within a fibrous capsule. Note the dilated excretory channels recognized by their lining membrane, ×70. *B* and *C*, Higher magnification of the parasites illustrating the solid nature and the scattered longitudinal muscle fibers, ×140. *D*, Even higher magnification showing the thick tegument of the parasite and the calcareous corpuscles, ×280. (Preparation courtesy of M.D. Little, Ph.D., Department of Tropical Medicine, School of Public Health and Tropical Medicine, Tulane University, New Orleans, Louisiana. In: Stiles, C.W. 1908. The occurrence of a proliferative cestode larva (*Sparganum proliferum*) in man in Florida. Hyg. Lab. Bull. No. 40, pp. 7–18.)

larvae in humans usually present with a mass in the lower part of the body, often involving the pelvic bone, pelvic organs, gluteal muscles, and, in one case, the cervical spinal canal (LaChance et al. 1983; Liao et al. 1984; Lin et al. 1978; Lo et al. 1987; Nakamura et al. 1990).

As stated, the nature of these acephalic larvae is unknown, and whether they are a *Cysticercus* of a species of *Taenia* or a *Tetrathyridium* of a species of *Mesocestoides* cannot be determined (Beaver, Rolon, 1981). The best way to refer to these parasites is to use the descriptive term *undifferentiated cestode larvae*.

Sparganum proliferum

Sparganum proliferum is a solid, cord-like, mobile worm with no bladder or lacuna, although on cross sections it may have dilated excretory channels lined with a membrane (Fig. 26–26 *A*). The distinct morphologic feature of this Pseudophyllidea larva consists of bundles of longitudinal muscle fibers scattered throughout the mesenchyme; in addition, the tegument is generally thick (Fig. 26–26 *A–D*). Descriptions of human infections with *S. proliferum* are few, mostly from Japan (Ijima, 1905; Morishita, 1972; Yoshida, 1914). One case each occurred in the United States (Gates, 1909; Stiles, 1908), Venezuela (Moulinier et al. 1982; Noya et al. 1992), and Paraguay (Beaver, Rolon, 1981). However, the Paraguayan case may turn out to be an undifferentiated Cyclophyllidea larva rather than *S. proliferum*.

The disease begins with a subcutaneous tumor in the thigh, shoulder, or neck and eventually spreads to other parts of the skin (Fig. 26–27 *A–B*), the muscles, and the internal viscera. It evolves over 5 to 25 years, and all patients die. All patients develop nodules throughout most of the skin, except for the face and head; the nodules may open due to ulceration or scarification, producing a motile worm up to 1.0 cm long (Fig. 26–27 *B*). Dissemination of the parasites to the internal organs involves mainly the abdomen, lungs, and brain. The parasites grow by budding and branching and apparently multiply by transverse fission of the buds (Fig. 26–28). Microscopically, the worms are solid, with abnormally dilated excretory channels, bundles of longitudinal muscles scattered throughout the body, and a thick tegument consistent with a *Sparganum* (Fig. 26–26 *A–D*). None of the organisms studied showed a scolex.

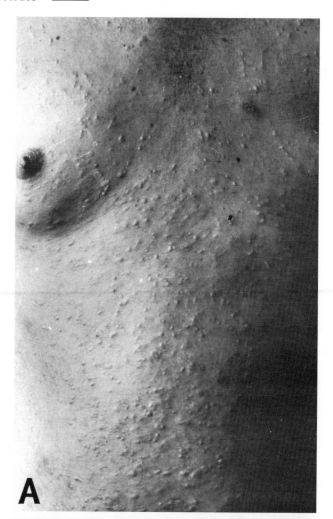

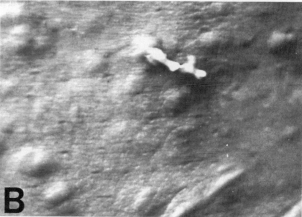

Fig. 26–27. *Sparganum proliferum* skin lesions. *A,* Involvement of a large area of the chest and abdomen. *B,* Detail of the lesions, one with a worm protruding from the skin. (In: Molinier, R., Martinez, E., Torres, J.R., et al. 1982. Human proliferative sparganosis in Venezuela: report of a case. Am. J. Trop. Med. Hyg. 31:358–363. Reproduced with permission.)

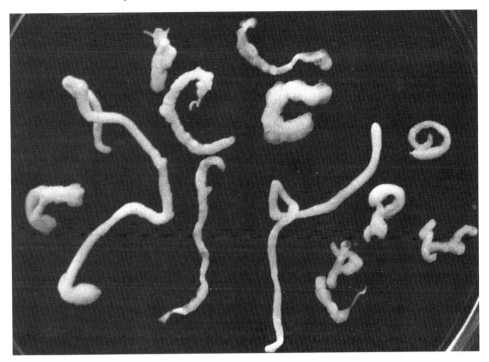

Fig. 26–28. *Sparganum proliferum*, gross appearance of parasites. Note the branching nature. (In: Noya, O.O., Noya, B.A., Arrechedera, H., et al. 1992. *Sparganum proliferum*: an overview of its structure and ultrastructure. Int. Parasitol. 22:631–640. Reproduced with permission.)

References

Acha PN, Aguilar FJ, 1964. Studies on cysticercosis in Central America and Panama. Am. J. Trop. Med. Hyg. 13:48–53

Afshar A, 1967. Cysticercosis in Iran. Ann. Trop. Med. Parasitol. 61:101–103

Akiguchi I, Fujiwara T, Matsuyama H, Muranaka H, Kameyama M, 1979. Intramedullary spinal cysticercosis. Neurology 29:1531–1534

Alagaratnam TT, Wing YK, Tuen H, 1988. Cysticercosis of the breast. Am. J. Trop. Med. Hyg. 38:601–602

Ali-Khan Z, Siboo R, Meerovitch E, Faubert G, Faucher MG, 1981. *Cysticercus racemosus* in an eosinophilic phlegmon in the brain. Trans. R. Soc. Trop. Med. Hyg. 75:774–779

Allan JC, Velasquez TM, Garcia NJ, Torres AR, Yurrita P, Fletes C, de Mata F, Soto de Altaro H, Craig PS, 1996. Epidemiology of intestinal taeniasis in four rural Guatemalan communities. Ann. Trop. Med. Parasitol. 90:157–165

Almeida AA de, Oliveira JEB de, 1971. Cisticercose ocular. Rev. Inst. Med. Trop. Sao Paulo 13:1–8

Anders K, Foley K, Stern E, Brown WJ, 1984. Intracranial sparganosis: an uncommon infection. Case report. J. Neurosurg. 60:1282–1286

Andrews R, Mason W, 1987. Cysticercosis presenting as acute scrotal pain and swelling. Pediatr. Infect. Dis. 6:942–943

Araki T, Nakazato H, Imaoka A, Fukunaga A, Osawa C, Matsuki N, Yasuhara M, 1976. Two cases of sparganosis *mansoni*: presumption of sub-pericardial parasitism and the movement of parasite during seven years. Jpn. J. Parasitol. 25:343–349

Arciniegas A, Gutierrez F, 1988. Our experience in the removal of intravitreal and subretinal cysticerci. Ann. Ophthalmol. 20:75–77

Arocker ME, Huber SV, Auer H, Grabner G, Stur M, 1992. *Taenia crassiceps* in the anterior chamber of the human eye. A case report. [in German. English summary]. Klin. Monatsbl. Augenheilkd. 201:34–37

Arora VK, Gupta K, Singh N, Bhatia A, 1994. Cytomorphologic panorama of cysticercosis on fine needle aspiration. A review of 298 cases. Acta Cytol. 38:377–380

Arriagada C, Matus C, Nogales-Gaete J, 1997. Tomografia computada en neurocisticercosis. In: Arriagada R, Nogales-Gaete J, Apt B (eds), *Neurocisticercosis: Aspectos epidemiologicos, patologicos, immunologicos, clinicos, imagenologicos y terapeuticos*. Santiago, Chile: Arrynog Ediciones, pp. 161–207

Arriagada V, Arriagada C, Terra E, Manen R, Julio D, 1997. Imagen de resonancia magnetica en neurocisticercosis. In: Arriagada R, Nogales-Gaete J, Apt B (eds), *Neurocisticercosis: Aspectos epidemiologicos, patologicos, immunologicos, clinicos, imagenologicos y terapeuticos*. Santiago, Chile: Arrynog Ediciones, pp. 209–278

Baily GG, Levy LF, 1989. Racemose cysticercosis treated with praziquantel. Trans. R. Soc. Trop. Med. Hyg. 83:95–96

Barlow JF, Church BG, 1969. Coenurosis in the brain of a child from South Dakota. S.D. J. Med. 22:37–44

Beaver PC, Jung RC, Cupp EW, 1984. *Clinical Parasitology*. Philadelphia: Lea & Febiger

Beaver PC, Rolon FA, 1981. Proliferating larval cestode in a man in Paraguay. A case report and review. Am. J. Trop. Med. Hyg. 30:625–637

Berman JD, Beaver PC, Cheever AW, Quindlen EA, 1991. *Cysticercus* of 60–milliliter volume in human brain. Am. J. Trop. Med. Hyg. 30:616–619

Bickerstaff ER, Cloake PCP, Hughes B, Smith WT, 1952. The racemose form of cerebral cysticercosis. Brain 75:1–18

Bickerstaff ER, Small JM, Woolf AL, 1956. Cysticercosis of the posterior fossa. Brain 79:622–634

Binstock PD, Azimi PH, Williams RA, 1987. Cerebral cysticercosis in a 22-month-old infant. Am. J. Clin. Pathol. 88:655–658

Boase AJ, 1956. *Coenurus* cyst of the eye. Br. J. Ophthalmol. 40:183–185

Bonne C, 1930. A peculiar *Sparganum* infection. Geneeskd. Tijdschr. Ned. 70:1235–1238

Bonne C, 1942. Researches on sparganosis in the Netherlands East Indies. Am. J. Trop. Med. 22:643–645

Bonne C, Lie KJ, 1940. Darmwandhelminthiasis teweeggebratch door spargana. Geneeskd. Tijdschr. Ned. 80:2788–2792

Briceno CE, Biagi FF, Martinez B, 1961. Cisticercosis. Observaciones sobre 97 casos de autopsias. Prensa Med. Mexicana 26:193–197

Buckley JJC, 1947. *Coenurus* from human spinal cord. Trans. R. Soc. Trop. Med. Hyg. 41:7–7

Cabieses F, Vallenas M, Landa R, 1959. Cysticercosis of the spinal cord. Neurosurgery 16:337–341

Chamadol W, Tangdumrongkul S, Thanaphaisal C, Sithithaworn P, Chamadol N, 1992. Intracerebral hematoma caused by *Sparganum*: a case report. J. Med. Assoc. Thail. 75:602–605

Chang KH, Chi JG, Cho SY, Han MH, Han DH, Han MC, 1992. Cerebral sparganosis: analysis of 34 cases with emphasis on CT features. Neuroradiology. 34:1–8

Chernette R, Bussieras J, Marionneau J, Boyer E, Roubin C, Prophette B, Naillard H, Fabiani B. 1995. Cysticercose envahissante a *Taenia crassiceps* chez un patient atteint de sida. Bull. Acad. Natl. Med. 179:777–783

Chi HS, Chi JG, 1978. A histopathological study on human cysticercosis. Korean J. Parasitol. 16:123–133

Chi JG, Chi HS, Lee SH, 1980. Histopathologic study on human sparganosis. Korean J. Parasitol. 18:15–23

Cho KJ, Lee HS, Chi JG, 1987. Intramural sparganosis manifested as intestinal obstruction—a case report. J. Korean Med. Sci. 2.137–139

Cho SY, Bae J, Seo BS, Lee SH, 1975. Some aspects of human sparganosis in Korea. Korean J. Parasitol. 13:60–77

Chopra JS, Nand N, Jain K, Mittal R, Abrol L, 1986. Generalized muscular pseudohypertrophy in cysticercosis. Postgrad. Med. J. 62:299–300

Chuck RS, Olk RJ, Weil GJ, Akduman L, Benenson IL, Smith ME, Kaplan HJ, 1997. Surgical removal of a subretinal proliferating cysticercus of taeniaeformis *crassiceps*. Arch. Ophthalmol. 115:562–563

Clapham PA, 1941. An English case of *Coenurus cerebralis* in the human brain. J. Helminthol. 19:84–86

Clapham PA, Peters BG, 1941. The differentiation of *Coenurus* species by hook measurements. J. Helminthol. 19:75–84

Colli BO, Assirati JJ, Machado HR, dos Santos F, Takayanagui OM, 1994. Cysticercosis of the central nervous system. II. Spinal cysticercosis. Arq. Neuropsiquiatr. 52.187–199

Connor DH, Sparks AK, Strano AJ, Neafie RC, Juvelier B, 1976. Disseminated parasitosis in an immunosuppressed patient. Possibly a mutated sparganum. Arch. Pathol. Lab. Med. 100:65–68

Corkum KC, 1966. Sparganosis in some vertebrates of Louisiana and observations on a human infection. J. Parasitol. 52:444–448

Correa FMA, Ferriolli P Jr, Forjaz S, Martelli N, 1962. Cenurose cerebral. A proposito de un caso humano. Rev. Inst. Med. Trop. 4:38–45

Cruz I, Cruz ME, Teran W, Schantz PM, Tsang V, Barry M, 1994. Human subcutaneous *Taenia solium* cysticercosis in an Andean population with neurocysticercosis. Am. J. Trop. Med. Hyg. 51:405–407

De Rivas D, 1937. *Cysticercosis bovis* in man. In: *Commemoration of the 30th Year Jubileum in Honor of K. J. Skrjabin*, pp. 569–570

Del Brutto OH, 1995. Single parenchymal brain cysticercus in the acute encephalitic phase: definition of a distinct form of neurocysticercosis with a benign prognosis. J. Neurol. Neurosurg. Psychiatry 58:247–249

Del Brutto OH, Quintero LA, 1995. Cysticercosis mimicking brain tumor: the role of albendazole as a diagnostic tool. Clin. Neurol. Neurosurg. 97:256–258

Diaz JF, Verastegui M, Gilman RH, Tsang VCW, Pilcher JB, Gallo C, Garcia HH, Torres P, Montenegro T, Miranda E, 1992. Immunodiagnosis of human cysticercosis (*Taenia solium*): a field comparison of an antibody-enzyme-linked immunosorbent assay (elisa), an antigen-elisa, and an enzyme-linked immunoelectrotransfer blot (EITB) assay in Peru. Am. J. Trop. Med. Hyg. 46:610–615

Dixon HBF, Smithers DW, 1934. Epilepsy in cysticercosis (*Taenia solium*) study of seventy-one cases. Q.J. Med. 3:603–616

Duplay J, Berard-Badier M, Cossa P, Ranque J, 1955. A propose d'un cas de cenurose cerebrale. Presse Med. 63:625–626

Earnest MP, Reller LB, Filley CM, Grek AJ, 1987. Neurocysticercosis in the United States: 35 cases and a review. Rev. Infect. Dis. 9:961–979

Epstein E, Proctor NSF, Heinz HJ, 1959. Intraocular *Coenurus* infestation. S. Afr. Med. J. 33:602–604

Fain A, 1956. *Coenurus* of *Taenia brauni* Setti parasitic in man and animals from the Belgian Congo and Ruanda-Urundi. Nature 178:1353

Fain A, Denisoff N, Homans L, Questlaux G, Van Laere L, Vincent M, 1956. Cenurose chez l'homme et les animaux due a *Taenia brauni* Setti, au congo Belge et au Ruanda-Urundi. II. Relation de huit cas humaines. Ann. Soc. Belge Med. Trop. 36:679–696

Fan KJ, Pezeshkopur GH, 1986. Cerebral sparganosis. Neurology 36:1249–1251

Faust EC, Campbell EH, Kellog CR, 1929. Morphological and biological studies on the species of *Diphyllobothrium* in China. Am. J. Hyg. 9:560–583

Fontan C, 1919. Csticercus bovis chez l'homme. Localise a la region mammaire. *Taenia inerme* de l'intestin. Parasitisme adulte et larvaire chez le meme sujet. Gaz. Hop. 92:183–184

Francois A, Favennec L, Cambon-Michot C, Gueit I, Biga N, Tron F, Brasseur P, Hemet J, 1998. *Taenia crassiceps* invasive cysticercosis. A new human pathogen in acquired immunodeficiency syndrome? Case reports. Am. J. Surg. Pathol. 22:488–492

Freeman RS, Fallis AM, Shea M, Maberley AL, Walters J, 1973. Intraocular *Taenia crassiceps* (Cestoda): Part II. The parasite. Am. J. Trop. Med. Hyg. 22:493–495

Fung CF, Ng TH, Wong WT, 1989. Sparganosis of the spinal cord. Case report. J. Neurosurg. 71:290–292

Gajdusek DC, 1978. Introduction of *Taenia solium* into West New Guinea with a note on an epidemic of burns from *Cysticercus* epilepsy in the Ekari people of the Wissel Lakes area. Papua New Guinea Med. J. 21:39–342

Gates H, 1909. Larval tapeworm in human flesh, or *Sparganum proliferum gatesius* (Stiles). Gulf States J. Med. Surg. Mobile Med. Surg. J. 15:543–553

Hermos JA, Healy GR, Schultz MG, Barlow J, Church WG, 1970. Fatal human cerebral coenurosis. JAMA 213:1461–1464

Holodniy M, Almenoff J, Loutit J, Steinberg GK, 1991. Cerebral sparganosis: case report and review. Rev. Infect. Dis. 13:155–159

Holtzman RN, Hughes JE, Sachdev RK, Jarenwattananon A, 1986. Intramedullary cysticercosis. Surg. Neurol. 26:187–191

Ibechukwu BI, Onwukeme KE, 1991. Intraocular coenurosis: a case report. Br. J. Ophthalmol. 75:426–431

Ijima I, 1905. On a new cestode larva parasitic in man (*Plerocercoides prolifer*). J. College Surg. Imperial Univ. Tokyo 20(Art 7), 21 pp

Ishii I, Ikejiri M, 1959. A case of scrotal tumor caused by the larval form of *Diphyllobothrium mansoni*. Igaku Kenkyu 29:156–159

Iwata S, 1972. Experimental and morphological studies on Manson's tapeworm *Diphyllobothrium erinacei* (Rudolphi). Special reference with its scientific name and relationship with *Spargana proliferum*. In: Morishita K, Komiya Y, Matsubayashi H (eds), *Progress of Medical Parasitology in Japan*, Vol. 4. Tokyo: Meguro Parasitological Museum, pp. 533–590

Jafri HS, Torrico F, Noh JC, Bryan RT, Balderrama F, Pilcher JB, Tsang VC, 1998. Application of the enzyme-linked immunoelectrotransfer blot to filter paper blood spots to estimate seroprevalence of cysticercosis in Bolivia. Am. J. Trop. Med. Hyg. 58:313–315

Johnstone HG, Jones OW Jr, 1950. Cerebral coenurosis in an infant. Am. J. Trop. Med. 30:431–441

Jones DWE, 1962. Ocular sparganosis in an African woman. Br. J. Ophthalmol. 46:123–125

Joyeux C, Houdemer E, Baer JG, 1944. Recherches sur la biologie des *Sparganum* et l'etiologie de la sparganose oculaire. Bull. Soc. Pathol. Exot. 27:70–78

Jung RC, Rodriquez MA, Beaver PC, Schenthal JE, Levy RW, 1981. Racemose cysticercus in human brain. A case report. Am. J. Trop. Med. Hyg. 30:620–624

Kamal MM, Grover SV, 1995. Cytomorphology of subcutaneous cysticercosis: a report of 10 cases. Acta Cytol. 39:809–812

Kaminsky RG, Gatei DG, Zimmermann RR, 1978. Human coenurosis from Kenya. E. Afr. Med. J. 55:355–359

Keane JR, 1984. Death from cysticercosis. West. J. Med. 140:787–789

Khamboonruang C, Premasathian D, Little MD, 1974. A case of intra-abdominal sparganosis in Chiang Mai, Thailand. Am. J. Trop. Med. Hyg. 23:538–539

Kim HW, Kim JH, 1970. A case of sparganosis infesting with stone in human ureter. Korean J. Urol. 11:23–25

Kimura M, Kimura H, Fukuchi T, 1967. A case of sparganosis resembling a breast tumor. Yonago Acta Med. 11:127–129

Kittiponghansa S, Tesana S, Ritch R, 1988. Ocular sparganosis: a cause of subconjunctival tumor and deafness. Trop. Med. Parasitol. 39:247–248

Klinker H, Tintelnot K, Joeres R, Muller J, Gross U, Schmidt Rotte H, Landwehr P, Richter E, 1992. *Taenia-crassiceps*-infektion bei AIDS. Dtsch. Med. Wochenschr. 117:133–138

Kron MA, Guderian R, Guevara A, Hidalgo A, 1991. Abdominal sparganosis in Ecuador: a case report. Am. J. Trop. Med. Hyg. 44:146–150

Kruskal BA, Moths L, Teele DW, 1993. Neurocysticercosis in a child with no history of travel outside the continental United States. Clin. Infect. Dis. 16:290–292

Kung IT, Lee D, Yu HC, 1989. Soft tissue cysticercosis. Diagnosis by fine-needle aspiration. Am. J. Clin. Pathol. 92:834–835

Kunkel JM, Hawksley CA, 1987. Correspondence. Cysticercosis presenting as a solitary dominant breast mass. Hum. Pathol. 18:1190–1191

Kurtycz DF, Alt B, Mack E, 1983. Incidental coenurosis: larval cestode presenting as an axillary mass. Am. J. Clin. Pathol. 80:735–738

LaChance MA, Clark RM, Connor DH, 1983. Proliferating

larval cestodiasis: report of a case. Acta Trop. 40:391–397

Lachberg S, Thompson RC, Lymbery AJ, 1990. A contribution to the etiology of racemose cysticercosis. J. Parasitol. 76:592–594

Landells JW, 1949. Intra-medullary cyst of the spinal cord due to the cestode *Multiceps multiceps* in the *Coenurus* stage. Report of a case. J. Clin. Pathol. 2:60–63

Leelachaikul P, Chuahirun S, 1977. Cysticercosis of the thyroid gland in severe cerebral cysticercosis: report of a case. J. Med. Assoc. Thail. 60:405

Lenczner M, Wollin DG, 1958. Cysticercosis: multiple infarcts and necrosis in bone. Can. Med. Assoc. J. 78:344–345

Liao SW, Lee TS, Shih TP, Ho WL, Chen ER, 1984. Proliferating sparganosis in lumbar spine: a case report. J. Formosan Med. Assoc. 83:603–611

Lin TP, Su IJ, Lu SC, Yang SP, 1978. Pulmonary proliferating sparganosis. A case report. J. Formosan Med. Assoc. 77:467–472

Lo YK, Chao D, Yan SH, Liu HC, Chu FL, Huang CI, Chang T, 1987. Spinal cord proliferative sparganosis in Taiwan: a case report. Neurosurgery 21:235–238

Loo L, Braude A, 1982. Cerebral cysticercosis in San Diego. A report of 23 cases and a review of the literature. Medicine 61:341–359

Lotz J, Hewlett R, Alheit B, Bowen R, 1988. Neurocysticercosis: correlative pathomorphology and MR imaging. Neuroradiology 30:35–41

Lucas SB, Hassounah O, Muller R, Doenhoff MJ, 1980. Abnormal development of *Hymenolepis nana* larvae in immunosuppressed mice. J. Helminthol. 54:75–82

Lucas SB, Hassounah O, Doenhoff M, Muller R, 1979. Aberrant form of *Hymenolepis nana*: possible opportunistic infection in immunosuppressed patients. Lancet 2:1372–1373

Manschot WA, 1976. *Coenurus* infestation of the eye and orbit. Arch. Ophthalmol. 94:961–964

Marquez-Monter H, Aguirre-Garcia J, Biagi FF, 1963. Cisticercosis del miocardio. Informe de cuatro casos con estudio necropsico. Rev. Fac. Med. 5:401–411

Matson DO, Rouah E, Lee RT, Armstrong D, Parke JT, Baker CJ, 1988. *Acanthameba* meningoencephalitis masquerading as neurocysticercosis. Pediatr. Infect. Dis. J. 7:121–124

McCormick GF, Giannotta S, Zee C, Fisher M, Zee CS, 1983. Carotid occlusion in cysticercosis. Neurology 33:1078–1080

Menon TB, Veliath GD, 1940. Tissue reactions to *Cysticercus cellulosae* in man. Trans. R. Soc. Trop. Med. Hyg. 33:537–544

Min HK, Han SH, Yoon SO, Oh CH, 1976a. Intestinal perforation due due to *Sparganum mansoni*. A case of sparganosis. Yonsei Rep. Trop. Med. 7:118

Min HK, Han SH, Yoon SO, Oh CH, 1976b. Intestinal perforation due to infection of *Sparganum mansoni*. Korean J. Parasitol. 14:61–64

Moreira MA, de-Freitas JR, Gerais BB, 1997. Granulomatous mastitis caused by sparganum. A case report. Acta Cytol. 41:859–862

Morishita K, 1972. Rare human tapeworms reported from Japan. In: Morishita K, Komiya Y, Matsubayashi H (eds), *Progress of Medical Parasitology in Japan*, Vol. 4. Tokyo: Meguro Parasitological Museum, pp. 465–488

Moulinier R, Martinez E, Torres JR, Noya O de N, Reyes O, 1982. Human proliferative sparganosis in Venezuela: report of a case. Am. J. Trop. Med. Hyg. 31:358–363

Mueller JF, 1974. The biology of *Spirometra*. J. Parasitol. 60:3–14

Nakamura T, Hara M, Matsuoka M, Tsuji M, 1990. Human proliferative sparganosis. A new Japanese case. Am. J. Clin. Pathol. 94:224–228

Nam JM, Kim BS, 1968. A case of sparganosis in the human epididymis. Korean J. Urol. 9:37–39

Noya OO, Noya BA, Arrechedera H, Torres JR, Arguello C, 1992. *Sparganum proliferum*: an overview of its structure and ultrastructure. Int. J. Parasitol. 22:631–640

Oh SJ, Chi JG, Lee SE, 1993. Eosinophilic cystitis caused by vesical sparganosis: a case report. J. Urol. 149:581–583

Orihel TC, Gonzalez P, Beaver PC, 1970. *Coenurus* from neck of Texas woman. Am. J. Trop. Med. Hyg. 19:255–257

Ortega E, Torres P, 1991. Un caso de infeccion humana por cisticerco racemoso de localizacion parenquimatosa en Valdivia, Chile. Rev. Inst. Med. Trop. Sao Paulo 33:227–231

Park YS, Cho CY, Kim KH, 1964. A case of sparganosis forming giant hematoma in scrotum. Korean J. Urol. 5:121–123

Pau A, Turtas S, Brambilla M, Leoni A, Rosa M, Viale GL, 1987. Computed tomography and magnetic resonance imaging of cerebral coenurosis. Surg. Neurol. 27:548–552

Pittella JE, 1997. Neurocysticercosis. Brain Pathol. 7:681–693

Prosser PR, Wilson CB, Forsham PH, 1978. Intrasellar cysticercosis presenting as a pituitary tumor: successful transsphenoidal cystectomy with preservation of pituitary function. Am. J. Trop. Med. Hyg. 27:976–979

Puppin D Jr, Cavegn BM, Delmaestro D, 1993. Subcutaneous cysticercosis of the tongue mimicking a tumor. Int. J. Dermatol. 32:818–819

Rabiela Cervantes MT, Rivas Hernandez A, Castillo Medina S, Gonzalez Angulo A, 1985. Morphological evidence indicating that *C. cellulosae* and *C. racemosus* are larval stages of *Taenia solium*. Arch. Invest. Med. Mex. 16:81–92

Rabiela Cervantes MT, Rivas Hernandez A, Flisser A, 1989. Morphological types of *Taenia solium* cysticerci. Parasitol. Today 5:357–359

Raina UK, Taneja S, Lamba PA, Bansal RL, 1996. Spontaneous extrusion of extraocular *Cysticercus* cysts. Am. J. Ophthalmol. 121:438–441

Rajshekhar V, Chandy MJ, 1994. Enlarging solitary cysticercus granulomas. J. Neurosurg. 80:840–843

Rangel R, Torres B, Del Brutto OH, Sotelo J, 1987. Cysticercotic encephalitis: a severe form in young females. Am. J. Trop. Med. Hyg. 36:387–392

Rao CM, Sattar SA, Gopal PS, Reddy CCM, Sadasivudu B, 1972. Cysticercosis resembling myopathy. Indian J. Med. 26:841–843

Rey L, Barbosa De Oliveira NR, Faure R, 1969. Bone cysticercosis caused by *Cysticercus racemosus*. Rev. Latinoam. Microbiol. Parasitol. 11:61–67

Richards FO Jr, Schantz PM, 1991. Laboratory diagnosis of cysticercosis. Clin. Lab. Med. 11:1011–1028

Richards FO Jr, Schantz PM, Ruiz Tiben E, Sorvillo FJ, 1985. Cysticercosis in Los Angeles County. JAMA 254:3444–3448

Rocca ED, Neira B, 1980. Cysticercosis of the rachis. Int. Surg. 65:31–35

Rudacki MA, Detoni XA, Teixeira WR, Boer VH, Oliveira GG, 1989. CT features of cellulosae and racemosus neurocysticercosis. J. Comput. Assist. Tomogr. 13:1013–1016

Sanson JG, Bode MJ, 1972. Human sparganosis: report of case in Wisconsin. Wisconsin Med. J. 71:164–166

Santamaria-Fries M, Fajardo L-G LF, Sogin ML, Olson PD, Relman DA, 1996. Lethal infection by a previously unrecognised metazoan parasite. Lancet 347:1797–1801

Sapunar J, Valenzuela H, Aracena M, 1982. Cisticercosis subconjuntival curada espontaneamente. Bol. Chil. Parasitol. 371:21–22

Sarti E, Schantz PM, Plancarte A, Wilson M, Gutierrez IO, Lopez AS, Roberts J, Flisser A, 1992. Prevalence and risk factors for *Taenia solium* taeniasis and cysticercosis in humans and pigs in a village in Morelos, Mexico. Am. J. Trop. Med. Hyg. 46:677–685

Saxena H, Samuel KC, Singh B, 1972. Cysticercosis of the heart. Indian Heart J. 24:313–315

Schenone H, Letonja T, 1974. Cisticercosis porcina y bovina en Latinoamerica. Bol. Chil. Parasitol. 29:90–95

Schenone H, Ramirez R, Rojas A, 1973. Aspectos epidemiologicos de la neurocisticercosis en America Latina. Bol. Chil. Parasitol. 28:61–72

Scholtz L, Mentis H, 1987. Pulmonary cysticercosis. S. Afr. Med. J. 72:573–574

Sen DK, 1980. *Cysticercus cellulosae* in the lacrimal gland, orbit, and eyelid. Acta Ophthalmol. 58:144–147

Sen DK, Muller R, Gupta VP, Chilana JS, 1989. Cestode larva (*Sparganum*) in the anterior chamber of the eye. Trop. Geogr. Med. 41:270–273

Sharma BS, Banerjee AK, Kak VK, 1987. Intramedullary spinal cysticercosis. Case report and review of literature. Clin. Neurol. Neurosurg. 89:111–116

Shea M, Maberley AL, Walters J, Freeman RS, Fallis AM, 1973. Intraocular *Taenia crassiceps* (Cestoda). Trans. Am. Acad. Ophthalmol. Otolaryngol. 77:778–783

Silver SA, Erozan YS, Hruban RH, 1996. Cerebral cysticercosis mimicking malignant glioma: a case report. Acta Cytol. 40:351–357

Slais J, 1970. *The Morphology and Pathogenicity of the Bladder. Cysticercus cellulosae and Cysticercus bovis*. La Hague, The Netherlands: Dr. W. Junk N.

Sorvillo FJ, Waterman SH, Richards FO, Schantz PM, 1992. Cysticercosis surveillance: locally acquired and travel-related infections and detection of intestinal tapeworm carriers in Los Angeles County. Am. J. Trop. Med. Hyg. 47:365–371

Sotelo J, Guerrero V, Rubio F, 1985. Neurocysticercosis: a new classification based on active and inactive forms. A study of 753 cases. Arch. Intern. Med. 145:442–445

Sotelo J, Marin C, 1987. Hydrocephalus secondary to cysticercotic arachnoiditis. A long-term follow-up review of 92 cases. J. Neurosurg. 66:686–689

Stiles CW, 1908. The occurrence of a proliferative cestode larva (*Sparganum proliferum*) in man in Florida. Hyg. Lab. Bull. No 40, pp. 7–18

Subianto DB, Tumada LR, Margono SS, 1978. Burns and epileptic fits associated with cysticercosis in mountain people of Irian Jaya. Trop. Geogr. Med. 30:275–278

Suzuki N, Kamazawa H, Hasogi H, Nakagawa O, Kumazawa H, Hosogi H, Nakagawa O, 1982. A case of human infection with the adult of *Spirometra erinacei*. Jpn. J. Parasitol. 31:23–26

Tami TA, Parker GS, Wong RT, 1987. Laryngeal cysticercosis. Otolaryngol. Head Neck Surg. 96:289–291

Templeton AC, 1968. Human *Coenurus* infection. A report of 14 cases from Uganda. Trans. R. Soc. Trop. Med. Hyg. 62:251–255

Templeton AC, 1971. Anatomical and geographical location of human coenurus infection. Trop. Geogr. Med. 23:105–108

Tsai MD, Chang CN, Ho YS, Wang AD, 1993. Cerebral sparganosis diagnosed and treated with stereotactic techniques. Report of two cases. J. Neurosurg. 78:19–132

Turner M, Leiper RT, 1919. On the occurrence of *Coenurus glomeratus* in man in West Africa. Trans. R. Soc. Trop. Med. Hyg. 13:23–24

Vanderick P, Fain A, Langi S, Balen H von, 1964. Deux nouveaux cas de cenurose humaine a *Taenia brauni* au Rwanda, avec une localisation orbitaire du cenure. Ann. Soc. Belge Med. Trop. 44:1077–1079

Venkataraman S, Vijayan GP, 1983. Uncommon manifestation of human cysticercosis with muscular pseudohypertrophy. Trop. Geogr. Med. 35:75–77

Vinken PJ, Garcia HH, Herrera G, Gilman RH, Tsang VCW, Pilcher JB, Diaz JF, Candy EJ, Miranda E, Naranjo J, Cysticercosis Working Group in Peru, 1994. Discrepancies between cerebral computed tomography and Western blot in the diagnosis of neurocysticercosis. Am. J. Trop. Med. Hyg. 50:152–157

Walts AE, Nivatpumin T, Epstein A, 1995. Distinctive case pulmonary cysticercus. Mod. Pathol. 8:299–302

Webb J, Seidel J, Correll RW, 1986. Multiple nodules on the tongue of a patient with seizures. J. Am. Dent. Assoc. 112:701–702

Welsh NH, Peters AL, Crewe Brown W, Blignaut P, Donnoli P, da Souza BS, Javary Y, 1987. Ocular cysticercosis. A report of 13 cases. S. Afr. Med. J. 71:719–722

Wilber RR, King EB, Howes EL, 1980. Cerebrospinal fluid cytology in five patients with cerebral cysticercosis. Acta Cytol. 24:421–426

Williams PH, Templeton AC, 1971. Infection of the eye by tapeworm Coenurus. Br. J. Ophthalmol. 55:766–769

Yamane Y, Okada N, Takihara M, 1975. On a case of long term migration of *Spirometra erinacei* larva in the breast of a woman. Yonago Acta Med. 19:207–213

Yoshida SO, 1914. On a second and third case of infection with *Plerocercoides prolifer* Ijima, found in Japan. Semin. Respir. Infect. 7:219–225

Zavala-Velazquez J, Bolio-Cicero A, Suarez Hoil G, 1984. Cisticercosis por *Cysticercus racemosus* de localizacion muscular. Patol. Rev. Lat. Am. 22:99–103

Zhong HL, Shao L, Lian DR, Deng ZF, Zhao SX, Gao PZ, He LY, Yung CF, Pan JY, 1983. Ocular sparganosis caused blindness. Chinese Med. J. 96:73–75

27

ECHINOCOCCUS—HYDATID DISEASE

The genus *Echinococcus* has four species—*E. granulosus, E. multilocularis, E. vogeli,* and *E. oligarthrus*—the adult stages of which are parasites in wild and domestic dogs and cats (Thompson, Lymbery, 1995). The larval stages, known as *hydatid cysts,* occur in many species of ungulates, rodents, and other animals, including humans. The infection produced by adult *Echinococcus* organisms in their definitive hosts is *echinococcosis,* and the infection produced by the larvae in animals and humans is *hydatid disease* or *hydatid cyst.* The term *hydatidosis,* as defined by some investigators, is the uncontrolled spread of a hydatid cyst, as in bone or as in secondary hydatidosis. However, these four terms are used interchangeably by most clinicians to refer to the human disease. The morphology and biologic behavior of the hydatid larvae are different for each of the four species of *Echinococcus,* resulting in different pathologic and clinical manifestations.

The classic species of *Echinococcus* in humans, based on morphologic criteria, are *E. granulosus* and *E. multilocularis,* but from the 1960s on, two species indigenous to Central and South America, *E. vogeli* and *E. oligarthrus,* have been recognized. However, it has

become apparent that geographic strains of a given species of *Echinococcus* have a marked genetic heterogeneity, which in some cases explains the differences in the epidemiology and the disease they produce. These differences resulted in much confusion in the past, which led to the description of numerous species (a total of 16 species and 13 subspecies). At present only the four previously mentioned species are accepted, but several *strains,* named either after the animal or after the geographic area where they occur, are recognized and are being intensively studied (Thompson, Lymbery, 1988, 1995). Whether some of these strains will eventually be classified as separate species, based on molecular taxonomic features, is now being decided.

In general, the life cycles of the four species of *Echinococcus* have enough similarities to allow generalizations; however, their geographic distribution, their biology, and the diseases they produce are diverse enough to require separate discussion. The importance of hydatidosis in humans rests on the wide distribution of the parasite, the large number of cases, and the morbidity it produces. In animals, hydatidosis is important because of the economic losses that the infection produces in livestock.

Morphology. The adult *Echinococcus* is less than 4 mm long and lives buried in the crypts of the small intestinal mucosa of its definitive hosts. It has a scolex with four suckers and a rostellum with two rows of hooklets; the size of the hooklets allows discrimination of the four species (Fig. 27–14). Moreover, the size of the hooklets is constant, whether in the larval or the adult stage, a feature that permits speciation of the larval stage. Behind the scolex is the strobila, composed of the neck of the parasite, the area where the proglottids grow and begin differentiation, followed by three proglottids. The anterior proglottid is immature, the middle one is mature, and the terminal one is gravid (Fig. IV–1). Gravid proglottids detach from the body and enter the intestinal contents to release the eggs, which are evacuated with the feces into the environment.

Life Cycle and Biology. The eggs of *Echinococcus* are morphologically similar to those of other taeniids and, like them, have a hexacanth embryo (three pairs of hooks) at the time of evacuation in the feces. Ingestion of eggs by the appropriate intermediate hosts or by humans results in the development of a hydatid larva in the tissues. Ingestion of the hydatid larva by dogs or cats produces the intestinal infection, usually with thousands of worms (Fig. 27–1).

The events following ingestion of an *Echinococcus* egg by the intermediate host or by humans, and the subsequent development of a hydatid cyst, are important to the student of medicine. In the stomach and small intestine the external envelope of the egg disaggregates and frees the *onchosphere* (embryo), which becomes activated (exhibits rhythmic movements) and soon makes contact with the microvilli of the epithelial cells of the intestine. The onchosphere, which measures up to 30 μm, rapidly migrates into the tissues and reaches the lamina propria 30 to 120 minutes after hatching, producing microscopic degeneration of host tissue in its vicinity. Penetration and movement of the onchosphere through the tissues probably occurs with the help of enzymes secreted by the parasite or by mechanical movement with assistance of the onchosphere hooks. Once the onchosphere reaches the lamina propria it finds a vessel and, traveling through the blood or lymphatic circulation, locates in the tissue, where further differentiation and growth occurs.

Experimental studies have shown that ingestion and contact with the gastrointestinal juices are not necessary for hatching and activation of the onchosphere. *Echinococcus granulosus* eggs placed directly in liver tissue, pleural and peritoneal cavities, and lungs of animals hatch and develop into hydatid cysts.

Once the onchosphere reaches an organ, it begins to develop into a hydatid cyst. First, the onchosphere rapidly undergoes a series of changes, beginning with the atrophy of hooks and muscle cells and the formation of a central cavity. In this cavity, the germinal membrane and the laminated layer (see the introduction to Part IV) start developing from divisions of five pairs of primary germinal cells of the onchosphere. The germinal membrane grows and apparently secretes the laminated layer. The smallest cyst with a recognizable central cavity is 40 μm in diameter; it grows to about 250 μm in 3 weeks and to 1 cm in 6 months to 1 year. During its early development (formation of a central cavity), the cyst elicits an inflammatory reaction that determines its fate. If the reaction is too intense, it causes death and degeneration of the cyst; if it occurs in the appropriate amount, it lays the foundation for the fibrous capsule necessary for the support and integrity of the cyst. Thus, the intensity of the inflammatory response to the early stage of a hydatid cyst determines the suitability of the intermediate host.

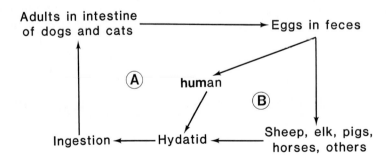

Fig. 27–1. *Echinococcus*, schematic life cycle. (*A*) **The cycle as it occurs among animals. (*B*) Ingestion by humans of eggs evacuated in the feces of dogs and cats, resulting in hydatid disease.**

Growth of the cyst continues at a rate influenced by the type of host, the tissue where the cyst is located, and both the species and the strain of *Echinococcus*. At certain point, cells of the germinal membrane begin proliferating starting as an anlage of cells (Fig. IV–7) that soon forms a protoscolex. The larva is sometimes limited by germinal membrane cells, from which additional protoscolices begin differentiating. This is a *brood capsule*, which often remains attached by a delicate stalk to the germinal membrane (IV–8). Inside the brood capsule protoscolices develop. Afterward, the brood capsule may detach and remain as such in the cyst, or it may break and liberate the protoscolices in the hydatid fluid. The freed protoscolices in the hydatid fluid make up the *hydatid sand*. Often, brood capsules in the cyst cavity continue growing and differentiating and form their own acellular membrane, to become *daughter cysts* (Fig. 27–2 A–D). All protoscolices in the cyst are the infective stages for the natural definitive hosts (dogs and cats). Some cysts never develop protoscolices (sterile cysts); others degenerate and calcify.

The germinal layer of hydatid cysts is formed by a syncytium of several kinds of cells, some of which, the undifferentiated cells, proliferate and differentiate into brood capsules and form protoscolices (Fig. IV–7). In addition, the germinal layer regulates the passage of macromolecules into the cyst. The germinal layer is supported externally by the laminated layer (Fig. IV–7), which probably controls the passage of immunologically active cells into the cyst. The fibrous or adventitial layer forms as a reaction of the host to the cyst (Fig. 27–3 C–D). It is the most external layer of the cyst, and its primary function is to support and maintain the structure of the cyst.

The following discussion covers the different types of hydatid disease separately because their epidemiologic, biologic, morphologic, and pathologic characteristics are very different from each other. *Echinococcus granulosus* produces *unilocular hydatid disease, E. multilocularis* produces *alveolar hydatid disease*, and *E. vogeli* and *E. oligarthrus* are responsible for *polycystic hydatid disease*.

Echinococcus granulosus— Unilocular Hydatid Disease

Unilocular hydatid disease is an important parasitic zoonotic infection with a wide distribution, producing significant morbidity and mortality. In those areas of the world where the disease is endemic, any patient of any age who presents with a mass anywhere in the body is first suspected of having a hydatid cyst. The morbidity produced by *E. granulosus* differs with the strain of the parasite; usually the strains affecting wild animals are less virulent than those occurring in domestic animals. The morphology, life cycle, and biology of *E. granulosus* are as outlined above; other aspects of the parasite and the disease it produces are discussed below.

Geographic Distribution and Epidemiology. *Echinococcus granulosus* is widely distributed in animals throughout the world (Fig. 27–4), and human infections occur in most of these areas. At least two patterns of transmission are recognized. One pattern involves wolves and wild intermediate hosts (deer, elk, and others), mostly in the arctic regions of North America and Eurasia. The other pattern is between domestic dogs and domestic intermediate hosts (sheep, goats, cows, and pigs). The first pattern of transmission, called the *sylvatic cycle*, produces accidental infections in humans, usually of low morbidity (Wilson et al. 1968). The second, or *pastoral cycle*, results in higher endemicity in the human populations at risk, and the infection causes higher morbidity and mortality.

Humans acquire hydatid disease by ingesting eggs passed in the feces of wild and domestic dogs, as do the animals that act as the natural intermediate hosts of the parasite. Intermediate hosts for *E. granulosus* are many domestic and wild animals, such as sheep, goats, cattle, pigs, camels, and horses. These hosts have different abilities to support the development of the cysts, making some of them poor intermediate hosts and others excellent intermediate hosts. For example, in most areas, cattle are poor hosts because the cysts they contain are rarely fertile. Humans are generally considered terminal hosts for the parasite. There are rare exceptions, such as the Turkana tribesmen of Kenya, who have a high incidence of the disease and the custom of not burying their dead (Fig. 27–5). The cysts they harbor are fertile, and dogs and other animals feed on the abandoned dead corpses, perpetuating the cycle in nature (MacPherson, 1983).

The hydatid larva of *E. granulosus* in humans is prevalent in South America, especially Argentina, Uruguay, Paraguay, Chile, southern Brazil, Peru, and Ecuador (Williams et al. 1971). The distribution in Central America is less well known, with the sporadic cases reported (WHO, 1979) probably not being due to *E. granulosus*. In Europe, the infection extends from the Iberian Peninsula to the Balkans, and in some areas (Bulgaria, Corsica, southern France, Italy, Greece, Portugal, Romania, Sicily, Spain, and Yugoslavia) it is

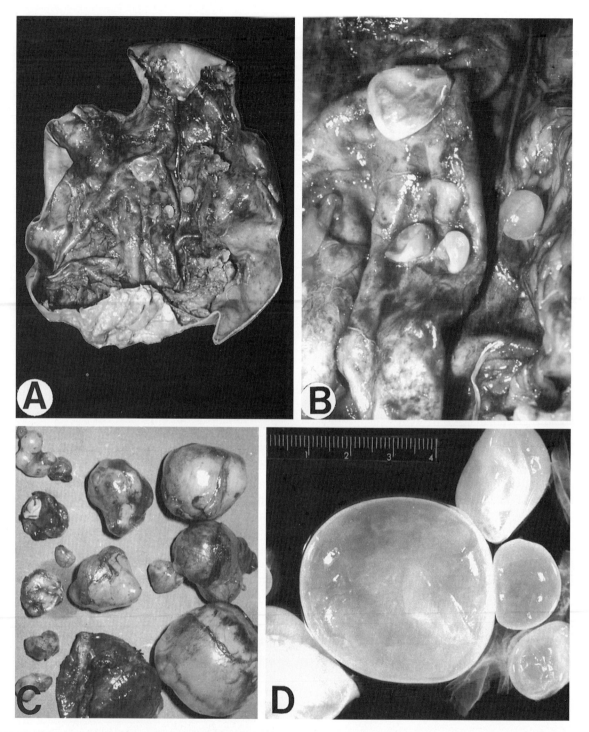

Fig. 27–2. *Echinococcus granulosus* of abdomen, gross morphology. *A,* Opened cyst showing the internal surface with brood capsules attached. *B,* Higher magnification of brood capsules. *C,* Daughter cysts found floating inside the cyst. *D,* Higher magnification of daughter cysts showing the egg white–colored laminated membrane. (Specimen courtesy of A. Gutierrez-Hoyos, M.D., Servicio de Patologia, Hospital Aranzazu, San Sebastian, Universidad del Pais Vasco, Spain.)

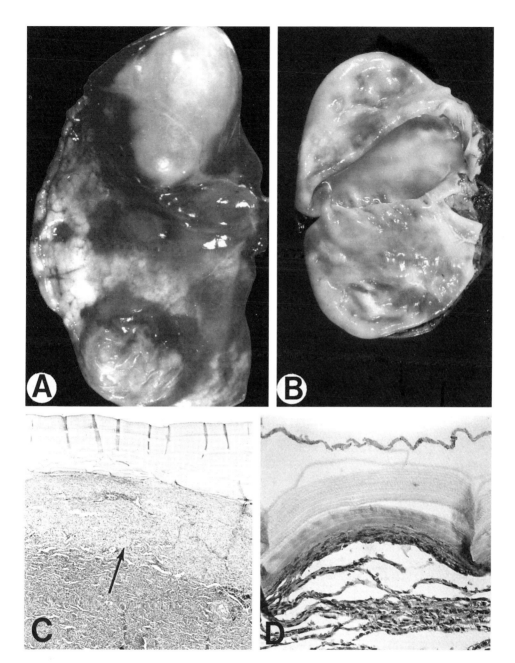

Fig. 27–3. *Echinococcus granulosus* cyst in lung. *A* and *B*, Gross picture of a cyst removed with a portion of lung (*A*); cyst isolated and opened (*B*). Note the laminated membrane. (Courtesy of H. Kim, M.D., Department of Pathology, Yonsei University College of Medicine, Seoul, Korea). *C* and *D*. Two other cases, sections stained with hematoxylin and eosin stain. *C*, Low-power view of a pulmonary cyst showing all the layers, including a thick, fibrous layer (arrow), ×19. *D*, Higher magnification of another pulmonary hydatid cyst, lacking a fibrous wall, removed from a 3-year-old child, ×187. (Courtesy of A. Gutierrez-Hoyos, M.D., Servicio de Patologia, Hospital Aranzazu, San Sebastian, Universidad del Pais Vasco, Spain.)

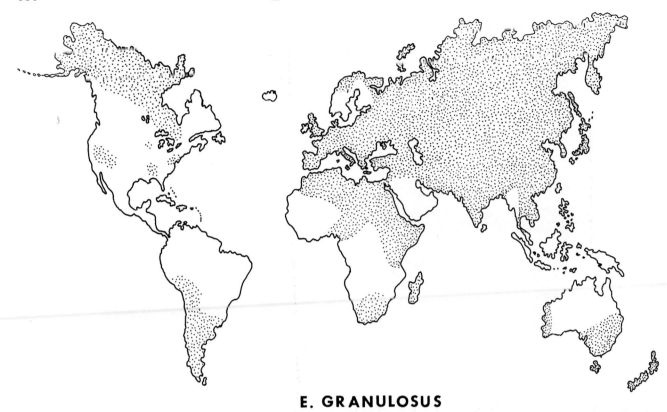

E. GRANULOSUS

Fig. 27–4. *Echinococcus granulosus*, geographic distribution.

hyperendemic. It is also present in southern England. In the Middle East, the infection is found in Turkey, Iraq, Iran, Saudi Arabia, Lebanon, Jordan, Syria, Oman, Israel, and the Islamic countries of the former Soviet Union. In the Asian continent, the infection occurs in Siberia, Afghanistan, Pakistan, Bangladesh, India, Sri Lanka, peninsular Malaya, Indonesia, Thailand, Vietnam, and Japan. In China it occurs mainly in the northeastern provinces (Craig et al. 1991). In Australia, Tasmania, and New Zealand the infection is also endemic. In the African continent, hydatid cyst occurs in Algeria, Morocco, Tunisia, Libya, Egypt, and several countries of eastern and central Africa, as well as in South Africa (Matossian et al. 1977). In at least two island countries, Iceland and Cyprus, the disease has been eradicated by active public health programs, mainly involving the control of dogs, education, and disposal of infected animal carcasses (Polydorou, 1984).

Unilocular hydatid disease occurs in the North American continent, where both types of transmission take place. In Alaska the infection occurs naturally in wild animals, the wolf being the main definitive host and moose, caribou, and reindeer the intermediate hosts; the dog–human cycle is also present to a lesser degree. This sylvatic strain produces an infection in humans characterized by low morbidity; clinically, it is managed conservatively (Wilson et al. 1968). The Canadian strain is also sylvatic but produces a more aggressive disease in humans (Meltzer et al. 1956). In the continental United States, the infection occurs mostly in immigrants from endemic areas; it is also acquired locally, but its frequency has declined to the point where it is now rare. Endemic areas of autochthonous infections in the United States have evolved during the last century. At first, they existed in Virginia, maintained principally by pigs as intermediate hosts and disappearing by 1947. By 1920, autochthonous infections began appearing in the lower Mississippi Valley, also maintained by pigs (Magath, 1954) and apparently disappearing by the early 1960s. A third focus of transmission, maintained by sheep, developed in the 1940s in the western states. At present, populations at risk for contracting unilocular hydatid disease in the United States are Basque-Americans in California, Mormons in central Utah, and Navajo and Zumi Indians in New Mexico (Pappaioanou et al. 1977).

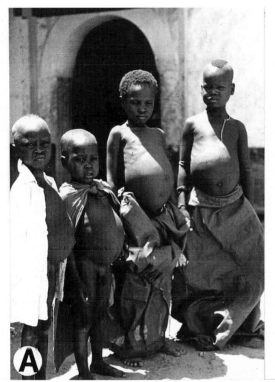

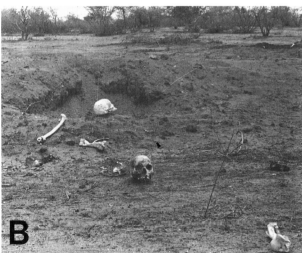

Fig. 27–5. *Echinococcus granulosus*, epidemiology among the Turkana people in Kenya, Africa. *A*, Four Turkana children with large hydatid cysts. *B*, Shallow Turkana grave that has been opened, presumably by dogs, wild carnivores, or both, perpetuating a cycle in which humans are intermediate hosts. (In: McPherson, C.N.L. 1983. An active intermediate host role for man in the life cycle of *Echinococcus granulosus* in Turkana, Kenya. Am. J. Trop. Med. Hyg. 32:397–404. Reproduced with permission.)

The prevalence of hydatid cyst in animal and human populations varies across the endemic areas. In Uruguay, a country of high endemicity, the prevalence of hydatid cysts was 67% in sheep and 60% in cattle in 1987. A serologic survey of the rural population showed a prevalence of over 1% (Bonifacino et al. 1991). A population survey in eastern African countries, using ultrasonography, revealed prevalence rates of up to 6% in Kenya, 3% in southern Sudan, and 2% in southern Ethiopia (MacPherson et al. 1989). A similar survey in Libya demonstrated a 2% prevalence rate (Shambesh et al. 1992).

Immunity. When considering the immunologic aspects of *Echinococcus* in humans, one must focus on the infective onchosphere (the embryo released from the egg in the intestine) that enters the tissues to form the cyst and the mature cyst. The onchospheres of several taeniids studied elicit a strong immunity that makes the host resistant to reinfection. In other words, animals exposed to onchospheres or onchosphere antigens show strong resistance to a challenge with the parasite. The result of this resistance is seen in animals maintained under conditions of heavy transmission, which usually have a single cyst. Humans in endemic areas often have specific antibodies directed against onchospheres, and under in vitro conditions these immune sera are capable of lysing the parasites. Moreover, as described above, the early development of hydatid cysts elicits an inflammatory reaction in the host consisting of eosinophils, polymorphonuclear cells and mononuclear cells.

Once the hydatid cyst develops in the tissues, it does not seem to be affected by the immunologic response of the host. Under normal conditions, established, mature cysts are not in contact with the immunologic system of the host, only those that rupture will have their fluid and protoscolices spilled in the tissues, where immune cells will act on them. About 70% of infected individuals are seropositive to the cysts; the immunoglobulins found in the sera of these individuals are IgG, IgM, and IgE. Why 30% of individuals with mature hydatid cysts do not have circulating antibodies is unknown; two explanations involve antigen-specific tolerance or an excess of antigen that effectively removes circulating antibodies. No studies have been done on the cell composition of the immune response in hydatid disease, but the elevation of circulating antibodies points to a Th2 cell-dominated response. Studies of the cytokine profiles of antigen-stimulated cells from infected individuals show production of interleukin-4 (IL-4), IL-10, and gamma interferon. This finding also supports a Th2 cell-mediated response, probably with Th0 and Th1 cell involvement. Some studies have involved experimental animals infected intraperitoneally with protoscolices, a mechanism that does not occur under natural conditions but does mimic rupture of a cyst. Under these conditions, the majority of protoscolices inoculated into the peritoneal cavity are destroyed by the inflammatory reaction, usually within 2 weeks postinfection. The killing of protoscolices under these experimental conditions is a cellular response. It does not occur if the protoscolices are placed in diffusion chambers that allow free passage of antibodies.

Clinical Findings. As described, the unilocular hydatid cyst develops slowly, requiring several years to reach 5 cm in diameter in most organs. Under special conditions, for example in richly vascularized organs such as the spleen and the lung, growth of the cyst may be rapid. In one case, a cyst in the lung grew up to 7 cm per year (Stermam, Brown, 1958). Hydatid cysts in humans 20 cm in diameter are common. The clinical manifestations of unilocular hydatid disease are therefore those of a slowly growing mass. Cysts in locations that expand easily can attain large sizes without interfering with vital functions. However, small cysts in locations that do not expand can produce significant mechanical compression of vital structures or interfere with function, resulting in early symptoms. Two examples are cysts in the fourth ventricle, producing obstruction of the aqueduct of Sylvius (Gokalp, Erdogan, 1988), and cysts in the eye (*color plate* XVI C).

As stated above, the onchospheres of *E. granulosus* usually enter the venules of the intestinal mucosa and lodge in the liver in about 75% of cases; in about 9% they reach the lung. Still others enter the arterial circulation to reach other organs: muscles 5%, spleen and kidney about 2% each, brain 1.5%, bones 1%, heart less than 1%, and other sites 3.5%.

Liver. Hydatid cysts in the liver occur roughly six times more often in the right lobe than in the left lobe. Often the cyst grows to a large size, making it difficult to determine in which lobe it was first located. Hydatid cysts of the liver usually are asymptomatic. They are diagnosed incidentally on routine x-ray films of the abdomen or when they grow large enough to be noted by the patient or the physician. The symptoms produced by the cyst depend on its exact location in the liver, its extension to adjacent structures, secondary bacterial infection, or other less common complications. Often, only poorly defined hepatic or biliary symptoms are the main complaint in some individuals; these symptoms

sometimes recur for many years. Cysts growing toward the thoracic cavity usually produce symptoms referred to the lower lobe of the right lung, with a chronic dry cough and pain. Cysts growing toward the peritoneal cavity can attain an enormous size and produce epigastric or right abdominal pain. In some individuals, a sensation of fullness, dyspeptic symptoms, and colicky pain may be the main complaints. Others have well-defined biliary colic. Compression of the portal vein may result in portal hypertension of varying degrees. Allergic symptoms, recurrent urticaria, pain, and vomiting are common; sometimes these symptoms are due to rupture of the cyst, which produces leakage of small amounts of fluid. In some previously asymptomatic patients, anaphylactic symptoms and signs may suddenly develop (Mooraki et al. 1996).

The main complications of hepatic hydatid cysts are rupture and secondary bacterial infection. The cysts may rupture into the pleural cavity, the abdominal cavity, the biliary system, or the circulatory system. Rupture to the pleural cavity (Freixinet et al. 1988; Rakower, Milwidsky, 1964) and the peritoneal cavity (Placer et al. 1988) with seeding of protoscolices produces secondary echinococcosis, often a fatal complication. It is estimated that over 3% of hepatic cysts rupture into the peritoneal cavity, producing acute abdominal pain that varies in location and intensity, nausea, vomiting, and peritoneal irritation, sometimes with shock. In some cases, a history of abdominal trauma is elucidated (Placer et al. 1988). In one case, the presentation suggested pelvic carcinomatosis (Mousa et al. 1987).

Rupture of the cyst into the biliary tree results in evacuation of cyst elements in the bile, from which hooklets and fragments of laminated membrane can be recovered. Acute cholecystitis and cholangitis resulted from secondary cyst growth in the cystic duct, producing obstruction after rupture into the gallbladder (Abou et al. 1996). Rupture into the bile ducts and the bronchi occurrred in one patient, with expectoration of bile (Sapunar et al. 1984). This complication can be diagnosed with ultrasography and computed tomography (CT) scans, which demonstrate fragments of the membranes in the bile ducts or communication between the cyst and the bile ducts (Marti-Bonmati et al. 1988). Rupture into the circulatory system is unusual and produces emboli to lungs and other organs, which in one case was fatal (Rakower, Beller, 1961). Secondary bacterial infection of hepatic hydatid cysts presents with symptoms of a liver abscess (Blenkharn et al. 1987). Infection occurs more often in cysts that rupture and communicate with other structures, such as the biliary tree or the thoracic cavity, and that rupture into a bronchus. Blood-borne infection is also possible. The fibrous capsule of the cyst usually keeps the infection contained within the cyst; surrounding tissues are not infected.

The diagnostic modalities of choice for hepatic hydatid disease include CT scans (Fig. 27–6 *A* and *color plate* XV *E*) and magnetic resonance imaging (MRI). These techniques provide the best studies of the size of the cyst, extension to other organs, and the integrity of the cyst.

Thoracic Cavity. Hydatid cysts in the thoracic cavity are located in the pulmonary parenchyma, the mediastinum (Rakower, Milwidsky, 1960), the pleural cavity, or the thoracic wall (Fig. 27–6 *B*). In a series of 20 individuals with thoracic cysts, 16 had cysts in the parenchyma, and 4 had extension of an infected hepatic cyst to the pleura and the right lower lobe of the lung (Novick et al. 1987). Cysts in the lung are often large, measuring more than 10 cm in diameter (Halezeroglu et al. 1997).

Pulmonary hydatid cysts (Fig. 27–3 *A–D*) are more important than cysts in the liver because of the complications they produce. Worldwide, the incidence of pulmonary hydatidosis has been increasing relatively in proportion to the decrease in hepatic cysts (Schenone et al. 1971). Approximately 90% of pulmonary hydatid cysts are solitary; the remainder occur concomitantly with a cyst in the liver (Imari, 1962). Pulmonary hydatid disease is more common in men than in women and occurs between 25 and 40 years of age. About one-third of individuals with pulmonary hydatid cysts are asymptomatic. The rest have chest pain, cough, expectoration, and sometimes severe hemoptysis. Infected cysts usually result in symptoms of chronic infection. Helpful laboratory tests include Cassoni's intradermal test, which is positive in over 85% of cases, and x-ray films. Absolute peripheral eosinophilia of over 400 eosinophils per cubic millimeter is found in one out of every five cases. Serologic tests are usually not helpful (Novick et al. 1987).

If the cyst ruptures, copious coughing with expectoration of cyst elements may follow (Imari, 1962). Ruptured large pulmonary cysts may be acutely fatal if enough fluid fills the respiratory tree (Fig. 27–7 *A–B*). Rupture of smaller cysts produces seeding of protoscolices to distal areas of the respiratory tree, with development of numerous cysts (secondary hydatidosis), a condition that is usually fatal. Cysts that rupture into the pleural cavity result in pleuritic pain, friction rub, and shortness of breath. Often the manifestations of pulmonary hydatid cysts are allergic symptoms such as urticaria, itching, and asthma. The diagnosis of pulmonary hydatid disease is usually based on the clinical presentation, x-ray films, and CT or MRI scans.

Heart. Cysts in the heart are asymptomatic in about 22% of cases, but in some persons, they may produce sudden death (Buris et al. 1987). The symptoms are usually precordial pain in 43% of cases, followed by dyspnea in 22%, fever in 13%, severe abdominal pain in 12%, and palpitations and congestive heart failure in 11% (Heyat et al. 1971). X-ray films of the heart and other imaging techniques are the best modalities

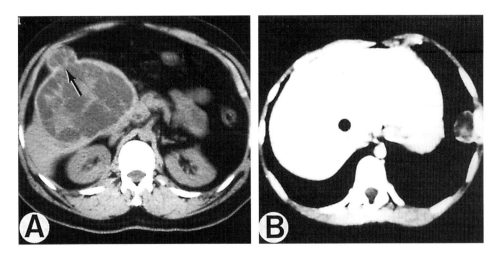

Fig. 27–6. *Echinococcus granulosus*, CT scan films. *A*, Hydatid cyst of the liver containing daughter cysts and an outpouching (arrow). *B*, Hydatid cyst of the thoracic wall (arrow).

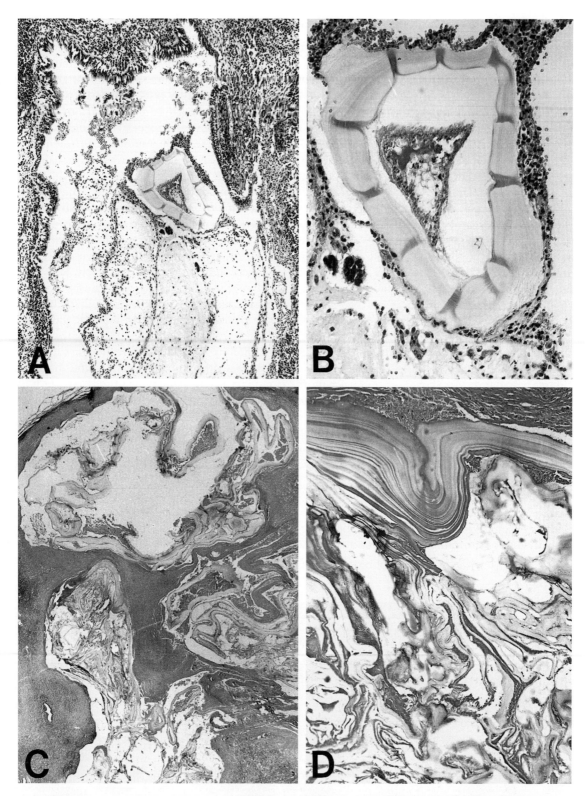

Fig. 27–7. *Echinococcus granulosus* in lung, sections stained with hematoxylin and eosin stain. *A*, Low-power view of a bronchus containing a small hydatid cyst with laminated and germinal membrane, in a person with a ruptured cyst and disseminated secondary echinococcosis, ×55. *B*, Higher magnification showing the laminated membrane and the inflammatory reaction, ×180. *C*, Low-power view of a pulmonary hydatid cyst from a person with several cysts. This cyst is dead and shows collapse and disorganization of the central cavity, with fragmentation of the laminated membrane, ×9. *D*, Higher magnification illustrating the fragmentation of the laminated membrane, simulating an *E. multilocularis* cyst. However, in one area, the laminated membrane is still intact and shows its normal thickness (top), ×70. (Preparation courtesy of K. Jiraki, M.D., American University Hospital, Beirut, Lebanon.)

for diagnosis (Alfonso et al. 1987). They often show excentric enlargement of the heart (Papo, Savic, 1962) or bulging of the wall. Cardiac hydatid cysts are usually located in the wall of the left ventricle, growing intramurally or extending to the subendocardium or the epicardium. Development of a myocardial hydatid cyst is restricted by the density of the cardiac muscle and results in morphologic variants of the cyst, often with multiple chambers (Canabal et al. 1955). Rupture of cardiac cysts into the pericardium produces pericarditis and seeding with protoscolices, as well as rupture into the chambers of the heart and embolism to either the lung (Buris et al. 1987) or the general circulation, with a fatal outcome (Keil et al. 1997). A degenerated, calcified hydatid cyst in the myocardium probably produces more harm than an alive, slow-growing cyst.

Central Nervous System. The occurrence of hydatid cysts in the central nervous system varies in different series, but it is uniformly low. In one series of 17 cases, the cyst was located in the brain, in 10, in the ventri-

cles in 4, in an extradural location in 2, and in an infratentorial area in 1 (Kaya et al. 1975). It presents in adults with focal neurologic signs such as hemiparesis, hemianopsia, speech disorders, and seizures. In children, who often are more commonly affected, the symptoms and signs are those of intracranial pressure (Karak et al. 1992), and the cysts may attain a large size, especially in infants. In one adult patient, a large cyst in the frontal area produced headaches, amenorrhea, galactorrhea, secondary sterility, and weight gain (Tiberin et al. 1984). X-ray films, CT scans, and MRI scans are the best methods for diagnosis. Laboratory tests are usually not helpful.

Other Sites. Hydatid cysts can occur in any tissue or organ; in the skeletal muscles, they produce symptoms of a slowly growing mass (Fig. 27–8 *B*). Those in the spleen (Fig. 27–8 *A*) and pancreas (*color plate* XVI *B*) may be silent for many years. In the spleen, the cysts may attain a large size (Gandhi, Bain, 1962) and often are asymptomatic (*color plate* XV *F*). When symptoms

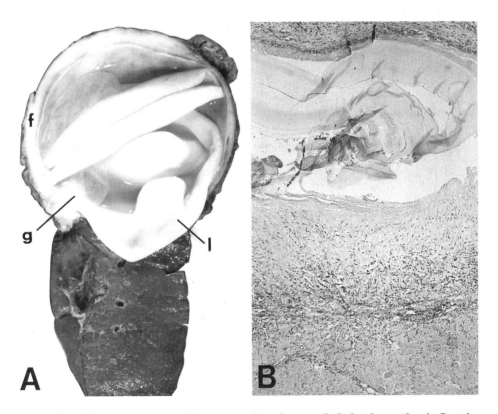

Fig. 27–8. *Echinococcus granulosus* **cysts in spleen and skeletal muscle.** *A,* **Cyst in the spleen showing the different layers: fibrous (f), laminated (l), and germinal (g).** *B,* **Cyst in skeletal muscle, section stained with hematoxylin and eosin stain, showing the fibrous layer and the scant inflammatory reaction, ×47. (Gross specimen and preparation courtesy of A. Gutierrez-Hoyos, M.D., Servicio de Patologia, Hospital Aranzazu, San Sebastian, Universidad del Pais Vasco, Spain.)**

occur, the main manifestation is that of a painful mass in the left upper abdominal quadrant (Uriarte et al. 1991). Cysts in the kidneys may also be silent or may produce nonspecific symptoms and are always difficult to diagnose (*color plate* XV *H*; Angulo et al. 1997). The most common symptoms are a palpable abdominal mass, flank pain, gross hematuria, and albuminuria (Angulo et al. 1997). In the eye, cysts produce symptoms early in their development (*color plate* XVI *C*). In bone, a hydatid cyst grows in a disorganized manner because no adventitial fibrous layer is formed. On x-ray films, the cyst appears as multiple small cavities (Fig. 27–9); clinically, it often presents as a spontaneous fracture (Rollinson, Geytenbeek, 1987). One cyst in the pelvic peritoneum created a fistula to the rectum, and the cyst membranes were passed through the anus; the recovered membranes corresponded to a cyst 8 cm in diameter (Apt et al. 1969). Cysts may occur in the sub-

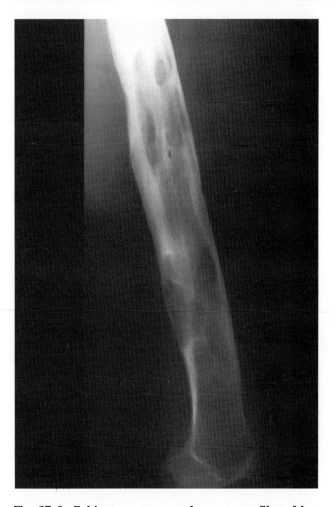

Fig. 27–9. *Echinococcus granulosus*, **x-ray film of hydatid cyst of bone. Note the multiple cystic lesions characteristic of bone hydatidosis.**

cutaneous tissues (Ishii et al. 1986) and sometimes rupture spontaneously to the outside, with evacuation of their contents (Calderon, 1959). In the skeletal muscles, hydatid cysts are easily diagnosed with imaging techniques (Carpintero et al. 1997; Casero et al 1996) A cyst with a maximum diameter of 7 cm was excised from the pterygopalatine-infratemporal fossa of a 23-year-old woman (Gangopadhyay et al. 1996).

Pathology. The cyst of *E. granulosus* is typically unilocular, spherical, or subspherical and is filled with clear fluid. It often consists of a single chamber (unilocular) that grows by expansion or by concentric enlargement. In some cases, pouching of the cyst produces secondary chambers, which may communicate with the central cavity or may be separated by incomplete septae (Fig. 27–3 *A*). In other cases, several cysts growing in close proximity may coalesce to form a cluster of cysts. In spite of its multilocular appearance in all of these cases, the cyst is still a unilocular cyst produced by *E. granulosus*. The anatomic changes produced by unilocular hydatid cysts depend on the organ involved, the size of the cyst, and whether it is intact or ruptured.

The gross appearance of hydatid cysts is characteristic, and on examination of the anatomic specimen their diagnosis is relatively easy (Figs. 27–2 and 27–3 *A–B*). Viable cysts characteristically have two layers and a fibrous or adventitial layer outside of the cyst; the thickness of the fibrous layer varies, depending on the size of the cyst and the organ in which it is located (Fig. 27–8 *A*). The acellular or laminated membrane is easily recognized by its ivory white color; it is friable and is easy to separate from the fibrous capsule (Figs. 27–3 *B* and 27–8 *A*). Finally, the germinal membrane is semitransparent and delicate, with a clear white-yellowish color. It has numerous brood capsules attached to the internal surface and can be separated easily from the laminated layer (Fig. 27–8 *A*). In larger cysts, daughter cysts may be present in the clear hydatid fluid (Fig. 27–2 *C–D*). If the fluid is collected, a granular sediment, the hydatid sand, deposits rapidly at the bottom of the container. This sediment is composed of protoscolices, brood capsules, and hooklets, all recognized on microscopic examination (Fig. 27–10 *A–B*).

In general, the inflammatory tissue reaction to viable, nonruptured hydatid cysts is minimal, with only scant mononuclear cell infiltration in the area where the affected organ is close to the cyst (Fig. 27–3 *C*). Degenerating and calcified cysts have a similar or sometimes a more intense infiltrate if the cyst is intact. Seepage of fluid and cyst contents or secondary bacterial infection of the cyst results in a marked inflammatory

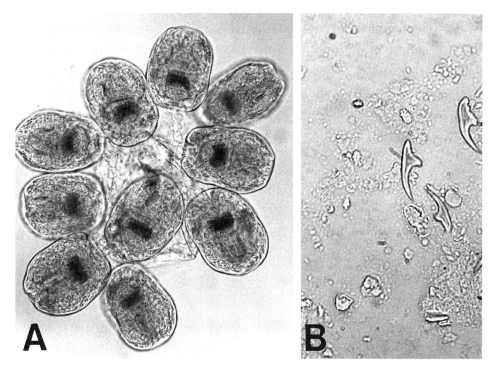

Fig. 27–10. *Echinococcus granulosus*, **hydatid sand, unstained.** *A*, **Medium-power magnification showing a collapsed brood capsule with 10 protoscolices still attached to the capsule,** ×180. *B*, **Squash preparation to isolate and study the hooklets,** ×705.

reaction with polymorphonuclear cells, mostly eosinophils, and a granulomatous inflammation with histiocytes, giant cells, and fibrous tissue around parasitic fragments. If viable protoscolices drain into the surrounding tissues or to distant tissues, they begin differentiating rapidly into new cysts. In these cases the infection is infiltrative, producing marked inflammation with numerous lymphocytes, plasma cells, and eosinophils.

Diagnosis. The diagnosis of hydatid cysts is often made on clinical grounds, based on the presentation of the disease and the history of exposure to the infection. Plain x-ray films, other imaging techniques, and ultrasound are the best methods of demonstrating the cyst, its exact location, its size, the presence or absence of calcification, and its relationship or drainage to other organs or structures. In a study of 273 patients, the radiologic diagnosis was false positive in 11% (Babra et al. 1994). Commonly used serologic tests are the latex agglutination test, counterimmunoelectrophoresis, and the enzyme-linked immunosorbent assay, with either whole hydatid fluid as antigen or with a thermolabile lipoprotein (antigen 5). Of these tests, which were compared in one study, the enzyme-linked immunosorbent assay was best, with about 85% positivity (Babra et al. 1994). Detection of hydatid antigen in the urine, using countercurrent immunoelectrophoresis, was done in about one-half of infected patients (Parija et al. 1997).

The histologic diagnosis is the best method, usually done on material obtained during surgery or at autopsy. Hydatid cysts removed during surgery usually consist of fragments mixed with the cyst fluid; the cyst is rarely intact. All tissues should be examined grossly for the presence of laminated membrane and daughter cysts. The specimens submitted for histologic diagnosis are necessary for assessment of the cyst's viability. During removal of a hydatid cyst, the surgeon usually instills hypertonic saline solution or formalin to sterilize the cyst (kill the protoscolices); often the surgeon requires feedback on the effectiveness of the sterilization technique. Dead cysts are necrotic, and their contents are often semisolid (Fig. 27–7 *C–D*). Calcified cysts are also dead and are removed only if infected secondarily (Fig. 27–11 *A* and *D*). They are received by the pathologist intact or in fragments. Fragments usually do not reveal the nature of the specimen on gross examination; multiple histologic sections of cyst contents are required for proper identification. Partially

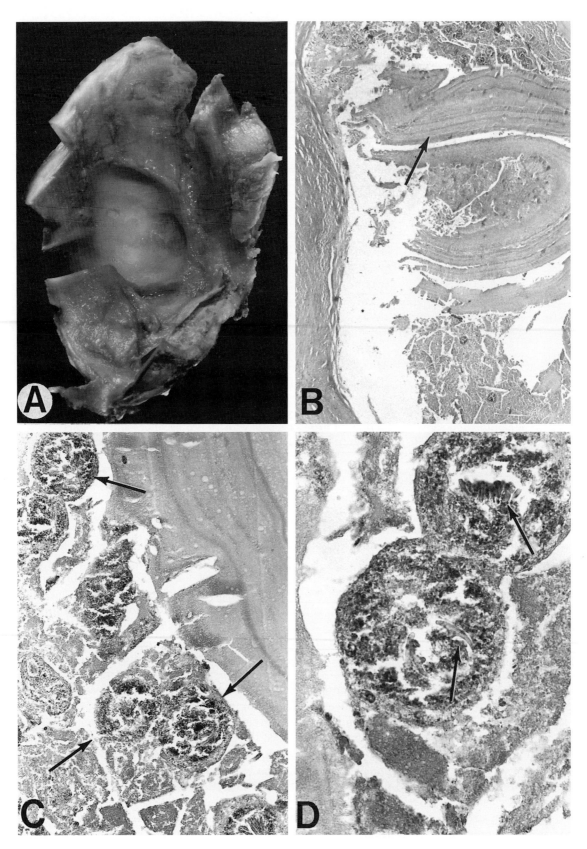

Fig. 27–11. *Echinococcus granulosus* of liver, calcified. A, Calcified wall of the cyst. B–D. Sections stained with hematoxylin and eosin stain. B, Low-power view of the cyst wall shows degenerated remnants of the cyst. Note the granular and swollen fragment of the laminated membrane (arrow), ×28. C, Higher magnification showing calcified protoscolices (arrows) and part of the laminated membrane, ×180. D, Higher magnification illustrating the calcified protoscolices with intact hooklets (arrows), ×450.

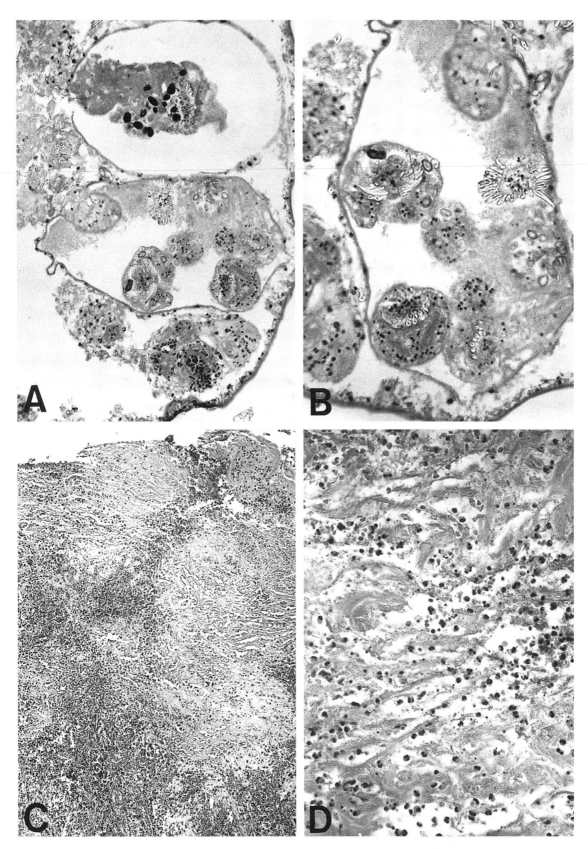

Fig. 27–12. *Echinococcus granulosus*, example of a recently dead cyst, section stained with hematoxylin and eosin stain. *A*, Medium-power view of the cyst with three dead brood capsules still recognizable as such, ×280. *B*, Higher magnification of one brood capsule showing dead protoscolices, most with their crown of hooklets, seen as highly refractile structures, ×450. *C*, Low-power view of the wall of the cysts (host) showing the inflammatory reaction, ×70. *D*, Higher magnification showing the infiltrating polymorphonuclear cells and necrotic tissue, ×270.

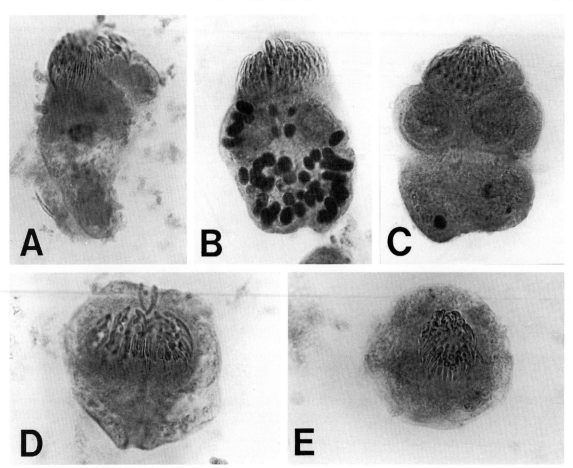

Fig. 27–13. *Echinococcus granulosus*, in a smear from a fine needle aspirate, stained with Papanicolaou stain. *A–E*, Different appearances of protoscolices due to artifact produced while making the smear. Note that the protoscolices in *D* and *E* are perpendicular to the slide. The constant feature is the presence of the scolex with the hooklets. Some protoscolices have calcareous corpuscles (dark bodies in *B*), all ×450. (Courtesy of C. Nunez, M.D., Department of Pathology, The Cleveland Clinic Foundation, Cleveland, Ohio.)

calcified cysts often have viable protoscolices in some areas because the cyst dies slowly and piecemeal.

Viable cysts have the characteristic three layers, and all the cellular elements appear to be well preserved, as judged by their staining characteristics (Fig. 29–7 *A–B*). The laminated membrane is positive with periodic acid–Schiff stain, a feature that is a histologic marker of hydatid cysts (Fig. 27–16 *D*). The laminated membrane of the *E. granulosus* cyst is approximately 10 times as thick as the germinal membrane (Figs. IV–7 *A–B* and 27–7 *C–D*). The protoscolices have hooklets, which appear in some histologic sections. They are of taxonomic value if studied on smears consisting of squashed protoscolices to free the hooklets and take accurate measurements (Fig. 27–10 *B*).

On histologic sections of degenerated cysts, the acellular membrane appears granular, and sometimes edematous and swollen; it stains amphophilic with hematoxylin and eosin stain (Fig. 27–11 *B–C*) and is positive with periodic acid–Schiff stain. Moreover, if the cyst is fragmented by the inflammatory reaction, fragments of acellular membrane can be demonstrated in the interstitium or phagocytized by macrophages and giant cells in preparations stained with periodic acid–Schiff stain. The protoscolices may be degenerated, but the hooklets remain intact for a long time (Figs. 27–11 *D* and 27–12 *A–D*). When parasitic elements are not recognized in histologic sections, examination of fresh or stained sediments from the formalin in which the specimen was received may reveal hooklets, protoscolices, or fragments of laminated membrane. One diagnostic modality for *Echinococcus* cysts studied by the anatomic pathologist is fine needle aspiration of smears stained with Papanicolaou stain.

Cysts located anywhere in the body are aspirated for diagnostic purposes, often without the suspicion of their being an *Echinococcus* cyst. The typical finding is protoscolices in a stage of preservation representative of the cyst. These protoscolices are often distorted and damaged, which occurs during preparation of the smears. The main characteristic is the presence of protoscolices, with their rostellum containing hooks (Fig. 27–13 *A–E*), or free hooklets somewhere in the smear. Study of the hooklets and careful measurement of a good number of them are required if the species of *Echinococcus* in the histologic sections is not evident. The size and shape of the hooklets alone permit identification of the species of *Echinococcus* in clinical material (Fig. 27–14)

Echinococcus multilocularis— Alveolar Hydatid Disease

Far fewer individuals are infected with *E. multilocularis* than with *E. granulosus*. However, the disease caused by *E. multilocularis* is important because of the greater morbidity and mortality it produces. This zoonosis is restricted mostly to the arctic and temperate regions of the world, where it usually occurs in wild animals. The morphologic and biologic characteristics of *E. multilocularis* are generally similar to those of other member of the genus discussed above. The adult *E. multilocularis* superficially resembles the adult *E. granulosus* in size and shape; microscopically, however, sufficient morphologic differences exist to allow their distinction. The life cycle of *E. multilocularis* differs from that of *E. granulosis* in that its definitive hosts are arctic foxes and its intermediate hosts are mostly small rodents, in which the cyst develops in about 2 months. This is an adaptation of the parasite to the shorter life span of the intermediate hosts. However, development of *E. multilocularis* cysts in humans is slow, and infections acquired in childhood manifest many years later.

Geographic Distribution and Epidemiology. In many places, the endemic area for *E. multilocularis* in the

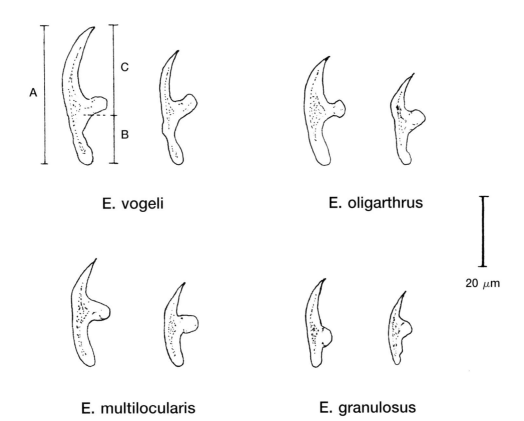

E. vogeli

E. oligarthrus

20 μm

E. multilocularis

E. granulosus

Fig. 27–14. Drawing at scale of the hooklets of the four species of *Echinococcus. A,* Total length of hooklet. *B,* Length of the handle. *C,* Length of the blade.

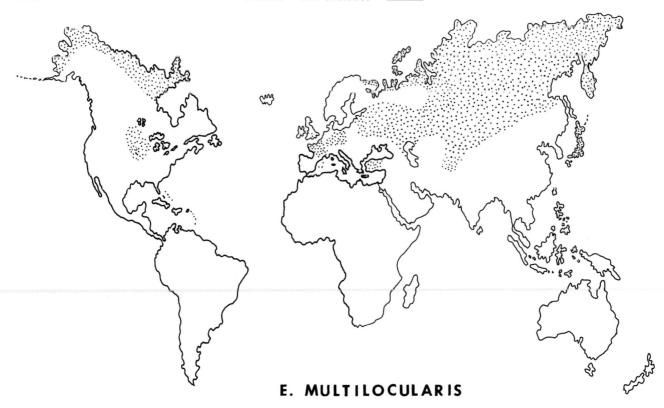

E. MULTILOCULARIS

Fig. 27–15. *Echinococcus multilocularis*, **geographic distribution.**

Northern Hemisphere overlaps that of *E. granulosus* (Fig. 27–15; Eckert, 1996). In Europe it occurs in southern Germany, eastern France, and parts of Switzerland and Austria. In Russia, *E. multilocularis* is widely distributed in the tundra, extending south to Turkey, northern Iran, northern India, and some parts of Japan. In China, its distribution occupies an area in the northern part of the country larger than that of *E. granulosus* (Craig et al. 1991). Sporadic cases reported in Italy, northern Africa, India, New Zealand, Uruguay, and Argentina are doubtful. In the American continent, *E. multilocularis* is found in Alaska and most of central Canada, extending from the Arctic to North Dakota in the United States, where it was first described (Leiby, Olsen, 1964). Later, *E. multilocularis* was found in the seven states adjacent to North Dakota (Leiby et al. 1970), as well as in Nebraska and Illinois (Ballard, Vande Vusse, 1983). More recently, the parasite was found in Indiana and Ohio (Storandt, Kazacos, 1993). This is an indication that peripheral spread from North Dakota is taking place on the American continent (Ballard, Vande Vusse, 1983). In Alaska numerous human infections have been reported (Wilson, Rausch, 1980), and at least one case is known in the continental United States (Gamble et al. 1979).

The definitive hosts of *E. multilocularis* are arctic foxes of the genera *Vulpis* and *Alopex*, which evacuate the worm eggs in their feces. These eggs are morphologically indistinguishable from other taeniid eggs, but they are resistant to cold temperatures and freezing. As stated, the natural intermediate hosts of *E. multilocularis* are rodents, the most common one being the northern vole (*Microtus oeconomus*); other mice, shrews, squirrels, and hamsters are also good hosts. Under experimental conditions, deer mice acquired the infection after being fed ground beetles previously exposed to fresh feces from infected foxes (Kriteky, Leiby, 1978). Moreover, in certain areas of France (Petavy et al. 1990, 1991), Central Europe, and North America, dogs and cats maintain a domestic life cycle (Leibby, Kritsky, 1972), facilitating human contact with the parasite. The infection in humans is accidental. It is thought to occur by the ingestion of wild berries contaminated with the eggs of the parasite, but other foods or water may carry the infection as well. Once the hexacanth embryo is free in the intestine, it enters the intestinal wall and travels to the liver, where it develops.

Estimates of the prevalence of alveolar hydatid disease are few. A seroepidemiologic survey of about 8000 people in eastern France showed 8 cases, or 1 per 1000

(Bresson-Hadni et al. 1994). Other estimates of prevalence based on the number of patients seeking medical help in some areas of Germany were about 3.1 cases per 100,000 and, in Switzerland, less than 1 per 100,000 (Lucius, Bilger, 1995). Until 1984, the known number of cases in France since 1930 was estimated to be 200 (WHO, 1984).

Clinical Findings. The clinical manifestations of *E. multilocularis* cyst or alveolar hydatid disease are similar to those of a slow-growing malignant tumor in the liver. The growth of the parasite is infiltrative, destroying the liver parenchyma, bile ducts, and blood vessels, resulting in symptoms of biliary obstruction and portal hypertension. Necrosis of the central portion of the cyst with abscess formation occurs in most cases. Emaciation, ascites, and esophageal varices may develop in the terminal stages of the disease, which consists of irreversible liver failure. Growth of the germinal membrane into blood vessels produces metastasis to almost any organ, but most commonly in the lungs and brain; eosinophilia may be present. The disease may first manifest as an extrahepatic syndrome produced by a metastasis. In one patient, the first manifestation of the infection took the form of cutaneous and subcutaneous nodules in the abdominal skin (Bresson-Hadni et al. 1996). In another patient, the first manifestation was involvement of the seventh dorsal vertebral body, with cord compression (Gaucher et al. 1983). The infiltrative nature of the disease often precludes resection of the tumor even in some asymptomatic cases (Stehr-Green et al. 1988). The mortality due to the infection is high; in Alaska, of the first 33 patients diagnosed with the disease, 67% died (Wilson, Rausch, 1980). In Europe, especially in Germany and Switzerland, the mortality was even higher; however, new imaging diagnostic modalities, awareness of the disease, and new surgical techniques have reduced the mortality considerably (Gottstein, 1992).

The clinical diagnosis is difficult, and the condition is often mistaken for a carcinoma. X-ray films and other imaging techniques reveal the lesion, usually with areas of calcification that often have a characteristic alveolar pattern consisting of small calcified rings 0.5 cm in diameter. Other imaging techniques, such as ultrasonography and CT, show a solid mass, often with a central area of necrosis. CT scans are also useful in follow-up studies of patients under treatment; MRI is also useful, especially in detecting extrahepatic metastasis. Serologic tests, mostly the enzyme-linked immunosorbent assay (ELISA) using *E. multilocularis* antigens, appear to give excellent results and differen-

tiate this species from *E. granulosus* (Gottstein et al. 1983). The original ELISA test has been refined by the use of specific fractions of the parasite as the antigen (Em2 fraction), which gives better results (Gottstein, 1992; Gottstein et al. 1989). Another modification of the ELISA, using another parasite epitope (Em18), appears useful in distinguishing active from inactive disease (Ito et al. 1995). Other serologic techniques are also available, such as indirect hemagglutination and the double diffusion test, but they are inferior to the ELISA with Em2 antigen (Lanier et al. 1987). A polymerase chain reaction probe for detecting parasite DNA in fine needle aspiration biopsy specimens and other samples is also in use (Gottstein, 1992).

Alveolar hydatid disease was once regarded as an invariably deadly infection, with most deaths occurring within 1 year of diagnosis (Mossiman, 1980). As stated above, surgical techniques such as liver transplantation are being used as treatment modalities (Gillet et al. 1988). Long-term follow-up of the success of liver transplantation is lacking, but one individual was well and disease free 6 years later (Mboti et al. 1996). Another important biologic aspect of the infection, recently discovered, is the spontaneous death of the cyst (mostly during the early stages of development) in persons with an asymptomatic infection in Alaska (Rausch et al. 1987). A similar finding was reported later from France (Bresson-Hadni et al. 1994). These asymptomatic individuals, diagnosed serologically, were studied to ascertain the viability of the cysts. Portions of surgically resected cysts inoculated into animals did not grow into cysts, confirming that the cysts were dead. In these patients the lesion was usually less than 2 cm in diameter; one lesion was 9.5 cm in one dimension. The World Health Organization (WHO, 1996) summarized the guidelines for treatment of alveolar hydatid disease, which results in 90% mortality if untreated. Radical surgery is recommended for all operable patients, followed by chemotherapy for at least 2 years; those with nonradical liver resection or with liver transplants should have chemotherapy for life. Recently, a large alveolar cyst described in a 6-year-old girl with acquired immune deficiency syndrome (AIDS), was diagnosed with fine needle aspiration (Sailer et al. 1997).

Pathology. The pattern of growth and development of alveolar echinococcosis in humans is different from that in their natural intermediate hosts (see the introduction to Part IV; Fig. IV–8 *A–B*). Structurally, these cysts are more complex (multivesicular), with infiltrative rather than expansive growth. The cyst in humans does not lead to the formation of a limiting fibrous layer (adventitial layer) or a host-tissue barrier but rather to an intense desmoplastic reaction. In this mass of fibrous tissue, the germinal and laminated membranes appear disorganized and distorted among focal calcification The normal pattern of multiple small cysts seen in the natural intermediate hosts does not develop in humans. The germinal cells infiltrate surrounding tissues, forming small exogenous and endogenous vesicles enmeshed in the dense connective tissue (Fig. 27–16). If the germinal cells enter blood or lymphatic vessels, metastatic growth occurs in distant organs. The cyst does not contain fluid but rather a semisolid (gelatinous) matrix.

As stated, the liver is the primary site for development of *E. multilocularis* (Fig. 27–17 A–D). The right lobe is involved in 28% of cases, the left lobe in 9%, and both lobes in 63%. Extension to contiguous structures occurs in 16% of cases, and metastatic lesions develop in 19%. Metastases to the brain are found in 13% of cases, to the lungs in 9% (Fig. 27–18 A–D), and to the mediastinum in 3%. In one patient, supraumbilical skin nodules developed (Bresson-Hadni et al. 1996). The gross lesion does not appear cystic but rather a hard, infiltrative mass resembling a malignant tumor (Fig. 27–18 A). The lesion is gray-whitish in color and is usually single, but several identical lesions may be present in the liver, mimicking metastatic disease. The central portion of the tumor is often cavitated because of necrosis, and sometimes it is filled with thick fluid or with pus-like material. The most characteristic part of the lesion is at the edge, close to the normal tissue, where there are 2 to 3 mm "microcysts" filled with clear fluid.

Microscopically, the lesion is composed of abundant collagenous tissue with foci of calcification throughout (Fig. 27–17 A–B). Among the collagen are spaces of different shapes, some containing laminated and germinal membranes growing in disarray (Fig. 27–17 C–D). Protoscolices and hooklets usually are not seen. However, if fragments of these apparently sterile cysts are inoculated into the peritoneal cavity of a natural intermediate host, the fragments will develop into normal viable alveolar cysts (Rausch et al. 1987). The tissue surrounding the cyst has a marked granulomatous inflammatory reaction, with abundant infiltration by polymorphonuclear cells (eosinophils), lymphocytes, histiocytes, and multinucleated giant cells (Fig. 27–21). The lesion has abundant granulation tissue, and cyst elements are not readily recognized on hematoxylin and eosin stains (Fig. 27–19 B–C). However, a periodic acid–Schiff stain usually reveals numerous fragments of laminated membrane (Figs. 27–18 D and 27–19 D). Metastatic lesions to lung (Fig. 27–18) and brain (Fig. 27–19 A–D) have identical gross and histologic characteristics. In at least one instance, the eye was involved by a metastasis (Figs. 27–20 A–B and 27–21 A–B; Williams et al. 1987).

Diagnosis. The clinical diagnosis of alveolar hydatid disease is difficult, often impossible. A suspicion of the disease may arise when the physician examines persons with chronic liver disease from endemic areas and with high-risk factors. In the Alaskan patients, these risk factors consisted of owning and living near dogs all of their lives and inhabiting houses built directly on the tundra rather than on a permanent foundation (Stehr-Green et al. 1988).

Serologic tests, such as the ELISA (Gottstein et al. 1985; Rausch et al. 1987) and others, appear to give good results. Biopsy and fine needle aspiration specimens (Ciftcioglu et al. 1997) or autopsy material requires careful examination because the cyst has sometimes been confused with a neoplastic lesion. The histologic pattern of the lesion is as described above; the presence of laminated membrane is easily demonstrated with a periodic acid–Schiff stain, and microscopic calcification is abundant. The protoscolices are rarely seen, but strands of

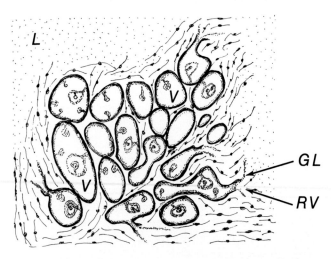

Fig. 27–16. *Echinococcus multilocularis,* **schematic representation of a larva growing abnormally in humans. The vesicles (V) grow a few protoscolices, which usually die. Some vesicles rupture (RV) and the germinal layer (GL) infiltrates the surrounding tissue, forming other vesicles. Parts of the germinal layer enter blood vessels to produce distant metastases. (Redrawn from: Thompson, R.C.A. 1995. Biology and systematics of** *Echinococcus.* **In: R.C.A. Thompson and A.J. Lymbery (eds.).** *The Biology of Echinococcus and Hydatid Disease.* **London: CAB Institute. Reproduced with permission.)**

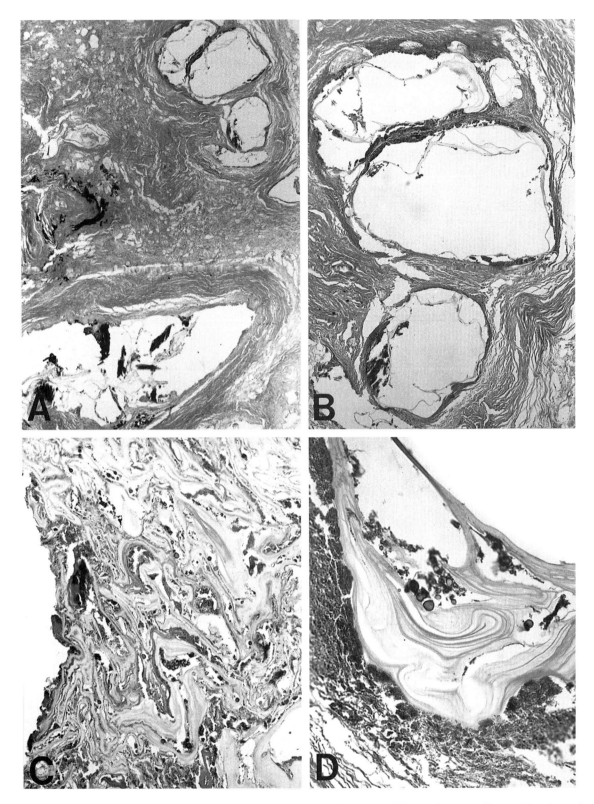

Fig. 27–17. *Echinococcus multilocularis* in liver, section stained with hematoxylin and eosin stain. *A*, Low-power view of the cyst illustrating a few vesicles enmeshed in a dense fibrous connective tissue. Note the areas of calcification (dark), ×11. *B*, Slightly higher magnification showing three vesicles lined with a thin, broken laminated layer, ×22. *C*, Medium magnification of another area illustrating a collapsed laminated membrane forming many disorganized layers among areas of calcium deposition, ×70. *D*, Higher magnification showing the convoluted laminated membrane with calcium and an apparent lack of the germinal membrane, ×180. (Preparation courtesy of A.F. Petay, M.D., Universite Claude Bernard, Lyon, France.)

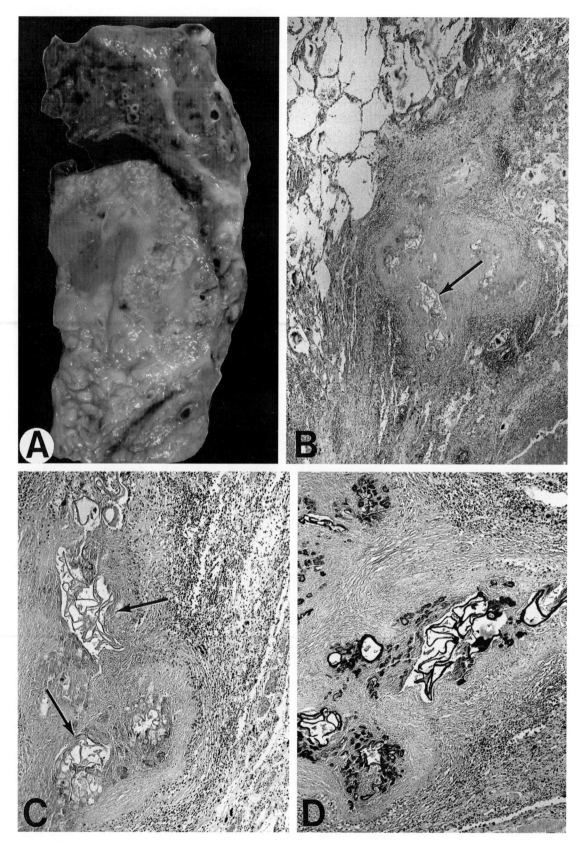

Fig. 27–18. *Echinococcus multilocularis* of lung. *A*, Gross appearance of a metastasis to the lung. Note the areas of calcification throughout the mass. *B* and *C*, Section stained with hematoxylin and eosin stain. *B*, Low-power view of a small satellite lesion showing a marked inflammatory reaction, fibrosis, and areas of central necrosis (cavitation) with a laminated membrane (ar-row), which is barely visible at this power, ×22. *C*, Higher magnification illustrating the greatly convoluted laminated membrane (arrows), ×55. *D*, Similar section, stained with periodic acid–Schiff stain, highlighting the laminated membrane, ×55. (Gross photograph and preparations courtesy of J.F. Wilson, M.D., Alaska Native Medical Center, Anchorage, Alaska.)

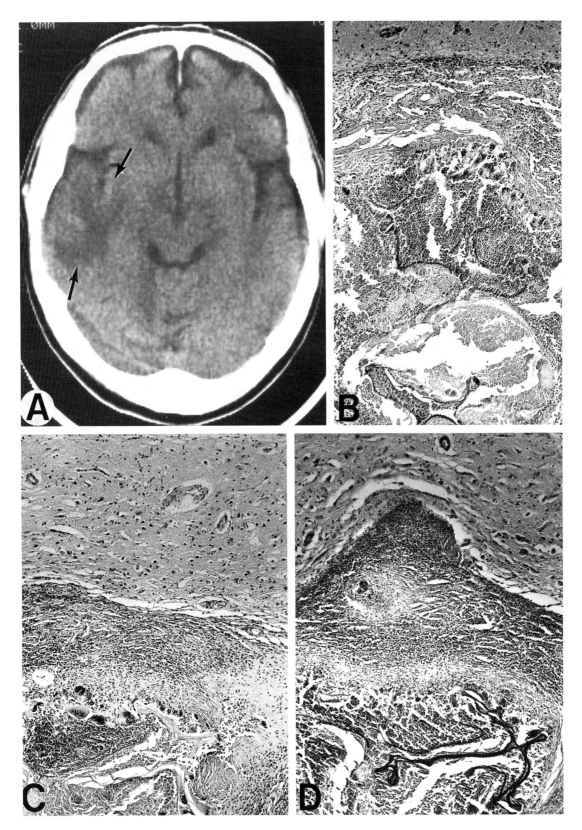

Fig. 27–19. *Echinococcus multilocularis* metastatic to brain. *A*, Computed tomogram of brain showing the lesion in the right temporal lobe (arrows). (Courtesy of G.A. Williams, M.D., Department of Ophthalmology, Eye Institute, Medical College of Wisconsin, Milwaukee, Wisconsin. In: Williams, D.F., Williams, G.F., Caya, J.G., et al. 1987. Intraocular *Echinococcus multilocularis.* Arch. Ophthalmol. 105:1106–1109. Reproduced with permission.) *B–D*, Histologic appearance of the lesion. Note the inflammatory reaction in some areas with multinucleated giant cells. The periodic acid–Schiff stain (*D*) clearly shows the laminated membrane, all ×55. (Preparation courtesy of J.F. Wilson, M.D., Alaska Native Medical Center, Anchorage, Alaska.)

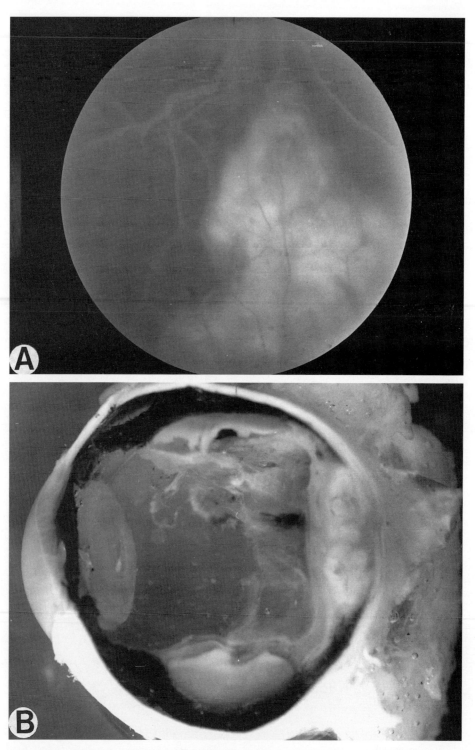

Fig. 27–20. *Echinococcus multilocularis* metastatic to the eye. *A*, Late phase of a fluorescent angiogram showing staining of the subintimal mass. *B*, Gross specimen corresponding to the bisected eye, with the cyst at the posterior pole. The tumor is located within the choroid and retina. *A*, Courtesy of G.A. Williams, M.D., and *B* courtesy of J.G. Caya, M.D., Department of Ophthalmology, Eye Institute, Medical College of Wisconsin, Milwaukee, Wisconsin. In: Williams, D.F., Williams, G.F., Caya, J.G., et al. 1987. Intraocular *Echinococcus multilocularis*. Arch. Ophthalmol. 105:1106–1109. Reproduced with permission.)

germinal membrane are closely associated with the acellular membrane. Careful measurements of hooklets are often the best way of identifying the parasite (Fig. 27–14). An avidin-biotin immunohistochemical method for detection of parasite antigens in tissue sections has given good results (Condon et al. 1988).

Echinococcus vogeli and Echinococcus oligarthrus— Polycystic Hydatid Disease

For many years, sporadic cases of hydatid cyst occurring in South and Central America, in areas not endemic for *E. granulosus*, appeared in the literature. Some of these cases occurred in immigrants from known endemic areas of *E. granulosus*, but others were found in indigenous inhabitants and had been acquired locally. One species, *E. oligarthrus*, had been known in some of these areas since the 1850s as a neotropical species in animals. This species became the prime suspect as the agent for the indigenous cases in Colombia and Panama (Thatcher, 1972; Thatcher, Sousa, 1966), but later it was recognized that these infections were not produced by *E. oligarthrus*. Rather, a different species undescribed at the time, *E. vogeli* (D'Alessandro et al. 1978, 1979; Rausch et al. 1978), was the responsible agent. Only in recent years have proven cases of *E. oligarthrus* been recognized in humans. This infection also pro-

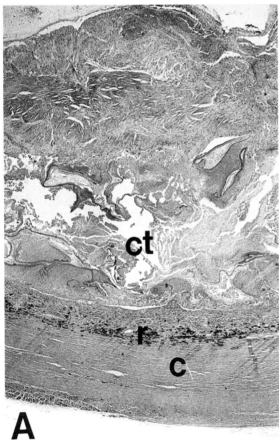

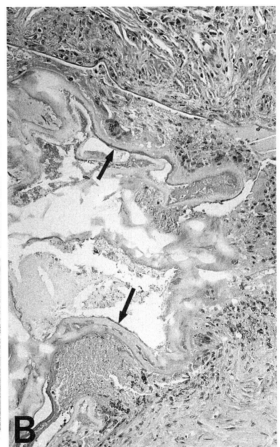

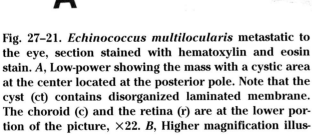

Fig. 27–21. *Echinococcus multilocularis* metastatic to the eye, section stained with hematoxylin and eosin stain. *A*, Low-power showing the mass with a cystic area at the center located at the posterior pole. Note that the cyst (ct) contains disorganized laminated membrane. The choroid (c) and the retina (r) are at the lower portion of the picture, ×22. *B*, Higher magnification illustrating the granulomatous reaction to fragments of the laminated membrane (arrows), ×140. (Preparation courtesy of J.G. Caya, M.D., Department of Ophthalmology, Eye Institute, Medical College of Wisconsin, Milwaukee, Wisconsin. Reported by: Williams, D.F., Williams, G.F., Caya, J.G., et al. 1987. Intraocular *Echinococcus multilocularis*. Arch. Ophthalmol. 105:1106–1109.)

duces a polycystic cyst (D'Alessandro, 1997; D'Alessandro et al. 1995; Lopera et al. 1989).

Geographic Distribution and Epidemiology. *Echinococcus vogeli* occurs naturally in wild bush dogs (*Speothos venaticus*) found in areas of Panama, Colombia, Venezuela, the Guianas, Ecuador, Peru, Bolivia, Paraguay, and southern Brazil. The intermediate hosts are "pacas" (*Cuniculus paca*), large rodents that occur in the same areas as the bush dog and, in addition, in Central America and southern Mexico. *Echinococcus oligarthrus* is found in the same areas where *E. vogeli* occurs, but in addition, it is present in northern Mexico (Salinas et al. 1996) and extends south to all the countries of Central America. The definitive hosts of *E. oligarthrus* are wild cats, especially jaguarundis (*Felis yagouaroundi*), pumas (*Felis concord*), and others. The intermediate hosts are rodents such as pacas, rabbits, agoutis (*Dasyproctata* species), rats, and opossums (Melendez et al. 1984).

The adults of *E. vogeli* and *E. oligarthrus* have morphologic characteristics that differentiate them from the other species of *Echinococcus* (Rausch, Bernstein, 1972); their life cycles are similar to that of other species, as described above. The growth pattern of the larvae differs in their natural intermediate hosts and in humans (Rausch et al. 1981). The only known modality of natural transmission is among wild animals; human infections are thus sporadic zoonotic infections. At present, 72 cases of polycystic hydatid cyst are known in 11 countries ranging from Nicaragua to Argentina. Of these, 31 cases are due to *E. vogeli* and 3 to *E. oligarthrus*; in the others, the species remains undetermined (D'Alessandro, 1997; D'Alessandro et al. 1996). Cases occurring outside the natural range of the bush dog are probably due to *E. oligarthrus* (D'Alessandro, 1997). *Echinococcus oligarthrus* was described in Brazil in 1863 as the first of the two species of *Echinococcus* in neotropical America; both species are unknown outside the American continent. Thus, cases of *E. oligarthrus* reported from India are at best misdiagnoses (Kini et al. 1997).

Clinical Findings. Infection with *E. vogeli* and *E. oligarthrus* occurs at all ages, with the median age being

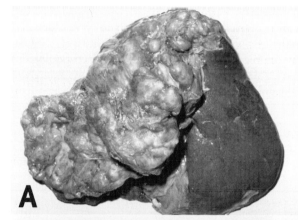
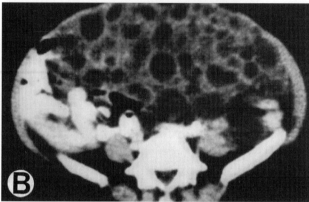

Fig. 27–22. *Echinococcus vogeli* in humans. *A*, Gross picture of the liver with a cyst. *B*, Computed tomogram of an abdominal cyst. (Courtesy of A. D'Alessandro, M.D., Department of Tropical Medicine, School of Public Health and Tropical Medicine, Tulane University, New Orleans, Louisiana.)

44 years; there is no gender difference. In 80% of cases the lesions are found in the liver alone or in combination with other organs, followed by the lung and other sites. Polycystic hydatid disease usually presents as a hard, painful tumor in the right hypochondrium (Fig. 27–22 *A–B*) or as a hepatic abscess; signs of portal hypertension are present in 25% of the cases (D'Alessandro, 1997). The evolution of the infection varies. Some patients recover after surgical treatment, others may have spontaneous remission of the cyst (D'Alessandro

Fig. 27–23. *Echinococcus vogeli. A*, Gross specimen from the peritoneal cavity of an experimentally infected animal. Note the polycystic nature of the larva. *B–D*. Histologic appearance of a cyst from an infected individual, hematoxylin and eosin stain. *B*, Low-power view of a degenerating cyst showing smaller cysts with collapsed membranes, ×11. *C*, Medium-power magnification illus-

trating one cavity, ×22. *D*, Higher-power magnification of degenerating protoscolices. Note the calcareous corpuscles (black) and some hooklets (arrows), ×280. (Gross specimen and preparation are courtesy of A. D'Alessandro, M.D., Department of Tropical Medicine, School of Public Health and Tropical Medicine, Tulane University, New Orleans, Louisiana.)

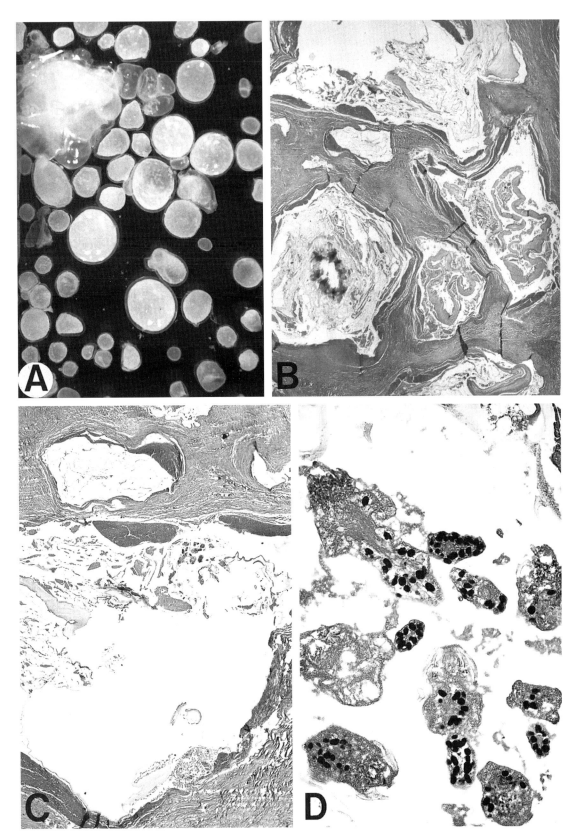

Fig. 27–23.

et al. 1979), and those who present with portal hypertension usually die (D'Alessandro, 1997).

On physical examination, most patients have a palpable, rounded mass in the right hypochondrium or epigastrium. The mass is sometimes fluctuant; it is often associated with the liver or the stomach and, on occasion, with the thoracic wall. Pulmonary cysts may present with expectoration, fever, and chills. Routine laboratory tests are unremarkable, and peripheral eosinophilia is rare. Serologic tests for hydatid cyst disease are usually positive. The main modalities of diagnosis are ultrasonography and CT, which usually demonstrate the polycystic nature of the mass; plain radiograms do not. The demonstration of a polycystic mass narrows the clinical diagnosis to a few entities, which, in conjunction with the patient's geographic area, usually provide the clinical diagnosis (D'Alessandro, 1997). Of the three known cases of *E. oligarthrus*, two had masses in the orbit and one had a mass in the heart. In all cases, the clinical diagnosis is confirmed by examination of tissue samples.

Pathology. The cysts of *E. vogeli* and *E. oligarthrus* are intermediate between those of *E. granulosus* and *E. multilocularis*. Growth occurs by internal division of small, fluid-filled cysts, resulting in the formation of separate chambers with a polycystic configuration (Fig. 27–23 *A* and *color plate* XVI *A*). The individual cysts measure 0.2 to 8.0 cm in diameter and occur in small or large groups; each cyst is separated from the others by its own adventitial layer. Polycystic hydatid disease occurs mostly in the liver, often extending to adjacent organs. In the majority of cases the cyst is visible on the surface of the liver, extending deep into the parenchyma. In other cases, the mesentery, omentum, intercostal muscles, diaphragm, lungs, pleura, pericardium, and heart are involved, due to extension of the primary liver cyst. The aggregation of individual cysts results in an enormous gray-white to ivory-white mass filled with a gelatinous substance (Fig. 27–23 *A*).

Microscopically, polycystic hydatid cysts in humans correlate with the gross morphology, consisting of multiple cavities ranging from a few millimeters to several centimeters (Fig. 27–23 *B*). Each cavity usually is composed of a germinal membrane, a laminated membrane, and a fibrous capsule, but degenerated vesicles show disorganization and collapse of the membranes into the cavity. The germinal membrane is 3 to 13 μm thick, and the laminated layer is 8 to 65 μm thick. Similar to other *Echinococcus* species, the laminated membrane stains deeply positively with periodic acid–Schiff stain. In the internal surface of the germi-

nal membrane, spherical brood capsules with several protoscolices are present (Fig. 27–23 *D*). Inconspicuous calcareous corpuscles and some foci of calcification are also seen. In some areas of the fibrous capsule, a granulomatous reaction is sometimes present, especially around degenerated vesicles.

The larva of *E. vogeli* in humans grows by both endogenous and exogenous proliferation of the membrane. The endogenous proliferation results in accumulation of membrane elements in the cystic cavity (Fig. 27–23 *C*). The exogenous proliferation is more important because it is invasive, similar to that of *E. multilocularis*. However, polycystic cysts exhibit a more controlled spread, do not produce metastasis, and thus are less pathogenic. In both *E. multilocularis* and *E. vogeli*, the pathogenicity of the larva in unnatural intermediate hosts is related to their abnormal growth, probably due to host–parasite incompatibility.

Diagnosis. The clinical diagnosis of polycystic hydatid disease is difficult. In most patients the disease is mistaken for another condition, most commonly hepatoma, cholangiocarcinoma, cirrhosis, abscess, cholecystitis, or abdominal tumors. In all cases, the diagnosis is based on examination of tissue samples. In tissue sections, the cyst is characterized by its polycystic nature, its germinal membrane with calcareous corpuscles, developed protoscolices, and thin, laminated membrane. Identification of the species is based on the study of rostellar hooklets found in the gelatinous fluid or in tissues (Fig. 27–14). Small portions of the cyst's germinal membrane, with protoscolices, should be used for squash preparations between a glass slide and a cover slip. The protoscolices are compressed and damaged and the hooklets separate, allowing careful measurements, which permits identification of the species of *Echinococcus* (Fig 28–14; Rausch et al. 1978).

References

Abou KS, Smith BM, MacLean JD, Poenaru D, Fried GM, Bret P, Barkun AN, 1996. Acute cholecystitis and cholangitis caused by *Echinococcus granulosus*. Am. J. Gastroenterol. 91:805–807

Alfonso F, Rey M, Balaguer J, Artiz V, Rabago G, 1987. Hydatid cyst of the right atrium diagnosed by echocardiography. Am. J. Cardiol. 60:931–932

Angulo JC, Sanchez CM, Diego A, Escribano J, Tamayo JC, Martin L, 1997. Renal echinococcosis: clinical study of 34 cases. J. Urol. 157:787–794

Apt W, Von Loebenstein R, Manubens S, 1969. Eliminacion de hidatide por via rectal. Bol. Chil. Parasitol. 24:142–145

Babra H, Messedi A, Masmoudi S, Zribi M, Grillot R, Ambroise-Thomas P, Beyrouti I, Sahnoun Y, 1994. Diagnosis of human hydatidosis: comparison between imagery and six serologic techniques. Am. J. Trop. Med. Hyg. 50:64–68

Ballard NB, Vande Vusse FJ, 1983. *Echinococcus multilocularis* in Illinois and Nebraska. J. Parasitol. 69:790–791

Blenkharn JI, Benjamin IS, Blumgart LH, 1987. Bacterial infection of hepatic hydatid cysts with *Haemophilus influenzae*. J. Infect. 15:169–171

Bonifacino R, Malgor R, Barbeito R, Balleste R, Rodriguez MJ, Botto C, Klug F, 1991. Seroprevalence of *Echinococcus granulosus* infection in a Uruguayan human population. Trans. R. Soc. Trop. Med. Hyg. 85:769–772

Bresson-Hadni S, Humbert P, Paintaud G, Auer H, Lenys D, Laurent R, Vuitton DA, Miguet JP, 1996. Skin localization of alveolar echinococcosis of the liver. J. Am. Acad. Dermatol. 34:873–877

Bresson-Hadni S, Laplante JJ, Lenys D, Rohmer P, Gottstein B, Jacquier P, Mercet P, Meyer JP, Miguet JP, Vuitton DA, 1994. Seroepidemiologic screening of *Echinococcus multilocularis* infection in a European area endemic for alveolar echinococcosis. Am. J. Trop. Med. Hyg. 51:837–846

Buris L, Takacs P, Varga M, 1987. Sudden death caused by hydatid embolism. J. Rechtsmed. 98:125–128

Calderon E, 1959. Hidatidosis subcutanea—ruptura espontanea de un quiste lumbar izquierdo. Bol. Chil. Parasitol. 14:85–86

Canabal EJ, Aguirre OV, Dighiero J, Purcallas J, Baldomir JM, Suzacq CV, 1955. *Echinococcus* disease of the left ventricle. A clinical, radiologic and electrocardiographic study. Circulation 12:520–529

Carpintero P, Kindelan J, Montero R, Carpintero A, 1997. Primary hydatidosis of the peripheral muscles: treatment with albendazole. Clin. Infect. Dis. 24:85–86

Casero RD, Costas MG, Menso E, 1996. An unusual case of hydatid disease: localization to the gluteus muscle. Clin. Infect. Dis. 23:395–396

Ciftcioglu MA, Yildirgan MI, Akcay MN, Reis A, Safali M, Aktas E, 1997. Fine needle aspiration biopsy in hepatic *Echinococcus multilocularis*. Acta Cytol. 41:649–652

Condon J, Rausch RL, Wilson JF, 1988. Application of the avidin-biotin immunohistochemical method for the diagnosis of alveolar hydatid disease from tissue sections. Trans. R. Soc. Trop. Med. Hyg. 82:731–735

Craig PS, Deshan L, Zhaoxun D, 1991. Hydatid disease in China. Parasitol. Today 7:46–50

D'Alessandro A, 1997. Polycystic echinococcosis in tropical America: *Echinococcus vogeli* and *E. oligarthrus*. Acta Trop. 67:43–65

D'Alessandro A, Moraes MAP, Raick AN, 1996. Polycystic hydatid disease in Brazil. Report of five new human cases and a short review of other published observations. Rev. Soc. Bras. Med. Trop. 29:219–228

D'Alessandro A, Ramirez LE, Chapadeiro E, Lopes ER, Mesquita PM de, 1995. Second recorded case of human infection by *Echinococcus oligarthrus*. Am. J. Trop. Med. Hyg. 52:29–33

D'Alessandro A, Rausch RL, Cuello C, Aristizabal N, 1979. *Echinococcus vogeli* in man, with a review of polycystic hydatid disease in Colombia and neighboring countries. Am. J. Trop. Med. Hyg. 28:303–317

D'Alessandro A, Rausch RL, Morales G, 1978, *Echinococcus vogeli* and *E. oligarthrus* in man and animals in Colombia. Fourth International Congress of Parasitology, Warsaw, Aug. 19–26. Abstracts, Sect. C, pp. 124–125

Eckert J, 1996. Der "gefährliche Fuchsbandwurm" (*Echinococcus multilocularis*) und die alveolare Echinokokkose des Menschen in Mitteleuropa. Berl. Munch. Tierarztl. Wochenschr. 109:202–210

Freixinet JL, Mestres CA, Cugat E, Mateu M, Gimferrer JM, Catalan M, Callejas MA, Letang E, Sanchez-Lloret J, 1988. Hepaticothoracic transdiaphragmatic echinococcosis. Am. Thorac. Surg. 45:426–429

Gamble WG, Segal M, Schantz PM, 1979. Alveolar hydatid disease in Minnesota: first human case acquired in the contiguous United States. JAMA 241:904–907

Gandhi RK, Bain AD, 1962. A large unilocular cyst of the spleen in a child. Br. J. Surg. 49:601–603

Gangopadhyay K, Abuzeid MO, Kfoury H, 1996. Hydatid cyst of the pterygopalatine-infratemporal fossa. J. Laryngol. Otol. 110:978–980

Gaucher A, Vinet E, Pere P, Plenat F, Ethgen D, Pourel J, 1983. Echinococcose alveolaire a localisation vertebrale. Presse Med. 12:1366

Gillet M, Miguet JP, Mantion G, Bresson-Hadni S, Becker MC, Rouget C, Christophe JL, Roullier M, Landecy G, Guerder L, Bechtel P, Vuitton-Drouhard D, 1988. Orthotopic liver transplantation in alveolar echinococcosis of the liver: analysis of a series of six patients. Transplant. Proc. 20:573–576

Gokalp HZ, Erdogan A, 1988. Hydatid cyst of the aquaduct of Sylvius. Clin. Neurol. Neurosurg. 90:83–85

Gottstein B, 1992. *Echinococcus multilocularis* infection: immunology and immunodiagnosis. Adv. Parasitol. 31:322–380

Gottstein B, Eckert J, Fey H, 1983. Serological differentiation between *Echinococcus granulosus* and *E. multilocularis* infections in man. Z. Parasitenk. 69:347–356

Gottstein B, Schantz PM, Wilson JF, 1985. Serological screening for *Echinococcus multilocularis* infections with ELISA. Lancet 1:1097–1098

Gottstein B, Tschudi K, Eckert J, Ammann R, 1989. Em2-ELISA for the follow-up of alveolar echinococcosis after complete surgical resection of liver lesions. Trans. R. Soc. Trop. Med. Hyg. 83:389–393

Halezeroglu S, Celik M, Uysal A, Senol C, Keles M, Arman B, 1997. Giant hydatid cysts of the lung. J. Thorac. Cardiovasc. Surg. 113:712–717

Heyat J, Nokhtari H, Hajaliloo J, Shakibi J, 1971. Surgical treatment of echinococcal cyst of the heart. Report of a case and review of the world literature. J. Thorac. Surg. 61:755–764

Imari AJ, 1962. Pulmonary hydatid disease in Iraq. Am. J. Trop. Med. Hyg. 11:481–490

Ishii Y, Fujino T, Weerasooriya MV, Kanematsu T, Imayama S, Miyaoka T, Sakamoto T, 1986. Subcutaneous echinococcosis: a case report from Kyushu. Jpn. J. Parasitol. 35:269–272

Ito A, Schantz PM, Wilson JF, 1995. Em18, a new serodiagnostic marker for differentiation of active and inactive cases of alveolar hydatid disease. Am. J. Trop. Med. Hyg. 52:41–44

Karak PK, Mittal M, Bhatia S, Mukhopadhyay S, Berry M, 1992. Isolated cerebral hydatid cyst with pathognomonic CT sign. Neuroradiology 34:9–10

Kaya U, Ozden B, Turker K, Tarcan B, 1975. Intracranial hydatid cysts. Study of 17 cases. J. Neurosurg. 42:580–584

Keil W, Pankratz H, Szabados A, Baur C, 1997. [Sudden death caused by an arterial hydatid embolism] Plotzlicher Tod durch arterielle Hydatidenembolie. Dtsch. Med. Wochenschr. 122:293–296

Kini U, Shariff S, Nirmala V, 1997. Aspiration cytology of *Echinococcus oligarthrus*. A case report. Acta Cytol. 41:544–548

Kriteky DC, Leiby PD, 1978. Studies on sylvatic echinococcosis. V. Factors influencing prevalence of *Echinococcus multilocularis* Leuckart 1863 in red foxes from North Dakota, 1965–1972. J. Parasitol. 64:625–634

Lanier AP, Trujillo DE, Schantz PM, Wilson JF, Gottstein B, McMahon BJ, 1987. Comparison of serologic tests for the diagnosis and follow-up of alveolar hydatid disease. Am. J. Trop. Med. Hyg. 37:609–615

Leiby PD, Carney WP, Woods CE, 1970. Studies on sylvatic echinococcosis. III. Host occurrence and geographic distribution of *Echinococcus multilocularis* in the north central United States. J. Parasitol. 56:1141–1150

Leibby PD, Kritsky DC, 1972. *Echinococcus multilocularis*: a possible domestic life cycle in Central North America and its public health implications. J. Parasitol. 58:1213–1215

Leiby PD, Olsen OW, 1964. The cestode *Echinococcus multilocularis* in foxes in North Dakota. Science 145:1066

Lopera RD, Melendez RD, Fernandez I, Sirit J, Perera MP, 1989. Orbital hydatid cyst of *Echinococcus oligarthrus* in a human in Venezuela. J. Parasitol. 75:467–470

Lucius R, Bilger B, 1995. *Echinococcus multilocularis* in Germany: increased awareness or spreading of a parasite? Parasitol. Today 11:430–434

MacPherson CNL, 1983. An active intermediate host role for man in the life cycle of *Echinococcus granulosus* in Turkana, Kenya. Am. J. Trop. Med. Hyg. 32:397–404

MacPherson CNL, Spoerry A, Zeyhle E, Romig T, Gorfe M, 1989. Pastoralists and hydatid disease: an ultrasound scanning prevalence survey in East Africa. Trans. R. Soc. Trop. Med. Hyg. 83:243–247

Magath TB, 1954. The importance of sylvatic hydatid disease. JAVMA 125:411

Marti-Bonmati L, Menor F, Ballesta A, 1988. Hydatid cyst of the liver: rupture into the biliary tree. Am. J. Radiol. 150:1051–1053

Matossian RM, Rickard MD, Smyth JD, 1977. Hydatidosis: a global problem of increasing importance. Bull. WHO 55:499–507

Mboti B, Van de Stadt J, Carlier Y, Peny M, Jacobs F, Bourgeois N, Adler M, Gelin M, 1996. Long-term disease-free survival after liver transplantation for alveolar echinococcosis. Acta Chir. Belg. 96:229–232

Melendez RD, Yepez MS, Coronado A, 1984. *Echinococcus oligarthrus* cysts of rabbits in Venezuela. J. Parasitol. 70:1004–1005

Meltzer H, Kovacs L, Orford T, Matas M, 1956. Echinococcosis in North American Indians and Eskimos. Can. Med. Assoc. J. 75:121–128

Mooraki A, Rahbar MH, Bastani B, 1996. Spontaneous systemic anaphylaxis as an unusual presentation of hydatid cyst: report of two cases. Am. J. Trop. Med. Hyg. 55:302–303

Mossiman F, 1980. Is alveolar hydatid disease of the liver incurable? Ann. Surg. 118:118–123

Mousa AM, Mehrez MG, Muhtaseb SA, 1987. Disseminated pelvic hydatidosis presenting as ovarian carcinomatosis: successful post-operative treatment with mebendazole. Int. J. Gynaecol. Obstet. 25:473–478

Novick RJ, Tchervenkov CI, Wilson JA, Munro DD, Mulder DS, 1987. Surgery for thoracic hydatid disease: a North American experience. Ann. Thorac. Surg. 43:681–686

Papo I, Savic S, 1962. Hydatid disease of the heart. A report on 2 cases treated surgically. Br. J. Surg. 49:598–600

Pappaioanou M, Schwabe CW, Sard DM, 1977. An evolving pattern of human hydatid disease transmission in the United States. Am. J. Trop. Med. Hyg. 26:732–742

Parija SC, Ravinder PT, Rao KS, 1997. Detection of hydatid antigen in urine by countercurrent immunoelectrophoresis. J. Clin. Microbiol. 35:1571–1574

Petavy AF, Deblock S, Walbaum S, 1990. The house mouse: a potential intermediate host for *Echinococcus multilocularis* in France. Trans. R. Soc. Trop. Med. Hyg. 84:571–572

Petavy AF, Seblock S, Walbaum S, 1991. Life cycles of *Echinococcus multilocularis* in relation to human infection. J. Parasitol. 77:133–137

Placer C, Martin R, Sanchez E, Soleto E, 1988. Rupture of abdominal hydated cysts. Br. J. Surg. 75:157

Polydorou K, 1984. How echinococcosis was conquered in Cyprus. World Health Forum 5:160–164

Rakower J, Beller A, 1961. Cerebral and pulmonary emboli from a ruptured hydatid cyst of the liver. Am. J. Trop. Med. Hyg. 10:208–214

Rakower J, Milwidsky H, 1960. Primary mediastinal echinococcosis. Am. J. Med. 29:73–83

Rakower J, Milwidsky H, 1964. Hydatid pleural disease. Am. Rev. Respir. Dis. 90:623–631

Rausch RL, Bernstein JJ, 1972. *Echinococcus vogeli* sp. n. (Cestoda: Taeniidae) from the bush dog, *Speothus venaticus* (Lund.). Z. Tropenmed. Parasitol. 23:25–34

Rausch RL, Rausch VR, D'Alessandro A, 1981. Characteristics of the larval *Echinococcus vogeli* Rausch and Bernstein, 1972 in the natural intermediate host, the paca, *Cuniculus paca* L. (Rodentia: Dasyproctidae). Am. J. Trop. Med. Hyg. 30:1043–1052

Rausch RL, Rausch VR, D'Alessandro A, 1978. Discrimination of the larval stages of *Echinococcus oligarthrus* (Diesing, 1863) and *E. vogeli* Rausch and Bernstein, 1972 (Cestoda: Taeniidae). Am. J. Trop. Med. Hyg. 27:1195–1202

Rausch RL, Wilson JF, Schantz PM, McMahon BJ, 1987. Spontaneous death of *Echinococcus multilocularis*: cases diagnosed serologically (by EM2ELISA) and clinical significance. Am. J. Trop. Med. Hyg. 36:576–585

Rollinson PD, Geytenbeek RJ, 1987. Hydatid disease of bone: a case report. S. Afr. Med. J. 71:727–728

Sailer M, Soelder B, Allerberger F, Zaknun D, Feichtinger H, Gottstein B, 1997. Alveolar echinococcosis of the liver in a six-year-old girl with acquired immunodeficiency syndrome. J. Pediatr. 130:320–323

Salinas LN, Jimenez GF, Cruz RA, 1996. Presence of *Echinococcus oligarthrus* (Diesing, 1863) Luhe, 1910 in *Lynx rufus texensis* Allen, 1895 from San Fernando, Tamaulipas state, in north-east Mexico. Int. J. Parasitol 26:793–796

Sapunar J, Parada M, Sapunar (hijo) J, Araya MV, Arroyo A, Rolle A, 1984. Quiste hidatidico hepatico abierto a vias biliares y a bronquios. Bol. Chil. Parasitol. 39:54–59

Schenone H, Rojas A, Cerpa M, Perez C, 1971. El problema de la frecuencia de las localizaciones del quiste hidatidico en el hombre. Bol. Chil. Parasitol. 26:106–114

Shambesh MK, MacPherson CNL, Beesley WN, Gusbi A, El-sonosi T, 1992. Prevalence of human hydatid disease in northwestern Libya: a cross-sectional ultrasound study. Ann. Trop. Med. Parasitol. 86:381–386

Stehr-Green JK, Stehr-Green PA, Schantz PM, Wilson JF, Lanier A, 1988. Risk factors for infection with *Echinococcus multilocularis* in Alaska. Am. J. Trop. Med. Hyg. 38:380–385

Stermam MM, Brown HW, 1958. *Echinococcus* in man and dog in the same household in New York City. JAMA 169:938–940

Storandt ST, Kazacos KR, 1993. *Echinococcus multilocularis* identified in Indiana, Ohio and east-central Illinois. J. Parasitol. 79:301–305

Thatcher VE, 1972. Neotropical echinococcosis in Colombia. Ann. Trop. Med. Parasitol. 66:99–105

Thatcher VE, Sousa OE, 1966. *Echinococcus oligarthrus* Diesing, 1863, in Panama and a comparison with a recent human hydatid. Ann. Trop. Med. Parasitol. 60:405–416

Thompson RCA, Lymbery AJ, 1988. The nature, extent and significance of variation within the genus *Echinococcus granulosus*. Adv. Parasitol. 27:210–256

Thompson RCA, Lymbery AJ, 1995. *Echinococcus and Hydatid Disease*. Oxford: CAB International

Tiberin P, Heilbronn YD, Hirsch M, Barmeir E, 1984. Giant cerebral *Echinococcus* cyst with galactorrhea and amenorrhea. Surg. Neurol. 21:505–506

Uriarte C, Pomares N, Martin M, Conde A, Alonso N, Bueno MG, 1991. Splenic hydatidosis. Am. J. Trop. Med. Hyg. 44:420–423

WHO, 1979. Hydatidosis in Latin American countries. Weekly Epidemiol. Rec. WHO No. 54, 41

WHO, 1984. Parasitic disease surveillance. Weekly Epidemiol. Rec. WHO No. 21, 160–164

WHO, 1996. Guidelines for treatment of cystic and alveolar echinococcosis in humans. WHO Informal Working Group on Echinococcosis. Bull. WHO 74:231–242

Williams DF, Williams GA, Caya JG, Werner RP, Harrison TJ, 1987. Intraocular *Echinococcus multilocularis*. Arch. Ophthalmol. 105:1106–1109

Williams JF, Lopez Aderos H, Trejos A, 1971. Current prevalence and distribution of hydatidosis with special reference to the Americas. Am. J. Trop. Med. Hyg. 20:224–236

Wilson JF, Diddams AC, Rausch RL, 1968. Cystic hydatid disease in Alaska. Am. Rev. Respir. Dis. 98:1–15

Wilson JF, Rausch RL, 1980. Alveolar hydatid disease. A review of clinical features of 33 indigenous cases of *Echinococcus multilocularis* infection in Alaskan Eskimos. Am. J. Trop. Med. Hyg. 29:1340–1355

Part V

The Arthropods

The arthropods of medical importance belong to several zoological groups. The great majority of them are responsible for the transmission of numerous biologic agents of human disease, for which most of them serve as obligatory intermediate hosts. Some arthropods, however, invade human tissues, producing infections that may cause important morbidity and sometimes mortality. Other arthropods live on their hosts, producing infestations that result in some morbidity. In human medicine, the main role of arthropods is the transmission of infectious agents, as stated above, usually by those arthropods that feed on blood. Mosquitoes transmit the viruses that produce viral encephalitis and yellow fever, the protozoa that cause malaria, and the nematodes that cause filariasis. Ticks transmit the rickettsial organisms that produce typhus, Rocky Mountain spotted fever, and Lyme disease, as well as the protozoa of babesiosis. Sand flies are responsible for transmission of bacteria—for example, the agent of bartonellosis and the protozoan that causes leishmaniasis. Lice transmit the spirochetes that produce relapsing fever; fleas, the bacillus responsible for plague. Beetles and cockroaches transmit the cestodes that produce hymenolepiasis. Some crustaceans are intermediate hosts of nematodes and tapeworms—for example, *Diaptomus* and *Cyclops* for *Dracunculus*, *Spirometra*, and *Diphyllobothrium*.

The study of arthropods as vectors of infections, as producers of allergies or allergic systemic reactions, or as nuisances is outside the scope of this book. Textbooks of medical parasitology and entomology, which discuss these subjects, are widely available. Only a few arthropods seen in tissue sections that produce a recognizable histologic reaction are discussed in Chapter 28.

28

PENTASTOMES, *DEMODEX* MITES, SCABIES, FLIES, AND FLEAS

Pentasomes

The Pentastomida, a class of the Arthropoda, is difficult to place within the zoologic hierarchy. The parasites in this class are considered by some as highly modified annelids and by others as being closer to the crustaceans (Riley et al. 1978). The all-inclusive name *pentastomes* refers to this group of parasites and the infection they produce as *pentastomiasis* (often as *porocephalosis*). However, because there is no conclusively documented infection in humans with a species of *Porocephalus* (Fain, 1975), the term *porocephalosis* should not be used. The species *Linguatula serrata*, which is responsible for human infections, produces *linguatulosis*, the name applied when the parasites recovered are conclusively identified. Pentastomes, or pentastomids, are a small group of arthropods (endoparasites) with worldwide distribution parasitizing the lungs and upper respiratory tract of many vertebrates, including dogs, snakes, and humans. The adult females, which are up to 10 cm long, are rounded or flattened, sometimes with a leaf-like or linguiform appearance. The males are one-half to one-third the size of the females (Fig. 28–1). The adult parasite in the upper respiratory tract passes eggs, which gain access to the environment in mucus, sputum, or feces. The intermediate hosts ingest the eggs, which free a four- or six-legged larva in the intestine. The larva, or nymph, enters the mucosa and migrates to the liver, spleen, lymph nodes, omentum, lungs, and other organs, where it molts several times, transforming into an infective nymph that encapsulates in the tissues. Ingestion of encapsulated nymphs by the predator definitive host results in the infection with adult parasites in the upper respiratory tract. Humans may suffer infections with either the adult or the larval stage of pentastomids.

Classification of the pentastomids is difficult, and its systematics is not well established (Riley, 1986; Self, 1969). Two of the accepted genera, *Linguatula* and *Armillifer*, have species that are important in human medicine; *Linguatula* has one species, *L. serrata*, and *Armillifer* has three, *A. armillatus*, *A. grandis*, and *A. moniliformis*. *Linguatula serrata* and *A. armillatus* produce about 99% of the human infections (Self, 1969), which usually occur in two ways. One way is by the ingestion of infective *eggs* passed with the mucus or feces of dogs, which results in the development of a larva in the tissues (visceral pentastomiasis) produced by *Linguatula* and *Armillifer*. The other way is by inges-

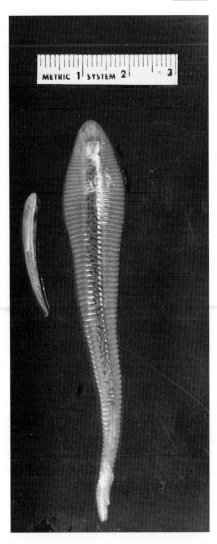

Fig. 28–1. *Linguatula serrata*, adults. Compare the size of the female (right) to that of the male (left). (In: Beaver, P.C., Jung, R.C. and Cupp, E.W. 1984 *Clinical Parasitology*, 9th ed. Philadelphia: Lea & Febiger. Reproduced with permission.)

tion of *larvae* in tissues of goats and other animals, which results in an infection with the adults in the upper respiratory tract (nasopharyngeal pentastomiasis) by *Linguatula* (Beaver et al. 1984; Schacher et al. 1969).

Linguatula serrata

Linguatula serrata produces a common infection of the upper respiratory tract of wild and domestic dogs in many areas. In Lebanon, the infection rate in the nares of stray dogs is over 43% (Khalil, Schacher, 1965a; Schacher et al. 1965). In the United States the infection in dogs is rare; it has been described in the Midwest and Georgia. In the intermediate hosts (rabbits) it is known in Oklahoma, Alabama, Mississippi, Georgia, and Maryland (Gardiner et al. 1984). The most important intermediate hosts of *Linguatula* are cows, sheep, and goats, but rabbits and other herbivorous animals also play a role in its transmission. Cases of *Linguatula* infection in humans have occurred in Africa, Europe, the Middle East, South America, Cuba, and the United States (Virginia, Mississippi, Michigan, and Texas). In the Middle East, the epidemiology of *Linguatula* parallels that of *E. granulosus*. Domestic dogs caring for a herd of goats or sheep are the infected definitive hosts, and herbivorous animals are the intermediate hosts.

The Visceral Form. Clinically, visceral linguatulosis (or pentastomiasis) is usually silent, like other pentastomid infections (see below). This infection is usually an incidental finding at autopsy (Tobie, 1957). It has also been found during abdominal surgery when the larva is noticed, either alive (Callard et al. 1976) or as a small nodule that is resected for diagnosis. The parasite is usually located in the omentum, the peritoneum, or the surface of any of the viscera. Many visceral *Linguatula* infections are diagnosed on the basis of findings in tissue sections (Fig. 28–2 *A–B*). Most of these reports do not include specific diagnostic characteristics, such as the presence of spines, and therefore are not credible; unquestionably, they are pentastomids in most instances. The best way to identify the parasite is by studying it in toto.

Unusual Locations. In some cases, the nymphs of *L. serrata* occur outside of their usual location in the abdominal cavity, producing unusually severe morbidity. The most important organ involved is the eye, where the parasite produces serious symptoms (*color plate* XVI *D*; Hunter, Higgins, 1960; Lang et al. 1987; Rendtorff et al. 1962). It also occurs in the prostate, producing granulomatous inflammation (Symmers, 1957). The infection in a Mexican child caused by the parasite in the pleura produced pleuropulmonary symptoms and required a lobectomy (de Leon Bojorge, Chacon, 1984).

The Nasopharyngeal Form. The nasopharyngeal form of linguatulosis presents with chronic upper respiratory

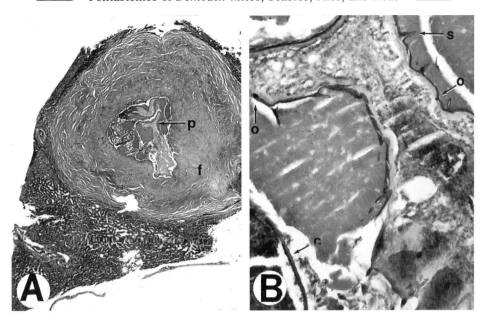

Fig. 28–2. *Linguatula* in liver, section stained with hematoxylin and eosin stain. *A*, Low-power view of the granuloma, ×25. *B*, Higher magnification shows some of the identifiable structures, ×250. Abbreviations: c, cuticle from previous molt; f, hyalinized granuloma; o, sclerotized openings of the cuticle; p, degenerated parasite; s, spines. (In: Gardiner, C.H., Dyke, J.W., and Shirley, S.F. 1984. Hepatic granuloma to a nymph of *Linguatula serrata* in a woman from Michigan: a case report and review of the literature. Am. J. Trop. Med. Hyg. 33:187–189. Reproduced with permission.)

tract symptoms. In these cases, the adult "worms" are visualized in the nasal or pharyngeal mucosa, from which they are recovered with forceps or other instruments. This method permits study of the nymphs and adults for proper identification. In chronic infections, the eggs are usually found in nasal secretions. In one patient, adults of *Linguatula* were isolated from the pulmonary parenchyma, where they had produced cavitating disease (Sagredo, 1924).

Halzoun or Parasitic Pharyngitis. Parasitic pharyngitis is a clinical syndrome consisting of allergic manifestations in the throat. There is pruritus in the throat extending to the ear, followed by congestion and edema of the buccopharyngeal mucosa, including the uvula, tonsils, larynx, eustachian tubes, conjunctivae, and lips. In addition, these patients may have unilateral conductive deafness, tinnitus, and facial palsy (Yagi et al. 1996). The symptoms invariably follow the consumption of raw animal viscera, though often they begin as the infectious meal is consumed. The duration of symptoms is variable. In mild cases it is 2 to 3 days; in moderate forms it is 5 to 8 days (Khouri, 1905; Watson, Abdel Kerim, 1956). In more severe cases there is

swelling of the neck and face, with dyspnea, dysphagia, and dysphoria, progressing to acute asphyxiation and death. Surveys of persons with symptoms of the disease in Sudan have shown that up to 20% of the population has experienced the disease (Yagi et al. 1996).

The viscera usually consumed is raw liver of sheep, goats, or cows, which are often infected with *F. hepatica*, *D. dendriticum*, or both. For this reason, a cause–effect connection between these two trematodes and halzoun was generally accepted. However, experiments with human volunteers have not demonstrated a relationship between consumption of liver infected with the trematodes and production of the disease (Azar, 1964). Similar results were obtained in experimental animals (Khalil, Schacher, 1965b).

The name *halzoun* ("snail" in Arabic) is given to the condition in the Middle East, especially in Lebanon. Another name, *marrara*, is used in Sudan for a similar syndrome because it follows the consumption of marrara, a delicacy consisting of the raw liver, lungs, trachea, and rumen of goats, cattle, camel, or sheep seasoned with chilies and lemon. The name *"alack"* is used in other places for infections producing similar oropharyngeal symptoms. In either case, the consumption of either raw liver or marrara results in ingestion of the two previously mentioned trematodes and, in addition, ingestion of *L. serrata* larvae (El-Hassan et al. 1991; Khalil, Schacter, 1965b). The larvae of *L. serrata* were isolated from a patient in Sudan who presented with marrara syndrome (El-Hassan et al. 1991). Ingestion of encapsulated nymphs of *Linguatula* frees the parasites either in the mouth (in which case they attach immediately to the oropharynx) or in the stomach. If freed in the stomach, the larvae migrate upward in the esophagus to the upper respiratory tract and attach to the mucosa. *Linguatula* is the only pentastomid capable of attaining adulthood in humans (Fain, 1975). The parasites in the oropharynx and nasal mucosa produce acute itching, edema, and sneezing that is sometimes paroxysmal. The violent sneezing and coughing may dislodge the parasites, which are expelled and sometimes are recovered by the victim. In most cases, expulsion of the "worms" relieves the acute symptoms within 30 minutes (Khalil, Schacher, 1965b). It is not rare for an infected individual to expel up to 20 *Linguatula* nymphs, and infected mesenteric lymph nodes from goats may contain up to 150 nymphs (Khalil, Schacher, 1965b). As stated, the symptoms of parasitic pharyngitis are allergic, produced by sensitization to the parasite antigens. In severe cases, the result is death due to anaphylaxis with acute edema of the vocal cords and larynx, producing asphyxiation.

The specific identification of the larvae (nymphs) of *Linguatula* is difficult in tissue sections. The parasites must be isolated from tissues and studied in toto. In some cases, the organisms have been dissected for identification from formalin-fixed tissues after first being observed in tissue sections (Tobie, 1957).

Armillifer

Armillifer is the most common genus of pentastomes; the species of this genus always produce infections in humans as larval (visceral) stages. *Armillifer armillatus* is known only in tropical Africa, where the adults inhabit the lungs of large snakes, such as pythons. *Armillifer moniliformis* occurs in Asiatic snakes and *A. grandis* in snakes of the Democratic Republic of Congo. Cases have been reported from Africa (Egypt, Gambia, Senegal, Ghana, Zimbabwe, Cameroon, and the Democratic Republic of Congo; Self et al. 1975), the Philippines, Indonesia, Tibet, and Malaya. *Armillifer grandis* has been reported in humans in the Democratic Re-

public of Congo (Fain, Salvo, 1966) and the Ivory Coast (Cagnard et al. 1979).

In humans, *A. armillatus* nymphs is usually located in the peritoneal cavity and the thorax. In the peritoneal cavity, the nymphs are encysted beneath the liver capsule and beneath the surface of the liver, as well as within the omentum, mesentery, intestinal walls, and other intestinal organs. *Armillifer moniliformis* is found in the liver and lungs. It was reported from Malaya as *Porocephalus moniliformis* in 46% of a series of autopsies in aborigines (Prathap et al. 1968, 1969). *Armillifer grandis* is usually found in the mesenteries (Fain, 1975).

The symptoms produced by infections with *Armillifer* are usually minimal. In some cases, after ingestion of eggs, migration of the young parasites from the intestine to the viscera produces severe abdominal pain and jaundice. In other cases, the presentation is that of an acute abdomen (Herzog et al. 1985). Once the nymphs grow to their normal size and encapsulate in the tissues, they become asymptomatic. The nymphs measure up to several centimeters in length and are curled on their ventral surface in the shape of a tightly closed letter **C**. Most human infections with *Armifiller* are found at autopsy and sometimes are discovered incidentally during abdominal surgery (Donges, 1966). Calcified larvae appear rarely (3 of 70,00) on plain radiograms of the abdomen (Fain, 1975). One larva studied in France had rings 4 to 5 mm in diameter and 1 to 2 mm thick. Inside the ring, the larva is 2 to 3 mm in diameter and is seen as a dark disc (Brochery et al. 1976). Calcified nymphs observed longitudinally have the typical appearance of a letter **C** (Fain, 1975; Herzog et al. 1985).

Unusual Locations. In one case, a large number of nymphs in the wall of the intestine produced obstruction and death; the parasites were classified as *A. armillatus* (Cannon, 1942). In addition, *A. armillatus* occurred in a lacrimal caruncle (Polderman, Manschot, 1979). A nymph of a species of *Armillifer* was also recovered from the eye (Gratama, Van Thiel, 1957) and a nymph of *A. grandis* from the eyelid (Fain, 1975).

Grossly, the larvae are recognized on the serosal surfaces, but they are usually found in other organs, forming nodules less than 1 cm in diameter. A nodule often has the characteristic **C** shape of the nymph and consists of a fibrous capsule from which the parasite is released easily for study. The larvae of *A. armillatus* are larger than those of *A. grandis* and have fewer circular exoskeletal thickenings (Fain, 1975). On microscopic examination, the intact, dead, or degenerated organism can be demonstrated (Fig. 28–3 *A–D*). Intact

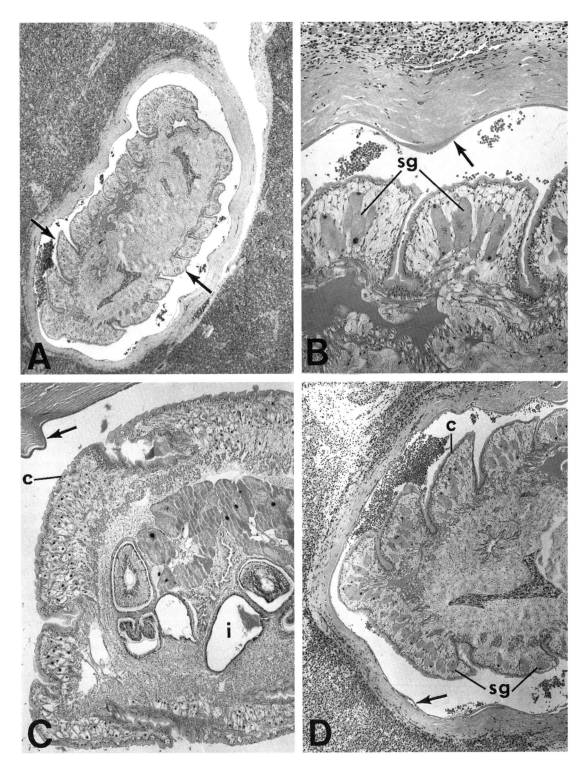

Fig. 28–3. Pentastomid larva in liver, section stained with hematoxylin and eosin stain. *A*, Low-power view showing an oblique section of a well-preserved, encapsulated larva in the liver; contrast this with Figure 28–2. Note the annulations of the body, seen on the section as deep folds of the cuticle (arrows), ×22. *B*, Higher magnification illustrating a detail of the larva, the fibrous capsule, the scant inflammatory reaction, and liver tissue. Note the previously molted cuticle of the larva against the fibrous wall (arrow). Subcuticular glands (sg),

×140. *C* and *D*, Medium-power magnification of larvae in liver on transverse (*C*) and oblique (*D*) sections. Note the cuticle (c), the subcuticular glands (sg), the shed or molted cuticle (arrow), and the intestine (i), ×55. (Preparations courtesy of K. Prathap, M.D., Department of Pathology, Faculty of Medicine, University of Malaya, Kuala Lumpur, Malaysia. Reported by: Prathap, K., Lau, K.S., and Bolton, J.M. 1969. Pentastomiasis: a common finding at autopsy among Malaysian aborigines. Am. J. Trop. Med. Hyg. 18:20–27.)

parasites are usually found inside a fibrous wall, with little or no inflammatory infiltration. Dead and degenerated ones occur within necrotic tissue surrounded by an acute or chronic inflammatory reaction, sometimes with granulomas (Drabick, 1987; Prathap et al. 1969). On cross sections, the parasite has a characteristic chitinous exoskeleton, a large intestine, and striated muscles. The diagnosis of a species is not possible, and only study of larvae recovered in toto allows classification of the organism.

Demodex—Demodiciosis

Two species of *Demodex*, *D. folliculorum* and *D. brevis*, are obligatory parasites of the human pilosebaceous follicles of the nose, as well as adjacent areas of the face, forehead, and scalp. The infection appears to be universal in humans, but reports of less than 100% prevalence exist, probably due to the sampling method used. It is estimated that every person carries a colony of 1000 to 2000 *Demodex* mites. The infection is acquired soon after birth because it is present in young infants.

Demodex folliculorum is less than 0.4 mm long and inhabits the hair follicles (Fig. 28–4 *A–B*). *Demodex brevis* is shorter and inhabits the sebaceous glands (Fig. 28–4 *C–D*). Thus, these two species have different ecologic niches in the skin. At present there is no conclusive evidence that *Demodex* has a harmful effect on humans, but the species in dogs, *D. caninum*, produces red mange in puppies, an often fatal disease.

In recent years, a fair number of reports have been published attributing a pathogenic role to *Demodex* in humans. *Demodex* has been found in 72% of patients attending a dermatology clinic in Brazil (Madeira, Sogayar, 1993) and in 29% of the scalps of 100 unselected autopsy patients in Germany (Hellerich, Metzelder, 1994). Another survey, in Poland, showed that the presence of the mites in hair follicles of the eyelid increased with age to 86% in the 26- to 34-year age group (Humiczewska et al. 1994). Although blepharitis was once attributed to the mite, careful studies of the incidence of mites and associated bacteria have not shown a clear association in these patients (Demmler et al. 1997). *Demodex* is also implicated as the etiologic agent of rosacea, a chronic inflammation of the face characterized by erythematous papules, telangiectasia, and pustules (Amichai et al. 1992; Forton, 1986; Forton, Seys, 1993). In some studies of patients with rosacea and controls matched for age and sex, there

was a significant increase in the number of mites in the patients (Bonnar et al. 1993). These authors concluded that there was a cause–effect relationship between the mite and the disease, but they did not consider the possibility that rosacea may be the cause of the population increase in the mites. Other authors have concluded that *Demodex* has no role in the development of rosacea (Burns, 1992; Sibenge, Gawkrodger, 1992). In one patient with rosacea, histologic examination of the skin showed an acute granulomatous inflammation around the mites (Hoekzema et al. 1995). One child had marked parakeratosis of the scalp, which was also associated with numerous *Demodex* mites (Pietrini et al. 1995). Skin biopsy specimens from areas inhabited by the mites, taken for unrelated medical reasons, invariably show this organism (Fig. 28–4 *A–D*).

The most interesting reports on *Demodex* as the cause of skin disease concern immune suppressed individuals, in whom the mites are sometimes found in lesions in areas other that their natural location. In a patient with mycosis fungoides, the lesions were located in the trunk (Nakagawa et al. 1996). A child with leukemia developed 1 to 2 mm erythematous papules and pustules in the face, with numerous mites (Sahn, Sheridan, 1992). In both of these patients, specific therapy resulted in regression of the lesions. In patients with acquired immune deficiency syndrome (AIDS), a papular pruritic eruption accompanied numerous *Demodex* mites has been described (Barrio et al. 1996; Jaureguiberry et al. 1993). The lesions sometimes extend to the skin of the neck (Dominey et al. 1989) and trunk (Redondo Mateo et al. 1993). The inflammation clears rapidly with specific treatment (Ashack et al. 1989; Dominey et al. 1989).

Sarcoptes scabiei—Scabies

The genus *Sarcoptes* has not been well studied, and the taxonomic status of the different species or strains occurring in animals and humans is uncertain. One species, *S. scabiei* var. *hominis*, also referred to as *S. sarcoptes scabiei*, occurs in humans. *Sarcoptes* and other related genera of acarid mites produce skin infestations generally known as *mange* in animals and as *scabies* in humans. Under both experimental and natural conditions, some of the *Sarcoptes* from animals can infect other species of animals and humans. For example, animal handlers often acquire the mites of the animals they work with, such as pigs (pig-handler's itch) and horses (cavalryman's itch), but usually the

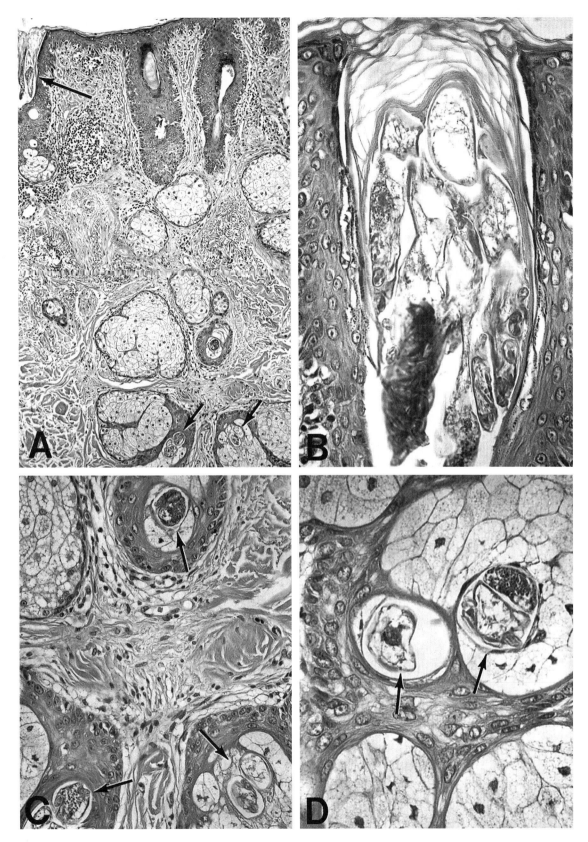

Fig. 28–4. *Demodex* in skin, section stained with hematoxylin and eosin stain. *A*, Low-power view of a skin section illustrating the location of *D. folliculorum* (long arrow) in the hair follicles and *D. brevis* (short arrows) deep in the sebaceous glands, ×70. *B*, High-power magnification of a hair follicle with several *D. folliculorum* (arrows), ×350. *C* and *D*, Higher magnification illustrates *D. brevis* (arrows), *C* ×220, *D* ×450.

717

mites survive for only a few days (Burgess, 1994). The infection is also acquired from dogs infected with *S. canis*, a different species that is morphologically similar to *S. scabiei*; the mite of pigs, *S. sarcoptes suis*, is considered a subspecies (Lee, Cho, 1995).

Sarcoptes inhabits the upper layers of the epidermis, where it makes a burrow and feeds on cells and juices oozing from chewed epithelium. The stage of *Sarcoptes* most commonly identified in humans is the adult female, which is about 350 to 450 μm in length by 250 to 350 μm in breadth. The males are slightly over one-half the size of the females. After the parasites in their burrows copulate, the females develop one to two eggs and deposit them in the burrow as they continue digging, often for several centimeters. The life span of a *Sarcoptes* female is about 6 to 8 weeks. Eggs are laid every 2 to 3 days, and hatching occurs in approximately 5 days. Development from egg to adult takes 10 to 13 days. (Arlian, Vyszenski-Moher, 1988).

Sarcoptes and the clinical lesions they produce are usually found in the skin of the hands and wrists in over 60% of cases, followed by the elbows, feet, penis, scrotum, and, to a lesser extent, the buttocks and axilla in 10% to 12%. Infections with species of animal *Sarcoptes* usually show a distribution different from that of *S. scabiei*. The predilection of *S. scabiei* for the skin of the wrist is remarkable; adult females deposited on the necks of volunteers reach the wrist a few hours later and begin digging. The actual number of mites producing clinical symptoms in individuals with scabies is important. In over 50% of cases, only 1 to 5 adult females are present; in 20%, 5 to 10 females occur; and the percentage of infestations with more than 10 females decreases rapidly.

The geographic distribution of *S. scabiei* is worldwide. In the United States, cases are frequent but data on their incidence are lacking. In the 1950s the infection was considered rare in most places, but the number of cases increased worldwide to pandemic proportions (Orkin, Maibach, 1978). The number of cases of scabies in the United States and other places is rising due to sexual transmission because the parasite is acquired by prolonged contact with infected individuals (Mellanby, 1985; Routh et al. 1994). The transmission of species of *Sarcoptes* from animals to humans has also been documented (Mitra et al. 1995). Fomites are relatively unimportant in transmission of the infection. The infection is common in residential homes for the elderly (Burns, 1987; CDC, 1988) and in hospices for human immune deficiency virus (HIV)-infected individuals (Moss, Salisbury, 1991). In hospital settings, outbreaks sometimes occur after treatment of patients with Norwegian scabies (Cardenes Santana et al. 1993; Hsueh et al. 1992).

Clinical Findings. The main clinical symptom of scabies is symmetrical itching on the skin of the finger webs (Fig. 28–5 A–B), sides of the digits, and especially the flexor surface of the wrist, usually at night. The hands are often the first area involved, frequently with eczematous lesions on the finger webs and the sides of the digits. From these areas the lesions may extend to the elbows, buttocks, and upper thighs. In females the breast, and in males the penis and scrotum, may be involved. In infants the disease affects the face and the soles of the feet (Epstein, Orkin, 1985).

The most common lesion produced by *Sarcoptes* is a burrow, seen grossly as a wavy line in the epidermis, at the end of which is the female in a small blister (Fig. 28–5 A–B). Small, erythematous, often excoriated papules with minor inflammatory changes are common in other areas of the body. Scratching usually leads to denudation of the epithelium and secondary infection that usually outlines the typical burrows. In some cases, nodular lesions and eczematous plaques develop in the elbows and genitals, usually appearing as small, firm masses. In clean persons, the infection presents with minimal symptoms that are difficult to diagnose; topical or systemic corticosteroids ameliorate the symptoms and signs. In small children, burrows are often not seen and the dominant picture is eczematiform; the distribution of the lesions is usually different from the norm.

One complication of scabies observed especially in developing countries is acute glomerulonephritis due to secondary infection of the skin lesions with nephritogenic strains of beta-hemolytic streptococci. Another superimposed bacterial infection is *Staphylococcus aureus*; in an elderly patient, this infection simulated a drug-induced erythroderma (Shelley et al. 1988).

Norwegian Scabies. One form of scabies, known as *Norwegian* or *crusted scabies*, is an opportunistic, disseminated disease with numerous exfoliating scales and a large number of mites (Fig. 28–5 C–D). The disease occurs in hosts who are immune-suppressed after organ transplantation (Espy, Jolly, 1976; Paterson et al. 1973) and for other reasons (Anolik, Rudolph, 1976), such as disseminated lupus (Chutimunt, 1996; Wanke et al. 1992); in patients with leukemia and in those with disorders such as mental retardation, senile dementia, and various neurologic diseases (Barnes et al. 1987); and at least once during pregnancy (Judge, Kobza-Black, 1995). Infants 2 to 9 months old

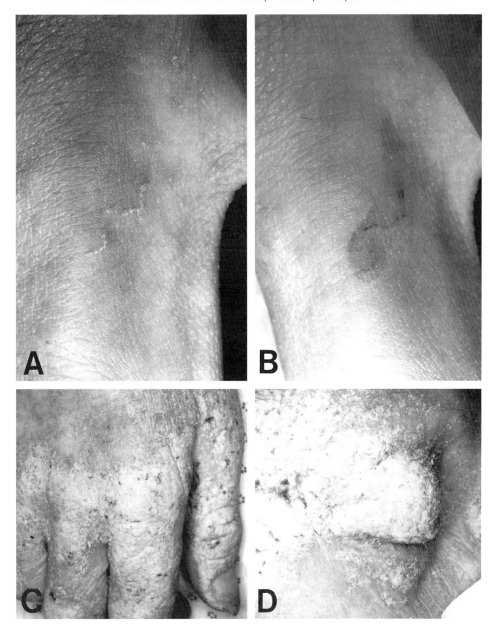

Fig. 28–5. *Sarcoptes*, **clinical lesions.** *A*, **The typical burrow in the skin.** *B*, **The same lesion after being stained with India ink stain to visualize the burrow.** *C* **and** *D*, **Hand and face of an individual with Norwegian scabies. (Courtesy of B.C. Lamkin, M.D., Department of Dermatology, University Hospitals of Cleveland and Case Western Reserve University School of Medicine, Cleveland, Ohio.)**

and some receiving prolonged topical steroid therapy also develop the disease (Camassa et al. 1995). Norwegian scabies also occurs in individuals with HIV infection (Ferrer et al. 1994; Glover et al. 1987; Sadick et al. 1986). This form of the infestation is highly contagious and often results in small epidemics (Orkin, 1985).

Pathology. The histologic changes due to scabies often affect all layers of the skin and sometimes the subcutaneous tissues. In histologic sections the burrows usually appear as empty holes in the cornified layer of the epidermis, with their roofs usually composed of orthokeratotic and parakeratotic cells. Occasionally, the female is found in the burrow (Fig. 28–6 *A–D*), but

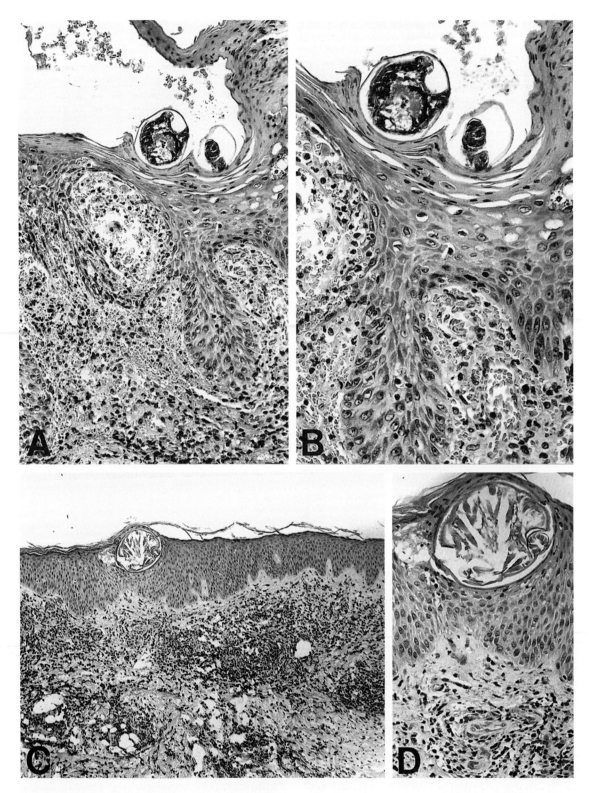

Fig. 28–6. *Sarcoptes*, microscopic lesion, sections stained with hematoxylin and eosin stain. *A*, Medium-power view of a section from a skin biopsy specimen shows a tunnel with two parasites. Note the inflammatory reaction, ×180. *B*, Higher magnification, ×280. *C*, Low-power view of another section from another biopsy specimen showing the marked lymphocytic inflammatory reaction; in some areas the infiltrate is perivascular. Note the tunnel with a female parasite, ×70. *D*, Higher magnification, ×180. (Courtesy of T.M. Zaim, M.D., Department of Dermatology and Pathology, University Hospitals of Cleveland, Case Western Reserve University School of Medicine, Cleveland, Ohio.)

more often the eggs occur in different stages of development. If the mite is found, several structures of the exoskeleton and the internal organs can be identified (Head et al. 1990). The dermis has an inflammatory infiltrate composed of lymphocytes, histiocytes, and eosinophils (Fig. 28–6 *A–B*). The papular lesions sometimes do not have burrows, but the cellular infiltrate is identical to that caused by lesions with burrows.

Nodular scabies has a dense inflammatory infiltrate of the dermis (Fig. 28–6 *C*). Most of the cells are lymphocytes, mixed with small numbers of plasma cells, eosinophils, and atypical mononuclear cells, some of which are found in mitosis. These changes have been confused with reticulosis (Cochran et al. 1976). Often the infiltrate extends down to the subcutaneous fat. A perivascular infiltrate is sometimes prominent, as is a vasculitis with fibrin and inflammatory cells in the walls. The epidermis is often hyperkeratotic; mites or their eggs are usually absent.

Norwegian scabies is characterized histologically by a massive orthokeratosis and parakeratosis with abundant mites, nymphs, and eggs in different stages of development (Fig. 28–7 *A–B*). The burrows are often stacked on top of each other and the dermis is thick, with a psoriatic appearance. The rete ridges are elongated, and the space between them has abundant collagen and an inflammatory infiltrate with lymphocytes and plasma cells.

Diagnosis. The diagnosis of scabies is usually clinical, based on the history and the typical appearance of the lesions. Examination of epidermal scrapings rarely reveals the organisms because their number is low. In Norwegian scabies, the number of *Sarcoptes* organisms is higher and they are easy to demonstrate. Biopsy specimens are rarely taken for the sole purpose of diagnosing scabies and only in cases where the infection is not suspected clinically. The mites are rarely present in sections of biopsy specimens; more often, only empty burrows are found. The infiltrate and the burrows are suggestive of scabies, but they are not diagnostic. If they

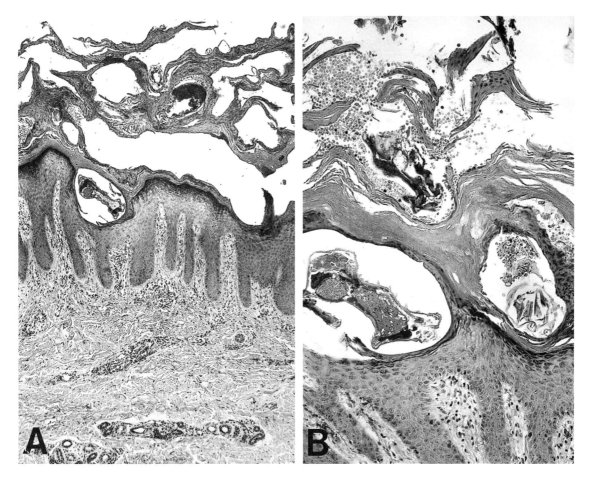

Fig. 28–7. *Sarcoptes*, **Norwegian scabies, sections stained with hematoxylin and eosin stain. *A*, Low-power view showing thickening of the squamous epithelium and numerous burrows with parasites, ×55. *B*, Higher magnification, ×140.**

are found, a search should be made for the mites in skin scrapings

In histologic sections, the mites are identified on the basis of their chitinous exoskeleton, the presence of legs, and some internal structures (Fig. 28–6 D; Head et al. 1990). The location of the tunnels in the epidermis and the size of the mite suggest *Sarcoptes*, but even if the adults are found, the species cannot be determined in tissue sections. A generic identification, such as "*Sarcoptes* species," is best, taking into consideration that other species from animals also infect humans.

Flies—Myiasis

A large group of insects (arthropods with three pairs of legs and usually wings), classified under the suborder Cyclorrhapha, comprise most of the organisms commonly known as *flies*. In general, flies have a worldwide distribution and play an important role in medical and veterinary medicine, both as vectors of numerous pathogenic agents and as producers of diseases. Flies that are vectors of pathogenic agents belong to two groups. One group feeds on blood or secretions of hosts that contain pathogenic organisms; in the fly, these organisms develop into infective stages that are inoculated into or deposited on the new host. The other group of flies acts as mechanical transporters or carriers of biologic agents transmitted by contamination directly to the new host or indirectly to its food.

The life cycle of flies is generally similar to that of other arthropods. Some flies lay eggs that develop into larvae (maggots), while others lay the larvae directly. The larvae develop into pupae and finally into the adult flies. Each species of fly has larvae or maggots that require distinct biologic conditions for development. If the larvae use an animal or a human host, the result is a condition known as *myiasis* (from the Greek *myia* = "fly"). In general, larvae living on feces or decaying dead bodies are scavengers and produce *accidental myiasis*; larvae living on necrotic tissue (involving wounds) produce *semispecific myiasis*; and those that require living tissues for their development produce *obligatory myiasis*. Although these three forms of myiasis occur in humans, a classification based on the organ system in which they occur is often more useful: intestinal, ocular, urinary, pulmonary, and cutaneous myiasis.

Reports of myiasis in different tissues and organs are relatively common throughout the world, and more often than not, cases of myiasis are seen by surgical pathologists as *maggots*. Maggots submitted for diagnosis come from dead tissues (accidental myiasis), from

wounds or from individuals in coma (semispecific myiasis), or from healthy individuals (obligatory myiasis). Classification of the maggot in these cases is often difficult and requires a specialist. Sometimes maggots are alive when submitted; in these cases, under suitable conditions, they complete their life cycle in the laboratory. Exact classification is possible based on the characteristics of the adult fly. There are several classic books dealing extensively with myiasis in humans, and the reader who wishes to learn more about this subject should consult them (James, 1948; Zumpt, 1965).

The cases of myiasis studied by the anatomic pathologist at the surgical desk are usually based on larva or several larvae (maggots) received for examination. The larvae are often retrieved from a comatose person or a dead body; sometimes they are removed surgically from a patient. These larvae are gray to white, have some segmentation of the body, and measure 0.8 to 1.5 cm in length. Often the larva is cylindrical, uniform in diameter, or tapering slightly toward one or both ends; at other times, the larva is more globose. Some larvae have circumferential rows of dark spines; at one end, the larva has a pair of chitinous structures, the spiracles, which are used for breathing. The spiracles have a characteristic morphology that allows some classification, usually to the group or genus level.

The larvae of flies that produce myiasis in humans belong to many genera that are found worldwide. Although myiasis is more common in the tropical areas, many species of flies in the temperate and arctic zones also produce infections. A discussion of some of the biologic characteristics of the flies that produce myiasis, their anatomic location in the host, and their clinicopathologic manifestations follows.

Cutaneous Myiasis

Cutaneous myiasis is perhaps the most common form of myiasis in animals and humans; it is produced by many species of flies belonging to several genera. These flies have different types of development (life cycles), and thus the manner in which they become parasites varies. In general, there are two types of cutaneous myiasis.

1. Invasion of the epidermis or upper dermis by several species of *Gasterophilus* (*G. intestinalis, G. nasalis,* and *G. hemorrhoidalis*) produces a form of cutaneous larva migrans described originally as *creeping eruption* or *myiasis linearis* (see Chapter 16).

The species of *Gasterophilus* are flies commonly known as *horse botflies*. The female attaches the eggs to the hair shafts of horses near the mouth. The eggs hatch, and the larvae are licked off by the horse and ingested. The larvae develop attached to the intestine, after which they are passed with feces to pupate in soil and transform into adults. In its natural hosts, *Gasterophilus* sometimes burrows into the skin and migrates toward the stomach to continue its development.

Human infections with *Gasterophilus* are unusual and have been reported less often in recent decades (Heath et al. 1968). In humans, the larvae enter the skin and produce the typical serpiginous migration of cutaneous larva migrans. The difference is that the *Gasterophilus* larva is larger and is easily recognized at the end of the tunnel, removed, and identified (see Chapter 14). On occasion, *Gasterophilus* has produced intestinal and ocular myiasis in humans (see below).

2. Invasion of the dermis and subcutaneous tissues by many species belonging to the genera *Hypoderma*, *Dermatobia*, *Cordylobya*, *Auchmeromya*, *Wohlfahrtia*, and *Cuterebra* produces lesions resembling a furuncle that contains the maturing larva. In its natural host the larva eventually leaves the skin, drops to the ground, pupates, and develops to adulthood.

The eggs of flies producing this form of cutaneous myiasis arrive in the skin in different ways. Species of *Hypoderma* (*H. bovis* and *H. lineatum*), or *cattle botflies*, and *H. tarandi*, the reindeer warble fly, attach their eggs to hairs of their hosts. The larvae hatch and penetrate the skin, usually through a hair follicle, and grow slowly up to 2.5 cm in length within about 6 months; they usually occur in the temperate zones. Species of *Hypoderma* are the most important flies producing cutaneous myiasis in Europe (Doby et al. 1985; Kearney et al. 1991). Species of *Dermatobia* (*D. hominis*) attach their eggs to the ventral surface of the abdomen of a mosquito, and the larvae drop on the skin while the mosquito feeds. The larvae then penetrate the skin and develop in a manner similar to that of *Hypoderma*; the distribution of *D. hominis* is tropical. Many cases occur in the United States and in European countries in travelers to tropical areas (Caumes et al. 1991; Chelmowski, Troy, 1991; Dondero et al. 1979). Several days after they return, patients present with the typical furuncle, which contains the larva (Arya et al. 1988). Species of *Cordylobya* (*C. anthropophaga* and *C. rodhaini*), the *tumbu flies*, deposit their eggs in decaying matter (feces), where they hatch; the larvae penetrate the skin when the host makes contact with them. These two species

occur in tropical Africa. *Cordylobya antropophaga* also occurs in northern Europe (Baily, Moody, 1985). *Auchmeromya* (*A. senegalensis*) also occurs in tropical Africa and is perhaps the only known blood-sucking fly in this group adapted to feed on humans. The eggs deposited on the skin grow into larvae that penetrate and develop in the subcutaneous tissues. Species of *Wohlfahrtia* (*W. vigil vigil* and *W. vigil opaca*) are larviparous and deposit larvae on the skin, which penetrate to the subcutaneous tissues. *Wohlfahrtia vigil vigil* occurs in Canada and the northern United States and *W. vigil opaca* in Utah, Colorado, and California. Both species are especially attracted to children and are responsible for most cases of cutaneous myiasis in children in North America. *Cuterebra* has more than 20 known species in North America, which deposit their eggs in vegetation. The eggs hatch in response to a warm-blooded animal and usually enter through the mucous membranes or cuts in the skin to develop in the subcutaneous tissues. Cases of *Cuterebra* are reported sporadically in almost every state in the eastern half of the United States; cases also occur in Canada and Central America (Baird et al. 1982). Identification of the species is difficult because the immature stages of most members of *Cuterebra* have not been described (Baird et al. 1982, 1989).

The general clinical and pathologic characteristics of the lesions produced by these flies are similar. Once the larva contacts the skin, it burrows and produces small tracks in the dermis. Soon the larva becomes stationary or burrows perpendicularly to the epidermis and begins to grow slowly in the dermis and the subcutaneous tissues. At first, there is a small blister or papule, that sometimes itches intensely. As growth progresses, the larva molts several times and the lesion becomes larger, developing the characteristics of a furuncle (Cogen et al. 1987; Grogan et al. 1987; Lane et al. 1987). Movements of the larva can be felt, and there is usually an opening on the epidermis, through which the posterior end of the parasite protrudes slightly, on which the spiracles of the larva can be seen as two dark dots. The inflammatory reaction around the parasite and the itching become more intense (Grogan et al. 1987), and the affected individual usually seeks medical attention. In some cases, especially in young children, the larva may burrow deeper into the tissues and organs. In at least one case, *D. hominis* entered the fontanelle of an infant and migrated to the brain, with fatal consequences (Rossi, Zucoloto, 1973). Surgical removal of the larva is the treatment of choice, and the specimen is usually sent to the laboratory for examination (*color plate* XVI *E* and Fig. 28–8 *A–B*).

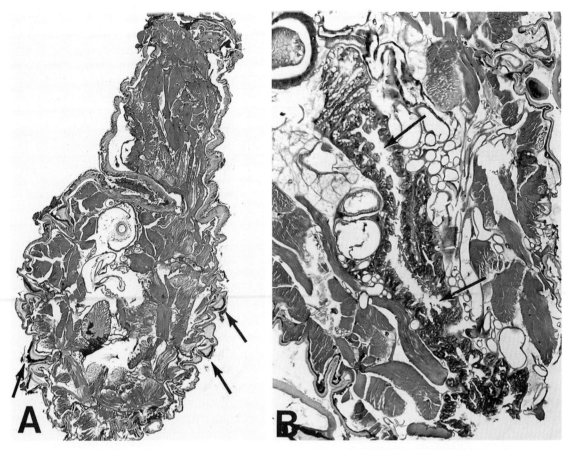

Fig. 28–8. Myiasis of the scalp of a woman who traveled to Belize and returned with a lesion (furuncle), from which a fly larva was removed and submitted for histologic examination, hematoxylin and eosin stain. *A,* Longitudinal section illustrating the general shape of the larva. Note the spines on the cuticle (arrows). The place where it was acquired, the size and shape of the larva, and the morphologic characteristics are those of *Dermatobia hominis,* ×22. *B,* Higher magnification of another section from the same larva showing the intestine (arrows), ×52. (From J.V. Suarez-Hoyos, M.D., Patterson and Coleman Labs, Tampa, Florida.)

One recommended form of therapy for furuncular myiasis is the application of raw bacon on the furuncle, where the larva with its two dark spiracles is visible. Within a few hours the larva migrates into the bacon deeply enough to be removed with tweezers, after which the lesion heals without complications (Bernhard, 1993; Brewer et al. 1993). The bacon interrupts airflow to the larva, which stimulates its migration; other similar products, such as petrolatum, will do just as well (Campos et al. 1994).

Myiasis of Wounds, Ulcers, and Moribund Flesh

Many flies producing myiasis deposit their eggs or larvae on wounds (Magnarelli, Andreadis, 1981), ulcers, or moribund flesh (comatose individuals). In these circumstances, the larvae feed on bacteria or necrotic tissue (Fig. 28–9 *A–D*). Contamination of wounds by maggots to produce a therapeutic effect (clearing the infection and allowing granulation tissue to develop) is a practice known for centuries and used in modern medicine. Some species of maggots may penetrate the wound and produce lesions similar to the ones described above.

The larvae of flies commonly infesting wounds, ulcers, and moribund flesh include *Chrysomia* (*C. bezziana*), which also lays its eggs in normal skin and may invade other sites (see below; it occurs only in Africa and Asia), *Calliphora* (*C. vomitoria* and *C. vicina*), *Phaenicia* (*P. sericata* and *P. cuprina*), *Cochliomya* (*C. macellaria* and *C. hominivorax*), and *Phormia* (*P. regina*). *Phormia regina* occurs in the United States and produced extensive lesions in the scalp of a terminally

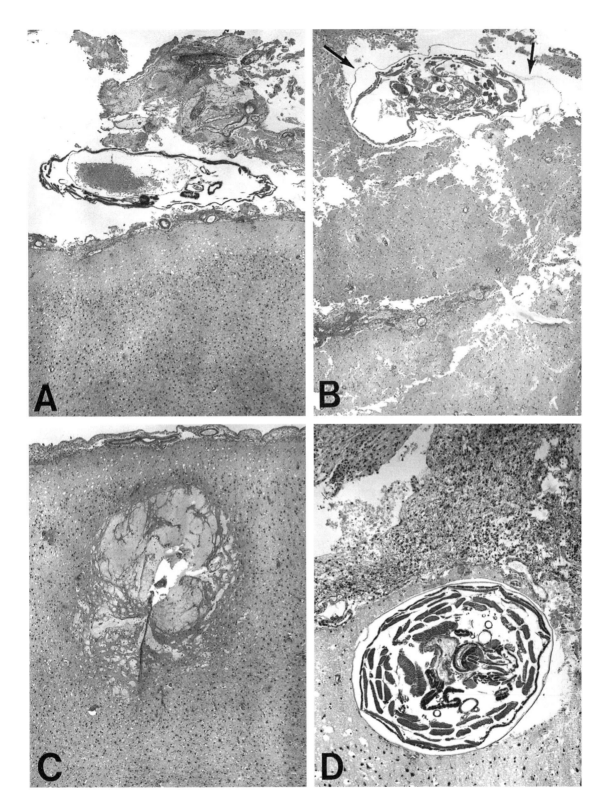

Fig. 28–9. Myiasis of moribund flesh, section stained with hematoxylin and eosin stain. Maggots found in the central nervous system of a young woman with a crushing wound of the skull; she remained unconscious for 2 days in the woods before dying. *A*, Longitudinal section of a larva in the meninges, ×22. *B*, Another larva in the brain tissue, recently molted, as indicated by the shed cuticle (arrows), ×213. *C*, Track left by one larva migrating postmortem through the brain. Note the lack of inflammation, ×28. *D*, The larva on cross section. Note the inflammatory infiltrate in *A* and *D*, ×70. (Preparations courtesy of A. Chang, M.D., Cuyahoga County Coroner's Office, Cleveland, Ohio.)

ill woman (Alexis, Mittleman, 1988). It deposits eggs in the wounds, while species of *Sarcophaga* (*S. hemorrhoidalis, S. fuscicauda,* and *S. carnaria*) and *Wohlfahrtia* (*W. magnifica*) deposit larvae. Cases of deep skin ulcers infested with maggots of *Musca domestica* (Burgess, Davies, 1991) and *Parasarcophaga argyrostoma* in England (Burgess, Spraggs, 1992) are also on record.

These types of myiasis usually present clinically as maggots on a wound (Fig. 28–10; Alexis, Mittleman, 1988; Arbit et al. 1986) or on an unconscious individual. The latter happens even in clean, well-maintained hospitals (Smith, Clevenger, 1986). Sometimes the maggots crawl out of the nose or other body cavities or out of tracheostomy tubes (Josephson, Krajden, 1993). Maggots occur most commonly in corpses left unattended in the environment and usually autopsied for medicolegal reasons. In these cases, maggots may be found anywhere on the outside of the body or, if there is a wound, in cavities or internal organs (*color plate* XVI *F–G*).

Ocular Myiasis

Invasion of the eye and eye structures by maggots sometimes occurs. Maggots invade most ocular structures, including the conjunctiva, cornea, anterior chamber,

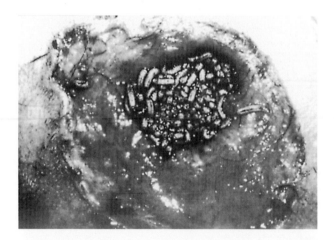

Fig. 28–10. Maggots in a scalp wound. This individual had an ulcerating squamous cell carcinoma of the scalp in an area of previous surgery for craniopharyngioma treated with radiation therapy. The ulcer was infested by larvae of *Sarcophaga*. (In: Arbit, E., Varim, R.E., and Brem, S.S. 1986. Myiatic scalp and skull infection with Diptera *Sarcophaga*: case report. Neurosurgery 18:361–362. Reproduced with permission.)

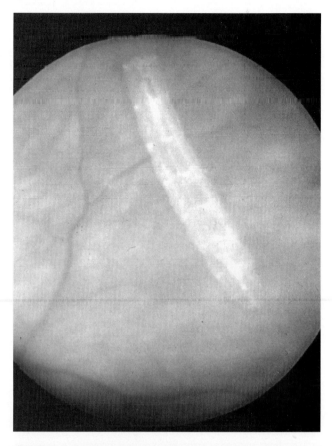

Fig. 28–11. Maggot (fly larva) in the posterior chamber of a patient. Note that the identification here cannot go beyond "maggot" based on the shape and segmentation of the body. (Courtesy of M.D. Little, Ph.D., Department of Tropical Medicine, School of Public Health and Tropical Medicine, Tulane University, New Orleans, New Orleans.)

lens, and vitreous. In any of these structures, the larva may cause significant damage. In general, the parasites occur either outside the eye (external ophthalmomyiasis; Fig. 28–12 *A–B*) or inside (internal ophthalmomyiasis; Fig. 28–11). Most species of maggots recovered from the eye are the same species found in subcutaneous tissues, or in wounds and ulcers, for example *Hypoderma, Chrysomia, Sarcophaga, Cuterebra, Cochliomya,* and *Wohlfahrtia* (*W. magnifica*). In addition, *Oestrus* (*O. ovis*), the sheep bot or nasal bot fly, and *Rhinostrus* (*R. purpureus*), the Russian gadfly, have both been isolated from the eye in many places (Dar et al. 1980). External ocular myiasis caused by *O. ovis* occurs worldwide, is common in the Middle East (Hira et al. 1993), and is reported sporadically in the United States (Heyde et al. 1986).

In cases of internal ocular invasion, the species of the larva is generally difficult to identify because it is

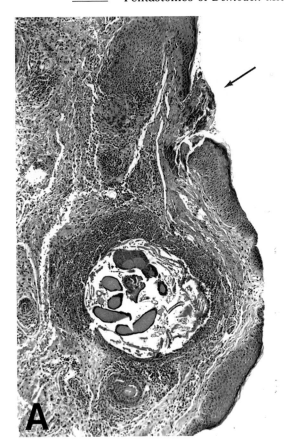
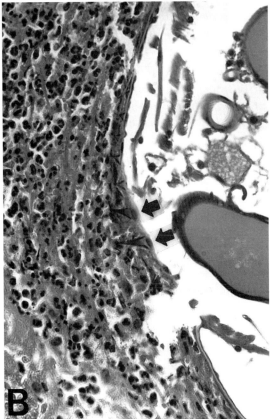

Fig. 28–12. Myiasis of the skin, probably due to *Oestrus ovis*, the sheep bot fly, in a woman from northwestern Ohio. This person felt a sharp pain in the left lower eyebrow and developed conjunctivitis within 24 hours. Examination revealed a foreign object partially buried in the dermis of the eyebrow. Sections of a biopsy specimen showed a fly larva tentatively identified as *O. ovis*, sec- **tion stained with hematoxylin and eosin stain. *A*, Low-power view of the histologic section showing the area of penetration (arrow), a cross section of the larva, and the marked acute inflammatory reaction, ×70. *B*, Higher magnification illustrating some internal structures of the parasite, a row of sharply pointed spines on the surface (arrows), and the polymorphonuclear cell infiltrate, ×450.**

usually destroyed (Currier et al. 1995). The general name *maggot*, *fly larva*, or *ocular myiasis* often suffices (Chaine, Bayen, 1986; Chodosh, Clarridge, 1992). In the Middle East, external ophthalmomyiasis produced by the nasal bot fly is common (Amr et al. 1993), often occurring in the conjunctiva (Cameron et al. 1991). *Gasterophilus intestinalis* has been found in one case of internal ophthalmomyiasis (Anderson, 1935). In the retina, the larva produces a marked inflammatory reaction (Gass, Lewis, 1976).

Intestinal Myiasis

Intestinal myiasis is the invasion of the stomach or intestinal mucosa by fly larva. Exact proof of coloniza- tion of the intestine by the larva is difficult, and therefore the majority of reported cases are doubtful. This is especially true when the report involves a species other than *Gasterophilus* (Arya et al. 1988; Barkin et al. 1983; CDC, 1985). Most reported cases of "intestinal myiasis" are due to larvae of species that oviposit or larviposit on food destined for consumption. Although most larvae and eggs ingested in this manner are destroyed in the stomach and the intestine, some may survive and are evacuated in the stools without producing symptoms (Cheong et al. 1973). Rarely do larvae invade the intestinal wall; *Gasterophilus* has been found in the stomachs of humans. Some families and genera of flies with species reported from the gastrointestinal tract are Muscidae, Calliphoridae, Phoridae, and *Clogmia*. The main symptoms of these infections are abdominal pain and vomiting; larvae are sometimes found in the vomitus (Smith, Thomas, 1979). In rare cases the larvae of *Gasterophilus* occur in the lungs, producing coin lesions (Ahmed, Miller, 1969).

Urogenital Myiasis

This form of myiasis is also difficult to document because the larvae recovered in urine samples often result from contamination of the container or the sample in the laboratory. The larvae invade the labia and the vagina, from which they are easily retrieved for examination and identification (Biery et al. 1979; Cilla et al. 1992). A species of *Chrysomia* produced the infection in a woman in Thailand (Koranantakul et al. 1991). In women, urinary myiasis is due to larvae entering the bladder through the urethra (Disney, Kurahashi, 1978).

In men, urinary myiasis is also acquired through the urethra. In some cases, the lesion is purely urethral (Gupta et al. 1983); in others, the larva migrates to the urinary bladder. A single *Chrysomia bezziana* was recovered from the urethra of a 36-year-old woman with severe abdominal pain and slight dysuria (Jdalayer et al. 1978). Another patient, in India, presented with acute urine retention and was treated; 2 weeks later, the patient passed about 10 to 15 maggots with each urine void several times; the species was *Magaselia scalaris* (Singh, Rana, 1989). A larva from a species of *Eristalis* was recovered from a patient who presented with symptoms of ureterolithiasis that subsided after the larva was passed with the urine (Korzets et al. 1993).

Myiasis of the Ears

The larvae of flies that usually invade the ears are the same species that occur on the skin or in wounds, ulcers, and moribund flesh (see above). This form, which is more common in children than in adults, presents as restlessness, a foul-smelling mucopurulent discharge, otalgia, and itching. Sometimes there is a history of small worms crawling out of the ear. In Australia, some cases involved the larvae of *Calliphora nociva* (Morris, Weinstein, 1986) and *Parasarcophaga crassipalpis* (Morris, 1987); in Israel, the parasite was *Sarcophaga hemorrhoidalis* (Braverman et al. 1994).

Other Sites

Another anatomic site susceptible to invasion by the larvae of flies is the gums (Anil et al. 1989; Sahba et al. 1984). The nasal sinuses may also be colonized (Magnarelli, Andreadis, 1981; Nevill et al. 1969; Smith, Clevenger, 1986). In some cases, invasion of the nasal cavity by the larvae of *O. ovis* (nasal bot fly) requires surgery to extract the maggots (Badia, Lund, 1994); in others, the maggots are sneezed out (Lucientes et al. 1997). The nasopharynx is sometimes involved (Mohammed, Smith, 1976). A species of *Magaselia* infected a boy's throat in Texas; he expectorated several larvae after feeling a crawling sensation (Carpenter, Chastain, 1992). Invasion of the brain by *Hypoderma* (François et al. 1987; Kalelioglu et al. 1989) and *Dermatobia* (Rossi, Zucoloto, 1973) has also occurred, especially in children; the larvae may enter through the eye. Diagnosis and identification of fly larvae in the brain, based on positive serologic reactions to larval antigens, without recovery or visualization of the parasite, are not credible (Danjou et al. 1975; Labbe et al. 1983).

Diagnosis. As stated above, the diagnosis of myiasis is based mostly on recognition of the larva. The parasite is identified by the morphologic characteristics of the larva studied in toto under a stereoscope. Often the species cannot be determined, but only the general group, such as the family or the genus—a task carried out by a specialist. Rarely, sections of the larva appear in tissue sections, most commonly in tissues retrieved during medicolegal autopsies performed on bodies left in the environment (Fig. 28–9 and *color plate* XVI *E–G*). Usually the only possible diagnosis in tissue sections is that of a maggot or fly larva (Fig. 28–8).

Tunga penetrans—Tungiasis

Fleas are usually vectors of important human pathogens, such as plague and murine typhus; sometimes they also produce dermatitis. *Tunga penetrans* is the only flea capable of invading the epidermis and producing lesions sometimes encountered by the anatomic pathologist. Known also as the *sandflea*, *T. penetrans* probably originated in the American continent and was introduced to Africa sometime after the discovery of America

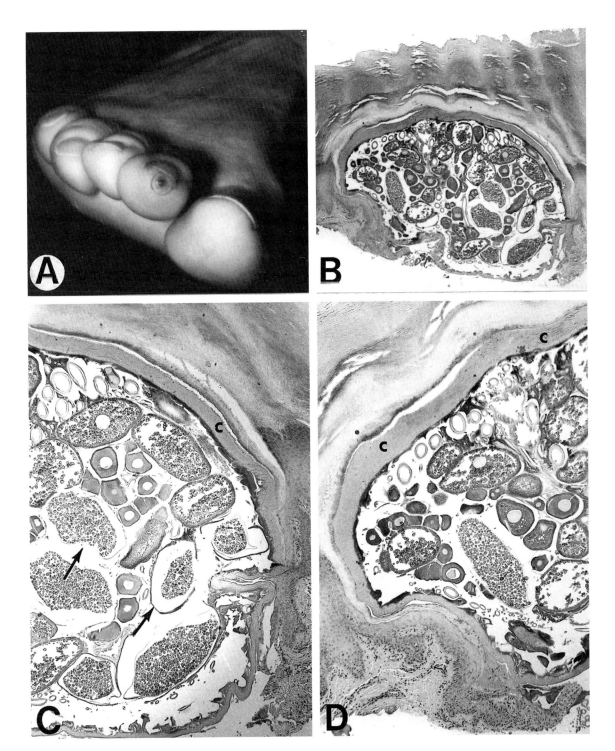

Fig. 28–13. *Tunga penetrans* in human skin. *A*, Gross photograph illustrating the typical appearance of tungiasis in a person who visited an endemic area. (Courtesy of B. Michel, M.D., Cleveland, Ohio.) *B–D*. Histologic sections of a specimen removed from another patient, stained with hematoxylin and eosin stain. *B*, Low-power view of epidermis shows the parasite. The section is off-center; thus the opening on the skin, by which the parasite communicates with the outside, is not seen. Note the typical intradermal location, ×22. *C* and *D*, Higher magnification illustrating the female with numerous developing eggs (arrows), the exoskeleton of the parasite (c), the squamous epithelium, and the minimal inflammatory infiltrate, ×55.

729

(Hoeppli, 1963). It is now widely prevalent in rural areas of both tropical America and Africa. Cases of *Tunga* infection imported from endemic areas occur in Europe (Bolzinger et al. 1994; Schmidt et al. 1993; Wardhaugh, Norris, 1994). They are also seen in the United States (Spielman et al. 1986; Vennos et al. 1995) and Australia (Spradbery et al. 1994), often baffling both dermatologists and pathologists.

The life cycle of *Tunga* is similar to that of other arthropods. The female is buried in the epidermis, where it lays eggs that are passed to the environment through an opening in the skin. The eggs hatch and produce larvae that eventually form pupae and later become adults. After copulation, the female has a phase of obligatory parasitism in the skin of humans or other animals, where the eggs are laid (Fig. 28–14). The adult female is less than 1 mm when it first enters the skin; it grows to 8 mm when fully developed and gravid.

Clinical Findings. The main symptoms of tungiasis are intense pruritus of the affected area, with continuous scratching. The parasite usually enters the skin between the toes, the soles of the feet, or, less frequently, other areas, usually those exposed to contact

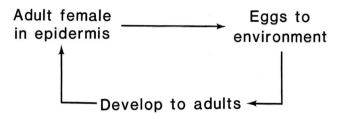

Fig. 28–14. *Tunga penetrans*, schematic representation of the life cycle.

with the organisms in soil. At first, the female causes irritation at the site of penetration, where a slight elevation begins forming. Ulceration of the central portion of this lesion follows, with formation of a small amount of pus. The lesion grows larger as the gravid female develops in the epidermis. A small, ulcerated portion of the epidermis shows the posterior end of the parasite exposed for breathing, evacuation of ejecta, and laying of eggs (Fig. 28–13 A). Scratching of the lesion may produce secondary bacterial infections, and many *Tunga* located close together result in confluent areas of ulceration. In some patients with heavy infections, the lesions extend to the fingers, elbows, and knees (Fig. 28–15 A–B).

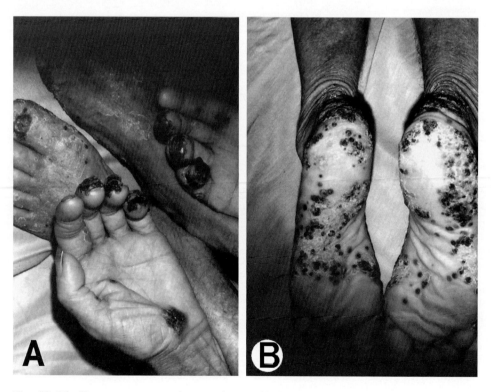

Fig. 28–15. *Tunga penetrans* in a patient suffering from a heavy infection. *A*, Note the invasion of the fingers and palm of the hand. *B*, The soles of the feet are heavily parasitized.

Pathology. In endemic areas where both physicians and the public are familiar with tungiasis, the pathologist almost never receives skin biopsy specimens from affected persons. In countries where the infestation is unknown, *Tunga* is usually seen in travelers to endemic areas. These lesions are usually excised and submitted for histologic examination.

The gross specimen is a rounded or ellipsoidal portion of skin, sometimes with the central superficial ulceration, which is seen as a dark or grayish area (Fig. 28–13 *A*). The tissue around the ulceration is whitish, sometimes glistening. If the tissue is cut and embedded to obtain sections perpendicular to the central area of necrosis, the appearance of the lesion and the parasite correlates with the clinical description. Off-center or tangential sections do not show the opening in the epidermis (Fig. 28–13 *B*).

Microscopically, the flea is seen within the epidermis, not in a burrow but "enveloped" by hypertrophied squamous epithelium, with elongated papillae that grow to the base of the parasite (Fig. 28–13 *B–C*). Any inflammatory infiltrate is usually minimal, consisting mainly of mononuclear cells, unless a superimposed bacterial infection is present (Fig. 28–13 *D*). The characteristic exoskeleton, striated muscles, intestine, and eggs are diagnostic features of the parasite. For practical purposes, the location in the epidermis and the size of the parasite are diagnostic (Fig. 28–13 *C–D*).

References

Ahmed MJ, Miller A, 1969. Pulmonary coin lesion containing a horse bot, *Gasterophilus*. Report of a case of myiasis. Am. J. Clin. Pathol. 52:414–419

Alexis JB, Mittleman RE, 1988. An unusual case of *Phormia regina* myiasis of the scalp. Am. J. Clin. Pathol. 90:734–737

Amichai B, Grunwald MH, Avinoach I, Halevy S, 1992. Granulomatous rosacea associated with *Demodex folliculorum*. Int. J. Dermatol. 31:718–719

Amr ZS, Amr BA, Abo Shehada MN, 1993. Ophthalmomyiasis externa caused by *Oestrus ovis* L. in the Ajloun area of northern Jordan. Ann. Trop. Med. Parasitol. 87:259–262

Anderson WB, 1935. Ophthalmomyiasis: a review of the literature and a report of a case of opthalmomyiasis interna posterior. Am. J. Ophthalmol. 18:699–705

Anil S, Jacob OA, Hari S, 1989. Oral myiasis: a case report. Ann. Dent. 48:28–30

Anolik MA, Rudolph RI, 1976. Scabies simulating Darier disease in an immunosuppressed host. Arch. Dermatol. 112:73–74

Arbit E, Varon RE, Brem SS, 1986. Myiatic scalp and skull infection with Diptera: *Sarcophaga*: case report. Neurosurgery 18:361–362

Arlian LG, Vyszenski-Moher DL, 1988. Life cycle of *Sarcoptes scabiei* var. *canis*. J. Parasitol. 74:427–430

Arya TV, Sehgal R, Bhandari S, Virk K, 1988. Human intestinal myiasis. J. Assoc. Physicians India. 36:168–169

Ashack RJ, Frost ML, Norins AL, 1989. Papular pruritic eruption of *Demodex* folliculitis in patients with acquired immunodeficiency syndrome. J. Am. Acad. Dermatol. 21:306–307

Azar JE, 1964. An unsuccessful trial on production of parasitic pharyngitis (Halzoun) in human volunteers. Am. J. Trop. Med. Hyg. 13:582–583

Badia L, Lund VJ, 1994. Vile bodies: an endoscopic approach to nasal myiasis. J. Laryngol. Otol. 108:1083–1085

Baily GG, Moody AH, 1985. Cutaneous myiasis caused by larvae of *Cordylobia anthropophaga* acquired in Europe. Br. Med. J. Clin. Res. Ed. 290:1473–1474

Baird CR, Podgore JK, Sabrosky CW, 1982. *Cuterebra* myiasis in humans: six new case reports from the United States with a summary of known cases (Diptera: Cuterebridae). J. Med. Entomol. 19:263–267

Baird JK, Baird CR, Sabrosky CW, 1989. North American cuterebrid myiasis. Report of seventeen new infections of human beings and review of the disease. J. Am. Acad. Dermatol. 21:763–772

Barkin JS, MacLeod C, Hamelik P, 1983. Intestinal myiasis. Am. J. Gastroenterol. 78:560–561

Barnes L, McCallister RE, Lucky AW, 1987. Crusted (Norwegian) scabies. Arch. Dermatol. 123:95–97

Barrio J, Lecona M, Hernanz JM, Sanchez M, Gurbindo MD, Lazaro P, Barrio JL, 1996. Rosacea-like demodicosis in an HIV-positive child. Dermatology 192:143–145

Beaver PC, Jung RC, Cupp EW, 1984. *Clinical Parasitology*. Philadelphia: Lea & Febiger

Bernhard JD, 1993. Bringing on the bacon for myiasis. Lancet 342:1377–1378

Biery TL, Clegern RW, Hart WW, 1979. Two cases of phorid (Diptera: Phoridae) myiasis in Texas. J. Med. Entomol. 15:122–123

Bolzinger T, Beylot-Barry M, Babin B, Beylot C, 1994. Cas pour diagnostic. Ann. Dermatol. Venerol. 121:55–56

Bonnar E, Eustace P, Powell FC, 1993. The *Demodex* mite population in rosacea. J. Am. Acad. Dermatol. 28:443–448

Braverman I, Dano I, Saah D, Gapany B, 1994. Aural myiasis caused by flesh fly larva, *Sarcophaga haemorrhoidalis*. J Otolaryngol. 23:204–205

Brewer TF, Wilson ME, Gonzalez E, Felsenstein D, 1993. Bacon therapy and furuncular myiasis. JAMA 270:2087–2088

Brochery J-L, Djian A, Somia A, Rousset J-J, 1976. Un cas de porocephalose nymphale radiologique d'origine senegalaise. Nouv. Presse Med. 5:1755

Burgess I, 1994. *Sarcoptes scabiei* and scabies. Adv. Parasitol. 33:235–292

Burgess I, Davies EA, 1991. Cutaneous myiasis caused by the housefly, *Musca domestica*. Br. J. Dermatol. 125:377–379

Burgess I, Spraggs PD, 1992. Myiasis due to *Parasarcophaga argyrostoma*—first recorded case in Britain. Clin. Exp. Dermatol. 17:261–263

Burns DA, 1987. An outbreak of scabies in a residential home. Br. J. Dermatol. 117:359–361

Burns DA, 1992. Follicle mites and their role in disease. Clin. Exp. Dermatol. 17:152–155

Cagnard V, Nicolas-Randegger J, Dago A, 1979. Pentastomose generalisee et mortelle a *Armillifer grandis* (Hett, 1915). Bull. Soc. Pathol. Exot. 72:345–352

Callard P, Champault G, Krivitzky A, Penalba C, Rousset JJ, 1976. Nymphe vivante de porocephale decouverte en cours d'intervention. Nouv. Presse Med. 5:1756

Camassa F, Fania M, Ditano G, Silvestris AM, Lomuto M, 1995. Neonatal scabies. Cutis 56:210–212

Cameron JA, Shoukrey NM, al Garni AA, 1991. Conjunctival ophthalmomyiasis caused by the sheep nasal botfly (*Oestrus ovis*). Am. J. Ophthalmol. 112:331–334

Campos JM, Araripe AL, Pone MV, Carvalho LM, 1994. Correspondence. Furuncular myiasis. Pediatr. Infect. Dis. J. 13:937

Cannon DA, 1942. Linguatulid infestation of man. Ann. Trop. Med. Parasitol. 36:160–166

Cardenes Santana MA, Suarez Ortega S, Jimenez Santana P, Carretero Hernandez G, Artiles Vicaino J, Melado Sanchez P, 1993. Brote epidemico de escabiosis en relacion con un paciente con infeccion por el virus de la inmunodeficiencia humana y sarna noruega. Rev. Clin. Esp. 193:155–158

Carpenter TL, Chastain DO, 1992. Facultative myiasis by *Megaselia* sp. (Diptera: Phoridae) in Texas: a case report. J. Med. Entomol. 29:561–563

Caumes E, Belanger F, Brucker G, Danis M, Gentilini M, 1991. Pathologie observee au retour de voyages en dehors de l'Europe. 109 observations. Presse Med. 20:1483–1486

CDC, 1985. Intestinal myiasis—Washington. Morb. Mort. Weekly Rep. 34:141–142

CDC, 1988. Scabies in health-care facilities—Iowa. Morb. Mort. Weekly. Rep. 37:178–179

Chaine G, Bayen MC, 1986. Myiase intravitreenne. A propos d'un cas. Bull. Mem. Soc. Fr. Ophthalmol. 97:40–42

Chelmowski MK, Troy JL, 1991. But it just looked like an insect bite. . . . A case of myiasis in Wisconsin. Wis. Med. J. 90:627–628

Cheong WH, Mahadevan S, Lie KJ, 1973. A case of intestinal myiasis in Malaysia. Southeast Asian J. Trop. Med. Public Health 4:281

Chodosh J, Clarridge J, 1992. Ophthalmomyiasis: a review with special reference to *Cochliomyia hominivorax*. Clin. Infect. Dis. 14:444–449

Chutimunt N, 1996. Crusted scabies associated with systemic lupus erythematosus: response to benzyl benzoate therapy. J. Med. Assoc. Thai. 79:65–68

Cilla G, Pico F, Peris A, Idigoras P, Urbieta M, Perez Trallero F, 1992. Miasis genital humana por *Sarcophaga*. Rev. Clin. Esp. 190:189–190

Cochran T, Thomson J, Fleming KA, 1976. Histology simulating reticulosis in secondary syphilis. Br. J. Dermatol. 95:251–254

Cogen MS, Hays SJ, Dixon JM, 1987. Cutaneous myiasis of the eyelid due to *Cuterebra* larva. JAMA 258:1793–1796

Currier RW, Johnson WA, Rowley WA, Laudenbach CW, 1995. Internal ophthalmomyiasis and treatment by laser photocoagulation: a case report. Am. J. Trop. Med. Hyg. 52:311–313

Danjou R, Badinand P, Madelpech S, Garin JP, Marcon G, Mojon M, 1975. Meningite a eosinophiles: un nouveau cas d'hypodermose a *Hypoderma lineatum*. Acta Trop. 32:389–391

Dar MS, Amer MB, Dar FK, Papazotos V, 1980. Ophthalmomyiasis caused by the sheep nasal bot, *Oestrus ovis* (Oestridae) larvae, in the Benghazi area of eastern Libya. Trans. R. Soc. Trop. Med. Hyg. 74:303–306

de Leon Bojorge B, Chacon RA, 1984. Subpleural linguatulid in a Mexican child. Incidental finding in a lobectomy specimen. Patologia 22:393–398

Demmler M, de Kaspar HM, Mohring C, Klauss V, 1997. Blepharitis. *Demodex folliculorum*, associated pathogen spectrum and specific therapy. [in German English summary]. Ophthalmologe. 94:191–196

Disney RHL, Kurahashi H, 1978. A case of urogenital myiasis caused by a species of *Megaselia* (Diptera: Phoridae). J. Med. Entomol. 14:717

Doby JM, Deunff J, Couatarmanac'h A, Guiguen C, 1985. L'hypodermose humaine en France en 1984: 266 cas inventories a ce jour. Repartition des origines geographiques connues. Bull. Soc. Pathol. Exot. 78:205–215

Dominey A, Rosen T, Tschen J, 1989. Papulonodular demodicidosis associated with acquired immunodeficiency syndrome. J. Am. Acad. Dermatol. 20:197–201

Dondero T Jr, Schaffner W, Athanasiou R, Maguire W, 1979. Cutaneous myiasis in visitors to Central America. South. Med. J. 72:1508–1511

Donges J, 1966. Parasitare Abdominalcysten bei Nigerianern. Z. Tropenmed. Parasitol. 17:252–256

Drabick JJ, 1987. Pentastomiasis. Rev. Infect. Dis. 9:1087–1094

El-Hassan AM, Eltoum IA, el-Asha BM, 1991. The Marrara syndrome: isolation of *Linguatula serrata* nymphs from a patient and the viscera of goats. Trans. R. Soc. Trop. Med. Hyg. 85:309

Epstein ES, Orkin M, 1985. Scabies: clinical aspects. In: Orkin M, Maibach HI (eds), *Cutaneous Infestations and Insect Bites*. New York: Marcel Dekker, Inc., pp. 19–24

Espy PD, Jolly HW Jr, 1976. Norwegian scabies: occurrence in a patient undergoing immunosuppression. Arch. Dermatol. 112:193–196

Fain A, 1975. The pentastomida parasitic in man. Ann. Soc. Belge Med. Trop. 55:59–64

Fain A, Salvo G, 1966. Pentastomose humaine produite par des nymphes d'*Armillifer grandis* (Hett) en republique democratique du Congo. Ann. Soc. Belge Med. Trop. 46:676–681

Ferrer E, Serrano C, Drobnic L, Moiset I, Jeremias J, 1994. Correspondencia. Dermatitis hiperqueratosica en un paciente con infeccion por VIH. Enferm. Infecc. Microbiol. Clin. 12:47–48

Forton F, 1986. *Demodex* et inflammation perifolliculaire chez l'homme. Ann. Dermatol. Venereol. 113:1047–1058

Forton F, Seys B, 1993. Density of *Demodex folliculorum* in rosacea: a case-control study using standardized skin-surface biopsy. Br. J. Dermatol. 128:650–659

Francois P, Martin G, Goullier A, Plasse M, Beaudoing A, 1987. Hypodermose neuromeningee compliquee d'hydrocephalie. Interet de l'imagerie par resonance magnetique nucleaire. Presse Med. 16:1231–1233

Gardiner CH, Dyke JW, Shirley SF, 1984. Hepatic granuloma due to a nymph of *Linguatula serrata* in a woman from Michigan: a case report and review of the literature. Am. J. Trop. Med. Hyg. 33:187–189

Gass JDM, Lewis RA, 1976. Subretinal tracks in ophthalmomyiasis. Trans. Am. Acad. Ophthalmol. Otolaryngol. 81:483–490

Glover R, Young L, Goltz RW, 1987. Norwegian scabies in acquired immunodeficiency syndrome: report of a case resulting in death from associated sepsis. J. Am. Acad. Dermatol. 16:396–399

Gratama S, Van Thiel PH, 1957. Ocular localization of *Armillifer armillatus*. Doc. Med. Geogr. Trop. 9:374–376

Grogan TM, Payne CM, Payne TB, Spier C, Cromey DW, Rangel C, Richter L, 1987. Cutaneous myiasis. Immunohistologic and ultrastructural morphometric features of a human botfly lesion. Am. J. Dermatopathol. 9:228–239

Gupta SC, Kumar S, Srivastava A, 1983. Urethral myiasis. Trop. Geogr. Med. 35:73–74

Head ES, Macdonald EM, Ewert A, Apisarnthanarax P, 1990. *Sarcoptes scabiei* in histopathologic sections of skin in human scabies. Arch. Dermatol. 126:1475–1477

Heath ACG, Elliott DC, Dreadon RG, 1968. *Gasterophilus intestinalis*, the horse bot-fly as a cause of cutaneous myiasis in man. N.Z. Med. J. 68:31–32

Hellerich U, Metzelder M, 1994. Incidence of scalp involvement by *Demodex folliculorum* Simon ectoparasites in a pathologic-anatomic and forensic medicine autopsy sample [in German]. Arch. Kriminol. 194:111–118

Herzog U, Marty P, Zak F, 1985. Pentastomiasis: case report of an acute abdominal emergency. Acta Trop. 42:261–271

Heyde RR, Seiff SR, Mucia J, 1986. Ophthalmomyiasis externa in California. West. J. Med. 144:80–81

Hira PR, Hajj B, al Ali F, Hall MJ, 1993. Ophthalmomyiasis in Kuwait: first report of infections due to the larvae of *Oestrus ovis* before and after the Gulf conflict. J. Trop. Med. Hyg. 96:241–244

Hoekzema R, Hulsebosch HJ, Bos JD, 1995. Demodicidosis or rosacea: what did we treat? Br. J. Dermatol. 133:294–299

Hoeppli R, 1963. Early references to the occurrence of *Tunga penetrans* in tropical Africa. Acta Trop. 20:143–153

Hsueh PR, Lin BH, Hwang CC, Hsieh BL, Liu JC, Lin M, 1992. Nosocomial outbreak of scabies. J. Formos. Med. Assoc. 91:228–232

Humiczewska M, Kuzna W, Hermach U, 1994. Frequency of occurrence of symptomatic and asymptomatic eyelid mite infestations among inhabitants of Szczecin [in Polish. English summary]. Wiad. Parazytol. 40:69–71

Hunter WS, Higgins RP, 1960. An unusual case of human porocephalosis. J. Parasitol. 46:68

James MT, 1948. *The Flies That Cause Myasis in Man*. Washington, D.C.: Department of Agriculture Miscellaneous Pub. No. 631

Jaureguiberry JD, Carsuzaa F, Pierre C, Arnoux D, Jaubert D, 1993. Correspondence. Folliculite a *Demodex*: une cause de prurit au cours de l'infection par le virus de l'immunodeficience humaine. Ann. Med. Interne Paris 144:63–64

Jdalayer T, Maleki M, Moghtaderi M, 1978. Human urogenital myiasis caused by *Chrysomyia bezziana*. Iranian. J. Public Health 7:116–119

Josephson RL, Krajden S, 1993. An unusual nosocomial infection: nasotracheal myiasis. J. Otolaryngol. 22:46–47

Judge MR, Kobza-Black A, 1995. Crusted scabies in pregnancy. Br. J. Dermatol. 132:116–119

Kalelioglu M, Akturk G, Akturk F, Komsuoglu SS, Kuzeyli K, Tigin Y, Karaer Z, Bingol R, 1989. Intracerebral myiasis from *Hypoderma bovis* larva in a child. Case report. J. Neurosurg. 71:929–931

Kearney MS, Nilssen AC, Lyslo A, Syrdalen P, Dannevig L, 1991. Ophthalmomyiasis caused by the reindeer warble fly larva. J. Clin. Pathol. 44:276–284

Khalil GM, Schacher JF, 1965a. *Linguatula serrata* in relation to halzoun and the marrara syndrome. Am. J. Trop. Med. 14:736–746

Khalil GM, Schacher JF, 1965b. Experimental studies on the etiology of Halzoun and the Marrara syndrome I. *Fasciola hepatica* and *Dicrocoelium dendriticum*. Middle East Med. J. 2:103–110

Khouri A, 1905. Le halzoun. Arch. Parasitol. 9:78–94

Koranantakul O, Lekhakula A, Wansit R, Koranantakul Y, 1991. Cutaneous myiasis of vulva caused by the muscoid fly (*Chrysomyia* genus). Southeast Asian J. Trop. Med. Public Health 22:458–460

Korzets Z, Bernheim J, Lengy J, Gold D, 1993. Human urogenital myiasis due to *Eristalis* larva: an unusual cause of ureteric obstruction. Nephrol. Dial. Transplant. 8:874–876

Labbe A, Desvignes V, Meyer M, Campagne D, Cohen F, Dechelotte P, 1983. Meningite a *Hypoderma bovis*. A propos d'un nouveau cas pediatrique. Ann. Pediatr. Paris 30:277–280

Lane RP, Lowell CR, Griffiths WA, Sonnex TS, 1987. Human cutaneous myiasis—a review and report of three cases due to *Dermatobia hominis*. Clin. Exp. Dermatol. 12:40–45

Lang Y, Garzozi H, Epstein Z, Barkay S, Gold D, Lengy J, 1987. Intraocular pentastomiasis causing unilateral glaucoma. Br. J. Ophthalmol. 71:391–395

Lee WK, Cho BK, 1995. Taxonomical approach to scabies mites of humans and animals and their prevalence in Korea. Korean J. Parasitol. 33:85–94

Lucientes J, Clavel A, Ferrer-Dufol M, Valles H, Peribanez MA, Gracia-Salinas MJ, Castillo JA, 1997. Short report: one case of nasal human myiasis caused by third stage instar larvae of *Oestrus ovis*. Am. J. Trop. Med. Hyg. 56:608–609

Madeira NG, Sogayar MI, 1993. Prevalencia de *Demodex folliculorum* e *Demodex brevis* em uma amostra da populacao de Botucatu, Sao Paulo, Brasil. Rev. Soc. Bras. Med. Trop. 26:221–224

Magnarelli LA, Andreadis TG, 1981. Human cases of furuncular trauma and nasal myiasis in Connecticut. Am. J Trop. Med. Hyg. 30:894–896

Mellanby K, 1985. Biology of the parasite. In: Orkin M, Maibach HE (eds), *Cutaneous Infestations and Insect Bites*. New York: Marcel Dekker, Inc., pp. 9–18

Mitra M, Mahanta SK, Sen S, Ghosh C, Hati AK, 1995. Transmission of *Sarcoptes scabiei* from animal to man and its control. J. Indian Med. Assoc. 93:142–143

Mohammed N, Smith KGV, 1976. Nasopharyngeal myiasis in man caused by larvae of *Clogmia* (= *Telmetoscopus*) *albipunctatus*. Trans. R. Soc. Trop. Med. Hyg. 70:91

Morris B, 1987. First reported case of human aural myiasis caused by the flesh fly *Parasarcophaga crassipalpis* (Diptera: Sarcophagidae). J. Parasitol. 73:1068–1069

Morris B, Weinstein P, 1986. A case of aural myiasis in Australia. Med. J. Aust. 145:634–635

Moss VA, Salisbury J, 1991. Scabies in an AIDS hospice unit. Br. J Clin. Pract. 45:35–36

Nakagawa T, Sasaki M, Fujita K, Nishimoto M, Takaiwa T, 1996. *Demodex* folliculitis on the trunk of a patient with mycosis fungoides. Clin. Exp. Dermatol. 21:148–150

Nevill EM, Basson PA, Schoonraad JH, Swanepoel K, 1969. A case of nasal myiasis caused by the larvae of *Telmatoscopus albipunctatus* (Williston) 1893 (Diptera: Psychodidae). S. Afr. Med. J. 43:512–534

Orkin M, 1985. Special forms of scabies. In: Orkin M, Maibach HI (eds), *Cutaneous Infestations and Insect Bites*. New York: Marcel Dekker, Inc., pp. 25–30

Orkin M, Maibach HI, 1978. Current concepts in parasitology: This scabies pandemic. N. Engl. J. Med. 298:496–498

Paterson WD, Allen BR, Beveridge GW, 1973. Norwegian scabies during immunosuppressive therapy. Br. Med. J. 4:211–212

Pietrini P, Favennec L, Brasseur P, 1995. Correspondence. *Demodex folliculorum* in parakeratosis of the scalp in a child. Parasite 2:94

Polderman AM, Manschot WA, 1979. *Armillifer armillatus* located within the lacrimal caruncle. Acta Leidensia 47:71–77

Prathap K, Lau KS, Bolton JM, 1969. Pentastomiasis: a common finding at autopsy among Malaysian aborigines. Am. J. Trop. Med. Hyg. 18:20

Prathap K, Ramachandran CP, Haug N, 1968. Hepatic and pulmonary porocephaliasis in a Malaysian orang asli (aborigine). Med. J. Malaya 23:92–95

Redondo Mateo J, Soto Guzman O, Fernandez Rubio E, Dominguez Franjo F, 1993. *Demodex*-attributed rosacea-like lesions in AIDS. Acta Derm. Venereol. 73:437

Rendtorff RC, Deweese MW, Murrah W, 1962. The occurrence of *Linguatula serrata*, a pentastomid, within the human eye. Am. J. Trop. Med. Hyg. 11:762–764

Riley J, 1986. The biology of pentastomids. Adv. Parasitol. 25:46–128

Riley J, Banaja AA, James JL, 1978. The phylogenetic relationships of the Pentastomida. The case for their inclusion within the Crustacea. Int. J. Parasitol. 8:245–254

Rossi MA, Zucoloto S, 1973. Fatal cerebral myiasis caused by the tropical warble fly, *Dermatobia hominis*. Am. J. Trop. Med. Hyg. 22:267–269

Routh HB, Mirensky YM, Parish LC, Witkowski JA, 1994. Ectoparasites as sexually transmitted diseases. Semin. Dermatol. 13:243–247

Sadick N, Kaplan MH, Pahwa SG, Sarngadharan MG, 1986. Unusual features of scabies complicating human T-lymphotropic virus type III infection. J. Am. Acad. Dermatol. 15:482–486

Sagredo N, 1924. *Linguatula-rhinaria*-Larve (*Pentastoma denticulatum*) in den Lungen des Menschen. Virchows Arch. Pathol. Anat. 251:608–615

Sahba GH, Sahba SS, Seyed M, Ghaemmachami AA, 1984. Case of gingival myiasis caused by *Wohlfahrtia magnifica* and a review of myiasis in man and animals in Iran. Proceedings of the XI International Congress of Tropical Medicine Mal., Calgary, Canada, Sept. 16–22. p. 131

Sahn EE, Sheridan DM, 1992. Demodicidosis in a child with leukemia. J. Am. Acad. Dermatol. 27:799–801

Schacher JF, Khalil GM, Salman S, 1965. A field study of halzoun (parasitic pharyngitis) in Lebanon. J. Trop. Med. Hyg. 68:226–230

Schacher JF, Saab S, Germanos R, Boustany N, 1969. The aetiology of halzoun in Lebanon: recovery of *Linguatula serrata* nymphs from two patients. Trans. R. Soc. Trop. Med. Hyg. 63:854–858

Schmidt C, Ulrich G, Bersch W, 1993. Tungiasis—eine in Mitteleuropa seltene Hautparasitose. Ein kasuisticher Beitrag. Pathologe 14:221–222

Self JT, 1969. Biological relationships of the Pentastomida; a bibliography on the Pentastomida. Exp. Parasitol. 24:63–119

Self JT, Hopps HC, Williams AO, 1975. Pentastomiasis in Africans. Trop. Geogr. Med. 27:1–13

Shelley WB, Shelley ED, Burmeister V, 1988. *Staphylococcus aureus* colonization of burrows in erythrodermic Norwegian scabies. A case study of iatrogenic contagion. J. Am. Acad. Dermatol. 19:673–678

Sibenge S, Gawkrodger DJ, 1992. Rosacea: a study of clinical patterns, blood flow, and the role of *Demodex folliculorum*. J. Am. Acad. Dermatol. 26:590–593

Singh TS, Rana D, 1989. Urogenital myiasis caused by *Megaselia scalaris* (Diptera: Phoridae): a case report. J. Med. Entomol. 26:228–229

Smith DR, Clevenger RR, 1986. Nosocomial nasal myiasis. Arch. Pathol. Lab. Med. 110:439–440

Smith KGV, Thomas V, 1979. Correspondence. Intestinal myiasis in man caused by larvae of *Clogmia* (= *Telmatoscopus*) *albipunctatus* Williston (Psychodidae, Diptera). Trans. R. Soc. Trop. Med. Hyg. 73:349–350

Spielman MI, Potter GK, Taubman SM, Hodge WR, 1986. Pain, pruritus, and swelling localized to two toes. Arch. Dermatol. 122:330

Spradbery JP, Bromley J, Dixon R, Tetlow L, 1994. Correspondence. Tungiasis in Australia: an exotic disease threat. Med. J. Aust. 161:173

Symmers WSC, 1957. Two cases of eosinophilic prostatitis due to metazoan infestation (with *Oxyuris vermicularis* and with a larva of *Linguatula serrata*). J. Pathol. Bacteriol. 73:549–555

Tobie JE, 1957. Tongue worm (*Linguatula serrata*) infestation in a patient with acute leukemia. Am. J. Clin. Pathol. 28:628–633

Vennos E, Burke E, Johns C, Miller S, 1995. Tungiasis. Cutis 56:206–207

Wanke NC, Melo C, Balassiano V, 1992. Crusted scabies in a child with systemic lupus erythematosus. Rev. Soc. Bras. Med. Trop. 25:73–75

Wardhaugh AD, Norris JF, 1994. A case of imported tungiasis in Scotland initially mimicking verrucae vulgaris. Scott. Med. J. 39:146–147

Watson JM, Abdel Kerim R, 1956. Observations on forms of parasitic pharyngitis known as "Halzoun" in the Middle East. J. Trop. Med. Hyg. 59:147–154

Yagi H, el Bahari S, Mohamed HA, Ahmed-el RS, Mustafa B, Mahmoud M, Saad MB, Sulaiman SM, el Hassan AM, 1996. The Marrara syndrome: a hypersensitivity reaction of the upper respiratory tract and buccopharyngeal mucosa to nymphs of *Linguatula serrata*. Acta Trop. 62:127–134

Zumpt F, 1965. *Myiasis in Man and Animals in the Old World*. London: Butterworths

Part VI

Differential Diagnosis

29

A GUIDE TO DIFFERENTIAL DIAGNOSIS BY ORGAN SYSTEMS AND TISSUES, WITH A LISTING OF PARASITES

Following is a summary of the parasites that occur in different tissues and organ systems. This summary is provided as a guide for the anatomic pathologist who encounters a protozoan, a helminth, or an arthropod in a tissue section. It attempts to be as comprehensive as possible; in some places, it is repetitious for the sake of completeness. It is hoped that this summary will provide a quick reference and a checklist for identification of organisms in tissue sections. The summary consists of tables arranged alphabetically by organ system. Each organ is subdivided into its main parts, and a list of parasites following the general phylogenetic organization of the text is provided for each part.

A. Central Nervous System

Anatomic Site and Parasite	Comments
Brain, Cerebellum, and Spinal Cord	
E. cuniculi	Intracellular
T. hominis	Intracellular

Anatomic Site and Parasite	Comments
T. anthropophthera	Intracellular
Thelohania	Intracellular
Leishmania	In macrophages
T. cruzi	Intracellular amastigotes
T. rhodesiense	Trypomastigotes in interstitium
T. gambiense	Trypomastigotes in interstitium
Acanthamoeba	Abscesses
Hartmannella	Abscesses
Naegleria	In brain tissues
E. histolytica	Abscesses
Toxoplasma	Trophozoites and cysts
Strongyloides	Larvae
Halicephalobus	Adult females, eggs, and larvae
A. cantonensis	Larvae
Baylisascaris	Larvae
Toxocara	Larvae
Dracunculus	Adult in spinal canal, ectopic
Gnathostoma	Larvae
Loa	Microfilariae in blood vessels
Trichinella	Larvae, encephalitis
Schistosoma	Adult and eggs, ectopic

Anatomic Site and Parasite	Comments
Fasciola	Adult, ectopic
Heterophyes	Adults and eggs in granulomas
Paragonimus	Adult, eggs, ectopic
Alaria	Mesocercariae
Cysticercus	In brain tissue
Coenurus	In brain tissue and ventricles
Sparganum	In brain tissue
E. granulosus	Cyst in brain tissue
E. multilocularis	Cyst in brain tissue
Maggots	Larva in brain tissue

Meninges

Naegleria	Trophozoites, meningitis
A. cantonensis	Larvae
Gnathostoma	Larvae
Meningonema	In cysterna magna
Paragonimus	Adult, eggs, ectopic
Cysticercus	In meningeal spaces
Coenurus	In meningeal spaces
E. granulosus	Cyst
Maggots	Larva in meningeal spaces

Spinal Fluid

Leishmania	In macrophages
T. cruzi	Trypomastigotes
T. rhodesiense	Trypomastigotes
T. gambiense	Trypomastigotes
Acanthamoeba	Trophozoites and cysts
Hartmannella	Trophozoites and cysts
Naegleria	Trophozoites
Toxoplasma	Trophozoites
A. cantonensis	Larval stages
Meningonema	Adult worm

B. Circulatory System

Anatomic Site and Parasite	Comments

Heart

Right ventricular cavity

D. immitis	Adult worms
Sparganum	Larva

Myocardium

T. anthropophthera	Intracellular
Thelohania	Intracellular
L. donovani	In macrophages, in interstitial infiltrate

Anatomic Site and Parasite	Comments
T. cruzi	Muscle fibers, myocarditis
T. gondii	Muscle fibers, myocarditis
P. falciparum	Capillaries, endothelial cells
Baylisascaris	Encapsulated larvae
Toxocara	Granulomas, encapsulated in pericardium
Trichinella	Myocarditis
Metagonimus	Adults, eggs
Paragonimus	Adults, eggs
Alaria	Mesocercariae
Cysticercus	Intermuscular tissues
E. granulosus	Cyst
E. oligarthrus	Cyst
Maggots	Postmortem invasion

Pericardium

E. histolytica	Left liver abscess, ruptured
Dracunculus	Adult, ectopic
M. ozzardi	Adults
M. perstans	Adults
Cysticercus	Larva
E. granulosus	Cyst

Pericardial effusion

Leishmania	Amastigotes in macrophages
E. histolytica	Trophozoites in pus
Strongyloides	Larvae in serous fluid
E. granulosus	Larval elements
All blood parasites	When effusion is hemorrhagic

Pulmonary Artery

A. cantonensis	Adults
Angiostrongylus spp.	Adults
D. immitis	Juveniles and adults
Wuchereria	Adults
Brugia	Adults
Schistosoma	Adults, eggs (embolized)
Sparganum	Larva
E. granulosus	Embolized ruptured cyst

Blood Vessels

P. falciparum	Endothelia of small vessels and capillaries
A. costarricensis	Ileocecal arteries (others in ectopic locations)
D. immitis	Adult worms
Schistosoma	Adult worms
Cysticercus	Producing obstruction
E. granulosus	Embolized ruptured cyst

C. Digestive System

Anatomic Site and Parasite	Comments
Mouth	
E. cuniculi	Intracellular, ulcerations
T. tenax	Trophozoite in saliva, gums
Leishmania	In macrophages
E. gingivalis	Trophozoite in saliva, gums
Anisakis	Larval stages
Gongylonema	Adults and eggs in squamous epithelium
Trichinella	In tongue muscle
Fasciola	Adults, while eating raw liver
Dicrocoelium	Adults, while eating raw liver
Sparganum	In issues
Cysticercus	In issues and subepithelial
Linguatula	Larvae, while eating raw animal viscera
Maggots	Larva in tissues or in oral cavity
Esophagus	
Leishmania	In macrophages, ulcers, growths
T. cruzi	Amastigotes, intracellular
Cryptosporidium	In brush border of cells of lower esophagus
P. falciparum	In blood vessels, capillaries
Balantidium	Ulcers
Gongylonema	Adults and eggs in squamous epithelium
Schistosoma	Eggs in granulomas
Fasciola	Adults, ectopic or after ingestion of raw liver
Stomach Wall	
N. connori	In epithelial cells, vessels
T. cruzi	Amastigotes, intracellular
Cryptosporidium	In brush border of epithelial cells
P. falciparum	In vessels and capillaries
Balantidium	Ulcerations
Strongyloides	Adult females, eggs and larvae
Ascaris	Adults, ectopic in lumen
Anisakis	Larvae in mucosa
Gnathostoma	Larvae in wall
Physaloptera	Adults, anterior end buried in mucosa
Schistosoma	Eggs in granulomas

Anatomic Site and Parasite	Comments
Fasciola	Adults, ectopic in wall
Alaria	Mesocercaria, in wall
Sparganum	In wall
E. granulosus	Cyst in wall
Maggots	Larva in mucosa
Gastric juice	
Giardia	Trophozoites and cysts
Strongyloides	Adults, larvae and eggs
Loa	Microfilariae
Small Intestine	
Enterocytozoon	Intracellular in epithelial cells, endothelium
E. cuniculi	Intracellular in epithelial cells, macrophages
E. intestinalis	Intracellular in epithelial cells, endothelial cells, macrophages
E. hellem	Intracellular in epithelial cells, endothelial cells, macrophages
N. connori	In vessels, epithelial cells
Leishmania	In macrophages, in interstitial infiltrate
T. cruzi	Amastigotes, intracellular
E. histolytica	Terminal ileum, mucosal ulcers
Cryptosporidium	In brush border of epithelial cells
Isospora	In epithelial cells
Cyclospora	In epithelial cells
Sarcocystis	In cells of lamina propria
Toxoplasma	Intracellular
P. falciparum	In vessels and capillaries
Balantidium	Ulcers
Strongyloides	Adult females, larvae and eggs in crypts
Hookworms	Adults attached to mucosa
Oesophagostomum	In nodules, mucosa, submucosa, serosa
Trichostrongylus	In mucosa, jejunum and ileum
A. costaricensis	Adults in ileocecal arteries; eggs and larvae in tissues
E. vermicularis	Adults in wall
Ascaris	Adults in duodenum; ectopic elsewhere
Anisakis	Larvae in wall
Gnathostoma	Adults in wall
Trichinella	Adults and larvae, small intestinal crypts
Aonchoteca	Adults, eggs and p. larvae in mucosa

Anatomic Site and Parasite	Comments
Schistosoma	Adults and eggs in wall
Fasciola	Adults in wall, ectopic
Fasciolopsis	Adults in lumen
N. salmincola	Adults in crypts
Heterophyids	Adults in crypts
Other intestinal trematodes	Adults in crypts
Paragonimus	Adult in wall, ectopic
Taenia	Adults in lumen
Diphyllobothrium	Adults in lumen
Hymenolepis	Adults in lumen and larvae in mucosa
Dipylidium	Adults in lumen
Other intestinal cestodes	Adults in lumen
Sparganum	In wall
E. granulosus	Cyst in wall
Maggots	Larva in mucosa

Appendix

T. cruzi	Amastigotes, intracellular
E. histolytica	Ulcers
P. falciparum	In vessels and capillaries
Balantidium	Ulcers
Oesophagostomum	In nodules, submucosal, subserosal
A. costarricensis	Adults in blood vessels; eggs and larvae in tissues
E. vermicularis	Adult in lumen; in mucosa
Ascaris	Adult
Anisakis	Larval stage in mucosa
Gnathostoma	Larva in wall
Rictularia	Adult in lumen
Trichuris	Adults in lumen and mucosa
Schistosoma	Eggs in tissues
Fasciola	Adult in wall, ectopic
Paragonimus	Adult in wall
Taenia	Proglottid in lumen
Other intestinal cestodes	Proglottids in lumen
Sparganum	In wall

Colon

Enterocytozoon	Intracellular in epithelial cells, endothelium
E. cuniculi	Intracellular in epithelial cells, macrophages
E. intestinalis	Intracellular in epithelial cells, endothelial cells, macrophages

Anatomic Site and Parasite	Comments
E. hellem	Intracellular in epithelial cells, endothelial cells, macrophages
Leishmania	In macrophages in interstitial infiltrate
T. cruzi	Amastigotes in cells
E. histolytica	In ulcers
Cryptosporidium	In brush border of epithelial cells
P. falciparum	In blood vessels and capillaries
Balantidium	In ulcers
Strongyloides	Infective larvae in wall
Oesophagostomum	Submucosal, subserosal nodules
Ternidens	Adults attached to mucosa
A. costarricensis	In vessels of ileocecal valve
Enterobius	In mucosa, lumen
Ascaris	Adults, ectopic
Anisakis	Larvae in mucosa
Gnathostoma	Larvae in wall
M. perstans	Adults, rectum wall
Trichuris	Adults in lumen and mucosa
Eustrongylides	Larva in wall, perforation
Schistosoma	Adults in vessels, eggs in tissues
Fasciola	Adults in wall, ectopic
Paragonimus	Adults in wall, ectopic
Sparganum	In all
E. granulosus	Cyst in wall

Liver

Parenchyma

T. anthropophthera	Intracellular
Leishmania	In macrophages
T. cruzi	In hepatocytes and macrophages
E. histolytica	Abscesses
Toxoplasma	In cells
P. falciparum	Blood vessels and sinusoids
Balantidium	Abscesses
Strongyloides	Larvae, sometimes in granulomas
A. costarricensis	Adults, ectopic
Enterobius	Adults, ectopic
Ascaris	Adults, eggs, ectopic
Baylisascaris	Larvae
Toxocara	Larvae
Gnathostoma	Larvae, migrating
M. perstans	Adults
C. hepatica	Adults, eggs
Schistosoma	Eggs in granulomas, adults

Anatomic Site and Parasite	Comments
Fasciola	Adults, eggs in abscesses
Clonorchis	Adults, eggs in abscesses
Opistorchis	Adults, eggs in abscesses
Sparganum	Larva
E. granulosus	Cyst
E. multilocularis	Cyst
E. vogeli	Cyst
Pentastomids	Encapsulated nymphs
Maggots	Larva in dead corpses
Biliary Tree—Gallbladder	
Enterocytozoon	Intracellular in epithelial cells
E. cuniculi	Intracellular in epithelial cells
E. intestinalis	Intracellular in epithelial cells
E. hellem	Intracellular in epithelial cells
Cryptosporidium	In brush border of epithelium
Ascaris	Adults, ectopic
Fasciola	Adults, eggs
Clonorchis	Adults, eggs
Opistorchis	Adults, eggs
Amphimerus	Adults, eggs
Dicrocoelium	Adults, eggs
E. granulosus	Protoscolices from ruptured cyst

Pancreas

T. anthropophthera	Intracellular
Thelohania	Intracellular
Leishmania	In macrophages in interstitial infiltrate
Cryptosporidium	In brush border of epithelial cells
Toxoplasma	Intracellular in parenchymal cells
Ascaris	Adults in duct, ectopic
M. perstans	Adults
Schistosoma	Eggs in granulomas; adults, ectopic
Clonorchis	Adults, eggs
Opistorchis	Adults, eggs
Amphimerus	Adults, eggs
Eurythrema	Adults, eggs
Alaria	Mesocercariae
E. granulosus	Cyst in parenchyma

Peritoneum

Leishmania	In macrophages infiltrating interstitium
T. cruzi	Intracellular amastigotes
E. histolytica	In peritonitis, usually bowel perforation

Anatomic Site and Parasite	Comments
Toxoplasma	Intracellular
Balantidium	In peritonitis, usually bowel perforation
Strongyloides	In tissues, in disseminated infection
Oesophagostomum	In nodules, larvae on surface
A. costarricensis	In blood vessels of ileocecal region
Enterobius	In nodules
Ascaris	Adults and eggs, ectopic
Anisakis	Larvae on surface; bowel perforation
Baylisascaris	Larvae in granuloma
Toxocara	Larvae in granuloma
Dracunculus	Larvae, adults, mostly in retroperitoneum
Gnathostoma	Larvae migrating in abscess
M. ozzardi	Adults
M. perstans	Adults
D. immitis	Larval stages
Eustrongylides	Larva
Schistosoma	Nodules and eggs
Fasciola	Adults, ectopic
Paragonimus	Adults, eggs, ectopic
Achillurbainia	Adults and eggs
Alaria	Mesocercariae
Cysticercus	Cyst
Coenurus	Cyst
Sparganum	Larvae, migrating; in abscess
E. granulosus	Cyst
E. vogeli	Cyst
Maggots	Larva in dead bodie.
Peritoneal fluid	
Leishmania	Amastigotes in macrophages
T. cruzi	In cells, amastigotes
E. histolytica	Trophozoites
Balantidium	Trophozoites
Toxoplasma	In cells
Strongyloides	Larvae
Mansonella	Adults, microfilariae
Loa	Microfilariae
E. granulosus	Cyst elements
Maggots	Larva in corpses
All blood parasites in hemorrhagic effusions	

Abdominal Wall

E. histolytica	In bowel perforations to outside
Acanthamoeba	In skin
Sarcocystis	In skeletal muscle

Anatomic Site and Parasite	Comments
Toxoplasma	Intraocular
P. falciparum	In capillaries and small blood vessels
Baylisascaris	Encapsulated in tissues
Toxocara	Encapsulated in tissues
Gnathostoma	Larvae, migrating; in abscess
Loa	Adults
Trichinella	In skeletal muscle
Fasciola	Adults, ectopic
Paragonimus	Adults, ectopic
Alaria	Mesocercariae
Cysticercus	Cyst
Coenurus	Cyst
Sparganum	Larvae, abscesses
E. granulosus	Cyst
Maggots	In skin, subcutaneous tissue

D. Endocrine System

Anatomic Site and Parasite	Comments
Testis	
Leishmania	In macrophages, in interstitial infiltrate
T. cruzi	Intracellular
Acanthamoeba	In abscesses
Toxoplasma	Intracellular
P. falciparum	In small vessels and capillaries
A. costarricensis	Adult, ectopic
Dracunculus	Adult, ectopic
Gnathostoma	Larvae, abscess
Wuchereria	Adult, lymphatics
Brugia	Adult, lymphatics
Schistosoma	Eggs, ectopic
Fasciola	Adult, ectopic
Sparganum	Larva
E. granulosus	Cyst
Ovaries	
P. falciparum	In small vessels and capillaries
Enterobius	Adults, ectopic; granulomas
E. granulosus	Cyst
Loa	Microfilariae
Adrenals	
Leishmania	In macrophages, interstitial infiltrate

Anatomic Site and Parasite	Comments
T. cruzi	Intracellular
E. histolytica	Disseminated infection
Toxoplasma	Intracellular; trophozoites and cysts
P. falciparum	In small blood vessels and capillaries
E. granulosus	Cyst
Thyroid	
T. anthropophthera	Intracellular
Thelohania	Intracellular
Leishmania	Intracellular in macrophages
T. cruzi	Intracellular
Toxoplasma	Intracellular in interstitial cells
P. falciparum	In small blood vessels and capillaries
E. granulosus	Cyst
Parathyroid	
T. anthropophthera	Intracellular
Pituitary	
Leishmania	In macrophages, in interstitial infiltrate
T. cruzi	Intracellular
Toxoplasma	Intracellular
Cysticercus	Cyst

E. Female Genital System

Anatomic Site and Parasite	Comments
Uterus	
Leishmania	In macrophages, in interstitial infiltrate
T. cruzi	Intracellular
E. histolytica	In abscesses, ulcers
Toxoplasma	Intracellular
P. falciparum	In small blood vessels and capillaries
Enterobius	Granulomas with adult worm, ectopic
Gnathostoma	Larvae in abscess
Schistosoma	Adults in blood vessels; eggs in granulomas
Fasciola	Adult, ectopic in abscess
Paragonimus	Adult, ectopic in abscess

Anatomic Site and Parasite	Comments
Sparganum	Larvae
E. granulosus	Cyst

Cervix

T. vaginalis	Trophozoites
T. cruzi	Intracellular
E. histolytica	In ulcers
Balantidium	In ulcers
Toxoplasma	Intracellular
P. falciparum	In small blood vessels and capillaries
Enterobius	Eggs in granulomas
Gnathostoma	Larvae
Schistosoma	Adults
Fasciola	Adult, ectopic in abscess
Paragonimus	Adult, ectopic in abscess
Sparganum	Larvae
E. granulosus	Cyst
Cervical smears	
T. vaginalis	Trophozoites
Acanthamoeba	Trophozoites
E. histolytica	Trophozoites
Toxoplasma	Intracellular trophozoites
Strongyloides	Larvae
Enterobius	Eggs, adults, ectopic
Ascaris	Eggs (contamination)
Loa	Microfilariae
Wuchereria	Microfilariae
Brugia	Microfilariae
Onchocerca	Microfilariae
Schistosoma	Eggs
All blood parasites in hemorrhagic smears	

Fallopian Tubes

E. histolytica	Abscess
P. falciparum	In small vessels and capillaries
Enterobius	Granulomas with adult, ectopic; eggs on serosa
Ascaris	Eggs on peritoneal surface, ectopic
Baylisascaris	Encapsulated larvae
Fasciola	Adult, ectopic
Schistosoma	Eggs in granulomas
E. granulosus	Cyst

Vagina

T. vaginalis	Trophozoites
E. histolytica	Ulcers

Anatomic Site and Parasite	Comments
Enterobius	Adult, ectopic
Ascaris	Adults, eggs
Maggots	Larva

Vulva

All skin and subcutaneous tissue parasites	
Enterobius	Adults in glands, abscess

Ovaries
See Endocrine System

Breast

Wuchereria	Adults
Brugia	Adults
All skin and subcutaneous tissue parasites	

F. Hemolymphatic System

Anatomic Site and Parasite	Comments

Bone Marrow

N. conori	Intracellular
T. anthropophthera	Intracellular
Leishmania	Intracellular in macrophages
T. cruzi	Intracellular
T. rhodesiense	In interstitium, trypomastigotes
T. gambiense	In interstitium, trypomastigotes
Acanthamoeba	Trophozoites, abscesses
E. histolytica	Trophozoites, abscesses
Hartmannella	Trophozoites, abscesses
Toxoplasma	Intracellular
P. falciparum	In small blood vessels and capillaries
E. granulosus	Cyst

Blood

Leishmania	Macrophages, rarely in polymorphonuclear cells
T. cruzi	Trypomastigotes
T. rangeli	Trypomastigotes
T. rhodesiense	Trypomastigotes
T. gambiense	Trypomastigotes
Plasmodium	In red blood cells
Babesia	In red blood cells
Entopolypoides	In red blood cells
Microfilariae	All except M. streptocerca

Lymph Nodes

T. anthropophthera	Intracellular

Anatomic Site and Parasite	Comments
Leishmania	In macrophages
T. cruzi	Intracellular
T. rhodesiense	In interstitium, trypomastigotes
T. gambiense	In interstitium, trypomastigotes
E. histolytica	Ulcers
Toxoplasma	Intracellular
P. falciparum	In small vessels and capillaries
Wuchereria	Adults
Brugia	Adults
M. perstans	Adults
Schistosoma	Eggs, ectopic
Alaria	Mesocercariae
Cysticercus	Cyst
E. granulosus	Cyst
Pentastomids	Encapsulated nymphs

Spleen

T. anthropophthera	Intracellular
Leishmania	In macrophages
T. cruzi	Intracellular
T. rhodesiense	In interstitium, trypomastigotes
T. gambiense	In interstitium, trypomastigotes
E. histolytica	Abscess
Toxoplasma	Intracellular
P. falciparum	In sinusoids
A. costarricensis	Adult, ectopic
Loa	Microfilariae
Schistosoma	Eggs
Fasciola	Adult, ectopic
Alaria	Mesocercariae
E. granulosus	Cyst

G. Male Genital System

Anatomic Site and Parasite	Comments

Scrotum

Dracunculus	Adult, ectopic
Wuchereria	Adults
Brugia	Adults
E. granulosus	Cyst
All other skin and subcutaneous parasites	

Penis

E. histolytica	Ulcers in skin, glans
Loa	Adult in skin
All skin and subcutaneous parasites	

Anatomic Site and Parasite	Comments

Prostate

E. hellem	Intracellular, abscess
Leishmania	In macrophages, in interstitial infiltrate
E. histolytica	Abscess
Toxoplasma	Intracellular
P. falciparum	In vessels and capillaries
Enterobius	Adult, ectopic
Wuchereria	Adult, in lymphatics
Brugia	Adult in lymphatics
Schistosoma	Eggs
Fasciola	Adult, ectopic
Paragonimus	Adult, ectopic
E. granulosus	Cyst
Linguatula	Larva

Semen and Urethral Secretions

T. vaginalis	Trophozoites
S. haematobium	Eggs, with sperm
S. intercalatum	Eggs with sperm

Testes

See Endocrine System

H. Musculoskeletal

Anatomic Site and Parasite	Comments

Skeletal Muscles

N. conori	Intracellular, muscle cells
Pleistophora	Intracellular
T. hominis	Intracellular
Thelohania	intracellular
T. cruzi	Intracellular, muscle cells
Acanthamoeba	Abscesses
E. histolytica	Abscesses
Sarcocystis	Intracellular, cysts, muscle cells
Toxoplasma	Intracellular, muscle cells
P. falciparum	In small vessels and capillaries
Strongyloides	Larvae
Hookworms	Larvae, intracellular; muscle cells
Baylisascaris	Larvae, encapsulated
Toxocara	Larvae, encapsulated
Gnathostoma	Larvae in abscess
Loa	Adult
Trichinella	Larvae, encapsulated
Fasciola	Adult, ectopic
Paragonimus	Adult, ectopic

Anatomic Site and Parasite	Comments
Cysticercus	Intermuscular tissues
C. longicollis	Intermuscular tissues
Coenurus	Cyst, intermuscular tissues
Sparganum	Larvae
E. granulosus	Cyst
Maggots	In living or dead persons

Bones

Acanthamoeba	Abscesses
E. histolytica	Abscesses
E. granulosus	Cyst

Joints

Dracunculus	Adults, calcified
Loa	Microfilariae in fluid
E. granulosus	Cyst
All blood parasites in hemorrhagic joint fluids	

I. Placenta and Fetus

Anatomic Site and Parasite	Comments

Placenta

T. cruzi	Intracellular, villi, membranes, cord
Toxoplasma	Intracellular, villi, membranes, cord
Plasmodium	In maternal circulation

Amniotic Fluid

T. cruzi	Trypomastigotes
Toxoplasma	Intracellular

Fetus

T. cruzi	Disseminated infection
T. rhodesiense	Disseminated infection
T. gambiense	Disseminated infection
Toxoplasma	Disseminated infection

J. Respiratory System

Anatomic Site and Parasite	Comments

Lungs

Parenchyma

N. conori	Intracellular

Anatomic Site and Parasite	Comments
Leishmania	In macrophages
T. cruzi	Intracellular amastigotes
Acanthamoeba	Abscess
Hartmannella	Abscess
E. histolytica	Abscess
P. falciparum	In capillaries
Strongyloides	Larvae in tissues
Hookworms	Larvae in tissues (?)
Enterobius	Adults in granuloma
Ascaris	Larvae; adults in abscesses; eggs
Baylisascaris	Encapsulated larvae
Toxocara	Encapsulated larvae
Gnathostoma	Larvae, migrating
Dracunculus	Adults, ectopic location
Wuchereria	Tropical eosinophilia
Brugia	Tropical eosinophilia
Eucoleus	Granulomas
Schistosoma	Adults, ectopic; eggs; pulmonary hypertension
Fasciola	Adults, ectopic
Paragonimus	Adults, eggs, granulomas
Alaria	Mesocercariae
Cysticercus	Larva
Sparganum	Adults
E. granulosus	Cyst
E. multilocularis	Cyst
Pentastomids	Encapsulated nymphs
Pleura	
E. histolytica	In abscesses of lungs
Baylisascaris	Encapsulated larvae
Gnathostoma	Larvae
M. ozzardi	Adults
M. perstans	Adults
Fasciola	Adult, ectopic
Sparganum	Larva
E. granulosus	Cyst
Pentastomids	Encapsulated nymphs
Upper respiratory tract	
E. cuniculi	Epithelial cells, intracellular
E. hellem	Epithelial cells, intracellular
N. conori	Intracellular
T. hominis	Epithelial cells, intracellular
T. tenax	Saprophyte; vaginalis in abscess (?)
Leishmania	Nasopharyngeal
Naegleria	Olfactory mucosa
Acanthamoeba	Olfactory mucosa
Cryptosporidium	Brush border, respiratory epithelium
Strongyloides	Larvae
Hookworms	Larvae
Mammomonogamus	Adults

Anatomic Site and Parasite	*Comments*
Ascaris	Larvae; adults, ectopic
Anisakis	Larva
Gnathostoma	Larva
Eustrongylides	Larva, expectorated
Fasciola	Adults, expectorated
Dicrocoelium	Adults, expectorated
Cysticercus	Larva
Linguatula	Adults, nymphs, expectorated
Maggots	Larva
Lower respiratory tract	
E. cuniculi	Epithelial cells, intracellular
E. hellem	Epithelial cells, intracellular
Enterocytozoon	Epithelial cells, intracellular
N. conori	Intracellular
Acanthamoeba	Abscesses
Hartmannella	Abscesses
E. histolytica	Abscesses
Cryptosporidium	Brush border, respiratory epithelium
Strongyloides	Larvae; adults, eggs
Hookworms	Larvae
Ascaris	Larvae; adults, ectopic; eggs
Eucoleus	Aerophila, granulomas, adults
E. granulosus	Cysts, other parasitic elements

Mediastinum

E. histolytica	Abscess
Ascaris	Adults, ectopic, rupture from liver
Gnathostoma	Larvae
Fasciola	Adult, ectopic
Sparganum	Larvae
E. granulosus	Cysts

Thoracic Wall

E. histolytica	In fistulas
Sarcocystis	In skeletal muscles
P. falciparum	In blood vessels and capillaries
Gnathostoma	Larvae
Trichinella	In skeletal muscle
Fasciola	Adults, ectopic
Cysticercus	Larvae
Coenurus	Larvae
Sparganum	Larvae
E. granulosus	Cysts
All skin and subcutaneous parasites	

Anatomic Site and Parasite	*Comments*
Sputum	
E. cuniculi	Spores, intracellular
Enterocytozoon	Spores, intracellular
E. histolytica	In abscesses ruptured to bronchial tree
Trichomonas	Tenax from oral cavity
Cryptosporidium	In pulmonary infections
Strongyloides	In disseminated infection
Hookworms	Larvae, Loeffler's syndrome
Mammomonogamus	Eggs, adults
Ascaris	Larvae, Loeffler's syndrome
Gnathostoma	Larvae
Fasciola	Adults, after eating raw liver
Dicrocoelium	Adults, after eating raw liver
Paragonimus	Eggs
E. granulosus	Ruptured cyst into bronchial tree

Pleural Fluid	
Leishmania	In macrophages
T. cruzi	Intracellular
E. histolytica	Trophozoites in ruptured abscesses
Acanthamoeba	Trophozoites in ruptured abscesses
Toxoplasma	Intracellular
Strongyloides	Larvae, disseminated infection
E. granulosus	Ruptured cyst to pleura
All blood parasites in hemorrhagic effusion	

K. Sensory Organs

Anatomic Site and Parasite	*Comments*
Eye	
Conjunctiva	
E. cuniculi	Intracellular, epithelial cells
E. hellem	Intracellular, epithelial cells
E. intestinalis	Intracellular, epithelial cells
V. corneae	Intracellular, epithelial cells
T. hominis	Intracellular, epithelial cells
Leishmania	In macrophages, in interstitial infiltrate
Acanthamoeba	Trophozoites

Anatomic Site and Parasite	Comments
E. histolytica	Trophozoites, ulcers
Toxoplasma	Intracellular
Onchocerca	Microfilariae
Loa	Adult
Dirofilaria	Adult in nodule
Dipetalonema	Adult in nodule
Schistosoma	Eggs, ectopic
Cysticercus	Cyst
Sparganum	Larvae
E. granulosus	Cyst
Pentastomids	Larvae
Maggots	Surface, periorbital tissues
Cornea	
T. hominis	Intracellular
E. cuniculi	intracellular, epithelial cells
E. hellem	Intracellular epithelial cells
E. intestinalis	Intracellular epithelial cells
V. corneae	Intracellular epithelial cells
Pleistophora	Intracellular, epithelial cells
T. rhodesiense	Trypomastigotes
T. gambiense	Trypomastigotes
Acanthamoeba	Trophozoites, keratitis
Hookworm	Larvae
Uveal tract and retina	
Leishmania	In macrophages, in interstitial infiltrate
Acanthamoeba	Trophozoites and cysts
E. histolytica	Trophozoites
Toxoplasma	Intracellular, granulomas
P. falciparum	In small vessels and capillaries
A. cantonensis	Larval stage
Toxocara	Larvae
Gnathostoma	Larvae
Filariae	Adults (?), larval
Onchocerca	Microfilariae
Schistosoma	Eggs, ectopic
Cysticercus	Cyst
C. longicollis	Cyst
Coenurus	Cyst
Sparganum	Larvae
E. granulosus	Cyst
Pentastomids	Encapsulated nymphs
Maggots	Larva
Anterior and posterior chambers	
Acanthamoeba	Trophozoites and cysts
E. histolytica	Trophozoites
Gnathostoma	Larvae
Angiostrongylus	Larvae
Onchocerca	Microfilariae

Anatomic Site and Parasite	Comments
Dipetalonema	Adult
Cysticercus	Cyst
Coenurus	Cyst
Sparganum	Larvae
E. granulosus	Cyst
E. multilocularis	Cyst
Maggots	Larva
Eyelids	
All skin and subcutaneous parasites	
Orbital tissues	
Leishmania	In macrophages, in interstitial infiltrate
Acanthamoeba	Trophozoites
E. histolytica	Trophozoites
Toxoplasma	Intracellular
D. immitis	Abscess
Dracunculus	Adult, ectopic
Gnathostoma	Larvae
Dirofilaria	In nodules
Loa	In tissues, adult
Trichinella	In ocular muscles
Schistosoma	Eggs, ectopic
Cysticercus	Cyst
Sparganum	Larvae
E. granulosus	Cyst
E. oligarthrus	Cyst
Maggots	Larva

Ear

Acanthamoeba	Trophozoites, cyst, otitis media
Ascaris	Adult in eustachian tubes
E. granulosus	Cyst
Maggots	Larva
Other arthropods	In external ear canal

L. Skin and Subcutaneous Tissues

Anatomic Site and Parasite	Comments

Epidermis

N. conori	In ulcers
Leishmania	In macrophages (cutaneous leishmaniasis)
T. rhodesiense	Trypomastigotes in interstitium
T. gambiense	Trypomastigotes in interstitium
Acanthamoeba	Trophozoites and cysts in ulcers

Anatomic Site and Parasite	Comments
E. histolytica	Trophozoites in ulcers
Toxoplasma	Intracellular
P. falciparum	In small vessels and capillaries
Strongyloides	In hair follicles (penetrating skin)
Hookworms	In tunnels (cutaneous larva migrans)
Gnathostoma	In tunnels (cutaneous larva migrans)
Anatrichosoma	Adults
Gasterophilus	In tunnels (cutaneous larva migrans)
Hypoderma	Producing myiasis
Demodex	In hair follicles and sebaceous glands
Sarcoptes	In tunnels (scabies)
Tunga	Intraepidermal (usually toes and feet)

Dermis

N. conori	In ulcers
Acanthamoeba	In ulcers, trophozoites, and cysts
Leishmania	In macrophages (cutaneous leishmaniasis)
T. rhodesiense	Trypomastigotes in interstitium
T. gambiense	Trypomastigotes in interstitium
Acanthamoeba	In ulcers, trophozoites, and cysts
E. histolytica	In ulcers, trophozoites
Toxoplasma	Intracellular
P. falciparum	In small vessels and capillaries
Pelodera	In granulomatous inflammation
Strongyloides	Larvae (cutaneous larva migrans)
Hookworms	Larvae (cutaneous larva migrans)
Gnathostoma	Larvae (cutaneous larva migrans)
M. streptocerca	Adults and microfilaria
Onchocerca	Adults in nodules, microfilaria in interstitium
Schistosoma	Eggs, ectopic
Gasterophilus	Larvae (cutaneous larva migrans)
Hypoderma	Larvae, myiasis (cutaneous larva migrans)

Subcutaneous Tissues

N. conori	In ulcers
Leishmania	In macrophages p. (cutaneous leishmaniasis)
T. cruzi	Intracellular
T. rhodesiense	Trypomastigotes in interstitium
T. gambiense	Trypomastigotes in interstitium
Acanthamoeba	Trophozoites, cysts, ulcers
E. histolytica	Trophozoites, ulcers
Toxoplasma	Intracellular
P. falciparum	In small vessels and capillaries
Strongyloides	Larvae in hyperinfections
Pelodera	Larvae

Anatomic Site and Parasite	Comments
Gnathostoma	Larvae
Wuchereria	In lymphatics (nodules), adults
Brugia	In lymphatics (nodules), adults
Onchocerca	Adults in nodules, microfilariae
Loa	Adults
M. streptocerca	Adults, microfilariae
D. repens	In nodules
D. tenuis	In nodules
D. striata	In nodules
D. ursi-like	In nodules
D. immitis-like	In nodules
Dioctophyme	Larvae
Schistosoma	Eggs, adults, ectopic
Fasciola	Adults, ectopic
Paragonimus	Adults, ectopic
Achillurbainia	Adults and eggs
Cysticercus	Cysts
Coenurus	Cysts
Sparganum	Larvae
E. granulosus	Cysts
Maggots	Larva

M. Urinary System

Anatomic Site and Parasite	Comments

Kidneys

E. cuniculi	Epithelial cells, intracellular
E. hellem	Epithelial cells, intracellular
T. anthropophthera	Intracellular
T. hominis	Epithelial cells, intracellular
Leishmania	In macrophages, in interstitial infiltrate
Acanthamoeba	In abscesses, trophozoites, cysts
E. histolytica	In abscesses, trophozoites
P. falciparum	In small vessels and capillaries
Strongyloides	Larvae in hyperinfection
Micronema	Adults, eggs, and larvae
Ascaris	Adults, ectopic
Gnathostoma	Larvae
M. perstans	Adults
Dioctophyme	Adults
Schistosoma	Eggs in granulomas
Fasciola	Adults, ectopic
Paragonimus	Adults, ectopic
Alaria	Mesocercariae
E. granulosus	Cysts

Anatomic Site and Parasite	*Comments*
Urinary Bladder	
E. hellem	Epithelial cells, intracellular
Toxoplasma	Intracellular
P. falciparum	In small vessels and capillaries
Diploscapter	Adults
Enterobius	Adults in females
Gnathostoma	Larvae
Fasciola	Adults, ectopic
Paragonimus	Adults, ectopic

Anatomic Site and Parasite	*Comments*
Schistosoma	Adults, eggs
Sparganum	Larvae
E. granulosus	Cysts
Maggots	Larva
Ureters	
E. hellem	Epithelial cells, intracellular
Schistosoma	Eggs, in granulomas
Sparganum	Larva

INDEX